SIDE EFFECTS OF DRUGS
ANNUAL 30

Side Effects of Drugs Annual 30

HONORARY EDITOR

Prof. M.N.G. Dukes, Oslo, Norway

ADVISORY EDITORIAL BOARD

Prof. F. Bochner, Adelaide, Australia
Prof. I.R. Edwards, Uppsala, Sweden
Prof. G.P. Velo, Verona, Italy

SIDE EFFECTS OF DRUGS ANNUAL 30

A worldwide yearly survey of new
data and trends in adverse drug reactions and
interactions

EDITOR

J. K. ARONSON MA, DPhil, MBChB, FRCP, FBPharmacolS, FFPM(Hon)

Reader in Clinical Pharmacology
University Department of Primary Health Care
Rosemary Rue Building, Old Road Campus, Headington, Oxford OX3 7LF

ELSEVIER

Amsterdam – Boston – Heidelberg – London – New York – Oxford
Paris – San Diego – San Francisco – Singapore – Sydney – Tokyo

Elsevier
Radarweg 29, PO Box 211, 1000 AE Amsterdam, The Netherlands
The Boulevard, Langford Lane, Kidlington, Oxford OX5 1GB, UK

First edition 2008

Notice
No responsibility is assumed by the publisher for any injury and/or damage to persons or property
as a matter of products liability, negligence or otherwise, or from any use or operation of any methods,
products, instructions or ideas contained in the material herein. Because of rapid advances in the medical
sciences, in particular, independent verification of diagnoses and drug dosages should be made

Library of Congress Cataloging-in-Publication Data
A catalog record for this book is available from the Library of Congress

British Library Cataloguing in Publication Data
A catalogue record for this book is available from the British Library

ISBN-13:   978-0-444-52767-7
ISSN: 0378-6080 (Series)

For information on all Elsevier publications
visit our website at books.elsevier.com

Printed and bound in Hungary

07 08 09 10 11   10 9 8 7 6 5 4 3 2 1

Contributors

M.C. ALLWOOD, BPHARM, PHD
  Pharmacy Academic Practice Unit, Faculty of Education, Health and Science, University of Derby, Kedleston Road, Derby, UK. E-mail: M.C.Allwood@derby.ac.uk

BRIAN J. ANGUS, BSC, MBCHB, DTM&H, MD, FRCP, FFTM(GLAS)
  Nuffield Department of Medicine, University of Oxford, John Radcliffe Hospital, Headington, Oxford, OX3 9DU, UK. E-mail: brian.angus@ndm.ox.ac.uk

J.K. ARONSON, MA, MBCHB, DPHIL, FRCP, FBPHARMACOLS, FFPM(HON)
  University Department of Primary Health Care, Rosemary Rue Building, Old Road Campus, Headington, Oxford OX3 7LF, UK. E-mail: jeffrey.aronson@clinpharm.ox.ac.uk

I. AURSNES, MD
  University of Oslo, Department of Pharmacology, P.O. Box 1057 Blindern, N-0316 Oslo, Norway. E-mail: i.a.aursnes@medisin.uio.no

PATRICK A. BALL
  Charles Sturt University, Correspondence Locked Bag 588, Wagga Wagga, New South Wales 2678, Australia. E-mail: pball@csu.edu.au

V.V. BANU REKHA, MBBS
  Tuberculosis Research Centre, Mayor VR Ramanathan Road, Chetpet, Chennai 600031, India. E-mail: bannu24@yahoo.com

M. BEHREND, MD, PHD, FACS
  Klinik für Viszeral-, Gefäß-, Thorax-, und Kinderchirurgie, Klinikum Deggendorf, Perlasberger Str. 41, D-94469 Deggendorf, Germany. E-mail: matthias.behrend@klinikum-deggendorf.de

STEFAN BEYENBURG, MD
  Service de Neurologie, rue Barblé 4, L-1210 Luxembourg, Luxembourg.
  E-mail: Beyenburg.Stefan@chl.lu

KRISTIEN BOELAERT, MRCP, PHD
  Division of Medical Sciences, IBR Building, 2nd floor, The Medical School, University of Birmingham, Birmingham, B15 2TH, UK. E-mail: k.boelaert@bham.ac.uk

F. BRAUN, MD
  Klinik für Allgemeine Chirurgie und Thoraxchirurgie, Zentrum Chirurgie, Universität Schleswig-Holstein, Campus Kiel, Arnold-Heller Strasse 7, 24105 Kiel, Germany.
  E-mail: felix.m.braun@gmx.de

ANDREW BYRNE, BA, MBBCH, BAO, MRCPSYCH, DIPMEDSC
  Fieldhead Hospital, South West Yorkshire Mental Health NHS Trust, Ouchthorpe Lane, Wakefield, WF1 3SP, UK. E-mail: andrew.byrne@swyt.nhs.uk

ALFONSO CARVAJAL, MD, PHD
  Instituto de Farmacoepidemiología, Facultad de Medicina, 47005 Valladolid, Spain.
  E-mail: carvajal@ife.uva.es

J.A. CENTENO, PHD, FRSC
  Division of Biophysical Toxicology, Department of Environmental & Infectious Disease Sci-
  ences, Armed Forces Institute of Pathology, Building 54, 14th Street & Alaska Avenue NW,
  Washington, DC 20306-6000, USA. E-mail: centeno@afip.osd.mil

N.H. CHOULIS, MD, PHD
  LAVIPHARM Research Laboratories, Agias Marinas Street, 19002 Peania (Attika), Greece.
  E-mail: nchoulis@lavipharm.gr

J.J. COLEMAN, MBCHB, MRCP(UK)
  Department of Clinical Pharmacology, Divison of Medical Sciences, University of Birmingham,
  Edgbaston, Birmingham, B15 2TT, UK. E-mail: j.j.coleman@bham.ac.uk

NATASCIA CORTI, MD
  University Hospital Zurich, Department of Medicine, Division of Infectious Diseases and Hospital Epidemiology, Rämistrasse 100, CH-8091 Zürich, Switzerland. E-mail: natascia.corti@usz.ch

J. COSTA, MD
  Clinical Pharmacology Department, Hospital Universitari Germans Trias i Pujol, Universitat
  Autònoma de Barcelona, Ctra de Canyet s/n, 08916 Badalona, Spain. E-mail: jcosta@menta.net

P.J. COWEN, MD
  University Department of Psychiatry, Warenford Hospital, Oxford, OX3 7JX, UK.
  E-mail: phil.cowen@psych.ox.ac.uk

STEPHEN CURRAN, BSC, MBCHB, MMEDSC, MRCPSYCH, PHD
  Fieldhead Hospital, South West Yorkshire Mental Health NHS Trust, Ouchthorpe Lane, Wakefield, WF1 3SP, UK. E-mail: s.curran@hud.ac.uk

H.R. DALTON, BSC, DPHIL, FRCP, DIPMEDED
  Department of Gastroenterology, Royal Cornwall Hospital, Truro, Cornwall, TR1 3LJ, United
  Kingdom. E-mail: Harry.Dalton@rcht.cornwall.nhs.uk

A. DEL FAVERO, MD
  Istituto di Medicina Interna e Science Oncologiche, Policlinico Monteluce, 06122 Perugia, Italy.
  E-mail: misoseg@unipg.it

S. DITTMANN, MD, DSCMED
  19 Hatzenporter Weg, 12681 Berlin, Germany. E-mail: sd.internat.immun.consult@t-online.de

M.N.G. DUKES
  Trosterudveien 19, 0778 Oslo, Norway. E-mail: mngdukes@online.no

RIF S. EL-MALLAKH
  Director, Mood Disorders Research Program, Department of Psychiatry and Behavioral Sciences, School of Medicine, University of Louisville, MedCenter One, 501 E Broadway, Suite
  340, Louisville, KY 40292, USA. E-mail: rselma01@louisville.edu

E. ERNST, MD, PHD, FRCP, FRCP (ED)
  Complementary Medicine, Peninsula Medical School, Universities of Exeter & Plymouth,
  25 Victoria Park Road, Exeter, EX2 4NT, UK. E-mail: Edzard.Ernst@pms.ac.uk

M. FARRÉ, MD
Unitat de Farmacologia, Institut Municipal d'Investigació Mèdica (IMIM)-Hospital del Mar, Universitat Autònoma de Barcelona, Doctor Aiguader 88, 08003 Barcelona, Spain. E-mail: mfarre@imim.es

H.J. FELLOWS, BSc, MRCP
Department of Gastroenterology, Royal Cornwall Hospital, Truro, Cornwall, TR1 3LJ, United Kingdom. E-mail: hfellows@hotmail.com

M.G. FRANZOSI, PhD
Department of Cardiovascular Research, Istituto di Ricerche Farmacologiche "Mario Negri", Via Giuseppe La Masa 19, 20156 Milan, Italy. E-mail: franzosi@marionegri.it

SUSANNA GALEA, MD, MRCPsych, MSc (Addictive Behaviour), Dip. (Forensic Mental Health), Associate Fellow ICDP
International Centre for Drug Policy, St George's, University of London, 6th Floor, Hunter Wing, Cranmer Terrace, London, SW17 0RE UK. E-mail: suegalea23@yahoo.co.uk

A.H. GHODSE, MD, PhD, FRCP, FRCPsych
International Centre for Drug Policy, St. George's, University of London, 6th Floor, Hunter Wing, Cranmer Terrace, London, SW17 0RE, UK. E-mail: h.ghodse@sghms.ac.uk

AN E. GOOSSENS, RPharm, PhD
Department of Dermatology, University Hospital, Catholic University of Leuven, Kapucijnenvoer 33, 3000 Leuven, Belgium. E-mail: an.goossens@uz.kuleuven.ac.be

ANDREAS H. GROLL, MD
Infectious Diseases Research Program, Center for Bone Marrow Transplantation and Department of Hematology/Oncology, University Children's Hospital, Muenster, Germany. E-mail: grollan@ukmuenster.de

SARAH GUZOFSKI, MD
University of Massachusetts, Medical School, Department of Psychiatry, 361 Plantation Street, Worcester, Massachusetts 01605, USA. E-mail: guzofsks@ummhc.org

JOB HARENBERG, MD
Institute of Experimental and Clinical Pharmacology, Faculty of Medicine Mannheim, Ruprecht-Karls-University Heidelberg, Theodor-Kutzer-Ufer 1-3, D-68167 Mannheim, Germany. E-mail: job.harenberg@med.ma.uni-heidelberg.de

J.T. HARTMANN, PhD, MD
Department of Hematology/Oncology/Immunology/Rheumatology/Pneumology, Eberhard Karls University Tübingen, UKT - Medical Center II, Department of Hematology, Oncology, Immunology, Rheumatology, Otfried-Müller-Strasse 10, 72076 Tübingen, Germany. E-mail: joerg.hartmann@med.uni-tuebingen.de

KATHARINA HARTMANN, MScPharm
Berna Biotech Ltd, Head Global Pharmacovigilance, 3000 Berne, Switzerland. E-mail: hartka@bluewin.ch

ALEXANDER IMHOF, MD
University Hospital Zurich, Department of Medicine, Division of Infectious Diseases and Hospital Epidemiology, Rämistrasse 100, CH-8091 Zürich, Switzerland. E-mail: alexander.imhof@usz.ch

NATALIA JIMENO, MD, PhD
  Instituto de Farmacoepidemiología, Facultad de Medicina, 47005 Valladolid, Spain.
  E-mail: najimeno@med.uva.es

MARKUS JOERGER, MD, PhD
  Department of Oncology & Hematology, Cantonal Hospital, Rorschacherstr 95, 9007 St. Gallen,
  Switzerland. E-mails: markus.joerger@kssg.ch, markus.joerger@gmail.com

MAX KUHN, MD
  Department of Internal Medicine, Division of Pneumology, Kantonsspital, Loestrasse 170, 7000
  Chur, Switzerland. E-mail: max.kuhn@scag.gr.ch

R. LATINI, MD
  Department of Cardiovascular Research, Istituto di Ricerche Farmacologiche "Mario Negri",
  Via Giuseppe La Masa 19, 20156 Milan, Italy. E-mail: latini@marionegri.it

MARTIN LEUWER, MD
  School of Clinical Science, University of Liverpool, The Duncan Building, Daulby Street, Liverpool, L69 3GA, UK. E-mail: mleuwer@liv.ac.uk

H.-P. LIPP, PhD
  Eberhard-Karls-University Tübingen, Department of Clinical Pharmacy, Röntgenweg 9, 72076
  Tübingen, Germany.

P. MAGEE, BSc, MSc, MRPharmS
  Director of Pharmaceutical Sciences, University Hospitals Coventry and Warwickshire, Clifford
  Bridge Road, Coventry, CV2 2DX, UK. E-mail: Pam.Magee@uhcw.nhs.uk

A.P. MAGGIONI, MD
  ANMCO Research Center, Via La Marmora 34, 50121 Florence, Italy.
  E-mail: maggioni@anmco.it

LUIS H. MARTÍN ARIAS, MD, PhD
  Instituto de Farmacoepidemiología, Facultad de Medicina, 47005 Valladolid, Spain.
  E-mail: lmartin@ife.uva.es

U. MARTIN, PhD, FRCP
  Department of Clinical Pharmacology, Divison of Medical Sciences, University of Birmingham,
  Edgbaston, Birmingham, B15 2TT, UK. E-mail: u.martin@bham.ac.uk

R.H.B. MEYBOOM, MD, PhD
  Department of Pharmacoepidemiology and Pharmacotherapy, Faculty of Pharmacy, Utrecht University, P.O. Box 80082, 3508 TB Utrecht, The Netherlands. E-mail: r.meyboom@who-umc.org

T. MIDTVEDT
  Department of Microbiology, Tumor and Cell Biology (MTC), Karolinska institutet, S 17177,
  Stockholm, Sweden. E-mail: tore.midtvedt@ki.se

SAMEH K. MORCOS, FRCS, FFRRCSI, FRCR
  Department of Diagnostic Imaging, Northern General Hospital, Sheffield Teaching Hospitals
  (NHS) Trust, Sheffield, S5 7AU, UK. E-mail: Sameh.Morcos@sth.nhs.uk

SHABIR MUSA, MBCHB, MRCPSYCH
  Fieldhead Hospital, South West Yorkshire Mental Health NHS Trust, Ouchthorpe Lane, Wakefield, WF1 3SP, UK. E-mail: shabir.musa@swyt.nhs.uk

R.C.L. PAGE, MD, FRCP, MA(ED)
  Endocrine Unit, Dundee House, City Hospital, Hucknall Road, Nottingham, NG5 1PB, UK.
  E-mail: renee.page@nuh.nhs.uk

JAYENDRA K. PATEL, MD
  University of Massachusetts, Medical School, Department of Psychiatry, 361 Plantation Street, Worcester, MA 01605, USA. E-mail: patelj@ummhc.org

M.H. PITTLER, MD, PHD
  Complementary Medicine, Peninsula Medical School, Universities of Exeter & Plymouth, 25 Victoria Park Road, Exeter, EX2 4NT, UK. E-mail: Max.Pittler@pms.ac.uk

B.C.P. POLAK, MD
  VU University Medical Center, Department of Ophthalmology, P.O. Box 7057, 1007 MB Amsterdam, The Netherlands. E-mail: bcp.polak@vumc.nl

ALAGARISAMY RAAJKUMAR, FCARCSI
  Department of Anaesthesia and Pain Medicine, Royal Perth Hospital, Perth, WA 6847, Australia.
  E-mail: araajkumar@yahoo.com

M. SCHACHTER, MD
  Department of Clinical Pharmacology, National Heart and Lung Institute, Imperial College, St. Mary's Hospital, London, W2 1NY, UK. E-mail: m.schachter@imperial.ac.uk

DIETER SCHMIDT, MD
  Epilepsy Research Group Berlin, Goethestr. 5, D-14163 Berlin, Germany.
  E-mail: dbschmidt@t-online.de

STEPHAN A. SCHUG, MD, FANZCA, FFPMANZCA
  Pharmacology and Anaesthesiology Unit, School of Medicine and Pharmacology, University of Western Australia, MRF Building G Block, Royal Perth Hospital, GPO Box X2213, Perth, WA 6847, Australia. E-mail: stephan.schug@uwa.edu.au

R.P. SEQUEIRA, PHD, FCP
  Department of Pharmacology & Therapeutics, College of Medicine & Medical Sciences, Arabian Gulf University, P.O. Box 22979, Manama, Bahrain. E-mail: Sequeira@agu.edu.bh

DOMENIC A. SICA, MD
  Section of Clinical Pharmacology and Hypertension, Division of Nephrology, Medical College of Virginia of Virginia Commonwealth University, Box 980160 MCV Station, Richmond, VA 23298-0160, USA. E-mail: dsica@mcvh-vcu.edu

OSCAR OZMUND SIMOOYA, BSC, MBCHB, MSC
  The Copper Belt University Health Services Division, P.O. Box 21692, Kitwe, Zambia, Central Africa. E-mail: cbumed@zamnet.zm

P.F.W. STRENGERS, MD
  Sanquin, Plesmanlaan 125, 1066 CX Amsterdam, The Netherlands.
  E-mail: p.strengers@sanquin.nl

SOUMYA SWAMINATHAN, MD
Tuberculosis Research Centre, Mayor VR Ramanathan Road, Chetpet, Chennai 600031, India.
E-mail: doctorsoumya@yahoo.com

GIJSBERT B. VAN DER VOET, PhD, ERT
Toxicology Laboratory, Department of Clinical Pharmacy and Toxicology, Leiden University
Medical Center, Building 1, Albinusdreef 2, 2333 ZA Leiden, The Netherlands.
E-mails: Gijsbert.VanderVoet@afip.osd.mil, G.B.van_der_Voet@lumc.nl

P.J.J. VAN GENDEREN, MD, PhD
Havenziekenhuis and Institute of Tropical Diseases, Department of Internal Medicine, Harbour
Hospital, Haringvliet 2, 3011 TD Rotterdam, The Netherlands.
E-mail: p.van.genderen@havenziekenhuis.nl

E. VAN TWUYVER, PhD
Sanquin, Plesmanlaan 125, 1066 CX Amsterdam, The Netherlands.
E-mail: e.vantwuyver@sanquin.nl

P. VERHAMME, MD
Center for Molecular and Vascular Biology, Catholic University of Leuven, Herestraat, 49, 3000
Leuven, Belgium. E-mail: Peter.Verhamme@uz.kuleuven.ac.be

R. VERHAEGHE, MD
Center for Molecular and Vascular Biology, Catholic University of Leuven, Herestraat, 49, 3000
Leuven, Belgium. E-mail: Raymond.Verhaeghe@uz.kuleuven.ac.be

G.M. WALSH, MSc, PhD
School of Medicine, Institute of Medical Sciences Building, University of Aberdeen, Forester-
hill, Aberdeen, AB25 2ZD, UK. E-mail: g.m.walsh@abdn.ac.uk

INGEBORG WELTERS, MD, PhD
School of Clinical Medicine, University of Liverpool, The Duncan Building, Daulby Street,
Liverpool, L69 3GA, UK. E-mail: I.Welters@liv.ac.uk

THOMAS J. WALSH, MD
Immunocompromised Host Section, Pediatric Oncology Branch, National Cancer Institute,
National Institutes of Health, Bethesda, MD, USA. E-mail: walsht@mail.nih.gov

EILEEN J. WONG, MD
Harvard Medical School, Massachusetts Mental Health Center, Department of Psychiatry, Ja-
maica Plain, MA 02130, USA. E-mail: ewong88@juno.com

OLIVER ZUZAN, MD
Department of Anaesthesia, 12th Floor, Royal Liverpool University Hospital, Prescot Street,
Liverpool, L7 8XP, UK. E-mail: oliver.zuzan@btinternet.com

Contents

Contributors   v

Special reviews   xv

Cumulative indexes of special reviews, Annuals 13–29   xvii

Table of Essays, Annuals 1–29   xxv

DoTS classification of adverse drug reactions   xxvii

How to use this book   xxix

Drug withdrawals because of adverse effects   xxxi
J.K. Aronson

1. Central nervous system stimulants and drugs that suppress appetite   1
   R.P. Sequeira

2. Antidepressant drugs   15
   P.J. Cowen

3. Lithium   23
   R.S. El-Mallakh

4. Drugs of abuse   31
   E. Wong, J.K. Patel, and S. Guzofski

5. Hypnosedatives and anxiolytics   49
   S. Musa, A. Byrne, and S. Curran

6. Antipsychotic drugs   56
   A. Carvajal, L.H. Martín Arias, and N. Jimeno

7. Antiepileptic drugs   78
   D. Schmidt and S. Beyenburg

8. Opioid analgesics and narcotic antagonists   106
   A.H. Ghodse and S. Galea

9. Anti-inflammatory and antipyretic analgesics and drugs used in gout   125
   A. Del Favero

10. General anesthetics and therapeutic gases   137
    I.D. Welters and M. Leuwer

11. Local anesthetics   152
    S.A. Schug and A. Raajkumar

12. Neuromuscular blocking agents and skeletal muscle relaxants   164
    O. Zuzan and M. Leuwer

13. Drugs that affect autonomic functions or the extrapyramidal system   170
    M. Schachter

14. Dermatological drugs, topical agents, and cosmetics   180
    A.E. Goossens and J.K. Aronson

15. Antihistamines (H$_1$ receptor antagonists)   189
    G.M. Walsh

16. Drugs acting on the respiratory tract   193
    M. Joerger, K. Hartmann, and M. Kuhn

17. Positive inotropic drugs and drugs used in dysrhythmias   209
    J.K. Aronson

18. Beta-adrenoceptor antagonists and antianginal drugs   223
    A.P. Maggioni, M.G. Franzosi, and R. Latini

19. Drugs acting on the cerebral and peripheral circulations   231
    R. Verhaeghe and P. Verhamme

20. Antihypertensive drugs   234
    J.J. Coleman and U. Martin

21. Diuretics   252
    D.A. Sica

22. Metals   262
    G.B. van der Voet and J.A. Centeno

23. Metal antagonists   273
    R.H.B. Meyboom

24. Antiseptic drugs and disinfectants   278
    P. Magee

25. Penicillins, cephalosporins, other beta-lactam antibiotics, and tetracyclines   280
    T. Midtvedt

26. Miscellaneous antibacterial drugs   297
    N. Corti and A. Imhof

27. Antifungal drugs   316
    A.H. Groll and T.J. Walsh

28. Antiprotozoal drugs   336
    O.O. Simooya

29. Antiviral drugs   343
    B.J. Angus

30. Drugs used in tuberculosis and leprosy   357
    V.V. Banu Rekha and S. Swaminathan

31. Antihelminthic drugs   364
    P.J.J. van Genderen

32. Vaccines   369
    S. Dittmann

33. Blood, blood components, plasma, and plasma products   381
    P.F.W. Strengers and E. van Twuyver

34. Vitamins, intravenous solutions, and drugs and formulations used in nutrition   394
    M.C. Allwood and P.A. Ball

35. Drugs affecting blood coagulation, fibrinolysis, and hemostasis   399
    J. Harenberg

36.   Gastrointestinal drugs   423
      H.J. Fellows and H.R. Dalton

37.   Drugs that act on the immune system: cytokines and monoclonal antibodies   435
      F. Braun and M. Behrend

38.   Drugs that act on the immune system: immunosuppressive and immunostimulatory
      drugs   452
      F. Braun and M. Behrend

39.   Corticotrophins, corticosteroids, and prostaglandins   463
      J. Costa and M. Farré

40.   Sex hormones and related compounds, including hormonal contraceptives   468
      M.N.G. Dukes

41.   Thyroid hormones, iodine, and antithyroid drugs   490
      K. Boelaert

42.   Insulin, other hypoglycemic drugs, and glucagon   494
      R.C.L. Page

43.   Miscellaneous hormones   507
      R.C.L. Page

44.   Drugs that affect lipid metabolism   515
      I. Aursnes

45.   Cytostatic and cytotoxic drugs   520
      H.-P. Lipp and J.T. Hartmann

46.   Radiological contrast agents   533
      S.K. Morcos

47.   Drugs used in ocular treatment   544
      B.C.P. Polak

48.   Treatments used in complementary and alternative medicine   551
      M.H. Pittler and E. Ernst

49.   Miscellaneous drugs, materials, medical devices, and techniques   561
      N.H. Choulis

50.   Medication errors   576
      J.K. Aronson

Address list of national centers that participate in the WHO Drug Monitoring Programme   582

Index of drugs   596

Index of adverse effects   611

Special reviews

The efficacy of lithium and comparisons with alternative agents 23
Fetotoxicity of cocaine 35
Epidemiology of the use of ecstasy 37
Khat 43
Antipsychotic drugs in elderly patients 59
Pregabalin 86
Routes of administration of opioids 106
Strategies to reduce upper gastrointestinal tract damage caused by non-steroidal anti-inflammatory drugs (NSAIDs) 125
Paracetamol and the risk of asthma 129
Prevention of pain due to propofol injection 143
Pathological gambling and dopamine receptor agonists 174
Susceptibility factors for the adverse effects of budesonide in children and very young children 194
Ciclesonide 196
Mometasone furoate 197
Respiratory adverse effects of long-acting beta$_2$-adrenoceptor agonists 198
Genetic susceptibility factors that affect the use of long-acting beta$_2$-adrenoceptor agonists 199
Angioedema due to angiotensin II receptor antagonists 238
Direct renin inhibitors—a new class of antihypertensive drugs but the same adverse effects? 242
Hypersensitivity reactions to sulfonamide derivatives 252
Cross-reactivity in penicillin and cephalosporin hypersensitivity reactions 280
Tetracyclines, chemically-modified tetracyclines, and their non-antimicrobial properties 288
Muscle damage from daptomycin 309
Drug–drug interactions with antifungal azoles 320
Combination regimens in the eradication of *Helicobacter pylori* 340
The combined effects of ribavirin + interferon 344
Ethambutol-induced optic neuropathy 358
Combination vaccines/multiple immunizations 369
Interactions of herbal medicines with warfarin 400
Heparin-induced thrombocytopenia 404
Hepatotoxicity of ximelagatran 411
Orlistat 429
Tamoxifen versus aromatase inhibitors 475
Finasteride 480
Administration of insulin by inhalation 495
Dipeptidyl peptidase IV inhibitors 498
Drug interactions with statins 517
Tyrosine kinase inhibitors 520

Contrast medium-induced nephrotoxicity	535
Gadolinium-based contrast agents and nephrogenic systemic fibrosis	538
Verteporfin and photodynamic therapy	545
Bisphosphonates and fractures	561
Bisphosphonates and osteonecrosis of the jaw	562
Interaction of methylthioninium chloride with selective serotonin reuptake inhibitors	569

Cumulative indexes of special reviews, Annuals 13–29

Index of drugs

Note: the format 29.460 refers to SEDA-29, p. 460.

Abetimus, drug development, 29.460
ACE inhibitors
    acetylsalicylic acid, interaction, 28.124
    angioedema, 22.225, 29.207
    cough, 19.211
    indications, 24.233
Acetaminophen, *see* Paracetamol
Acetylsalicylic acid, 21.100
    ACE inhibitors, interaction, 28.124
    benefit to harm balance in preventing strokes and
        heart attacks, 27.109
    co-medication, 26.423
    gastrointestinal effects, 17.95, 18.90
    Reye's syndrome, 15.85
    rhinosinusitis/asthma, 17.94
Acupuncture
    incidence of adverse effects, 29.589
    traumatic effects, 29.590
Aerosols, delivery, 27.172
Albumin, human, anaphylaxis, 14.296
Alcohol, vitamin A, beta-carotene, interaction,
    24.442
Aldosterone antagonists, in heart failure, 24.246
Aluminium, in albumin solutions, 23.359
Aminoglycoside antibiotics, 17.304
    contact dermatitis, 13.225
    dosage regimens, 20.234, 21.265, 23.264
    nephrotoxicity, 15.268, 17.305
    ototoxicity, 14.222, 18.268
    and ribostamycin, 15.270
Amiodarone, dysrhythmias, 25.211
    respiratory toxicity, 15.168
    thyroid disease, 27.192
Amphetamines, 29.3
Amphotericin, liposomal, 17.319
    nephrotoxicity, 13. 231, 14.229, 27.276
Anabolic steroids, abuse in sport, 29.508
Analgesics
    headache, 21.95
    headaches in children, 23.114
    nephropathy, 21.98
Androgens, in women, 24.477
Anesthesia, dental, safety of, 16.122
Anesthetics
    halogenated, renal damage, 20.106

    local, combinations, 20.121
    local, neurotoxicity, 21.129, 25.152
    ocular, 17.542
Anorectic drugs
    cardiac valvulopathy 22.3, 23.2, 24.4, 25.5
    primary pulmonary hypertension, 18.7, 21.2, 23.2,
        25.5
Anthracyclines, 25.533
Anticancer antimetabolites, 29.531
Anticholinergic drugs, 22.507
Anticoagulants, oral, skin necrosis, 29.358
Anticonvulsants, *see* Antiepileptic drugs
Antidepressants, *see also individual agents*
    during and after pregnancy, 21.17
    mania, 29.18
    overdose, 28.14
Antidysrhythmic drugs
    in atrial fibrillation, 24.197
    prodysrhythmic effects, 17.218, 23.196
Antiepileptic drugs
    bone loss, 27.74
    comparison, 25.78
    death, 23.83
    overdosage, 22.84
    psychiatric effects, 22.82, 27.72
Antiestrogens, genotoxicity and tumorigenicity,
    27.429
Antifungal drugs
    drug interactions (azoles), 24.318, 28.299, 29.282
    Pneumocystis jiroveci (carinii) pneumonia, 18.289
Antihistamines
    cardiovascular adverse effects, 17.196, 22.176,
        25.183, 26.180
    drowsiness/sedation, 21.170, 23.171, 26.182
Antihypertensive drugs, 19.209
    in diabetes mellitus, 28.226
    fixed-dose combinations, 22.224
    individualizing therapy, 17.246
Antimalarial drugs, 14.237, 17.325, 20.257
    adjunctive treatments, 24.330
    prophylaxis, 13.239, 23.304
Antimicrobial drugs
    allergic reactions, 23.251
    coagulation disorders, 18.258
    colitis, 17.303
    intestinal motility, 13.220
    male fertility, 16.262

new, 13.210
new, with adjuvants, 17.296
the pill and pregnancy, 24, 274
policies and politics, 16.273
prescribing, 15.254
preterm infants, 21.258
prudent use, 25.279 , 27.242, 28.265
resistance, 13.210, 19.237, 20.228, 21.257,
    22.265, 23.250, 24.273, 29.244
seizures, 18.261
side chains, 16.264
Antioxidant vitamins, 20.363
Antiprotozoal drugs
    African trypanosomiasis, 18.293
    toxoplasmosis, 20.262
Antipsychotic drugs
    comparisons of different types 25.53, 27.50
    diabetes mellitus, 28.60
    use in conditions other than schizophrenia, 27.49
    weight gain, 26.56
Antiretroviral drugs, metabolic complications,
    28.329
Antithyroid drugs, pregnancy, 13.377
Antituberculosis drugs, 16.341
    genetic susceptibility, 28.342
    liver damage, 25.363, 26.339
    Mycobacterium avium–complex infection, 20.278
Appetite suppressants
    cardiac valvulopathies, 22.3, 23.2, 24.4, 25.5
    primary pulmonary hypertension, 18.7, 21.2, 23.2,
        25.5
Aspirin, *see* Acetylsalicylic acid
Asthma medications, exacerbation of asthma, 20.165
Atovaquone, 19.266
Avoparcin
    lessons from, 27.242
    resistance, 29.244
Azoles, *see* Antifungal drugs

Baclofen, withdrawal syndrome, 26.152
Bambuterol, cardiac failure, 23.181
Benzodiazepines
    brain damage, 14.36
    depression, 17.43
    medicolegal aspects, 13.33
Beta$_2$-adrenoceptor agonists, 18.159
    asthma, 19.178, 21.179
    asthma deaths, 17.164
Beta-adrenoceptor antagonists, sexual function,
    15.188
Beta-carotene, *see also* Vitamin A
    alcohol, vitamin A, interaction, 24.442
    tumorigenicity, 25.454
Beta-lactam antibiotics
    effects on eukaryotic cells, 13.212
    immediate hypersensitivity reactions, 14.211
    pregnancy, 25.280
Botulinum toxin A, use in primary axillary hyper-
    hidrosis, 27.161

Calcium antagonists, long-term safety, 20.185,
    21.208, 22.214
Carnitine, 13.269
Carotenoids, tumorigenicity, 25.454

Ceftriaxone, 15.258
    nephrolithiasis, 29.246
Cephalosporins, immunological reactions, 28.267
Charcoal, activated, in digitalis overdose, 24.201
Chloramphenicol, children, 15.267
Chloroquine, 15.286
Chondroprotective agents, 14.439
Chymopapain, 14.264
Ciclosporin, urinary system, 19.348
Clozapine, 15.50
    agranulocytosis, 22.1359
Cocaine
    cardiovascular effects, 18.5
    fetotoxicity, 29.41
    prenatal exposure and perinatal effects, 27.1
    second-generation effects, 20.24
Cocamidopropylbetaine, allergy, 19.151
Complementary and alternative therapies, indirect
    risks, 27.521
    esophagus, adverse effects on, 14.442
Contrast media
    adverse effects, 13.431, 24.525
    anaphylactoid and allergic reactions, 20.422
    delayed reactions, 26.513
    in magnetic resonance imaging, 20.419
    nephrotoxicity, 27.500, 28.556, 29.575
Corticosteroids, *see* Glucocorticoids
Cosmetics
    adverse effects, 13/117
    contact allergy, 16.150, 19.151
    ingredient labeling 22.159
Co-trimoxazole, hypersensitivity reactions, 20.264
COX2 inhibitors, 24.115, 25.126, 26.116
    vascular disease, 29.116

Deferiprone, cardiac siderosis, 29.235
Deferoxamine, 16.247
    bone dysplasia, 23.241
    cardiac siderosis, 29.235
    bone dysplasia, 23.241
    cardiac siderosis, 29.235
Diamorphine, progressive spongiform leukoen-
    cephalopathy, 24.40
Diclofenac, liver damage, 20.91
Digitalis, in atrial fibrillation, 24.197
Digoxin, compared with other drugs in heart failure
    in sinus rhythm, 14.141
    compared with other drugs in chronic uncompli-
        cated atrial
fibrillation, 14.144
    in heart failure in sinus rhythm, 18.196
Diuretics
    diabetes mellitus, electrolyte abnormalities, and
        the ALLHAT trial, 27.219
    hyponatremia, 29.219
    renal cell carcinoma, 23.225
    renal insufficiency, 25.250
Dofetilide, 26.208
Dopamine receptor agonists, sleep disorders, 26.160,
    27.149

Ecstasy, *see* MDMA
EDTA, pseudothrombocytopenia, 21.250
Endothelin receptor antagonists, in hypertension,
    26.233

Enzyme inhibitors, 15.337
Erythromycin, versus the new macrolides, 21.269
Erythropoietin, pure red cell aplasia, 27.348
　status and safety, 16.400
Etoposide, 27.477
Euxyl K 400, contact allergy, 16.150

Felbamate
　aplastic anemia, 19.68, 22.86
　risk/benefit ratio, 23.86
Fenfluramine
　cardiac valvulopathies, 22.3, 23.2, 24.4, 25.5
　primary pulmonary hypertension, 18.7, 21.2, 23.2,
　　25.5
Fenoterol, safety in severe asthma, 23.182
Fentanyl, buccal and transdermal administration,
　20.77
Fertility drugs
　malignant melanoma, 26.434
　ovarian cancer, 24.474
Fish oil, 13.460
Flecainide, in supraventricular dysrhythmias, 21.200
Fluoroquinolones, 18.271
Fluorouracil, adverse effects, 23.476
Folic acid, dietary supplementation, 19.369
　safety aspects, 27.407
Formoterol, tolerance, 24.187
Fragrances, contact allergy, 20.149

Gadolinium salts, nephrotoxicity, 28.561
General anesthetics, *see* Anesthetics
Germanium, 16.545
Glucocorticoids
　bone, 16.447, 22.182, 25.195
　contact allergy, 15.139, 21.158
　effective dose and therapeutic ratio, 23.175
　and eyes, 29.481
　and growth, 14.335
　inhaled, effects on mouth and throat, 29.168
　inhaled, effects on skin, 29.169
　inhaled, growth inhibition, 26.186
　inhaled, risks in children, 27.174
　inhaled, systemic availability, 24.185, 26.187
　musculoskeletal adverse effects, 21.417
　osteoporosis and osteonecrosis, 16.447, 19.377,
　　20.374, 21.417, 22.182, 28.473
　preterm infants, 17.445
Grapefruit juice, drug interactions 23.519
Growth hormone
　adults, 16.501
　insulin resistance, 24.504
　malignancy, 23.468

Hepatitis B vaccine, demyelinating diseases, 21.331,
　22.346, 24.374
Heroin, *see* Diamorphine
Histamine (H$_2$) receptor antagonists, 13.330, 15.393
HIV-protease inhibitors
　insulin resistance, 22.317
　lipodystrophy, 22.317
HMG Co-A reductase inhibitors, interactions, 25.530
Hormones, sex, tumors, 22.465
5-HT, *see* Serotonin

Hypnotics, 20.30
　avoiding adverse effects, 21.37
Hypoglycemic drugs, combinations of, 27.458,
　28.521

Immunization
　adverse effects, 24.364
　and autoimmune disease, 27.336
　bioterrorism, 25.378, 26.354
　multiple, 27.334
　surveillance after, 15.340, 22.333, 23.335, 24.364,
　　25.376, 26.353, 27.334
Immunotherapy, in leishmaniasis, 15.299
Incretin mimetics, 29.528
Indometacin, fetal and neonatal complications,
　18.102
Influenza vaccine, 29.332
Insulin
　human, and hypoglycemia, 15.452
　modes of administration, 26.464
　resistance, and growth hormone, 24.504
　synthetic analogs, 24.489
Interferons, psychological and psychiatric effects,
　29.384
Interleukin-2, 14.325
Irinotecan, 27.477
Isoniazid, prophylactic, toxicity, 24.352

Kava kava
　liver damage, 27.518
　adverse effects, 28.579
Ketorolac, risk of adverse effects, 17.110

Lamotrigine, skin rashes, 20.62, 24.88
Laxatives, abuse, 13.336
Leflunomide, 29.435
Leukotriene receptor antagonists, Churg–Strauss
　syndrome, 24.183, 27.177, 29.174
Lipid-lowering drugs, 13.402, 15.479
Lithium
　adverse effects, prevention and treatment, 13.17,
　　17.28
　beneficial uses other than in bipolar disorder,
　　27.19
　interactions, 16.13, 18.30
　intoxication, prevention and treatment, 17.29
　monitoring therapy, 18.25
　mortality, 19.14
　urinary system, 14.18, 19.16
Local anesthetics, *see* Anesthetics
Loop diuiretics, *see* Diuretics
Lorenzo's oil, 27.475
Lyme disease vaccine, autoimmune disease, 24.366

Macrolides, drug interactions, 14.220
　intestinal motility, 18.269
Malaria vaccines, 22.306
Mannitol, 28.236
MAO inhibitors, *see* Monoamine oxidase inhibitors
MDMA
　cognitive effects, 26.32
　deaths, 24.32
Measles immunization
　autism, 23.350

Crohn's disease, 23.350
  neurological adverse effects, 23.348
  subacute sclerosing panencephalitis, 29.335
Melatonin, 25.523
Metamfetamine, 29.3
Metformin
  contraindications, 28.515
  lactic acidosis, 23.459, 29.526
Methyldibromoglutaronitrile, contact allergy, 16.150,
    19.151
Mibefradil, drug interactions, 23.210
Midazolam, 15.112
Midodrine, 26.159
Milrinone, intravenous, acute heart failure, 21.196
MMR immunization
  autism, 23.350, 25.387, 28.363
  Crohn's disease, 23.350, 25.387
Monoamine oxidase inhibitors, 13.6, 17.361
Morphine, managing adverse effects, 26.98
Muscle relaxants
  emergency medicine, 20.133
  eyes, 21.145
  hypersensitivity reactions, 27.138
  intensive care, 19.140

Niacin, extended-release, 16.440
Neuromuscular blocking agents, anaphylaxis, 29.145
  non-depolarizing neuromuscular blockers, 15.127
  residual paralysis, 27.139
NSAIDs, *see also* COX2 inhibitors
  acute renal insufficiency, 28.122
  blood pressure, 19.92, 27.102
  children, 19.96
  current controversies, 17.102
  COX2 inhibitors, 24.115, 25.126, 26.116
  dyspepsia, 28.120
  gastrointestinal adverse effects, 14.79, 17.95,
    18.90, 18.99, 20.86, 21.96, 22.108, 23.114
  gastrointestinal damage, role of *Helicobacter py-
    lori*, 27.105
  gastrointestinal toxicity, prevention, 19.93
  inflammatory bowel disease, 25.131
  inhibiting cardioprotective effects of acetylsali-
    cylic acid, 28.118
  intracerebral hemorrhage, 28.119
  necrotizing fasciitis, 28.121
  nephrotoxicity, 18.100, 20.89, 24.120, 26.111
  skin reactions, 13.72
  topical, 18.163

Ocular drugs
  allergic reactions, 21.486
  geriatric patients, 16.542
  risk factors for adverse effects, 22.507
Omeprazole, tumors, 16.423
Opioids
  abuse, 29.44
  adverse effects, prevention, 24.100
  death, 25.37
  obstetric use, 24.102
  tolerance in neonates, 23.97
Oral contraceptives
  antimicrobial drugs, and pregnancy, 24.274
  and breast cancer, 15.426

  formulations, 24.472
  third-generation, 25.484, 26.442
  venous thromboembolism, 23.442

Paclitaxel, adverse effects, 21.463
Pancreatic enzyme supplements, fibrosing colonopa-
    thy, 20.322
Paracetamol
  liver damage, 17.98, 18.94
  overdose, 13.68, 23.117
Parenteral nutrition
  bone effects, 22.378
  cholestasis, 22.376
  infections, 22.379
Penicillins
  acute desensitization, 23.252
  immunological reactions, 28.267
Peritoneal dialysis fluids, effects on peritoneum,
    22.381
Phentermine, cardiac valvulopathies, 24.4
Platinum compounds, 26.490
Polio vaccine, AIDS, 23.352
Polyaspartic acid, protective against nephrotoxicity,
    17.305
Polyethylene glycol, electrolyte, mineral, metal, and
    fluid balance, 29.376
Polystyrene sulfonates, 25.271
Polyvinylpyrrolidone, storage disease, 22.522
Propofol, infusion syndrome, 26.135
Propolis, allergy, 17.181
Proton pump inhibitors, tumors, 23.383
PUVA, malignant melanoma, 22.166
Pyrazinamide, in latent pulmonary tuberculosis,
    27.323

Quinidine, versus quinine, 15.295
Quinine, versus quinidine, 15.295

Rhesus anti-D, prophylaxis, 13.297
Ribostamycin, and aminoglycosides, 15.270
Rocuronium, allergic reactions, 26.150
Rotashield, intussusception, 23.354

Salbutamol, adrenoceptor genotypes, 29.173
Salmeterol, tolerance, 24.187
Sedatives, 29.128
Sex hormones, tumors, 22.465
Serotonin
    receptor antagonists, 15.391
    selective serotonin reuptake inhibitors, drug inter-
      actions, 22.13
    selective serotonin reuptake inhibitors, suicidal be-
      havior, 29.19
Smallpox vaccination, 27.339
Somatostatin, 15.468
Spinal manipulation, adverse effects, 29.591
Statins, *see* HMG Co-A reductase inhibitors
Steroids, *see* Glucocorticoids
Sumatriptan, 17.171
Suramin, patients with prostate cancer, 20.283
Suxamethonium, postoperative myalgia, 28.155

Teniposide, 27.477
Tetracyclines
    adverse effects, 26.268
    comparative toxicity, 22.268
    and metalloproteinases, 26.266
    in pregnancy, 25.280
    in rheumatology, 23.255
    therapeutic effects, 24.278
Theophylline, asthma, 17.2, 18.1, 18.2
Thiazides, *see* Diuretics
Thiazolidinediones, peripheral edema, 29.531
Thiomersal, in vaccines, 28.357
Thyroid hormones, 29.464
Thyroxine, drug interactions, 24.484
Tiaprofenic acid, cystitis, 18.106
Toiletries, *see* Cosmetics
Topiramate, cognitive effects, 26.81
Topoisomerase inhibitors, 27.477
Topotecan, 27.477
Tretinoin, topical, teratogenicity, 18.164
Triazolam, 16.33
Tricyclic antidepressants, mania, 13.8
L-tryptophan, eosinophilia-myalgia syndrome, 15.514
Tumor necrosis factor antagonists, infection risk, 29.395

Vaccines, *see also individual agents*
    combinations, 29.327
    poliomyelitis, 22.352
    thiomersal in, 28.357
Valproate, polycystic ovary syndrome, 26.81
Vancomycin
    lessons from, 27.242
    resistance, 29.244
Vigabatrin
    psychosis and abnormal behavior, 18.71
    visual field defects, 21.78, 24.95, 25.98, 26.82
Vinca alkaloids, 28.538
Vitamin A, 17.436
    alcohol, beta-carotene, interaction, 24.442
    hypervitaminosis, 15.411
    in pregnancy, 21.405
    and prostate cancer, 13.346
Vitamin B_6, debate, 23.420
Vitamin E, co-medication, 26.423
Vitamin K
    cancer, 23.424
    skin reactions, 25.461
Vitamins, in old age, 22.431
Zidovudine, 13.246

Index of adverse effects

Cardiovascular
atrial fibrillation, antidysrhythmic drugs, 24.197
atrial fibrillation, digitalis, 24.197
cardiac failure, aldosterone antagonists, 24.246
cardiac failure, bambuterol, 23.181
cardiac siderosis, deferoxamine/deferiprone, 29.235
cardiotoxicity, antihistamines, 17.196, 25.183, 26.180
cardiotoxicity, calcium antagonists, 20.185
cardiotoxicity, cocaine, 18.5
cardiotoxicity, coxibs, 29.116
cardiotoxicity, propofol, 26.135
dysrhythmias, antihistamines, 22.176
dysrhythmias, amiodarone, 25.211
heart attacks, acetylsalicylic acid, 27.109
hypertension, NSAIDs, 19.92, 27.102
prodysrhythmic effects, antidysrhythmic drugs, 17.218, 23.196
QT interval prolongation, 24.54
valvulopathies, fenfluramine, 22.3, 23.2, 24.4, 25.5
valvulopathies, phentermine, 24.4, 25.5
venous thromboembolism, oral contraceptives, 23.442

Respiratory
amiodarone, 15.168
asthma, acetylsalicylic acid, 17.94
asthma, fenoterol, 23.182
asthma, in pregnancy, 28.186
asthma deaths, beta$_2$-adrenoceptor agonists, 17.164
asthma exacerbation, asthma medications, 20.165
bronchoconstriction, paradoxical, nebulizer solutions, 13.134

Churg–Strauss syndrome, leukotriene receptor antagonists, 24.183, 27.177, 29.174
cough, ACE inhibitors, 19.211
primary pulmonary hypertension, appetite suppressants, 18.7, 21.2, 23.2, 25.5
rhinosinusitis, acetylsalicylic acid, 17.94

Ear, nose, throat
glucocorticoids, inhaled, 29.168

Nervous system
brain damage, benzodiazepines, 14.36
demyelinating diseases, hepatitis B vaccine, 21.331, 22.346, 24.374
drowsiness/sedation, antihistamines, 21.170, 23.171, 26.182
headache, analgesics, 21.95, 23.114
intracerebral hemorrhage, NSAIDs, 28.119
neuroleptic malignant syndrome, 20.41
neurotoxicity, anesthetics, local, 21.129
neurotoxicity, measles immunization, 23.348
overdosage, antiepileptic drugs, 22.84
poliomyelitis, vaccines, 22.352
progressive spongiform leukoencephalopathy, diamorphine, 24.40
seizures, antimicrobial drugs, 18.261
sleep disorders, dopamine receptor agonists, 26.160, 27.149
strokes, acetylsalicylic acid, 27.109
strokes, risperidone, 28.76
subacute sclerosing panencephalitis, measles vaccine, 29.335
tardive dyskinesia, 14.47, 20.38
tardive syndromes, 17.54
transient symptoms, intrathecal anesthetics, 25.152

Neuromuscular
  residual paralysis, neuromuscular blocking drugs,
    27.139
Sensory systems
  eye effects, glucocorticoids, 29.481
  eye effects, muscle relaxants, 21.145
  ototoxicity, aminoglycosides, 14.222, 18.268
  visual field defects, vigabatrin, 21.78, 24.95,
    25.98, 26.82
Psychological
  cognitive effects, MDMA, 26.32
  cognitive effects, metamfetamine, 29.3
  cognitive effects, topiramate, 26.78
  interferons, 29.384
Psychiatric
  antiepileptic drugs, 22.82, 27.72
  autism, MMR/measles immunization, 23.350,
    25.387, 28.363
  depression, benzodiazepines, 17.43
  mania, antidepressants, 13.8, 29.18
  interferons, 29.384
  psychosis and abnormal behavior, vigabatrin,
    18.71
  suicidal behavior, SSRIs, 29.19
Endocrine
  diabetes mellitus, antihypertensive drugs, 28.226
  diabetes mellitus, antipsychotic drugs, 28.60
  diabetes mellitus, diuretics, 27.219
  insulin resistance, growth hormone, 24.504
  insulin resistance, HIV-protease inhibitors, 22.317
  ovarian hyperstimulation syndrome, valproate,
    26.477
  polycystic ovary syndrome, valproate, 26.81
  thyroid disease, amiodarone, 27.192
Metabolism
  antiretroviral drugs, 28.329
  hyperlactatemia, 29.302
  hypoglycemia, insulin, 15.452
  lactic acidosis, metformin, 23.459, 29.526
  lipoatrophy, 29.302
  lipodystrophy, HIV-protease inhibitors, 22.317
  metabolic acidosis, propofol, 26.135
  mitochondrial toxicity, 29.302
  polyvinylpyrrolidone storage disease, 22.522
  weight gain, antipsychotic drugs, 26.56
Electrolyte balance
  electrolyte abnormalities, diuretics, 27.219,
    29.219
  polyethylene glycol, 29.376
Mineral balance
  polyethylene glycol, 29.376
Metal balance
  polyethylene glycol, 29.376
Fluid balance
  peripheral edema, thiazolidinediones, 29.531
  polyethylene glycol, 29.376
Hematologic
  agranulocytosis, clozapine, 22.59
  aplastic anemia, felbamate, 19.68, 22.86
  coagulation disorders, beta-lactam antibiotics,
    18.258
  eosinophilia-myalgia syndrome, tryptophan,
    15.514
  pseudothrombocytopenia, EDTA, 21.250
  pure red cell aplasia, erythropoietin, 27.348

Mouth
  Glucocorticoids, inhaled, 29.168
Gastrointestinal
  bleeding, acetylsalicylic acid, 17.95, 18.90
  cholestasis, total parenteral nutrition, 22.376
  colitis, antimicrobial drugs, 17.303
  Crohn's disease, MMR/measles immunization,
    23.350, 25.387
  dyspepsia, NSAIDs, 28.120
  fibrosing colonopathy, pancreatic enzyme supple-
    ments, 20.322
  inflammatory bowel disease, NSAIDs, 25.131
  intestinal motility, antimicrobial drugs, 13.220
  intestinal motility, macrolides, 18.269
  intussusception, Rotashield, 23.354
  ulceration, bleeding and perforation, NSAIDs,
    14.79, 16.103, 17.95, 18.90, 18.99, 19.93,
    20.86, 21.96, 22.108, 23.114, 27.105
Liver
  hepatotoxicity, alcohol/vitamin A/beta-carotene,
    24.442
  hepatotoxicity, antituberculosis drugs, 25.363,
    26.339
  hepatotoxicity, diclofenac, 20.91
  hepatotoxicity, kava kava, 27.518
  hepatotoxicity, paracetamol, 17.98, 18.94
  Reye's syndrome, acetylsalicylic acid, 15.85
Urinary tract
  acute renal insufficiency, NSAIDs, 28.122
  cystitis, tiaprofenic acid, 18.106
  nephrolithiasis, ceftriaxone, 29.246
  nephrotoxicity, aminoglycosides, 15.268, 17.305
  nephrotoxicity, amphotericin, 13.231, 14.229,
    27.276
  nephrotoxicity, analgesics, 21.98
  nephrotoxicity, anesthetics, halogenated, 20.106
  nephrotoxicity, ciclosporin, 19.348
  nephrotoxicity, contrast media, 27.500, 28.556,
    29.575
  nephrotoxicity, gadolinium salts, 28.561
  nephrotoxicity, lithium, 14.18, 19.16
  nephrotoxicity, NSAIDs, 18.100, 20.89, 24.120,
    26.111
  renal cell carcinoma, diuretics, 23.225
  renal insufficiency, diuretics, 25.250
Skin
  contact allergy, 23.160
  contact allergy, glucocorticoids, 15.139
  contact dermatitis, aminoglycosides, 13.225
  cutaneous reactions, NSAIDs, 13.72
  glucocorticoids, inhaled, 29.169
  necrosis, oral anticoagulation, 29.358
  rashes, lamotrigine, 20.62, 24.88
  vitamin K$_1$, 25.461
Serosae
  peritoneum, peritoneal dialysis, 22.381
  pleurodesis, 25.189
Musculoskeletal
  bone, total parenteral nutrition, 22.378
  bone dysplasia, deferoxamine, 23.241
  bone loss, antiepileptic drugs, 27.74
  bone mineral density, glucocorticoids, 25.195
  eosinophilia-myalgia syndrome, tryptophan,
    15.514

growth in children, inhaled glucocorticoids, 26.186
growth in children, oral glucocorticoids, 14.335
osteoporosis and osteonecrosis, glucocorticoids, 16.447, 19.377, 20.374, 21.417, 22.182, 28.473
rhabdomyolysis, propofol, 26.135
postoperative myalgia, suxamethonium, 28.155
Sexual function
and beta-adrenoceptor antagonists, 15.188
Immunologic
allergic reactions, antimicrobial drugs, 23.251
allergic reactions, rocuronium, 26.150
anaphylaxis, human albumin, 14.296
anaphylaxis, neuromuscular blocking agents, 29.145
angioedema, ACE inhibitors, 22.225, 29.207
autoimmune disease, immunizations, 27.336
autoimmune disease, Lyme disease vaccine, 24.366
cocamidopropylbetaine, 19.151
contrast agents, 20.422
cosmetics, 16.150, 19.151
co-trimoxazole, 20.264
desensitization, penicillin, 23.252
Euxyl K 400, 16.150
fragrances, 20.149
glucocorticoids, 21.158
hypersensitivity reactions, beta-lactam antibiotics, 14.211
hypersensitivity reactions, muscle relaxants, 27.138
immune reconstitution disease, 29.315
methyldibromoglutaronitrile, 16.150, 19.151
ocular drugs, 21.486
propolis, 17.181
red man syndrome, 17.312
Infection risk
AIDS, polio vaccine, 23.352
necrotizing fasciitis, NSAIDs, 28.121
total parenteral nutrition, 22.379
tumor necrosis factor antagonists, 29.395
Body temperature
malignant hyperthermia, 18.112
Trauma
acupuncture, 29.590
Death
antiepileptic drugs, 23.83
calcium antagonists, 22.214
ecstasy, 24.32
lithium, 19.14
opiates, 25.37, 29.44
Drug abuse
anabolic steroids in sport, 29.508
Drug tolerance
antimicrobial drug resistance, 19.237, 20.228, 21.257, 22.265, 23.250, 24.273, 25.279, 29.244
opioids in neonates, 23.97
Drug withdrawal
baclofen, 26.152
Genotoxicity
antiestrogens, 27.429
Tumorigenicity
alcohol/vitamin A/beta-carotene, 24.442

antiestrogens, 27.429
beta-carotene, 25.454
carotenoids, 25.454
fertility drugs, 24.474, 26.434
growth hormone, 23.468
omeprazole, 16.423
oral contraceptives, 15.426
proton pump inhibitors, 23.383
PUVA, malignant melanoma, 22.166
sex hormones, 22.465
vitamin K, 23.424
Fertility
fertility, male, antimicrobial drugs, 16.262
Pregnancy
affective disorders in, 21.17
antimicrobial drugs and the pill, 24.274
antithyroid drugs, 13.377
asthma, 28.186
beta-lactams, 25.280
cocaine, 27.1
opioids, 24.102
tetracyclines, 25.280
vitamin A, 21.405
Teratogenicity
tretinoin, topical, 18.164
Fetotoxicity
cocaine, 20.24, 27.1, 29.41
indometacin, 18.102
Susceptibility factors
children, inhaled glucocorticoids 27.174
children, NSAIDs, 19.96
genetic susceptibility, antituberculosis drugs, 28.342
genetic susceptibility, beta-adrenoceptor agonists, 29.173
intensive care, muscle relaxants, 19.140
neonatal complications, indometacin, 18.102
ocular drugs, 22.507
old age, vitamins, 22.431
preterm infants, beta-lactam antibiotics, 21.258
Drug administration
delivery of aerosols, 27.172
dosage regimens, aminoglycosides, 23.264
errors, 28.587, 29.596
formulations, oral contraceptives, 24.472
inhaled glucocorticoids, systemic availability, 24.185
intravitreal and parabulbar injection, 29.581
labeling problems, cosmetics, 22.159
Drug overdose
antidepressants, 28.14
digitalis, charcoal, 24.201
paracetamol, 23.117
Drug formulations
enantiomers and racemates, 13.442
Drug-drug interactions
acetylsalicylic acid ACE inhibitor, 28.124
acetylsalicylic acid/NSAIDs, 28.118
alcohol/vitamin A/beta-carotene, 24.442
antimicrobial drugs/the pill, 24.274
antifungal azoles, 24.318, 28.299, 29.282
grapefruit juice, 23.519
HMG Co-A reductase inhibitors, 25.530
lithium, 16.13

lithium/specific serotonin reuptake inhibitors, 18.30
macrolides, 14.220
mibefradil, 23.210
monoamine oxidase inhibitors/foods, 13.6
NSAIDs/ACE inhibitors, 28.122
paracetamol, 13.68
specific serotonin reuptake inhibitors, 22.13
thyroxine, 24.484

Methods
ethnopharmacology, 14.429
eukaryotic cells, effects of beta-lactams, 13.212
hemolytic disease of the newborn, prophylaxis, 13.297
onchocerciasis, treatment, 14.261
post-marketing surveillance, 14.210, 15.266, 24.274

Table of Essays, Annuals 1–29

SEDA	Author	Country	Title
1	M.N.G. Dukes	The Netherlands	The moments of truth
2	K.H. Kimbel	Germany	Drug monitoring: why care?
3	L. Lasagna	USA	Wanted and unwanted drug effects: the need for perspective
4	M.N.G. Dukes	The Netherlands	The van der Kroef syndrome
5	J.P. Griffin, P.F. D'Arcy	UK	Adverse reactions to drugs—the information lag
6	I. Bayer	Hungary	Science vs practice and/or practice vs science
7	E. Napke	Canada	Adverse reactions: some pitfalls and postulates
8	M.N.G. Dukes	Denmark	The seven pillars of foolishness
9	W.H.W. Inman	UK	Let's get our act together
10	S. Van Hauen	Denmark	Integrated medicine, safer medicine and "AIDS"
11	M.N.G. Dukes	Denmark	Hark, hark, the fictitious dogs do bark
12	M.C. Cone	Switzerland	Both sides of the fence
13	C. Medawar	UK	On our side of the fence
14	M.N.G. Dukes, E. Helsing	Denmark	The great cholesterol carousel
15	P. Tyrer	UK	The nocebo effect—poorly known but getting stronger
16	M.N.G. Dukes	Denmark	Good enough for Iganga?
17	M.N.G. Dukes	Denmark	The mists of tomorrow
18	R.D. Mann	UK	Databases, privacy, and confidentiality the effect of proposed legislation on pharmacoepidemiology and drug safety monitoring
19	A. Herxheimer	UK	Side effects: freedom of information and the communication of doubt
20	E. Ernst	UK	Complementary/alternative medicine: what should we do about it?
21	H. Jick	USA	Thirty years of the Boston Collaborative Drug Surveillance Program in relation to principles and methods of drug safety research
22	J.K. Aronson, R.E. Ferner	UK	Errors in prescribing, preparing, and giving medicines: definition, classification, and prevention
23	K.Y. Hartigan-Go, J.Q. Wong	Philippines	Inclusion of therapeutic failures as adverse drug reactions
24	I. Palmlund	UK	Secrecy hiding harm: case histories from the past that inform the future
25	L. Marks	UK	The pill: untangling the adverse effects of a drug
26	D.J. Finney	UK	From thalidomide to pharmacovigilance: a personal account
26	L.L. Iversen	UK	How safe is cannabis?
27	J.K. Aronson	UK	Louis Lewin—Meyler's predecessor
27	H. Jick	USA	The General Practice Research Database
28	J.K. Aronson	UK	Classifying adverse drug reactions in the 21st century
29	M. Hauben, A. Bate	USA/Sweden	Data mining in drug safety

DoTS classification of adverse drug reactions

Adverse drug reactions have been classified in these volumes since SEDA-28 according to the DoTS system (SEDA-28, xxvii–xxxiii; Br Med J 2003;327:1222–5). In this system adverse reactions are classified according to the **Dose** at which they usually occur, the **Time-course** over which they occur, and the **Susceptibility factors** that make them more likely, as follows:

- **Relation to dose**
  - Toxic reactions (reactions that occur at supratherapeutic doses)
  - Collateral reactions (reactions that occur at standard therapeutic doses)
  - Hypersusceptibility reactions (reactions that occur at subtherapeutic doses in susceptible individuals)
- **Time course**
  - Time-independent reactions (reactions that occur at any time during a course of therapy)
  - Time-dependent reactions
    * Immediate or rapid reactions (reactions that occur only when a drug is administered too rapidly)
    * First-dose reactions (reactions that occur after the first dose of a course of treatment and not necessarily thereafter)
    * Early reactions (reactions that occur early in treatment then either abate with continuing treatment, owing to tolerance, or persist)
    * Intermediate reactions (reactions that occur after some delay but with less risk during longer term therapy, owing to the "healthy survivor" effect)
    * Late reactions (reactions the risk of which increases with continued or repeated exposure)
    * Withdrawal reactions (reactions that occur when, after prolonged treatment, a drug is withdrawn or its effective dose is reduced)
    * Delayed reactions (reactions that occur some time after exposure, even if the drug is withdrawn before the reaction appears)
- **Susceptibility factors**
  - Genetic
  - Age
  - Sex
  - Physiological variation
  - Exogenous factors (for example drug–drug or drug–food interactions, smoking)
  - Diseases

The following reactions have been classified in SEDA using this system:

ACE inhibitors: angioedema	29.207
Adrenaline: hypertension	30.170
Angiotensin II receptor antagonists: angioedema	30.238
Anticoagulants, oral: skin necrosis	29.358
Antipsychotic drugs: diabetes mellitus	28.60
Bisphosphonates: osteonecrosis of the jaw	30.562

Cocaine: myocardial infarction	29.38
Contrast media: nephrotoxicity	29.575, 30.535
Diuretics, loop and thiazide: hyponatremia	29.219
Dopamine receptor agonists: pathological gambling	30.174
Dopamine receptor agonists: sleep attacks	28.162
Ephedrine: vasospasm	30.171
Ergot-derived dopamine receptor agonists: fibrotic reactions	30.176
Ethambutol: optic neuropathy	30.358
Exenatide: nausea	30.499
Gadolinium salts: nephrotoxicity	28.561
Glucocorticoids: osteoporosis	28.185
Heparin: type II thrombocytopenia	30.404
Nitrofurantoin: lung disease	30.303
Pseudoephedrine: toxic epidermal necrolysis	30.172
SSRIs: suicidal behavior	29.19
Statins: myopathy and rhabdomyolysis	30.516
Thionamides: agranulocytosis	29.520, 30.490
Vigabatrin: visual field loss	28. 101, 29.99, 30.98
Ximelagatran: liver damage	30.411

How to use this book

THE SCOPE OF THE ANNUAL

The *Side Effects of Drugs Annual* has been published every year since 1977. It is designed to provide a critical and up-to-date account of new information relating to adverse drug reactions and interactions from the clinician's point of view. It complements the standard encyclopedic work in this field, *Meyler's Side Effects of Drugs: The International Encyclopedia of Adverse Drug Reactions and Interactions*, the 15th edition of which was published in 2006.

PERIOD COVERED

The present *Annual* reviews all reports that presented significant new information on adverse reactions to drugs during 2005. During the production of this *Annual*, some more recent papers have also been included; older literature has also been cited when it is relevant. Special reviews (see below) often cover a much wider range of literature.

SELECTION OF MATERIAL

In compiling the *Side Effects of Drugs Annual* particular attention is devoted to publications that provide essentially new information or throw a new light on problems already recognized. Some confirmatory reports are also described. In addition, some authoritative new reviews are listed. Publications that do not meet these criteria are omitted. Readers anxious to trace all references on a particular topic, including those that duplicate earlier work, or to cross-check an electronic search, are advised to consult *Adverse Reactions Titles,* a monthly bibliography of titles from about 3400 biomedical journals published throughout the world, compiled by the Excerpta Medica International Abstracting Service.

℞ *SPECIAL REVIEWS*

The special reviews deal in more detail with selected topics, often interpreting conflicting evidence, providing the reader with clear guidance. They are identified by the traditional prescription symbol and are printed in italics. This volume includes a Cumulative Index of the Special Reviews that were published in SEDA-13 to SEDA-29 (page xvii) and a list of the Special Reviews that appear in the current Annual (page xv).

CLASSIFICATION OF DRUGS

Drugs are classified according to their main field of use or the properties for which they are most generally recognized. In some cases a drug is included in more than one chapter (for example, lidocaine is mentioned in Chapter 11 as a local anesthetic and in Chapter 17 as an antidysrhythmic drug). Fixed combinations of drugs are dealt with according to their most characteristic component or as a combination product.

DRUG NAMES

Drugs are usually called by their recommended or proposed International Non-proprietary Names (rINN or pINN); when these are not available, chemical names have been used. If a fixed combination has a generic combination name (e.g. co-trimoxazole for trimethoprim + sulfamethoxazole) that has been used; in some cases brand names have been used instead.

SYSTEM OF REFERENCES

References in the text are tagged using the following system, which was introduced in SEDA-24:

M   A meta-analysis or other form of systematic review;
A   An anecdote or set of anecdotes (i.e. case histories);
R   A major review, including non-systematic statistical analyses of published studies;
r   A brief commentary (e.g. an editorial or a letter);
C   A major randomized controlled trial or observational study;
c   A minor randomized controlled trial or observational study or a non-randomized study;
H   A hypothesis article;
E   An experimental study (animal or in vitro);
S   Official (e.g. Governmental, WHO) statements.

The various editions of *Meyler's Side Effects of Drugs* are cited in the text as SED-l4, SED-15, etc; the *Side Effects of Drugs Annuals 1–29* are cited as SEDA-1, SEDA-2, etc.

INDEXES

Index of drugs: this index provides a complete listing of all references to a drug for which adverse effects and/or drug interactions are described.

Index of adverse effects: this index is necessarily selective, since a particular adverse effect may be caused by very large numbers of compounds; the index is therefore mainly directed to adverse effects that are particularly serious or frequent, or are discussed in special detail; before assuming that a given drug does not have a particular adverse effect, consult the relevant chapters.

American spelling has been used, e.g. anemia, estrogen rather than anaemia, oestrogen.

Jeffrey K. Aronson

SIDE EFFECTS OF DRUGS ESSAY

Drug withdrawals because of adverse effects

The life cycle of a therapeutic agent is a long and convoluted one. It usually starts with an anecdotal report of some sort (for example, the results of a screening test or a single clinical observation), which leads to a hypothesis. That hypothesis is then tested in what is nowadays called "proof of concept". If such proof is obtained, further evidence of efficacy is sought, in the form of observational studies (Phase I studies) and then small and large randomized trials (Phase II and III studies). If these are successful, the drug will receive a marketing authorization, but its life cycle is by no means over. More evidence of benefit in different circumstances will be obtained and postmarketing surveillance and informal observations will start to yield reports of suspected adverse reactions that were not recorded during the premarketing phases. Systematic reviews of beneficial and harmful effects will increase knowledge about the favourability or otherwise of the balance between those effects. Then, if the balance between benefit and harm becomes unfavourable, because of the emergence of a serious adverse effect, the drug will be reviewed by the Marketing Authorisation Holder and regulatory authorities, and in the worst case its authorization may be revoked, although before that happens other courses of action are possible.

Adverse effects are much more difficult to assess than beneficial ones for many well-known reasons. A major method for garnering information about them is voluntary organized reporting, in systems such as the Yellow Card scheme in the UK and the Adverse Event Reporting System in the USA, the primary surveillance database used by the Food and Drug Administration (FDA) for identifying postmarketing drug safety problems. Recently all reports of suspected adverse drug reactions submitted to the FDA from the inception of the Adverse Event Reporting System database in 1969 to December 2002 have been analysed, and drug withdrawals and restricted distribution programs based on concerns about safety have been documented (1).

During the 33-year period from 1969, when the reporting of so-called "adverse drug events" (a meaningless term—it should be "suspected adverse drug reactions" (2)) was initiated, to 2002, about 2.3 million case reports for a cumulative number of about 6000 marketed drugs were entered into the database. Most reports were for female patients. During this period, many suspected or proven adverse reactions were identified (Table 1), some of which led to important changes to the product labelling, in the forms of boxed warnings, other warnings, precautions, contraindications, and statements about adverse reactions. More than 75 drugs/drug products were removed from the market because of safety problems. In addition, 11 drugs had special requirements for prescriptions added or had restricted distribution programs. Drugs withdrawn or restricted represented a small proportion (about 1%) of all marketed drugs.

The cumulative numbers of reports in this database are shown in Figure 1. Although the numbers of reports had been on the increase, since 1999 the numbers of reports have been falling, from a maximum of 225 247 in 1999 to 178 542 in 2002. Of course, this may be because of worsening reporting rather than safer drugs.

However, the database of drugs that have been withdrawn from the market world wide, or whose labelling has been changed, is much larger. Drugs may be withdrawn, never to return. Others are withdrawn but then reappear,

Table 1. *The top 20 adverse events overall and the top 20 adverse events with a serious outcome reported to the FDA from 1969 to 2002 (1)*

Adverse event (all reports)	Number of reports	Adverse event with a serious outcome	Number of reports
Drug ineffective	151 431	Pyrexia	41 529
Dermatitis	122 171	Dyspnea	35 717
Headache	80 308	Vomiting	28 928
Nausea	76 900	Hypotension	24 977
Pruritus	74 869	Condition worsened	23 156
Pyrexia	74 817	Death	20 991
Dyspnea	74 205	Weakness	20 268
Dizziness (excluding vertigo)	72 995	Pneumonia	19 146
Vomiting	69 818	Convulsions	19 043
Urticaria	61 965	Cardiac arrest	18 295
Weakness	59 607	Chest pain	17 847
Pain	57 635	Pain	57 635
Abdominal pain	56 400	Nausea	17 841
Condition worsened	55 659	Thrombocytopenia	17 820
Diarrhea	53 959	Abdominal pain	16 803
Chest pain	44 077	Myocardial infarction	16 742
Hypotension	41 931	Dermatitis	15 778
Alopecia	39 062	Diarrhea	15 454
Sedation	36 830	Sepsis	15 133
Convulsions	35 813	Confusion	14 764

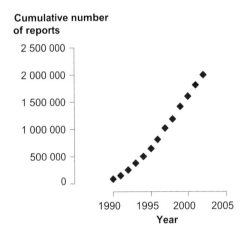

Fig. 1. Cumulative numbers of reports of suspected adverse drug reactions in the FDA's Adverse Event Reporting System database, 1990–2002.

with a risk management plan (for example clozapine (3), alosetron (4)) or for a new indication (for example bupropion (5), thalidomide (6)). Yet others have their label changed (for example aspirin (7)). In some cases a new formulation is withdrawn but the drug itself continues to be made available (for example indometacin as Osmosin® (8)); in some cases it is the route of administration that is abandoned (for example topical penicillins (9)). I have analysed 284 drugs that have been affected in

one of these ways. Most of these examples have been summarized in Stephens's textbook (10), which I have supplemented from the list of cases that I have been collecting for many years. The earliest drug on the list is chloroform (introduced in 1847 and banned by the FDA in 1976); the earliest in modern times is chloramphenicol, which dates from 1950 and whose use was restricted in the UK in 1967 to the treatment of typhoid and *Haemophilus influenzae* meningitis (11); the latest is rosiglitazone, whose label has recently been changed (12). The results of this analysis are shown in Tables 2–5.

Table 2 shows the numbers of drugs affected by changes in the last five decades and the current one. The numbers have increased with time and although the number seems to have fallen during the current decade, this may simply reflect the fact that many fewer drugs are now being marketed than before. Alternatively, better premarketing risk management, such as screening compounds for inhibitory effects on hERG channels as a way of avoiding the adverse effect of QT interval prolongation (13) or for inhibition of cytochrome P450 isozymes in order to avoid drug interactions (14), may have produced a real reduction. These data are similar to those of a previous analysis of 121 drugs from 1960 to 1999 (15), also shown in Table 2.

Table 2. *The numbers of drugs affected by changes in licensing or labelling by decade since the 1950s*

Decade	Number of drugs affected (%)	Data of Fung et al. (15) (%)
1950s	5 (0.02)	–
1960s	29 (10)	12
1970s	53 (19)	17
1980s	84 (30)	40
1990s	87 (31)	31
2000s	26 (9)	–

Table 3 shows the top 14 systems involved by the adverse effects reported, using the systems headings customary in the Side Effects of Drugs Annuals. Since some drugs affected more than one system, the number of cases adds up to considerably more than 284. The liver was most commonly affected, by a long way, followed by the cardiovascular, haematological, and nervous systems and the skin. These results are comparable to those of a previous analysis of 121 drugs from 1960 to 1999 (15), also shown in Table 3. There were no consistent patterns of changes in the systems affected with time. However, there may have been an increase in the number of drugs that caused serious adverse effects on the liver, from 13% of all reports in the 1960s and 1970s to 15% in the 1980s and 20% in the 1990s. Conversely,

Table 3. *The top 14 systems affected by adverse reactions to the 284 drugs in the database; other systems were affected by fewer than eight drugs each*

System affected by adverse drug reaction	Number of drugs affected (%)	Data of Fung et al. (15) (%)
Liver	74 (16)	26
Cardiovascular	40 (8.7)	8.7
Hematologic	39 (8.5)	11
Nervous system	36 (7.9)	
Skin	34 (7.4)	6.3
Tumorigenicity*	28 (6.1)	6.3
Urinary tract	28 (6.1)	
Immunologic	27 (5.9)	
Drug abuse	23 (5.0)	
Psychiatric	17 (3.7)	
Sensory systems†	15 (3.3)	
Gastrointestinal	12 (2.6)	
Drug–drug interactions	11 (2.4)	
Respiratory	11 (2.4)	

*Mostly in animals.

†Eyes and ears in about equal proportions.

Table 4. *The top 20 classes of drug that contributed to the adverse effects of the 284 drugs in the database; other classes contributed under four drugs each*

Class of drug affected	Number (%)	Data of Fung et al. (15) (%)
Anti-infective drugs	32 (11)	
NSAIDs	26 (9.2)	13
Hypnosedatives	18 (6.3)	
Antidepressants	16 (5.6)	7.4
Appetite suppressants	13 (4.6)	4.1
Hormones	10 (3.5)	
Analgesics	9 (3.2)	8.3
Beta-blockers	7 (2.5)	
Herbal drugs	6 (2.1)	
Hypoglycemic drugs	6 (2.1)	
Laxatives	6 (2.1)	
Lipid modulators	6 (2.1)	
Anesthetics	5 (1.8)	
Antiarrhythmic drugs	5 (1.8)	
Antipsychotic drugs	5 (1.8)	
Diuretics	5 (1.8)	
Vasodilators	5 (1.8)	5.8
Antianginal drugs	4 (1.4)	
Antitussive drugs	4 (1.4)	
Contrast media	4 (1.4)	

the risk of serious haematological damage may have decreased with time, from 11% in the 1970s and 13% in the 1980s to 7.8% in the 1990s. Despite screening for effects on hERG channels, there was no obvious fall in the risk of serious cardiovascular adverse effects, the incidence of which may even have increased with time. The numbers of reports for other systems were too small and variable to make any conclusions.

Table 4 shows the types of drugs affected. Anti-infective agents (a class that includes antibacterial, antiviral, antiprotozoal, antifungal drugs, vaccines, and disinfectants) topped the list, followed closely by non-steroidal anti-inflammatory drugs, as might be expected. These results do not bear a close resemblance to those previously obtained by Fung et al. (15), also shown in Table 4, but there may have been differences in the methods of classification.

Table 5 shows the time between the year in which the drug was marketed and the time at which its licensing or labelling status was changed, arranged by decade. With successive decades the time from marketing to the change in status has become progressively shorter. This must be because during this time pharmacovigilance methods have improved and regulatory requirements have become progressively

Table 5. *The time between marketing of the drug and the time at which its licensing or labelling status was changed*

Decade during which change occurred (n = 190)	Number within 1 year (%)	Number at 1–2 years (%)	Number at 3–5 years (%)	Number within 5 years (%)	Number later than 5 years (%)
Pre-1950s (25)	0	0	0	0	25 (100)
1950s (20)	0	1 (5)	3 (15)	4 (20)	16 (80)
1960s (36)	5 (14)	3 (8)	3 (8)	11 (31)	25 (69)
1970s (43)	3 (7)	1 (2)	6 (14)	10 (23)	33 (77)
1980s (37)	10 (27)	3 (8)	12 (32)	25 (64)	12 (32)
1990s (29)	12 (41)	8 (28)	3 (10)	23 (79)	6 (21)

more stringent, although it is possible that companies are taking greater risks and being caught out sooner than they have been in the past.

There are lessons to be learned from this analysis. Firstly, although the liver is the most common organ to be affected by drugs whose licensing or labelling status is subsequently changed, effects on the liver do not have strong predictive value of the risk of such changes, since other systems are also often affected. Similarly, there is no one group of drugs that emerges as being particularly likely to suffer, although one should perhaps be more cautious with new NSAIDs and psychotropic drugs, which feature commonly. The attrition rate for anti-infective drugs is disappointing, given the increasing emergence of resistant microbial strains and the relative lack of new effective drugs.

Next, the delay in discovering serious adverse effects of new drugs is becoming encouragingly shorter, which suggests that pharmacovigilance techniques are paying off, at least where serious adverse effects are concerned. However, other adverse effects are still not being followed up as assiduously as might be, judging from a recent study of 63 case reports of suspected adverse reactions that were newly described in 1997, 83% of which were not subjected to further detailed evaluation (16).

Finally, the importance of encouraging physicians, pharmacists, other health-care professionals, and patients to continue to report serious suspected adverse drug reactions, whether unknown or known, to manufacturers and their local regulatory agencies cannot be overemphasized.

Drug development is becoming increasingly difficult. Continued attrition of potentially useful drugs because of serious unwanted effects will not help. Careful premarketing screening should reduce the problem but may also reduce the number of potentially useful drugs available for full development and subsequent licensing. Better risk management strategies are needed to handle problems when they arise, by means other than revocation of licences (17, 18).

Acknowledgement

I am grateful to John Talbot for helpful comments on an early version of this essay.

References

1. Wysowski DK, Swartz L. Adverse drug event surveillance and drug withdrawals in the United States, 1969–2002. The importance of reporting suspected reactions. Arch Intern Med 2005;165:1363–9.

2. Aronson JK, Ferner RE. Clarification of terminology in drug safety. Drug Saf 2005;28(10):851–70.

3. Bastani B, Alphs LD, Meltzer HY. Development of the Clozaril Patient Management System. Psy-

chopharmacology (Berl) 1989;99 Suppl:S122–5.

4. Miller D, Bennett L, Hollis K, Tennis P, Cook S, Andrews E. A patient follow-up survey programme for alosetron: assessing compliance to and effectiveness of the risk management programme. Aliment Pharmacol Ther 2006;24(5):869–78.

5. Spriet-Pourra C, Auriche M. Drug withdrawal from sale. 2nd ed. Richmond: PJB Publications Ltd; 1994.

6. Annas GJ, Elias S. Thalidomide and the Titanic: reconstructing the technology tragedies of the twentieth century. Am J Public Health 1999;89(1):98–101.

7. Macdonald S. Aspirin use to be banned in under 16 year olds. BMJ 2002;325(7371):988.

8. Laidler P, Maslin SC, Gilhome RW. What's new in Osmosin and intestinal perforation? Pathol Res Pract 1985;180(1):74–6.

9. Lerman SJ. Why not use topical penicillin? Pediatrics 1976;58(2):302.

10. Stephens MDB. Appendix I: Drug products withdrawn from the market for safety reasons. In: Talbot J, Waller P, editors. Stephens' detection of new adverse drug reactions. 5th ed. Chichester: John Wiley & Sons Ltd; 2004, p. 667–702.

11. Anonymous. Chloramphenicol. Br Med J 1967;1(5538):484.

12. Rosen CJ. The rosiglitazone story—lessons from an FDA Advisory Committee meeting. N Engl J Med 2007;357(9):844–6.

13. Shah RR. Drug-induced QT interval prolongation—regulatory guidance and perspectives on hERG channel studies. Novartis Found Symp 2005;266:251–80.

14. Brown HS, Ito K, Galetin A, Houston JB. Prediction of in vivo drug–drug interactions from in vitro data: impact of incorporating parallel pathways of drug elimination and inhibitor absorption rate constant. Br J Clin Pharmacol 2005;60(5):508–18.

15. Fung M, Thornton T, Mybeck K, Hsiao-Hui J, Hornbuckle K, Muniz E. Evaluation of the characteristics of safety withdrawal of prescription drugs from worldwide pharmaceutical markets–1960 to 1999. Drug Inf J 2001;35:293–317.

16. Loke YK, Price D, Derry S, Aronson JK. Case reports of suspected adverse drug reactions—systematic literature survey of follow-up. BMJ 2006;332(7537):335–9.

17. Aronson JK. Classifying adverse drug reactions in the 21st century. In: Aronson JK, editor. Side effects of drugs, annual 28. Amsterdam: Elsevier; 2005. p. xxvii–xxxiii.

18. Committee for Medicinal Products for Human Use (CHMP). Guideline on risk management systems for medicinal products for human use. 14 November 2005: EMEA/CHMP/96268/2005.

Reginald P. Sequeira

1 Central nervous system stimulants and drugs that suppress appetite

AMPHETAMINES *(SED-15, 180; SEDA-27, 29; SEDA-28, 4, 28; SEDA-29, 1)*

Note on spelling: In International Non-proprietary Names (INNs) the digraph -ph- is usually replaced by -f-, although usage is not consistent, and -ph- is used at the beginnings of some drug names (for example, compare fenfluramine and phentermine) or when a name that begins with a ph- is modified by a prefix (for example, chlorphentermine). For the amphetamines the spellings that are used in SEDA are as follows: amfetamine, benzfetamine, dexamfetamine, metamfetamine (methylamphetamine), and methylenedioxymetamfetamine (ecstasy); however, for the general term for the group of drugs the more common spelling "amphetamines" is used.

Amfetamine *(SEDA-29, 2)*

Cardiovascular During short-term treatment with a modified-release formulation of mixed amfetamine salts in children with ADHD, *changes in blood pressure, pulse, and QT_c interval* were not statistically significantly different from the changes that were seen in children with ADHD taking placebo (1^C). Short-term cardiovascular effects were assessed during a 4-week, double-blind, randomized, placebo-controlled, forced-dose titration study with once-daily mixed amfetamine salts 10, 20,

and 30 mg ($n = 580$). Long-term cardiovascular effects were assessed in 568 subjects during a 2-year, open extension study of mixed amfetamine salts 10–30 mg/day. The mean increases in blood pressure after 2 years of treatment (systolic 3.5 mmHg, diastolic 2.6 mmHg) and pulse (3.4/minute) were clinically insignificant. These findings differ from previously reported linear dose–response relations with blood pressure and pulse with immediate-release methylphenidate during short-term treatment (2^C). These differences may be attributable to differences in timing between dosing and cardiovascular measurements or to differences in formulations. Both amphetamine and methylphenidate have sympathomimetic effects that can lead to increases in systolic blood pressure and diastolic blood pressure at therapeutic doses, although the effect size on blood pressure may differ (3^C).

Nervous system *Working memory performance* may be improved or impaired by amfetamine, depending on dosage and baseline working memory capacity. There was an inverted U-shaped relation between the dose of D-amfetamine and working memory efficiency in 18 healthy people (mean age 24 years, 6 women) who were randomized single-blind to either amfetamine ($n = 12$) or placebo ($n = 6$) (4^c). The primary outcome measures were self-administered questionnaires and blood-oxygenation-level-dependent (BOLD) functional magnetic resonance imaging. Given the overlap between neurochemical systems affected by amfetamine and those disordered in schizophrenia, the effect of amfetamine on working memory in healthy individuals may provide insight into the memory deficits that occur in schizophrenia.

Side Effects of Drugs, Annual 30
J.K. Aronson (Editor)
ISSN: 0378-6080
DOI: 10.1016/S0378-6080(08)00001-9

Drug–drug interactions   Amfetamine reduces regional brain activation during the performance of several cognitive tasks (5[c]). The results of a double-blind, placebo-controlled study in healthy volunteers suggested that both *lithium* and *valproate* can significantly attenuate dexamfetamine-induced changes in brain activity in a task-dependent and region-specific manner (6[c]). There is also good evidence that dexamfetamine stimulates the phosphatidylinositol (PI) cycle in vivo (7[c]) and in vitro (8[E]), and this may be the mechanism responsible for its effect on brain activation; both lithium and valproate can attenuate the PI-cycle, probably through different mechanisms (9[R]).

Ecstasy (3,4-methylenedioxymetamfetamine, MDMA)

See Chapter 4.

Metamfetamine   *(SEDA-29, 3)*

Nervous system   *Chronic cerebral vasculitis* and *delayed ischemic stroke* due to metamfetamine has been reported (10[A]).

- A 19-year-old woman used metamfetamine intravenously four times over 2 months and had a headache on each occasion, except the second. She stopped using it, but the headache continued, and about 3 months later she developed severe right-sided headache. She also noticed blurred vision on the left side and numbness of the left arm and leg. She denied any other drug use, including oral contraceptives. Her blood pressure was 110/70 mmHg. Magnetic resonance angiography showed bleeding of the right posterior cerebral artery and characteristic features of vasculitis. Her symptoms gradually improved.

Delayed-onset stroke due to metamfetamine is rare, but is associated with the use of other sympathomimetics, such as ephedrine and cocaine.

Drug abuse   Concerns have been raised in an editorial about the effects on children, through abuse and neglect, of metamfetamine abuse in parents (11[r]). The author provocatively suggested that the drug users are not victims but rather violators of the law and thus criminals who needed to be confined when necessary and rehabilitated to protect society and families. Indeed, in some regions in the USA more than 50% of the inmates are being held on metamfetamine-related crimes. One rural county of 11 000 people in Colorado had more than 4 dozen children placed in foster care in just 1 year because of metamfetamine-related abuse and neglect. The health-care costs for dentistry, psychiatry, and social services are substantial and increasing in this group, and violence is also on the increase. This epidemic has led the US Congress to form a Meth Caucus to consider legislation to chart an effective course of action.

Susceptibility factors

Genetic   Metamfetamine is reported to be the most popular drug among young abusers in Japan (10[A], 12[c]), where genetic factors have been studied and may contribute to vulnerability to the effects of metamfetamine. Methamphetamine-associated psychosis resembles paranoid schizophrenia. Oxidative stress in dopaminergic pathways is postulated to underlie this neurotoxicity, and polymorphisms in the quinone oxidoreductase (NQO2) gene may contribute (12[C]). In 191 Japanese subjects polymorphisms in the NQO1 and NQO2 genes were determined. The genotype and allele frequencies for the polymorphism (Pro 187 Ser) of the NQO1 gene did not differ across the subgroups of patients and controls. In contrast, the genotype frequency for the insertion/deletion polymorphism was significantly different in patients with prolonged-type metamfetamine psychosis. If this is confirmed, the insertion/deletion polymorphism in the promoter region of the NQO2 gene would be a specific mechanism by which genetic variation leads to a risk of metamfetamine-induced psychosis. There is evidence for dopamine–quinone mediated metamfetamine psychosis (13[E]), and detoxification of dopamine–quinones is catalysed by the quinoreductases, NQO1 and NQO2 (14[E], 15[E]).

Glutathione S-transferases also play an important role in the defense against oxidative stress due to metamfetamine. The genes encoding glutathione S-transferases, and specifically the GSTP1 gene, may have a role in inducing genetic vulnerability (16^C). Genotyping in 189 metamfetamine abusers and 199 controls showed that a functional polymorphism on exon 5 of the GSTP1 gene, especially the G allele of the GSTP1 polymorphism, may contribute to a vulnerability to psychosis associated with metamfetamine abuse in the Japanese population. Specifically, variant GSTP1 genes may lead to an excess of metabolic products of the oxidative process induced by metamfetamine and may lead to metamfetamine-induced neurotoxicity, including damage to dopamine neurons.

Six single nucleotide polymorphisms (SNPs) in the GABA$_A$ receptor $\gamma 2$ subunit gene (GABRG2), three of which are new, have been identified (17^c). Two of these SNPs, 315C>T and 1128+99C>A, were used as representatives of the linkage disequilibrium blocks for further case-control association analysis. No associations were found in either allelic or genotype frequencies. There was a haplotypic association in GABRG2 with metamfetamine use disorder. These findings suggest that GABRG2 may be one of the susceptibility genes for metamfetamine use disorder.

Drug–drug interactions When *bupropion* and metamfetamine were co-administered to 26 subjects, 20 of whom completed the protocol, there was no evidence of additive cardiovascular effects (18^c). The subjects received metamfetamine 0, 15, and 30 mg intravenously before and after randomization to bupropion 150 mg bd in a modified-release formulation or matched placebo. There was a non-significant trend for bupropion to reduce metamfetamine-associated increases in blood pressure and a significant reduction in the metamfetamine-associated increase in heart rate. Bupropion reduced the plasma clearance of metamfetamine and the appearance of amfetamine in the plasma. Metamfetamine did not alter the peak and trough concentrations of bupropion or its metabolites. These findings are relevant to the potential use of bupropion in ameliorating acute abstinence in metamfetamine users. However, the risk of seizures during bupropion treatment for metamfetamine abuse has not been estimated.

Management of adverse reactions Many have raised concerns about the public health problem created by the use of metamfetamine, especially in urban gay and bisexual men. Some communities have prevalences of metamfetamine use 20 times that in the general population. High-risk sexual behaviors facilitated by metamfetamine has been consistently associated with a high rate of HIV infection. Cognitive behavioral therapy and contingency management techniques have been used in the treatment of cocaine dependence and are now being tried for metamfetamine dependence. In a randomized controlled trial of four behavioral treatments (cognitive behavioral therapy, contingency management, cognitive behavioral therapy + contingency management, and gay-specific cognitive behavioral therapy) for 16 weeks with follow-up for 1 year in 162 treatment-seeking, metamfetamine-dependent gay and bisexual men, 61% of whom were HIV-positive, treatments that included contingency management produced maximum suppression of metamfetamine use (19^C). The contingency management therapy included an operant reinforcement schedule that provided increasingly valuable incentives delivered in the form of vouchers for consecutive urine samples that documented abstinence; these vouchers could be exchanged for goods or services promoting an addiction-free lifestyle. Heavy users were excluded. Maximum reductions in unprotected receptive anal intercourse resulted from the gay-specific cognitive behavioral therapy, which also produced the fastest rate of reduction in reported unprotected receptive anal intercourse. Cognitive behavioral therapy + contingency management significantly reduced metamfetamine use (measured using urine drug screens) and increased attendance at therapy sessions over standard cognitive behavioral therapy. Extent of drug use and psychiatric problems reduced during the treatment period across conditions, with maintenance of improvements up to 1 year after randomization, suggesting that the specific treatments delivered to gay and bisexual men seeking treatment for metamfetamine dependence are less important than that they receive significant exposure to some treatment. The structural effects of regular clinic visits, urine screens, etc., may contribute towards maintenance. Thus, drug abuse treatments merit consideration as a primary strategy for preventing HIV infection in this population.

Lobeline   *(SED-15, 2116)*

Respiratory Lobeline-induced *cough* is evoked reflexively and its magnitude in the conscious state may be subject to subjective variation. It is likely that it originates from juxtapulmonary capillary receptors, based on a study of the cough response to lobeline in either comatose patients ($n = 4$) or anesthetized subjects ($n = 5$) (20^c).

Methylphenidate   *(SED-15, 2307; SEDA-29, 10)*

Considering the widespread usage of methylphenidate in children, the availability of studies on developmental effects in children, and public concern about the effects of methylphenidate (and other stimulants) on child development, the National Toxicology Program and the National Institute of Environmental Health Sciences Expert Panel commissioned a comprehensive review, and their report has been published (21^{RS}). The neurobiology and advances in the pharmacology of psychostimulants, including their long-term effects, have been reviewed (22^R). A review of the published literature has shown no reliable evidence of harms from long-term treatment with methylphenidate, for at least 1 year, in children and adolescents with ADHD (23^M).

Comparative studies Risperidone produces greater reductions in ADHD total score than methylphenidate in children with moderate mental retardation. Co-morbidity and adverse effects, especially on body weight, are important in choosing between these medications and it is prudent to use atypical antipsychotic drugs. However, children with moderate mental retardation and solely symptoms of inattention may be appropriate candidates for a therapeutic trial with methylphenidate (24^C).

Placebo-controlled studies Large doses of methylphenidate are effective in the treatment of adult ADHD (25^C). Methylphenidate 1.1 mg/kg/day has been evaluated in a randomized, 6-week, placebo-controlled, parallel study in 146 adults with DSM-IV ADHD, using standardized instruments for diagnosis and separate assessment of ADHD and symptoms of depression and anxiety. Methylphenidate produced marked improvement in the symptoms of ADHD compared with placebo (76 versus 19%), with an effect size of 1.41. There were significant random effects of drug-by-time interactions for inattentive symptoms and hyperactive/impulsive symptoms. Of individual adverse effects reported, only methylphenidate-associated *appetite suppression, dry mouth*, and *mild moodiness* reached the threshold for statistical significance. There were no serious cardiovascular adverse effects, but there was a small but statistically significant *increase in pulse rate* associated with methylphenidate. Serum concentrations of methylphenidate 1 hour after dosing averaged 10 (range 1.0–26) ng/ml at an average daily dose of 1.1 mg/kg. Concentrations of methylphenidate did not correlate with dose, adverse effects, changes in depression and anxiety scores, or ADHD-CGI scores at week 6, but they did correlate with a 30% reduction in ADHD symptoms. The investigators emphasized that a comparison of the effect size of a single-site study with those of multi-site studies should be made with caution owing to lack of rating uniformity. The results of this study suggest that the response to methylphenidate is independent of psychiatric co-morbidity. The relatively short exposure to treatment also needs to be considered, because in clinical practice more gradual dose escalation is the rule. It is possible that continued exposure would lead to altered effectiveness of long-term methylphenidate treatment. Open-ended questioning of adverse events limits precision.

Methylphenidate significantly improved motor planning and response inhibition in both subtypes of ADHD—combined and inattentive (26^c). There is a debate about two questions: (a) whether combined ADHD and inattentive ADHH are subtypes of the same disorder or two different disorders; (b) whether there are cognitive differences between children with combined ADHD and inattentive ADHD. In boys aged 11.5–14 years with combined ADHD ($n = 10$) or inattentive ADHD ($n = 12$) or controls ($n = 10$) the oculomotor test was used to investigate executive functions (which involve frontal–striatal functioning) and the response to methylphenidate (27^c). Methylphenidate produced significant cognitive benefit in both forms of ADHD, suggesting that the two are possibly aspects of the same condition.

Susceptibility factors

Genetic Homozygosity in the 10-repeat allele of the dopamine transporter gene (DAT1) seems to be associated with a poor response to methylphenidate in children with ADHD. There was an association between DAT density, measured using single-photon emission-computed tomography, and homozygosity in the 10-repeat allele at DAT1 and the response to methylphenidate in 11 Korean children with ADHD (28[c]). The authors suggested that a larger dose of methylphenidate is needed in children with this genotype compared with those without, and that the 10-repeat allele at DAT1 gene could be used as a predictor of the response to methylphenidate. However, the number of subjects in this study was small, and it would be wrong to generalize the results to a hypothesis about predicting the response to methylphenidate in ADHD. Also, the ADHD rating scale (ARS) score of the severity of ADHD symptoms before methylphenidate treatment was significantly greater in the children without the 10-repeat allele homozygosity than in those with, which could also have accounted for the better treatment response. Moreover, no data were provided from age-matched healthy controls. Despite these limitations, this study is the first to have examined the relation between the variable-number tandem repeats (VNTR) genotype at DAT1 and DAT density using neuroimaging in children with ADHD, and the relation to the response to methylphenidate. It would be interesting to examine the relation between DAT density and the VNTR polymorphism of various dopamine-related genes, in particular the dopamine receptor gene (DRD4).

Drug overdose Exposure to methylphenidate rarely produces major outcomes (29[R], 30[cR], 31[cR]). Preschool children who take less than 1 mg/kg of methylphenidate regularly can be safely managed at home, despite the fact that about one-third will develop minor symptoms (32[R]). Over the 3 years between April 2000 and March 2003, unintentional overdoses of methylphenidate in 49 children aged under 6 years were evaluated (33[c]). The children (28 boys and 21 girls, aged 11–60 months) took a total median dose of 0.9 (range 0.3–12) mg/kg. In all cases the medication had been

prescribed for an older sibling. Symptoms occurred in 24 (49%): agitation/irritability (35%), somnolence (20%), abdominal pain (4%), vomiting (4%), tachycardia (4%). It is unclear if referral to a health-care facility is required after ingestion of more than 1 mg/kg, because most have minor neurological symptoms with very few life-threatening cardiovascular events. Also, symptoms are three times more likely to develop after intentional exposure to methylphenidate than after unintentional exposure.

METHYLXANTHINES *(SEDA-27, 1; SEDA-28, 1; SEDA-29, 1)*

Caffeine *(SED-15, 588; SEDA-29, 1)*

Drug overdose In 14 deaths, the mean caffeine concentration in blood was 183 (range 79–344) mg/l (34[A]). Death due to intoxication with caffeine has also been reported in two adults (35[A]). Caffeine was found in their femoral blood in concentrations of 192 and 567 mg/l, and the authors suggested that since caffeine is often used as a cutting agent or diluent for illicit drugs, overdosage may have been unintentional in these cases.

Theophylline *(SED-15, 3361; SEDA-29, 1)*

Nervous system *Stuttering* is a rare adverse effect of theophylline (36[A], 37[A]) and provides interesting clues to the pharmacological mechanisms involved (38[H]). Theophylline-induced stuttering may involve disruption of the optimal balance between excitatory and inhibitory neurotransmission in the brain by inhibiting GABA receptors. This disruption might also cause dysfunction in white matter fiber tracts, such as those that connect Broca's area to the motor cortex. This leads to hyperexcitation of the motor cortex, which may mimic the motor cortex hyperexcitability that occurs in developmental stuttering. Theophylline also enhances dopaminergic neurotransmission by antagonism at adenosine receptors, and this may mimic the hyperdopaminergic state that occurs in the brain of developmental stutterers. Pharmacological enhancement of dopaminergic neurotransmission by other drugs has been reported to cause stuttering in fluent individuals and to aggravate dysfluency in stutterers (39[C]).

Modafinil   *(SED-15, 2369; SEDA-29, 10)*

Placebo-controlled studies   Modafinil 200 mg/day reduced extreme sleepiness in patients with shift-work sleep disorder (SWSD) and resulted in a small but significant improvement in performance compared with placebo (40[c]). However, several considerations limit the interpretation and applicability of these findings. Validated criteria and instruments are needed for assessing excessive sleepiness in SWSD. Although the Multiple Sleep Latency Test used in this study is sensitive to changes in sleepiness during the night, it has not been specifically validated as a clinical instrument for measuring night-time sleepiness, particularly in the absence of objectively monitored sleep in the laboratory on the day before testing. Instead, the researchers used psychomotor vigilance tests to assess alertness at night. Actual work performance was not evaluated.

While studies to date have shown that modafinil improves wakefulness in patients with excessive sleepiness associated with obstructive apnea/hypopnea syndrome, narcolepsy, and shift-work sleep disorder (41[c]), it would be of interest to establish if it also reduces the adverse outcomes that are associated with these disorders, for example *motor vehicle accidents* in patients with obstructive sleep apnea/hypopnea, and job errors and/or accidents in patients with shift-work sleep disorder. There is some evidence that suggests that modafinil improves quality of life (42[c], 43[c]).

Modafinil 400 mg/day for 8 weeks, along with psychosocial treatment, significantly improved cocaine abstinence in 62 consecutive predominantly Afro-American cocaine-dependent patients (aged 25–63 years) in a randomized, double-blind, placebo-controlled trial at a university out-patients center (44[c]). The primary measure was cocaine abstinence based on urinary benzylecgonine concentrations. Secondary measures were craving, cocaine withdrawal, retention, and adverse events. Those who took modafinil provided significantly more benzylecgonine-negative urine samples and were more likely to achieve a protracted period ($\geqslant$3 weeks) of cocaine abstinence. There were no serious medication-related adverse events, and none of the patients discontinued modafinil because of adverse events. Adverse events that occurred in at least 5% of those who took modafinil and with at least twice the incidence in those who took placebo were: *nausea* (23%), *upper respiratory symptoms* (17%), *anxiety* (13%), *tachycardia* (13%), *urinary tract infection* (10%), *dizziness* (7%), *dry mouth* (7%), *reduced appetite* (7%), and *racing thoughts* (7%). None of the patients ascribed euphoria or cocaine-like effects to the study medications. In six of 30 patients who took modafinil, dosage reductions were required because of adverse events, from the initial dose of 400 mg/day to either 300 mg/day (*n* = 2) or 200 mg/day (*n* = 4); the adverse events resolved in each case. The results of this study were limited by the small sample size, the subjective nature of the questionnaires used to assess craving and withdrawal, and the fact that a substantial proportion of patients had a cocaine-negative sample at baseline. It is possible that the steady improvement seen in those who took modafinil reflected the effect of diminished reward from the use of cocaine.

Drug–drug interactions

Clozapine   Weight loss associated with modafinil has been reported in a man with a schizoaffective disorder who took clozapine (45[c]).

- A 33-year-old African-American man with a 10-year history of bipolar schizotype disorder was treated with clozapine. He experienced severe sedation, fatigue, and weight gain. After 6 months he was given modafinil 200 mg/day and had no adverse effects for 3 years. During the first year his weight fell and his BMI was reduced by 5.1 kg/m^2 (from 35.5 to 30.4 kg/m^2); he had not altered his diet or increased his physical activity. After 3 years his BMI had stabilized at 29.6 kg/m^2. Modafinil was withdrawn because of Medicaid Formulary restrictions, and his weight rose by 27 kg over 6 months. Modafinil was restarted and he lost 9 kg over 6 weeks.

The authors of this paper suggested that modafinil may help in reducing or reversing weight gain and associated morbidity in patients taking antipsychotic drugs.

Cocaine   There is no evidence of a harmful pharmacokinetic interaction of modafinil with cocaine. In 12 subjects who were given intravenous cocaine 20 or 40 mg on consecutive days before and after modafinil 400 and 800 mg/day for 7 days, there were no significant changes in the total AUC, clearance, or half-life of cocaine (46[c]). The most common adverse events were headache and insomnia and other adverse events included dyspepsia, nasal congestion, constipation, urinary urgency, and dysphoria after cocaine administration; there were no serious or unexpected adverse events. One subject had a brief period of hypotension and nausea after cocaine 40 mg on two occasions.

DRUGS THAT SUPPRESS APPETITE   *(SEDA-27, 4; SEDA-28, 6; SEDA-29, 11)*

An international group of experts from nine countries from four continents have developed a consensus statement addressing the prevalence, causes, risks, prevention, diagnosis, treatment, and psychology of childhood obesity (47[S]). According to these guidelines, the decision to intervene with pharmacotherapy or bariatric surgery must be made on a case-by-case basis. The authors emphasized that although somewhat encouraging, there is only limited and short-term evidence to support the use of selected drugs or surgical procedures to alleviate morbid obesity in this population.

Fenfluramines   *(SED-15, 1333; SEDA-29, 11)*

Drug contamination   Poisoning from the ingestion of a herbal weight loss product adulterated with fenfluramine has been reported (48[A]).

- A previously healthy 31-year-old woman was found comatose beside an empty bottle of a herbal weight loss product (name not specified), with 120 tablets missing. She was febrile, with a heart rate of 120/minute, a blood pressure of 80/60 mmHg, and in need of airway protection. There was bilateral pupillary dilatation and horizontal nystagmus.

Her limbs were hypertonic and rigid. Serum concentrations of fenfluramine and norfenfluramine were 2480 and 330 ng/ml respectively. She had an uncomplicated course and recovered.

Legislation supporting the screening of herbal supplement for synthetic drugs may avert potentially serious harm to consumers.

Sibutramine   *(SED-15, 3131; SEDA-28, 8; SEDA-29, 11)*

Sibutramine 10 mg/day for 6 months plus diet and exercise produced significant weight loss (10.3 versus 2.4 kg) in 60 obese Brazilian adolescents aged 14–17 years in a randomized, double-blind, placebo-controlled trial (49[c]). The reduction in mean body mass index (BMI) was greater with sibutramine than placebo (3.6 versus 0.9 kg/m^2). No participant withdrew because of adverse events. There were no differences in blood pressure or heart rate between the groups and no echocardiographic changes. *Constipation* was more common with sibutramine (40 versus 13%). Obese patients lost more weight in this study than in a previous study (50[C]), even without behavioral intervention. Differences in ethnicity, cultural influences, and the small sample size may have contributed to the observed differences. Although short-term treatment with sibutramine does not seem to be associated with morphological valvular abnormalities, its long-term safety has yet to be established.

Cardiovascular   Reversible *cardiomyopathy* has been reported in a patient taking sibutramine (51[A]).

- A month after starting to take sibutramine 15 mg/day, a 36-year-old obese man (BMI 38 kg/m^2) developed an upper respiratory tract infection. He developed progressively increasing fatigue and weight gain, and congestive heart failure was diagnosed. He had normal coronary arteries, a dilated left ventricle, and a low ejection fraction. Echocardiography showed some hypokinetic segments. Sibutramine was withdrawn and he was given diuretics, metoprolol, digoxin, ramipril, and low-dose aspirin. His clinical status improved but he continued to have NYHA class 1 symptoms.

A cause-and-effect relation could not be substantiated in this case, because there were other confounders, such as the upper airway infection 3 weeks before the onset of heart failure.

Nervous system   In men with obstructive sleep apnea/hypopnea, treatment with sibutramine 15 mg ($n = 11$) or placebo ($n = 9$) at bedtime for 1 month did not worsen sleep or breathing during sleep (52^c). At baseline, the patients had an apnea–hypopnea index greater than 10 AH/hour. Each underwent overnight polysomnography both before entering the study and at the end of 1 month. During the study two patients withdrew prematurely, one because of headache. There were no significant differences between the groups in measures of sleep efficiency, respiratory disturbance, body weight, blood pressure, or cardiac or respiratory frequency. There was a significant *reduction in the amount of rapid eye movement sleep* with sibutramine, from 19 to 13%, and in Epworth sleepiness score with placebo and sibutramine. The size of the sample in this study was too small and the results did not provide enough evidence to support the conclusions.

Pregnancy and teratogenicity   Pregnancy and fetal outcomes have been reported in two patients who used sibutramine during early pregnancy (53^A).

- A healthy 22-year-old G1P1A0, who had had a spontaneous vaginal delivery of a healthy boy 14 months before, took sibutramine 10 mg/day for 30 days for the purpose of weight reduction, not knowing that she was pregnant again. Sibutramine was withdrawn. She had an uneventful pregnancy and at 39 weeks of gestation delivered an infant weighing 3450 g with an Apgar score of 10. There were no gross malformations. Follow up for 2.5 years showed adequate growth and development.
- A 30-year-old G2P1A0 took sibutramine throughout the first 5 weeks of pregnancy and developed vaginal bleeding at 13 weeks gestation. Ultrasonography showed a singleton intrauterine pregnancy consistent with dates. The fetal nuchal translucency was within the reference range. The bleeding resolved spontaneously and 10 days later she had a spontaneous abortion. Although the fetus was grossly normal, the placenta showed signs of chromosomal anomalies. Autopsy of the fetus was not performed.

These data are insufficient to demonstrate the effects of sibutramine on the unborn child.

In 10 parturients who took sibutramine during the first trimester of pregnancy, two suffered a spontaneous abortion, while seven delivered healthy neonates (54^A). There were favorable

outcomes in two pregnant women who took sibutramine during the first trimester (55^A).

Pending more information, women should be advised to notify their physician if they intend to become pregnant or if they become pregnant during therapy with sibutramine, and to use appropriate contraception while taking sibutramine.

DRUGS USED IN ALZHEIMER'S DISEASE   *(SEDA-27, 7; SEDA-28, 9; SEDA-29, 12)*

Donepezil   *(SED-15, 1179; SEDA-28, 9; SEDA-29, 12)*

Observational studies   There was partial improvement in cognitive measurements with donepezil after 6–8 months in three patients with Wernicke–Korsakoff syndrome (56^c). Previous reports have suggested promising results (57^c, 58^{cr}, 59^c). However, the extent of benefit in each case is hard to interpret, because of a variety of confounding factors, including short treatment periods, lack of reporting of sequential cognitive testing, and variables such as the spontaneous partial recovery that occurs in the first few months after diagnosis of Wernicke–Korsakoff syndrome and treatment with thiamine. No clear conclusions can therefore be drawn from these case reports.

Comparative studies   In a double-blind study 769 subjects with an amnestic subtype of mild cognitive impairment, a transitional state between the cognitive changes of normal aging and early Alzheimer's disease, were randomly assigned to receive vitamin E 2000 IU/day, donepezil 10 mg/day, or placebo for 3 years (60^C). Possible or probable Alzheimer's disease developed in 211 subjects. Compared with placebo, there were no significant differences in the probability of progression to Alzheimer's disease in the vitamin E group (hazard ratio = 1.02; 95% CI = 0.74, 1.41) or in the donepezil group (hazard ratio = 0.80; 95% CI = 0.57, 1.13) during the 3 years of treatment. However, during the first 12 months donepezil reduced the likelihood of progression to Alzheimer's disease, a finding that was supported by secondary outcome measures. Among carriers of one or more Apo-E ε4 alleles, the benefit of donepezil was evident throughout the 3-year follow up. There were no significant differences in the rates of progression to Alzheimer's disease between the vitamin E and placebo groups at any time, either among all patients or among Apo-E ε4 carriers. Vitamin E produced no benefit in patients with mild cognitive impairment. Although donepezil was associated with a lower rate of progression to Alzheimer's disease during the first 12 months of treatment, the rate of progression to Alzheimer's disease after 3 years was not lower among patients who took donepezil than among those who took placebo.

Placebo-controlled studies A meta-analysis of randomized, double-blind, placebo-controlled, multicenter, multinational trials of donepezil (5 and 10 mg/day) in patients with probable Alzheimer's disease ($n = 2376$) or probable/possible vascular dementia ($n = 1219$) according to NINCDS–ADRDA criteria and NINDS–AIREN criteria respectively (10 studies lasting 12–24 weeks) has been published (61^M). In both conditions the percentage of withdrawals from the donepezil 10 mg/day group was higher than from the donepezil 5 mg/day and placebo groups. Withdrawals because of adverse events were higher in all those with vascular dementia than in those with Alzheimer's disease, perhaps because of inappropriate polypharmacy (patients with vascular dementia took on average eight other medications). Cardiovascular events were more common in those with vascular dementia but were not increased by donepezil. In both Alzheimer's disease and vascular dementia, donepezil produced significant benefits compared with placebo on measures of cognition and global function. Placebo-treated patients with Alzheimer's disease had reduced cognition and global function, whereas placebo-treated patients with vascular dementia remained stable, suggesting that the effects of donepezil in vascular dementia were driven by improvement rather than stabilization or reduced decline.

In a double-blind, randomized, placebo-controlled trial, 69 patients with multiple sclerosis and cognitive impairment were treated with donepezil (10 mg/day) or placebo for 24 weeks (62^C). Of those treated with donepezil,

65% had significant improvement on a test of verbal learning and memory, compared with 50% of those given placebo. The patients and clinicians judged that there was significantly greater memory improvement in those who took donepezil. *Unusual dreams* occurred more frequently with donepezil (34%) than placebo (8.8%). Although these results are encouraging, the therapeutic efficacy of donepezil was not particularly impressive. The study did not include assessment by care givers, who would have provided more reliable information on patients' cognitive status. Moreover, since the evaluating physician was the treating physician, bias may have been introduced. The sample size was small and randomization resulted in unequal representation of patients for disease course and disability. The reported adverse effects, such as *abnormal dreams* (34%), *diarrhea* (26%), *nausea* (26%), *spasticity* (17%), and *numbness* (17%), were more common than in trials in Alzheimer's disease. In patients with multiple sclerosis and cognitive impairment there is little justification for off-label use of donepezil since the benefit to harm balance is unfavorable (63^r).

Cardiovascular The causes of *syncope* in patients with Alzheimer's disease treated with donepezil have been reported in 16 consecutive patients (12 women, 4 men) with Alzheimer's disease, mean age 80 years, who underwent staged evaluation, ranging from physical examination to electrophysiological testing (64^C). The mean dose of donepezil was 7.8 mg/day and the mean duration of donepezil treatment at the time of syncope was 12 months. Among the causes of syncope, carotid sinus syndrome ($n = 3$), complete atrioventricular block ($n = 2$), sinus node dysfunction ($n = 2$), and paroxysmal atrial fibrillation ($n = 1$) were diagnosed. No cause of syncope was found in six patients. Non-invasive evaluation is recommended before withdrawing cholinesterase inhibitors in patients with Alzheimer's disease and unexplained syncope.

Endocrine In healthy men aged 61–70 years, donepezil 5 mg/day ($n = 12$) or placebo ($n = 12$) for 4 weeks, followed by donepezil 10 mg/day for another 4 weeks reversed age-related *down-regulation of the growth hormone/insulin-like growth factor-1 (IGF-1) axis* (65^c).

In view of this, it would be important to investigate whether donepezil or other cholinesterase inhibitors, such as rivastigmine or galantamine, can restore the senile decline of growth hormone secretion in the long term, and to evaluate the benefit to harm balance as an intervention for the somatopause.

Susceptibility factors   *Down's syndrome* was associated with higher plasma donepezil concentrations than in healthy volunteers, and patients with higher concentrations developed adverse reactions more often (66^c). In 14 patients (9 men) aged 15–37 years and six healthy controls aged 21–27 years, the mean plasma donepezil concentrations were 18 and 28 ng/ml at doses of 3 and 5 mg/day respectively in those with Down's syndrome and 7.8 and 18 ng/ml respectively in healthy volunteers taking 2 and 5 mg/day. Although slightly different dosages were used in the two groups, making a comparison of low dosages inappropriate, nevertheless at a dose of 5 mg/day there was a clear difference in plasma concentrations. Considering the potential use of donepezil in peoples with Down's syndrome (67^{cr}, 68^c) and the serious adverse effects of donepezil in these patients (69^c), this difference in pharmacokinetics of donepezil is important. The authors proposed that the usual maintenance dose of 10 mg/day in the USA and EU is probably too much for patients with Down's syndrome; they recommended 3–5 mg/day instead.

Memantine   *(SED-15, 2250)*

Memantine, a non-competitive antagonist at the N-methyl-D-aspartate (NMDA) glutamate receptor, significantly attenuates the progression of Alzheimer's disease from moderate to severe (70^{cr}) and has an additive effect when co-administered with donepezil (71^c). Considering that memantine can provide protection against the neurotoxic effect of the HIVgp120 protein, it is being evaluated for the treatment of HIV-associated dementia (72^r).

Rivastigmine   *(SED-15, 3072)*

Comparative studies   Dual cholinesterase inhibitors, such as rivastigmine, may be neuropro-

tective in Alzheimer's disease (73^c). Brain grey matter density changes were measured using voxel-based morphometry in 26 patients with minimal to mild Alzheimer's disease treated with donepezil, rivastigmine, or galantamine for 20 weeks. Patients whose drug treatment inhibited both acetylcholinesterase and butyrylcholinesterase, i.e. rivastigmine, did not have the widespread cortical atrophic changes in parietotemporal regions that are invariably reported in untreated patients, and that were detectable in those who took selective cholinesterase inhibitors, such as donepezil and galantamine. A strength of this study was its combined clinical, neuropsychological, and neuroimaging characterization of small groups of carefully screened patients, a powerful means of assessing specific drug effects in neuropsychiatric disorders. However, residual neurobiological and genetic heterogeneity in small groups of patients, despite careful selection, might have influenced the findings. None of the patients had the wild type butyrylcholinesterase variant, Apo-E status was not a significant co-variate in any analysis, and there were no interactions between Apo-E status and drug groups.

Placebo-controlled studies   Using the data from two pooled open extensions of four 6-month, randomized, placebo-controlled trials, projections of decline, had the patients not been treated, were made using a baseline-dependent mathematical model (74^C). MMSE data were available for 1998 rivastigmine-treated patients with Alzheimer's disease and 657, 298, and 83 were still taking it at 3, 4, and 5 years respectively. According to the global deterioration scale (GDS), the severity of dementia was as follows: very mild 2%, mild 27%, moderate 38%, moderately severe 30%, severe 4%. Projected mean scores in untreated patients with Alzheimer's disease fell below 10 points in the mini-mental state examination (MMSE) at about 3 years, while the mean MMSE score of patients who continued to take rivastigmine stayed above 10 points for 5 years. The most common adverse event was *nausea*, at least once during the open extensions in 865 patients (40%), followed by *vomiting* ($n = 560$; 28%), *agitation* ($n = 504$; 25%), *accidental trauma* ($n = 422$; 21%), *dizziness* ($n = 421$; 21%), and *diarrhea* ($n = 379$; 19%). In most cases, these events were mild or moderate, although in 451 patients (22%) withdrawal was required. These adverse events during long-term exposure to rivastigmine are similar in type and severity to those observed with rivastigmine and other cholinesterase inhibitors during short-term use. The incidence of new adverse events and the rate of withdrawal due to adverse events fell with treatment duration.

The neural correlates of the effects of rivastigmine given as add-on therapy to patients with schizophrenia taking antipsychotic drugs who displayed moderate cognitive impairment on visual sustained attention have been studied in a double-blind, placebo-controlled, longitudinal design using BOLD functional magnetic resonance imaging (75[c]). Rivastigmine improved attention and was associated with increased activity in the neural regions that are involved in visual processing and attention systems, namely the occipital/fusiform gyrus and the frontal regions. The 12-week study initially involved 36 patients, but only 20 completed it. Unwillingness to continue with the study was not because of adverse effects of rivastigmine. The dosage of rivastigmine was 1.5 mg bd orally for 2 weeks, 3 mg bd for 2 weeks, 4.5 mg bd for 2 weeks, and 6 mg bd thereafter. In line with previous data (76[c], 77[c]), the results of this study suggested that rivastigmine increases cerebellar activity and influences, albeit non-significantly, attentional processes in schizophrenia. There were no differences between the groups in tardive dyskinesia, other adverse effects, or symptoms.

Evaluation of short-latency afferent inhibition (SAI) may be useful in identifying patients with Alzheimer's disease who are likely to respond to cholinesterase inhibitors (78[c]). In 14 patients with Alzheimer's disease, pathologically reduced short-latency afferent inhibition was increased by a single oral dose of rivastigmine, and the baseline value and the change were associated with a response to long-term treatment. About two-thirds of the patients had an abnormal baseline value. In contrast, normal baseline short-latency afferent inhibition, or an abnormal value that was not greatly increased by a single dose of rivastigmine, was invariably associated with a poor response to long-term treatment.

References

1. Findling RL, Biederman J, Wilens TE, Spencer TJ, McGrough JJ, Lopez FA, Tulloch SJ. Short- and long-term cardiovascular effects of mixed amphetamine salts extended release in children. J Pediatr 2005;147:348–54 [on behalf of the SL1381.301 and .302 Study Groups].
2. Findling RL, Short EJ, Manos MJ. Short-term cardiovascular effects of methylphenidate and adderall. J Am Acad Child Adolesc Psychiatry 2001;40:525–9.
3. Gutgesell H, Atkins D, Barst R, Buck M, Franklin W, Humes R, Ringel R, Shaddy R, Taubert KA. AHA scientific statement: cardiovascular monitoring of children and adolescents receiving psychotropic drugs. J Am Acad Child Adolesc Psychiatry 1999;38:1047–50.
4. Tipper CM, Cairo TA, Woodward TS, Phillips AG, Liddle PF, Ngan ET. Processing efficiency of a verbal working memory system is modulated by amphetamine: an fMRI investigation. Psychopharmacology 2005;180:634–43.
5. Willson MC, Wilman AH, Bell EC, Asghar SJ, Silverstone PH. Dextroamphetamine causes a change in regional brain activity in vivo during cognitive tasks: an fMRI study utilizing BOLD. Biol Psychiatry 2004;56:284–91.
6. Bell EC, Willson MC, Wilman AH, Dave S, Asghar SJ, Silverstone PH. Lithium and valproate attenuate dextroamphetamine-induced changes in brain activation. Hum Psychopharmacol 2005;20:87–96.
7. Silverstone PH, O'Donnell T, Ulrich M, Asghar S, Hanstock CC. Dextroamphetamine increases phosphoinositol cycle activity in volunteers: an MRS study. Hum Psychopharmacol 2002;17:425–9.
8. Yu M-F, Lin W-W, Li L-T, Yin H-S. Activation of metabotropic glutamate receptor 5 is associated with effect of amphetamine on brain neurons. Synapse 2003;50:333–44.
9. Gurvich N, Klein PS. Lithium and valproic acid: parallels and contrasts in diverse signaling contexts. Pharmacol Ther 2002;96:45–66.
10. Ohta K, Mori M, Yoritaka A, Okamoto K, Kishida S. Delayed ischaemic stroke associ-

ated with methamphetamine use. J Emerg Med 2005;28:165–7.

11. Assael LA. Methamphetamine: an epidemic of oral health neglect, loss of access to care, abuse and violence. J Oral Maxillofac Surg 2005;63:1253–4.

12. Ohgake S, Hashimoto K, Shimizu E, Koizumi H, Okamura N, Koike K, Matsuzawa D, Sekine Y, Inada T, Ozaki N, Iwata N, Harano M, Komiyama T, Yamada M, Sora I, Ujike H, Shirayama Y, Iyo M. Functional polymorphism of the NQO2 gene is associated with methamphetamine psychosis. Addict Biol 2005;10:145–8.

13. Hashimoto S, Tsukada H, Nishiyama S, Fukumoto D, Kakiuchi T, Shimizu E, Iyo M. Protective effects of N-acetyl-L-Cysteine on the reduction of dopamine transporters in the striatum of the monkeys treated with methamphetamine. Neuropsychopharmacology 2004;29:2018–23.

14. Ross D, Kepa JK, Winski SL, Beall HD, Anwar A, Siegel D. NAD(P)H: Quinone oxidoreductase 1 (NQO1): chemoprotection, bioactivation, gene regulation and genetic polymorphism. Chem Biol Interact 2000;129:77–97.

15. Long II DJ, Jaiswal AK. NRH: Quinone oxidoreductase 2 (NQO2). Chem Biol Interact 2000;129:99–112.

16. Hashimoto T, Hashimoto K, Matsuzawa D, Shimizu E, Sekine Y, Inada T, Ozaki N, Iwata N, Harano M, Komiyama T, Yamada M, Sora I, Ujike H, Iyo M. A functional glutathione S-transferase P1 gene polymorphism is associated with methamphetamine-induced psychosis in Japanese population. Am J Med Gen Part B (Neuropsych Genet) 2005;135B:5–9.

17. Nishiyama T, Ikeda M, Iwata N, Suzuki T, Kitajima T, Yamanouchi Y, Sekine Y, Iyo M, Harano M, Komiyama T, Yamada M, Sora I, Ujike H, Inada T, Furukawa T, Ozaki N. Haplotype association between GABAA receptor $\gamma 2$ subunit gene (GABRG2) and methamphetamine use disorder. Pharmacogenomics J 2005;5:89–95.

18. Newton TF, Roache JD, De la Garza II R, Fong T, Wallace CL, Li S-H, Elkashef A, Chiang N, Kahn R. Safety of intravenous methamphetamine administration during treatment with bupropion. Psychopharmacology 2005;182:426–35.

19. Shoptaw S, Reback CJ, Peck JA, Yang X, Rotheram-Fuller E, Larkins S, Veniegas RC, Freese TE, Hucks-Ortiz C. Behavioral treatment approaches for methamphetamine dependence and HIV-related sexual risk behaviors among urban gay and bisexual men. Drug Alcohol Depend 2005;78:125–34.

20. Raj H, Bakshi GS, Tiwari RR, Anand A, Paintal AS. How does lobeline injected intravenously produce a cough? Resp Physiol Neurobiol 2005;145:79–90.

21. Golub M, Costa L, Crofton K, Frank D, Fried P, Gladen B, Henderson R, Liebelt E, Lusskin S, Marty S, Rowland A, Scialli J, Vore M. NTP-CERHR expert panel report on the reproductive and developmental toxicity of methylphenidate. Birth Defects Res (Part B) 2005;74:300–81.

22. Fone KCF, Nutt DJ. Stimulants: use and abuse in the treatment of attention deficit hyperactivity disorder. Curr Opin Pharmacol 2005;5:87–93.

23. Hazell PL. In children with attention-deficit hyperactivity disorder who have been taking methylphenidate for at least 1 year, is there any evidence of harmful effects? Evidence-Based Health Care Public Health 2005;9:10–5.

24. Correia Filho AG, Bodanese R, Silva TL, Alvares JP, Aman M, Rohde LA. Comparison of risperidone and methylphenidate for reducing ADHD symptoms in children and adolescents with moderate mental retardation. J Am Acad Child Adolesc Psychiatry 2005;44:748–55.

25. Spencer T, Biederman J, Wilens T, Doyle R, Surman C, Prince J, Mick E, Aleardi M, Herzig K, Faraone S. A large, double-blind, randomized clinical trial of methylphenidate in the treatment of adults with attention-deficit/hyperactivity disorder. Biol Psychiatry 2005;57:456–63.

26. O'Driscoll GA, De'patie L, Holahan A-L, Savion-Lemieux T, Barr RG, Jolicoeur C, Doughlas VI. Executive functions and methylphenidate response in subtypes of attention-deficit/hyperactivity disorder. Biol Psychiatry 2005;57:1452–60.

27. Milich R, Balentine AC, Lynam D. ADHD combined type and ADHD predominantly inattentive type are distinct and unrelated disorders. Clin Psychol Sci Pract 2001;8:463–8.

28. Cheon K-A, Ryle Y-H, Kim JW, Cho D-Y. The homozygosity for 10-repeat allele at dopamine transporter gene and dopamine transporter density in Korean children with attention deficit hyperactivity disorder: relating to treatment response to methylphenidate. Eur Neuropsychopharmacol 2005;15:95–101.

29. White SR, Yadao CM. Characterization of methylphenidate exposures reported to a regional poison control center. Arch Pediatr Adolesc Med 2000;154:1199–203.

30. Klein-Schwartz W. Pediatric methylphenidate exposures: 7-year experience of poison centers in the United States. Clin Pediatr (Phila) 2003;42:159–64.

31. Watson WA, Litovitz T, Rodgers Jr GC, Klein-Schwartz W, Youniss J, Rose SR, Borys D, May ME. 2002 Annual report of the American Association of Poison Control Centers Toxic Exposure Surveillance System. Am J Emerg Med 2003;21:353–421.

32. Bailey B, Letarte A, Abran M-C. Methylphenidate unintentional ingestion in preschool children. Ther Drug Monit 2005;27:284–6.

33. Foley R, Mrvos R, Krenzelok EP. A profile of methylphenidate exposures. J Toxicol Clin Toxicol 2000;38:625–30.

34. Moffatt AC, Osselton MD, Widdop B, Galichet LY. Clarke's Analysis of Drugs and Poisons in Pharmaceuticals, Body Fluids and Postmortem Material. 3rd ed. London: Pharmaceutical Press; 2004:736–8.

35. Kerrigan S, Lindsey T. Fatal caffeine overdose: two case reports. Forensic Sci Int 2005;153:67–9.
36. Gerard JM, Delecluse F, Robience Y. Theophylline induced stuttering. Mov Disord 1998;1:847–8.
37. Rosenfield DB, McCarthy M, McKinney K, Viswanath NS, Nudelman HB. Stuttering induced by theophylline. Ear Nose Throat J 1994;73:914, 918–20.
38. Movsessian P. Neuropharmacology of theophylline induced stuttering: the role of dopamine, adenosine and GABA. Med Hypotheses 2005;64(2):290–7.
39. Stager SV, Calis K, Grothe D, Bloch M, Berensen NM, Smith PJ, Braun A. Treatment with medications affecting dopaminergic and serotonergic mechanisms: effects on fluency and anxiety in persons who stutter. J Fluency Disord 2005;30(4):319–35.
40. Czeisler CA, Walsh JK, Roth T, Hughes RJ, Wright KP, Kingsbury L, Arora S, Schwartz JRL, Niebler GE, Dinges DF, for the US Modafinil in Shift Work Sleep Disorder Study Group. Modafinil for excessive sleepiness associated with shift-work sleep disorder. N Engl J Med 2005;353:476–86.
41. Becker PM, Schwartz JR, Feldman NT, Hughes RJ. Effect of modafinil on fatigue, mood and health-related quality of life in patients with narcolepsy. Psychopharmacology 2004;171:133–9.
42. Keating GM, Raffin MJ. Modafinil. A review of its use in excessive sleepiness associated with obstructive sleep apnea/hypopnea syndrome and shift work sleep disorder. CNS Drugs 2005;19:785–803.
43. Rosenberg R, Erman M, Emsellem H. Modafinil improves quality of life and is well tolerated in shift work sleep disorder. Sleep 2005;26(Suppl):A112–3.
44. Dackis CA, Kampman KM, Lynch KG, Pettinati HM, O'Brien CP. A double-blind, placebo-controlled trial of modafinil for cocaine dependence. Neuropsychopharmacology 2005;30:205–11.
45. Henderson DC, Louie PM, Koul P, Namey L, Daley TB, Nguyen DD. Modafinil-associated weight loss in a clozapine-treated schizoaffective disorder patients. Ann Clin Psychiatry 2005;17:95–7.
46. Donovan JL, DeVane CL, Malcolm RJ, Mojsiak J, Chiang N, Elkashef A, Taylor RM. Modafinil influences the pharmacokinetics of intravenous cocaine in healthy cocaine-dependent volunteers. Clin Pharmacokinet 2005;44:753–65.
47. Speiser PW, Rudolf NCJ, Anhalt H, Camacho-Hubner C, Chiarelli F, Eliakim A, Freemark M, Gruters A, Hershkovitz E, Iughetti L, Krude H, Latzer Y, Lustig RH, Pescovitz OH, Pinhas-Hamiel O, Rogol AD, Shalitin S, Sultan C, Stein D, Vardi P, Werther GA, Zadik Z, Zukerman-Levin N, Hochberg Z, on behalf of the Obesity Consensus Work-

ing Group. Childhood obesity. J Clin Endocrinol Metab 2005;90:1871–87.
48. Bryant SM, Lozada C, Wahl M. A Chinese herbal weight loss product adulterated with fenfluramine. Ann Emerg Med 2005;46:208.
49. Godoy-Matos A, Carraro L, Viera A, Oliveira J, Guedes EP, Mattos L, Rangel C, Moreira RO, Coutinho W, Appolinario JC. Treatment of obese adolescents with sibutramine: a randomized, double-blind, controlled study. J Clin Endocrinol Metab 2005;90:1460–5.
50. Berkowitz RI, Wadden TA, Tershakovec AM, Cronquist JL. Behavior therapy and sibutramine for the treatment of adolescent obesity: randomized controlled trial. JAMA 2003;289:1805–12.
51. Sayin T, Güidal M. Sibutramine: Possible cause of a reversible cardiomyopathy. Int J Cardiol 2005;99:481–2.
52. Martinez D, Basile BR. Sibutramine does not worsen sleep apnea syndrome: a randomized double-blind placebo controlled study. Sleep Med 2005;6:467–70.
53. Ramzi F, Elias D, Mona S, Zreik TG. Sibutramine in pregnancy. Eur J Obstet Gynecol Reprod Biol 2005;122:243–4.
54. Einarson A, Bonari L, Sarkar M, Mckenna K, Koren G. Exposure to sibutramine during pregnancy: a case series. Eur J Obstet Gynecol Reprod Biol 2004;116:112.
55. Kadioglu M, Ulku C, Yaris F, Kesim M, Kalyoncu NI, Yaris E. Sibutramine use in pregnancy: a report of two cases. Birth Defects Res Clin Mol Teratol 2004;70:545–6.
56. Cochrane M, Cochrane A, Jauhar P, Ashton E. Acetylcholinesterase inhibitors for the treatment of Wernicke–Korsakoff syndrome – three further cases show response to donapezil. Alcohol Alcohol 2005;40:151–4.
57. Angunawela II, Barker A. Anticholinesterase drugs for alcoholic Korsakoff syndrome. Int J Geriatr Psychiatry 2001;16:338–9.
58. Casadevall CT, Pascual MLF, Fernandez TT, Escalza CI, Navas VI, Fanlo MC, Morales AF. Pharmacological treatment of Korsakoff psychosis: a review of the literature and experience in two cases. Rev Neurol 2002;35:341–5.
59. Sahin HA, Gurvit IH, Bilgic B, Hanagasi HA, Emre M. Therapeutic effects of an acetylcholinesterase inhibitor (donepezil) on memory in Wernicke–Korsakoff's disease. Clin Neuropharmacol 2002;25:16–20.
60. Petersen RC, Thomas RG, Grundman M, Bennett D, Doody R, Ferris S, Galasko D, Jis S, Kaye J, Levey A, Pfeiffer E, Sano M, Van Dyck CH, Thal LJ, for the Alzheimer's Disease Cooperative Study Group. Vitamin E and donepezil for the treatment of mild cognitive impairment. N Engl J Med 2005;352:2379–88.
61. Passmore AP, Bayer AJ, Steinhagen-Thiessen E. Cognitive, global, and functional benefits of donepezil in Alzheimer's disease and vascular

dementia: results from large-scale clinical trials. J Neurol Sci 2005:229–30, 141–6.

62. Krupp LB, Christodoulou C, Melville RN, Scherl WF, McAllister WS, Elkins LE. Donepezil improved memory in multiple sclerosis in a randomized clinical trial. Neurology 2004;63:1579–85.

63. Amato MP. Donepezil for memory impairment in multiple sclerosiss. Lancet Neurol 2005;4:72–3.

64. Bordier P, Lanusse S, Garrigue S, Reynard C, Robert F, Gencel L, Lafitte A. Causes of syncope in patients with Alzheimer's disease treated with donepezil. Drugs Aging 2005;22:687–94.

65. Obermayr RP, Mayerhofer L, Knechtelsorfer M, Mersich N, Huber ER, Geyer G, Trgl K-H. The age-related down-regulation of the growth hormone/insulin-like growth factor-1 axis in the elderly male is reversed considerably by donepezil, a drug for Alzheimer's disease. Exp Gerontol 2005;40:157–63.

66. Kondoh T, Nakashima M, Sasaki H, Moriuchi H. Pharmacokinetics of donepezil in Down's syndrome. Ann Pharmacother 2005;39:572–3.

67. Krishnani PS, Sullivan JA, Walter BK, Spiridiqliozzi GA, Doraiswami PM, Krishnan KR. Cholinergic therapy for Down's syndrome. Lancet 1999;353:1064–5.

68. Cipriani G, Bianchetti A, Trabucchi M. Donepezil use in the treatment of dementia associated with Down's syndrome. Arch Neurol 2003;60:292.

69. Hemigway-Eltomey JM, Lerner AJ. Adverse effects of donepezil in treating Alzheimer's disease associated with Down's syndrome. Am J Psychiatry 1999;156:1470.

70. Reisberg B, Doody R, Stoffler A, Schmitt F, Ferris S, Mobius HJ, Memantine Study Group. Memantine in moderate-to-severe Alzheimer's disease. N Engl J Med 2003;348:1333–41.

71. Tarriot PN, Farlow MR, Grossberg GT, Graham SM, McDonald S, Gergel I, Memantine Study Group. Memantine treatment in patients with moderate to severe Alzheimer's disease already receiving donepezil: a randomized controlled trial. JAMA 2004;291:317–24.

72. Alisky JM. Could cholinesterase inhibitors and memantine alleviate HIV dementia? J Acquir Immune Defic Syndr 2004;38:113–4.

73. Venneri A, McGeown WJ, Shanks MF. Empirical evidence of neuroprotection by dual cholinesterase inhibition in Alzheimer's disease. Neuroreport 2005;16:107–10.

74. Small GW, Kaufer D, Mendiondo MS, Quarg P, Spiegel R. Cognitive performance in Alzheimer's disease patients receiving rivastigmine for up to 5 years. Int J Clin Pract 2005;59:473–7.

75. Aasen I, Kumari V, Sharma T. Effects of rivastigmine on sustained attention in schizophrenia. An fMRI study. J Clin Psychopharmacol 2005;25:311–7.

76. Schmahmann JD. The role of the cerebellum in affect and psychosis. J Neurolinguist 2000;13:189–214.

77. Friedman JI. Cholinergic targets for cognitive enhancement in schizophrenia: focus on cholinesterase inhibitors and muscarinic agonists. Psychopharmacology 2004;174:45–53.

78. Di Lazzaro V, Oliviero A, Pilato F, Saturno E, Dileone M, Marra C, Ghirlanda S, Ranieri F, Gainotti G, Tonali P. Neurophysiological predictors of long term response to AChE inhibitors in AD patients. J Neurol Neurosurg Psychiatry 2005;76:1064–9.

P.J. Cowen

2 Antidepressant drugs

GENERAL

Psychiatric Antidepressant drug treatment is sometimes associated with *mania*, particularly in patients with bipolar disorder (SEDA-29, 18). However, patients with bipolar disorder often suffer from depression, which makes balancing benefits and harms of antidepressant medication difficult. It is particularly relevant to know whether any specific class of antidepressants is more likely than another to trigger mania.

Evidence from 12 trials has been assessed in a systematic review, in which 1088 patients with bipolar depression were randomized to different kinds of antidepressant medication or placebo (1[M]). A high proportion of patients (75%) were taking concomitant therapy with a mood stabilizer or an atypical antipsychotic drug. Overall, antidepressant treatment did not increase the risk of switching to mania relative to placebo (3.8 versus 4.7%, difference = 0.9%, CI = −2.0, 3.8). However, patients who were taking tricyclic antidepressants had a higher rate of manic switching compared with other antidepressants (mainly SSRIs and MAOIs). The rate of manic switch on tricyclics was 10% and for other antidepressants 3.2% (absolute risk difference of 6.8%, CI = 1.7, 12%).

These findings suggest that tricyclic antidepressants should not be used in depressed patients with bipolar disorder unless it is essential and that SSRIs should probably be first-line treatment. However, the data are derived from short-term studies (up to 10 weeks) and the course of the bipolar disorder during longer-term treatment with antidepressants is unclear. Also most of the patients in the systematic review were taking other drugs (mood stabilizers

and antipsychotic drugs), which would be expected to lessen the risk of mania. Hence, the rate of manic switching in patients taking antidepressants as sole therapy could be higher.

TRICYCLIC ANTIDEPRESSANTS
(SED-15, 3489; SEDA-27, 11; SEDA-28, 15; SEDA-29, 19)

Drug overdose Accidental or intentional overdose with tricyclic antidepressants continues to claim lives. Death after tricyclic overdose is associated with seizures, coma, and ventricular dysrhythmias. Even in an intensive care unit, treatment can be very challenging (2[A]).

- A 17-month-old girl took about 750 mg of amitriptyline (usual adult daily dose 150 mg). Two hours later she was comatose with minimal response to painful stimuli. She also had multifocal clonic seizures. Her blood pressure was 70/40 mmHg and heart rate 140/minute. Arterial pH was 7.24. Electrocardiography showed a ventricular tachycardia and wide QRS complexes. She was treated with intravenous fluids for circulatory support, diazepam (0.3 mg/kg/hour) for seizures, intravenous lidocaine (20 µg/kg/minute), and sodium bicarbonate (2 mmol/kg). There was no response to this therapy; and she remained in a deep coma with persistent cardiac dysrhythmias and seizures. Ten hours after admission, hemoperfusion was started and continued for 2 hours. Just before and during hemoperfusion, she had several episodes of ventricular fibrillation, which were treated successfully with cardioversion. After hemoperfusion her cardiac rhythm returned to normal and the seizures stopped. Her serum amitriptyline concentration fell from 1299 to 849 µg/l. Her cardiovascular and neurological status returned to normal the next day.

This case vividly illustrates the life-threatening consequences of tricyclic antidepressant overdose, in which serum concentrations of more than 1000 µg/l carry a high risk of mortality. Because of the high toxicity of tricyclic anti-

Side Effects of Drugs, Annual 30
J.K. Aronson (Editor)
ISSN: 0378-6080
DOI: 10.1016/S0378-6080(08)00002-0

depressants, children are particularly at risk from accidental ingestion of tablets from inadequately secured containers, a point worth making when prescribing tricyclic antidepressant for patients who have young children. The value of hemoperfusion in tricyclic antidepressant overdose has been debated. General opinion is that it is unlikely to be helpful, because the large volume of distribution of tricyclic antidepressants means that relatively little drug will be removed.

SELECTIVE SEROTONIN RE-UPTAKE INHIBITORS (SSRIs)
(SED-15, 3109; SEDA-27, 12; SEDA-28, 15; SEDA-29, 19)

Liver   There are rare reports of *hepatotoxicity* in association with SSRIs (SEDA-28, 17; SEDA-29, 21), but establishing causality is often difficult.

- A 39-year-old woman with a severe depressive illness took fluvoxamine in increasing doses, but after 9 days reported upper quadrant pain and vomiting (3^A). Her liver enzymes were raised (aspartate transaminase 609 µmol/l, previously 11 µmol/l). Tests for hepatitis and HIV were negative, but hepatic biopsy showed cholestasis and hepatocytolysis with possible duct damage. The liver enzymes fell when fluvoxamine was withdrawn but increased again 4 days after fluvoxamine re-challenge. They continued to rise when citalopram was substituted for fluvoxamine but fell when citalopram was withdrawn. She eventually responded to ECT and was discharged with normal liver function tests. However, 10 months later she was again admitted with a depressive psychosis. Olanzapine was started and 7 days later citalopram added; 4 days later this she again developed upper quadrant pain and raised aspartate transaminase activity (251 µmol/l). Citalopram was withdrawn and the liver enzymes gradually returned to normal over the next 3 weeks. She eventually responded well to olanzapine alone.

In this case the hepatotoxicity with citalopram and fluvoxamine appears to have been confirmed by re-challenge. Sometimes patients who have experienced hepatotoxicity with one SSRI can apparently be treated with a different SSRI without recurrence. However, this did not seem to be the case here because the patient had the same adverse hepatic reaction to two structurally unrelated SSRIs.

Teratogenicity   The safety of SSRIs in pregnancy continues to be debated. In a summary of systematic reviews of the safety of SSRIs in pregnancy and lactation the authors concluded that thus far there is little evidence that SSRIs cause birth defects (4^M) (but see Paroxetine below).

Fetotoxicity   There are concerns that the use of SSRIs in later pregnancy may be associated with *persistent pulmonary hypertension* in the newborn (5^S).

When mothers take SSRIs during the later stages of pregnancy, their newborn infants are at risk of serotonin-related symptoms, including *jitteriness, hypoglycemia, hypothermia*, and *convulsions* (SEDA-28, 17). Of 93 cases of neonatal symptoms associated with the use of SSRIs in mothers around the time of delivery 64 were associated with paroxetine but reactions were also reported in infants whose mothers had taken citalopram, fluoxetine, and sertraline (6^c). It is unclear from these data whether paroxetine is actually most likely to provoke the neonatal syndrome, but in adults its use is associated with more severe withdrawal reactions than other SSRIs. It should also be noted that it is not clear whether the syndrome described in neonates is due to SSRI withdrawal or a form of serotonin toxicity.

Lactation   All SSRIs are excreted in breast milk to some extent, there is little evidence that infants who are breast-fed by mothers who are taking SSRIs suffer acute adverse effects (4^c), although there have been case reports of possible transient reactions, such as crying, poor food intake, and sleep disturbance (SEDA-28, 17). Whether the small amounts of SSRI ingested by infants in breast milk can cause longer-term developmental problems is uncertain.

Drug–drug interactions   SSRIs increase the risk of bleeding, probably through an effect on platelet function, and the risk of gastrointestinal bleeding is increased three-fold in people taking SSRIs (SEDA-28, 16). Concomitant treatment with *aspirin* or *NSAIDs* increased the risk five and twelve times respectively. An interaction might also be expected with *warfarin*, not only because SSRIs and warfarin can cause bleeding, but also because SSRIs that inhibit CYP2C9 (fluoxetine and fluvoxamine) might inhibit the metabolism of warfarin and prolong its activity. The risk of gastrointestinal bleeding during combined treatment of SSRIs with warfarin has been studied in 98 784 patients aged 65 years or older who had used warfarin for at least a year (7[C]). Of these patients 1538 were admitted to hospital with gastrointestinal bleeding. The risk of exposure to fluoxetine or fluvoxamine did not differ from that of a nested case–control group (1.2, CI = 0.8, 1.7) and the risk with other SSRIs was similar (1.1, CI = 0.9, 1.4). These data are reassuring, but people who take combined treatment with SSRIs and anticoagulants need careful monitoring (SEDA-27, 14).

Citalopram and escitalopram

(SED-15, 794)

Escitalopram is the active S-enantiomer of citalopram (8[R]). One would therefore expect escitalopram to be twice as potent as citalopram but otherwise not to differ significantly from the racemic mixture. However, escitalopram is marketed as being more efficacious than citalopram because, it is argued, the inactive R-isomer present in the racemate actually inhibits binding of the S-enantiomer to its site of action, the serotonin transporter. In some, but not all, clinical trials escitalopram has been statistically superior to citalopram in terms of speed of onset of therapeutic action and improvement on depression rating scales. The clinical significance of these differences is debatable (9[M]).

In terms of adverse effects escitalopram appears to be equivalent to citalopram. For example, in placebo-controlled trials, escitalopram produced unwanted effects typical of the SSRI class, including *nausea* (15%), *ejaculation disorders* (9%), *insomnia* (9%), *diarrhea* (8%), *somnolence* (7%), *dry mouth* (6%), and *dizziness* (6%).

Escitalopram is extensively metabolized in the liver by CYP2C19, CYP3A4, and CYP2D6, and its blood concentrations are increased by drugs that inhibit one or more of these enzymes. In vitro, escitalopram is a weak inhibitor of CYP2D6. Drugs that are substrates for CYP2D6 and that have a narrow therapeutic index (for example, flecainide and metoprolol)

should be prescribed with caution in conjunction with escitalopram. As with other SSRIs, escitalopram should not be co-administered with monoamine oxidase inhibitors.

Nervous system Sudden-onset *diplopia* can be an alarming symptom and can be associated with serious underlying disorders, such as cranial nerve lesions, orbital disease, intranuclear ophthalmoplegia, and vertebrobasilar insufficiency.

- A 28-year-old medical student developed major depression and was given citalopram (20 mg/day) (10[A]). After 12 days he described incapacitating diplopia which resolved when he closed one eye. Neurological and ophthalmic examination was normal and no structural lesion was detected with brain magnetic resonance imaging. The citalopram was withdrawn and the diplopia resolved within 3 days.

The fact that withdrawal of citalopram led to rapid resolution of the diplopia suggests that it was due to the citalopram, but the mechanism of this rare adverse effect is unclear.

The *rabbit syndrome* is a movement disorder characterized by involuntary perioral movements that mimic the chewing movements of a rabbit. The condition is distinguished from tardive dyskinesia by the lack of tongue involvement. Rabbit syndrome is usually associated with antipsychotic drug treatment, but two cases have been associated with escitalopram and citalopram; both resolved when the antidepressant was withdrawn (11[A]). SSRIs can rarely cause extrapyramidal movement disorders (SEDA-22, 23), probably through indirect interaction with dopaminergic pathways, and this is presumably the mechanism here. Venlafaxine did not produce the rabbit syndrome in either patient, even though venlafaxine is a potent serotonin re-uptake inhibitor. This suggests that rabbit syndrome may be more specifically associated with citalopram and escitalopram than with SSRIs in general. Alternatively, the concomitant noradrenergic potentiation produced by venlafaxine may have prevented expression of the movement disorder.

Psychological SSRIs are generally thought to have relatively little effect on tasks of psychological performance in comparison to tricyclic antidepressants and agents such as mirtazapine (SEDA-28, 19). In 24 healthy men and

women aged 30–50 years who were randomized to receive citalopram (40 mg/day), sertraline (100 mg/day), and placebo for 14 days in
a crossover, within-subject design, citalopram
but not sertraline caused *impaired vigilance* on
the Mackworth clock task (12[c]). The same authors have previously reported similar deficits
after fluoxetine, paroxetine, and venlafaxine,
suggesting that impairment of vigilance might
be a general consequence of drugs that potently
block serotonin re-uptake. In contrast to other
SSRIs, sertraline did not apparently impair vigilance in the Mackworth clock task. The authors
speculated that this might be due to its concomitant dopamine re-uptake blocking properties.
This study has a certain ecological validity because it investigated the effects of subchronic
treatment with SSRIs rather than the more common approach of using single doses. However,
it is not clear how far the reduction in vigilance that the authors detected would lead to
deficits in performance of real-world tasks such
as driving (see below). Also we do not know
how SSRI treatment might alter psychological performance in depressed patients, many of
whom have pre-existing cognitive deficits due
to the depressive disorder.

The effects of both acute and subchronic
mirtazapine and escitalopram on *driving performance* in a specially adapted vehicle have
been studied in 18 healthy participants (9 men
and 9 women, mean age 31.4 years) (13[c]). They
were randomly assigned to escitalopram (increasing to 20 mg/day over 15 days), mirtazapine (increasing to 45 mg/day over 15 days), and
placebo in a double-blind crossover design. Escitalopram did not alter driving performance at
any time, whereas mirtazapine impaired driving
after 2 days but not after 9 and 16 days. These
data suggest that escitalopram in standard clinical doses does not alter driving performance in
healthy volunteers. The effects of mirtazapine,
even at the highest dose, were fairly transient;
however, it seems sensible to warn patients
starting mirtazapine treatment to be cautious
about driving until they have adapted to the
sedative effects of the drug.

Fluvoxamine   *(SED-15, 1430)*

Drug–drug interactions   Sexual dysfunction
is a common adverse effect of SSRIs and

various treatments have been proposed, of
which *sildenafil* is the only strategy with consistent support from controlled trials. Sildenafil is metabolized by CYP3A4, which is
inhibited by fluvoxamine. The effects of fluvoxamine (100 mg/day for 10 days) on the
pharmacokinetics of sildenafil (50 mg orally)
has been evaluated in 12 healthy men (mean
age 25 years) using a double-blind, placebo-
controlled, crossover design (14[c]). Fluvoxamine increased the AUC of sildenafil by about
40% and prolonged its half-life by about 20%.
This suggests that patients taking fluvoxamine should use lower doses of sildenafil for
the treatment of SSRI-induced sexual dysfunction. A similar but smaller effect might occur
with co-prescription of sildenafil and fluoxetine, which is a weaker inhibitor of CYP3A4
than fluvoxamine.

Paroxetine   *(SED-15, 2722)*

Metabolism   *Increases in cholesterol* are most
commonly reported in association with atypical antipsychotic drugs, such as olanzapine;
however, similar reactions have been reported
with some antidepressants, including mirtazapine and doxepin (SEDA-29, 19), which cause
significant weight gain, probably through histamine H_1 receptor blockade. Serum cholesterol
concentrations have been measured in 38 patients (23 men and 15 women) suffering from
panic disorder before and after 3 months of
treatment with paroxetine (20–40 mg/day)
(15[c]). At baseline the mean total cholesterol
concentrations of the patients did not differ
from those of controls (4.06 versus 4.29 mmol/l;
156 versus 165 mg/dl). However, after paroxetine the cholesterol concentrations rose significantly to 4.55 mmol/l (175 mg/dl).

Of the SSRIs, paroxetine is the agent most
likely to cause *weight gain*; however, in this
study the authors reported no change in body
mass index during the 3 months of treatment,
suggesting a more direct effect of paroxetine on
metabolism. Further work will be needed to see
if similar metabolic effects are associated with
other SSRIs and in patients with other treatment
indications.

Teratogenicity   In a recent guideline the National Institute for Health and Clinical Excellence has suggested that the use of paroxetine in the first trimester of pregnancy could be associated with an increased risk of *fetal heart defects* (5[S]).

SEROTONIN AND NORADRENALINE RE-UPTAKE INHIBITORS (SNRIs)

Duloxetine   *(SEDA-29, 23)*

Cardiovascular   Early descriptions of duloxetine suggested that it might be less likely than venlafaxine to cause *increased blood pressure*. The cardiovascular profile of duloxetine has been reviewed from a database of eight double-blind randomized trials in depression, in which 1139 patients took duloxetine (40–120 mg/day) and 777 took placebo (16[M]). Relative to placebo, duloxetine produced a small but significant increase in heart rate (about 2/minute). Duloxetine produced a greater rate of sustained increase in systolic blood pressure than placebo (1 versus 0.4%, relative risk 2.1) but no difference in diastolic blood pressure. There were also significantly more instances of significantly increased systolic blood pressure in patients taking duloxetine than placebo at any clinic visit (19 versus 13%). These findings suggest that duloxetine can produce increases in blood pressure in some people, presumably through its potentiation of noradrenaline function. How the effect of duloxetine compares with that of venlafaxine remains to be established.

Venlafaxine   *(SED-15, 3614; SEDA-27, 16; SEDA-28, 19; SEDA-29, 24)*

Nervous system   Venlafaxine as monotherapy has been associated with both the *serotonin syndrome* (SEDA-28, 20) and the *neuroleptic malignant syndrome* (SEDA-25, 18), which can be difficult to distinguish.

• A 40-year-old woman took venlafaxine 150 mg bd for a severe depressive disorder and after 12 days developed a tremor, posturing, confusion, muscular rigidity, a mask-like facies, dysphagia, hypertension, and tachycardia (17[A]). The venlafaxine was withdrawn and she improved. The next day the venlafaxine was re-started and the symptoms returned more severely, this time accompanied by a pyrexia of 38 °C and a dramatically raised creatine kinase activity (2097 U/l, reference range 0–190 U/l). A brain scan and cerebrospinal fluid were normal. There were no myoclonic movements and no sweating. Venlafaxine was again withdrawn and she recovered over the following week. She was then given mirtazapine without recurrence of the abnormal neurological state and her depression remitted within the next month.

The authors described this as a case of serotonin syndrome rather than neuroleptic malignant syndrome, because no dopamine receptor blocking drug was involved. However, drugs other than antipsychotic agents have sometimes been implicated in neuroleptic malignant syndrome (SEDA-25, 18) and it is well established that drugs that potentiate serotonin can indirectly affect dopamine pathways. In this case the reported symptoms, including muscular rigidity, change in conscious state, hyperthermia, autonomic instability, and increased creatine kinase activity are more consistent with neuroleptic malignant syndrome than the serotonin syndrome.

Sexual function   Drugs that potentiate serotonin function can cause *ejaculatory delay* in men, and this has led to the use of SSRIs to treat premature ejaculation (SEDA-26, 13). Venlafaxine is also reported to cause problems with ejaculation during routine use and its efficacy has been studied in a placebo-controlled, crossover study in 31 men with ejaculation latencies of less than 2 minutes (18[c]). Both placebo and venlafaxine (75 mg/day of the XL formulation) significantly increased latency to ejaculation over baseline, placebo by 2 minutes and venlafaxine by 3 minutes; there was no difference between the two treatments. The authors concluded that venlafaxine is not effective for the management of premature ejaculation. However, the small number of subjects studied and the large placebo effect makes this conclusion tentative. It does appear, however, that the effect of venlafaxine on ejaculation delay is probably less striking than, for example, that of paroxetine.

Drug–drug interactions   Some SSRIs can increase blood concentrations of co-administered *clozapine*, presumably by inhibition of CYP1A2 (SEDA-25, 16). The effect of venlafaxine on *clozapine* concentrations has been studied in 11 in-patients with chronic schizophrenia (19[c]). Clozapine concentrations were not altered by venlafaxine. This is consistent with relative lack of inhibition of CYP enzymes by venlafaxine; however the doses of venlafaxine were modest (maximum 150 mg/day) and it is possible that higher doses might alter clozapine concentrations.

OTHER ANTIDEPRESSANTS

Bupropion (amfebutamone)
(SED-15, 108; SEDA-27, 14; SEDA-28, 18; SEDA-29, 24)

Psychiatric   Bupropion can cause *delirium* and *seizures* in susceptible individuals, usually those with a history of major psychiatric disorder (SEDA-24, 16).

- A 35-year-old woman with no history of a psychiatric disorder was given bupropion 300 mg/day for smoking cessation (20[A]). After 5 days she developed an acute paranoid state with ideas of reference and fixed convictions concerning her partner's fidelity. She was also irritable and slightly grandiose. Bupropion was withdrawn and she was given benzodiazepines. She recovered over the next 2 days.

This case suggests that bupropion can rarely cause psychotic symptoms even in people without susceptibility factors, although it is conceivable that this patient might, for example, have had a family history of psychiatric disorder. Amfebutamone is believed to enhance dopaminergic function, and the psychiatric phenomena experienced by the patient, principally paranoid delusions and elevated mood, are consistent with a hyperdopaminergic state.

Electrolyte balance   *Hyponatremia* with SSRIs is well described (SEDA-27, 12) but has also been reported with other antidepressants, including the selective noradrenaline re-uptake inhibitor reboxetine.

- A 49-year-old woman, who was taking oxcarbazepine for bipolar disorder, developed hyponatremia after also taking bupropion (21[A]).

Oxcarbazepine can also cause hyponatremia, but in this case the hyponatremia appeared to correlate with the prescription of bupropion rather than oxcarbazepine and was also reproduced by amfebutamone re-challenge. This case suggests that amfebutamone can also cause hyponatremia, although it is possible that the presence of oxcarbazepine was necessary for the adverse effect to occur.

Drug–drug interactions   While in vitro studies have suggested that amfebutamone (bupropion) is a weak inhibitor of CYP2D6, case reports suggest that it may in fact have cause significant drug interactions though inhibition of CYP2D6 (SEDA-29, 25). In 21 subjects, mean age 40 years, 48% female, who were randomly assigned to receive either amfebutamone 300 mg/day for 17 days or placebo in a parallel group design, amfebutamone, but not placebo, produced a substantial increase in the dextromethorphan/dextrorphan ratio, showing that it is an effective inhibitor of CYP2D6 in vivo (22[c]).

Mirtazapine   *(SED-15, 2356; SEDA-27, 16; SEDA-28, 19)*

Hematologic   Mianserin, an analogue of mirtazapine, has been associated with an increased risk of *agranulocytosis*, but the risk with mirtazapine is not well-established.

- A 44-year-old woman with major depression was given mirtazapine 30 mg/day. She had a normal white blood cell count (6.8×10^9/l) (23[A]). After 3 weeks she complained of a sore throat, difficulty in swallowing, and an aphthous ulcer in the mouth. Her temperature was slightly raised (37.7 °C) and her white cell count was 2.2×10^9/l, with a granulocyte count of 1.1×10^9/l. Mirtazapine was withdrawn and she was given sultamicillin 375 mg bd. Within 2 weeks her white cell count had risen to 3.8×10^9/l, with a granulocyte count of 3.2×10^9/l. Four weeks later she was treated successfully with sertraline while her white count continued to rise.

The neutropenia in this case was consistent with an effect of mirtazapine. This is presumably an uncommon adverse effect, but this case reinforces advice given in the *British National Formulary* that patients taking mirtazapine should be advised to report any sore throat, fever, or stomatitis.

Reboxetine　*(SED-15, 3028; SEDA-27, 16)*

Metabolism　The noradrenaline re-uptake inhibitor, reboxetine, does not cause weight gain during routine clinical use and indeed has been advocated as an adjunctive treatment in the management of olanzapine-induced weight gain.

- A 44-year-old woman with bipolar disorder took lamotrigine 100 mg/day and reboxetine 12 mg/day (24[A]). She noted a loss of appetite but continued to eat three meals a day. However, over the next year her weight fell from 55 to 43 kg. There seemed to be no psychiatric explanation for the weight loss and no medical cause could be discovered. The reboxetine and lamotrigine were withdrawn and her weight returned to baseline over the next 3 months. Around that time she again took reboxetine, this time as a sole agent, and once again her weight started to fall.

The loss of weight in this patient did not seem to be due her to psychiatric condition. The authors speculated that reboxetine might have some serotonergic activity, which could have accounted for a reduction in appetite and concomitant weight loss. However, drugs that potentiate noradrenaline activity can also reduce hunger, so this adverse effect could be due to the well characterized noradrenergic effects of reboxetine.

Gastrointestinal　In six children aged 6–15 years with co-morbid enuresis and attention deficit/hyperactivity disorder (ADHD), which had failed to respond to methylphenidate, reboxetine 4–8 mg/day for 6 weeks reduced the frequency of bedwetting from an average of five times a week to once a week (25[c]). Reboxetine was generally well-tolerated, although three of the children reported *anorexia*. It is difficult to draw firm conclusions from this small open study. However, the effect of reboxetine on enuresis would be consistent with its inhibitory effect on micturition, which has been noted before (SEDA-27, 16). If reboxetine does prove effective for this indication it would probably be safer than the standard drug management, which is imipramine. However, psychological approaches, such as behavior therapy, are first-line treatments.

References

1. Gijsman HJ, Geddes JR, Rendell JM, Nolen WA, Goodwin GM. Antidepressants for bipolar depression: a systematic review of randomized, controlled trials. Am J Psychiatry 2004;161:1537–47.
2. Donmez O, Cetinkaya M, Canbek R. Hemoperfusion in a child with amitriptyline intoxication. Pediatr Nephrol 2005;20:105–7.
3. Solomons K, Gooch S, Wong A. Toxicity with selective serotonin re-uptake inhibitors. Am J Psychiatry 2005;162:1225–6.
4. Hallberg P, Sjoblom V. The use of selective serotonin reuptake inhibitors during pregnancy and breast-feeding: a review and clinical aspects. J Clin Psychopharmacol 2005;25:59–73.
5. National Institute for Health and Clinical Excellence. Antenatal and postnatal mental health: clinical management and service guidance— NICE Guidance. February 2007; http://guidance.nice.org.uk/CG45.
6. Sanz EJ, De Las-Cuevas C, Bate A, Edwards R. Selective serotonin reuptake inhibitors in pregnant women and neonatal withdrawal syndrome: a database analysis. Lancet 2005;365:482–7.
7. Kurdyak PA, Juurlink DN, Kopp A, Hermann N, Mamdani MM. Antidepressants, warfarin and risk of hemorrhage. J Clin Psychopharmacol 2005;25:561–4.
8. Murdoch D, Keam SJ. Escitalopram: a review of its use in the management of major depressive disorder. Drugs 2005;65:2379–404.
9. National Institute for Health and Clinical Excellence. CG23. Depression: management of depression in primary and secondary care— NICE Guidance. December 2005; http://guidance.nice.org.uk/CG23.

10. Mowla A, Ghanizadeh AG, Ashkani HA. Diplopia with citalopram. J Clin Psychopharmacol 2005;25:623–4.

11. Parvin M, Swatz CM. Dystonic rabbit syndrome from citalopram. Clin Neuropharmacol 2005;28:289–91.

12. Riedel WJ, Eikmans K, Heldens A, Schmitt JAJ. Specific serotonergic reuptake inhibition impairs vigilance performance acutely and after subchronic treatment. J Psychopharmacol 2005;19:12–20.

13. Wingen M, Bothmer J, Langer S, Ramaekers G. Actual driving performance and psychomotor function in healthy subjects after acute and subchronic treatment with escitalopram, mirtazapine, and placebo: a crossover trial. J Clin Psychiatry 2005;66:436–43.

14. Hesse C, Siedler H, Burhenne J, Riedel K-D, Haefeli WE. Fluvoxamine affects sildenafil kinetics and dynamics. J Clin Psychopharmacol 2005;25:589–92.

15. Kim EJ, Yu B-H. Increased cholesterol levels after paroxetine treatment in patients with panic disorder. J Clin Psychopharmacol 2005;25:597–9.

16. Thase ME, Tran PV, Curtis W, Pangallo B, Mallinckrodt C, Detke MJ. Cardiovascular profile of duloxetine, a dual re-uptake inhibitor of serotonin and norepinephrine. J Clin Psychopharmacol 2005;25:132–40.

17. Montanes-Rada F, Bilbao-Garay J, de Lucas-Taracena MT, Ortzi-Ortiz ME. Venlafaxine, serotonin syndrome and differential diagnosis. J Clin Psychopharmacol 2005;25:101–2.

18. Kilic S, Ergin H, Baydinc YC. Venlafaxine extended release for the treatment of patients with premature ejaculation: a pilot, single-blind, placebo-controlled, fixed dose crossover study on short-term administration of an antidepressant drug. Int J Androl 2005;28:47–52.

19. Repo-Tiihonen E, Eloranta A, Hallikainen T, Tiihonen J. Effects of venlafaxine treatment on clozapine plasma levels in schizophrenia patients. Neuropsychobiology 2005;51:173–6.

20. Khazaal Y, Kolly S, Zullino DF. Psychotic symptoms associated with bupropion treatment for smoking cessation. J Subst Use 2005;10:62–4.

21. Bagley SC, Yaeger D. Hyponatremia associated with bupropion, a case verified by rechallenge. J Clin Psychopharmacol 2005;1:98–9.

22. Kotlyar M, Brauer LH, Tracey TS, Hatsukami DK, Harris J, Bronanrs CA, Adson DE. Inhibition of CYP2D6 activity by bupropion. J Clin Psychopharmacol 2005;25:226–9.

23. Ozcanli T, Unsalver B, Ozdemir S, Ozmen M. Sertraline and mirtazapine-induced severe neutropenia. Am J Psychiatry 2005;162:1386.

24. Lu TY-T, Kupa A, Easterbrook G, Mangoni AA. Profound weight loss associated with reboxetine use in a 44 year old woman. Br J Clin Pharmacol 2005;60:218–20.

25. Toren P, Ratner S, Laor N, Lerer-Amisar D, Weizman A. A possible antienuretic effect of reboxetine in children and adolescents with attention deficit/hyperactivity disorder: case series. Neuropsychobiol 2005;51:239–42.

Rif S. El-Mallakh

3

Lithium

℞ **The efficacy of lithium and comparisons with alternative agents**

Bipolar illness appears to be a changing illness. A comparison of psychiatric services in North-West Wales in the 1890s and the 1990s has shown that the rate of admissions increased from 4.0 every 10 years to 6.3 every 10 years (1[R]). Similarly, the daily hospital occupancy rate for patients with bipolar affective disorder rose from 16 per million to 24 per million. While acknowledging that there have been many social changes that may have contributed to these differences, the authors suggested that current treatments leave much to be desired. Reviews of lithium treatment have reached similar conclusions, particularly regarding the effect of lithium in acute episodes (2[R]).

A review of treatment guidelines has shown that there is great variability in the various recommendations, despite the claim that they are all evidence-based (3[R]). Nevertheless, there are foundational recommendations that seem to be consistent, which include the use of lithium and valproate for most patients with bipolar affective disorder.

There are several reasons for the perception that lithium may not be as effective as initially believed. Among these are questions about study design and diagnostic drift (i.e. changes in how bipolar illness is diagnosed over time) (4[R]). Many maintenance studies involve enrichment of the sample for alternative agents, which reduces the apparent effect of lithium. In addition, many factors are associated with a good response to lithium. These include a family history of a response to lithium (5[R]), higher social status, social support, and compliance with medication (6[R]). Predictors of a poor response to lithium include stress, high expressed emotion, neurotic personality traits, unemployment, and a high number of previous episodes (5[R]). It is likely that most of these factors are simply predictors of a good prognosis rather than lithium-specific factors.

Pharmacogenetics   Individuals with the short form of the serotonin transporter have a poorer response to lithium (7[E]). The short form of the serotonin transporter is a genetic polymorphism that increases the risk of depression in the setting of adversity (8[E], 9[E], 10[E]) and reduces the likelihood of a response to antidepressant treatment, and is therefore associated with a poorer outcome (11[E], 12[E], 13[E], 14[E]). Similarly, a single nucleotide polymorphism (SNP) in the gene that encodes brain-derived neurotrophic factor (the val66met SNP of BDNF) has been associated with a poor response to lithium (15[E]). This SNP is over-represented among patients with rapid cycling (16[E]), who are less likely to respond well to lithium.

Clinicians have some control of a few factors that are associated with a poor response to lithium. For example, a psychoeducational program can have a dramatic effect on compliance with lithium, reflected in more stable lithium concentrations (17[C]).

Placebo-controlled studies   A systematic review of controlled trials has shown that lithium + haloperidol is superior to placebo in the control of manic symptoms (18[M]).

Lithium is also effective in individuals with co-morbid pathological gambling and a mood disturbance. In a randomized, 10-week, placebo-controlled study in 40 subjects randomly assigned to modified-release lithium or placebo, 83% of those who took lithium responded compared with only 29% of those who took placebo (19[C]).

Comparative studies   While the efficacy of lithium alone or in combination continues to be

Side Effects of Drugs, Annual 30
J.K. Aronson (Editor)
ISSN: 0378-6080
DOI: 10.1016/S0378-6080(08)00003-2

reconfirmed, drawbacks related to adherence to therapy or genetic links to poorer outcomes have also been highlighted. For those reasons, alternatives to lithium, such as anticonvulsants and antipsychotic drugs, have often been discussed (20[R]). However, several studies have reconfirmed the efficacy of lithium in acute mania and its equivalence to some of the newer options.

Lamotrigine   *In a subanalysis of two 18-month maintenance studies of the use of lithium, lamotrigine, or placebo in delaying relapse in subjects with type I bipolar illness, 98 subjects 55 years of age or older were identified (21[C]). Lithium delayed the time to mania compared with placebo, but lamotrigine also delayed the time to either mania or depression compared with placebo.*

Olanzapine   *In a 12-month relapse prevention comparison of olanzapine and lithium in subjects initially stabilized on the combination, each was efficacious in preventing relapse into either mania or depression (22[C]). Olanzapine was significantly better than lithium in preventing relapse into mania or mixed mania, but lithium was better than olanzapine in preventing relapse into depression.*

Quetiapine   *In acute non-mixed mania, lithium was significantly more effective than placebo and equivalent to quetiapine in reducing manic symptoms, as measured by the Young Mania Rating Scale (23[C]). In addition, a larger fraction of subjects taking lithium or quetiapine remained in the study compared with those taking placebo. The effect was evident in the first week of treatment and was maintained throughout the 3 months of the study.*

Valproate and divalproex   *In relapse prevention studies, valproate was superior to lithium in the prevention of recurrences over 1 year in subjects who initially presented with a dysphoric manic episode (24[C]).*

However, lithium was equivalent to divalproex in the prevention of relapse in rapid cycling subjects over 20 months (25[C]). It was also equivalent to divalproex in youths aged 5–17 years with type I or II bipolar illness, randomly assigned to either agent and followed for 76 weeks (26[C]).

Cardiovascular   In two studies lithium treatment was associated with *prolongation of the corrected QT interval* (QT_c). A retrospective analysis of the records of 76 patients taking lithium showed that intervals of over 440 msec were significantly more common in subjects with lithium concentrations over 1.2 mmol/l than in those with concentrations in the usual target range (55 versus 8%); T wave inversion was also more common in subjects with high lithium concentrations (73 versus 17%) (27[c]).

Similar results have been reported in 39 in-patients with either bipolar illness or schizophrenia; the duration of the QT_c interval correlated significantly with lithium concentrations and those with the longest QT_c intervals had the highest lithium concentrations (28[c]).

Nervous system   In a review of published cases of the *syndrome of irreversible lithium-induced neurotoxicity* (SILENT), *cerebellar dysfunction* was the most commonly reported long-lived outcome (29[R]).

Psychiatric

Delirium and dementia   The incidence of delirium in elderly subjects (over 65 years old) taking lithium does not appear to be higher than in those who are taking valproate (30[C]). Among 5360 subjects with a mood disorder who had taken lithium or valproate in the previous year, the incidence of delirium with valproate was very similar to that of lithium (4.1 versus 2.8 cases/100 person-years; HR $=$ 1.36; 95% CI $=$ 0.94, 1.97). Both of these rates were significantly lower than the rates observed with the anticholinergic drug benzatropine.

Actually, lithium has been associated with many effects that are believed to be neuroprotective (31[R]). Most importantly, it reduces the activity of glycogen synthase kinase-3 (GSK-3), which leads to reduced production of the tau protein (32[E], 33[E]). This effect suggests that lithium may reduce degenerative processes in a wide variety of illnesses (31[R], 33[E]). However, lithium may actually increase the production of amyloid beta (34[E]), although previous reports have suggested that lithium reduces amyloid beta and its consequent toxicity (35[E], 36[c]).

Clinically, lithium may protect patients against dementia, although it has been reported that patients who take lithium are actually at a higher risk of developing dementia (37[E]). However, in truth, patients with bipolar affective disorder are at a higher risk of dementia, and lithium treatment reduces the relative risk nearly to that of the general population (38[E]).

Suicide   In a systematic review of 32 randomized trials in which 1389 patients took lithium and 2069 took another agent (carbamazepine, divalproex, lamotrigine, or the antidepressants amitriptyline, fluvoxamine, mianserin, and maprotiline), among the seven studies that reported suicides, lithium-treated patients had significantly fewer completed events (39[M]). These included two suicides on lithium (out of 503, 0.4%) and 11 suicides on other agents (two placebo, two amitriptyline, six carbamazepine, and one lamotrigine, out of a total of 601, 1.8%) (OR = 0.26; 95% CI = 0.09, 0.77).

The lower rate of completed suicides in those taking lithium is of particular note, since suicidal ideation may actually be more common in lithium-treated patients. In 128 patients followed prospectively for an average of 13 years suicidal ideation was non-significantly higher in lithium-treated patients than in those taking valproate or carbamazepine (40[C]). This may be related to clinician preference, since among patients with bipolar affective disorder and suicidal ideation in the Systematic Treatment Enhancement Program for Bipolar Disorder (STEP-BD) clinicians were more likely to prescribe antidepressants and second-generation antipsychotic drugs, while they reserved lithium for more severely ill individuals (41[C]).

There was a similar pattern in an observational study of all lithium prescriptions and recorded suicides in Demark from 1995 to1999 inclusive (42[C]). Purchasing lithium was associated with a higher rate of suicide, but purchasing lithium at least twice was associated with a significantly lower risk (0.44; 95% CI = 0.28, 0.70). In other words, lithium is prescribed for patients who are at high risk of suicide, but continuing to take lithium appears to be protective. These studies have laid the foundations for a current adequately powered, prospective study of the purported anti-suicide effect of lithium (43[r]).

Endocrine

Thyroid   In a controlled, cross-sectional comparison of 100 patients with mood disturbance who had taken lithium for at least 6 months and 100 psychiatrically normal controls, lithium did not increase the prevalence of thyroid autoimmunity; a minimally larger number of control subjects had antithyroid peroxidase antibodies (11 controls versus 7 patients with mood disorders) and anti-thyroglobulin antibodies (15 versus 8) (44[C]).

However, lithium is associated with hypothyroidism. In 1705 patients, aged 65 years or over, who had recently started to take lithium, identified from the 1.3 million adults in Ontario receiving universal health care coverage, the rate of treatment with thyroxine was 5.65 per 100 person-years, significantly higher that the rate of 2.70/100 person-years found in 2406 new users of valproate (45[C]). Of 46 adults taking lithium in a psychiatric clinic, 17% developed overt hypothyroidism while 35% had subclinical hypothyroidism (raised concentrations of thyroid stimulating hormone, TSH) (46[c]).

The antithyroid effect of lithium has occasionally been used to benefit patients. In a case of amiodarone-induced thyrotoxicosis that did not respond to antithyroid drugs and glucocorticoids, low-dose lithium normalized thyroid function (47[A]).

Parathyroid   Of 12 patients who underwent parathyroid gland resection while maintaining their intake of lithium, only eight remained normocalcemic (48[c]). Nevertheless, the authors recommended that surgery should be considered if there is hyperparathyroidism.

Urinary tract   Cases of lithium-induced *nephrogenic diabetes insipidus* continue to appear (49[A], 50[A]). This effect is clearly distinct from bipolar illness, as non-psychiatric subjects taking lithium develop a reduced response to desmopressin and a reduced ability to concentrate their urine during water deprivation (51[c]). Diabetes insipidus in lithium-treated subjects appears to be mediated by second messengers (51[c]) with consequent effects on cytoplasmic aquaporin 2 (51[c], 52[E]), or cyclo-oxygenase 1 and 2 (COX-1, COX-2) (53[E], 54[E]).

Musculoskeletal Lithium may increase the production of parathyroid hormone, subclinical increases in which may underlie the observation that lithium is associated with a reduced risk of bone fractures. In a case-control study of 124 655 individuals who suffered a bone fracture matched with 373 962 subjects who had not had any bone injury, the relative risk of a bone fracture was significantly lower in those who took lithium, both before and after correction for psychotropic drug use (OR = 0.67; 95% CI = 0.55, 0.81) (55[C]).

Death There were significantly fewer deaths from all causes in lithium-treated patients (9 out of 696, 1.3%) compared with those who took other agents (22 out of 788, 2.8%; OR = 0.42; 95% CI = 0.21, 0.87) (39[M]). Individuals with bipolar illness have a doubled standardized mortality ratio compared with the general population (56[M]). This difference appears to be due to factors such as frequent depressive episodes, co-morbidity with substance abuse, and lifestyle problems, such as reduced exercise, poor diet, and a lower quality of medical care (56[M]). The use of lithium may reduce overall mortality (39[M], 56[M]).

Teratogenicity *Anencephaly* in the child of a woman taking lithium appears to have been co-incidental (57[A]).

Fetotoxicity In a prospective study of 10 pregnant women who were taking lithium before delivery lithium equilibrated completely across the placenta (ratio of umbilical cord lithium concentration to maternal blood = 1.05) across a wide range of maternal lithium serum concentrations (0.2–2.6 mmol/l); infant serum concentrations exceeding 0.64 mmol/l were associated with *lower Apgar scores, longer hospital stays*, and *higher rates of neuromuscular complications* (58[cr]).

Drug overdose A brief review of cases of lithium toxicity has suggested that there is no clinical evidence that gastric lavage is useful in lithium overdose (59[r]). However, an anecdote is of interest, since it suggests that gastric lavage soon after ingestion may be beneficial (60[A]).

• A 32-year-old man took 50 modified-release tablets of lithium carbonate and arrived at the emergency services soon after ingestion. Gastric lavage

yielded several tablet fragments. Associated with other supportive measures, his serum lithium concentration never exceeded 0.75 mmol/l.

However, the more problematic cases of lithium poisoning are those in which the lithium concentration increases slowly.

• A 42-year-old woman who presented with a change in mental status and rapidly decompensated into respiratory failure and required ventilatory assistance for 2 months had not taken an overdose—her lithium concentration had increased slowly (61[A]).

Drug–drug interactions

ACE inhibitors There have been scattered reports of lithium toxicity associated with the use of ACE inhibitors and attributed to reduced lithium excretion; however, this is not a predictable interaction (SED-15, 2096).

• Lithium toxicity occurred in a 46-year-old man when his antihypertensive agent was changed from fosinopril to lisinopril (62[A]).

Antiepileptic drugs Priapism was associated with co-administration of lithium, oxcarbazepine, and aripiprazole in a 16 year-old boy (63[A]). It started soon after oxcarbazepine 300 mg bd had been added to lithium 1200 mg/day and resolved without recurrence after oxcarbazepine was withdrawn.

Antimicrobial drugs In a case-control study in subjects whose lithium concentration exceeded 1.3 mmol/l, initiation of a concomitant medication (OR = 2.70, 95% CI = 0.78, 9.31) and particularly antibiotics (OR = 3.14, 95% CI = 1.15, 8.61) were associated with potential toxicity (64[c]). Parenthetically, high temperature can precipitate lithium toxicity (65[A]).

Minocycline The co-administration of lithium and minocycline in an adolescent was associated with pseudotumor cerebri (66[A]), although minocycline can do this on its own (SED-15, 2349).

Non-steroidal anti-inflammatory drugs Non-steroidal anti-inflammatory drugs can increase lithium concentrations (67[c]). Nimesulide increased lithium concentrations in a crossover study (68[c]).

Olanzapine Lithium toxicity in a 62-year-old woman, in whom lithium concentrations peaked at 3.0 mmol/l and who presented with delirium and extrapyramidal symptoms, was attributed to the combination of lithium with olanzapine, but the course was what one would expect with lithium toxicity alone (69[A]).

Risperidone Co-administration of lithium and risperidone has been associated with the rabbit syndrome (70[A]). This reaction was probably caused by the risperidone, and the role of lithium was not clear.

Ziprasidone Two patients with schizoaffective illness developed new signs of mild lithium toxicity after intramuscular injections of ziprasidone (71[A]).

Drug–procedure interactions A seizure induced by transcranial magnetic stimulation (TMS) in a patient with bipolar affective disorder taking maintenance lithium (72[A]), may not have been related to lithium, since therapeutic concentrations of lithium can actually increase the seizure threshold (73[R]). A case series of patients who underwent *electroconvulsive therapy* (ECT) while taking lithium, suggested that concern about the concomitant use of lithium and ECT may be exaggerated (74[c]).

Monitoring therapy Lithium concentrations are important predictors of outcome, but can also be associated with the type of outcome. Low lithium concentrations (<0.6 mmol/l) are associated with a low likelihood of depressive relapse (12%), while higher concentrations (>0.8 mmol/l) are associated with a higher likelihood of depressive relapse (64%) (75[C]). This has been interpreted as showing that low concentrations, rather than higher concentrations, of lithium are more effective in preventing depressive relapse; however, the difference in concentrations may be reflections of more problematic illness in which the clinician has maximized lithium treatment.

References

1. Harris M, Chandran S, Chakraborty N, Healy D. The impact of mood stabilizers on bipolar disorder: the 1890s and 1990s compared. Hist Psychiatry 2005;16:423–34.
2. Carney SM, Goodwin GM. Lithium—a continuing story in the treatment of bipolar disorder. Acta Psychiatr Scand Suppl 2005;426:7–12.
3. Fountoulakis KN, Vieta E, Sanchez-Moreno J, Kaprinis SG, Goikolea JM, Kaprinis GS. Treatment guidelines for bipolar disorder: a critical review. J Affect Disord 2005;86:1–10.
4. Deshauer D, Fergusson D, Duffy A, Albuquerque J, Grof P. Re-evaluation of randomized control trials of lithium monotherapy: a cohort effect. Bipolar Disord 2005;7:382–7.
5. Alda M, Grof P, Rouleau GA, Turecki G, Young LT. Investigating responders to lithium prophylaxis as a strategy for mapping susceptibility genes for bipolar disorder. Prog Neuropsychopharmacol Biol Psychiatry 2005;29:1038–45.
6. Kleindienst N, Engel RR, Greil W. Psychosocial and demographic factors associated with response to prophylactic lithium: a systematic review for bipolar disorders. Psychol Med 2005;35:1685–94.
7. Rybakowski JK, Suwalska A, Czerski PM, Dmitrzak-Weglarz M, Leszczniska-Rodziewicz A, Hauser J. Prophylactic effect of lithium in bipolar affective illness may be related to serotonin transporter genotype. Pharmacol Rep 2005;57:124–7.
8. Caspi A, Sugden K, Moffitt TE, Taylor A, Craig IW, Harrington H, McClay J, Mill J, Martin J, Braithwaite A, Poulton R. Influence of life stress on depression: moderation by a polymorphism in the 5-HTT gene. Science 2003;301:386–9.
9. Jacobs N, Kenis G, Peeters F, Deron C, Vlietinck R, van Os J. Stress-related negative affectivity and genetically altered serotonin transporter function: evidence of synergism in shaping risk of depression. Arch Gen Psychiatry 2006;63:989–96.
10. Wilhelm K, Mitchell PB, Niven H, Finch A, Wedgwood L, Scimone A, Blair IP, Parker G, Schofield PR. Life events, first depression onset and the serotonin transporter gene. Br J Psychiatry 2006;188:210–5.
11. Murphy GM, Hollander SB, Rodrigues HE, Kremer C, Schatzberg AF. Effects of the serotonin trasporter gene promoter polymorphism on mir-

trazapine and paroxetine efficacy and adverse events in geriatric major depression. Arch Gen Psychiatry 2004;61:1163–9.

12. Pollock BG, Ferrell RE, Mulsant BH, Mazundar S, Miller M, Sweet RA, Davis S, Kirshner MA, Houck PR, Stack JA, Reynolds III CF, Kupfer DJ. Allelic variation in the serotonin transporter promoter affects onset of paroxetine treatment response in late-life depression. Neuropsychopharmacology 2000;23:587–90.

13. Durham LK, Webb SM, Milos PM, Clary CM, Seymour AB. The serotonin transporter polymorphism, 5HTTLPR, is associated with a faster response time to sertraline in an elderly population with major depressive disorder. Psychopharmacology (Berl) 2004;174(4):525–9.

14. Yu YW, Tsai SJ, Chen TJ, Lin CH, Hong CJ. Association study of the serotonin transporter promoter polymorphism and symptomatology and antidepressant response in major depressive disorders. Mol Psychiatry 2002;7:1115–9.

15. Rybakowski JK, Suwalska A, Skibinska M, Szczepankiewicz A, Leszczniska-Rodziewicz A, Permoda A, Czerski PM, Hauser J. Prophylactic lithium response and polymorphism of the brain-derived neurotrophic factor gene. Pharmacopsychiatry 2005;38:166–70.

16. Muller DJ, de Luca V, Sicard T, King N, Strauss J, Kennedy JL. Brain-derived neurotrophic factor (BDNF) gene and rapid-cycling bipolar disorder: family-based association study. Br J Psychiatry 2006;189:317–23.

17. Colom F, Vieta E, Sánchez-Moreno J, Martínez-Arán A, Reinares M, Gokolea JM, Scott J. Stabilizing the stabilizer: group psychoeducation enhances the stability of serum lithium levels. Bipolar Disord 2005;7(Suppl 5):32–6.

18. Cipriani A, Rendell JM, Geddes JR. Haloperidol alone or in combination in acute mania. Cochrane Database Syst Rev 2006;3:CD004362.

19. Hollander E, Pallanti S, Allen A, Sood E, Baldini Rossi N. Does sustained-release lithium reduce impulsive gambling and affective instability versus placebo in pathological gamblers with bipolar spectrum disorders? Am J Psychiatry 2005;162:137–45.

20. Dunner DL. Safety and tolerability of emerging pharmacological treatments for bipolar disorder. Bipolar Disord 2005;7:307–25.

21. Sajatovic M, Gyulai L, Calabrese JR, Thompson TR, Wilson BG, White R, Evoniuk G. Maintenance treatment outcomes in older patients with bipolar I disorder. Am J Geriatr Psychiatry 2005;13:305–11.

22. Tohen M, Greil W, Calabrese JR, Sachs GS, Yatham LN, Oerlinghausen BM, Koukopoulos A, Cassano GB, Grunze H, Licht RW, Dell'Osso L, Evans AR, Risser R, Baker RW, Crane H, Dossenback MR, Bowden CL. Olanzapine versus lithium in the maintenance treatment of bipolar disorder: a 12-month, randomized double-blind, controlled clinical trial. Am J Psychiatry 2005;162:1281–90.

23. Bowden CL, Grunze H, Mullen J, Brecher M, Paulsson B, Jones M, Vågerö M, Svensson K. A randomized, double-blind, placebo-controlled efficacy and safety study of quetiapine or lithium as monotherapy for mania in bipolar disorder. J Clin Psychiatry 2005;66:111–21.

24. Bowden CL, Collins MA, McElroy SL, Calabrese JR, Swann AC, Weisler RH, Wozniak PJ. Relationship of mania symptomatology to maintenance treatment response with divalproex, lithium, or placebo. Neuropsychopharmacology 2005;30:1932–9.

25. Calabrese JR, Shelton MD, Rapport DJ, Youngstrom EA, Jackson K, Bilali S, Ganocy SJ, Findling RL. A 20-month, double-blind, maintenance trial of lithium versus divalproex in rapid cycling bipolar disorder. Am J Psychiatry 2005;162:2152–61.

26. Findling RL, McNamara NK, Youngstrom EA, Stansbrey R, Gracious BL, Reed MD, Calabrese JR. Double-blind 18-month trial of lithium versus divalproex maintenance treatment in pediatric bipolar disorder. J Am Acad Child Adolesc Psychiatry 2005;44:409–17.

27. Hsu CH, Liu PY, Chen JH, Yeh TL, Tsai HY, Lin LJ. Electrocardiographic abnormalities as predictors for over-range lithium levels. Cardiology 2005;103:101–6.

28. Mamiya K, Sadanaga T, Sekita A, Nebeyama Y, Yao H, Yukawa E. Lithium concentration correlates with QTc in patients with psychosis. J Electrocardiol 2005;38:148–51.

29. Adityanjee, Munshi KR, Thampy A. The syndrome of irreversible lithium-effectuated neurotoxicity. Clin Neuropharmacol 2005;28:38–49.

30. Shulman KI, Sykora K, Gill SS, Mamdani M, Bronskill S, Wodchis WP, Anderson G, Rochon P. Incidence of delirium in older adults newly prescribed lithium or valproate: a population-based cohort study. J Clin Psychiatry 2005;66:424–7.

31. Wada A, Yokoo H, Yanagita T, Kobayashi H. Lithium: potential therapeutics against acute brain injuries and chronic neurodegenerative diseases. J Pharmacol Sci 2005;99(4):307–21.

32. Nakashima H, Ishihara T, Suguimoto P, Yokota O, Oshima E, Kugo A, Terada S, Hamamura T, Trojanowski JQ, Lee VM, Kuroda S. Chronic lithium treatment decreases tau lesions by promoting ubiquitination in a mouse model of tauopathies. Acta Neuropathol (Berl) 2005;110(6):547–56.

33. Noble W, Planel E, Zehr C, Olm V, Meyerson J, Suleman F, Gaynor K, Wang L, LaFrancois J, Feinstein B, Burns M, Krishnamurthy P, Wen Y, Bhat R, Lewis J, Dickson D, Duff K. Inhibition of glycogen synthase kinase-3 by lithium correlates with reduced tauopathy and degeneration in vivo. Proc Natl Acad Sci USA 2005;102:6990–5.

34. Feyt C, Kienlen-Campard P, Leroy K, N'Kuli F, Courtoy PJ, Brion JP, Octave JN. Lithium chloride increases the production of amyloid-beta peptide independently from its inhibition of glycogen synthase kinase 3. J Biol Chem 2005;280:33220–7.

35. Su Y, Ryder J, Li B, Wu X, Fox N, Solenberg P, Brune K, Paul S, Zhou Y, Liu F, Ni B. Lithium,

a common drug for bipolar disorder treatment, regulates amyloid-beta precursor protein processing. Biochemistry 2004;43:6899–908.

36. Wei H, Leeds PR, Qian Y, Wei W, Chen R, Chuang D. Beta-amyloid peptide-induce death of PC12 cells and cerebellar granule cell neurons is inhibited by long-term lithium treatment. Eur J Pharmacol 2000;392:117–23.

37. Dunn N, Holmes C, Mullee M. Does lithium therapy protect against the onset of dementia? Alzheimer Dis Assoc Disord 2005;19(1):20–2.

38. Nunes PV, Forlenza OV, Gattaz WF. Lithium and risk for Alzheimer's disease in elderly patients with bipolar disorder. Br J Psychiatry 2007;190:359–60.

39. Cipriani A, Pretty H, Hawton K, Geddes JR. Lithium in the prevention of suicidal behavior and all-cause mortality in patients with mood disorders: a systematic review of randomized trials. Am J Psychiatry 2005;162(10):1805–19.

40. Born C, Dittmann S, Post RM, Grunze H. New prophylactic agents for bipolar disorder and their influence on suicidality. Arch Suicide Res 2005;9(3):301–6.

41. Goldberg JF, Allen MH, Miklowitz DA, Bowden CL, Endick CJ, Chessick CA, Wisniewski SR, Miyahara S, Sagduyu K, Thase ME, Calabrese JR, Sachs GS. Suicidal ideation and pharmacology among STEP-BD patients. Psychiatr Serv 2005;56(12):1534–40.

42. Kessing LV, Søndergård L, Kvist K, Andersen PK. Suicide risk in patients treated with lithium. Arch Gen Psychiatry 2005;62(8):860–6.

43. Lauterbach E, Ahrens B, Felber W, Oerlinghausen BM, Kilb B, Bischof G, Heuser I, Werner P, Hawellek B, Maier W, Lewitzka U, Pogarell O, Hegerl U, Bronisch T, Richter K, Niklewski G, Broocks A, Hohagen F. Suicide prevention by lithium SUPLI—challenges of a multicenter prospective study. Arch Suicide Res 2005;9(1):27–34.

44. Baethge C, Blumentritt H, Berghöfer A, Bschor T, Gleen T, Adli M, Schlattmann P, Bauer M, Finke R. Long-term lithium treatment and thyroid antibodies: a controlled study. J Psychiatry Neurosci 2005;30:423–7.

45. Shulman KI, Sykora K, Gill SS, Mamdani M, Anderson G, Marras C, Wodchis WP, Lee PE, Rochon P. New thyroxine treatment in older adults beginning lithium therapy: implications for clinical practice. Am J Geriatr Psychiatry 2005;13:299–304.

46. Aliasgharpour M, Abbassi M, Shafaroodi H, Razi F. Subclinical hypothyroidism in lithium-treated psychiatric patients in Tehran, Islamic Republic of Iran. East Mediterr Health J 2005;11:329–33.

47. Boeving A, Cubas ER, Santos CM, Carvalho GA, Graf H. O uso de carbonato de lítio no tratamento da tireotoxicose induzida por amiodarona (Use of lithium carbonate for the treatment of amiodarone-induced thyrotoxicosis). Arq Bras Endocrinol Metabol 2005;49:991–5.

48. Hundley JC, Woodrum DT, Saunders BD, Doherty GM, Gauger PG. Revisiting lithium-associated hyperparathyroidism in the era of intraoperative parathyroid hormone monitoring. Surgery 2005;138:1027–31.

49. Di Paolo A. Complications during lithium maintenance therapy. Rev Med Brux 2005;26:173–7.

50. Imam SK, Hasan A, Shahid SK. Lithium-induced nephrogenic diabetes insipidus. J Pak Med Assoc 2005;55:125–7.

51. Walker RJ, Weggery S, Bedford JJ, McDonald FJ, Ellis G, Leader JP. Lithium-induced reduction in urinary concentrating ability and urinary aquaporin 2 (AQP2) excretion in healthy volunteers. Kidney Int 2005;67:291–4.

52. Rojek A, Nielsen J, Brooks HL, Gong H, Kim YH, Kwon TH, Frokiaer J, Nielsen S. Altered expression of selected genes in kidney of rats with lithium-induced NDI. Am J Physiol Renal Physiol 2005;288(6):F1276–89.

53. Kotnik P, Nielsen J, Kwon TH, Krzisnik C, Frøkiaer J, Nielsen S. Altered expression of COX-1, COX-2, and mPGES in rats with nephrogenic and central diabetes insipidus. Am J Physiol Renal Physiol 2005;288:F1053–68.

54. Rao R, Zhang MZ, Zhao M, Cai H, Harris RC, Breyer MD, Hao CM. Lithium treatment inhibits renal GSK-3 activity and promotes cyclooxygenase 2-dependent polyuria. Am J Physiol Renal Physiol 2005;288:F642–9.

55. Vestergaard P, Rejnmark L, Mosekilde L. Reduced relative risk of fractures among users of lithium. Calcif Tissue Int 2005;77:1–8.

56. Morriss R, Mohammed FA. Metabolism, lifestyle and bipolar affective disorder. J Psychopharmacol 2005;19(6 Suppl):94–101.

57. Grover S, Gupta N. Lithium-associated anencephaly. Can J Psychiatry 2005;50(3):185–6.

58. Newport DJ, Viguera AC, Beach AJ, Ritchie JC, Cohen LS, Stowe AN. Lithium and placental passage and obstetrical outcome: implications for clinical management during late pregnancy. Am J Psychiatry 2005;162(11):2162–70.

59. Teece S, Crawford I. Best evidence topic report: no clinical evidence for gastric lavage in lithium overdose. Emerg Med J 2005;22:43–4.

60. Borrás Blasco J, Murcia López A, Romero Crespo I, Sirvent Pedreño A, Navarro Ruiz A. Intoxicación aguda por comprimidos de liberación sostenida decarbonato de litio. A propósito de un caso clínico (Acute intoxication with sustained-release lithium carbonate tablets. A propos of a case). Farm Hosp 2005;29:140–3.

61. Toronjadze T, Polena S, Santucci T, Naik S, Watson C, Lakovou C, Babury MA, Gintautas J. Prolonged requirement for ventilatory support in a patient with Eskalith overdose. Proc West Pharmacol Soc 2005;48:148–9.

62. Meyer JM, Dollarhide A, Tuan IL. Lithium toxicity after switch from fosinopril to lisinopril. Int Clin Psychopharmacol 2005;20:115–8.

63. Negin B, Murphy TK. Priapism associated with oxcarbazepine, aripiprazole, and lithium. J Am Acad Child Adolesc Psychiatry 2005;44:1223–4.

64. Wilting I, Movig KL, Moolenaar M, Hekster YA, Brouwers JR, Heerdink ER, Nolen WA, Egberts AC. Drug–drug interactions as a determinant of elevated lithium serum levels in daily clinical practice. Bipolar Disord 2005;7:274–80.

65. Cebezón Pérez N, García Lloret T, Redondo de Pedro M. Intoxicación por litio desencadenada por un proceso febril. A propósito de un caso (Lithium intoxication triggered by a process of high temperature. Concerning a case). Aten Primaria 2005;36:344–5.

66. Jonnalagadda J, Saito E, Kafantaris V. Lithium, minocycline, and pseudotumor cerebri. J Am Acad Child Adolesc Psychiatry 2005;44:209.

67. Phelan KM, Mosholder AD, Lu S. Lithium interaction with the cyclooxygenase 2 inhibitors rofecoxib and celecoxib and other nonsteroidal anti-inflammatory drugs. J Clin Psychiatry 2003;64:1328–34.

68. Sidhu S, Kondal A, Malhotra S, Garg SK, Pandhi P. Effect of nimesulide co-administration on pharmacokinetics of lithium. Indian J Exp Biol 2004;42:1248–50.

69. Tuglu C, Erdogan E, Abay E. Delirium and extrapyramidal symptoms due to a lithium–olanzapine combination therapy: a case report. J Korean Med Sci 2005;20:691–4.

70. Mendhekar DN. Rabbit syndrome induced by combined lithium and risperidone. Can J Psychiatry 2005;50:369.

71. Miodownik C, Hausmann M, Frolova K, Lerner V. Lithium intoxication associated with intramuscular ziprasidone in schizoaffective patients. Clin Neuropharmacol 2005;28:295–7.

72. Tharayil BS, Gangadhar BN, Thirthalli J, Anand J. Seizure with single pulse transcranial magnetic stimulation in a 35-year-old otherwise-healthy patient with bipolar disorder. JECT 2005;21:188–9.

73. El-Mallakh RS. Acute lithium neurotoxicity. Psychiatr Develop 1986;4:311–28.

74. Dolenc TJ, Rasmussen KG. The safety of electroconvulsive therapy and lithium in combination: a case series and review of the literature. JECT 2005;21:165–70.

75. Kleindienst N, Severus WE, Möller HJ, Greil W. Is polarity of recurrence related to serum lithium level in patients with bipolar disorder? Eur Arch Psychiatry Clin Neurosci 2005;255:72–4.

Eileen Wong, Jayendra K. Patel, and Sarah Guzofski

4

Drugs of abuse

CANNABINOIDS (SED-15, 614; SEDA-27, 32; SEDA-28, 36; SEDA-29, 35)

Cardiovascular   Cardiovascular complications can be caused by smoking cannabis, which has been identified as a susceptibility factor in some young cardiac patients.

- Two young men, aged 18 and 30 years, developed retrosternal pain with shortness of breath, attributed to acute coronary syndrome (1[A]). Each had smoked marijuana and tobacco and admitted to intravenous drug use. Urine toxicology was positive for tetrahydrocannabinol. Aspartate transaminase and creatine kinase activities and troponin-I and C-reactive protein concentrations were raised. Echocardiography in the first patient showed hypokinesia of the posterior and inferior walls and in the second hypokinesia of the basal segment of the anterolateral wall. Coronary angiography showed normal coronary anatomy with coronary artery spasm. Genetic testing for three common genetic polymorphisms predisposing to acute coronary syndrome was negative.

The authors suggested that marijuana had increased the blood carboxyhemoglobin concentration, leading to reduced oxygen transport capacity, increased oxygen demand, and reduced oxygen supply.

Two other cases have been reported (2[A]).

- A 48-year-old man, a chronic user of cannabis who had had coronary artery bypass grafting 10 years before and recurrent angina over the past 18 months, developed chest pain. An electrocardiogram showed intermittent resting ST segment changes and coronary angiography showed that of the three previous grafts, only one was still patent. There was also sub-total occlusion of a stent in the left main stem. After 24 hours he had a cardiac arrest while smoking cannabis and had multiple episodes of ventricular fibrillation, requiring both electrical and pharmacological cardioversion. He

then underwent urgent percutaneous coronary intervention which involved stenting of his left main stem. He eventually stabilized and recovered for discharge 11 weeks later.

- A 22-year-old man had two episodes of tight central chest pain with shortness of breath after smoking cannabis. He had been a regular marijuana smoker since his mid-teens and had used more potent and larger amounts during the previous 2 weeks. An electrocardiogram showed ST segment elevation in leads V1-5, with reciprocal ST segment depression in the inferior limb leads. A provisional diagnosis of acute myocardial infarction was made. Thrombolysis was performed, but the electrocardiographic changes continued to evolve. Angiography showed an atheromatous plaque in the left anterior descending artery which was dilated and stented. There was early diffuse disease in the cardiac vessels.

The authors suggested that in the first case *ventricular fibrillation* had been caused by increased myocardial oxygen demand in the presence of long-standing coronary artery disease. In the second case, they speculated that chronic cannabis use may have contributed to the unexpectedly severe *coronary artery disease* in a young patient with few risk factors.

In terms of its potential for inducing cardiac dysrhythmias, cannabis is most likely to cause palpitation due to a dose-*related sinus tachycardia*. Other reported dysrhythmias include *sinus bradycardia, second-degree atrioventricular block*, and *atrial fibrillation*. Also reported are *ventricular extra beats* and other *reversible electrocardiographic changes*. *Supraventricular tachycardia* after the use of cannabis has been reported (3[A]).

- A 35-year-old woman with a 1-month history of headaches was found to be hypertensive, with a blood pressure of 179/119 mmHg. She smoked 20 cigarettes a day and used cannabis infrequently. Her family history included hypertension. Electrocardiography suggested left ventricular hypertrophy but echocardiography was unremarkable. She was given amlodipine 10 mg/day and the blood pressure improved. While in the hospital, she smoked marijuana and about 30 minutes later developed palpitation, chest pain, and shortness of

Side Effects of Drugs, Annual 30
J.K. Aronson (Editor)
ISSN: 0378-6080
DOI: 10.1016/S0378-6080(08)00004-4

breath. The blood pressure was 233/120 mmHg and the pulse rate 150/minute. Electrocardiography showed atrial flutter with 2 : 1 atrioventricular block. Cardiac troponin was normal at 12 hours. Urine toxicology was positive for cannabis only. Two weeks later, while she was taking amlodipine 10 mg/day and atenolol 25 mg/day, her blood pressure was 117/85 mmHg.

The authors reviewed the biphasic effect of marijuana on the autonomic nervous system. At low to moderate doses it causes *increased sympathetic activity*, producing a tachycardia and increase in cardiac output; blood pressure therefore increases. At high doses it causes *increased parasympathetic activity*, leading to bradycardia and hypotension. They thought that this patient most probably had adrenergic atrial flutter.

Nervous system   *Extrapyramidal effects* have been reported for the first time in a patient taking neuroleptic drugs who smoked cannabis (4[A]).

- A 20-year-old man with no previous movement disorders, who had smoked marijuana for 4 years was given risperidone 9 mg/day and clorazepate 10–20 mg/day for paranoid schizophrenia. After 4 weeks he started using marijuana again and had at least two episodes of cervical and jaw dystonia with oculogyric crises, for which intramuscular biperiden was effective. He acknowledged heavy marijuana use before each episode. He was then given oral biperiden 2–4 mg/day and risperidone was replaced by olanzapine 30 mg/day. He again started smoking marijuana and had similar episodes of dystonia and oculogyric crises. No other causes of secondary extrapyramidal disorders were found.

The authors suggested a causal association between use of marijuana and extrapyramidal disorders. The research literature contains evidence that the endogenous cannabinoid system plays a role in basal ganglia transmission circuitry, possibly by interfering with dopamine reuptake. Furthermore, central cannabinoid receptors are located in two areas that regulate motor activity, the lateral globus pallidus and substantia nigra (5[AR]).

Cerebrovascular disease due to marijuana is infrequent but has again been reported.

- A 36-year-old man developed acute aphasia followed by a convulsive seizure a few hours later after heavy consumption of hashish and 3–4 alcoholic beverages at a party (6[A]). He had no previous vascular risk factors. His blood pressure was

120/80 mmHg. An MRI scan showed two ischemic infarcts, one in the left temporal lobe and one in the right parietal lobe. Magnetic resonance angiography of the head and neck showed narrowing of the distal temporal branches of the left middle cerebral artery without involvement of its proximal segment. There was no evidence of diffuse atherosclerotic disease. There was tetrahydrocannabinol in the urine. Electroencephalography and transesophageal echocardiography were normal. He was given ticlopidine. A year later, he had a second episode of aphasia and right hemiparesis immediately after smoking marijuana. His blood pressure was 140/80 mmHg. An MRI scan showed acute left and right frontal cortical infarctions. He had a third stroke 18 months later, when he developed auditory agnosia after heavy use of hashish and 3–4 drinks of alcohol. On this occasion he was normotensive. An MRI scan showed acute infarcts in the right posterior temporal lobe and lower parietal lobe.

The authors discussed the importance of the close temporal relation between the use of cannabis and alcohol and the episodes of stroke. The mechanism was unclear. However, they speculated that a vasculopathy, either toxic or immune inflammatory, was the most likely mechanism.

In another case a cannabis smoker had recurrent *transient ischemic attacks*.

- A 50-year-old male cigarette smoker with hypertension had episodes of transient right-sided hemisensory loss lasting only a few minutes (7[A]). Coughing while smoking marijuana was the apparent trigger. Electroencephalography was negative. An MRI scan of the brain showed chain-like low-flow infarctions in the white matter of the left parietal subcortex. Duplex sonography and digital subtraction angiography showed a subocclusive stenosis of the left internal carotid artery. Blood flow to the left middle cerebral artery was reduced and delayed and there was steal by the right middle cerebral artery. Endarterectomy of the left internal carotid resolved the symptoms.

The authors suggested that marijuana may increase the risk of reduced cerebral perfusion. Coughing may have contributed by reduced flow velocity within arteries supplying the brain and by a sudden increase in intracranial pressure.

Psychological   Marijuana *impairs memory*, although it is not clear which components of memory are affected. Memory involves two components: an initial delay-independent discrimination or "encoding" and a second delay-dependent discrimination or "recall" of information. In five subjects tetrahydrocannabinol acutely impaired delay-dependent discrimination but not delay-independent discrimination (8[c]). In other words, smoking marijuana increased the rates of forgetting but did not alter initial discriminability.

The use of marijuana is related to risky behaviors that may result in other drug use, high-risk sexual activity, risky car driving, traffic accidents, and crime. The acute effects of marijuana on human risk taking has been investigated in a laboratory setting in 10 adults who were given three doses of active marijuana cigarettes (half placebo and half 1.77, 1.77, and 3.58% tetrahydrocannabinol) and placebo cigarettes (9[C]). There were measurable changes in risky decisions after marijuana. Tetrahydrocannabinol 3.58% increased selection of the risky response option and also caused shifts in trial-by-trial response probabilities, suggesting altered sensitivity to both reinforced and losing risky outcomes. The authors suggested that the effect on risk taking was possibly seen only at the 3.58% dose because it created a requisite level of impairment to disrupt inhibitory processes in the mesolimbic-prefrontal cortical network.

The neurocognitive effects of marijuana have been studied in 113 young adults (10[C]). Marijuana users, identified by self-reporting and urinalysis, were categorized as light users (<5 joints per week) or heavy users (5 or more joints per week) and current users or former users, the latter having used the drug regularly in the past (1 or more joint per week) but not for at least 3 months. IQ, memory, processing speed, vocabulary, attention, and abstract reasoning were assessed. Current regular heavy users performed significantly worse than non-users beyond the acute intoxication period. Memory, both immediate and delayed, was most strongly affected. However, after 3 months abstinence, there were no residual effects of marijuana, even among those who had formerly had heavy use.

Psychiatric   Cannabis is commonly used by people with schizophrenia, and there is a possible association between the drug and the presentation, symptoms, and course of the illness. The effects of marijuana on *psychotic symptoms and cognitive deficits* in schizophrenia have been studied in 13 medicated stable patients and 13 healthy subjects in a double-blind, placebo-controlled randomized study using 2.5 and 5 mg of intravenous delta-9-tetrahydrocannabinol (THC) (11[C]). Tetrahydrocannabinol transiently worsened cognitive deficits, perceptual alterations, and a range of positive and negative symptoms in those with schizophrenia. There were no positive effects. These results suggest a role for cannabinoid receptors in the pathophysiology of schizophrenia.

Respiratory   A recent reviewer has commented that the most serious adverse effects of smoked cannabis are on the respiratory system (12[R]), and, as noted in SEDA-29 (p. 35), cannabis smoking can cause pneumothorax. The term *"Bong lung"* is used to refer to a histological change that occurs in the lungs of chronic cannabis smokers (13[c]). Patients with cannabis-induced recurrent *pneumothorax* often undergo resection of bullae. In Australia, the histopathology of resected lung was examined in 10 cannabis smokers, 5 heavy tobacco smokers, and 5 non-smokers. All marijuana smokers had irregular emphysema with cystic blebs and bullae in the lung apices. There was also massive accumulation of intra-alveolar pigmented histiocytes or "smoker's macrophages" throughout the pulmonary parenchyma, but sparing of the peribronchioles, similar to desquamative interstitial pneumonia.

Ear, nose, throat   Bilateral *angle-closure glaucoma* has been reported after combined consumption of ecstasy and cannabis (14[A]).

- A 29-year-old woman developed severe headaches, blurred vision, and malaise. Her visual acuity was <20/400 in the right eye and 20/40 in the left eye. Intraocular pressures were raised at 38 and 40 mmHg. Slit lamp examination showed bilateral conjunctival hyperemia, corneal edema, and shallow anterior chambers. Gonioscopy showed bilateral circular closed angles. The pupils were mid-dilated and non-reactive to light. The optic nerve heads in both eyes had slightly enlarged cups. She admitted to recreational use of ecstasy and marijuana before this ophthalmic crisis and also 2 years earlier, when she had had an episode of ophthalmic migraine with headache and transient blurred vision. Ophthalmic examination showed a narrow anterior chamber angle in both eyes.

The authors suggested that the bilateral angle-closure glaucoma had been precipitated by a combined mydriatic effect of ecstasy and cannabis.

Tumorigenicity Three different associations of cannabinoids with cancer have been discussed (15[R]). Firstly, there is a possible direct carcinogenic effect. In in vitro studies and in mice tetrahydrocannabinol alone does not seem to be carcinogenic or mutagenic. However, cannabis smoke is both carcinogenic and mutagenic and contains similar carcinogens to those in tobacco smoke. Cannabis is possibly linked to digestive and respiratory system cancers. Case reports support this association but epidemiological cohort studies and case-control studies have provided conflicting evidence. Secondly, there is conflicting evidence on the beneficial effects of tetrahydrocannabinol and other cannabinoids in patients with cancer. In some in vitro and in vivo studies, tetrahydrocannabinol and synthetic cannabinoids had antineoplastic effects, but in others tetrahydrocannabinol had a negative effect on the immune system. No anticancer effects of tetrahydrocannabinol in humans have so far been reported. Thirdly, cannabis may palliate some of the symptoms and adverse effects of cancer. Cannabis may improve appetite, reduce nausea and vomiting, and alleviate moderate neuropathic pain in patients with cancer. The authors defined the challenge for the medical use of cannabinoids as the development of safe, effective, and therapeutic methods of using it that are devoid of the adverse psychoactive effects. Lastly, they discussed the possible associations between cannabis smoking and tumors of the prostate and brain, noting the need for larger, controlled studies.

Fetotoxicity Cannabis is the illicit drug that is most commonly used by young women and they are not likely to withdraw until the early stages of pregnancy. The effects of early maternal marijuana use on fetal growth have been reported in pregnant women who elected voluntary saline-induced abortion at mid-gestation (weeks 17–22) (16[C]). Marijuana ($n = 44$) and non-marijuana exposed fetuses ($n = 95$) were compared and adjusted for maternal alcohol and cigarette use. Both fetal foot length and body weight were significantly reduced by marijuana. Fetal growth impairment was greatest in the group with moderate, regular exposure to about 3–6 joints/week and not in those with heavy maternal marijuana use. There was no significant effect on fetal body length and head circumference due to prenatal marijuana exposure.

COCAINE *(SED-15, 848; SEDA-27, 33; SEDA-28, 38; see also Chapter 11)*

Ear, nose, throat *Cochleovestibular deficit* has been attributed to intralabyrinthine hemorrhage after cocaine consumption (17[A]).

- A 43-year-old man taking maintenance methadone used intranasal cocaine and drank alcohol and suddenly developed tinnitus in the left ear and progressive giddiness. He had left deafness, right spontaneous horizontal nystagmus, and left areflexia on caloric stimulation. A diagnosis of cochleovestibular deficit was made. A week later the right spontaneous horizontal nystagmus had resolved but was elicitable by a head-shaking maneuver. An MRI scan showed blood in the left labyrinth. Neurological and ophthalmological examinations were normal. The giddiness resolved after several weeks but his hearing did not recover.

The authors presumed that this disorder was due to cocaine-induced vascular effects. As cocaine prevents reuptake of amines by presynaptic receptors, increased concentrations of amines may lead to abruptly altered circulation.

Nervous system The adverse effect of cocaine on the clinical course in *subarachnoid hemorrhage* has been studied in a retrospective review of the medical records of 151 patients with intracranial aneurysms treated at a Taiwanese hospital between January 1996 and December 2001 (18[A]). Of 108 patients who had subarachnoid hemorrhage, 36 had used cocaine within the previous 24 hours and 20 of them had subarachnoid hemorrhages of greater severity (Hunt and Hess grade of IV or V) compared with eight of 72 non-cocaine users. There was significant angiographically confirmed vasospasm in 28 of the cocaine users and 20 of the non-users. There was a 2.8-fold greater risk of vasospasm associated with cocaine use. Cocaine has vasoactive properties that both influence and increase the occurrence of cerebral vasospasm, the main cause of morbidity and mortality in patients with subarachnoid hemorrhage who survive the initial event.

Liver   Cocaine has been separately associated with *acute hepatitis* and *thrombotic micro-angiopathy*. In one case both conditions occurred simultaneously (19[A]).

- A 22-year-old woman, with a 3-year history of alcohol and intravenous cocaine abuse and chronic hepatitis C virus infection, developed fever, jaundice, vomiting, and weakness. She was jaundiced, with markedly raised transaminases (aspartate transaminase 1264 U/l, alanine transaminase 1305 U/l) increased alkaline phosphatase, and normal gamma-glutamyltransferase and serum total bilirubin. Partial thromboplastin time was 33 seconds. A complete blood count and renal function were normal. Urine screen was positive for cocaine. Over the next 48 hours she developed acute respiratory and renal failure, hypotension, and tonic-clonic seizures. She also developed severe thrombocytopenia (platelet cell count 21×10^9/L), impaired coagulation, and a hemolytic anemia with 6–7 schistocytes per microscopic field. A chest X-ray showed bilateral alveolar infiltrates compatible with acute respiratory distress syndrome. An electrocardiogram showed an acute inferior myocardial infarction. Liver biopsy showed multifocal hepatic necrosis and microvesicular steatosis, consistent with toxic hepatitis. She recovered after plasma exchange, blood transfusions, and hemodialysis.

The authors noted that thrombotic microangiopathy due to cocaine is fairly rare. Its pathogenesis is unclear, possible mechanisms being an immune reaction or direct damage to the vascular endothelium. Cocaine-induced acute hepatitis has been linked to several toxic metabolites, including norcocaine and N-hydroxynorcocaine, which are produced by cytochrome P450 enzymes.

℞ *Fetotoxicity of cocaine*

The current view is that in utero exposure to cocaine has a subtle impact on offspring development and functioning (SEDA-28, 43; SEDA-29, 41). The Maternal Lifestyle Study, a prospective randomized study, has followed 717 infants exposed only to cocaine and 7442 non-exposed infants from birth to hospital discharge at 12 network sites (20[C], 21[C]). Cocaine-exposed infants were younger (1.2 weeks), weighed less (536 g), and were smaller (2.6 cm shorter and head circumference 1.5 cm smaller). Congenital anomalies were not increased. Acute

subtle changes in central and autonomic nervous system function, such as irritability, jitteriness, tremors, high pitched crying, and excessive suck, were more common in the cocaine-exposed group. There was a significantly increased prevalence of infection in the infants of cocaine-using mothers. Hepatitis was 42 times more common, syphilis was 15 times as common, and human immunodeficiency virus positivity was 16 times more common (although the overall prevalence was only 0.1%). Exposure to cocaine increased the likelihood of involvement with social services such as child protection agencies.

The preliminary results of the Meconium Project, a study done in Barcelona between October 2002 and February 2004, have been reported (22[c]). The findings were based on the first 830 meconium samples and 549 mother–infant pairs. Overall drug use was 7.9%, and drug screens detected 6-monoacetymorphine and cocaine. There was under-reporting of drug abuse. The self-reporting rates in interviews were opiates 1.3%, cocaine 1.8%, and both drugs 1.3%; meconium analysis showed higher rates (8.7, 4.4, and 2.2% respectively). One declared case of ecstasy consumption was confirmed. Arecoline, the main alkaloid in areca nuts, was found in meconium samples from four Asian neonates whose mothers had consumed betel nuts. The use of opiates and cocaine during pregnancy was associated with active use of cannabis, tobacco smoking, and a higher number of cigarettes smoked. Lower birth weight in newborns was associated with mothers who used cocaine only and both cocaine and opiates. One of the four infants exposed to arecoline had a low birth weight, hypotonia, and hyporeflexia.

Motor development   *A second report from the Maternal Lifestyle Study focused on motor development in 392 children prenatally exposed to cocaine and 776 non-exposed control infants who were identified by meconium assay and mothers' self-reporting (23[C]). Motor skills were assessed at 1 month with the NICU Network Neurobehavioral Scale (NNNS), at 4 months with the posture and fine motor assessment of infants (PFMAI), at 12 months with the Bayley Scales of Infant Development-2nd edition (BSID-II), and at 18 months with the Peabody Developmental Motor Scales (PDMS). The infants with prenatal cocaine exposure had motor skill deficits at 1 month, but normal function at 18 months. Heavy cocaine use was associated with poorer motor performance. Both lower and higher nicotine exposures related to poorer motor performance.*

Behavior   *Prenatal exposure to cocaine is associated with behavioral problems in children of school age. The degree to which sex-specific effects can be identified in relation to prenatal cocaine exposure was the focus of two studies by the same group of researchers. In the first study 499 subjects, who had been prospectively followed since pregnancy, were evaluated in a laboratory at 7 years (24[C]). The findings support sex- and alcohol-moderated effects on prenatal cocaine exposure. Among boys with prenatal alcohol exposure, those with significant cocaine exposure had significantly higher levels of Delinquent Behavior than the boys with no cocaine exposure. Prenatal cocaine exposure in the alcohol-exposed boys doubled the likelihood of clinically significant Externalizing Behavior scores compared with controls. In the absence of prenatal alcohol exposure, prenatal cocaine exposure alone in boys had no significant effect. In contrast, among girls with no prenatal alcohol exposure, the presence of prenatal cocaine exposure correlated with significant Externalizing Behaviors and Aggressive Behaviors compared with controls. Clinically significant Externalizing Behavior scores were almost five times as likely in this group. In contrast, among girls with prenatal alcohol exposure, no association was found. Prenatal cocaine exposure in the alcohol-exposed group of boys doubled the likelihood of clinically significant Externalizing Behavior scores compared with controls. In contrast, among girls with prenatal alcohol exposure, there was no association between prenatal cocaine exposure and behavior.*

In the second study the same group evaluated the effects of prenatal cocaine exposure on child behavior in 506 African–American mother–child pairs (25[C]). The mothers were identified as cocaine users and non-users during the initial prenatal visits with urine screen confirmation. Offspring behavior was assessed 6–7 years later using caregiver reports with the Achenbach Child Behavior Checklist (CBCL). Analyses stratified by sex and prenatal alcohol exposure showed that behaviors in girls

without prenatal alcohol exposure but with prenatal cocaine exposure were adverse: 6.5% of the unique variance in behavior was related to prenatal cocaine exposure. Among these girls, the likelihood of scoring in the abnormal range for Aggression was 17 times control.

Neurodevelopment   *Neurodevelopmental and cognitive outcomes among prenatally cocaine exposed children have been documented by measuring school performance in 62 cocaine-exposed and 73 control children who were students at an American inner-city school (26[C]). The children were followed prospectively from birth to the end of the 4th grade. Their report cards, standardized test results, teacher and parent reports, and birth and early childhood data were studied. Both groups had poor grade progression from grades 1 to 4 (71 versus 84%), low Grade Point averages, reading skills below grade level (30 versus 28%), and below-average standardized test scores. The children with higher Full Scale Intelligence Quotients and better home environments, regardless of drug status, had successful progression.*

Drug overdose   Body packing is an important differential diagnosis in patients who present with symptoms of acute drug toxicity (SEDA-18, 38; SEDA-21, 32; SEDA-27, 36; SEDA-29, 43). Successful management of a cocaine body packer after endoscopic removal has been reported (27[A]).

- A 55-year-old man was found unconscious at Al Doha airport in Qatar later had a generalized seizure. He was unconscious, afebrile, and tachypneic. His blood pressure was 150/90 mmHg and his pulse rate 105/minute. His pupils were fixed and dilated. A brain CT scan was unremarkable. A plain X-ray of the abdomen showed two packets in the stomach and one in the rectum. The packets, each of which weighed about 80 g, were removed by endoscopy, and he recovered consciousness after five days of conservative treatment.

In this case cocaine was found in the urine and the packets contents were also identified as cocaine.

Ecstasy (3,4-methylenedioxymet-amfetamine, MDMA) *(SED-15, 180;*
SEDA-27, 29; SEDA-28, 4, 28; SEDA-29, 1;
for other amphetamines see Chapter 1)

℞ *Epidemiology of the use of ecstasy*

"Club drugs", which are used primarily by young adults at all night "raves", dance parties, including ecstasy, have been frequently reviewed (28^R, 29^R, 30^R). Ecstasy is classified as an empathogen or enactogen, as the subjective experience has been described by users as intensely emotional and as creating a perception that one can experience the emotions of others.

Recent US data suggest a decline in the use of ecstasy. Programs sponsored by the US Drug Enforcement Administration have systematically collected results from toxicological analyses conducted by state and local forensic laboratories on substances seized by law enforcement operations. The numbers of seizures of ecstasy in 2003 were down from a peak in 2001. These data are concordant with other surveys done in the USA, including a decline in the prevalence of use by students in secondary schools, which appears to be related to reduced availability and perceptions of the risks associated with its use. The percentage of 12th graders who said that there was a great risk of harm associated with using ecstasy increased from 38% in 2000 to 58% in 2004. The perceived availability of ecstasy by students fell from 62% in 2001 to 48% on 2004. Moreover, the disapproval of people who tried ecstasy once or twice increased from 81% in 2001 to 88% in 2004.

Surveys conducted by the Office of Applied Studies of the Substance Abuse and Mental Health Services Administration (SAMHSA) on the prevalence, patterns, and consequences of the use and abuse of alcohol, tobacco, and illegal drugs in the general US civilian non-institutionalized population in 2003 showed that 4.6% of the US population aged 12 and above had ever used ecstasy, 0.9% had used it in the past year, and 0.2% had used it in the past month. About 2.4% of those aged 12–17 years had ever used ecstasy compared with 15% of those aged 18–25 years and 3.1% of those aged 26 and over. However, the trend was different in

Australia, where a national survey showed an increase in lifetime use of ecstasy from 2.4% in 1998 to 6.1% in 2001, with past year use rising from 0.9 to 2.4%. Furthermore, 10% of teenage ecstasy users and 6.9% of users in their twenties used ecstasy daily or weekly. Lifetime use of ecstasy among 10th grade students in Turkey rose from 2.7% in 1998 to 3.3% in 2001.

New data suggest that use of ecstasy occurs in a variety of settings and is not any more restricted to raves. Amongst US university undergraduate students, the number of sexual partners increased the likelihood of ecstasy use, as did self-reported sexual identity. Gay, lesbian, and bisexual students were more than two times as likely to have used ecstasy in the past year. Polysubstance use amongst ecstasy users was the norm (29^R).

In an epidemiological study of 2000 randomly selected individuals in West Germany and 1000 in East Germany in 2001, the lifetime prevalences of ecstasy and amfetamine use were about 4 and 3% respectively. The percentage of people who reported that "one should never try (ecstasy) at all" increased from 72% in 1993 to 87% in 2001. In another epidemiological study in Germany involving 8139 randomly selected adults aged 18–59, 46% responded. In West Germany, 1.5% reported having tried ecstasy at least once. The younger subjects were more experienced—5.2 and 5.7% of the 18–20 and 21–24 year-olds respectively reported using it; 1.8 and 3.7% of the 18–20 year-olds and 3.7% of the 21–24 year-olds had used ecstasy within the last 12 months. During the 30 days before the interview, 0.3% of the interviewees reported having used ecstasy. However, in East Germany, ecstasy was the only substance with a higher prevalence, which, when extrapolated, suggested that 1.2 million of the 18–59 year-olds reported having taken ecstasy within the 12-months before the interview.

The Early Developmental Stages of Psychopathology Study recruited a representative sample of 14–24 year olds from metropolitan Munich and its surrounds; the longitudinal analyses involved 2446 of the 3021 interviews done at baseline. The findings suggested that men use ecstasy more often than women. While the onset of use was unlikely before the age of 14, it was followed by a sudden surge in use, which appeared to stagnate at age 24 for women and 26 for men. The increase in use was in the younger cohort. Ecstasy users, compared with non-users, had a higher probability of using other illicit drugs. Use of ecstasy appeared to be a transient phenomenon—88% of the occasional users were non-users at follow-up and only 0.8% of the sample fulfilled the diagnostic criteria for a lifetime ecstasy-related substance use disorder. Moreover, increased proportions of the subjects in the group of lifetime ecstasy users had at least one mental disorder besides abuse or dependency. In most of the cases (88%), the onset of mental disorders occurred before the first use of ecstasy or a related substance. There were no significant differences in the incidence of mental disorders prospectively between the baseline ecstasy abstainers and ecstasy users in the follow-up period.

In the 1990s, a new dance and music culture called "techno" emerged in many European countries. Techno music was often associated with raves, which were also known as Techno raves. Around the same time, in Berlin, the Love Parade movement, ardent techno fans, started and attracted 1.5 million people in 1999. This caught the attention of the leisure industry, and magazines, music, and other paraphernalia were aimed at the adolescents and young adults involved in the techno scene. The use of club drugs is closely associated with this culture. In a study of 1664 adolescents and young adults designed to investigate the phenomenon of ecstasy use in the "techno party scene" in 1996, cannabis was the most commonly used drug in this group. About 50% of the group had used ecstasy once in their life and 44% had used speed; the 12-month and last-month usage rates were 40 and 28% respectively for ecstasy and 46 and 35% for speed. Ecstasy users were likely to have used combination drugs, the most prevalent sequences being "cannabis–ecstasy–speed" (10%) followed by "cannabis–ecstasy–speed–hallucinogens" (8%). The authors reported that the exclusive use of ecstasy in the techno party scene was almost non-existent. In the "Techno Study", in which 1412 persons were interviewed, the variability and stability of ecstasy use behavior in the techno party scene were explored. This study found even more drug use in 1998–9. Again cannabis was the more commonly used drug. The lifetime, 12-month, and last-month prevalences were respectively 40, 30, and 20% for ecstasy and 41, 31, and 21% for speed.

During 19 in-depth interviews, with a response rate of 46%, exploring the reasons for ecstasy use, the three main explanations identified were (a) affiliation, (b) stimulation, and (c) relaxation (30^R). Ecstasy was perceived as being extremely helpful in stimulating interactions with people and stimulating effects were mentioned, especially in combination with music. "Feeling good" or "a desire to feel good" were the most commonly cited reasons for using ecstasy. Fear of reduced efficiency (75%) and fear of damage to health (62%) and developing addiction (36%) were common reasons for quitting. However, 44% stated that "ecstasy did nothing to me". The author concluded that ecstasy is second only to cannabis in illegal drug preferences among adolescents and young adults in Germany. Increased rates of ecstasy use in East Germany paralleled increases in ecstasy-related crimes by 60% in that area. Moreover, ecstasy users were more often polydrug users with increase degrees of psychopathology; the existence of mental illness increased the likelihood of future use of ecstasy. According to the author, ecstasy does not seem to determine substance-specific drug-use-related behavior. It rather seems to be yet another substance in the youth-related illicit substance carousel. Most people who begin to use a variety of illicit substances for whatever reasons, stop on their own without treatment of any sort.

Many large metropolitan areas saw a surge in the use of ecstasy among its young adults during the late 1990s. In the USA, Seattle reported high levels of club drug use compared with the national average and increases in problematic behavior and morbidity/mortality associated with the use of these drugs. Seattle also had a history of providing permits for large rave dance parties. Those who had ever used ecstasy were much more likely to use almost all other drugs; 26% of ecstasy users at rave parties mentioned ever using "research chemicals" (a broad array of poorly studied psychoactive chemicals used to explore new psychedelic experiences) compared with 1% of non-ecstasy users. At raves, behaviors associated with the use of ecstasy in the prior 6 months included unprotected sex by nearly one-third and driving under the influence of ecstasy by 38%. The proportion who reported having "overdosed, passed out, or had a bad experience" caused by ecstasy was 15%; 6% agreed that their use had been out of control in the previous 6 months. About 26% said that they worried that they might later have problems with health and memory. The use of adulterated ecstasy was reported by respondents in all groups, from 29 to 59% at rave parties. About 12–18% of those who had ever used ecstasy reported that they had used antidepressants to control its effects; 16% took vitamins and 11% took 5-hydroxytryptophan to protect against the depressant effects of ecstasy. Lifetime ecstasy use was 11% among 12th graders nationally, compared with 16% in Seattle; usage during the prior 30 days was 2% nationally and 6% locally. Use of ecstasy was second only to use of cannabis among illicit drugs used by school children. About 50% of all those surveyed who had ever used ecstasy had not used it in the past 6 months and most of those who had used it reported using it less than monthly. Not only were ecstasy users less likely to be active users than active drinkers, but those who did use it did so much less frequently.

Among men who have sex with men, drug use and sexual activity were inextricably connected for all participants who also reported strong expectations that ecstasy and other drugs lowered inhibitions and increased courage in finding sex partners, trying new sexual experiences, or going to gay venues they might not otherwise visit. All except African–Americans described ecstasy as a commonly used drug. Those who had ever used ecstasy were more likely to report unprotected anal sex and were more likely to have a sexually transmitted disease than those who had never used ecstasy.

Of 13 deaths in which ecstasy was identified, three were determined to have resulted at least partly from ecstasy. Nine out of 10 cases in which ecstasy was present but was ruled as not having directly caused the death were due to gun shot wounds or motor vehicle accidents. There was one case of overdose with ecstasy and metamfetamine. In four of 10 cases, ecstasy concentrations were above the concentration associated with recreational use, but death was ruled to be caused by physical trauma. There were three suicides with gun shot wounds to the head, of whom two were positive for ecstasy.

Community surveys have shown that Latinos report significantly lower levels of lifetime use of ecstasy, while STD clinic data point to significantly lower ecstasy use among African–Americans. Thus, ecstasy users were primarily

Caucasians and men in their late teens or twenties (31^C). Most people who have ever used ecstasy either no longer continue to use it or use it infrequently, so opportunities for acute negative consequences are infrequent compared with alcohol. Acute toxicity due to moderate doses of ecstasy appears to be low, based on self-reporting and low mortality rates in the community. Rates of emergency department admissions and student use of ecstasy were higher in Seattle than the national average. Among men who have sex with men, ecstasy use was higher than among heterosexual men and was associated with higher levels of both unprotected sex and sexually transmitted diseases.

In a report from Korea, hair and urine samples were collected from 791 subjects aged 20–62 years suspected of drug use (32^C). Ecstasy and/or MDA (its main metabolite) were found in 5.6%. Only four subjects were positive for MDA alone. However, only 9 subjects had both ecstasy and MDA in the urine. Abuse of ecstasy or MDA was found principally among young adults, of whom 73% were aged 20–29 and 27% aged 30–39; in this group 88% of men and 18% of women had positive hair samples. The concentrations of ecstasy and MDA in the hair of male abusers were higher than in female abusers. The authors speculated that it may be difficult to detect ecstasy or MDA in urine samples from occasional abusers. They also observed that polydrug use was not common among the Korean users of ecstasy.

Cardiovascular   Of 50 participants, randomly recruited on four different nights from a popular night club, users of ecstasy, alcohol, cannabis, and other psychostimulants did not have significant differences in their body temperature despite increases in environmental temperature and period of dancing (33^C). However, *increased blood pressure* was predicted by the number of ecstasy tablets ingested and the amount of cocaine used. There were significant differences in both heart rate and blood pressure between polysubstance users compared with the alcohol and cannabis users. The authors suggested that polysubstance users may be at higher risk of cardiovascular toxicity. However, more data are needed to confirm these observations.

Coronary spasm has been attributed to ecstasy (34^A).

- A previously healthy 20-year-old Caucasian woman developed intermittent left-sided chest tightness associated with palpitation but no dyspnea, hemoptysis, calf pain, or swelling. She had been out the night before with her friends to a club, since when she had become more restless, anxious, and unable to sleep. She was very talkative, but cold and sweaty and had dilated pupils. She had normal heart sounds and sinus rhythm. An electrocardiogram showed ischemia, with wide spread ST segment depression and T wave inversion, consistent with coronary artery spasm. Her creatine kinase and troponin T concentrations were not raised and an echocardiogram was normal. She made a complete recovery with standard intravenous doses of nitrates. Amphetamine derivatives, presumed to have been from a drink laced with ecstasy, were found in her urine.

The authors speculated that the mechanism of action was endothelial dysfunction, similar to that postulated for cocaine-induced coronary spasm.

Psychological Concerns have been raised about the effect of long-term ecstasy use on *cognition*. Visual evoked potentials have been studied during digit discrimination in eight heavy ecstasy users, 8 moderate ecstasy users, and 18 drug-free controls (35[c]). Only one subject had used ecstasy in the previous 6 months. The heavy users made significantly more errors than the other two groups. They had reduced amplitude but not latency of visual evoked potentials at both the occipital (Oz) and frontal (Fz) leads during the task. The effect in the occipital leads was present in P200 for heavy users only and in P300 components for both groups of users. In the frontal leads the amplitude effect was present in N250 for heavy users only and in P300 components for both groups. These results suggest that ecstasy consumption affects cortical activity, reflected in both exogenous and endogenous aspects of information processing, especially those components that affect attentional demands. Long-term exposure to ecstasy causes long-term electroencephalographic deficits suggesting altered cortical activity.

Ecstasy-related deficits in cognitive functioning, such as shifting, inhibition, updating, and access to long-term memory elements of the central executive functions, have been evaluated in two studies, one of which focused on updating and access to long-term memory, and the other on switching and inhibition (36[C]). The first study supported an ecstasy-related deficit in memory updating and access to long-term memory that was not related to sex, intelligence, amphetamine use, or sleep quality. Access to long-term memory, as indexed by word fluency scores, was more related to aspects of cocaine use than to equivalent indices of ecstasy use. Contrary to the investigators' expectations, updating executive component process was influenced by cannabis. In the second study, there was no evidence of any ecstasy-related deficit on inhibition and switching measures. Thus, ecstasy/polydrug users reached a lower level on the computation span task and recalled fewer letters correctly on the letter-updating task. Ecstasy/polydrug users scored higher on an intelligence test and significantly higher on a sleep questionnaire, and the main effect remained significant after controlling for these co-variates. Contrary to expectations, ecstasy/polydrug users actually performed better than controls on the random letter generation task used to measure inhibition. There were no significant ecstasy/polydrug-related effects on the tasks used to measure switching. Thus, both studies provide support for ecstasy/polydrug-related deficits in memory updating and access to semantic memory, but not shifting or inhibition. The authors questioned the unanticipated effects of ecstasy in producing more letters and caution in over-interpreting these findings, saying that on other similar measures these differences did not exist. As ecstasy users were frequently polydrug users, and since the impact of concurrently used drugs in ecstasy users appears to be significantly large, the contribution of other drug use cannot be minimized. Effects of ecstasy/polydrug use on executive functions are not uniform—ecstasy/polydrug users perform worse on updating and access tasks, but not shifting and inhibition tasks, which appear to be relatively unaffected.

Psychiatric National drug information strategies convey the message that the use of ecstasy is associated with an increase in both the incidence and severity of *major affective disorder*. However, very little research supports this. Many reviewers have felt that the use of ecstasy results in a depressed mood. In a meta-analysis of 22 studies of self-reported depressive symptoms in ecstasy users there was a significant but small effect size of 0.31 (95% CI = 0.17, 0.37) (37[M]). Estimated lifetime ecstasy use, but not duration of use, usual dose per episode, or abstention, predicted the effect size. Although the effect size was small, it contrasted with most published literature, which has generally shown no association between the use of ecstasy and depressive symptoms. It is possible that individual studies were not statistically powerful enough to detect effects that only emerged through meta-analysis. However, the authors noticed that smaller studies produced larger effect sizes. Furthermore, they questioned the quality of the primary data sources. Only nine of the 23 studies controlled for use of cannabis between the groups, and only eight of these recorded use parameters. This meant that it was not possible to differentiate the effects of ecstasy accurately from those of cannabis. Very few studies reported wider drug histories. The authors cited the example of a study that showed that although most of the volunteers self-reported a preference for using ecstasy, their actual behavior was discrepant and they valued intoxication over the effects of individual drugs. A posteriori classification of most ecstasy-using populations would more accurately define them as having a preference for alcohol and cannabis. There was no association between effect size and abstention from ecstasy. The authors suggested that although use of ecstasy may have been postponed or stopped, other substance misuse had continued, preventing a linear relation between abstention and effect size. They mentioned problems with the measuring scales used and heterogeneity amongst the ecstasy users. Specifically, self-reported scales may be heavily confounded by the somatic effects of substance misuse. Interpretation is further complicated by the high prevalence of psychiatric co-morbidity amongst drug users. The observed effects may be common to polysubstance misuse in general rather than to the use of ecstasy per se. The authors recommended that drug users should be informed that substance misuse has both acute and subacute effects that may have negative effects on health, work, and relationships.

Immunologic   *Immunosuppression* has been attributed to ecstasy (38[A]).

- A 24-year-old African–American man developed a vesicular rash on his left forehead and eyelids consistent with herpes zoster ophthalmicus. He reported safe sexual practices and no intravenous drug use, but had used ecstasy three times a day for 4 days before the onset of symptoms. He slowly improved with intravenous aciclovir.

Varicella zoster reactivation is a potential complication of immunosuppression and is uncommon under the age of 50. After ruling out all the potential causes for the infection, the authors speculated that ecstasy had caused immunosuppression, leading to the infection. In support of this they invoked previous reports of immunosuppression with ecstasy.

Body temperature   Abuse of ecstasy occurs in a variety of settings. Six new cases of severe *hyperthermia* over 2 months have been reported (39[A]).

- A 20-year-old woman was found unresponsive at a rave. She was hot to the touch and on the way to hospital had a tonic–clonic seizure and became pulseless and apneic. Aggressive resuscitation was unsuccessful. An autopsy showed gross pulmonary congestion and edema. She had acute neuronal ischemia and mild hepatic steatosis, without any evidence of myocardial damage. Her blood ecstasy concentration was 1.21 mg/l. Death was reported to have been secondary to ecstasy toxicity.
- A 20-year-old man, a previously healthy student, became agitated within 4 hours of ingesting two tablets of ecstasy at the same rave. His friends reported previous uneventful use of similar amounts. He was comatose and had minimal purposeful movements and a temperature of 41.5 °C. His heart rate was 200/minute and his BP 123/57 mmHg. He had hot dry skin and diffuse intermittent myoclonus. Urine toxicology was positive for ecstasy only. His glucose was 2.5 mmol/l (42 mg/dl), platelets 80×10^9/l, sodium 148 mmol/l, creatinine 186 μmol/l (2.1 mg/dl), and total bilirubin 34 μmol/l (2.0 mg/d; peak creatine kinase activity was 17 000 iu/l. He recovered with cooling.
- An 18-year-old man at the same rave developed an altered mental state after taking two "tulips" (slang for ecstasy tablets, which contained pure ecstasy). He was alert but disoriented in person, place, and time. His rectal temperature was 40.7 °C. His heart rate was 177/minute, sodium 144 mmol/l, creatine 175 μmol/l (2.3 mg/dl), blood urea nitrogen 6.4 mmol/l (18 mg/dl), and peak creatine kinase activity 4964 iu/l. His urine was positive for ecstasy only. He recovered as his core temperature fell with treatment.
- A 20-year-old man became unconscious and had generalized tonic–clonic seizures 2 hours after taking one ecstasy tablet. He had a rectal temperature of 40.6 °C, a heart rate of 170/minute, and a blood pressure of 92/21 mmHg. He had roving eye movements and myoclonus. His blood pH was 6.92, the serum sodium was 144 mmol/l, and his urine was positive for ecstasy. He recovered with cooling.

- A 22-month-old boy took a pill from a "Tic-Tac" container that had been filled with ecstasy tablets by his parents. Two hours later he was responsive to only painful stimuli and had roving eye movements. He had a rectal temperature of 39.3 °C and a heart rate of 190/minute. He had bruxism, sweating, and rigid limbs with intermittent writhing. His urine was positive for ecstasy only. He gradually improved with cooling.
- A 27-year-old quadriplegic man became unconscious 2 hours after taking one tablet of ecstasy for recreational purposes. He had a rectal temperature of 41.3 °C, a heart rate of 130/minute, and a blood pressure of 120/58 mmHg. He had roving eye movements with 5 mm equal reactive pupils. His urine was positive for ecstasy and cannabinoids. He recovered with cooling.

The authors observed that three of the six patients had been exposed to ecstasy outside of a rave and had hyperthermia despite not having vigorous muscle activity, thereby questioning previous assumptions about pathogenesis. There were no contaminants in the tablets, based on laboratory analyses. The authors speculated that another cause of hyperthermia and acute toxicity could be a genetic predisposition to defective metabolism of ecstasy, especially CYP2D6 deficiency. They postulated that hyperthermia in ecstasy users could be heterogeneous and was more likely to be due to a combination of causes.

Death   A fatal outcome after the use of ecstasy in a private setting rather than at a rave has been reported (40[A]).

- A 19-year-old woman consumed beer, cannabis, and four ecstasy tablets with friends in her apartment. Two hours later, she suddenly jumped up and made some uncontrolled movements. She had cramps, was unable to speak, and needed support to walk. Following bouts of trembling and sweating she seemed to fall asleep, and her colleagues left her in her bedroom. An hour later they found that she had vomited and was trembling and barely conscious. She could not be resuscitated. At autopsy, there was cerebral edema and massive pulmonary edema and her distal bronchi were filled with gastric contents. The right ventricle was dilated and filled with blood. Histologically, there was generalized vascular congestion, perivascular edema of the brain, and pulmonary edema with focal atelectasis. There were no signs of disseminated intravascular coagulation. There was fatty degeneration of the liver. These findings were consistent with asphyxiation, hypoxia, shock, and cardiopulmonary failure. No ethanol was detected in the blood or cerebrospinal fluid but the urine concentration was 100 mg/l. There were cannabinoids and amphetamines in the urine and blood.

The authors bemoaned the fact that ecstasy is still falsely considered to be harmless by most users. They emphasized that the classic user profile has changed over recent years, with non-rave party use increasing, as ecstasy is more readily available. They also observed that a quieter environment, which is supposed to reduce the risk of adverse effects, did not prevent this woman's death. According to her friends, who had ingested similar amounts of ecstasy from the same supply without any untoward effects, this had been her first experience with ecstasy. Her blood ecstasy concentration of 3.8 mg/l was highly toxic. As her friends did not have any untoward reactions, the authors proposed that different people have different sensitivity. Ecstasy probably had a direct toxic effect on vital centers in the brain stem, leading to central nervous impairment after a short initial state of excitation. Cannabinoid concentrations did not suggest a likely contribution to death.

Drug tolerance   Ecstasy can release large amounts of serotonin in the synaptic cleft, with an 80% loss of brain serotonin and its metabolites within 4 hours of an injection of ecstasy. However, ecstasy inhibits monoamine oxidases A and B, leading to an increase in serotonin and other catecholamines (41[R]). Chronic tolerance to ecstasy in humans is a robust empirical phenomenon, which leads to dosage escalation and bingeing. Tolerance to ecstasy develops rapidly; many users describe their first experience as their best, and with repeated use its positive effects subside rapidly. Many predicted that ecstasy would not become a drug of abuse, specifically because of the early reduction in subjective efficacy. This is opposite to cocaine. Many recreational users increase the dosage; however, taking a double dose does not double the supposedly beneficial effects but increases the negative effects. Chronic bingeing is statistically linked to higher rates of drug-related psychobiological problems. Thus, the authors suggested that regular ecstasy users should balance their desire for an optimal on-drug experience with the need to minimize the post-drug consequences. Some individuals intensify their use to maximize the on-drug experience, while others use it sparingly to minimize the long-term consequences. The rate of development of chronic tolerance can be variable, even with regular ecstasy use. The authors postulated that serotonergic mechanisms may partly explain the unusual pattern of chronic tolerance with ecstasy.

Susceptibility factors

Infants   The effects of ingestion, accidental or otherwise, of ecstasy in infants continue to be reported (42[Ar]).

- An 11-month-old, breast-fed boy of Argentinian–Italian origin developed generalized seizures, depressed consciousness (Glasgow coma scale 12), repetitive and jerky movements of limbs with associated hyper-reflexia and muscle rigidity, dilated non-reactive pupils, and perioral cyanosis. He had a sinus tachycardia of 190/minute and pulse oximetry of 83%. There was ecstasy 11.7 mg/l and its metabolite MDA 1.2 mg/l in the urine. Cocaine 1.3 mg/l and benzoylecgonine 0.4 mg/l were found in a proximal hair sample and cocaine 4.6 mg/l and benzoylecgonine 0.5 mg/l in a distal segment. His mother's hair was negative. He recovered completely within 24 hours.

This infant appeared to have accidentally ingested ecstasy. The extremely high urinary concentration of the parent drug and metabolites excluded the possibility of intoxication through breast-feeding. The urine concentration of ecstasy was in the range encountered in acute intoxication and adult deaths. The child's symptoms were consistent with cardiovascular and autonomic effects and acute toxic effects of ecstasy. The hair analysis showed chronic exposure to cocaine, which could have been through passive inhalation of cocaine, ingestion of powder residues, or intentional administration/exposure through breast milk. This case highlighted the importance of drug testing in unusual cases, even in infants.

- A 15-month-old infant developed seizures (43[Ar]). Her heart rate was 200/minute, her peripheries were cyanosed, and she had labored breathing, dilated pupils reacting sluggishly to light, and a temperature of 37.3 °C. There was a rash over the right iliac fossa. Her neck and back were arched. Her liver was enlarged. There was no response to rectal diazepam, rectal paraldehyde, or intravenous lorazepam, but she responded to phenytoin and anesthesia with thiopental and suxamethonium. Amphetamine was detected in her urine.

Discussion with parents revealed that accidental ingestion of ecstasy may have occurred after a teenaged uncle's party.

Khat

℞

Khat, or qat, is a stimulant commonly used in East Africa, Yemen, and Southern Saudi Arabia. Khat leaves from the evergreen bush Catha edulis are typically chewed while fresh, but can also be smoked, brewed in tea, or sprinkled on food. Its use is culturally based.

The major effects of khat on the central nervous system can be attributed to cathinone (S-[-]-alpha-aminopropriophenone) in fresh khat leaves and cathine (norpseudoephedrine) in dried khat leaves and stems. Cathinone, a phenylalkylamine, is the major active component and is structurally similar to amfetamine. It degrades to norpseudoephedrine and norephedrine within days of leaf picking. Cathinone increases dopamine release and reduces dopamine re-uptake (44[R]).

Khat is often used in social gatherings called "sessions", which can last 3–4 hours. They are generally attended by men, although khat use among women is growing. Men are also more likely to be daily users. Users pick leaves from the khat branch, chew them on one side of the mouth, swallowing only the juice, and adding fresh leaves periodically. The khat chewer may experience increased alertness and euphoria. About 100–300 grams of khat may be chewed during each session, and 100 grams of khat typically contains 36 mg of cathinone.

Khat has been recognized as a substance of abuse with increasing popularity. It is estimated that 10 million people chew khat worldwide, and it is used by up to 80% of adults in Somalia and Yemen. It now extends to immigrant African communities in the UK and USA. It is banned in Saudi Arabia, Egypt, Morocco, Sudan, and Kuwait. It is also banned in the USA and European countries. However, in Australia, its importation is controlled by a licence issued by the Therapeutic Goods Administration, which allows up to 5 kg of khat per month per individual for personal use.

There have been several review articles describing khat and its growth (44[R]). The World Health Organization Advisory Group's 1980 report reviewed the pharmacological effects of khat in animals and humans (45[R]). The societal context of khat use has also been reviewed (46[R]).

Cardiovascular *Khat is a sympathomimetic amine and increases blood pressure and heart rate. Limited evidence suggests that khat increases the risk of acute myocardial infarction. In Yemen 100 patients admitted to an intensive care unit with an acute myocardial infarction were compared with 100 sex- and age-matched controls recruited from an ambulatory clinic (47^C). They completed a questionnaire on personal habits, such as khat use and cigarette smoking, past medical history, and a family history of myocardial infarction. Use of khat was an independent risk factor for acute myocardial infarction, with an odds ratio of 5.0 (95% CI = 1.9, 13). The relation was dose-related: "heavy" khat users were at higher risk than "moderate" users, although the extent of use and the potency of khat used were estimated, being hard to quantify. To explain the increased risk of acute myocardial infarction, the authors suggested that it may have been related to increased blood pressure and heart rate, with a resultant increase in myocardial oxygen demand. They also suggested that khat could have acted via the mechanisms proposed to explain acute myocardial infarction after the use of amphetamines, such as catecholamine-induced platelet aggregation and coronary vasospasm.*

Nervous system *The prevalence and health effects of headache in Africa have been reviewed (48^R). In 66 khat users 25% reported headaches (49^c) and in people with migraine 12% reported using khat (50^c).*

Psychiatric *In addition to the acute stimulant effects of euphoria and alertness caused by khat, there is the question of whether continued khat use alters mood, behavior, and mental health.*

- *A 33-year-old unemployed Somali man with a 10-year history of khat chewing, who had lived in Western Australia for 4 years, and who was socially isolated, started to sleep badly, and had weight loss and persecutory delusions (51^A). His mental state deteriorated over 2–3 months and he thought that his relatives were poisoning him and that he was being followed by criminals. He had taken rifampicin and ethambutol for pulmonary tuberculosis for 1 year but became non-compliant for 2 months before presentation. He had reportedly chewed increasing amounts of khat daily from his backyard for last 2 years. There was no history of*

other drug use and his urine drug screen was negative. He responded well to olanzapine 20 mg/day and was discharged after 4 weeks, as his psychosis was gradually improving.

The impact of khat use on psychological symptoms was one of several factors considered in a study in which 180 Somali refugees were interviewed about psychiatric symptoms and about migration-related experiences and traumas (52^C). Suicidal thinking was more common among those who used khat (41 of 180) after migration compared with those who did not (21 of 180). However, a causal relationship cannot be deduced from these data.

The authors raised the concern that khat psychosis could be increasing in Australia because of a growing number of African refugees. Furthermore, factors related to immigration, such as social displacement and unemployment, may predispose to abuse, especially as khat is easily available in Australia.

In a cross-sectional survey of Yemeni adults the self-reported frequency of khat use and psychological symptoms was assessed using face-to-face interviews with members from a random sample of urban and rural households (53^C). Of 800 adults surveyed, 82% of men and 43% of women had used khat at least once. There was no association between khat and negative adverse psychological symptoms, and khat users had less phobic anxiety (56%) than non-users (38%). The authors were surprised by these results and offered several explanations: that the form of khat used in Yemen is less potent than in other locations; that prior reports of khat-related psychosis occurred in users in unfamiliar environments; that the sampling procedure may have under-represented heavier khat users; and that their measurement tool was not sensitive enough to detect psychological symptoms.

In Hargeisa, Somalia, trained local interviewers screened 4854 individuals for disability due to severe psychiatric problems and identified 169 cases (137 men and 32 women) (54^C). A subset of 52 positive screening cases was randomly selected for interview and were matched for age, sex, and education with controls. In all, 8.4% of men screened positive and 83% of those who screened positive had severe psychotic symptoms. Khat chewing and the use of greater amounts of khat were more common in this group. Khat users were also more likely to have had active war experience. Only 1.9% of women had positive screening. Khat use starting at an earlier age and in larger amounts (in "bundles" per day) correlated positively with psychotic symptoms.

Gastrointestinal Constipation is a common physical complaint among khat users (46[R]). The World Health Organization Advisory Group attributed this adverse effect to the tannins and norpseudoephedrine found in khat (45[r]).

Anorexia due to khat is probably due to norephedrine (45[r]).

The tannins in khat have been associated with delayed intestinal absorption, stomatitis, gastritis, and esophagitis observed with khat use (45[r]).

Khat chewing may be a risk factor for duodenal ulcer. In a case-control study 175 patients with duodenal ulceration (all diagnosed by endoscopy) and 150 controls completed a questionnaire about their health habits (55[c]). Khat use, defined as chewing khat at least 14 hours/week, was significantly more common among the cases (76 versus 35%). Potential confounding variables, including smoking, use of alcohol or NSAIDs, a family history, and chronic hepatic and renal disease, were not significantly different between the two groups. The authors postulated several mechanisms, including a physiological reaction to the stress response to cathine or exposure to chemicals, such as pesticides.

Drug dependence Khat use can lead to dependence, which is more important because of its social consequences than because of the effects of physical withdrawal. Khat users may devote significant amounts of time to acquiring and using khat, to the detriment of work and social responsibilities. The physical effects of early khat withdrawal are generally mild. Chronic users may experience craving, lethargy, and a feeling of warmth during early khat abstinence.

Tumorigenicity Three studies of the association of khat with head and neck cancers have been reviewed (56[M]). The studies showed a trend towards an increased risk of oral cancer and head and neck cancer with the use of khat, but there were too few data for a definitive conclusion. Tobacco use, which is common among

khat users, and alcohol use were confounding factors.

A possible association of cancer of the oral cavity with khat has been studied in exfoliated buccal and bladder cells from healthy male khat users; the cells were examined for micronuclei, a marker of genotoxic effects (57[c]). Of 30 individuals who did not use cigarettes or alcohol, 10 were non-users of khat and the other 20 used 10–60 g/day. The 10 individuals who used more than 100 g/day had an eight-fold increase in the frequency of micronuclei compared with non-users. There was a statistically significant dose-response relation between khat use and the number of micronuclei in oral mucosal cells but not urothelial cells. In a separate set of samples taken from khat users and non-users who also used cigarettes and alcohol, alcohol and cigarette use caused a 4.5-fold increase in the frequency of micronuclei and use of khat in addition to alcohol and cigarettes further doubled the frequency. In buccal mucosal cells from four individuals who ingested 100 g/day for 3 days, the maximum frequency of micronuclei occurred at 27 days after chewing and returned to baseline after 54 days. These data together suggest that khat, especially in combination with alcohol and smoking, may contribute to or cause oral malignancy.

However, in a small study of biopsies taken from the oral mucosa of 40 Yemeni khat users and 10 non-users there were no histopathological changes consistent with malignancy (58[c]). In the khat users, there were changes such as acanthosis, orthokeratosis, epithelial dysplasia, and intracellular edema on both the chewing and non-chewing sides of the oral mucosa. However, none of these lesions was malignant or pre-malignant. The authors thought that these changes were most probably due to mechanical friction or possibly due to chemical components of the khat or pesticides that had been used on the plants.

Fertility Reduced sperm count, semen volume, and sperm motility have been associated with khat dependence (46[R]).

Fetotoxicity Reduced infant birth weight has been reported in khat-using mothers (44[R]).

Lactation Reduced lactation has been reported in khat-using mothers (44[R]).

Drug contamination *Some khat leaves are grown with chemical pesticides. In 114 male khat users in two different mountainous areas of Yemen, users of khat that had been produced in fields in which chemical pesticides were used regularly had more acute gastrointestinal adverse effects (nausea and abdominal pain) and chronic body weakness and nasal problems (59ᶜ). The authors suggested that organic chemical pesticides such as dimethoate-cide can cause such adverse effects.*

Drug overdose *Acute toxicity requiring emergency medical treatment is rare. When it occurs there is a typical sympathomimetic syndrome, which should be treated with fluids, control of hyperthermia, bed rest, and, if necessary, sedation with benzodiazepines (44ᴿ).*

OPIOID ANALGESICS

See Chapter 8, in which both therapeutic and abuse aspects of the opioids are covered.

Psilocybin

Psychiatric *Hallucinogen persisting perception disorder* (HPPD) has been reported after the use of psilocybin (60ᴬ).

- An 18-year-old student, who had used cannabis moderately for many years developed perceptual impairment and dysphoric mood, which lasted for 8 months. The perceptual disturbances initially appeared after he took 40 hallucinogenic mushrooms in an infusion. He re-experienced the symptoms the following day after a cannabis snort. He reported visual disturbances such as distortion of objects, auditory disturbance with a sensation of resonance, depersonalization, derealization, changes in the perception of body weight, spatiotemporal disturbances, and inability to distinguish illusion from reality. These symptoms were similar to those experienced after initial intoxication with the mushrooms. Flashbacks occurred daily and got worse in the dark. Because these symptoms were distressing he stopped using cannabis 2 months later. The symptoms abated but then increased again 4 months later. An MRI scan, electroencephalography, and blood tests were normal. He was depressed and had a social phobia tendency but no thought disorder or hallucinations. He was initially treated with amisulpiride and then with olanzapine, to provide more sedation. However, this exacerbated his symptoms and was replaced by risperidone 2 mg/day. He was given sertraline for persistent dysphoric mood and anxiety. After 6 months, the flashbacks disappeared and his mood and social interactions improved.

This case suggests that HPPD can result from co-intoxication by psilocybin and cannabis and can persist after drug consumption has stopped.

References

1. Papp E, Czopf L, Habon T, Halmosi R, Horvath B, Marton Z, Tahin T, Komocsi A, Horvath I, Melegh B, Toth K. Drug-induced myocardial infarction in young patients. Int J Cardiol 2005;98:169–70.
2. Lindsay AC, Foale RA, Warren O, Henry JA. Cannabis as a precipitant of cardiovascular emergencies. Int J Cardiol 2005;104:230–2.
3. Fisher BAC, Ghuran A, Vadamalai V, Antonios TF. Cardiovascular complications induced by cannabis smoking: a case report and review of the literature. Emerg Med J 2005;22:679–80.
4. Altable CR, Urrutia AR, Martinez MIC. Cannabis-induced extrapyramidalism in a patient on neuroleptic treatment. J Clin Psychopharmacol 2005;25:91–2.
5. Arsenault L, Cannon M, Witton J. Causal association between cannabis and psychosis: examination of the evidence. Br J Psychiatry 2004;184:110–7.
6. Mateo I, Pinedo A, Gomez-Beldarrain M, Basterretxea JM, Garcia-Monco JC. Recurrent stroke associated with cannabis use. J Neurol Neurosurg Psychiatry 2005;76:435–7.
7. Haubrich C, Diehl R, Donges M, Schiefer J, Loos M, Kosinski C. Recurrent transient ischemic attacks in a cannabis smoker. J Neurol 2005;252:369–70.
8. Lane SD, Cherek DR, Lieving LM, Tcheremissine OV. Marijuana effects on human forgetting functions. J Exp Analysis Behav 2005;83:67–83.
9. Lane SD, Cherek DR, Tcheremissine OV, Lieving LM, Pietras CJ. Acute marijuana effects on human risk taking. Neuropsychopharmacology 2005;30:800–9.

10. Fried PA, Watkinson B, Gray R. Neurocognitive consequences of marihuana—comparison with pre-drug performance. Neurotoxicol Teratol 2005;27:231–9.

11. D'Souza DC, Abi-Saab WM, Madonick S, Forselius-Bielen K, Doersch A, Braley G, Gueorguieva R, Cooper TB, Krystal JH. Delta-9-tetrahydrocannabinol effects in schizophrenia: implications for cognition, psychosis and addiction. Biol Psychiatry 2005;57:594–608.

12. Iversen L. Long-term effects of exposure to cannabis. Curr Opin Pharmacol 2005;5:69–72.

13. Gill A. Bong lung: regular smokers of cannabis show relatively distinctive histologic changes that predispose to pneumothorax. Am J Surg Pathol 2005;29:980–1.

14. Trittibach P, Frueh BE, Goldblum D. Bilateral angle-closure glaucoma after combined consumption of "ecstasy" and marijuana. Am J Emerg Med 2005;23:813–4.

15. Hall W, Christie M, Currow D. Cannabinoids and cancer: causation, remediation and palliation. Lancet Oncol 2005;6:35–42.

16. Hurd YL, Wang X, Anderson V, Beck O, Minkoff H, Dow-Edwards D. Marijuana impairs growth in mid-gestation fetuses. Neurotoxicol Teratol 2005;27:221–9.

17. Nicoucar K, Sakbani K, Vukanovic S, Guyot J-P. Intralabyrinthine haemorrhage following cocaine consumption. Acta Oto-Laryngol 2005;125:899–901.

18. Tang BH. Cocaine and subarachnoid hemorrhage. J Neurosurg 2005;102:961–2.

19. Balaguer F, Fernandez J. Cocaine-induced acute hepatitis and thrombotic microangiopathy. JAMA 2005;293:797–8.

20. Bauer CR, Shankaran S, Bada HS, Lester B, Wright LL, Krause-Steinrauf H, Smeriglio VL, Finnegan LP, Maza PL, Verter J. The Maternal Lifestyle Study: drug exposure during pregnancy and short-term maternal outcomes. Am J Obstet Gynecol 2002;186:487–95.

21. Bauer CR, Langer JC, Shankaran S, Bada H, Lester B, Wright LL, Krause-Steinrauf H, Smeriglio VL, Finnegan LP, Maza PL, Verter J. Acute neonatal effects of cocaine exposure during pregnancy. Arch Pediatr Adolesc Med 2005;159:824–34.

22. Pichini S, Puig C, Zuccaro P, Marchei E, Pellegrini M, Murillo J, Vall O, Pacifici R, Garcia-Algar O. Assessment of exposure to opiates and cocaine during pregnancy in a Mediterranean city: Preliminary results of the "Meconium Project". Forensic Sci Int 2005;153:59–65.

23. Miller-Loncar C, Lester BM, Seifer R, Lagasse LL, Bauer CR, Shankaran S, Bada HS, Wright LL, Smeriglio VL, Bigsby R, Liu J. Predictors of motor development in children prenatally exposed to cocaine. Neurotoxicol Teratol 2005;27:213–20.

24. Nordstrom Bailey B, Sood BG, Sokol RJ, Ager J, Janisse J, Hannigan JH, Covington C, Delaney-Black V. Gender and alcohol moderate prenatal cocaine effects on teacher-report of child behavior. Neurotoxicol Teratol 2005;27:181–9.

25. Sood BG, Nordstrom Bailey B, Covington C, Sokol RJ, Ager J, Janisse J, Hannigan JH, Delaney-Black V. Gender and alcohol moderate caregiver reported child behavior after prenatal cocaine. Neurotoxicol Teratol 2005;27:191–201.

26. Hurt H, Brodsky N, Roth H, Malmud E, Giannetta J. School performance of children with gestational cocaine exposure. Neurotoxicol Teratol 2005;27(2):203–11.

27. Khan FY. The cocaine 'body-packer' syndrome: diagnosis and treatment. Indian J Med Sci 2005;59:457–8.

28. Britt GC, McCance-Katz EF. A brief overview of the clinical pharmacology of "club drugs". Subst Use Misuse 2005;40:1189–201.

29. Maxwell JC. Party drugs: properties, prevalence, patterns and problems. Subst Use Misuse 2005;40:1203–40.

30. Soellner R. Club drug use in Germany. Subst Use Misuse 2005;40:1279–93.

31. Banta-Green C, Goldbaum G, Kingston S, Golden M, Harruff R, Logan BK. Epidemiology of MDMA and associated club drugs in the Seattle area. Subst Use Misuse 2005;40:1295–315.

32. Han E, Yang W, Lee J, Park Y, Kim E, Lim M, Chung H. The prevalence of MDMA/MDA in both hair and urine in drug users. Forensic Sci Int 2005;152:73–7.

33. Cole JC, Sumnall HR, Smith GW, Rostami-Hodjegan A. Preliminary evidence of cardiovascular effects of polysubstance misuse in nightclubs. J Psychopharmacol 2005;19(1):67–70.

34. Bassi S, Ritto D. Ecstasy and chest pain due to coronary artery spasm. Int J Cardiol 2005;99:485–7.

35. Casco C, Forcella MC, Beretta G, Grieco A, Campana G. Long-term effects of MDMA (ecstasy) on the human central nervous system revealed by visual evoked potentials. Addict Biol 2005;10:187–95.

36. Montgomery C, Fisk JE, Newcombe R, Murphy PN. The differential effects of ecstasy/polydrug use on executive components: shifting, inhibition, updating and access to semantic memory. Psychopharmacology 2005; 182:262–76.

37. Sumnall HR, Cole JC. Self-reported depressive symptomatology in community samples of polysubstance misusers who report ecstasy use: a meta-analysis. J Psychopharmacol 2005;19(1):84–92.

38. Zwick OM, Fischer DH, Flanagan JC. "Ecstasy" induced immunosuppression and herpes zoster ophthalmicus. Br J Ophthalmol 2005;89:923–4.

39. Patel MM, Belson MG, Longwater AB, Olson KR, Miller MA. MDMA (ecstasy)-related hyperthermia. J Emerg Med 2005;29(4):451–4.

40. Libiseller K, Pavlic M, Grubwieser O, Rabl W. Ecstasy—deadly risk even outside rave parties. Forensic Sci Int 2005;153:227–30.

41. Parrott AC. Chronic tolerance to recreational MDMA (3,4-methlenedioxymethamphetamine) or ecstasy. J Psychopharmacol 2005;19(1):71–83.

42. Garcia-Algar O, Lopez N, Bonet M, Pellegrini M, Marchei E, Pichini S. 3,4-Methylenedioxymethamphetamine (MDMA) intoxication in an infant chronically exposed to cocaine. Ther Drug Monit 2005;27(4):409–11.
43. Campbell S, Qureshi T. Taking ecstasy…it's child's play! Pediatr Anesth 2005;15:256–60.
44. Haroz R, Greenberg MI. Emerging drugs of abuse. Med Clin N Am 2005;89:1259–76.
45. World Health Organization Advisory Group. Review of the pharmacology of khat. Bull Narcotics 1980;32:83–93.
46. Al-Motarreb A, Baker K, Broadley KJ. Khat: pharmacological and medical aspects and its social use in Yemen. Phytother Res 2002;16:403–13.
47. Al-Motarreb A, Briancon S, Al-Jaber N, Al-Adhi B, Al-Jailani F, Salek MS, Broadley KJ. Khat chewing is a risk factor for acute myocardial infarction: a case-control study. Br J Clin Pharmacol 2005;59:574–81.
48. Tekle Haimanot R. Burden of headache in Africa. J Headache Pain 2003;4:S47–54.
49. Mekasha A. The clinical effects of khat. Ethiopia 1984:77–81.
50. Tekle Haimanot R, Seraw B, Forsgren L, Ekbom K, Ekstedt J. Migraine, chronic tension-type headache, and cluster headache in an Ethiopian rural community. Cephalagia 1995;15:482–8.
51. Stefan J, Mathew B. Khat chewing: an emerging drug concern in Australia? Aust N Z J Psychiatry 2005;39:842–3.
52. Bhui K, Abdi A, Abdi M, Pereira S, Dualeh M. Traumatic events, migration characteristics and psychiatric symptoms among Somali refugees—preliminary communication. Soc Psychiatry Psychiatr Epidemiol 2003;38:35–43.
53. Numan N. Exploration of adverse psychological symptoms in Yemeni khat users by the Symptoms Checklist-90 [SCL-90]. Addiction 2004;99:61–5.
54. Odenwald M, Neuner F, Schauer M. Khat use as risk factor for psychotic disorders: a cross-sectional and case-control study in Somalia. BMC Med 2005;3:5.
55. Raja'a YA, Noma T, Warafi TA. Khat chewing is a risk factor for duodenal ulcer. Saudi Med J 2000;21:887–8.
56. Goldenberg D, Lee J, Koch WM, Kim MM, Trink B, Sidransky D, Moon CS. Habitual risk factors for head and neck cancer. Otolaryngol Head Neck Surg 2004;131:986–93.
57. Kassie F, Darroudi F, Kundi M, Schulte-Hermann R, Knasmuller S. Khat (*Catha edulis*) consumption causes genotoxic effects in humans. Int J Cancer 2001;92:329–32.
58. Ali AA, Al-Sharabi AK, Aguirre JM. Histopathological changes in oral mucosa due to takhzeen al-qat: a study of 70 biopsies. J Oral Pathol Med 2006;35:81–5.
59. Date J, Tanida N, Hobara T. Qat chewing and pesticides: a study of adverse health effects in people in the mountainous areas of Yemen. Int J Environ Health Res 2004;6:405–14.
60. Espiard ML, Lecardeur L, Abadie P, Halbecq I, Dollfus S. Hallucinogen persisting perception disorder after psilocybin consumption: a case study. Eur Psychiatry 2005;20:458–506.

Shabir Musa, Andrew Byrne, and Stephen Curran

5   Hypnosedatives and anxiolytics

BENZODIAZEPINES   *(SED-15, 429; SEDA-27, 43; SEDA-28, 52; SEDA-29, 51)*

Alprazolam

Comparative studies   In a randomized, cross-over, open study of the control of nausea and vomiting in 19 patients with operable breast cancer, granisetron alone was compared with granisetron plus alprazolam (1[c]). Alprazolam increased the efficacy of granisetron. The addition of alprazolam did not increase the incidence of adverse reactions to granisetron, but neither the adverse effects nor their frequencies were specified.

Psychological   In a placebo-controlled, within-subject, repeated-measures study of the effects of alprazolam on human risk-taking behavior, 16 adults were given placebo or alprazolam 0.5, 1.0, and 2.0 mg (2[C]). Alprazolam produced dose-related changes in subjective effects and response rates and dose-dependently increased selection of the risky response option. At a dose of 2.0 mg there was an increased probability of making consecutive risky responses following a gain on the risky response option. Thus, alprazolam *increased risk-taking* under laboratory conditions. In agreement with previous studies, the observed shift in trial-by-trial response probabilities suggested that sensitivity to consequences (for example oversensitivity to recent rewards) may be an important mechanism in the psychopharmacology of risky decision making. Additionally, risk-seeking personality traits may predict the acute effects of drugs on risk-taking behavior.

In a double-blind, crossover, placebo-controlled study in 12 healthy men of the impact of alprazolam 0.25 and 1.00 mg on aspects of action monitoring, i.e. the monitoring of response conflict and the detection and correction of errors by means of neurophysiological measures, alprazolam significantly reduced the amplitude of the error-related negativity (ERN) and therefore affected brain correlates of error detection (3[C]). It increased reaction time and the latencies of lateralized readiness potentials (LRP), thereby affecting motor preparation. It had no effect on amplitude differences in the N2 amplitude component between congruent and incongruent trials, and therefore did not disturb conflict monitoring on correct trials. Alprazolam did not disturb post-error adjustments of behavior.

The cognitive effects of a single dose of alprazolam 0.5 or 1 mg on measures of psychomotor function, visual attention, working memory, planning, and learning have been assessed in 36 healthy adults in a double-blind, parallel-group study (4[C]). Alprazolam 0.5 mg reduced only the speed of attentional performance, although the magnitude of this reduction was large ($d = 0.8$). At a dose of 1.0 mg, there was impairment of psychomotor function, equivalent to that seen for attentional function at the lower dose. In addition, there was moderate impairment ($d = 0.5$) in working memory and learning. These results suggest that low-dose alprazolam primarily alters visual attentional function. At the higher dose psychomotor functions also became impaired, and it is likely that a combination of these led to the observed moderate impairment of higher-level executive and memory processes.

Endocrine   In a parallel, double-blind, placebo-controlled study in 13 elderly women and 12 elderly men, alprazolam 0.5 mg bd for 3 weeks caused significant rises in inter-dose morning plasma cortisol concentrations in the women but not in the men (5[C]). In addition, higher morning plasma cortisol concentrations

Side Effects of Drugs, Annual 30
J.K. Aronson (Editor)
ISSN: 0378-6080
DOI: 10.1016/S0378-6080(08)00005-6

were significantly associated with better cognitive performance. The authors concluded that elderly women had greater inter-dose *activation of the hypothalamic–pituitary–adrenal axis* during treatment with therapeutic doses of alprazolam than men, but they stated that this could have been related to drug withdrawal.

In a double-blind, crossover, placebo-controlled study of the effects of alprazolam 5 mg and dehydroepiandrosterone (DHEA) 100 mg/day, alone and in combination, on hypothalamic–pituitary–adrenal axis activity in 15 men (aged 20–45 years; body mass index 20–25 kg/m^2), alprazolam significantly *increased basal growth hormone* and *blunted the responses to exercise of plasma cortisol, ACTH, AVP, and DHEA* (6^C). DHEA and alprazolam in combination significantly increased the growth hormone response to exercise. The authors concluded that DHEA and alprazolam up-regulate growth hormone during exercise, perhaps by blunting a suppressive (HPA axis) system and potentiating an excitatory (glutamate receptor) system.

Drug withdrawal   The potential interaction of paroxetine 20 mg/day and alprazolam 1 mg/day for 15 days on polysomnographic sleep and subjective sleep and awakening quality has been evaluated in a randomized, double-blind, double-dummy, placebo-controlled, repeated-dose, four-period, crossover study in 22 young subjects with no history of sleep disturbances (7^c). There were subjective withdrawal symptoms after abrupt discontinuation of alprazolam, including increased subjective sleep latency and reduced subjective sleep efficiency.

Brotizolam

Drug–drug interactions   Brotizolam is a triazolothienodiazepine used in the treatment of insomnia. *Erythromycin* 1200 mg/day or placebo for 7 days was given to 14 healthy men in a double-blind, randomized, crossover design (8^C). On the sixth day they took a single oral dose of brotizolam 0.5 mg and blood samples were taken for 24 hours. Erythromycin significantly increased the C$_{max}$, AUC, and half-life of brotizolam. This is *in vivo* evidence of the involvement of CYP3A4 in the metabolism of brotizolam.

Diazepam   (SED-15, 1103; SEDA-29, 54)

Placebo-controlled studies   In a double-blind, placebo-controlled, randomized trial in 120 children with spastic cerebral palsy received a bedtime dose of diazepam or placebo (9^C). A bedtime dose of diazepam to reduce hypertonia and muscle spasm, with passive stretching exercises, significantly improved behavior. The diazepam relaxed the muscles making the passive stretching easy, and the movements sustained muscle relaxation during the day. There was a significant improvement in wellbeing, improved activities of daily living, and reduced family burden of caring. There were fewer unwarranted crying spells during the day and less wakefulness during the night. There was no daytime sedation.

Psychological   Healthy men and women ($n = 46$) were randomly assigned to placebo or diazepam 5 or 10 mg in a double-blind, between-groups design to examine the effect of diazepam on *self-aggressive behavior* under controlled laboratory conditions (10^C). The participants were then provided with the opportunity to self-administer electric shocks during a competitive reaction time task. Self-aggression was defined by the intensity of shock chosen. Diazepam 10 mg was associated with higher average shocks than placebo and a greater likelihood of attempting to self-administer a shock that they were led to believe was severe and painful. There were sedative effects, but diazepam did not impair memory, attention, concentration, pain threshold, or reaction-time performance. The authors concluded that clinically relevant doses of diazepam may be associated with self-aggressive behavior without significantly impairing basic cognitive processes or psychomotor performance.

Endocrine   Acute diazepam administration causes a *reduction in plasma cortisol concentrations*, consistent with reduced activity of the hypothalamic–pituitary–adrenal axis, especially in individuals experiencing stress. However, the effects of chronic diazepam treatment on cortisol have been less well studied, and the relation to age, anxiety, duration of treatment, and dose are poorly understood. In a double-blind, placebo-controlled, crossover study, young (19–35 years, $n = 52$) and elderly (60–79 years, $n = 31$) individuals with and without generalized anxiety disorder took diazepam 2.5 or 10 mg for 3 weeks (11[C]). The elderly had significant reductions in plasma cortisol concentrations compared with placebo, both after the first dose and during chronic treatment, but the younger subjects did not. A final challenge with the same dose did not produce any significant cortisol effects in either group and the cortisol response in the elderly was significantly reduced compared with the initial challenge. These results are consistent with the development of tolerance to the cortisol-reducing effects of diazepam. The effect was more apparent in the elderly, was not modulated by generalized anxiety disorder or dosage, and was not related to drug effects on performance and on self-ratings of sedation and tension.

Genotoxicity   The possible genotoxic effects of propofol and diazepam have been investigated in 45 patients undergoing open heart surgery (12[c]). Peripheral blood samples were collected before and at the end of anesthesia the anesthesia with either diazepam 0.2 mg/kg + fentanyl 10 micrograms/kg ($n = 24$) or propofol 1 mg/kg + fentanyl 10 micrograms/kg ($n = 21$). Anesthesia was maintained by pancuronium and fentanyl plus diazepam 5 mg/kg or propofol 2–4 mg/kg/hour. The mean frequencies of chromosomal aberrations, before and at the end of the anesthesia, were not significantly different. Age, smoking, and sex were not confounding factors.

Lorazepam   *(SED-15, 2163;*
SEDA-29, 55)

Psychological   In a double-blind, placebo-controlled study of sex differences in the effects of lorazepam in trained social drinkers, lorazepam substituted for alcohol equally in both sexes and increased associated scores for *light-headedness* (13[C]). The women had much greater performance impairment in a digital symbol substitution test after lorazepam than the men. These results suggest that the stimulus and cognitive effects of benzodiazepine receptor agonists are modulated by different brain mechanisms.

The effects of lorazepam on the *allocation of study time, memory, and judgement of*

learning have been investigated in a cognitive task in which the repetition of word presentation was manipulated (14[C]). The study was placebo-controlled in 30 healthy volunteers. In a measure of the accuracy of delayed judgement of learning, all the participants benefited from word repetition; although lorazepam reduced overall performance, accuracy was not affected. All the participants then benefited from repetition of learning, although performance in those who took lorazepam remained lower than in those who took placebo. Repetition of learning had an effect on judgement of learning in both groups. Finally, study time fell significantly with the frequency of presentation an effect that was prevented by lorazepam. These findings suggest that lorazepam has a differential effect on the monitoring and the control processes involved in learning.

Lormetazepam

Psychological   In a randomized, double-blind, placebo-controlled, crossover study in 18 young adults (mean age, 27 years), a single dose of lormetazepam 1 mg had no significant effect on either visual simple reaction time or visual choice reaction time (15[c]). Lormetazepam caused mild *dizziness* in two subjects.

Midazolam   *(SED-15, 2337;*
SEDA-29, 56)

Observational studies   In 27 children with refractory generalized convulsive status epilepticus, midazolam 0.2 mg/kg as a bolus followed by 1–5 (mean 3.1) micrograms/kg/minute as a continuous infusion achieved complete control of seizures in 26 children within 65 minutes (16[c]). There were no adverse effects, such as hypotension, bradycardia, or respiratory depression. In one patient with acute meningoencephalitis, status epilepticus could not be controlled. Five patients died of the primary disorders, one with progressive encephalopathy.

Comparative studies   In a multicenter, randomized controlled comparison of buccal midazolam and rectal diazepam for emergency-room treatment of 219 separate episodes of active seizures in 177 children aged 6 months and older with and without intravenous access, the dose varied with age, from 2.5 to 10 mg (17[C]). The primary end point was therapeutic success—cessation of seizures within 10 minutes and for at least 1 hour without respiratory depression requiring intervention. The therapeutic response was 56% (61 of 109) for buccal midazolam and 27% (30 of 110) for rectal diazepam. When center, age, known diagnosis of epilepsy, use of antiepileptic drugs, prior treatment, and length of seizure before treatment were taken into account by logistic regression, buccal midazolam was more effective than rectal diazepam. The rates of respiratory depression did not differ.

Placebo-controlled studies   In a double-blind, randomized, placebo-controlled trial 130 patients were randomized to either midazolam 7.5 mg of orally ($n = 65$) or a placebo ($n = 65$) as premedication before upper gastrointestinal endoscopy (18[C]). The median anxiety score during the procedure was significantly reduced by midazolam. Significantly more of those who took midazolam graded overall tolerance as "excellent or good" and reported a partial to complete amnesia response. Those who took midazolam were more willing to repeat the procedure if necessary. Midazolam significantly prolonged the median recovery time. There were no significant effects on satisfaction score or hemodynamic changes.

Oxazepam

Tolerance   Additional doses of benzodiazepines in long-term users are commonly needed, but it is unknown whether these additional doses have any effect. The effects of an additional 20 mg dose of oxazepam has been assessed in a double-blind, balanced-order, crossover, randomized study in 16 long-term users of oxazepam and 18 benzodiazepine-naïve controls (19[C]). The effects of oxazepam 10 and 30 mg were assessed on: (a) saccadic eye movements as a proxy for the sedative effect; (b) the acoustic startle response as a proxy for the anxiolytic effects; (c) memory; (d) reaction time tasks; (e) subjective measurements. There were dose-related effects on the peak velocity of saccadic eye movement and response probability and on the peak amplitude of

the acoustic startle response. Comparison with the controls suggested that the sedative effects might be confounded with the suppression of sedative withdrawal symptoms, whereas the patients were as sensitive as the controls to the effects of an additional dose of oxazepam on the acoustic startle response. Neither 10 mg nor 30 mg of oxazepam affected the reaction time tasks in the patients, whereas the controls had dose-related impairment. The memory impairing effects did not differ significantly. In contrast to the controls, the patients could not discriminate between a 10 mg and a 30 mg dose, as assessed by visual analogue scales and the Spielberger State-Trait Anxiety Inventory Version 1, which might indicate a placebo effect of 10 mg in patients. The authors concluded that additional doses of oxazepam during long-term treatment have pronounced effects, even after daily use for more than 10 years.

Temazepam

Psychological   In a five-period crossover study in 15 healthy subjects aged 18–25 years, placebo, temazepam (15 and 30 mg), and clonidine (150 and 300 micrograms) were given orally in counterbalanced order in sessions at least 4 days apart (20[C]). Performance on a range of tasks aimed at assessing the role of central noradrenergic mechanisms in cognitive function was significantly impaired in a dose-related fashion, and both drugs caused subjective *sedation*. Clonidine did not affect the formation of new long-term memories, in contrast to temazepam, but did impair measures of working memory.

OTHER HYPNOSEDATIVES

Chloral hydrate   *(SED-15, 705; SEDA-27, 46)*

Susceptibility factors

Preterm infants   The degree of sedation (COMFORT), feeding behavior, and cardiorespiratory events (bradycardia, apnea) before and after oral chloral hydrate 30 mg/kg have been prospectively evaluated in 26 former preterm infants during procedural sedation at term post-conception age (21[c]). There was a significant increase in sedation up to 12 hours after administration and a minor but significant reduction in oral intake. There was a significant increase in the number of episodes of bradycardia and in the duration of the most severe. The study was therefore stopped when 26 neonates had been recruited. Infants who had severe bradycardia after chloral hydrate had a lower gestational age at birth but no difference in post-conceptional age at time of inclusion. Chloral hydrate was associated with an increase in unintended adverse effects in former preterm infants, probably reflecting differences in the pharmacodynamics and pharmacokinetics of chloral hydrate.

Zaleplon   *(SED-15, 3710; SEDA-27, 46; SEDA-28, 56; SEDA-29, 57)*

Observational studies   The results of a 1-year open extension of two randomized, double-blind studies of zaleplon have been reported (22[c]). In 316 older patients who took zaleplon nightly from 6 to 12 months and were then followed through a 7-day single-blind, placebo-controlled, run-out period, the safety profile was similar to that observed in a short-term trial in an equivalent population. The data also suggested that therapy for up to 12 months produced and maintained statistically significant improvement in time to persistent sleep onset, duration of sleep, and the number of nocturnal wakenings. Withdrawal was not associated with rebound insomnia. The authors concluded that placebo-controlled, double-blind trials are needed to confirm these results.

Zolpidem   *(SED-15, 3723; SEDA-28, 56; SEDA-29, 57)*

Nervous system   In a double-blind, placebo-controlled study in eight healthy men, zolpidem 10 mg produced statistically significant *postural sway* in the tandem stance test, and triazolam 0.25 mg was statistically significant only as defined by the polygonal area of foot pressure center (23[c]). Zolpidem, which has a minimal muscle-relaxant effect, produced more imbalance than triazolam, which is known for its muscle relaxant effect. The authors suggested that in the use of hypnotics, sway derives from suppression of the central nervous system relevant to awakening rather than from muscle relaxation.

Psychological   Following 8 hours of undisturbed night-time sleep, 80 subjects (50 men, 30 women) took oral zolpidem 0, 5, 10, or 20 mg at 1000 h (20 per group) and then oral melatonin 0 or 5 mg at 1030 h (thus, 10 subjects per drug combination) (24[c]). They napped from 1000 to 1130 h, after which they were given cognitive tests (Restricted Reminding, Paired-Associates, and Psychomotor Vigilance). They were tested again after a second nap from 1245 to 1600 h. Melatonin 5 mg plus zolpidem 0 mg enhanced daytime sleep, with no memory or performance impairment. Zolpidem 20 mg plus melatonin 0 mg also enhanced daytime sleep (non-significantly), but *memory and vigilance were impaired*. The authors concluded that there were no advantages to using melatonin plus zolpidem. Functional coupling of sleep-inducing and memory-impairing effects may be specific to benzodiazepine-receptor agonists such as zolpidem, suggesting potential advantages to using melatonin in the operational environment.

In a double blind, placebo-controlled study in 36 young healthy volunteers, zolpidem 5 or 10 mg increased N2 and P3 latencies and reduced N2 and P3 amplitudes (25[c]). However, contrary to expectations, there was no change in N1 while P2 amplitude was increased by the higher dose. The effects on N2 and P3 amplitudes and latencies were similar to those of other hypnosedatives. However, zolpidem unexpectedly increased P2 amplitude, which the authors attributed to its selective receptor binding profile.

In a double-blind, crossover, randomized, placebo-controlled study in 22 healthy volunteers, single doses of zolpidem 10 mg and triazolam 0.25 mg had no effect on the enhanced non-word recall observed after sleep or on improvement in the performance of a digit symbol substitution test in subjects who slept (26[c]). The authors concluded that the hypnotics did not interfere with nocturnal sleep-induced improvement in memory.

References

1. Abali H, Oyan B, Guler N. Alprazolam significantly improves the efficacy of granisetron in the prophylaxis of emesis secondary to moderately emetogenic chemotherapy in patients with breast cancer. Chemotherapy 2005;51(5):280–5.
2. Lane SD, Tcheremissine OV, Lieving LM, Nouvion S, Cherek DR. Acute effects of alprazolam on risky decision making in humans. Psychopharmacology 2005;181(2):364–73.
3. Riba J, Rodriguez-Fornells A, Munte TF, Barbanoj MJ. A neurophysiological study of the detrimental effects of alprazolam on human action monitoring. Cognitive Brain Res 2005;25(2):554–65.
4. Snyder PJ, Werth J, Giordani B, Caveney AF, Feltner D, Maruff P. A method for determining the magnitude of change across different cognitive functions in clinical trials: the effects of acute administration of two different doses alprazolam. Hum Psychopharmacol 2005;20(4):263–73.
5. Pomara N, Willoughby LM, Ritchie LC, Sidtis JJ, Greenblatt DJ, Nemeroff CB. Sex-related elevation in cortisol during chronic treatment with alprazolam associated with enhanced cognitive performance. Psychopharmacology 2005;182(3):414–9.
6. Deuster PA, Faraday MM, Chrousos GP, Poth MA. Effects of dehydroepiandrosterone and alprazolam on hypothalamic-pituitary responses to exercise. J Clin Endocrinol Metab 2005;90(8):4777–83.
7. Barbanoj MJ, Clos S, Romero S, Morte A, Giménez S, Lorenzo JL, Luque A, Dal-Ré R. Sleep laboratory study on single and repeated dose effects of paroxetine, alprazolam and their combination in healthy young volunteers. Neuropsychobiology 2005;51(3):134–47.
8. Tokairin T, Fukasawa T, Yasui-Furukori N, Aoshima T, Suzuki A, Inoue Y, Tateishi T, Otani K. Inhibition of the metabolism of brotizolam by erythromycin in humans: in vivo evidence for the involvement of CYP3A4 in brotizolam metabolism. Br J Clin Pharmacol 2005;60(2):172–5.
9. Mathew A, Mathew MC. Bedtime diazepam enhances well being in children with spastic cerebral palsy. Pediatr Rehabil 2005;8(1):63–6.
10. Berman ME, Jones GD, McCloskey MS. The effects of diazepam on human self-aggressive behaviour. Psychopharmacology 2005;178:100–6.
11. Pomara N, Willoughby LM, Sidtis J, Cooper TB, Greenblatt DJ. Cortisol response to diazepam: its relationship to age, dose, duration of treatment and presence of generalised anxiety disorder. Psychopharmacology 2005;178:1–8.
12. Karahalil B, Yagar S, Bahadir G, Durak P, Sardas S. Diazepam and propofol used as anaesthetics during open-heart surgery do not cause chromosomal aberrations in peripheral blood lymphocyctes. Mutat Res 2005;581:181–6.
13. Jackson A, Stephens D, Duka T. Gender differences in response to lorazepam in a human drug discrimination study. J Psychopharmacol 2005;19(6):614–9.
14. Izaute M, Bacon E. Specific effects of an amnesic drug: effect of lorazepam on study time allocation and judgement on learning. Neuropsychopharmacology 2005;30:196–204.
15. Fabbrini M, Fritelli C, Bonanni E, Maestri M, Mance ML, Iudice A. Psychomotor performance in healthy young adult volunteers receiving lormetazepam and placebo: A single-dose, randomised, double-blind, crossover trial. Clin Ther 2005;27(1):78–83.
16. Ozdemir D, Gulez P, Uran N, Yendur G, Kavakli T, Aydin A. Efficacy of continuous midazolam infusion and mortality in childhood refractory generalised convulsive status epilepticus. Seizure 2005;14:129–32.
17. McIntyre J, Robertson S, Norris E, Appleton R, Whitehouse WP, Phillips B, Martland T, Berry K, Collier J, Smith S, Choonara I. Safety and efficacy of buccal midazolam versus rectal diazepam for emergency treatment of seizures in children: a randomised controlled trial. Lancet 2005;366:205–10.
18. Mui L, Teoh AYB, Enders KWN, Lee Y, Au Yeung ACM, Chan Y, Lau JYW, Chung SCS. Premedication with orally administered midazolam in adults undergoing diagnostic upper endoscopy: a double-blind, placebo-controlled randomised trial. Gastrointest Endosc 2005;61(2):195–200.
19. Oude Voshaar RC, Verkes R-J, van Luijtelaar GLJM, Edelbroek PM, Zitman FG. Effects of additional oxazepam in long-term users of oxazepam. J Clin Psychopharmacol 2005;25(1):42–50.
20. Tiplady B, Bowness E, Stien L, Drummond G. Selective effects of clonidine and temazepam on attention and memory. J Psychopharmacol 2005;19(3):259–65.
21. Allegaert K, Daniels H, Naulaers G, Tibboel D, Devlieger H. Pharmacodynamics of chloral hydrate in former preterm infants. Eur J Pediatr 2005;164:403–7.
22. Ancoli-Israel S, Richardson GS, Mangano RM, Jenkins L, Hall P, Jones WS. Long-term use of sedative hypnotics in older patients with insomnia. Sleep Med 2005;6:107–13.
23. Nakamura M, Ishii M, Niwa Y, Yamazaki M, Ito H. Temporal changes in postural sway caused by ultrashort-acting hypnotics: triazolam and zolpidem. ORL 2005;67(2):106–12.
24. Wesensten NJ, Balkin TJ, Reichardt RM, Kautz MA, Saviolakis GA, Belenky G. Daytime sleep and performance following a zolpidem and melatonin cocktail. Sleep 2005;28(1):93–103.

25. Lucchesi LM, Braga NI, Manzano GM, Pompeia S, Tufik S. Acute neurophysiological effects of the hypnotic zolpidem in healthy volunteers. Prog Neuropsychopharmacol Biol Psychiatry 2005;29(4):557–64.

26. Melendez J, Galli I, Boric K, Ortega A, Zuniga L, Henriquez-Roldan CF, Cardenas AM. Zolpidem and triazolam do not affect the nocturnal sleep-induced memory improvement. Psychopharmacology 2005;181:21–6.

Alfonso Carvajal, Luis H. Martín Arias, and Natalia Jimeno

6   Antipsychotic drugs

GENERAL   (SED-15, 2438)

Comparative studies   The primary and main outcomes of the Clinical Antipsychotic Trials of Intervention Effectiveness both in schizophrenic patients and in patients with dementia have been released. In the first study, 1493 patients with schizophrenia recruited at 57 US sites were randomly allocated to olanzapine (7.5–30 mg/day), perphenazine (8–32 mg/day), quetiapine (200–800 mg/day) and ziprasidone (40–160 mg/day) for up to 18 months (1[C]). The main conclusion of the study was that patients with chronic schizophrenia discontinued their antipsychotic drug medication at a high rate, indicating substantial limitations in the effectiveness of the drugs. In fact, overall 74% of patients withdrew within 18 months; the time to withdrawal for any cause was significantly longer with olanzapine than quetiapine or risperidone but not perphenazine or ziprasidone. The time to withdrawal because of intolerable adverse effects was similar across the groups (olanzapine, 19%; quetiapine, 15%; risperidone, 10%; perphenazine, 16%; ziprasidone, 15%). The authors suggested that the ways in which clinicians, patients, families, and policymakers evaluate the trade-offs between efficacy and adverse effects, as well as drug prices, will determine future patterns of use.

Cardiovascular   Since the early 1960s, *sudden cardiac death* has been reported with antipsychotic drugs (SEDA-24, 54). In a population-based retrospective case–control study performed in the Integrated Primary Care Information project, a longitudinal observational database, the use of antipsychotic drugs, particularly haloperidol, was associated with a

significant increase in the risk of sudden death (adjusted OR = 5.0; 95% CI = 1.6, 15 for antipsychotic drugs as a whole; adjusted OR = 5.6; 95% CI = 1.6, 19 for haloperidol; number of cases and controls 775 and 6297 respectively; mean ages 71 and 69 years respectively) (2[C]). Sudden death was defined as a natural death due to cardiac causes heralded by abrupt loss of consciousness within 1 hour after the onset of acute symptoms or unwitnessed, or an unexpected death of someone seen in a stable medical condition under 24 hours before with no evidence of a non-cardiac cause. For each case of sudden death, up to 10 controls were randomly drawn from the source population matched for age, sex, and practice.

QT interval prolongation, torsade de pointes, and other *dysrhythmias* are a focus of particular interest (SEDA-27, 52; SEDA-28, 59, SEDA-29, 62). The authors of a new review identified 45 reports containing 70 cases of torsade de pointes, most associated with antipsychotic drugs (3[R]). Female sex, heart disease, hypokalemia, high doses of the offending agent, concomitant use of a QT interval prolonging agent, and a history of long QT syndrome were identified as susceptibility factors. A thorough review of antipsychotic drugs and QT prolongation included some practical observations and suggestions (4[R]):

- there are almost no antipsychotic drugs available that do not prolong the QT interval;
- thioridazine, mesoridazine, and pimozide should not be prescribed for patients with known heart disease, a personal history of syncope, a family history of sudden death under age 40 years, or congenital long QT syndrome;
- a baseline electrocardiogram should be obtained in all patients to determine the QT_c interval as well as the presence of other abnormalities suggesting a cardiac disorder.

Side Effects of Drugs, Annual 30
J.K. Aronson (Editor)
ISSN: 0378-6080
DOI: 10.1016/S0378-6080(08)00006-8

Brugada-like electrocardiographic abnormalities have occurred after thioridazine overdose (5[A]).

- A previously healthy 58-year-old woman whose blood concentration of thioridazine was 1480 µg/l (usual therapeutic concentrations are up to 200 µg/l) became comatose and had muscular rigidity. An electrocardiogram showed sinus rhythm with significant QT prolongation and 1 day later evolved into a Brugada-like pattern. Over the next 72 hours, both the electrocardiogram and the clinical abnormalities resolved.

Nervous system   When the potency and doses of antipsychotic drugs are considered, atypical antipsychotic drugs are not necessarily safer than typical antipsychotic drugs in relation to the development of *parkinsonism*, according to the results of a population-based retrospective cohort study in 57 838 adults with dementia aged 66 years and older (6[C]). There was incident parkinsonism (a new diagnosis of Parkinson's disease or the dispensing of an antiparkinsonian drug) in 4.3 per 100 person-years of follow-up in those taking typical antipsychotic drugs ($n = 14\,198$; adjusted HR = 1.3; 95% CI = 1.0, 1.6), in 3.5 per 100 person-years in those taking atypical antipsychotic drugs ($n = 11\,571$; adjusted HR = 1.0), and in 1.3 per 100 person-years in a control group taking non-antipsychotic drugs ($n = 32\,069$; adjusted HR = 0.4; 95% CI = 0.3, 0.4). Medium and high doses of higher-potency typical antipsychotic drugs accounted for adjusted HRs of 2.2 (95% CI = 1.5, 3.1) and 2.3 (95% CI = 1.4, 3.5) respectively; similarly, medium and high doses of atypical antipsychotic drugs accounted for adjusted HRs of 1.3 (95% CI = 0.9, 1.7) and 2.1 (95% CI = 1.4, 3.0) respectively. The authors stressed the importance of these findings, given that a quarter of older adults in the study were given a high-dose agent. Since risperidone was the most commonly used atypical drug, the results might not be generalizable to all atypical drugs. These results are similar to those of a meta-analysis in which there was no evidence that atypical antipsychotic drugs were less likely to produce extrapyramidal effects than low-potency conventional antipsychotic drugs (7[M]) (SEDA-28, 59).

The prevalence of *tardive dyskinesia* in a Xhosa population in South Africa was within the range reported in other studies, 29 of 102 patients using typical antipsychotic drugs (8[c])

(see SEDA-20, 38 for details of the prevalences of tardive dyskinesia in different populations). In-patients and out-patients from different clinics who had been exposed to typical antipsychotic drugs for at least 6 months and were currently taking an antipsychotic drug were screened for abnormal movements using the Abnormal Involuntary Movement Scale; other data were gathered from the patients and from a chart review. In a logistic regression model, years of treatment and total cumulative antipsychotic drug dose were significant predictors of tardive dyskinesia. Subjects with higher total consumption of foods containing antioxidants had lower rates of tardive dyskinesia; only consumption of onions was significantly associated with a reduced prevalence of tardive dyskinesia.

The incidence and severity of *neurological soft signs* have been assessed in schizophrenic patients taking haloperidol ($n = 37$), risperidone ($n = 19$), clozapine ($n = 34$), and olanzapine ($n = 18$) (9[c]). There were no significant differences across the four groups. The authors therefore suggested that neurological soft signs are independent of antipsychotic drug treatment. However, the cross-sectional character of the study, along with the small sample size, limited this conclusion.

Antipsychotic drug-induced *laryngeal dystonia* is a life-threatening adverse effect of both high-potency and low-potency antipsychotic drugs, and the diagnosis is often elusive (SEDA-22, 51). Two cases of acute laryngeal dystonia have been reported (10[Ar]).

- A 28-year-old man with auditory hallucinations was given haloperidol 5 mg/day, biperiden 4 mg/day and diazepam 6 mg/day. After 9 days, the dose of haloperidol was increased to 15 mg/day and biperiden to 6 mg/day. A day later he developed severe extrapyramidal signs. The haloperidol was withdrawn and switched to thioridazine 200 mg/day, which was followed by marked improvement. Five months later he relapsed and the dosage of thioridazine was increased to 300 mg/day. A month later, 4 hours after taking thioridazine 800 mg in an attempt to relieve anxiety, he developed severe respiratory distress; he was grasping his throat with his hands and his lips were slightly cyanotic. Laryngeal dystonia was suspected, based on the clinical presentation and on the previous history. He was given biperiden lactate 5 mg intramuscularly, which produced improvement; 10 minutes later he was given another dose and the dystonia resolved.
- A 35-year-old woman with schizophrenia developed acute respiratory distress and laryngeal stridor. Antipsychotic-induced laryngeal dystonia was

diagnosed. She was given biperiden lactate 10 mg intramuscularly and her symptoms resolved fully within 30 minutes. On the advice of a psychiatrist, and to sedate her for admission to a psychiatric hospital, her mother had secretly put 50 drops of haloperidol (10 mg/ml) in her food 1 hour before the symptoms appeared.

In addition, the authors reviewed 26 previously published cases of antipsychotic drug-induced laryngeal dystonia. They suggested that this condition could be the cause of unexpected deaths related to antipsychotic drug use. The differential diagnosis includes acute anaphylaxis, tardive laryngeal dystonia, airway obstruction, and respiratory dyskinesia. The diagnosis can be confirmed by laryngoscopy, which shows intermittent dystonic movements of the laryngeal musculature, with no edema. Anticholinergic drugs appear to be effective and, unlike benzodiazepines, do not compromise respiration.

Endocrine   Some antipsychotic drugs increase the serum prolactin concentration, increasing the risks of serious chronic medical problems, such as menstrual abnormalities, gynecomastia, galactorrhea, osteoporosis, and cardiovascular disease (SEDA-27, 53; SEDA-29, 63). The prevalence of *hyperprolactinemia* in patients with chronic schizophrenia taking long-term haloperidol has been studied in 60 patients in Korea (28 women; illness mean duration, 15.5 years) (11[c]). There was hyperprolactinemia, defined as a serum prolactin concentration over 20 ng/ml in men and 24 ng/ml in women, in 40; the prevalence of hyperprolactinemia in women (93%) was significantly higher than in men (47%). There was also a significant correlation between haloperidol dose and serum prolactin concentration in women, but not in men.

The relation between prolactin concentrations and osteoporosis has been studied by measuring prolactin concentrations and lumbar spine and hip bone mineral densities in women with schizophrenia taking so-called "prolactin-raising antipsychotic drugs" (*n* = 26; mean treatment duration, 8.4 years) or olanzapine (*n* = 12; mean treatment duration, 6.3 years) (12[c]). Prolactin concentrations were 1692 and 446 IU/l respectively (reference range 50–350 IU/l). Hyperprolactinemia was associated with low bone mineral density: 95% of women

with either osteopenia or osteoporosis had hyperprolactinemia, whereas only 11% of those with normal prolactin concentrations had abnormal bone mineral density.

The relation between antipsychotic drug-induced hyperprolactinemia and *hypoestrogenism* has been studied in 75 women with schizophrenia (13[c]). Serum estradiol concentrations were generally reduced during the entire menstrual cycle compared with reference values. There was hypoestrogenism, defined as serum estradiol concentrations below 30 pg/ml in the follicular phase and below 100 pg/ml in the periovulatory phase, in about 60%.

Metabolism   Atypical antipsychotic drugs have been linked to *obesity, hyperlipidemia, type 2 diabetes mellitus*, and *diabetic ketoacidosis* (SEDA-26, 56; SEDA-28, 60). While the incidence of new-onset diabetes mellitus appears to be increasing in patients with schizophrenia taking certain atypical antipsychotic drugs, it is unclear whether these agents directly affect glucose metabolism or simply increase risk factors for diabetes, such as obesity, lipid abnormalities, and reduced activity secondary to sedative effects. Glucose metabolism in 36 out-patients with schizophrenia aged 18–65 years taking clozapine (*n* = 12), olanzapine (*n* = 12), or risperidone (*n* = 12) has been examined in a cross-sectional study (14[c]). There was no significant difference in fasting baseline plasma glucose concentrations. Those taking clozapine or olanzapine had significant insulin resistance compared with those taking risperidone. There were no significant differences in total cholesterol, high-density lipoprotein cholesterol, low-density lipoprotein cholesterol, or serum triglyceride concentrations; however, controlling for sex, there was a significant difference (clozapine > olanzapine > risperidone). Insulin resistance is a major but not necessary risk factor for type 2 diabetes; leptin, in turn, is important for the control of body weight and the authors proposed that leptin could be considered to be a link between obesity, insulin resistance syndrome, and treatment with some antipsychotic drugs. However, consistent with other results, the small sample size, the cross-sectional design, and the exclusion of obese subjects may limit the generalizability of these findings.

In patients, particularly children, taking the new antipsychotic drugs, *obesity* is a focus of special interest. A thorough search for studies that addressed obesity in children and adolescents in relation to the new antipsychotic drugs showed that risperidone is associated with less weight gain than olanzapine (15[R]).

Antipsychotic drugs in elderly patients

Use and effectiveness Antipsychotic drugs are currently used to treat the psychiatric and behavioral symptoms that affect elderly patients with dementia (16[R]). This is an unlicensed indication, but 25% of elderly patients in nursing homes receive these drugs (17[c]). The main conclusions from a double-blind, placebo-controlled study (CATIE-AD) in 421 out-patients were that adverse effects offset the efficacy of atypical antipsychotic drugs in managing psychosis, aggression, or agitation in patients with Alzheimer's disease, who were randomly assigned to olanzapine (mean dose 5.5 mg/day), quetiapine (57 mg/day), risperidone (mean dose 1.0 mg/day), or placebo (18[C]). At 12 weeks there were no significant differences with regard to the time to withdrawal for any reason: olanzapine (median 8.1 weeks), quetiapine (median 5.3 weeks), risperidone (median 7.4 weeks), and placebo (median 8.0 weeks). Although the median time to withdrawal because of lack of efficacy favored olanzapine (22 weeks) and risperidone (27 weeks) compared with quetiapine (9.1 weeks) and placebo (9.0 weeks), the time to withdrawal because of adverse events or intolerability clearly favored placebo. Overall, 24% of patients who took olanzapine, 16% of those who took quetiapine, 18% of those who took risperidone, and 5% of those who took placebo withdrew because of intolerability. There were no significant differences among the groups with regard to improvements on the Clinical Global Impression of Change scale. Moreover, neither quetiapine nor rivastigmine was effective in agitation in people with dementia in institutional care.

In a double-blind, randomized, placebo-controlled study quetiapine was associated with significant cognitive decline in 93 patients with Alzheimer's disease, dementia, and clinically significant agitation (19[C]).

These results coincide with those of a recent review of evidence (20[R]) and a recent meta-analysis (21[M]), although early pivotal comparisons of risperidone, haloperidol, and placebo in agitated and demented patients did not find substantial differences when the evaluation was performed at 12 months (SEDA-25, 68).

Antipsychotic drugs and stroke in patients with dementia Different warnings to clinicians have been issued on the link between atypical antipsychotic drugs and cerebrovascular adverse events (SEDA-27, 52; SEDA-28, 59; SEDA-29, 62). The US Food and Drug Administration issued a similar warning in April 2003 (22[S]). These warnings have led to a controversy among doctors (23[r], 24[R]).

An early multicenter, double-blind, randomized, trial in Australia and New Zealand in 384 patients with dementia showed that risperidone caused more cerebrovascular events (9%; n = 167) than placebo (1.8%; n = 170) (SEDA-28, 75). Now, a meta-analysis of the effect of olanzapine for the behavioral and psychological symptoms of dementia has shown that olanzapine may also be associated with an increased risk of cerebrovascular adverse effects (25[M]). Nevertheless, several studies have not found any association between the use of atypical antipsychotic drugs and cerebrovascular events (26[C], 27[C]).

Neither of two observational studies of the relation between atypical antipsychotic drugs and the risk of ischemic stroke showed a similar significant risk. In the first, a population-based retrospective cohort study, patients over 65 years with dementia who took atypical antipsychotic drugs showed no significant increase in the risk of ischemic stroke compared with those who took typical antipsychotic drugs (adjusted hazard ratio = 1.0; 95% CI = 0.8, 1.3) (28[C]). The numbers of new admissions for ischemic stroke were 284 in those taking atypical antipsychotic drugs (n = 17 845) and 227 in those taking typical antipsychotic drugs (n = 14 865). In the second study, data from prescription-event monitoring of olanzapine (n = 8826), risperidone (n = 7684), and quetiapine (n = 1726) were examined (29[C]). The patients were mainly old (median ages 83, 81, and 69 years respectively; women 33, 74, and 70% respectively). Within 6 months of starting treatment, 10 patients had a first occurrence of *a stroke or a transitory ischemic attack with olanzapine (0.1%; five fatal), 23 with risperidone (0.3%; nine fatal), and six with quetiapine (0.3%; one fatal). After adjusting for three confounders (age, sex, and indication) there were no significant differences in the relative risks of stroke between olanzapine and either risperidone or quetiapine, or between risperidone and quetiapine (RR = 1.9; 95 % CI = 0.5, 2.9 and RR = 2.1; 95% CI = 0.6, 7.6).*

In another trial olanzapine 2.5–7.5 mg/day was not associated with a higher risk of adverse cardiovascular events compared to typical antipsychotic drugs (haloperidol or promazine chlorhydrate) in 346 patients aged 71–92 years with vascular dementia and behavioral problems (30[C]).

Antipsychotic drugs and venous thromboembolism *A possible association between venous thromboembolism and the use of antipsychotic drugs was first suggested in the 1950s after the introduction of the phenothiazines (31[A]). Later, a 7-fold increase in the risk of idiopathic venous thromboembolism was found among users of conventional antipsychotic drugs who were under 60 years of age and had no major risk factors (32[C]). More recently, a 6-month retrospective cohort study of residents of US nursing homes aged 65 years and over has shown that users of atypical but not typical antipsychotic drugs had an increased risk of hospitalization for venous thromboembolism compared with non-users (33[C]). The adjusted hazard ratio was 2.0 (95% CI = 1.4, 2.8) for risperidone (43 events; 3451 person-years); 1.9 (1.1, 3.3) for olanzapine (15 events; 1279 person-years); and 2.7 (1.1, 6.3) for clozapine and quetiapine (10 events; 443 person-years); there were 439 events in non-users (50 604 person-years). Since dementia was much more prevalent among users of atypical antipsychotic drugs, confounding by indication was possible; however, the findings were confirmed after excluding residents with severe cognitive decline.*

Antipsychotic drugs and ventricular dysrhythmias and cardiac arrest *In a retrospective case-control study in US residents of nursing homes aged 65 years and over, conventional (adjusted OR = 1.9; 95% CI = 1.3, 2.7) but not atypical antipsychotic drugs (adjusted*

OR = 0.9; 95% CI = 0.6, 1.3) were associated with an increased risk of hospitalization for ventricular dysrhythmias and cardiac arrest (34[C]). Among residents who took conventional antipsychotic drugs, those with cardiac disease were 3.3 times (95% CI = 1.9, 5.5) more likely to be hospitalized for ventricular dysrhythmias and cardiac arrest than non-users without cardiac disease. The number of patients hospitalized for ventricular dysrhythmias and cardiac arrest (cases) was 649, and 2962 controls were selected among in-patients in the inception cohort whose primary diagnosis at discharge was septicemia, gastrointestinal hemorrhage, rectal bleeding, gastritis with bleeding, duodenitis with bleeding, or influenza.

Atypical antipsychotic drugs and the risk of death *A thorough meta-analysis of published (n = 6) and unpublished (n = 9) double-blind, parallel-group, randomized, placebo-controlled trials has shown an increased risk of death in patients with dementia taking atypical antipsychotic drugs (35[M]). There were more deaths among patients randomized to drugs (118 out of 3353; 3.5%) than those who took placebo (40 out of 1757; 2.3%) (OR = 1.5; 95% CI = 1.1, 2.2). There were no differences in dropouts.*

In a recent retrospective cohort study conventional antipsychotic drugs (n = 9142) were at least as likely as atypical agents (n = 13 748) to increase the risk of death among elderly people; accordingly, conventional drugs should not be used to replace atypical agents withdrawn in response to the FDA warning (36[C]). The adjusted relative risk was significantly higher with conventional antipsychotic drugs (RR = 1.4; 95% CI = 1.3, 1.5) and in all subgroups defined according to the presence or absence of dementia or nursing home residency. Hence, the US Food and Drug Administration has newly issued a warning: "All of the atypical antipsychotic drugs are approved for the treatment of schizophrenia. None, however, is approved for the treatment of behavioral disorders in patients with dementia. Because of these findings, the Agency will ask the manufacturers of these drugs to include a Boxed Warning in their labeling describing this risk and noting that these drugs are not approved for this indication. Zambia, a combination product containing olanzapine and fluoxetine, approved for the treatment of depressive episodes associated with bipolar disorder, will also be included in the request. . . The Agency is also considering adding a similar warning to the labeling for older antipsychotic medications because the limited data available suggest a similar increase in mortality for these drugs" (37^S). Similarly, the European Agency for the Evaluation of Medicinal Products has underlined these risks in a public statement: "Neuroleptic drugs are known to be used in patients with dementia who experience psychotic symptoms and disturbed behavior. There are insufficient data to confirm any difference in the risk of mortality or cerebrovascular accidents among atypical neuroleptic drugs, including olanzapine, or between atypical and conventional neuroleptic drugs" (38^S).

INDIVIDUAL DRUGS

Aripiprazole

Placebo-controlled studies   In a 4-week, double-blind, randomized placebo-controlled study in 36 US centers 414 patients with schizophrenia or schizoaffective disorder were randomized to aripiprazole (15 or 30 mg/day) or haloperidol (10 mg/day) (39[c]). Haloperidol and both doses of aripiprazole produced statistically significant improvements from baseline compared with placebo. Unlike haloperidol, aripiprazole was not associated with significant extrapyramidal symptoms or raised prolactin at the endpoint. There were no statistically significant differences in mean changes in body weight and no patients who took aripiprazole had clinically significant increases in the QT_c interval.

Nervous system   *Oral dyskinesia* emerged after several months of treatment with haloperidol 7.5 mg/day and gradually disappeared within 2 months after therapy was changed to aripiprazole 10 mg/day (40[A]).

Endocrine   *Galactorrhea* has been attributed to aripiprazole after only 2 days of administration (41[A]).

- A 29-year-old woman with a schizoaffective disorder took haloperidol 5 mg/day and then 9 mg/day

because of acute psychotic episodes. She had no adverse effects such as amenorrhea or galactorrhea. Haloperidol was then replaced by aripiprazole 15 mg/day and on the evening of the second day she developed breast tenderness and marked galactorrhea. The serum prolactin concentration was 32 ng/ml (reference range 5–25 ng/ml). Aripiprazole was withdrawn and haloperidol restarted. The galactorrhea resolved in 1 week.

Drug formulations   In January 2005, an oral solution of aripiprazole was approved by the FDA, providing an option for adults with difficulty in swallowing (42^S, 43[R]).

Chlorpromazine   *(SED-15, 733; SEDA-28, 64)*

Sensory systems   *Deposits in the cornea and lens* can complicate long-term chlorpromazine therapy and *in vivo* confocal imaging of such deposits has now been reported, supposedly for the first time (44[A]).

- A 59-year-old woman who for 20 years had taken chlorpromazine up to 1200 mg/day (mean dose 400 mg/day) gradually developed blurred vision in her left eye. Slit-lamp biomicroscopy showed multiple fine creamy-white deposits on her corneal endothelium and anterior crystalline lens capsule bilaterally. Microstructural analysis of the corneal endothelium showed that there were no abnormalities in cellular morphology resulting from these deposits.

Clozapine   *(SED-15, 823; SEDA-26, 59; SEDA-27, 55; SEDA-28, 65; SEDA-29, 66)*

Susceptibility factors   The results of an observational, non-randomized, interethnic comparison of clozapine dosage, clinical response, plasma concentrations, and adverse effects profiles have been published (45[c]). Compared to Caucasian patients (*n* = 20), Asian patients (*n* = 20) appeared to have lower dosage requirements for clinical efficacy. The Asian patients scored significantly lower than the Caucasian patients on the Simpson and Angus Scale for extrapyramidal adverse effects, but there were no significant differences on the Abnormal Involuntary Movement Scale or the Liverpool University Neuroleptic Side-effect Rating

Scale. Since there was no difference between ethnic groups in clozapine concentrations, the authors concluded that the higher extrapyramidal adverse effects scores in the Caucasian group might be attributed to more chronic illness duration, more concomitant medications, and the lack of standardized rating training. Genetic differences between these ethnic groups were not analysed in this study. However, it should be emphasized that Asians are genetically heterogeneous and differences are found between various Asian ethnic groups.

Clinical predictors of response to clozapine have been previously examined (SEDA-27, 55) and the evidence on predictors and markers of clozapine response has been reviewed (46^M). Higher baseline clinical symptoms and functioning in the previous years and low cerebrospinal homovanillic acid/5-hydroxyindoleacetic acid concentrations were identified as reliable, and three potential measures were also identified: reduced frontal cortex metabolic activity, reduced caudate volume, and improvement in P50 sensory gating. The authors pointed out that none of these is specific to clozapine, but that this does not reduce their value, instead showing that they do not clarify why clozapine is different from other antipsychotic drugs, for example in terms of efficacy in treatment-resistant patients.

Observational studies   Catatonic schizophrenia is a controversial syndrome and there is debate about its etiology and treatment. There has been a report of two cases of catatonic schizophrenia successfully treated with clozapine: a 49-year-old woman and a 19-year-old man (47^A). Both responded to clozapine despite being resistant to several conventional and atypical antipsychotic drugs and, in the second case, a course of electroconvulsive therapy. These two cases are intriguing, because the dose of clozapine required to improve catatonia was about double the dose required to improve psychosis significantly (600 and 750 mg/day). The two patients had common adverse effects of clozapine; the first had mild *nocturnal hypersalivation* and mild/moderate *constipation*, and the second had moderate nocturnal hypersalivation.

Clozapine has been evaluated in patients with bipolar type or bipolar disorder with psychotic features (SEDA-28, 65).

• A 38-year-old woman with a 22-year history of resistant rapid-cycling bipolar I disorder finally responded well to a combination of clozapine 350 mg/day + topiramate 300 mg/day (48^A). Over 3 years of treatment she had no adverse effects, such as agranulocytosis, hyperglycemia, hyperlipidemia, or weight gain; in fact she had weight loss of 12 kg. She then developed daytime fatigue and palpitation, which resolved after she was given atenolol 100 mg/day.

Cardiovascular   *Cardiomyopathy* has been associated with clozapine, and partial data initially suggested an incidence of 1 in 500 (0.2%) in the first month (SED-15, 824). In a review of articles on adverse cardiac effects associated with clozapine, it has been estimated that clozapine is associated with a low risk of potentially fatal myocarditis or cardiomyopathy (0.01–0.19%), and that this low risk of serious adverse cardiac events should be outweighed by a reduction in suicide risk in most patients (49^M).

Nervous system   It is currently thought that clozapine causes less *tardive dyskinesia* than haloperidol and even that it can improve pre-existing dyskinesia (SEDA-27, 56). It also seems to have little or no potential to cause *tardive dystonia*, which is usually considered to be a variant of tardive dyskinesia; it has even been speculated that it may be effective in treating this adverse effect (SEDA-29, 67). Clozapine has now been evaluated in an open study in seven patients (mean age 29 years; mean dose 428 mg/day) with chronic exacerbated schizophrenia and severe tardive dyskinesia (50^c). Extrapyramidal Symptoms Rating Scale scores fell by 83% after 3 years and 88% after 5 years. None of the patients had adverse effects related to clozapine: their weight did not change significantly and their serum glucose, cholesterol, and triglyceride concentrations remained within the reference ranges.

Metabolism   *Weight gain* has been commonly associated with clozapine (SEDA-27, 56; SEDA-28, 66; SEDA-29, 66). Substantial interindividual and inter-racial differences suggest that genetic factors may be important. For example, the relation between genetic variants of the β_3 adrenoceptor and the G-protein β_3 subunit and clozapine-induced body weight change has been studied (SEDA-29, 67). Now, in a long-term follow-up study (14 months) of

93 patients with schizophrenia the possible relation between clozapine-induced weight gain and a genetic polymorphism in the alpha-2A adrenergic receptor, $-1291C>G$, has been examined (51[c]). The GG genotype was associated with a significantly higher mean body weight gain (8.4 kg) than the CC genotype (2.8 kg).

The effect of clozapine on *serum ghrelin concentrations* has been investigated in 12 patients over 10 weeks after the start of treatment (52[c]). In contrast to increased body mass indices and serum leptin concentrations, there were no significant changes in serum ghrelin concentrations. The authors claimed that these results do not support a causal involvement of ghrelin in clozapine-related weight gain.

Hyperlipidemia associated with antipsychotic drugs has been reviewed (SEDA-29, 64). Haloperidol and the atypical antipsychotic drugs ziprasidone, risperidone, and aripiprazole would be associated with lower risks of hyperlipidemia, whereas chlorpromazine, thioridazine, and the atypical drugs quetiapine, olanzapine, and clozapine would be associated with higher risks. However, severe clozapine-induced hypercholesterolemia and hypertriglyceridemia has been reported in a patient taking clozapine (53[A]).

- A 42-year-old man with a schizoaffective disorder had new-onset hyperlipidemia while taking clozapine (after failing therapy with traditional antipsychotic drugs). Before taking clozapine his total cholesterol measurements were 2.9–5.5 mmol/l and there were no triglyceride measurements. Despite treatment with various antihyperlipidemic agents, his total cholesterol concentration reached 12 mmol/l and his triglyceride concentration reached 54 mmol/l. His antipsychotic drug therapy was switched to aripiprazole and his lipid concentrations improved dramatically, to the point that antihyperlipidemic treatment was withdrawn. When he was given clozapine again his lipid concentrations again worsened.

Hematologic   *Neutropenia and agranulocytosis* associated with clozapine has been extensively studied and discussed (SED-15, 829); *agranulocytosis* after long-term clozapine therapy has also been reported (SEDA-27, 57). On the other hand, cases of negative or positive rechallenge in patients with agranulocytosis have been reported (SED-15, 830). Now clozapine rechallenge after delayed neutropenia has been reported, supposedly for the first time (54[A]).

- A 45-year-old woman developed neutropenia after taking clozapine 500 mg/day for 6 years combined with other agents (olanzapine 10 mg/day, benzopril hydrochloride 20 mg/day, and haloperidol 150 mg/day). Clozapine was withdrawn immediately and the granulocytes recovered within a few days. However, 10 weeks later clozapine was restarted and there was no recurrence over more than 3 years.

Salivary glands   *Hypersalivation* is a common and well-known adverse effect of clozapine, and the use of antimuscarinic agents, adrenoceptor antagonists, and adrenoceptor agonists has been proposed (SED-15, 831; SEDA-29, 68). In 12 patients clonidine 50–100 micrograms/day relieved clozapine-induced sialorrhea, with good results in three and partial results in eight (55[c]). Theoretically, the reduction in sialorrhea with clonidine could have been due to reduced plasma noradrenaline concentrations, resulting in less stimulation of unopposed β-adrenoceptors in the salivary glands.

Susceptibility factors

Infection   Clozapine toxicity has been attributed to the effects of cytokines during an acute infection (56[A]).

- A 51-year-old woman developed toxic serum concentrations of clozapine and N-desmethylclozapine (norclozapine) during an acute urinary tract infection and had a short period of aphasia and akinesia, followed by incoherence of speech and a gait disturbance.

The authors suspected that, since the prescribed antibiotics (trimethoprim, sulfamethoxazole, and ampicillin) did not seem to be responsible for the large rise in serum clozapine concentrations, the rise might have been secondary to cytokine-mediated inhibition of cytochrome P450.

Drug overdose   Fatal and non-fatal cases of overdose have been reported with clozapine (SED-15, 833; SEDA-27, 57) and suspected cases of poisoning in which blood clozapine and N-desmethylclozapine (norclozapine) were measured have been reviewed (57[R]). There were seven fatal and five non-fatal clozapine cases of overdose, and 54 other people died while taking clozapine. Clozapine poisoning could not be diagnosed on the basis of blood clozapine and norclozapine concentrations alone. Analysis of ante-mortem blood specimens collected for white cell count monitoring and the blood clozapine/norclozapine ratio may provide additional interpretative information.

Drug–drug interactions *Fluvoxamine* increases clozapine plasma concentrations (SEDA-27, 58).

- A 34-year-old man, who had taken clozapine for 3 years in a dose that had been gradually increased up to 900 mg/day, was also given fluvoxamine 100 mg/day and 6 days later developed dystonia, dysarthria, hypersalivation, and dizziness; fluvoxamine was withdrawn and the adverse effects abated completely within 1 week (58[A]).

Droperidol   *(SED-15, 1192; SEDA-27, 58; SEDA-28, 69; SEDA-29, 69)*

Droperidol 0.5 micrograms reduced the need for postoperative morphine delivered via a patient-controlled analgesia device (59[A]). At these doses it was non-sedating and caused no dyskinetic movements.

Olanzapine   *(SED-15, 2598; SEDA-26, 61; SEDA-27, 59; SEDA-28, 70; SEDA-29, 70)*

Observational studies   In a 7-month open study 39 patients (mean age 52 years; 26% men) taking olanzapine (mean dose 15 mg/day) had limited non-significant improvement in the Wisconsin Card Sorting Test for cognitive assessment (60[c]). The following adverse events were considered to have been treatment-related: *weight gain* (n = 6), *extrapyramidal disorders* (n = 2), and *increased appetite, weakness*, and *confusion* (n = 1 each).

Comparative studies   Olanzapine has been compared with other typical and atypical antipsychotic drugs in a 3-year prospective observational investigation, the European Schizophrenia Out-patient Health Outcomes (SOHO) study, sponsored by the market authorization holder of olanzapine, in 10 European countries (61[c]). From the initial sample of 10 972

patients who started or changed antipsychotic drug medication for schizophrenia, 8400 were given only one antipsychotic drug at the baseline visit and composed the reference sample (olanzapine 4636; risperidone 1671; quetiapine 651; amisulpride 278; clozapine 291; oral typical 499; and depot typical 374). There were significantly fewer patients with *extrapyramidal symptoms* in all treatment groups after 6 months, the largest improvements being observed in patients taking olanzapine or clozapine. Conversely, there were *increases in weight and body mass index* (BMI) in all treatment groups; these were significantly greater in patients taking olanzapine or clozapine (mean body weight increases 2.4 and 2.3 kg respectively; mean BMI changes 0.9 and 0.8 kg/m^2 respectively). In all groups the patients with a lower BMI at baseline had a greater increase in weight and BMI than patients with a higher BMI at baseline; there were no sex-related differences in weight or BMI. Mean doses of all the antipsychotic drugs increased from baseline to 6 months and most patients maintained treatment for 6 months with the single antipsychotic drug that was prescribed at baseline. Reasons for drop-outs (12%) were not given.

Olanzapine versus amisulpride   There were moderate but significant improvements in neurocognition (including executive function, working memory, and declarative memory) in a randomized, double-blind, 8-week study in 52 patients with schizophrenia assigned either to olanzapine (10–20 mg/day; n = 18) or amisulpride (400–800 mg/day; n = 18) (62[c]). Of 16 dropouts, six were due to adverse events: olanzapine—*sedation* (n = 2) and *increased transaminases* (n = 1); amisulpride—*rash, extrapyramidal symptoms*, and *galactorrhea* (n = 1 each).

Olanzapine versus haloperidol   There was a different adverse effects profile in a 16-week, double-blind study in 63 out-patients with schizophrenia, who had previously been receiving fluphenazine, when comparing olanzapine (n = 29; mean age 42 years; 22 men) and haloperidol (n = 34; mean age 46 years; 24 men) (63[c]). Patients taking olanzapine had significantly fewer *extrapyramidal symptoms* than those taking haloperidol. However, they had significantly *higher systolic, but not diastolic, blood pressure. Weight gain* was also greater in the patients taking olanzapine.

Olanzapine versus lithium   In a comparison of olanzapine and lithium in 87 patients with bipolar disorder in a 12-month, randomized, double-blind trial olanzapine was equally effective in preventing recurrence of depression and more effective than lithium in preventing recurrence of manic and mixed episodes (64[c]). *Weight gain* was significantly greater with olanzapine (mean 1.8 kg). One patient committed suicide during the initial open phase and two taking lithium died during the double-blind period.

Olanzapine versus risperidone   In an 8-week study, pre-school-age children with bipolar disorder (aged 4–6 years) took either olanzapine (*n* = 15; mean age 5.0 years; 10 boys; mean dose 6.3 mg/day) or risperidone (*n* = 16; mean age 5.3 years; 12 boys; mean dose 1.4 mg/day) (65[c]). There were significantly more dropouts with olanzapine (6 versus 1), including one patient who withdrew because of adverse events (*increased appetite and hand tremor*). The main adverse events, found with both treatments, were significant *increases in prolactin concentrations* and *weight gain*. With both treatments, *increased appetite, flu-like symptoms, headaches*, and *sedation* were the most commonly reported adverse effects.

Olanzapine versus ziprasidone   In a 28-week multicenter, randomized, double-blind, parallel-group study sponsored by Eli Lilly, the market authorization holder of olanzapine, in 548 patients with schizophrenia, 277 were assigned to olanzapine (mean 15.3 mg/day) and 271 to ziprasidone (mean 116 mg/day) (66[c]). The proportions of men in the two groups were similar (65 and 64% respectively) and the mean age was slightly higher in the olanzapine group (40 versus 38 years). Significantly more patients withdrew with ziprasidone than olanzapine (58 versus 41%). However, the patients who took olanzapine had significantly greater *weight gain* (13 versus 1.8%; mean changes 3.1 and −1.1 kg respectively) and *increased appetite* (7.2 versus 2.6%). There were significant *increases in total cholesterol and low-density lipoprotein cholesterol* in those who took olanzapine. On the other hand, those who took ziprasidone had more *insomnia* (22 versus 6.9%), *anorexia* (2.6 versus 0.4%), *dystonias* (2.2 versus 0%), and *hypotension* (1.8 versus 0%).

Patients taking olanzapine (mean dose 12.6 mg/day; *n* = 71) had significantly more *weight gain* than those taking ziprasidone (mean dose 135.2 mg/day; *n* = 55) in a 6-month, randomized, double-blind, multicenter study of 126 patients (67[c]). The mean changes in body weight and body mass index were 5.0 kg and 1.3 kg/m^2 respectively with olanzapine and −0.8 kg and −0.6 kg/m^2 with ziprasidone.

Placebo-controlled studies   In a 12-week, double-blind study 60 patients with borderline personality disorders were randomized to either olanzapine 5–20 mg/day (*n* = 30; mean age 26 years; five men) or placebo (*n* = 30; mean age 26 years; three men) (68[c]). Those who took olanzapine had significantly greater *weight gain* (mean increase with olanzapine 2.7 kg; range −9 to 7 kg) than those who took placebo (mean increase −0.05 kg; range −8 to 3 kg). Olanzapine was also associated with a small *increase in cholesterol concentration* (olanzapine 8 μmol/l, placebo 3 μmol/l).

Nervous system   *Akathisia* has previously been reported in 16% of patients taking olanzapine (SEDA-21, 56). Of 10 patients with refractory panic disorder (mean age 35 years; three men) who were given olanzapine (mean dose 12.3 mg/day) one (no age and sex data given) developed significant *akathisia* at week 4 while taking 17.5 mg/day; it did not resolve at a lower dose of 12.5 mg/day (69[A]).

Possible *neuroleptic malignant syndrome* (SED-15, 2601; SEDA-27, 60; SEDA-28, 71) has again been attributed to olanzapine (70[A]).

- A 39-year-old woman with no previous psychiatric history, who was given cefuroxime and gentamicin intravenously for a suspected pneumonia, became manic and delirious; she was given olanzapine 15 mg/day and then 30 mg/day and oxazepam 45 mg/day. During the next month she developed a fluctuating fever up to 40.9 °C, including a 10-day normothermic period; she also developed autonomic instability, with a labile blood pressure and slight rigidity. However, serum creatine kinase activity did not increase. The symptoms disappeared when olanzapine was withdrawn.

Seizures (SED-15, 2602; SEDA-27, 60; SEDA-28, 72) associated with olanzapine in premarketing studies have been estimated to occur in 0.9% of patients (SEDA-24, 67). Myoclonic status can be triggered in susceptible patients (71[A]).

- A 54-year-old woman, with probable Alzheimer's disease, who was taking citalopram 20 mg/day and donepezil 5 mg/day and had paranoid ideas and agitation, was also given olanzapine 5 mg/day. During the next 48 hours she developed spontaneous and action-induced myoclonus in the trunk and limbs, which responded to clonazepam 1 mg/day and stopped when olanzapine was withdrawn. Electroencephalography showed slower background activity, with high-amplitude generalized spikes and continuous spike–wave and polyspike–wave complexes. She remained seizure free after withdrawal of clonazepam and when 9 months later she was given haloperidol 3 mg/day for new neuropsychiatric symptoms.

A 30-year-old woman with a schizophrenic disorder had a recurrence of *tardive dystonia* while taking olanzapine and was successfully treated with clozapine 150 mg/day (72[A]).

Metabolism   There was significant *weight gain* (SED-15, 2605; SEDA-27, 61; SEDA-28, 72; SEDA-29, 74) in 12 drug-naive patients with a first-episode of psychosis who took olanzapine for 3–4 months (mean dose 10.7 mg/day) compared with a control group of four healthy volunteers (8.8 versus 1.2 kg) (73[c]).

In 55 subjects randomized to olanzapine 10 mg/day, risperidone 4 mg/day, or placebo for 2 weeks, there were significant increases in weight with olanzapine (2.25 kg) and risperidone (1.05 kg) (74[c]).

Immunologic   A Guillain–Barré-like syndrome has been associated with *olanzapine hypersensitivity* (SED-15, 2608) in a patient who already had an immunological disorder (75[A]).

- A 58-year-old man with Vogt–Koyanagi–Harada syndrome, alopecia, vitiligo, and poliosis started to take olanzapine 5 mg/day for hypomania; he was also taking clonazepam 6 mg/day, valproic acid 600 mg/day, and prednisone 5 mg/day. Three weeks later he developed rapidly progressive numbness and weakness culminating in paresis of all four limbs, a generalized erythematous macular rash on the trunk and limbs, and hepatic dysfunction. He improved after withdrawal of olanzapine and 5 courses of plasma exchange over 10 days, and 6 months later his strength had returned to normal.

Susceptibility factors

Genetic   Some studies have tried to identify genetic susceptibility factors for weight gain

with olanzapine (SEDA-27, 53, 57, and 62; SEDA-29, 64). The role of the −759C/T polymorphism in the $5HT_{2C}$ receptor gene, located at q24 of the X chromosome, has now been examined in 42 subjects (age data not provided; 34 men) with schizophrenia who took olanzapine 7.5–20 mg/day for 4 weeks (mean endpoint serum concentration 24 ng/ml) (76[C]). There was no difference in mean olanzapine dose between patients with the alleles T or C. Of the 42 patients, 15 gained more than 10% of their body weight and there were no T alleles in those subjects; of the other 27 patients without a 10% weight gain, 11 had a T allele (41%). Conversely, subjects with a C allele gained a mean of 12% over their initial body weight compared to those with a T allele, who gained a mean of 4.7%. These significant differences suggest a possible protective effect of the T allele on weight gain associated with olanzapine, although other confounding variables (such as diet and exercise) were not recorded in this study.

Drug–drug interactions

Fluvoxamine (SED-15, 2609; SEDA-28, 73; SEDA-29, 75)   To determine whether a subtherapeutic dose of fluvoxamine, a potent inhibitor of CYP1A2, could affect the metabolism of olanzapine, male smokers with stable psychotic illnesses taking olanzapine (mean dose 17.5 mg/day) were switched to a mean dose of 13.0 mg/day and were given fluvoxamine 25 mg/day (77[c]). At 2, 4, and 6 weeks there were no significant changes in olanzapine plasma concentration, antipsychotic response, or metabolic indices (for example serum glucose and lipids). The ratio of 4′-N-desmethyl-olanzapine:olanzapine fell from 0.45 at baseline to 0.25 at week 6, suggesting inhibition of CYP1A2-mediated olanzapine 4′-N-demethylation by fluvoxamine. In conclusion, these results suggested that a 26% reduction in olanzapine therapeutic dose requirement may be achieved by co-administration of a subtherapeutic oral dose of fluvoxamine.

Drug overdose (SED-15, 2608; SEDA-27, 62; SEDA-29, 75)   In a fatal case of olanzapine overdose a cardiac dysrhythmia, nonconvulsive status epilepticus, and persistent choreoathetosis occurred consecutively (78[A]).

- A 62-year-old man with bipolar disorder taking olanzapine 30 mg/day and lithium 1200 mg/day attempted suicide with an estimated 750 mg of olanzapine. He developed delirium, a ventricular tachycardia, and cardiac asystole, which responded to resuscitation. On day 3 electroencephalography showed generalized frequent small amplitude spike and wave complexes with no limb movements, which resolved with intravenous fosphenytoin. His consciousness improved over the next 2 weeks, but he then lapsed progressively into coma and had choreoathetosis and dystonia in his head and all limbs. He died on day 57 from congestive heart failure and pneumonia. Post-mortem findings showed bilateral bronchopneumonia, mild cortical atrophy, and enlargement of the lateral ventricles without other major lesions; at microscopy, there was reactive astrocytosis in the striatum, globus pallidus, and thalamus bilaterally.

Management of adverse drug reactions

Various therapies have been used to avoid or to control weight gain during olanzapine treatment, including nizatidine (SEDA-25, 65), famotidine (SEDA-29, 74), and behavioral therapy (SEDA-26, 58). Topiramate has now also been used to treat weight gain in 43 women who had taken olanzapine for at least 3 months in a 10-week, double-blind, placebo-controlled study (79[c]). Those who took topiramate lost on average 5.6 kg (95% CI = 3.0, 8.5).

Sibutramine up to 15 mg/day has also been assessed in 37 subjects with schizophrenia or schizoaffective disorder and olanzapine-associated weight gain in a 12-week, double-blind, randomized study (80[C]). Those who took sibutramine had significantly greater mean weight loss than those who took placebo (3.76 versus 0.82 kg). However, the patients who took sibutramine had a mean increase in systolic blood pressure of 2.1 mmHg, anticholinergic adverse effects, and sleep disturbances.

Monitoring therapy   In an open 2-week study in 54 in-patients with schizophrenia (aged 18–75 years; 38 men), olanzapine had a beneficial effect at a plasma concentration of 20–50 ng/ml (81[c]); the authors suggested that olanzapine plasma concentration measurement may be useful in optimizing acute treatment in some patients.

Quetiapine   *(SED-15, 2995; SEDA-26, 63; SEDA-27, 62; SEDA-29, 75; see also special review above)*

Observational studies   A post-hoc analysis of the Spectrum trial, an international open non-comparative study, sponsored by AstraZeneca Pharmaceutical, has recently been published; this study was purportedly carried out to evaluate improvements in efficacy and tolerability gained by switching to quetiapine in patients who had previously taken haloperidol ($n = 43$), olanzapine ($n = 66$), or risperidone ($n = 55$) (82[c]). Switching to quetiapine produced improvements from baseline in Positive and Negative Syndrome Scale and in Calgary Depression Scale for Schizophrenia scores. There were significant reductions in *extrapyramidal adverse effects* on the Simpson–Angus scale and Barnes Akathisia scale. Patients who switched to quetiapine from haloperidol had a mean weight gain of 2 kg, while those who switched from olanzapine had a mean loss of 1 kg and those who switched from risperidone had a mean gain of 0.7 kg.

In seven patients with refractory schizophrenia taking high-dose quetiapine 1200–2400 mg/day, there were mild to marked improvements in positive symptoms, violent behavior, behavioral disturbances, and sociability (83[A]). *Sedation, orthostasis, dysphagia,* and a *nocturnal startle reaction* were reported and were responsive to dosage reduction. *Weight gain* was 4.1 kg and there were no significant *electrocardiogram abnormalities*.

Placebo-controlled studies   In 542 outpatients with bipolar I or II disorder experiencing a major depressive episode, who were randomly assigned to 8 weeks of quetiapine (300 or 600 mg/day; $n = 181$ and $n = 180$ respectively) or placebo ($n = 181$), both doses produced statistically significant improvement in Montgomery–Asberg Depression Rating Scale (MADRS) total scores compared with placebo from week 1 onward (84[C]). There were *extrapyramidal symptoms* in 8.9% of those who took 600 mg/day, 6.7% of those who took 300 mg/day, and 2.2% of those who took placebo. Patients who took quetiapine 600 mg/day had a mean weight gain of 1.6 kg, compared with 1.0 kg in those who took 300 mg/kg and 0.2 kg in those who took placebo.

Nervous system   Quetiapine seems to cause a lower incidence of *extrapyramidal symptoms* than other antipsychotic drugs (SED-15, 2995). Two patients with schizophrenia who developed focal tardive dystonia with atypical antipsychotic drugs (risperidone and olanzapine) had marked sustained improvement when quetiapine was gradually introduced and the other antipsychotic drugs were withdrawn; there was no loss of control of psychotic symptoms (85[A]).

Psychiatric   Two patients developed resistant *auditory hallucinations* when taking quetiapine (86[A]). One of these patients, a 39-year-old woman who took 600 mg/day, developed mild sedation, which resolved spontaneously by week 4.

Drug abuse   An unusual case of quetiapine abuse has been reported (87[A]).

- A 34-year-old woman with a history of polysubstance dependence (alcohol, cannabis, and cocaine), depressive episodes associated with multiple suicide attempts, and borderline personality disorder, who had been incarcerated after conviction on charges of physical assault and possession of controlled substances, complained of difficulty in sleeping, poor impulse control, irritability, and depressed mood. She was given oral quetiapine 600 mg/day. On one occasion, she crushed two 300-mg tablets, dissolved them in water, boiled them, drew the solution through a cotton swab, and injected the solution intravenously. Apart from having "the best sleep I ever had" she described no dysphoric, euphoric, or other effects. She admitted to previous intranasal abuse of crushed quetiapine tablets.

Drug withdrawal   Incapacitating quetiapine withdrawal has been reported (88[A]).

- A 36-year-old woman with rapid-cycling bipolar II disorder and premenstrual mood exacerbation was treated as an out-patient with lamotrigine 400 mg/day, clonazepam 0.5 mg tds, and quetiapine 100 mg/day. She gained 9 kg in 6 months and was advised to reduce the dose of quetiapine to 50 mg/day. After 1 day, she reported nausea, dizziness, headache, and anxiety severe enough to preclude normal daily activities. She was instructed to take quetiapine 75 mg/day, but her symptoms continued and only resolved when she took 100 mg/day. Slower reduction in the dose of quetiapine (by 12.5 mg/day every 5 days) with an antiemetic, ondansetron, also failed. On a third attempt, prochlorperazine successfully reduced her withdrawal symptoms, although moderate nausea persisted for 2 days after complete withdrawal.

No other medications were changed, so quetiapine withdrawal was the most likely explanation for the symptoms in this case.

Drug–drug interactions

Escitalopram   Among the atypical antipsychotic drugs available in Europe, quetiapine seems to be associated with less weight gain. However, severe weight gain can occur and has been reported in a supposed interaction with escitalopram (89[A]).

- A 16-year-old adolescent girl was given quetiapine for a first psychotic episode for 5 months and had no weight gain. Because her depressive symptoms were pronounced after remission of her psychotic symptoms, she was given escitalopram and had a dramatic increase in weight (8 kg over 1 month). Quetiapine was replaced by amisulpride and there was a transient fall in weight. However, severe psychotic symptoms led to reintroduction of quetiapine, and her weight again rose dramatically (8 kg over 1 month). Withdrawal of escitalopram and replacement by topiramate was followed by weight stabilization.

The authors did not propose a mechanism for this supposed interaction.

Fluvoxamine   Concomitant administration of quetiapine and fluvoxamine reportedly caused neuroleptic malignant syndrome (90[A]).

- A 57-year-old man with major depression took fluvoxamine 150 mg/day for 1 year with no adverse effects and in remission stopped taking it. He later developed agitation and was given risperidone, and then, because of extrapyramidal symptoms, quetiapine 150 mg/day. However, 2 months later he again became depressed and fluvoxamine 100 mg/day was added. After 10 days, he stopped eating and drinking and developed muscle rigidity. On day 13 he had a fever, severe extrapyramidal symptoms, a high blood pressure, and a tachycardia, and was becoming stuporose. He had a raised creatine kinase activity (7500 IU/l) and leukocyte count (13×10^9/l). All psychotropic drugs were stopped and he was given dantrolene by intravenous infusion. His symptoms gradually improved.

The authors suggested that since the doses of quetiapine and fluvoxamine were relatively low and since they are metabolized by different CYP isozymes, this was probably not a pharmacokinetic interaction. Instead, they suggested that it may have been caused by dopamine–serotonin disequilibrium.

Risperidone   *(SED-15, 3052; SEDA-27, 62; SEDA-28, 74; SEDA-29, 76)*

Comparative studies   In a double-blind, randomized, controlled, flexible-dose trial of the Early Psychosis Global Working Group, 555 patients (mean age 25 years; 71% men; median treatment length 206 days) with first-episode psychosis were assigned either to haloperidol ($n = 277$; mean modal dose 2.9 mg/day) or risperidone ($n = 278$; mean modal dose 3.3 mg/day). Haloperidol caused significantly more frequent and severe *extrapyramidal symptoms* (mainly emergent dyskinesia, parkinsonism, parkinsonian dystonia, and akathisia) associated with more concomitant medication (mainly anticholinergic drugs and benzodiazepines) (91[C]). In contrast, risperidone caused significantly more *weight gain* than haloperidol at month 3 (4.6 versus 3.5 kg) but not at the end point (7.5 versus 6.5 kg); risperidone caused *higher prolactin concentrations* (women, $n = 73$, mean 74 ng/ml; men, $n = 185$, mean 34 ng/ml) than haloperidol (women, $n = 71$, mean 48 ng/ml; men, $n = 178$, mean 22 ng/ml) (reference prolactin concentrations in women <25 ng/ml, in men <18 ng/ml); haloperidol caused hyperprolactinemia in one patient and risperidone caused it in 14; risperidone also caused *galactorrhea* ($n = 6$), *gynecomastia* ($n = 3$), and moderate *hyperglycemia* ($n = 1$).

Similarly, risperidone caused *extrapyramidal symptoms* in fewer patients (24%) than haloperidol did (43%) in a two-phase study in patients with acute bipolar mania (phase I, 3 weeks, patients receiving either risperidone 1–6 mg/day, haloperidol 2–12 mg/day, or placebo (92[c]). Plasma prolactin concentration was higher with risperidone (no data provided); prolactin-related adverse events included non-puerperal lactation, breast pain, dysmenorrhea, and reduced libido or sexual dysfunction; these effects occurred in six patients on risperidone (4%) and in two on haloperidol (1.3%).

Placebo-controlled studies   In a 12-week, double-blind, randomized, placebo-controlled study in 40 patients with treatment-resistant schizophrenia (funded by Johnson & Johnson Pharmaceutical Research & Development), the addition of risperidone to clozapine improved overall symptoms and positive and negative symptoms (93[C]). The adverse events profile of clozapine + risperidone was similar to that of clozapine + placebo. Clozapine + risperidone did not cause additional weight gain, agranulocytosis, or seizures compared with clozapine + placebo. All the patients completed 12 weeks of treatment; however, the small sample size precluded definitive conclusions.

From an initial sample of 36 patients with autism spectrum disorder (aged 5–17 years) who started an 8-week open study with risperidone, responders continued treatment for another 16 weeks ($n = 26$); two children withdrew because of unacceptable weight gain and the other 24 entered a double-blind withdrawal phase and were assigned to either risperidone ($n = 12$) or placebo ($n = 12$). *Increased appetite* and *weight gain* were the most important adverse events (mean increase 5.7 kg during 6 months, expected developmental weight gain 2.4 kg) (94[c]).

In a two-phase placebo-controlled study with an initial sample of 45 patients, 39 of whom completed the study, the addition of low doses of risperidone (0.5 mg/day) appeared to improve symptoms in patients with obsessive–compulsive disorder taking fluvoxamine monotherapy (95[c]). The main adverse events included *transient sedation* and mildly *increased appetite*.

Of 65 men (mean age 52 years) with post-traumatic stress disorder randomized to risperidone ($n = 33$) or placebo ($n = 32$) in a 4-month double-blind study supported by the Janssen Research Foundation, 22 and 26 patients respectively completed the study (96[c]). There were no significant differences in weight.

The success of masking procedures in double-blind studies has recently been studied by the Research Units on Pediatric Psychopharmacology Autism Network following an 8-week placebo-controlled trial of risperidone in 101 autistic children (aged 5–17 years) (97[c]). Clinicians attributed improvement to risperidone and lack of improvement to placebo, whether the child was taking risperidone or placebo; in contrast, the parents attributed improvement to risperidone only in the placebo group. Although the parents reported that adverse events influenced their guesses, the presence of adverse events was not associated with correct guesses. Adverse events therefore did not threaten the blindness of the study.

Cardiovascular   The possible association of risperidone with QT_c *interval prolongation* is controversial (SEDA-24, 54). There were no significant changes in 73 patients with schizophrenia (mean age 34 years; 59% men) who took risperidone for 42 days (mean dose 3.7, range 4–6 mg/day) (98[c]).

Nervous system   Co-administration of lithium and risperidone has been associated with the *rabbit syndrome* (99[A]). This reaction was probably caused by the risperidone, and the role of lithium was not clear.

Endocrine   *Hyperprolactinemia* has already been associated with risperidone (SED-15, 3058; SEDA-28, 77; SEDA-29, 78). In a randomized, double-blind, 12-week study in 78 in-patients with schizophrenia assigned to either risperidone 6 mg/day (73% men; $n = 41$) or haloperidol 20 mg/day (81% men; $n = 37$), prolactin concentrations increased significantly in men in both groups (100[c]). Adjusted for haloperidol dose equivalents (risperidone 6 mg/day equivalent to haloperidol 12 mg/day), risperidone caused a significantly larger rise in prolactin than haloperidol. The study was limited by the small number of women in the sample, which allowed the comparison of prolactin concentrations by sex but without consideration of treatment; the women had a significantly larger rise in prolactin than the men.

Drug withdrawal   *Tardive dyskinesia* (SED-15, 3056) at multiple sites, including respiratory dyskinesia, has been associated with withdrawal of risperidone (101[A]).

- An 84-year-old Japanese woman with mixed dementia taking bromperidol and biperiden was switched to risperidone 2 mg/day. After several weeks she began to have limb and orofacial dyskinesia and staggered while walking. The risperidone was abruptly withdrawn. During the following days the previous abnormal movements increased and extended to the trunk. There was respiratory dyskinesia with dyspnea. The symptoms resolved completely in risperidone withdrawal and treatment with haloperidol and biperiden.

Susceptibility factors

Genetic   The effect of the Ser9Gly polymorphism of the dopamine D_3 receptor (DRD3) gene in responses to antipsychotic drugs has previously been studied (SEDA-26, 55). Its effect on the response to risperidone has been studied in 123 Han Chinese with acute schizophrenia treated for up to 42 days (102[c]). Compared with patients with the Gly9Gly genotype, after adjusting, those with Ser9Gly had significant better performance on negative symptoms and better functioning but not better positive symptoms.

Children   Risperidone has been assessed in children with autistic disorder and disruptive behavior in a multicenter, two-part, open study (103[c]). Part one consisted of a 4-month open phase in 63 children (aged 5–17 years; 49 boys) taking risperidone 2.0 mg/day; of the 12 dropouts, five were due to loss of efficacy and one to an adverse event (constipation); there was a mean weight gain of 5.1 kg, which was significantly greater than expected from developmental norms. Part two was a randomized, double-blind study in which risperidone was either substituted by placebo ($n = 16$) or continued ($n = 16$); there were more relapses in those who took placebo ($n = 10$) than in those who continued to take risperidone ($n = 2$). One of six dropouts in the first part of the study was due to an adverse event (constipation); over the 6 months of the study there was a mean weight gain of 5.1 kg.

Elderly subjects   In 129 patients (aged 18–93 years) patients over 40 years had higher risperidone total plasma concentrations (estimated as 35% per decade in patients over 42 years) (104[c]). According to the authors, this might lead to an increased incidence of adverse events in elderly subjects.

Drug formulations   A long-acting injectable formulation of risperidone (SEDA-29, 79) has been used in recent studies that showed significant symptomatic improvement as measured with the Positive and Negative Syndrome Scale.

In the first study, a multicenter trial across 22 European countries, a total of 715 stable patients (mean age 40 years; 63% men), most with schizophrenia, who had already participated in a run-in 6-month trial with the same medication, entered the 12-month extension phase (105[C]). The subjects received risperidone injections every 2 weeks; the initial dose was 25 mg in most cases (84%) and the rest were given

37.5 mg (9%) or 50 mg (7%); the end point dose was 25 mg in 39% of patients, 37.5 mg in 23%, and 50 mg in 37%. There were 207 dropouts (29% of the whole sample), adverse events being the reason for withdrawal in 20 patients (2.8%)—exacerbation of the disease ($n = 3$), delirium, relapse, and weight gain (all $n = 2$); one patient died with pneumonia. There was weight gain in 54 patients (8%), with significant increases in body weight (79.1 versus 80.4 kg) and body mass index (27.0 versus 27.5 kg/m^2); at endpoint, 20% of patients had an increase in body weight of 7% or more. One patient developed new-onset diabetes mellitus and one hyperglycemia. Other observed adverse events were anxiety ($n = 83$, 12%), insomnia ($n = 73$, 10%), depression ($n = 52$, 7%), headache ($n = 38$, 5%), and sexual dysfunction ($n = 12$, 1.7%).

A similar design was used in 249 patients with schizoaffective disorder who received injectable risperidone for 6 months (initial dose 25 mg in 82% of patients, end-point doses ranging from 25 mg in 49% of patients to 75 mg in one); oral risperidone supplementation was needed in 19% (mean modal dose 3 mg/day) (106[c]). Three patients died during the study with heart attack, stroke, and gastrointestinal bleeding; other important adverse events were increases in body weight and body mass index (mean increases 1.4 kg and 0.5 kg/m^2), sexual dysfunction (4%), and new-onset diabetes mellitus (0.4%).

In a third study, a 6-month multicenter open trial using risperidone injections in 382 patients in an early illness stage (mean age 29 years; 69% men), mainly with schizophrenia; non-adherence was the reason for medication change in 42% of the patients (107[C]). Of the whole sample, 88% received a starting dose of 25 mg every 2 weeks; at 6 months, 45% were still being treated with this dose, while 27% and 28% received larger parenteral doses (37.5 and 50 mg respectively), and oral risperidone was added in 19% of patients (mean modal dose 2.7 mg/day). A total of 278 subjects (78%) completed the study. Adverse events accounted for dropouts in 21 cases (6% of the whole sample). Treatment-related adverse events were reported by 217 patients (57%), the most frequent being insomnia (7%), exacerbation of disease (6%), depression (5%), anxiety (5%), weight increase (4%), and relapse and headache

(3% each); other observed events were injection site pain (2%), sexual dysfunction (2%), and new-onset diabetes mellitus, gynecomastia, hyperprolactinemia, and non-puerperal lactation (0.3% each); body weight and body mass index increased by 1.8 and 0.6 kg/m^2 respectively.

In a 12-week, double-blind study, 193 Caucasian, 174 African–American, and 72 subjects from other races, all of them with schizophrenia or schizoaffective disorder, were randomized to long-acting injectable risperidone (25, 50, or 75 mg every 2 weeks) or placebo (108[c]). Race influenced neither efficacy nor extrapyramidal symptoms nor body weight.

Finally, of 192 patients who had remained symptomatically stable for at least 1 month with another major second-generation antipsychotic drug, olanzapine (mean age 38 years; 63% men), 70% completed a 6-month study with injectable risperidone; treatment-related adverse events were reported by 121 patients (63%), mostly anxiety (12%), exacerbation of disease (10%), insomnia (9%), depression (6%), and akathisia (5%) (109[c]).

Drug dosage regimens   Of 82 subjects, those who initially took higher oral doses of risperidone were more likely to have extrapyramidal adverse effects (mean dose 4.3 mg/day) (110[c]).

Drug overdose   Delayed complications, including respiratory depression, can occur after risperidone overdose (111[A]).

- A 26-year-old woman with schizophrenia who had taken risperidone 6 mg/day for 3 months was found unconscious. She later reported having taken 30 mg of risperidone in a suicidal attempt. On day 3 she developed transient respiratory distress, with lethargy, tongue protrusion, and pharyngeal-laryngeal muscle spasm.

Drug–drug interactions

Thioridazine   Thioridazine 25 mg bd significantly increased the steady-state plasma concentration of risperidone (3 mg bd) and reduced 9-hydroxyrisperidone in 12 patients with schizophrenia (112[c]). Since risperidone mainly undergoes 9-hydroxylation yielding an active metabolite, 9-hydroxyrisperidone, metabolic inhibition could account for this increase. Moreover, there was a greater rise in risperidone concentrations in subjects with more capacity for CYP2D6-dependent 9-hydroxylation of risperidone.

Sertindole   *(SED-15, 3120; SEDA-26, 66)*

Metabolism   Four patients developed tardive dyskinesia while taking conventional antipsychotic drugs and were switched to sertindole (113[A]). Three apparently recovered from the movement disorder. In the other patient sertindole monotherapy was not sufficient to reduce the movement effects, but combination treatment with tetrabenazine resulted in a greater reduction in extrapyramidal symptoms. There was no evidence of QT_c prolongation in these patients, but one patient gained 8 kg in weight.

Ziprasidone   *(SED-15, 3721; SEDA-27, 66; SEDA-28, 79; SEDA-29, 81)*

Observational studies   In an open 12-week study of ziprasidone in 12 patients with Parkinson's disease and psychosis, two withdrew because of adverse effects; one had increased diurnal *sedation* on day 5 and the other had *deterioration of gait* at 1 week (114[c]). The other 10 patients reported significant improvement in psychiatric symptoms and no deterioration in motor symptoms. The small sample size and lack of a control group precluded definitive conclusions.

In an open study nine patients with treatment-resistant schizophrenia took clozapine + ziprasidone for 6 months (115[c]). Mental state improved in seven, with significant reductions in the mean Brief Psychiatric Rating Scale score. The combination allowed an 18% reduction in the daily dose of clozapine. All had some adverse effects before combination treatment (each had been unsuccessfully treated with at least two first-generation antipsychotic drugs and/or two second-generation drugs as monotherapy) and during combination treatment, but the co-administration of ziprasidone did not result in a corresponding increase in adverse effects; for example, there was neither further weight gain ($n = 5$) nor weight loss in patients with previous weight gain ($n = 2$). However, the small sample size and the lack of a control group precluded definitive conclusions.

Published and unpublished studies from 1995 to 2004, in which intramuscular ziprasidone was assessed, have been reviewed (116[R]). The most common adverse events in the 921 patients were *nausea, headache, dizziness, anxiety, somnolence, insomnia*, and *injection-site pain*; 1.1 to 6.1% withdrew because of treatment-related adverse events.

Comparative studies   Ziprasidone is the first atypical antipsychotic drug to be available in both intramuscular and oral formulations in the USA. These two formulations have been compared with haloperidol in a 6-week, multicenter, parallel-group, flexibly dosed study in patients with an acute exacerbation of schizophrenia or schizoaffective disorder (117[C]). They were randomized to ziprasidone ($n = 427$; intramuscularly for 3 days, then orally 40–80 mg bd) or haloperidol ($n = 138$; intramuscularly for 3 days, then orally 5–20 mg/day). At the end of the intramuscular phase the patients who had receiving ziprasidone had significantly better Brief Psychiatric Rating Scale Total scores than those who had received haloperidol, but at end point there were no significant between-group differences. However, ziprasidone produced significantly greater improvement in negative subscale scores, both at the end of the intramuscular phase and at the end of the study. Haloperidol caused more *extrapyramidal effects*, including akathisia and movement disorders. At end of the study, mean weight change in the ziprasidone group was 0.25 kg compared with -0.15 kg in the haloperidol group; mean QT_c changes from baseline were $+3.2$ ms versus -3.5 ms respectively.

In a double-blind study, 144 agitated patients who required emergency sedation were randomized to ziprasidone 20 mg ($n = 46$), droperidol 5 mg ($n = 50$), or midazolam 5 mg ($n = 48$) (118[C]). Those who were sedated with droperidol or ziprasidone required rescue medications to achieve adequate sedation less often than those who were sedated with midazolam; more remained agitated at 15 minutes after ziprasidone. There was *akathisia* in one patient who received droperidol, one who received midazolam (and subsequently droperidol rescue sedation), and four who received ziprasidone. There were no other adverse events.

Musculoskeletal   *Rhabdomyolysis* has previously been associated with ziprasidone (SEDA-27, 66).

- A 50-year-old man who was treated with ziprasidone 40 mg bd for 3 weeks had a substantial rise in creatine kinase activity without any evidence of muscle trauma, stiffness, or swelling or any signs of neuroleptic malignant syndrome (119[A]). There was no renal insufficiency or compartment syndrome.

The authors suggested that ziprasidone may enhance muscle cell permeability leading to rhabdomyolysis.

Drug overdose Various reports of ziprasidone overdose have been published (SEDA-28, 80). In a retrospective chart review of isolated cases reported to a Poisons Center during 2001 to 2003, 30 patients met the criteria among about 150 000 exposures that were reviewed (120[R]). Eight patients accidentally took ziprasidone and 22 intentionally. The average dose of ziprasidone was 205 mg (recommended dose 80–160 mg/day) and only one required significant medical intervention.

References

1. Lieberman JA, Stroup TS, McEvoy JP, Swartz MS, Rosenheck RA, Perkins DO, Keefe RSE, Davis SM, Davis CE, Lebowitz BD, Severe J, Hsiao JK. Effectiveness of antipsychotic drugs in patients with chronic schizophrenia. N Engl J Med 2005;353:1209–23.
2. Straus SM, Sturkenboom MC, Bleumink GS, Dieleman JP, van der Lei J, de Graeff PA, Kingma JH, Stricker BH. Non-cardiac QT$_c$-prolonging drugs and the risk of sudden cardiac death. Eur Heart J 2005;26:2007–12.
3. Justo D, Prokhorov V, Heller K, Zeltser D. Torsade de pointes induced by psychotropic drugs and the prevalence of its risk factors. Acta Psychiatr Scand 2005;111:171–6.
4. Stöllberger C, Huber JO, Finsterer J. Antipsychotic drugs and QT prolongation. Int Clin Psychopharmacol 2005;20:243–51.
5. Copetti R, Proclemer A, Pillinini PP. Brugada-like ECG abnormalities during thioridazine overdose. Br J Clin Pharmacol 2005;59:608.
6. Rochon PA, Stukel TA, Sykora K, Gill S, Garfinkel S, Anderson GM, Normand SL, Mamdani M, Lee PE, Li P, Bronskill SE, Marras C, Gurwitz JH. Atypical antipsychotics and parkinsonism. Arch Intern Med 2005;165:1882–8.
7. Leucht S, Wahlbeck K, Hamann J, Kissling W. New generation antipsychotics versus low-potency conventional antipsychotics: a systematic review and meta-analysis. Lancet 2003;361:1581–9.
8. Patterson BD, Swingler D, Willows S. Prevalence of and risk factors for tardive dyskinesia in a xhosa population in the eastern cape of south Africa. Schizophr Res 2005;76:89–97.
9. Bersani G, Gherardelli S, Clemente R, Di Giannantonio M, Grilli A, Conti CM, Exton MS, Conti P, Doyle R, Pancheri P. Neurologic soft signs in schizophrenic patients treated with conventional and atypical antipsychotics. J Clin Psychopharmacol 2005;25:372–5.
10. Christodoulou C, Kalaitzi C. Antipsychotic drug-induced acute laryngeal dystonia: two case reports and a mini review. J Psychopharmacol 2005;19:307–12.
11. Jung DU, Seo YS, Park JH, Jeong CY, Conley RR, Kelly DL, Shim JC. The prevalence of hyperprolactinemia after long-term haloperidol use in patients with chronic schizophrenia. J Clin Psychopharmacol 2005;25:613–5.
12. O'Keane V, Meaney AM. A new risk factor for osteoporosis in young women with schizophrenia? J Clin Psychopharmacol 2005;25:26–31.
13. Bergemann N, Mundt C, Parzer P, Jannakos I, Nagl I, Salbach B, Klinga K, Runnebaum B, Resch F. Plasma concentrations of estradiol in women suffering from schizophrenia treated with conventional versus atypical antipsychotics. Schizophr Res 2005;73:357–66.
14. Henderson DC, Cagliero E, Copeland PM, Borba CP, Evins E, Hayden D, Weber MT, Anderson EJ, Allison DB, Daley TB, Schoenfeld D, Goff DC. Glucose metabolism in patients with schizophrenia treated with atypical antipsychotic agents. Arch Gen Psychiatry 2005;62:19–28.
15. Vieweg WV, Sood AB, Pandurangi A, Silverman JJ. Newer antipsychotic drugs and obesity in children and adolescents. How should we assess drug-associated weight gain? Acta Psychiatr Scand 2005;111:177–84.
16. American Psychiatric Association. Practice guideline for the treatment of patients with Alzheimer's disease and other dementias of late life. Am J Psychiatry 1997;154(5 Suppl):1–39.
17. Katz IR, Rovner BW, Schneider L. Use of psychoactive drugs in nursing homes. N Engl J Med 1992;327:1392–3.
18. Schneider LS, Tariot PN, Dagerman KS, Davis SM, Hsiao JK, Ismail MS, Lebowitz BD, Lyketsos CG, Ryan JM, Stroup TS,

Sultzer DL, Weintraub D, Lieberman JA, for the CATIE-AD Study Group. Effectiveness of atypical antipsychotic drugs in patients with Alzheimer's disease. N Engl J Med 2006;355:1525–38.

19. Ballard C, Margallo-Lana M, Juszczak E, Douglas S, Swann A, Thomas A, O'Brien J, Everratt A, Sadler S, Maddison C, Lee L, Bannister C, Elvish R, Jacoby R. Quetiapine and rivastigmine and cognitive decline in Alzheimer's disease: randomised double blind placebo controlled trial. BMJ 2005;330:874–7.

20. Sink KM, Holden KF, Yaffe K. Pharmacological treatment of neuropsychiatric symptoms of dementia. JAMA 2005;293:596–608.

21. Schneider LS, Dagerman KS, Insel P. Efficacy and adverse effects of atypical antipsychotics for dementia: meta-analysis of randomized, placebo controlled trials. Am J Geriatr Psychiatry 2006;14:191–210.

22. US Food and Drug Administration. 2003 Safety alert: RISPERDAL (risperidone). http://www.fda.gov./medwatch/SAFETY/2003/risperdal.htm.

23. Mowat D, Fowlie D, MacEwan T. CSM warning on atypical antipsychotics and stroke may be detrimental for dementia. BMJ 2004;328:1262.

24. Smith DA, Beier MT. Association between risperidone treatment and cerebrovascular adverse events: examining the evidence and postulating hypotheses for an underlying mechanism. J Am Med Dir Assoc 2004;5:129–32.

25. Wooltorton E. Olanzapine (Zyprexa): increase incidence of cerebrovascular events in dementia patients. CMAJ Astron. J. 2004;170:1395.

26. Herrmann N, Mamdani M, Lanctôt KL. Atypical antipsychotics and risk of cerebrovascular accidents. Am J Psychiatry 2004;161:1113–5.

27. Liperoti R. Cerebrovascular events among elderly patients treated with conventional or atypical antipsychotics. 2004 Annual meeting of the American Geriatrics Society. http://www.americangeriatrics.org/news/meeting/schedule_events.pdf.

28. Gill SS, Rochon PA, Herrmann N, Lee PE, Sykora K, Gunraj N, Normand SLT, Gurwitz JH, Marras C, Wodchis WP, Mamdani M. Atypical antipsychotic drugs and risk of ischaemic stroke: population based retrospective cohort study. BMJ 2005;330:445.

29. Layton D, Harris S, Wilton LV, Shakir SA. Comparison of incidence rates of cerebrovascular accidents and transient ischaemic attacks in observational cohort studies of patients prescribed risperidone, quetiapine or olanzapine in general practice in England including patients with dementia. J Psychopharmacol 2005;19:473–82.

30. Moretti R, Torre P, Antonello RM, Cattaruzza T, Cazzato G. Olanzapine as a possible treatment of behavioral symptoms in vascular dementia: risks of cerebrovascular events. A controlled, open-label study. J Neurol 2005;252:1186–93.

31. Grahmann H, Suchenwirth R. Thrombosis hazard in chlorpromazine and reserpine therapy of endogenous psychoses. Nervenarzt 1959;30:224–5.

32. Zornberg GL, Jick H. Antipsychotic drug use and risk of first-time idiopathic venous thromboembolism: a case-control study. Lancet 2000;356:1219–23.

33. Liperoti R, Pedone C, Lapane KL, Mor V, Bernabei R, Gambassi G. Venous thromboembolism among elderly patients treated with atypical and conventional antipsychotic agents. Arch Intern Med 2005;165:2677–82.

34. Liperoti R, Gambassi G, Lapane KL, Chiang C, Pedone C, Mor V, Bernabei R. Conventional and atypical antipsychotics and the risk of hospitalization for ventricular arrhythmias or cardiac arrest. Arch Intern Med 2005;165:696–701.

35. Schneider LS, Dagerman KS, Insel P. Risk of death with atypical antipsychotic drug treatment for dementia. JAMA 2005;294:1934–42.

36. Wang PS, Schneeweiss S, Avorn J, Fischer MA, Mogun H, Solomon DH, Brookhart MA. Risk of death in elderly users of conventional vs. atypical antipsychotic medications. N Engl J Med. 2005;353:2335–41.

37. US Food and Drug Administration, FDA Public Health Advisory. Deaths with antipsychotics in elderly patients with behavioral disturbances. http://www.fda.gov/cder/drug/advisory/antipsychotics.htm.

38. EMEA. EMEA public statement on the safety of olanzapine (Zyprexa, Zyprexa Velotab). http://www.emea.europa.eu/pdfs/human/press/pus/085604en.pdf.

39. Kane JM, Carson WH, Saha AR, McQuade RD, Ingenito GG, Zimbroff DL, Ali MW. Efficacy and safety of aripiprazole and haloperidol versus placebo in patients with schizophrenia and schizoaffective disorder. J Clin Psychiatry 2002;63:763–71.

40. Grant MJ, Baldessarini RJ. Possible improvement of neuroleptic-associated tardive dyskinesia during treatment with aripiprazole. Ann Pharmacother 2005;39:1953.

41. Ruffatti A, Minervini L, Romano M, Sonino N. Galactorrhea with aripiprazole. Psychother Psychosom 2005;74:391–2.

42. Medical News. FDA approves oral solution formulation of Abilify (aripiprazole) for schizophrenia. http://www.medicalnewstoday.com/articles/18670.php.

43. Fleischhacker WW. Aripiprazole. Expert Opin Pharmacother 2005;6:2091–101.

44. Phua YS, Patel DV, McGhee CN. In vivo confocal microstructural analysis of corneal endothelial changes in a patient on long-term chlorpromazine therapy. Graefe's Arch Clin Exp Ophthalmol 2005;243:721–3.

45. Ng CH, Chong SA, Lambert T, Fan A, Hackett LP, Mahendran R, Subramaniam M, Schweitzer I. An inter-ethnic comparison study of clozapine dosage, clinical response

and plasma levels. Int Clin Psychopharmacol 2005;20:163–8.

46. Chung C, Remington G. Predictors and markers of clozapine response. Psychopharmacology 2005;179:317–35.

47. Dursun SM, Hallak JE, Haddad P, Leahy A, Byrne A, Strickland PL, Anderson IM, Zuardi AW, Deakin JF. Clozapine monotherapy for catatonic schizophrenia: should clozapine be the treatment of choice, with catatonia rather than psychosis as the main therapeutic index? J Psychopharmacol 2005;19:432–3.

48. Chen CK, Shiah IS, Yeh CB, Mao WC, Chang CC. Combination treatment of clozapine and topiramate in resistant rapid-cycling bipolar disorder. Clin Neuropharmacol 2005;28:136–8.

49. Merrill DB, Dec GW, Goff DC. Adverse cardiac effects associated with clozapine. J Clin Psychopharmacol 2005;25:32–41.

50. Louzã MR, Bassitt DP. Maintenance treatment of severe tardive dyskinesia with clozapine: 5 years' follow-up. J Clin Psychopharmacol 2005;25:180–2.

51. Wang YC, Bai YM, Chen JY, Lin CC, Lai IC, Liou YJ. Polymorphism of the adrenergic receptor alpha 2a −1291C>G genetic variation and clozapine-induced weight gain. J Neural Transm 2005;112:1463–8.

52. Theisen FM, Gebhardt S, Bromel T, Otto B, Heldwein W, Heinzel-Gutenbrunner M, Krieg JC, Remschmidt H, Tschop M, Hebebrand J. A prospective study of serum ghrelin levels in patients treated with clozapine. J Neural Transm 2005;112:1411–6.

53. Ball MP, Hooper ET, Skipwith DF, Cates ME. Clozapine-induced hyperlipidemia resolved after switch to aripiprazole therapy. Ann Pharmacother 2005;39:1570–2.

54. Small JG, Weber MC, Klapper MH, Kellams JJ. Rechallenge of late-onset neutropenia with clozapine. J Clin Psychopharmacol 2005;25:185–6.

55. Praharaj SK, Verma P, Roy D, Singh A. Is clonidine useful for treatment of clozapine-induced sialorrhea? J Psychopharmacol 2005;19:426–8.

56. Jecel J, Michel TM, Gutknecht L, Schmidt D, Pfuhlmann B, Jabs BE. Toxic clozapine serum levels during acute urinary tract infection: a case report. Eur J Clin Pharmacol 2005;60:909–10.

57. Flanagan RJ, Spencer EP, Morgan PE, Barnes TR, Dunk L. Suspected clozapine poisoning in the UK/Eire, 1992–2003. Forensic Sci Int 2005;155:91–9.

58. Peritogiannis V, Tsouli S, Pappas D, Mavreas V. Acute effects of clozapine–fluvoxamine combination. Schizophr Res 2005;79:345–6.

59. Lo Y, Chia Y-Y, Liu K, Ko N-H. Morphine sparing with droperidol in patient controlled analgesia. J Clin Anaesth 2005;17:271–2.

60. Stratta P, Donda P, Rossi A, Rossi A. Executive function assessment of patients with schizophrenic disorder residual type in olanzapine treatment: an open study. Hum Psychopharmacol 2005;20:401–8.

61. Lambert M, Haro JM, Novick D, Edgell ET, Kennedy L, Ratcliffe M, Naber D. Olanzapine vs. other antipsychotics in actual outpatient settings: six months tolerability results from the European Schizophrenia Out-patient Health Outcomes study. Acta Psychiatr Scand 2005;111:232–43.

62. Wagner M, Quednow BB, Westheide J, Schlaepfer TE, Maier W, Kuhn KU. Cognitive improvement in schizophrenic patients does not require a serotonergic mechanism: randomized controlled trial of olanzapine vs amisulpride. Neuropsychopharmacology 2005;30:381–90.

63. Buchanan RW, Ball MP, Weiner E, Kirkpatrick B, Gold JM, McMahon RP, Carpenter Jr WT. Olanzapine treatment of residual positive and negative symptoms. Am J Psychiatry 2005;162:124–9.

64. Tohen M, Greil W, Calabrese JR, Sachs GS, Yatham LN, Oerlinghausen BM, Koukopoulos A, Cassano GB, Grunze H, Licht RW, Dell'Osso L, Evans AR, Risser R, Baker RW, Crane H, Dossenbach MR, Bowden CL. Olanzapine versus lithium in the maintenance treatment of bipolar disorder: a 12-month, randomized, double-blind, controlled clinical trial. Am J Psychiatry 2005;162:1281–90.

65. Biederman J, Mick E, Hammerness P, Harpold T, Aleardi M, Dougherty M, Wozniak J. Open-label, 8-week trial of olanzapine and risperidone for the treatment of bipolar disorder in preschool-age children. Biol Psychiatry 2005;58:589–94.

66. Breier A, Berg PH, Thakore JH, Naber D, Gattaz WF, Cavazzoni P, Walker DJ, Roychowdhury SM, Kane JM. Olanzapine versus ziprasidone: results of a 28-week double-blind study in patients with schizophrenia. Am J Psychiatry 2005;162:1879–87.

67. Simpson GM, Weiden P, Pigott T, Murray S, Siu CO, Romano SJ. Six-month, blinded, multicenter continuation study of ziprasidone versus olanzapine in schizophrenia. Am J Psychiatry 2005;162:1535–8.

68. Soler J, Pascual JC, Campins J, Barrachina J, Puigdemont D, Alvarez E, Perez V. Double-blind, placebo-controlled study of dialectical behavior therapy plus olanzapine for borderline personality disorder. Am J Psychiatry 2005;162:1221–4.

69. Hollifield M, Thompson PM, Ruiz JE, Uhlenhuth EH. Potential effectiveness and safety of olanzapine in refractory panic disorder. Depress Anxiety 2005;21:33–40.

70. Nielsen J, Bruhn AM. Atypical neuroleptic malignant syndrome caused by olanzapine. Acta Psychiatr Scand 2005;112:238–40.

71. Camacho A, Garcia-Navarro M, Martinez B, Villarejo A, Pomares E. Olanzapine-induced myoclonic status. Clin Neuropharmacol 2005;28:145–7.

72. García-Lado I, García-Caballero A, Recimil MJ, Area R, Ozaita G, Lamas S. Reappearance of tardive dystonia with olanzapine treated with clozapine. Schizophr Res 2005;76:357–8.

73. Sengupta SM, Klink R, Stip E, Baptista T, Malla A, Joober R. Weight gain and lipid metabolic abnormalities induced by olanzapine in first-episode, drug-naive patients with psychotic disorders. Schizophr Res 2005;80:131–3.

74. Roerig JL, Mitchell JE, de Zwaan M, Crosby RD, Gosnell BA, Steffen KJ, Wonderlich SA. A comparison of the effects of olanzapine and risperidone versus placebo on eating behaviors. J Clin Psychopharmacol 2005;25:413–8.

75. Benito-Leon J, Mitchell AJ. Guillain–Barré-like syndrome associated with olanzapine hypersensitivity reaction. Clin Neuropharmacol 2005;28:150–1.

76. Ellingrod VL, Perry PJ, Ringold JC, Lund BC, Bever-Stille K, Fleming F, Holman TL, Miller D. Weight gain associated with the −759C/T polymorphism of the 5HT2C receptor and olanzapine. Am J Med Genet B Neuropsychiatr Genet 2005;134:76–8.

77. Albers LJ, Ozdemir V, Marder SR, Raggi MA, Aravagiri M, Endrenyi L, Reist C. Low-dose fluvoxamine as an adjunct to reduce olanzapine therapeutic dose requirements: a prospective dose-adjusted drug interaction strategy. J Clin Psychopharmacol 2005;25:170–4.

78. Davis LE, Becher MW, Tlomak W, Benson BE, Lee RR, Fisher EC. Persistent choreoathetosis in a fatal olanzapine overdose: drug kinetics, neuroimaging, and neuropathology. Am J Psychiatry 2005;162:28–33.

79. Nickel MK, Nickel C, Muehlbacher M, Leiberich PK, Kaplan P, Lahmann C, Tritt K, Krawczyk J, Kettler C, Egger C, Rother WK, Loew TH. Influence of topiramate on olanzapine-related adiposity in women: a random, double-blind, placebo-controlled study. J Clin Psychopharmacol 2005;25:211–7.

80. Henderson DC, Copeland PM, Daley TB, Borba CP, Cather C, Nguyen DD, Louie PM, Evins AE, Freudenreich O, Hayden D, Goff DC. A double-blind, placebo-controlled trial of sibutramine for olanzapine-associated weight gain. Am J Psychiatry 2005;162:954–62.

81. Mauri MC, Steinhilber CP, Marino R, Invernizzi E, Fiorentini A, Cerveri G, Baldi ML, Barale F. Clinical outcome and olanzapine plasma levels in acute schizophrenia. Eur Psychiatry 2005;20:55–60.

82. Larmo I, de Nayer A, Windhager E, Lindenbauer B, Rittmannsberger H, Platz T, Jones AM, Altman C, Spectrum Study Group. Efficacy and tolerability of quetiapine in patients with schizophrenia who switched from haloperidol, olanzapine or risperidone. Hum Psychopharmacol 2005;20:573–81.

83. Pierre JM, Wirshing DA, Wirshing WC, Rivard JM, Marks R, Mendenhall J, Sheppard K, Saunders DG. High-dose quetiapine in treatment refractory schizophrenia. Schizophr Res 2005;73:373–5.

84. Calabrese JR, Keck PE Jr., Macfadden W, Minkwitz M, Ketter TA, Weisler RH, Cutler AJ, McCoy R, Wilson E, Mullen J. A randomized, double-blind, placebo-controlled trial of quetiapine in the treatment of bipolar I or II depression. Am J Psychiatry 2005;162:1351–60.

85. Gourzis P, Polychronopoulos P, Papapetropoulos S, Assimakopoulos K, Argyriou AA, Beratis S. Quetiapine in the treatment of focal tardive dystonia induced by other atypical antipsychotics: a report of 2 cases. Clin Neuropharmacol 2005;28:195–6.

86. Mosolov SN, Kabanov S. Quetiapine in the treatment of patients with resistant auditory hallucinations: two case reports with long-term cognitive assessment. Eur Psychiatry 2005;20:430.

87. Hussain MZ, Waheed W, Hussain S. Intravenous quetiapine abuse. Am J Psychiatry 2005;162:1755–6.

88. Kim DR, Staab JP. Quetiapine discontinuation syndrome. Am J Psychiatry 2005;162:1020.

89. Holzer L, Paiva G, Halfon O. Quetiapine-induced weight gain and escitalopram. Am J Psychiatry 2005;162:192–3.

90. Matsumoto R, Kitabayashi Y, Nakatomi Y, Tsuchida H, Fukui K. Neuroleptic malignant syndrome induced by quetiapine and fluvoxamine. Am J Psychiatry 2005;162:812.

91. Schooler N, Rabinowitz J, Davidson M, Emsley R, Harvey PD, Kopala L, McGorry PD, Van Hove I, Eerdekens M, Swyzen W, De Smedt G, Early Psychosis Global Working Group. Risperidone and haloperidol in first-episode psychosis: a long-term randomized trial. Am J Psychiatry 2005;162:947–53.

92. Smulevich AB, Khanna S, Eerdekens M, Karcher K, Kramer M, Grossman F. Acute and continuation risperidone monotherapy in bipolar mania: a 3-week placebo-controlled trial followed by a 9-week double-blind trial of risperidone and haloperidol. Eur Neuropsychopharmacol 2005;15:75–84.

93. Josiassen RC, Joseph A, Kohegyi E, Stokes S, Dadvand M, Paing WW, Shaughnessy RA. Clozapine augmented with risperidone in the treatment of schizophrenia: a randomized, double-blind, placebo-controlled trial. Am J Psychiatry 2005;162:130–6.

94. Troost PW, Lahuis BE, Steenhuis MP, Ketelaars CE, Buitelaar JK, van Engeland H, Scahill L, Minderaa RB, Hoekstra PJ. Long-term effects of risperidone in children with autism spectrum disorders: a placebo discontinuation study. J Am Acad Child Adolesc Psychiatry 2005;44:1137–44.

95. Erzegovesi S, Guglielmo E, Siliprandi F, Bellodi L. Low-dose risperidone augmentation of fluvoxamine treatment in obsessive-compulsive disorder: a double-blind, placebo-controlled study. Eur Neuropsychopharmacol 2005;15:69–74.

96. Bartzokis G, Lu PH, Turner J, Mintz J, Saunders CS. Adjunctive risperidone in the treatment of chronic combat-related posttraumatic stress disorder. Biol Psychiatry 2005;57:474–9.

97. Vitiello B, Davies M, Arnold LE, McDougle CJ, Aman M, McCracken JT, Scahill L, Tierney E, Posey DJ, Swiezy NB, Koenig K. Assessment of the integrity of study blindness in a pediatric clinical trial of risperidone. J Clin Psychopharmacol 2005;25:565–9.

98. Chiu CC, Chang WH, Huang MC, Chiu YW, Lane HY. Regular-dose risperidone on QTc intervals. J Clin Psychopharmacol 2005;25:391–3.

99. Mendhekar DN. Rabbit syndrome induced by combined lithium and risperidone. Can J Psychiatry 2005;50:369.

100. Zhang XY, Zhou DF, Cao LY, Zhang PY, Wu GY, Shen YC. Prolactin levels in male schizophrenic patients treated with risperidone and haloperidol: a double-blind and randomized study. Psychopharmacology 2005;178:35–40.

101. Komatsu S, Kirino E, Inoue Y, Arai H. Risperidone withdrawal-related respiratory dyskinesia: a case diagnosed by spirography and fibroscopy. Clin Neuropharmacol 2005;28:90–3.

102. Lane HY, Hsu SK, Liu YC, Chang YC, Huang CH, Chang WH. Dopamine D3 receptor Ser9Gly polymorphism and risperidone response. J Clin Psychopharmacol 2005;25:6–11.

103. Research Units on Pediatric Psychopharmacology Autism Network. Risperidone treatment of autistic disorder: longer-term benefits and blinded discontinuation after 6 months. Am J Psychiatry 2005;162:1361–9.

104. Aichhorn W, Weiss U, Marksteiner J, Kemmler G, Walch T, Zernig G, Stelzig-Schoeler R, Stuppaeck C, Geretsegger C. Influence of age and gender on risperidone plasma concentrations. J Psychopharmacol 2005;19:395–401.

105. Kissling W, Heres S, Lloyd K, Sacchetti E, Bouhours P, Medori R, Llorca PM. Direct transition to long-acting risperidone—analysis of long-term efficacy. J Psychopharmacol 2005;19(5 Suppl):15–21.

106. Mohl A, Westlye K, Opjordsmoen S, Lex A, Schreiner A, Benoit M, Bräunig P, Medori R. Long-acting risperidone in stable patients with schizoaffective disorder. J Psychopharmacol 2005;19(5 Suppl):22–31.

107. Parellada E, Andrezina R, Milanova V, Glue P, Masiak M, Turner MS, Medori R, Gaebel W. Patients in the early phases of schizophrenia and schizoaffective disorders effectively treated with risperidone long-acting injectable. J Psychopharmacol 2005;19(5 Suppl):5–14.

108. Ciliberto N, Bossie CA, Urioste R, Lasser RA. Lack of impact of race on the efficacy and safety of long-acting risperidone versus placebo in patients with schizophrenia or schizoaffective disorder. Int Clin Psychopharmacol 2005;20:207–12.

109. Gastpar M, Masiak M, Latif MA, Frazzingaro S, Medori R, Lombertie ER. Sustained improvement of clinical outcome with risperidone long-acting injectable in psychotic patients previously treated with olanzapine. J Psychopharmacol 2005;19(5 Suppl):32–8.

110. Riedel M, Schwarz MJ, Strassnig M, Spellmann I, Muller-Arends A, Weber K, Zach J, Muller N, Moller HJ. Risperidone plasma levels, clinical response and side-effects. Eur Arch Psychiatry Clin Neurosci 2005;255:261–8.

111. Akyol A, Senel AC, Ulusoy H, Karip F, Erciyes N. Delayed respiratory depression after risperidone overdose. Anesth Analg 2005;101:1490–1.

112. Nakagami T, Yasui-Furukori N, Saito M, Mihara K, De Vries R, Kondo T, Kaneko S. Thioridazine inhibits risperidone metabolism: a clinically relevant drug interaction. J Clin Psychopharmacol 2005;25:89–91.

113. Perquin LN. Treatment with the new antipsychotic sertindole for late-occurring undesirable movement effects. Int Clin Psychopharmacol 2005;20:335–8.

114. Gómez-Esteban JC, Zarranz JJ, Velasco F, Lezcano E, Lachen MC, Rouco I, Barcena J, Boyero S, Ciordia R, Allue I. Use of ziprasidone in parkinsonian patients with psychosis. Clin Neuropharmacol 2005;28:111–4.

115. Ziegenbein M, Kropp S, Kuenzel HE. Combination of clozapine and ziprasidone in treatment-resistant schizophrenia: an open clinical study. Clin Neuropharmacol 2005;28:220–4.

116. Preskorn SH. Pharmacokinetics and therapeutics of acute intramuscular ziprasidone. Clin Pharmacokinet 2005;44:1117–33.

117. Brook S, Walden J, Benattia I, Siu CO, Romano SJ. Ziprasidone and haloperidol in the treatment of acute exacerbation of schizophrenia and schizoaffective disorder: comparison of intramuscular and oral formulations in a 6-week, randomized, blinded-assessment study. Psychopharmacology 2005;178:514–23.

118. Martel M, Sterzinger A, Miner J, Clinton J, Biros M. Management of acute undifferentiated agitation in the emergency department: a randomized double-blind trial of droperidol, ziprasidone, and midazolam. Acad Emerg Med 2005;12:1167–72.

119. Zaidi AN. Rhabdomyolysis after correction of hyponatremia in psychogenic polydipsia possibly complicated by ziprasidone. Ann Pharmacother 2005;39:1726–31.

120. LoVecchio F, Watts D, Eckholdt P. Three-year experience with ziprasidone exposures. Am J Emerg Med 2005;23:586–7.

Dieter Schmidt and Stefan Beyenburg

7 Antiepileptic drugs

GENERAL

Musculoskeletal Several types of centrally acting drugs, including benzodiazepines, anticonvulsants, antidepressants, and opioids, have been associated with increased risks of *fractures*. However, it is unclear whether this increase is related to an effect on bone mineral density or to other factors, such as an increased risk of falls. The relation between bone mineral density and the use of benzodiazepines, anticonvulsants, antidepressants, and opioids has been studied in US adults aged 17 years and older from the Third National Health and Nutrition Examination Survey (NHANES III, 1988–94) (1[C]). Total femoral bone mineral density in 7114 men and 7532 women was measured by dual-energy X-ray absorptiometry. In linear regression models, there was significantly reduced bone mineral density in subjects taking anticonvulsants (0.92 g/cm^2; 95% CI = 0.89, 0.94) and opioids (0.92 g/cm^2; 95% CI = 0.88, 0.95) compared with non-users (0.95 g/cm^2; 95% CI = 0.95, 0.95) after adjusting for several potential confounders. The anticonvulsants were carbamazepine, clonazepam, divalproex, ethosuximide, mephobarbital, methsuximide, phenobarbital, phenytoin, primidone, and valproic acid. There was reduced bone mineral density in patients who had taken carbamazepine, phenobarbital, or phenytoin for at least 2 years. There was a trend towards lower bone density with prolonged use. Other centrally acting drugs—benzodiazepines or antidepressants—were not associated with significantly reduced bone mineral density. These findings have implications for fracture-prevention strategies.

Drug–drug interactions Given the risk of teratogenicity associated with many antiepileptic drugs, effective contraception is particularly important (2[R]). Several commonly used antiepileptic drugs interfere with the *combined oral contraceptive*, either by induction of CYP isozymes or by other mechanisms. They include carbamazepine, oxcarbazepine, phenobarbital, phenytoin, primidone, and topiramate. However, use of the combined oral contraceptive may still be possible, with a combination that contains at least 50 micrograms of estrogen, although for maximal efficacy it should be combined with a barrier method. Breakthrough bleeding suggests that a higher dose of estrogen is necessary, although its absence does not guarantee contraceptive efficacy. Progesterone-only formulations, progesterone implants, and combined contraceptive patches are not recommended for women taking these antiepileptic drugs.

Carbamazepine *(SED-15, 627; SEDA-27, 76; SEDA-28, 88; SEDA-29, 88)*

Nervous system In a cross-sectional study from the Netherlands, the main complaints of patients taking carbamazepine monotherapy were: *fatigue* 15%, *tiredness* 18%, *memory loss* 20%, and *difficulty in concentrating* 16% (3[c]). However, complaints were not associated with continuing seizure activity or other treatment factors.

Coma due to carbamazepine intoxication in a pregnant woman (at 33 weeks gestation) has again been described, with a favorable outcome for both mother and child after charcoal administration and plasmapheresis (4[A]).

Electrolyte balance Carbamazepine can cause acute *hyponatremia* and subsequent tonic–clonic seizures; in another recent case the

Side Effects of Drugs, Annual 30
J.K. Aronson (Editor)
ISSN: 0378-6080
DOI: 10.1016/S0378-6080(08)00007-X

serum sodium concentration was 122 mmol/l (5^A). Several susceptibility factors increase the risk of hyponatremia, including age over 40 years, concomitant use of medications associated with hyponatremia, menstruation, psychiatric conditions, surgery, psychogenic polydipsia, and female sex.

Reproductive system   Male infertility with *asthenozoospermia* during long-term treatment with carbamazepine 400 mg/day has been reported in a 29-year-old man (6^A). After switching to another anticonvulsant sperm motility was improved. This single case report suggests a direct effect of carbamazepine on sperm function.

Immunologic   The risk of *erythema multiforme* (Stevens–Johnson syndrome or toxic epidermal necrolysis) associated with the use of carbamazepine has been confirmed in a case control study (7^C).

- A 63-year-old Japanese man with epilepsy developed skin eruptions, liver dysfunction, high fever, leukocytosis, and atypical lymphocytosis 4 weeks after he started taking carbamazepine (8^A). Titers of human herpesvirus 7 (HHV-7)-specific IgG antibodies were significantly increased and HHV-7 DNA was detected in his serum by polymerase chain reaction.

These findings suggest that reactivation of HHV-7 may contribute to the development of drug-induced hypersensitivity syndrome.

Susceptibility factors   In a retrospective study of 74 patients undergoing epilepsy surgery who were taking long-term carbamazepine, 51% of adults and 52% of children had raised drug concentrations (9^c). Among the children, 13% had symptoms of toxicity compared with 9.3% of the adults. Two variables that were significantly related to toxicity were the average postoperative dose of carbamazepine and the carbamazepine concentration of the day of surgery. Other major susceptibility factors were *the dose of fentanyl* (which inhibits CYP450 isozymes, especially CYP3A), *lower body weight, age*, and *blood loss*. The authors suggested that postoperatively reduced doses of carbamazepine should be considered.

Drug–drug interactions   The extent of acute co-prescribing in primary care to children taking long-term antiepileptic drugs, which could give rise to potentially harmful drug–drug interactions has been assessed in 178 324 children aged 0–17 years in 161 general practices throughout Scotland, of whom 723 (0.41%) were taking long-term antiepileptic drug therapy with 14 agents; sodium valproate (39%), carbamazepine (28%), and lamotrigine (12%) accounted for 80% of the total (10^c). The children also received 4895 acute co-prescriptions for 269 different medicines. The average numbers of acute co-prescriptions for non-antiepileptic drugs were 8, 11, 6, and 6 for those aged 0–1, 2–4, 5–11, and 12–17 years respectively. Of these acute co-prescriptions 72 (1.5%) prescribed for 22 children (3.0%) were identified as potential sources of clinically serious interactions. The antiepileptic drugs involved were carbamazepine, phenobarbital, and phenytoin. The age-adjusted prevalence rates for potentially serious co-prescribing were 86, 26, 22, and 33 per 1000 children in those aged 0–1, 2–4, 5–11, and 12–17 years respectively. The drugs most commonly co-prescribed that could have given rise to interactions were *antacids, erythromycin, ciprofloxacin, theophylline*, and low-dose *oral contraceptives*. In 10 of the 20 children who were at risk of a potentially clinically serious adverse drug interaction, the acute co-prescription was prescribed off-label because of age or specific contraindications or warnings. The authors concluded that in primary care, 3.0% of children taking long-term antiepileptic drugs are co-prescribed therapeutic agents that could give rise to clinically serious drug–drug interactions.

- A 37-year-old woman who took carbamazepine 1000 mg/day for neuropathic pain for 2 years without clinical or laboratory signs of toxicity developed symptoms of carbamazepine intoxication and a raised plasma carbamazepine concentration after taking *oxybutynin* and *dantrolene* (11^A).

Oxybutynin is metabolized by CYP3A, which also catalyses the metabolism of carbamazepine, and in rats dantrolene is metabolized by CYP1A1, CYP1A2, and CYP3A (12^E); the authors therefore suggested that this interaction was mediated by inhibition of carbamazepine metabolism.

Gabapentin   *(SED-15, 1465; SEDA-27, 77; SEDA-28, 89; SEDA-29, 89)*

Placebo-controlled studies   The effects of gabapentin (300 versus 600 mg/day; $n = 40$) on irritable bowel syndrome with visceral hypersensitivity have been evaluated in a randomized, double-blind, placebo-controlled study (13[C]). The most common adverse events in those taking gabapentin were *dizziness* and *somnolence* ($n = 4$ each).

The optimal pre-emptive dose of gabapentin for postoperative pain relief after lumbar diskectomy has been investigated in a randomized, double-blind, placebo-controlled study in 100 patients (14[C]). The most common adverse effects were *nausea and vomiting* (15 episodes) and the number of adverse events increased with increasing gabapentin doses from 300 to 1200 mg 2 hours before surgery. No patient reported vertigo, somnolence, ataxia, or headache.

The effect of gabapentin monotherapy on residual pain (maximum dose 500–1200 mg/day) has been evaluated in 10 patients with neuroborreliosis (15[c]). There were no severe adverse events. The only reported adverse effects were slight *headache, fatigue*, and initial *dizziness*.

Drug overdose   A 54-year-old white woman was found dead in her apartment (16[A]). Postmortem blood analysis identified paracetamol (97 mg/l), citalopram (0.4 mg/l), gabapentin (24 mg/l) and metaxalone (21 mg/l). The concentration of metaxalone was within the range of concentrations that have previously been reported in deaths involving metaxalone. The medical examiner ruled that the cause of death was suicidal intoxication with metaxalone and gabapentin.

Lamotrigine   *(SED-15, 1990; SEDA-27, 77; SEDA-29, 90)*

Observational studies   The effectiveness of lamotrigine therapy has been assessed during the first year of use in 360 patients with epilepsy who served as their own controls in 37 centers in the Netherlands; effectiveness could be assessed in 165 (17[c]). Lamotrigine was effective in 60% of the patients who started taking it because of adverse events with other antiepileptic drugs. Adverse events necessitated withdrawal of lamotrigine in 22%, the most common reason being rash (7%). Seven of the 53 patients who took lamotrigine because of adverse effects of previous medications had significant worsening of seizure control, while 33 patients responded well.

The roles of ethosuximide, sodium valproate, and lamotrigine have been evaluated in children and adolescents with typical absence seizures in a systematic review of randomized controlled trials (18[M]). Only four randomized controlled trials fulfilled the inclusion criteria. The authors could not find any reliable evidence to inform clinical practice (mainly because of heterogeneity). Only one study of lamotrigine was analysed. Adverse effects related to the nervous system were common (reported by 5% or more of participants): *weakness, headache, dizziness*, and *hyperkinesia*. Other reported complaints were *abdominal pain, nausea*, and *anorexia*. *Rash* was common, but in only one of the patients was it thought to be related to lamotrigine.

In a cross-sectional comparison of topiramate and lamotrigine in children lamotrigine caused adverse events less frequently; however, both medications were generally well tolerated and events were classified as mild to moderate (19[c]). One-third of the children ($n = 65$) who took lamotrigine had adverse events, mostly related to the central nervous system and early in treatment. *Rash* (6%), *headache* (5%), and *sleep disturbances* (8%) were observed only with lamotrigine; 11% of the children who took lamotrigine withdrew because of adverse events.

Comparative studies   Lamotrigine has been compared with carbamazepine and valproic acid in newly diagnosed focal and idiopathic generalized epilepsy in an open randomized multicenter 24-week monotherapy trial (20[c]). In those who took lamotrigine ($n = 121$) the five most frequent adverse drug reactions were *fatigue* (13%), *erythematous rash* (7.4%), *pruritus* and *dizziness* (5.8% each), and *nervousness* (5.0%). In 12 patients lamotrigine was withdrawn because of adverse events.

Placebo-controlled studies   In a small randomized double-blind, placebo-controlled 8-week study of lamotrigine in 24 women who met Structured Clinical Interview for DSM-IV (SCID) criteria for borderline personality disorder, all tolerated the drug relatively well (21[C]).

Respiratory   A patient taking sodium valproate developed an *interstitial pneumonitis* after taking lamotrigine 75 mg/day for 2 months (22[A]). It resolved after lamotrigine withdrawal. A pharmacodynamic interaction with sodium valproate might have been of importance.

Nervous system   Recurrent severe *aseptic meningitis* has been associated with lamotrigine (23[A]).

- A 16-year old girl with systemic lupus erythematosus, who had taken a stable dose of sodium valproate for idiopathic generalized epilepsy, had two episodes of severe aseptic meningitis after taking lamotrigine. Both episodes resolved after withdrawal. The first episode developed 10 days after the onset of lamotrigine add-on treatment and the second episode 1 hour after restarting lamotrigine 25 mg.

Rapid and full recovery on lamotrigine withdrawal and the greater severity of the second episode after repeated exposure strengthened the likelihood of a hypersensitivity reaction to lamotrigine, although the exact mechanism remains to be elucidated.

Sensory systems   The effects of lamotrigine on vision have been evaluated in 18 patients during routine ophthalmological examination, including visual acuity testing, tonometry, slit lamp examination, fundoscopy, automated kinetic perimetry, electro-oculography, and electroretinography (24[c]). There were no abnormalities. Four patients complained of *blurred vision*; one had visual field constriction in both eyes, which was of unclear clinical significance (poor compliance), and a reduced light/dark ratio on electro-oculography. Another patient with blurred vision had abnormal electro-oculography, but the visual fields were normal. Two patients had abnormal electro-oculography but no visual symptoms. Electroretinography was normal in all cases. However, in the whole group of those taking lamotrigine, the light/dark ratio was reduced dose-dependently. At the recommended dose no

effect on visual function could be demonstrated. The authors concluded that lamotrigine did not cause irreversible visual field impairment, although there may have been dose-dependent retinal toxicity. The cellular mechanism of the electrophysiological changes in patients taking lamotrigine remains to be elucidated.

Psychiatric   A 23-year-old woman with schizophrenia had *worsening of psychiatric symptoms* after exposure to lamotrigine (25[A]). This patient was taking quetiapine 400 mg/day and divalproex sodium 1500 mg/day. Because of excessive somnolence valproate was withdrawn and lamotrigine was started at 12.5 mg bd. On the second day the patient had worsening of psychotic symptoms, which the authors attributed to lamotrigine.

Two patients taking lamotrigine 225 and 200 mg/day developed forced normalization (26[c]). Lamotrigine led to seizure control and disappearance of interictal epileptiform discharges from the electroencephalogram. However, simultaneously they had de novo psychopathology and disturbed behavior. Reduction of the dose of lamotrigine led to disappearance of the symptoms and reappearance of the spikes but not the seizures.

Hematologic   Lamotrigine (mean daily dose 250 mg) did not change the concentrations of plasma total homocysteine, plasma and red cell folate, or plasma vitamin B_{12} after 32 weeks in 11 subjects (27[c]).

Skin   *Toxic epidermal necrolysis* has been associated with concomitant use of lamotrigine and carbamazepine (28[A]).

- A 25-year-old woman with epilepsy developed maculopapular eruptions on the skin with involvement of the mucous membrane 7 weeks after lamotrigine had been added to carbamazepine. She also had adult respiratory distress syndrome. After 3 days the skin lesions progressed to a generalized bullous eruption and desquamation. Lamotrigine and carbamazepine were withdrawn and she finally recovered completely.

Drug–drug interactions   In a review of the medical charts of 570 epilepsy outpatients 12 years and older co-medication with phenytoin, carbamazepine, and valproate sodium was the major predictor of lamotrigine serum concentrations (29[c]). Co-medication regimens with felbamate, oxcarbazepine, and phenobarbital were small but significant predictors. No other antiepileptic drugs (clobazam, gabapentin, levetiracetam, topiramate, vigabatrin, zonisamide), with the possible exception of oxcarbazepine, affected lamotrigine. Phenytoin increased lamotrigine clearance by about 125%, carbamazepine by about 30–50%, and oxcarbazepine slightly. Valproate reduced lamotrigine clearance by about 60%.

Levetiracetam *(SED-15, 2035;*
SEDA-27, 79; SEDA-28, 91; SEDA-29, 91)

Observational studies   The efficacy and tolerability of levetiracetam as add-on therapy in patients with refractory partial-onset seizures was evaluated in an open, single-arm study in 99 patients, in which an 8-week baseline period was followed by a 4-week titration period and a 12-week maintenance period (30[c]). The initial dosage was 1000 mg/day and it could be increased to 2000 mg/day after 2 weeks and to 3000 mg/day after another 2 weeks to obtain adequate seizure control; 1.2, 9.5, and 89% took the three doses respectively (mean daily dose 2373 mg). Mean treatment duration was 112 days. The most frequent drug-related adverse events (occurring in 5% or more of the 99 patients) were *fatigue* (27%), *somnolence* (11%), *headache* (8.1%), *dizziness* (8.1%), *nausea* (6.1%), and *lethargy* (6.1%). The most common adverse reactions (adverse events that were at least possibly related to the study drug) were *fatigue, somnolence*, and *dizziness*.

Levetiracetam has been evaluated in 285 children with refractory epilepsy in a prospective, multicenter, observational study, in which levetiracetam was used as an add-on open treatment (31[c]). The mean maximum dosage of levetiracetam was 48 mg/kg/day. Adverse effects occurred at a mean dosage of 46 mg/kg/day. There were no serious persistent adverse events. There was reversible *colitis* and an *apnea syndrome* in a child with phosphorylase-A kinase deficiency. Mild to moderate adverse effects were reported in 128 patients (45%): *somnolence* (24%), *general behavioral changes* (15%), *aggression* (11%), and *sleep disturbances* (3.2%). Mental retardation was associated with a poor response, more adverse effects, and earlier withdrawal.

In a multicenter, prospective, uncontrolled study of levetiracetam in 110 children with refractory epilepsy (21 patients under 4 years old) all were taking several other antiepileptic drugs when levetiracetam was started (32[c]). In general, levetiracetam was well tolerated. There were no significant laboratory anomalies. The main adverse events were *somnolence* and *irritability* (14%). In two patients treatment was withdrawn because of adverse effects. One patient developed severe acute *choreoathetosis* after a few days, reversible after levetiracetam withdrawal.

Levetiracetam 1000–3000 mg/day off label has been studied as a preventive agent in transformed migraine in an open study for 3 months in 36 patients aged at least 18 years (33[c]). Other preventive drugs were allowed if they had been used in a stable dose for over 30 days. Adverse events were reported by 18 patients. Eight patients withdrew because of adverse effects: *somnolence* ($n = 2$), *lack of concentration* ($n = 2$), and *chest tightness, constipation, anorgasmia,* and *ankle edema* (one each). The most common adverse events were *somnolence, weakness,* and *anxiety. Weight gain, depression,* and *emotional instability* also occurred.

Adults ($n = 16$) who met the DSM-IV criteria for social anxiety disorder were treated with either levetiracetam (500–3000 mg/day) or placebo for 7 weeks (34[C]). The mean dose of levetiracetam at the final visit was 2279 mg/day ($n = 9$). Two patients taking levetiracetam group withdrew, one because of severe *headache and drowsiness* and one because of *disinhibition and inebriation.*

In an open study in nine patients with Huntington's disease, levetiracetam up to 3000 mg/day for up to 48 days reduced the severity of the chorea as measured by the Unified Huntington's Disease Rating Scale (UHDRS) chorea subscore, but did not affect total motor scores (35[c]). *Somnolence* contributed to a 33% drop-out rate, and three patients developed *Parkinsonism.*

Of six patients given levetiracetam for essential tremor three withdrew, two because of *somnolence* (500 mg/day), one because of lack of efficacy (36[c]).

Comparative and placebo-controlled studies   Levetiracetam had a significantly lower withdrawal rate than topiramate (OR = 0.52;

95% CI = 0.29, 0.93) and oxcarbazepine (OR = 0.55; 95% CI = 0.33, 0.92), with comparable efficacy in patients with partial epilepsy (37[M]). Levetiracetam had a lower (but not significantly lower) withdrawal rate than tiagabine and zonisamide. Of the 672 patients who took levetiracetam 106 withdrew (16%) compared with 46 (13%) of 351 patients in the placebo groups. The Mantel–Haenszel Odds Ratios (95% CI) for withdrawal estimated from the meta-analysis of each drug compared with placebo were as follows: gabapentin 1.04 (0.67, 1.61), lamotrigine 1.16 (0.81, 1.66), levetiracetam 1.26 (0.86, 1.84), tiagabine 2.02 (1.30, 3.12), topiramate 2.42 (1.56, 3.74), oxcarbazepine 2.27 (1.62, 3.17), and zonisamide 1.78 (1.03, 3.08). The authors concluded that indirect comparisons based on meta-analysis showed that levetiracetam add-on therapy has a favorable responder and withdrawal rate relative to several other antiepileptic drugs in patients with partial epilepsy at the doses that are used in clinical trials.

Nervous system   Levetiracetam can cause *hypersomnia* (38[A]).

- A 65-year-old woman with focal symptomatic epilepsy that was difficult to treat developed increased sleep needs (hypersomnia) in the absence of subjective excessive disabling daytime sleepiness when the dosage of levetiracetam as add-on treatment to carbamazepine 1350 mg/day was increased to 2000 mg/day. Actigraphy, polysomnography, and multiple sleep latency tests showed that these symptoms may have been due an increase in sleep propensity.

The authors argued that increased sleep needs in the absence of subjective sleepiness may be due to an effect of levetiracetam on specific brain structures, although the exact mechanism by which levetiracetam causes hypersomnia is unclear.

- A 58-year old man with Huntington's disease took levetiracetam to reduce symptoms of chorea and developed parkinsonism, lethargy, and daytime somnolence after 6 weeks (39[A]). The dosage of levetiracetam was reduced from 750 to 500 mg/day but the symptoms and signs of parkinsonism (resting tremor, rigidity, increased dystonia, and gait difficulty) persisted. Levetiracetam was withdrawn; the adverse effects resolved completely within 7 days and the chorea returned to baseline.

Electrolyte balance   Levetiracetam has been associated with *hyponatremia* in a patient who was initially treated with carbamazepine and developed hyponatremia (sodium concentration 122 mmol/l) with complex partial status epilepticus (40[A]). Repeated introduction of levetiracetam 500 mg bd after withdrawal of carbamazepine resulted in a worsening of the hyponatremia (117 mmol/l). Levetiracetam was withdrawn and the sodium concentration normalized after 2 days.

Drug–drug interactions   The effect of levetiracetam on the pharmacokinetics of other antiepileptic drugs has been analysed using data from randomized clinical trials (41[C]). Serum concentrations were measured at baseline and after the addition of levetiracetam (1000–4000 mg/day) or placebo in four phase 3 studies in patients with refractory partial epilepsy receiving stable dosages of other antiepileptic drugs. Levetiracetam did not alter mean steady-state serum concentrations of carbamazepine, gabapentin, lamotrigine, phenobarbital, phenytoin, primidone, or valproic acid. For vigabatrin, there was no significant change in serum drug concentration after the addition of levetiracetam, but the number of observations was too small to allow a final conclusion.

Oxcarbazepine   (SED-15, 2646; SEDA-27, 79; SEDA-28, 94; SEDA-29, 93)

Observational studies   In an open study in 24 infants and young children (mean age 20 months; range 2–45) with partial seizures, the dosage of oxcarbazepine was titrated from 10 to 60 mg/kg/day (42[c]). The treatment phase of 30 days (completed by 19 patients) was followed by an extension phase of 6 months (completed by 13 patients). The most common adverse events during the treatment phase were *pyrexia* (n = 5), *irritability* (n = 5), and *somnolence* (n = 7). The most common adverse events during the extension phase were *pyrexia* (n = 9), *ear infections* (n = 9), *pharyngitis* (n = 5).

The effects of oxcarbazepine have been studied retrospectively in 175 Finnish patients, of whom 97 used oxcarbazepine as their first drug (Group I), and 78 as second monotherapy (Group II) after failure of a previous drug (43[c]).

The 1-year retention rates of oxcarbazepine treatment were 91% in Group I and 77% in Group II. Withdrawals were due to unspecified adverse effects in three patients in Group I and 11 in Group II, and due to lack of efficacy in two patients in Group I and six in Group II.

In 70 patients (aged 5–12 years) with newly diagnosed benign childhood epilepsy with centrotemporal spikes (BECTS) who took oxcarbazepine monotherapy for 18 months there was sustained cessation of seizures in 53% of patients (44[c]). A further 21% had some relapses but were subsequently rendered seizure free, 21% had a greater than 50% improvement, and 5% did not improve. Interictal epileptiform activity normalized in 58%, 35% had an improvement in the grade of electroencephalographic pathology, and 7% had no change at all. The initial mildly weak scores in isolated cognitive domains did not deteriorate, and even improved in some cases, with concomitant electroencephalographic improvement or normalization and effective seizure control. There were transient adverse effects, including *headache* ($n = 4$), *drowsiness* ($n = 3$), *weight gain* ($n = 3$), and *irritability, skin rash*, and *insomnia* (one each). One patient developed asymptomatic *hyponatremia* below 125 mmol/l, which normalized within 1 month while the patient continued to take the same daily dose. There were no intolerable adverse effects necessitating drug withdrawal.

Comparative studies   In a single-blind, randomized study oxcarbazepine and carbamazepine were compared in the treatment of alcohol withdrawal in 29 patients (45[c]). The carbamazepine group took 600 mg on days 1–3, 300 mg on day 4, and 100 mg on day 5. The oxcarbazepine group took 900 mg on days 1–3, 450 mg on day 4, and 150 mg on day 5. Those who took oxcarbazepine had significantly fewer withdrawal symptoms and reported significantly less "craving for alcohol". There was no difference in adverse effects, autonomic parameters, or cognition processing. The authors concluded that oxcarbazepine might be a useful alternative to carbamazepine in the treatment of alcohol withdrawal. Confirmation in a larger study is needed.

Electrolyte balance   Drug-induced *hyponatremia* is commonly attributed to the syndrome of inappropriate antidiuretic hormones

(SIADH). A 28-year-old woman with secondary antiphospholipid syndrome developed asymptomatic hyponatremia secondary to excessive water intake after using oxcarbazepine (46[A]). This suggests a new mechanism for oxcarbazepine-induced hyponatremia.

Sexual function   *Priapism* has been attributed to oxcarbazepine (47[A]).

• A 16-year-old boy with a bipolar disorder and pervasive developmental disorder, who was taking lithium 600 mg bd and aripiprazole 5 mg/day, became increasingly hypersexual and irritable. Oxcarbazepine 300 mg bd was added and on day 4 the dosage of oxcarbazepine was increased to 300 mg in the morning and 600 mg at night. Within 48 hours he had two discrete episodes of prolonged painless penile erection, each lasting about 30 minutes. Oxcarbazepine was withdrawn and he had no further episodes.

In the FDA labelling, priapism is listed as being associated with oxcarbazepine. The authors cautioned that lithium and atypical neuroleptic drugs have also been reported to be associated with prolonged penile erection.

Teratogenicity   Exposure to antiepileptic drugs during the first trimester of pregnancy has been associated with an increased risk of major congenital anomalies in the offspring. However, most studies have been fraught with methodological shortcomings, and differences in ascertainment methods and classifications prevent data pooling. Individual studies have lacked the statistical power to assess the risks associated with specific drugs. Information about drugs other than lamotrigine and oxcarbazepine is scant. Although the teratogenic effects of lamotrigine and oxcarbazepine have not been established with certainty, no investigations to date have identified any statistically significant difference in the rates of major congenital anomalies between infants exposed to lamotrigine or oxcarbazepine and infants exposed to carbamazepine (48[R]).

Susceptibility factors

Children   Relatively few well-designed studies have shown the long-term safety and tolerability of newer antiepileptic drugs in a large group of children. Extensive clinical data from the worldwide Clinical Development Program and a compassionate use program on the safety and tolerability of oxcarbazepine in children have been reported (49ᶜ). Oxcarbazepine is indicated for use as monotherapy and adjunctive therapy in children with partial epilepsy (in the USA at 4 years of age and in Europe at 6 years of age). The most common adverse events (10%) in the Clinical Development Program were *headache* (33%), *somnolence* (32%), *vomiting* (28%), and *dizziness* (23%), whereas in the compassionate use program the most common adverse events (1%) were *rash* (2.7%), *fatigue* (1.6%), *nausea* (1.2%), and *somnolence* (1.2%).

Phenobarbital   *(SED-15, 2798;*
SEDA-28, 95; SEDA-29, 95)

Susceptibility factors

Age   The effect of age on the pharmacokinetics of phenobarbital at steady state has been studied in 224 patients aged 65 years and older (mean 73) taking long-term phenobarbital using concentration measurements from the database of a monitoring service (50ᶜ). Controls aged 20–50 (mean 36) years were matched for sex, weight, and type of anticonvulsant co-medication. The apparent oral clearance of phenobarbital was significantly lower in the elderly patients. Co-medication with carbamazepine and phenytoin was associated with a moderate reduction in phenobarbital clearance. The authors concluded that age-related reduction in phenobarbital clearance may have clinical implications: elderly patients require smaller dosages, and monitoring the clinical response and serum concentrations may be of special importance in this age group. Besides age, co-medication is important in explaining some of the variation in phenobarbital pharmacokinetics.

Phenytoin and fosphenytoin
(SED-15, 2813; SEDA-27, 80; SEDA-28, 95;
SEDA-29, 95)

Nervous system   The hypothesis that routine use of phenytoin for seizure prophylaxis after subarachnoid hemorrhage may adversely affect neurological and cognitive recovery has been tested in 527 patients (51ᶜ). A so called "phenytoin burden" for each patient was calculated by multiplying the average serum phenytoin concentration by the time in days between the first and last measurements, up to a maximum of 14 days from ictus. Functional outcome at 14 days and 3 months was measured using the modified Rankin scale; a poor functional outcome was defined as dependence or worse (modified Rankin Scale 4 or more). Cognitive outcomes were assessed at 14 days and 3 months by telephone interview. Phenytoin burden was associated with a poor functional outcome at 14 days, but not at 3 months. Higher quartiles of phenytoin burden were associated with *worse cognitive status scores* at hospital discharge and at 3 months. 5% of the patients had seizures in the hospital and this was associated with a poor functional outcome at 14 days in a univariate analysis only.

In a small open pilot study phenytoin was associated with *changes in brain structure* in nine patients with post-traumatic stress disorder, with a significant 6% increase in right brain volume, as measured by a specific volumetric MRI method (52ᶜ). Increased hippocampal volume correlated with a reduction in symptom severity. Phenytoin did not have a significant effect on depression or anxiety. The authors speculated that the effect of phenytoin on glutamatergic function could have explained these findings.

Immunologic   Aromatic anticonvulsant agents, such as carbamazepine and phenytoin, can cause the *anticonvulsant hypersensitivity syndrome* (53ᴬ).

- A 53-year-old woman took phenytoin 300 mg/day for 1 month following a generalized tonic–clonic seizure. Because she developed symptoms and signs of phenytoin overdose and a rash the phenytoin was temporarily withdrawn and later restarted. A couple of days later she developed a fever, symptoms and signs of acute respiratory distress, a generalized maculopapular rash, vaginal bleeding, and multiorgan dysfunction, including rhabdomyolysis. Skin biopsy showed changes consistent with Stevens–Johnson syndrome. The lesions progressed to toxic epidermal necrolysis. After treatment with glucocorticoids and extubation she required intermittent hemodialysis and skin care for several weeks.

Teratogenicity Fragility in chromosome 10q23.3 was reported in a fetus exposed to phenytoin during pregnancy (54[A]).

Drug–drug interactions Phenytoin induces the metabolism of both *cyclophosphamide* and *thiotepa* (55[A]).

- A 42-year-old man with cancer was given two 4-day courses of high-dose chemotherapy with cyclophosphamide, thiotepa, and carboplatin, followed by peripheral blood progenitor cell support. From 5 days before the start of the second course the patient received phenytoin for epileptic seizures. Exposure to 4-hydroxycyclophosphamide (the active metabolite of cyclophosphamide) and tepa (the main active metabolite of thiotepa) during the second course increased by 51 and 115% respectively, compared with the first course, whereas exposure to cyclophosphamide and thiotepa was significantly reduced (67 and 29% respectively).

℞ *Pregabalin*   (SEDA-28, 56)

Like gabapentin, pregabalin (3-isobutyl GABA) binds to the alpha-2 delta subunit of voltage-gated calcium channels. It has been evaluated in patients with chronic post-herpetic neuralgia, painful diabetic peripheral neuropathy, generalized anxiety disorder, fibromyalgia syndrome, and refractory partial seizures. The usual dosage regimen is 150–600 mg/day. Pregabalin is eliminated unchanged by the kidneys. It does not induce CYP3A4, and no pharmacokinetic drug interactions have been reported.

Placebo-controlled trials

Generalized anxiety disorder In a double-blind, fixed-dose, parallel-group, placebo- and active-controlled, multicenter, 4-week study, 271 patients with generalized anxiety disorder were randomized to pregabalin 50 mg tds (n = 70), pregabalin 200 mg tds (n = 66), placebo (n = 67), or lorazepam 2 mg tds (n = 68), followed by a 1-week double-blind taper (56[C]). The adjusted mean change scores on the Hamilton Anxiety Scale were significantly improved by pregabalin 200 mg tds, and the most common adverse events were somnolence and dizziness, which were usually mild or moderate in intensity and were often transient.*

In a similar placebo-controlled study pregabalin 200, 400, or 450 mg/day, in two or three

divided doses, was generally well tolerated (57[C]). Dizziness, somnolence, dry mouth, euphoria, blurred vision, incoordination, and flatulence were the most common adverse events and were generally mild to moderate. The incidences of dizziness were 35, 49, and 42% with pregabalin 200, 400, and 450 mg/day (15% with placebo). The incidences of somnolence were 31, 37, and 24% (13% with placebo). The incidences of dry mouth were 24, 27, and 17% (2–10% with placebo). Withdrawals caused by adverse events occurred in 9–13% (8% with placebo). Twice-daily and thrice-daily dosing had similar efficacy and tolerability.

Post-herpetic neuralgia The safety of oral pregabalin 150–600 mg/day in three randomized, double-blind, placebo-controlled, multicenter studies in post-herpetic neuralgia lasting 8–13 weeks in a total of 779 evaluable patients has been reviewed (58[M]). Pregabalin was superior to placebo in relieving pain and improving pain-related sleep interference. It was generally well tolerated when force-titrated over 1 week to fixed dosages (maximum 600 mg/day) in trials that enrolled mostly elderly patients. Dizziness, somnolence, peripheral edema, headache, dry mouth, and diarrhea were the most common adverse events and were generally mild to moderate. The incidences of dizziness with pregabalin 150, 300, and 600 mg/day were 12, 28, and 28% respectively (12–15% with placebo). The incidences of somnolence were 15, 24, and 25% (7% with placebo). The incidences of peripheral edema were 3, 13, and 19% with pregabalin (0–2% with placebo). Withdrawal rates due to adverse effects were 11, 16, and 32% with pregabalin (5–10% with placebo). Somnolence was cited as the most common reason for discontinuing pregabalin.*

A fourth trial of pregabalin in chronic post-herpetic neuralgia has been presented in detail (59[C]). It was a 12-week randomized, double-blind, multicenter, placebo-controlled, parallel-group study in patients with chronic post-herpetic neuralgia or painful diabetic peripheral neuropathy. Patients were randomized to placebo (n = 65) or to one of two pregabalin regimens: a flexible schedule of 150, 300, 450, or 600 mg/day with weekly dose escalation based on patients' individual responses and tolerability (n = 141) or a fixed schedule of 300 mg/day for 1 week followed by 600 mg/day for 11 weeks (n = 132). The most common adverse events in those taking pregabalin were dizziness, peripheral edema, weight gain (not affecting diabetes control), and somnolence. The adverse events that most often led to withdrawal of pregabalin were dizziness (2–8%), nausea (1–6%), vertigo (2–3%), and somnolence (0–4%).

Painful diabetic neuropathy   In a 6-week, randomized, double-blind, multicenter placebo-controlled study of pregabalin, 246 men and women with painful diabetic neuropathy took pregabalin 150 or 600 mg/day; dizziness was the most common adverse effect (60[C]).

Fibromyalgia syndrome   In a multicenter, double-blind, 8-week, randomized, placebo-controlled trial of pregabalin 150, 300, and 450 mg/day on pain, sleep, fatigue, and health-related quality of life in 529 patients with fibromyalgia syndrome the most common adverse events with 150, 300, and 450 mg/day were dizziness (23, 32, 49%), somnolence (16, 28, 28%), headache (12, 28, 28%), dry mouth (6.8, 6.0, 13%), peripheral edema (5.3, 6.7, 11%), infection (8.3, 9.7, 9.8%), weakness (5.3, 9.0, 8.3%), euphoria (1.5, 8.2, 7.6%), abnormal thoughts (5.3, 3.7, 7.6%), and weight gain (7.6, 9.7, 6.8%) (61[C]). Rates of withdrawal because of adverse events were similar across all four treatment groups.

Seizures   Pregabalin for add-on treatment in refractory partial seizures has been evaluated in several trials (62[M]). In 758 patients in three fixed-dose studies the most common adverse effects were related to the central nervous system, and these were responsible for most withdrawals. Dizziness (29%), somnolence (21%), and ataxia (13%) were the most common. Other adverse effects that occurred in more than 10% of patients were weakness (11%) and weight gain (10 versus 1.4% with placebo). Weight gain, defined as a 7% or more increase from baseline, occurred in 18% of patients taking pregabalin and 2.2% of patients taking placebo when baseline was compared with the last visit carried forward. Overall, pregabalin caused a mean gain of 2.1 kg over 3 months. Pregabalin was withdrawn because of adverse effects in 5.3% for dizziness, 3.3% for somnolence, 3.0% for ataxia, 1.8% for weakness, and 0.4%

for weight gain. The profile of adverse effects was similar in longer open trials, in which the four most common adverse effects were dizziness (33 with 1.4% withdrawals), somnolence (27 with 1.6% withdrawals), accidental injury (26 with 0.3% withdrawals), and weight gain (22 with 2.0% withdrawals). Most adverse effects were mild to moderate. They were usually dose-related and started in the first 2 weeks of treatment. Pregabalin was also associated with weight gain, which appeared to be dose-related and was seen in up to 14% of patients taking 600 mg/day.

Pregabalin add-on treatment for refractory partial seizures was evaluated in a fixed-dose and a flexible-dose regimen in a double-blind evaluated, placebo-controlled study (63[C]). Most adverse events were mild or moderate. With the exception of weight gain, the adverse events tended to become less frequent or even to resolve during continued treatment. Adverse events that were reported by 10% or more of 131 patients taking a fixed dose of 600 mg/day compared with a flexible dose of 150–600 mg/day were dizziness (43 and 24%), ataxia (21 and 9.2%), weight gain of 7% or more (20 and 19%), weakness (18 and 17%), somnolence (18 and 19%), vertigo (14 and 11%), diplopia (12 and 6.1%), amblyopia and blurred vision (10 and 2.3%). Reasons for withdrawal were dizziness (14 and 5.3%), ataxia (13 and 3.1%), weight gain (0 and 0%), weakness (2.2 and 0.8%), somnolence (6.6 and 1.5%), vertigo (6.6 and 2.3%), diplopia (4.4 and 1.5%), amblyopia (1.5 and 0.8%), and headache (2.2 and 0%). There was a higher withdrawal rate in the first week of treatment in the fixed-dose group (24 versus 3%). Efficacy was better in the fixed-dose group but tolerability was better in the flexible-dose group.

In a 12-week multicenter, double-blind, randomized, parallel-group, placebo-controlled study of pregabalin 600 mg/day either twice or thrice daily in refractory partial epilepsy the four most common adverse events for the two respective regimens were dizziness (42 and 38%), somnolence (30 and 23%), ataxia (17 and 27%), and weight gain (20 and 15%) (64[C]).

Systematic review   Several of the studies quoted above, in post-herpetic neuralgia, peripheral neuropathy, generalized anxiety, and refractory partial epilepsy (four trials each), have been reviewed (65^M). Most of the reported adverse effects were mild to moderate, were usually dose-related, and started in the first 2 weeks of treatment. Up to 33% of patients taking pregabalin and 10% of those taking placebo withdrew because of adverse effects, which were most often related to the central nervous system. Somnolence and dizziness (in up to 50 and 42% of patients respectively) and peripheral edema in neuropathic pain (19%), ataxia in epilepsy (27%), and headache in anxiety (29%) were the most common adverse events. Other adverse effects that occurred in more than 10% of patients, in decreasing order, were abnormal thinking, weakness, nervousness, amblyopia, amnesia, diarrhea, and incoordination. Pregabalin was also associated with weight gain, which appeared to be dose-related and was seen in up to 14% of patients taking 600 mg/day. The mean weight gain from baseline was 0.50–2.28 kg. Four of 19 patients from one center had myoclonus associated with pregabalin. Severe adverse events were infrequent and were seen in both the pregabalin and the placebo groups; they included accidental injuries, rash, hemiparesis, ventricular asystole, and colitis. There were three deaths due to cardiac arrest, but one was in a patient taking placebo and the other two were not considered to be related to pregabalin. Rapid withdrawal of pregabalin resulted in anxiety, nervousness, and irritability in the anxiety trials; it is not known if similar withdrawal symptoms occur in patients using pregabalin for conditions other than anxiety.

Nervous system   The most frequent adverse effects of pregabalin in the treatment of neuropathic pain are dizziness (12–28%), somnolence (15–25%), and peripheral edema (3–13%) (66^R). These effects are dose-related in the therapeutic range of doses (i.e. are collateral effects) and are usually mild to moderate. Other nervous system adverse effects include weakness (6–10%), ataxia (3–10%), headache (6–9%), blurred vision (3–10%), tremor (3–11%), lack of coordination (2–10%), and confusion (incidence unreported).

Encephalopathy with focal brain edema has been described after pregabalin withdrawal in a patient who seems to have been reported twice (67^A, 68^A).

• An 80-year old woman with post-herpetic neuralgia abruptly stopped taking pregabalin and 30 hours later developed unexplained nausea, headache, and ataxia, progressing to delirium 8 days later. An MRI brain scan showed T2 hyperintense lesions in the splenium.

Similar MRI abnormalities, interpreted as focal vasogenic edema, develop in some patients with epilepsy after rapid withdrawal of anticonvulsants and patients with high-altitude cerebral edema have abnormalities and the same neurological symptoms. This case is the first to associate abnormalities in the splenium with neurological symptoms after withdrawal of a gabapentin-type anticonvulsant, and is among the first in a patient without epilepsy, suggesting that sudden anticonvulsant withdrawal alone, unaccompanied by seizures, can initiate symptomatic focal brain edema. The similarity of this syndrome to high-altitude cerebral edema suggests a possible common pathophysiology and offers potential therapies.

Of 19 patients with refractory partial epilepsy four had new-onset myoclonic seizures on starting pregabalin (69^c). One had focal myoclonic jerks of the left arm, and the others had multifocal myoclonus.

In other patients aggravation of seizures was dose-related; it reduced in intensity and frequency on dosage reduction and disappeared when pregabalin was withdrawn (70^c).

• An 89-year-old woman developed severe asterixis after taking pregabalin 150 mg/day for postherpetic pain (71^A). She had prominent negative myoclonus in all limbs, but slightly more in the arms. The asterixis severely impaired standing and walking and also led to recurrent falls. Other causes of asterixis, such as metabolic disorders, focal brain lesions, and inflammation, were excluded by laboratory tests, cerebrospinal fluid analysis, and CT scanning. Withdrawal led to rapid improvement.

Drug–drug interactions   Drug interactions with other antiepileptic drugs (carbamazepine, lamotrigine, phenytoin, and valproate) have been studied in patients taking pregabalin 600 mg/day (200 mg tds) for 7 days (72^c). Trough steady-state concentrations of the other drugs were not affected by pregabalin. Likewise, pregabalin steady-state pharmacokinetics were not affected by the other drugs and were similar to those previously observed in healthy subjects taking pregabalin alone. The combinations were generally well tolerated.

Tiagabine   *(SED-15, 3419; SEDA-29, 95)*

Observational studies   Tiagabine has been evaluated in a multicenter open study in 243 patients with uncontrolled partial seizures (73[c]). It was given as adjunctive therapy and titrated stepwise to a target of 40 mg/day, in two or three divided doses, during a 12-week fixed-schedule titration period, followed by a 12-week flexible continuation period. Adverse events were more frequent during the titration period than the continuation period. Most were mild and related to the nervous system. There were nine serious adverse events in those who took twice-daily tiagabine and two in those who took it thrice daily. Common adverse events (at least 5%) in the fixed-schedule titration period were *dizziness, somnolence, headache, tremor, weakness, ataxia, confusion, nausea, pharyngitis, infections, depression, myoclonus, amblyopia*, and *amnesia*. Events related to the nervous system, such as *dizziness* and *headache*, were generally mild. There were no clinically significant changes in clinical chemistry, hematology, or vital signs.

In an open study of tiagabine as augmentation therapy for anxiety (*n* = 18) *cognitive slowing* was the most common adverse event (in 44%) (74[c]). Other adverse events were *somnolence* (22%) and *headache, insomnia, rash, flu-like syndrome*, and *raised alanine transaminase activity* (11% each). These adverse events were mild to moderate and no serious adverse events were reported. Two patients withdrew because of adverse effects.

Gastrointestinal   In a 3-month open comparative study 91 patients with chronic pain were randomized to gabapentin (maximum dose 2400 mg/day) or tiagabine (24 mg/day) (75[c]). Four patients taking tiagabine *gastric disturbances* led to withdrawal from the study.

Topiramate   *(SED-15, 3447; SEDA-27, 81; SEDA-28, 96; SEDA-29, 96)*

Observational studies   In an open study in 211 patients with treatment-resistant focal epilepsy, topiramate was given in a target dosage of 200 mg/day over a 1-month titration period (76[c]). In the subsequent 6-month maintenance period, the dosage was varied according to the clinical effect (median topiramate dose 300 mg/day). Topiramate was generally well tolerated and adverse events were mild and transient. There was at least one adverse event in 107 patients (51%). The most common was *weight loss*, which occurred in 13%, followed by *somnolence* (11%), *paresthesia* (10%), *insomnia* (9%), *emotional lability* (9%), *dizziness* (8%), and *fatigue* (7%); other adverse effects, mostly affecting the nervous system, were rare. Few patients withdrew from the study because of adverse events (7%).

In an open study topiramate was used as monotherapy over 2 years in 692 adults and children with different types and syndromes of epilepsy (77[c]). The dosage was individually adjusted to a maximum of 400 (median 125) mg/day in adults or 9 (median 3.3) mg/kg/day in children under 12 years. There were adverse events in 65% and serious adverse events in 7.8%. The most frequent adverse event was *paresthesia* (16%). Other frequent adverse events (in at least 5%) were *headache* (13%), *anorexia* (8.4%), *weight loss* (8.4%), *nausea* (7.1%), *dizziness* (6.5%), and *somnolence* (5.2%). There were *kidney stones* in two patients (leading to withdrawal in one). Adverse effects were mostly mild. In 7.6% the dosage of topiramate was adjusted and in 9.2% topiramate was withdrawn; 8.8% withdrew from the study because of adverse events.

Comparative studies   In a randomized 12-week study 31 men with pathologic gambling were randomized to either topiramate (*n* = 15) or fluvoxamine (*n* = 16) (78[c]). Twelve of the 15 patients from the topiramate group completed the 12-week treatment. Two of the dropouts had topiramate-associated adverse events, such as *lack of concentration, dizziness*, and *vertigo*.

In a comparative cross-sectional study of the adverse effects of topiramate and lamotrigine in children, lamotrigine caused adverse effects less often than topiramate; however, both medications were generally well tolerated and events were classified as mild to moderate (19[c]). Half of the children who took topiramate had an adverse event, compared with one-third of the children who took lamotrigine. The adverse events were mostly related to the nervous system, occurred early in treatment, and were more frequent when topiramate was given as adjunctive therapy. *Poor appetite, drowsiness, speech difficulties*, and *weight loss* were observed only with topiramate, *rash* and *headaches* only with lamotrigine. *Nervousness* and *seizure aggravation* were more frequent with topiramate. There were *sleep disturbances* with lamotrigine.

Placebo-controlled studies　In a randomized, placebo-controlled study obese subjects with hypertension took topiramate 96 mg/day ($n = 175$) or 192 mg/day ($n = 178$) (79[C]). Adverse events were mostly related to the nervous system and included *paresthesia, fatigue, taste disturbance, loss of appetite*, and *difficulty in concentration and attention*. Paresthesia was the most common adverse event, in 33%, and was attributed to inhibition of carbonic anhydrase. The proportions of patients who withdrew because of adverse effects were 7% with placebo, 14% with topiramate 96 mg/day, and 15% with 192 mg/day. There were serious adverse events possibly related to topiramate in five patients: vertigo, hypesthesia, tremor, fatigue, psychomotor slowing, and renal pain.

In a 10-week, randomized, double-blind, placebo-controlled trial topiramate was evaluated in 30 patients with bulimia nervosa (80[C]). There were significant changes in the frequency of binging/purging, body weight, and quality of life compared with placebo. According to the authors all the patients tolerated topiramate well.

In a 4-week, multicenter, randomized, double-blind, placebo-controlled study in 65 children aged 6–17 years with bipolar disorder, the most common adverse events with topiramate included *reduced appetite* (28%), *nausea* (24%), *diarrhea* (14%), and *paresthesia* (14%) (81[C]). Of these, only reduced appetite and nausea were more common during topiramate therapy. One patient in each group withdrew because of adverse effects. Topiramate caused significant *weight loss* compared with placebo; the mean change in body weight from baseline to final visit was −1.76 compared with +0.95 kg with placebo; however, none withdrew because of weight loss.

Retrospective studies　Topiramate add-on treatment in juvenile myoclonic epilepsy has been evaluated post-hoc in a subgroup of 22 patients from two 20-week multicenter, double-blind, randomized, placebo-controlled studies (82[C]). The target dose of topiramate was 400 mg/day (adults) or 6 mg/kg/day (children). The most common adverse events in the topiramate-treated patients ($n = 11$) were *nausea* ($n = 5$), *insomnia* ($n = 3$), *upper respiratory tract infections* ($n = 3$), and *abnormal vision, reduced appetite, difficulty in concentration/attention, diarrhea, epistaxis*, and *flu-like symptoms* ($n = 2$ each). Two patients taking topiramate withdrew because of adverse events.

A retrospective parental survey of 21 children aged 6–18 years demonstrated the efficacy and safety of topiramate in the treatment of chronic daily headache (average dose 30 mg/day) (83[C]). In those who responded to treatment there were no adverse events. Of the eight non-responders, six discontinued topiramate because they thought it was ineffective. Another complained of *abdominal problems and mild paresthesia*, and another non-responder had *dysphoria and hallucinations* while taking only 25 mg/day.

The time course of adverse events in 264 patients with focal epilepsy taking topiramate 200 mg/day added to carbamazepine has been evaluated in a post hoc analysis of data from a 12-week multicenter, double-blind, placebo-controlled trial in three groups of adults with refractory focal epilepsy (84[C]). The only significant adverse events were *nervousness* and *paresthesia*, which were more frequent in those taking topiramate (9 versus 2%). The average adverse event time was longer with topiramate than with placebo. Of the 10 most common single adverse events when topiramate was gradually titrated to 200 mg/day, the daily incidence of seven adverse events (*somnolence, loss of appetite, nervousness, fatigue, dizziness, upper respiratory tract infection*, and *vertigo*) peaked during titration and then fell to rates similar to placebo. The daily incidence of paresthesia increased during titration and was maintained for the duration of the study. Relatively few patients had cognitive symptoms (9% with topiramate, 5% with placebo). However, *cognitive adverse effects* were the most common reason for withdrawal of treatment. In those taking topiramate there was average *weight loss* of 2.0 kg.

Sensory systems　Topiramate may be associated with *acute myopia* and *secondary angle* *closure glaucoma*. Up to March 2004 the Spanish System of Pharmacovigilance collected six reports of myopia and two of glaucoma in eight patients who had taken topiramate 25–100 mg/day (85[c]). These adverse events occurred early in the course of treatment and were reversible after withdrawal.

Psychiatric   Topiramate has been associated with several psychiatric adverse events, such as *nervousness, depression, behavioral problems, mood lability*, and *psychosis*. *Obsessive–compulsive disorder* has also been reported (86[A]).

- A 19-year-old man with focal epilepsy took carbamazepine 1000 mg/day and lamotrigine 300 mg/day. Because his seizures persisted topiramate was added up to 200 mg/day and the dose of carbamazepine was reduced to 300 mg/day. Behavioral problems started within a week and worsened over the following months. He finally developed obsessive-compulsive disorder. Citalopram was given in doses up to 60 mg/day and topiramate was tapered within 2 weeks. The symptoms improved.

The authors discussed the hypothesis of a coincidental finding as well as the development of an alternative psychosis but finally attributed the patient's psychiatric disorder to topiramate.

Three patients with *hypomania* associated with topiramate have been reported. All had chronic mood disorders and all developed symptoms of hypomania soon after starting to take topiramate titrated up to 100 mg/day in addition to pre-existing psychotropic drugs (87[c]). The authors speculated that the antidepressant effects of topiramate had caused hypomania by release of monoamine neurotransmitters.

Metabolism   Topiramate commonly causes *weight loss*. In an 8-week, double-blind, placebo-controlled study of topiramate 250 mg/day in the treatment of aggression in 42 men with borderline personality disorder there was significant weight loss of 5.0 kg (95% CI = 3.4, 6.5) (88[C]). There were no psychotic symptoms or other serious adverse events. Some patients complained of *fatigue, dizziness, headache*, or *paresthesia*.

In a 10-week randomized, double-blind, study in 64 women with recurrent major depressive disorder, the dosage of topiramate was titrated up to 200 mg/day (89[C]). There were

no serious adverse effects, including psychotic symptoms and suicidal acts. Adverse effects such as *headache, fatigue, dizziness*, and *paresthesia* were rated as mild. After 10 weeks there was *weight loss*, which was usually regarded as beneficial.

Acid-base balance   Since topiramate can be associated with *metabolic acidosis* in both children and adults the incidence and magnitude of the effect of topiramate on serum bicarbonate concentrations in an adult population have been evaluated in a retrospective cohort study in 54 patients (40 women), of whom 26 had low serum bicarbonate concentrations while taking topiramate (mean concentration 18.8 mmol/l, range 13–21) (90[c]). However, this was not associated with any clinically significant problems.

Sexual function   Topiramate can be associated with *erectile dysfunction* (91[A]).

- A 37-year-old man with cryptogenic frontal lobe epilepsy took topiramate up to 200 mg/day as adjunctive therapy while taking carbamazepine 1200 mg/day and valproate 900 mg/day. Two weeks after reaching the maximal dose of topiramate he complained of erectile dysfunction. After withdrawal of topiramate, sexual function was completely restored within 1 month.
- A 43-year-old man with cryptogenic temporal lobe epilepsy was randomized to topiramate during a multicenter study, and 4 weeks after the target dose of 100 mg/day had been reached reported erectile dysfunction. Withdrawal of topiramate resulted in normal sexual function within 2 weeks.

The authors speculated that erectile dysfunction with topiramate may be due to low concentrations of free testosterone after increased hepatic metabolism.

Body temperature   Severe *hyperthermia* resulting in residual cerebellar and cognitive dysfunction has been reported in a patient taking topiramate (92[A]).

- A 27-year-old man was found unconscious with generalized status epilepticus. His rectal temperature was 42.9 °C, blood pressure 94/42 mmHg, pulse 155/minute, and respiratory rate 30/minute. He was intubated and his epileptic seizures were controlled with different antiepileptic drugs. He developed acute renal insufficiency secondary to rhabdomyolysis and disseminated intravascular coagulation. One week after the episode of hyperthermia he developed action tremors of the hands, bilateral dysmetria, head tremor, and severe gait disturbances. He was unable to stand. He had been taking topiramate 200 mg bd for aggressive behavior for 2 years with lorazepam 1 mg bd. After withdrawal of topiramate he improved. However, 11 months later he was still having bilateral arm and head tremors and slurred speech.

The authors attributed severe heatstroke to topiramate and suggested that the underlying mechanism of disturbed thermoregulation may have been related to inhibition of carbonic anhydrase, which is involved in sweat production and thermoregulation.

Drug–drug interactions   *Enzyme-inducing co-medication* can reduce serum topiramate concentrations by about a half in children and one-third in adults. The steady-state pharmacokinetics of topiramate have been compared in 70 children and 70 adults with epilepsy (93[c]). In the absence of enzyme-inducing co-medications, the mean oral clearance of topiramate was 42% higher in children than in adults. Co-medication with enzyme-inducing antiepileptic drugs increased the apparent oral clearance of topiramate by about 1.5–2 times. The oral clearance of topiramate was highest in young children and fell progressively with age until puberty, presumably because of age-dependent changes in the rate of drug metabolism. The authors suggested that younger patients may require higher dosages to achieve serum topiramate concentrations comparable with those found in older children and adults.

The effect of enzyme induction by *carbamazepine* on the pharmacokinetics and metabolic profile of topiramate has been studied in 20 healthy volunteers who took a single oral dose of topiramate 200 mg on two randomized occasions, once alone and once on day 18 of a 24-day course of carbamazepine (maintenance dosage 600 mg/day) (94[c]). There were no serious adverse events. Those possibly related to topiramate alone (somnolence, taste alteration, and paresthesia in four subjects) were mild to moderate. Topiramate concentrations in the urine were unchanged by carbamazepine, although mean oral clearance increased twofold.

Valproate sodium and semisodium (divalproex)   *(SED-15, 3579; SEDA-27, 82; SEDA-28, 99; SEDA-29, 97)*

Observational studies   The tolerability of antiepileptic drugs has been examined in 780 adult and adolescent patients with newly diagnosed epilepsy presenting with a range of seizure types and epilepsy syndromes over 20 years period (95[c]). Sodium valproate (n = 315), carbamazepine (n = 312), and lamotrigine (n = 249) were the most common drugs prescribed as first monotherapy. Seizure freedom was achieved with modest or moderate daily doses (median carbamazepine 400 mg, valproate 1000 mg, lamotrigine 150 mg) in most of the patients who achieved remission. The time to the first seizure did not differ among the three drugs. Adverse effects leading to withdrawal were less common with valproate (7%) and lamotrigine (7%) than with carbamazepine (16%). Among the 178 patients taking valproate, 17 withdrew because of adverse effects—*rash, tiredness*, and *headache* in one patient each, *ataxia, weight gain*, and other adverse effects in two patients each, *tremor* in three patients, and *nausea or vomiting* in five. Sedation and mood changes were not seen.

In a community-based cross-sectional study using a questionnaire, patients with epilepsy were asked about complaints they had associated with the use of valproate and other antiepileptic drugs (3[c]). The complaints that were associated with valproate, with a threshold of 15% of patients were *weight gain* (22%), *fatigue and tremor* (21% each), *memory problems* (19%), and *tiredness* (19%).

Divalproex sodium and generic immediate-release valproic acid have been compared in a 6-year prospective clinical study of 9260 psychiatric admissions (96[c]). In-patients who initially took divalproex sodium had a 33% longer hospital stay and a 3.8% higher re-admission rate than patients who initially took valproic acid. Initial treatment with divalproex prolonged length of stay by 30% in patients taking divalproex and valproic acid during subsequent admissions. After other variables had been controlled by analysis of variance, the hospital stay of patients who continued to take the initial medication was 15% longer (2.0 days) for divalproex than valproic acid. Switching medications was more common for valproic acid, partly because of the study design. There was medication intolerance in about 6.4% more patients taking valproic acid than divalproex. However, switching from valproic acid to divalproex did not significantly prolong length of stay over that for continuous divalproex or increase the rehospitalization rate. The authors concluded that lower peak valproate concentrations with divalproex sodium may be associated with improved tolerance but less effectiveness. Modified-release divalproex could reduce effectiveness further and require higher doses. Thus, inpatients are better served by starting with generic valproic acid and by changing to modified-release divalproex only if intolerance occurs. This would save up to one-third of inpatient costs and two-thirds of a billion dollars yearly in medication costs.

Nervous system   Valproate causes postural tremor in 6–45% of patients. Its characteristics have not been quantitatively assessed, and it is not known whether the prevalence or severity of tremor is affected by the valproate formulation (modified-release versus conventional). In a prospective study, 18 consecutive patients with newly diagnosed focal or generalized epilepsy were assigned to valproate ($n = 10$) or modified-release valproate ($n = 8$) monotherapy (97^c). At baseline, the two groups had similar postural tremor amplitudes. At follow-up, after at least 8 weeks, those who had taken the modified-release formulation had remained at the same level, whereas those who had taken the conventional formulation had a significant *increase in tremor amplitude* despite comparable valproate doses and comparable plasma valproate concentrations. These results suggest that modified-release valproate may cause less tremor activity than conventional valproate. The mechanisms underlying this difference are unclear but may include greater peak:trough concentration variation.

The authors pointed out that reversible valproate-associated *parkinsonism*, which was originally reported in 1994, emerged only 4 years later in 1998 in the FDA's Adverse Event Reporting System (AERS). The apparent delay can be explained by the fact that the FDA adopted a new dictionary for coding adverse events in November 1997, before which extrapyramidal disorder, a more general term, was used for coding parkinsonism and Parkinson's

disease. These findings emphasize the need for clinicians to take the first step in post-marketing surveillance by reporting unanticipated possibly drug-related events to manufacturers and governmental agencies (98^{CR}).

Sensory systems   To investigate whether initial valproate monotherapy causes visual field defects and visual dysfunction, visual fields were examined in 18 patients with epilepsy (aged 18–50 years) who had taken valproate monotherapy for 2–20 years (99^c). None of the patients had vigabatrin-type concentric visual field defects. There were acquired color vision defects in two patients. All had normal contrast sensitivity. The authors concluded that valproate is not associated with visual field defects similar to vigabatrin, but can cause *abnormalities in color vision*.

Metabolism   The effects of valproate 2070 mg/day and lamotrigine 250 mg/day on total plasma homocysteine, plasma and erythrocyte folate, and plasma vitamin B_{12} concentrations have been studied in 20 patients with epilepsy before and after a 32-week period of monotherapy (27^c). Lamotrigine had no effect, but valproate caused a 57% *increase in plasma vitamin B_{12} concentrations* over baseline and a 27% *fall in plasma homocysteine concentrations*. The mechanisms of these changes are unknown. The data suggest that hyperhomocysteinemia may not be a serious clinical problem among patients with epilepsy taking lamotrigine or valproate.

Hematologic   *Fanconi syndrome* has been reported in a child taking valproate (100^A).

- A 2-year-old girl with mental retardation, quadriplegia, and epilepsy developed an autoimmune hemolytic anemia and renal Fanconi syndrome. She had been treated with zonisamide and clobazam from 3 months of age and valproic acid from 1 year. A Coombs' test was positive. She had a metabolic acidosis with hypernatremia, hyperchloremia, hypokalemia, hypophosphatemia, and hypouricemia. Although the serum concentration of valproate was within the reference range at 34 mg/l, the ammonia concentration was increased at 1140 (reference range 120–660) mg/l. Valproate was withdrawn, the anemia resolved, and the Coombs' test became negative 2 weeks later; she recovered completely within 3 months.

Although the pathogenetic mechanism involved in the development of valproate-associated Fanconi syndrome is unknown, immunological abnormalities caused by valproate were implicated by the authors.

Three cases of *acute leukemia* with features of secondary leukemia have been reported in patients taking valproic acid: two cases of acute myelogenous leukemia with multilineage dysplasia, one with trisomy 8 and one with monosomy 7, and one case of secondary acute lymphoblastic leukemia with del (7) (q22q34), del (9) (q21.11q22), del (11) (q12q23) (101[c]). One patient had a previous myelodysplastic syndrome while taking valproic acid. The authors proposed that valproic acid can cause secondary leukemia by increasing DNA damage through chronic inhibition of histone deacetylase. However, given that valproate has been available for many decades all over the world and is very widely used but an association with leukemia has not been reported before, this association may have been coincidental. The authors cautioned that it needs to be confirmed in larger prospective epidemiological studies to further elucidate the role of valproate, if any, and histone deacetylation in the development of leukemia.

Salivary glands   *Sialadenosis*, a non-inflammatory parenchymatous salivary gland disease that causes recurrent bilateral swelling of the salivary glands, is a very rare adverse effect of valproic acid that has been reported only once in the world literature to date.

- A 26-year-old woman with posttraumatic epilepsy developed bilateral swelling of her parotid glands (102[A]). She had initially taken phenytoin, but when the seizures persisted, valproate 300 mg tds was started. A few weeks later she noted increasing painless swellings in both parotid glands. She also became aware of a slight enlargement and induration in both submandibular glands. She developed a typical "hamster-like" facial expression, with pouched cheeks. In a biopsy from the right parotid gland there were no histological signs of inflammation. Light and electron microscopy of all the affected salivary glands showed granular sialadenosis with predominantly moderate electron-dense secretory cytoplasmic granules. There were no relevant degenerative alterations. There was no histological evidence of peripheral neuropathy of the nerve supply, leading to disordered activity of acinar cells by loss of neurosecretory granules. Withdrawal of valproate and switching to carbamazepine only slightly reduced the parotid gland swelling, although it was softer. Glucocorticoid therapy was ineffective and she had lateral parotidectomy, with a satisfactory outcome.

Liver   The use of valproate in bipolar disorder is associated with extremely low rates of hepatotoxicity (1/49 000) and pancreatitis (<1%), which are more common in younger patients and do not justify the routine monitoring of hepatic function and amylase activity (103[R]).

Hepatocellular carcinoma arising in non-alcoholic steatohepatitis has been reported in a patient taking valproic acid (104[A]).

- A 64-year-old man was incidentally found to have multiple tumors in the liver when he developed pneumonia. He was obese and had taken a standard dose of valproic acid since clipping surgery for subarachnoid hemorrhage 17 years before, since when he had not taken any alcohol. He had moderate hyperlipidemia and no evidence of diabetes mellitus or hepatitis B or C infection. He died of hepatic insufficiency and at autopsy a tumor, maximum 13 cm in diameter, occupied the entire left lobe and one-third of the right lobe of the liver. Histologically it was a moderately differentiated hepatocellular carcinoma with foci of poorly differentiated tumor. The non-malignant area showed non-alcoholic steatohepatitis with moderate bridging fibrosis, without interface hepatitis, hemochromatosis, or copper accumulation.

The authors speculated that obesity, hyperlipidemia, and long-term valproic acid could all have been associated with non-alcoholic steatohepatitis, which in turn may have contributed to the development of hepatocellular carcinoma.

Hair   *Thinning of the hair* has been attributed to valproate (105[A]).

- A 16-year-old girl took magnesium valproate 800 mg/day for 5 months and developed diffuse hair thinning, more evident in the frontal and parietal regions. Valproate was withdrawn and 2 months later the hair shedding stopped, and there was significant hair re-growth with no evidence of thinning.
- A 24-year-old woman taking magnesium valproate developed hair loss after the dose of adjunctive lamotrigine was increased to 100 mg/day. She continued to take the treatment because seizure control was stable; the hair loss persisted. Androgenetic hair loss was excluded on the basis of the clinical presentation and trichography.

Reproductive system   Women aged 18–45 years (n = 80) with bipolar disorder and not taking steroid contraceptives were recruited to complete questionnaires about their menstrual cycle and to provide blood samples for measurement of a range of reproductive endocrine and metabolic hormone concentrations

(106^C). There were current *menstrual abnormalities* in 52 of the 80 women, 40 of whom reported at least one menstrual abnormality that had preceded the diagnosis of bipolar disorder. Menstrual abnormalities had developed after treatment for bipolar disorder in 15, 14 of whom had developed the abnormalities after treatment with valproate. Of those 15, 12 reported changes in menstrual flow (heavy or prolonged bleeding) and five reported changes in cycle frequency. There were no significant differences between women who took or did not take valproate in mean free or total serum testosterone concentrations. However, among those who took valproate, the duration of use correlated significantly with free testosterone concentrations. Three of the 50 women taking valproate, and none of the 22 taking other antimanic medications, met the criteria for polycystic ovary disease. Other reproductive and metabolic values outside the reference ranges included raised 17-alpha-OH-progesterone, luteinizing hormone, follicle-stimulating hormone ratios, homeostatic model assessment (HOMA) values, and low estrogen and dehydroepiandrosterone sulfate (DHEAS) concentrations. Pre-existing menstrual abnormalities predicted higher concentrations of 17-alpha-OH-progesterone, free testosterone, and estrone, as well as the development of new menstrual abnormalities. Body mass index (BMI) was significantly positively correlated with free testosterone concentrations and insulin resistance across all subjects, regardless of medication. The authors concluded that menstrual disturbances are common in women with bipolar disorder and in many cases precede diagnosis and treatment. Treatment with valproate also contributes significantly to the development of menstrual abnormalities and increased testosterone concentrations over time. Some bipolar women, regardless of type of medication, have reproductive and metabolic hormonal abnormalities, but the causes of such abnormalities require further study. Women with pre-existing menstrual abnormalities may represent a group at risk for reproductive dysfunction while they are being treated for bipolar disorder.

Teratogenicity Neurological and cognitive functions in school-aged children exposed to valproate monotherapy in utero have been evaluated in a population-based, evaluator-blinded,

controlled study (107^C). The children ($n = 39$, aged 6.6–13 years) and their mothers were identified through a pregnancy registry. Mothers taking carbamazepine monotherapy and mothers with epilepsy but no antiepileptic drug treatment during pregnancy and their age- and sex-matched children served as controls. The prevalence of low intelligence (IQ < 80) was 19% and the prevalence of exceptionally low intelligence (IQ < 70) 10% in the children who had been exposed to valproate. In contrast, the children who had been exposed to carbamazepine and the children of women with epilepsy but without drug exposure during pregnancy all had at least low average intelligence. The mothers who had used valproate scored significantly lower in IQ tests and also had a significantly lower educational level. Altogether 21% of the children had minor neurological dysfunction. The authors cautioned that in a population-based setting, inheritance and environmental factors could have partly explained the increased prevalence of neurocognitive symptoms in children exposed to valproate in utero, although there is concern about possible long-term adverse effects of intrauterine valproate exposure.

Valproate embryopathy is a well recognized syndrome caused by prenatal exposure to the valproic acid. In five half-siblings with the same mother (four different fathers) who all had valproate embryopathy, valproic acid 500–2000 mg/day was the sole anticonvulsant in all five pregnancies (108^C). Mean birth weight at term was 2900 (range 2400–3400) g. Common features of valproate embryopathy in the five children included flat, broad nasal bridge (5/5), hypoplastic midface (4/5), hypertelorism/telecanthus (4/5), a smooth philtrum (4/5), a thin upper lip (5/5), and long thin tapering fingers (4/5). Other features were hypoplastic fifth toenails (2/5), irregularly placed toes (2/5), micro/brachycephaly (2/5), cleft palate (1/5), duplication cyst of small intestine (1/5), and hemangioma (1/5). None had a neural tube defect. Neuropsychological testing of the three children over 4 years of age showed cognitive ability in the low normal or borderline range (mean IQ = 83; range 75–86), with significantly lower scores of adaptive behavior and motor skills. Although fetal valproate embryopathy may at least in part have been responsible for the low normal or borderline IQ and the delay in early speech and motor development, the authors suggested that parental neglect may have contributed to the cognitive profile. In addition, documentation of valproate embryopathy in all five pregnancies lends further support to the speculation that as yet unspecified genetic factors may increase the risk of valproate embryopathy.

Drug dosage regimens   In a retrospective review of the medical records of 14 in-patients with acute mania whose treatment included divalproex ER 30 mg/kg/day (mean 2034, range 1500–3000 mg/day), two had documented adverse effects, none severe (109[c]). The results suggested that divalproex ER can be safely administered by oral loading and that using a standard loading protocol can result in therapeutic serum concentrations in most patients in 3 days or less.

Drug administration route   In 102 adult patients who took standardized high-dosage intravenous valproate in various emergencies, including status epilepticus, mild adverse effects occurred in seven (110[c]). They included a nonspecific feeling of warmth with dizziness for some seconds during fast bolus injection in three patients. One patient developed a moderate generalized allergic skin reaction, which disappeared within a few hours after withdrawal of therapy, one had nausea and vomiting, and one had mild fatigue plus a transient tremor of both hands. There were no reactions at injection sites. Serious adverse effects were not documented. In particular there was no evidence of sedation, cardiorespiratory disturbances, or hypotension, as are often seen with barbiturates and phenytoin.

Intravenous valproate is an emerging treatment option for acute migraine. Data in adults suggests both efficacy and tolerability of rapid infusion of valproate as abortive therapy, but there are few data in children. In a retrospective chart review of all children who received intravenous valproate (mean 976 mg infused over 12 minutes) valproate infusion was well tolerated (111[c]). Adverse events included cold sensation ($n = 1$), dizziness ($n = 3$), nausea ($n = 1$), a possible absence seizure ($n = 1$), paresthesia ($n = 2$), and tachycardia ($n = 2$).

Drug overdose   The clinical features, complications, and pharmacokinetics of valproic acid

after intentional acute overdose have been described in six patients (112[c]). The doses were 18, 24, 30, 50, and 60 g; in one case the dose was unknown. The nervous system was predominantly affected (6/6), followed by respiratory failure (5/6) and multiorgan failure (2/6). Mechanical ventilation was required in five of six patients because of respiratory depression or profound coma. Hemodialysis was used in 4/6 of the cases because of hyperammonemia, a worsening neurological condition, or organ dysfunction. Cerebral edema and hemorrhagic pancreatitis occurred in two patients and two died. The valproate peak concentration was 520–1700 mg/l (mean 1127 mg/l). Ammonia was raised in all cases (mean 5500 µg/l. All the patients had signs of impaired mitochondrial beta-oxidation, with increased serum concentrations of medium- and long-chain acylcarnitines.

Drug–drug interactions

Anticancer drugs   A pharmacokinetic interaction of valproic acid with anticancer drugs has been observed in a patient with epilepsy (113[A]).

• A 34-year-old man with epilepsy taking valproic acid underwent cisplatin-based chemotherapy for a testicular tumor. The first cycle of chemotherapy reduced the serum valproate concentration by about 50% and several generalized tonic–clonic seizures resulted. The next six cycles over 7 months also caused seizures in association with reduced serum valproate concentrations. In contrast, the serum concentration of phenytoin, which was given daily after the second cycle of chemotherapy, was unchanged. After the completion of chemotherapy, the serum concentration of a tumor marker, hCGbeta, fell to 1.2 ng/ml from more than 120 ng/ml.

The authors concluded that careful monitoring of valproate concentrations is necessary during cancer chemotherapy, because anticancer agents can reduce the serum concentration and antiepileptic activity of valproate.

Antiepileptic drugs   The effect of zonisamide on the steady-state pharmacokinetics of valproate sodium has been studied in 22 patients with epilepsy aged 18–55 years in an open study (114[c]). Steady-state zonisamide (200 mg bd) had no significant effect on the mean C_{max}, AUC, or other pharmacokinetic parameters of valproic acid. In the presence of valproic acid, mean zonisamide oral clearance (1.23 l/hour) and half-life (53 hours) were generally consistent with values reported in healthy volunteers taking zonisamide monotherapy. The authors concluded that there is no interaction of these two drugs.

Carbapenems   A probable interaction of meropenem with valproic acid resulted in epileptic seizures (115[A]).

- A 21-year-old woman had a generalized tonic–clonic seizure and was given a continuous intravenous infusion of valproic acid 1000 mg/day over 24 hours. On day 6, the serum valproic acid concentration was 53 µg/ml. On day 13, intravenous meropenem 1 g tds was started. On day 15, when she was afebrile, she had numerous myoclonic seizures involving her arms and face; the serum valproic acid concentration was 42 µg/ml. The dose of valproic acid was increased to 2880 mg. Two days later, she had a generalized tonic–clonic seizure despite the increased dosage, and the plasma concentration of valproic acid fell to 7 µg/ml. The dose of valproic acid was increased to 3600 mg/day but the serum concentration remained below 10 µg/ml. On day 19 meropenem was withdrawn. The serum valproic acid concentration rose to 52 µg/ml on day 27.

The authors reviewed the literature and found 11 cases of interactions of carbapenem antibiotics with valproic acid. A possible mechanism is increased glucuronidation of valproate, and a direct proconvulsant effect of the antibiotic may also contribute.

Oral contraceptives   An interaction of valproate with a combined oral contraceptive has been reported (116[A]).

- A 26-year-old woman had her first convulsion during her first menstrual cycle at age 13 years. Partial seizures began at age 23 years soon after the introduction of an oral contraceptive containing ethynodiol diacetate 1 mg and ethinylestradiol 35 micrograms. Her seizures occurred more often while she was taking active rather than inactive oral contraceptive formulations. Morning trough serum valproate concentrations were 54 µg/ml during the third week of active pill use and 139 µg/ml on days 5–7 of inactive pill use. Serum concentrations during subsequent cycles confirmed lower concentrations during the use of active pills (total 70 µg/ml, unbound 6.9 µg/ml) than inactive pills (total 110 µg/ml, unbound 12.8 µg/ml).

The authors suggested that oral contraceptives may have induced glucuronidation, which inactivates valproate.

Psychotropic drugs   Interactions of valproate with psychotropic medications of all types have been reviewed, with a particular focus on mechanisms and potential clinical consequences (117[R]). More specifically interactions caused by inhibition by valproate of uridine diphosphate glucuronyltransferases (UDPGT), which metabolizes lamotrigine and olanzapine. For other psychotropic drugs, such as chlorpromazine, clozapine, doxepin, imipramine, lorazepam, loxapine, oxazepam, and temazepam, inhibition of UDPGT is less likely to affect their metabolism. However, valproate also inhibits CYP isozymes. One example is CYP2C9, which is an important although not a major metabolic enzyme for olanzapine, phenobarbital, and thioridazine. Valproate also inhibits CYP2C19, which is important for the metabolism of olanzapine, methophenobarbital, and phenobarbital. These interactions can result in adverse effects (for example sedation when valproate is added to phenobarbital and hypersensitivity skin reactions when valproate is added to lamotrigine). When valproate is used, lower doses and slower titration is recommended for add-on treatment with phenobarbital or lamotrigine.

Management of adverse drug reactions   The use of carnitine in patients with acute valproate poisoning and a raised ammonia concentration has been reviewed in 674 patients, median age 26 (range 1–58) years (118[c]). Carnitine (55 doses) was given to 19 patients who had taken valproate alone and 196 doses of carnitine were given to patients with mixed overdoses that included valproate, all with raised ammonia concentrations. None had an allergic reaction or other adverse effects.

- A 19-year-old man had fatal cerebral edema after an overdose of valproic acid 20 g (333 mg/kg) modified-release tablets with risperidone 60 mg and venlafaxine 3 g (119[A]). He was awake but lethargic, and after 43 hours his mental status began to worsen and at 48 hours intubation was necessary. His serum ammonia concentration was 3380 µg/l (reference range 150–560 µg/l). At 65 hours the ammonia concentration was markedly increased at 11910 µg/l and the valproic acid concentration was moderately raised at 192 mg/l. By 90 hours the ammonia concentration had fallen to 1170 µg/l. By 110 hours he had fixed dilated pupils and bilateral extensor posturing. CT scans of the brain showed cerebral edema and possible tentorial herniation. Brain blood flow studies at 120 hours showed no cerebral perfusion and he was declared brain dead. The ammonia concentration at that time was 800 µg/l and the serum valproic acid concentration was 61 mg/l.

This case was unusual because of the modest quantity of valproic acid ingested and the similarly modest serum concentration of 305 mg/l with a very high ammonia concentration.

Vigabatrin   *(SED-15, 3623; SEDA-27, 83; SEDA-28, 101; SEDA-29, 99)*

Sensory systems

> **DoTS classification:**
> *Reaction*: Visual field loss from vigabatrin
> *Dose relation*: Collateral reaction
> *Time course*: Late
> *Susceptibility factors*: More common in adults

In patients with intractable partial epilepsy taking vigabatrin add-on treatment, there were *visual field defects* in at least one eye in 27 of 34 patients (120[c]). Of the subgroup of 27 patients who had both eyes reliably tested, 16 had bilateral defects, of whom seven were severely affected and had nasally dominant, crescentic, or concentric defects. Five had unilateral visual field defects. Four of the 27 affected patients reported blurred vision. There were no significant differences between patients with and without visual field defects in terms of age, sex, duration, or cause of the epilepsy, and duration, maximum daily dose, or cumulative dose of vigabatrin.

The effects of vigabatrin on visual function in children, particularly in those who have been exposed to vigabatrin in utero, are little studied. Visual function has been studied in two children who were exposed prenatally to vigabatrin and other antiepileptic drugs (121[A]). In the first case the mother had taken vigabatrin 1 g/day and carbamazepine; a concentric field defect was found. She also had a homonymous quadrantanopia after temporal lobe surgery for epilepsy. The child was examined at the age of 7 years and 9 months; standard ophthalmological examination, including static perimetry, was normal. In the second case the mother had

taken carbamazepine and valproate, and vigabatrin 3 g/day was added at week 16. Standard ophthalmological examination, including static perimetry, was normal. The child was examined at the age of 6 years and 10 months. Major and minor malformations were found, including left radius aplasia, a long philtrum, dextrocardia, two superior vena cavas, and hypospadias. Standard ophthalmological examination showed visual acuities of 0.8 and cycloplegic refraction sf + 0.75 D in both eyes. Kinetic perimetry was inconclusive and field-specific visual evoked potentials were normal, but there were early positive responses in peripheral recordings, the significance of which was unclear. The two children who had been exposed to vigabatrin in utero had no overt ophthalmic abnormalities. However, it is still unclear whether prenatal vigabatrin exposure carries a risk of visual dysfunction. There were no structural eye malformations, but there were borderline abnormalities of perimetry and field-specific visual evoked potentials.

Flash electroretinography has been recorded in 11 adults taking vigabatrin with other antiepileptic drugs, six of whom stopped taking vigabatrin, and nine children who took vigabatrin alone or with other antiepileptic drugs, five of whom discontinued vigabatrin (122[c]). Abnormal b-waves were found in 16%, 30 Hz flicker in 50%, and oscillatory potentials in 76%. Of the nine patients who continued to take vigabatrin (four children and five adults), one child had attenuated oscillatory potentials and two unchanged electroretinography; two of the adults had unchanged electroretinography, and two had changes in b-waves and/or flicker and/or oscillatory potentials. Electroretinography in 4/5 children greatly improved after withdrawal of vigabatrin and was unchanged in the fifth; there were mild to moderate improvements in flicker and oscillatory potentials in 4/6 adults after withdrawal of vigabatrin and no changes in two.

Contrast sensitivity and visual acuity have been studied in 28 children (mean age 4.9 years) with seizure disorders who had taken vigabatrin and 14 healthy children (mean age 3.1 years) (123[c]). Both were reduced in vigabatrin-treated children with infantile spasms compared with vigabatrin-treated children with other seizure disorders and the healthy subjects. The other factors examined had no significant effect on contrast sensitivity or visual acuity, with adjustment for seizure type. The reduced vision was probably associated with infantile spasms rather than with vigabatrin.

Zonisamide   *(SED-15, 3728; SEDA-27, 83; SEDA-28, 101; SEDA-29, 100)*

Placebo-controlled studies   Zonisamide has been assessed in 351 patients with refractory partial seizures taking a stable regimen of 1–3 antiepileptic drugs in a double-blind, placebo-controlled study (124[C]). The most common adverse events at respective doses of 100, 300, and 500 mg/day were *somnolence* (5.4, 3.6, 14%), *headache* (7.1, 13, 6.8%), *dizziness* (1.8, 7.3, 12%), and *nausea* (3.6, 11, 7.6%) during the titration phase and headache (11, 11, and 4.2%) and pharyngitis (11, 1.8, 2.5%) during the subsequent fixed-dose phase; zonisamide was withdrawn because of adverse effects in 1.8, 18, and 27%.

In an analysis of four randomized, placebo-controlled, add-on studies of zonisamide in patients with drug-resistant partial epilepsy the relative risk of withdrawal of zonisamide was 1.64 (1.20, 2.26) at a dosage of 300–500 mg/day, and 1.47 (1.07, 2.02) at a dosage of 100–500 mg/day. The following adverse effects were significantly associated with zonisamide compared with placebo: *ataxia* OR = 4.50 (99% CI = 1.05, 19.2); *dizziness* 1.77 (1.00, 3.12); *somnolence* 1.96 (1.12, 3.44); *agitation* 2.37 (1.00, 5.64); and *anorexia* 3.00 (1.31, 6.88) (125[M]).

In a chart review of 45 patients aged 8–18 years with absence seizures, 23 became free of seizures; two stopped taking zonisamide, one because of *increased seizures* and one because of *sleepiness* and inefficacy (126[c]).

Urinary tract   *Renal calculi* occur at a rate of about 1% in patients with bipolar disorder taking zonisamide, and the risk increases if zonisamide is given in combination with other carbonic anhydrase inhibitors, such as acetazolamide and topiramate (103[R]). The risk factors for crystalluria due to antiepileptic drugs has been studied in 278 urine specimens from patients with epilepsy aged between 7 months and 36 years, mean age 12 years (127[c]). The

antiepileptic drugs studied were valproate (174 urinary samples), zonisamide (139), carbamazepine (138), phenobarbital (65), phenytoin (52), acetazolamide (17), clonazepam (15), sultiame (6), ethosuximide (6), nitrazepam (4), and clobazam (4). Zonisamide, sultiame, and an alkaline urine were risk factors.

Susceptibility factors

Age   In a review of the charts of 50 children (mean age 9.1 years, range 9 months to 20 years) who received zonisamide (mean 16 mg/kg/day), eight were seizure-free and 11 others had a 50% or more improvement in seizure control, including 11 of 28 patients for whom treatment with six or more antiepileptic drugs was insufficient; 31 had at least one adverse event while taking zonisamide (128[c]). The most common adverse effects were reduced appetite (n = 14), weight loss (n = 5), and increased phenytoin concentrations (n = 5); 14 discontinued treatment because of adverse effects, including eight with reduced appetite, two with kidney stones, and two with behavioral problems.

Of 131 children aged 1–22 years with a broad spectrum of seizure types and epilepsy syndromes, 101 achieved a 50% or greater reduction in seizure frequency, including 39 who became free of seizures (129[c]). Adverse effects that were reported in more than one patient included reduced appetite (n = 12), weight loss (n = 9), insomnia (n = 7), sedation and sleepiness (n = 5), cognitive effects (n = 4), increased seizure activity (n = 3), weight gain (n = 1), and failure to gain weight (n = 1). Three patients stopped taking zonisamide because of adverse events, one with insomnia and increased seizure frequency, another with failure to gain weight, and a third with behavioral changes.

Drug dosage regimens   In 23 children with West syndrome different zonisamide titration protocols were used to raise the serum zonisamide concentration: (1) increase the dosage in three steps, from 3 to 10 mg/kg every 3 days (n = 8), (2) increase the dosage from 5 to 10 mg/kg over 3–7 days (n = 5), and (3) start with 10 mg/kg and maintain this dosage for 2 weeks (n = 10) (130[c]). The maximum serum zonisamide concentration was higher in those who had excellent or good responses (32 μg/ml; $n = 8$) than in those in whom it was ineffective (22 μg/ml; $n = 15$). The time required for cessation of spasms was shorter in the 3rd group (mean 5.7 days) than in the 1st and 2nd groups (mean 10 days). There were few adverse effects, except for transient hyperthermia and gastrointestinal symptoms. The authors concluded that a starting dose of 10 mg/kg of zonisamide is safe and effective.

Drug–drug interactions   In 56 patients who underwent intracarotid *amobarbital* infusion, there was reduced anesthetization in two and very rapid recovery in nine; 10 of the 11 were taking a medication with some carbonic anhydrase-inhibitory effects—topiramate ($n = 7$), zonisamide ($n = 2$), hydrochlorothiazide ($n = 1$), and furosemide ($n = 1$) (131[c]). Of 40 who were not taking a carbonic anhydrase inhibitor only one recovered early and that patient had recently stopped taking topiramate. The authors suggested that failure of anesthetization during intracarotid amobarbital infusion is associated with a possible interac-

tion of amobarbital and carbonic anhydrase and that intracarotid amobarbital infusion should not be performed until at least 8 weeks after withdrawal of a carbonic anhydrase inhibitor.

Several antiepileptic drugs have clinically significant pharmacokinetic interactions with *oral contraceptives*, which can result in contraceptive failure. The effects of zonisamide 400 mg/day on the pharmacokinetics of the individual components of a combination oral contraceptive (ethinylestradiol 35 micrograms and norethindrone 1 mg) and on pharmacodynamic variables that may be increased by reduced contraceptive efficacy (concentrations of serum luteinizing hormone, follicle-stimulating hormone, and progesterone) have been studied in an open crossover study in healthy premenopausal women who took a combination oral contraceptive during three 28-day cycles (132[c]). The C_{max} and AUC of ethinylestradiol and norethindrone were not altered and there were no changes in concentrations of luteinizing hormone, follicle-stimulating hormone, or progesterone.

References

1. Kinjo M, Setoguchi S, Schneeweiss S, Solomon DH. Bone mineral density in subjects using central nervous system-active medications. Am J Med 2005;118:1414.e7–12.
2. Hart Y. Contraception for women with epilepsy. Women's Health Med 2005;2:27–8.
3. Carpay JA, Aldenkamp AP, van Donselaar CA. Complaints associated with the use of antiepileptic drugs: results from a community-based study. Seizure 2005;14:198–206.
4. Saygan-Karamursel B, Guven S, Onderoglu L, Deren O, Durukan T. Mega-dose carbamazepine complicating third trimester of pregnancy. J Perinat Med 2005;33:72–5.
5. Kuz GM, Manssourian A. Carbamazepine-induced hyponatremia: assessment of risk factors. Ann Pharmacother 2005;39:1943–6.
6. Hayashi T, Yoshinaga A, Ohno R, Ishii N, Kamata S, Watanabe T, Yamada T. Asthenozoospermia: possible association with long-term exposure to an anti-epileptic drug of carbamazepine. Int J Urol 2005;12:113–4.
7. Lin MS, Dai YS, Pwu RF, Chen YH, Chang NC. Risk estimates for drugs suspected of being as-

sociated with Stevens–Johnson syndrome and toxic epidermal necrolysis: a case-control study. Intern Med J 2005;35:188–90.
8. Hara H, Kobayashi M, Yokoyama A, Tochigi M, Matsunaga A, Shimizu H, Goshima J, Suzuki H. Drug-induced hypersensitivity syndrome due to carbamazepine associated with reactivation of human herpesvirus 7. Dermatology 2005;211:159–61.
9. Hiremath GK, Kotagal P, Bingaman W, Hovinga C, Wyllie E, Morris H, Nelson D. Risk factors for carbamazepine elevation and toxicity following epilepsy surgery. Seizure 2005;14:312–7.
10. Novak PH, Ekins-Daukes S, Simpson CR, Milne RM, Helms P, McLay JS. Acute drug prescribing to children on chronic antiepilepsy therapy and the potential for adverse drug interactions in primary care. Br J Clin Pharmacol 2005;59:712–7.
11. Vander T, Odi H, Bluvstein V, Ronen J, Catz A. Carbamazepine toxicity following oxybutynin and dantrolene administration: a case report. Spinal Cord 2005;43:252–5.

12. Jayyosi Z, Villoutreix J, Ziegler JM, Batt AM, De Maack F, Siest G, Thomas PE. Identification of cytochrome P-450 isozymes involved in the hydroxylation of dantrolene by rat liver microsomes. Drug Metab Dispos 1993;21(5):939–45.

13. Lee KJ, Kim JH, Cho SW. Gabapentin reduces rectal mechanosensitivity and increases rectal compliance in patients with diarrhoea-predominant irritable bowel syndrome. Aliment Pharmacol Ther 2005;22(10):981–8.

14. Pandey CK, Navkar DV, Giri PJ, Raza M, Behari S, Singh RB, Singh U, Singh PK. Evaluation of the optimal preemptive dose of gabapentin for postoperative pain relief after lumbar diskectomy: a randomized, double-blind, placebo-controlled study. J Neurosurg Anesthesiol 2005;17:65–8.

15. Weissenbacher S, Ring J, Hofmann H. Gabapentin for symptomatic treatment of chronic neuropathic pain in patients with late-stage Lyme borreliosis: a pilot study. Dermatology 2005;211:123–7.

16. Moore KA, Levine B, Fowler D. A fatality involving metaxalone. Forensic Sci Int 2005;149:249–51.

17. Knoester PD, Keyser A, Renier WO, Egberts ACG, Hekster YA. Deckers CLP. Effectiveness of lamotrigine in clinical practice: results of a retrospective population-based study. Epilepsy Res 2005;65:93–100.

18. Posner EB, Mohamed K, Marson AG. A systematic review of treatment of typical absence seizures in children and adolescents with ethosuximide, sodium valproate or lamotrigine. Seizure 2005;14:117–22.

19. Shechter T, Shorer Z, Kramer U, Lerman-Sagie T, Ronen E, Rotem R, Gorodischer R. Adverse reactions of topiramate and lamotrigine in children. Pharmacoepidemiol Drug Saf 2005;14:187–92.

20. Steinhoff BJ, Ueberall MA, Siemes H, Kurlemann G, Schmitz B, Bergmann L, the LAM-SAFE Study Group. The LAM-SAFE Study: lamotrigine versus carbamazepine or valproic acid in newly diagnosed focal and generalised epilepsies in adolescents and adults. Seizure 2005;14:597–605.

21. Tritt K, Nickel C, Lahmann C, Leiberich PK, Rother WK, Loew TH, Nickel MK. Lamotrigine treatment of aggression in female borderline-patients: a randomized, double-blind, placebo-controlled study. J Psychopharmacol 2005;19:287–91.

22. Saravanan N, Otaiku OM, Namushi RN. Interstitial pneumonitis during lamotrigine therapy. Br J Clin Pharmacol 2005;60:666–7.

23. Kilfoyle DH, Anderson NE, Wallis WE, Nicholls DW. Recurrent severe aseptic meningitis after exposure to lamotrigine in a patient with systemic lupus erythematosus. Epilepsia 2005;46:327–8.

24. Arndt CF, Husson J, Derambure P, Hache JC, Arnaud B, Defoort-Dhellemmes S. Retinal electrophysiological results in patients receiving lamotrigine monotherapy. Epilepsia 2005;46:1055–60.

25. Chan Y-C, Miller KM, Shaheen N, Votolato NA, Hankins MB. Worsening of psychotic symptoms in schizophrenia with addition of lamotrigine: a case report. Schizophr Res 2005;78:343–5.

26. Clemens B. Forced normalisation precipitated by lamotrigine. Seizure 2005;14:485–9.

27. Gidal BE, Tamura T, Hammer A, Vuong A. Blood homocysteine, folate and vitamin B12 concentrations in patients with epilepsy receiving lamotrigine or sodium valproate for initial monotherapy. Epilepsy Res 2005;64:161–6.

28. Mansouri P, Rabiei M, Pourpak Z, Hallaji Z. Toxic epidermal necrolysis associated with concomitant use of lamotrigine and carbamazepine: a case report. Arch Dermatol 2005;141:788–9.

29. Weintraub D, Buchsbaum R, Resor Jr SR, Hirsch LJ. Effect of antiepileptic drug comedication on lamotrigine clearance. Arch Neurol 2005;62:1432–6.

30. Beran RG, Berkovic SF, Black AB, Danta G, Hiersemenzel R, Schapel GJ, Vajda FJE. Efficacy and safety of levetiracetam 1000–3000 mg/day in patients with refractory partial-onset seizures: a multicenter, open-label single-arm study. Epilepsy Res 2005;63:1–9.

31. Opp J, Tuxhorn I, May T, Kluger G, Wiemer-Kruel A, Kurlemann G, Gross-Selbeck G, Rating D, Brandl U, Bettendorf U, Hartel C, Korn-Merker E. Levetiracetam in children with refractory epilepsy: a multicenter open label study in Germany. Seizure 2005;14:476–84.

32. Grosso S, Franzoni E, Coppola G, Iannetti P, Verrotti A, Cordelli DM, Marchiani V, Pascotto A, Spalice A, Acampora B, Morgese G, Balestri P. Efficacy and safety of levetiracetam: an add-on trial in children with refractory epilepsy. Seizure 2005;14:248–53.

33. Rapoport AM, Sheftell FD, Tepper SJ, Bigal ME. Levetiracetam in the preventive treatment of transformed migraine: a prospective, open-label, pilot study. Curr Ther Res Clin Exp 2005;66:212–21.

34. Zhang W, Connor KM, Davidson JR. Levetiracetam in social phobia: a placebo controlled pilot study. J Psychopharmacol 2005;19:551–3.

35. Zesiewicz TA, Sullivan KL, Hauser RA, Sanchez-Ramos J. Open-label pilot study of levetiracetam (Keppra) for the treatment of chorea in Huntington's disease. Mov Disord 2005;20:1205–9.

36. Sullivan KL, Hauser RA, Zesiewicz TA. Levetiracetam for the treatment of essential tremor. Mov Disord 2005;20:640.

37. Otoul C, Arrigo C, Van Rijckevorsel K, French JA. Meta-analysis and indirect comparisons of levetiracetam with other second-generation antiepileptic drugs in partial epilepsy. Clin Neuropharmacol 2005;28:72–8.

38. Khatami R, Siegel AM, Bassetti CL. Hypersomnia in an epilepsy patient treated with levetiracetam. Epilepsia 2005;46:588–9.

39. Zesiewicz TA, Sanchez-Ramos J, Sullivan KL, Hauser RA. Levetiracetam-induced parkinsonism in a Huntington disease patient. Clin Neuropharmacol 2005;28:188–90.

40. Nasrallah K, Silver B. Hyponatremia associated with repeated use of levetiracetam. Epilepsia 2005;46:972–3.
41. Gidal BE, Baltes E, Otoul C, Perucca E. Effect of levetiracetam on the pharmacokinetics of adjunctive antiepileptic drugs: a pooled analysis of data from randomized clinical trials. Epilepsy Res 2005;64:1–11.
42. Northam RS, Hernandez AW, Litzinger MJ, Minecan DN, Glauser TA, Mangat S, Zheng C, Souppart C, Sturm Y. Oxcarbazepine in infants and young children with partial seizures. Pediatr Neurol 2005;33:337–44.
43. Rainesalo S, Peltola J, Auvinen A, Keränen T. Retention rate of oxcarbazepine monotherapy in an unselected population of adult epileptics. Seizure 2005;14:72–4.
44. Tzitiridou M, Panou T, Ramantani G, Kambas A, Spyroglou K, Panteliadis C. Oxcarbazepine monotherapy in benign childhood epilepsy with centrotemporal spikes: a clinical and cognitive evaluation. Epilepsy Behav 2005;7:458–67.
45. Schik G, Wedegärtner FR, Liersch J, Hoy L, Emrich HM. Oxcarbazepine versus carbamazepine in the treatment of alcohol withdrawal. Addict Biol 2005;10:283–8.
46. Mavragani CP, Vlachoyiannopoulos PG. Is polydipsia sometimes the cause of oxcarbazepine-induced hyponatremia? Eur J Intern Med 2005;16:296–7.
47. Negin B, Murphy TK. Priapism associated with oxcarbazepine, aripiprazole, and lithium. J Am Acad Child Adolesc Psychiatry 2005;44:1223–4.
48. Perucca E. Birth defects after prenatal exposure to antiepileptic drugs. Lancet Neurol 2005;4:781–6.
49. Bourgeois BFD, D'Souza J. Long-term safety and tolerability of oxcarbazepine in children: a review of clinical experience. Epilepsy Behav 2005;7:375–82.
50. Messina S, Battino D, Croci D, Mamoli D, Ratti S, Perucca E. Phenobarbital pharmacokinetics in old age: a case-matched evaluation based on therapeutic drug monitoring data. Epilepsia 2005;46:372–7.
51. Naidech AM, Kreiter KT, Janjua N, Ostapkovich N, Parra A, Commichau C, Connolly ES, Mayer SA, Fitzsimmons B-FM. Phenytoin exposure is associated with functional and cognitive disability after subarachnoid hemorrhage. Stroke 2005;36:583–7.
52. Bremner JD, Mletzko T, Welter S, Quinn S, Williams C, Brummer M, Siddiq S, Reed L, Heim CM, Nemeroff CB. Effects of phenytoin on memory, cognition and brain structure in post-traumatic stress disorder: a pilot study. J Psychopharmacol 2005;19:159–65.
53. Amato A, Marlowe KF. Severe case of phenytoin-induced anticonvulsant hypersensitivity syndrome. Am J Health-Syst Pharm 2005;62:2295–7.
54. Morel CF, Duncan AMV, Desilets V. A fragile site at 10q23 (FRA10A) in a phenytoin-exposed fetus: a case report and review of the literature. Prenat Diagn 2005;25:318–21.
55. De Jonge ME, Huitema ADR, Van Dam SM, Beijnen JH, Rodenhuis S. Significant induction of cyclophosphamide and thiotepa metabolism by phenytoin. Cancer Chemother Pharmacol 2005;55:507–10.
56. Feltner DE, Crockatt JG, Dubovsky SJ, Cohn CK, Shrivastava RK, Targum SD, Liu-Dumaw M, Carter CM, Pande AC. A randomized, double-blind, placebo-controlled, fixed-dose, multicenter study of pregabalin in patients with generalized anxiety disorder. J Clin Psychopharmacol 2003;23:240–9.
57. Pohl RB, Feltner DE, Fieve RR, Pande AC. Efficacy of pregabalin in the treatment of generalized anxiety disorder: double-blind, placebo-controlled comparison of BID versus TID dosing. J Clin Psychopharmacol 2005;25:151–8.
58. Frampton JE, Foster RH. Pregabalin: in the treatment of postherpetic neuralgia. Drugs 2005;65:111–8.
59. Freynhagen R, Strojek K, Griesing T, Whalen E, Balkenohl M. Efficacy of pregabalin in neuropathic pain evaluated in a 12-week, randomised, double-blind, multicentre, placebo-controlled trial of flexible- and fixed-dose regimens. Pain 2005;115(3):254–63.
60. Richter RW, Portenoy R, Sharma U, Lamoreaux L, Bockbrader H, Knapp LE. Relief of painful diabetic peripheral neuropathy with pregabalin: a randomized, placebo-controlled trial. J Pain 2005;6(4):253–60.
61. Crofford LJ, Rowbotham MC, Mease PJ, Russell IJ, Dworkin RH, Corbin AE, Young Jr JP, LaMoreaux LK, Martin SA, Sharma U. Pregabalin for the treatment of fibromyalgia syndrome: results of a randomized, double-blind, placebo-controlled trial. Arthritis Rheum 2005;52:1264–73.
62. Ryvlin P. Defining success in clinical trials-profiling pregabalin, the newest AED. Eur J Neurol 2005;12(Suppl 4):12–21.
63. Elger CE, Brodie MJ, Anhut H, Lee CM, Barrett J. Pregabalin add-on treatment in patients with partial seizures: a novel evaluation of flexible-dose and fixed dose regimens in a double-blind, placebo controlled study. Epilepsia 2005;46:1926–36.
64. Beydoun A, Uthman BM, Kugler AR, Greiner MJ, Knapp LE, Garofalo EA. Safety and efficacy of two pregabalin regimens for add-on treatment of partial epilepsy. Neurology 2005;64(3):475–80.
65. Shneker BF, McAuley JW. Pregabalin. A new neuromodulator with broad therapeutic indications. Ann Pharmacother 2005;39:2029–37.
66. Zareba G. Pregabalin: a new agent for the treatment of neuropathic pain. Drugs Today 2005;41:509–16.
67. Oaklander AL, Buchbinder BR. Pregabalin-withdrawal encephalopathy and splenial edema: a link to high-altitude illness? Ann Neurol 2005;58:309–12.

68. Ginsberg DL. Sudden pregabalin discontinuation associated with focal brain edema. Prim Psychiatry 2005;12:26–7.

69. Huppertz HJ, Feuerstein TJ, Schulze-Bonhage A. Myoclonus in epilepsy patients with anticonvulsive add-on therapy with pregabalin. Epilepsia 2001;42(6):790–2.

70. Chaves J, Sander JW, Sander L. Seizure aggravation in idiopathic generalized epilepsies. Epilepsia 2005;46(Suppl 9):133–9.

71. Heckmann JG, Ulrich K, Dutsch M, Neundörfer B. Pregabalin associated asterixis. Am J Phys Med Rehabil 2005;84(9):724.

72. Brodie MJ, Wilson EA, Wesche DL, Alvey CW, Randinitis EJ, Posvar EL, Hounslow NJ, Bron NJ, Gibson GL, Bockbrader HN. Pregabalin drug interaction studies: lack of effect on the pharmacokinetics of carbamazepine, phenytoin, lamotrigine, and valproate in patients with partial epilepsy. Epilepsia 2005;46:1407–13.

73. Arroyo S, Boothman BR, Brodie MJ, Duncan JS, Duncan R, Nieto M, Pita Calandre E, Forcadas I, Crawford PM. A randomised open-label study of tiagabine given two or three times daily in refractory epilepsy. Seizure 2005;14:81–4.

74. Schwartz TL, Azhar N, Husain J, Nihalani N, Simionescu M, Coovert D, Jindal S, Tirmazi S. An open-label study of tiagabine as augmentation therapy for anxiety. Ann Clin Psychiatry 2005;17:167–72.

75. Todorov AA, Kolchev CB, Todorov AB. Tiagabine and gabapentin for the management of chronic pain. Clin J Pain 2005;21:358–61.

76. Giannakodimos ST, Georgiadis G, Tsounis ST, Triantafillou N, Kimiskidis V, Giatas K, Karlovasitou A, Mitsikostas DD, Thodi E, Polychronopoulos P, Ramopoulos N, Michailidis K, Michalis N, Garganis K, Gatzonis ST, Balogiannis ST, Kazis AR, Milonas I, Van Oene JC. Add-on topiramate in the treatment of refractory partial-onset epilepsy: clinical experience of outpatient epilepsy clinics from 11 general hospitals. Seizure 2005;14:396–402.

77. Guerrini R, Carpay J, Groselj J, van Oene J, Schreiner A, Lahaye M, Schwalen S, TOP-INT-51 Investigators' Group. Topiramate monotherapy as broad-spectrum antiepileptic drug in a naturalistic clinical setting. Seizure 2005;14:371–80.

78. Dannon PN, Lowengrub K, Gonopolski Y, Musin E, Kotler M. Topiramate versus fluvoxamine in the treatment of pathological gambling: a randomized, blind-rater comparison study. Clin Neuropharmacol 2005;28:6–10.

79. Tonstad S, Tykarski A, Weissgarten J, Ivleva A, Levy B, Kumar A, Fitchet M. Efficacy and safety of topiramate in the treatment of obese subjects with essential hypertension. Am J Cardiol 2005;96:243–51.

80. Nickel C, Tritt K, Muehlbacher M, Gil FP, Mitterlehner FO, Kaplan P, Lahmann C, Leiberich PK, Krawczyk J, Kettler C, Rother WK, Loew TH, Nickel MK. Topiramate treatment in bulimia nervosa patients: a randomized, double-blind, placebo-controlled trial. Int J Eat Disord 2005;38:295–300.

81. Delbello MP, Findling RL, Kushner S, Wang D, Olson WH, Capece JA, Fazzio L, Rosenthal NR. A pilot controlled trial of topiramate for mania in children and adolescents with bipolar disorder. J Am Acad Child Adolesc Psychiatry 2005;44:539–47.

82. Biton V, Bourgeois BF, YTC/YTCE Study Investigators. Topiramate in patients with juvenile myoclonic epilepsy. Arch Neurol 2005;62:1705–8.

83. Borzy JC, Koch TK, Schimschock JR. Effectiveness of topiramate in the treatment of pediatric chronic daily headache. Pediatr Neurol 2005;33:314–6.

84. Majkowski J, Neto W, Wapenaar R, Van Oene J. Time course of adverse events in patients with localization-related epilepsy receiving topiramate added to carbamazepine. Epilepsia 2005;46:648–53.

85. Cereza G, Pedros C, Garcia N, Laporte J-R. Topiramate in non-approved indications and acute myopia or angle closure glaucoma. Br J Clin Pharmacol 2005;60:578–9.

86. Ozkara C, Ozmen M, Erdogan A, Yalug I. Topiramate related obsessive–compulsive disorder. Eur Psychiatry 2005;20:78–9.

87. Kaplan M. Hypomania with topiramate. J Clin Psychopharmacol 2005;25:196–7.

88. Nickel MK, Nickel C, Kaplan P, Lahmann C, Muhlbacher M, Tritt K, Krawczyk J, Leiberich PK, Rother WK, Loew TH. Treatment of aggression with topiramate in male borderline patients: a double-blind, placebo-controlled study. Biol Psychiatry 2005;57:495–9.

89. Nickel C, Lahmann C, Tritt K, Muehlbacher M, Kaplan P, Kettler C, Krawczyk J, Loew TH, Rother WK, Nickel MK. Topiramate in treatment of depressive and anger symptoms in female depressive patients: a randomized, double-blind, placebo-controlled study. J Affect Disord 2005;87:243–52.

90. Garris SS, Oles KS. Impact of topiramate on serum bicarbonate concentration in adults. Ann Pharmacother 2005;39:424–6.

91. Holtkamp M, Weissinger F, Meierkord H. Erectile dysfunction with topiramate. Epilepsia 2005;46:166–7.

92. Galicia SC, Lewis SL, Metman LV. Severe topiramate-associated hyperthermia resulting in persistent neurological dysfunction. Clin Neuropharmacol 2005;28:94–5.

93. Battino D, Croci D, Rossini A, Messina S, Mamoli D, Perucca E. Topiramate pharmacokinetics in children and adults with epilepsy: a case-matched comparison based on therapeutic drug monitoring data. Clin Pharmacokinet 2005;44:407–16.

94. Britzi M, Perucca E, Soback S, Levy RH, Fattore C, Crema F, Gatti G, Doose DR, Maryanoff BE, Bialer M. Pharmacokinetic and metabolic investigation of topiramate disposition in healthy subjects in the absence and in

the presence of enzyme induction by carbamazepine. Epilepsia 2005;46:378–84.

95. Mohanraj R, Brodie MJ. Pharmacological outcomes in newly diagnosed epilepsy. Epilepsy Behav 2005;6(3):382–7.

96. Wassef AA, Winkler DE, Roache AL, Abobo VB, Lopez LM, Averill JP, Mian AI, Overall JE. Lower effectiveness of divalproex versus valproic acid in a prospective, quasi-experimental clinical trial involving 9,260 psychiatric admissions. Am J Psychiatry 2005;162:330–9.

97. Rinnerthaler M, Luef G, Mueller J, Seppi K, Wissel J, Trinka E, Bauer G, Poewe W. Computerized tremor analysis of valproate-induced tremor: a comparative study of controlled-release versus conventional valproate. Epilepsia 2005;46:320–3.

98. Hauben M, Reich L. Valproate-induced Parkinsonism: use of a newer pharmacovigilance tool to investigate the reporting of an unanticipated adverse event with an "old" drug. Movement Disord 2005;20(3):387.

99. Sorri I, Rissanen E, Mäntyjärvi M, Kälviäinen R. Visual function in epilepsy patients treated with initial valproate monotherapy. Seizure 2005;14(6):367–70.

100. Watanabe T, Nakayasu K, Nagayama Y. Autoimmune hemolytic anemia and renal Fanconi syndrome caused by valproate therapy. Eur J Pediatr 2005;164:186–7.

101. Coyle TE, Bair AK, Stein C, Vajpayee N, Mehdi S, Wright J. Acute leukemia associated with valproic acid treatment: a novel mechanism for leukemogenesis? Am J Hematol 2005;78:256–60.

102. Mauz PS, Morike K, Kaiserling E, Brosch S. Valproic acid-associated sialadenosis of the parotid and submandibular glands: diagnostic and therapeutic aspects. Acta Oto-Laryngol 2005;125:386–91.

103. Singh V, Muzina DJ, Calabrese JR. Anticonvulsants in bipolar disorder. Psychiatr Clin N Am 2005;28:301–23.

104. Sato K, Ueda Y, Ueno K, Okamoto K, Iizuka H, Katsuda S. Hepatocellular carcinoma and nonalcoholic steatohepatitis developing during long-term administration of valproic acid. Virchow's Archiv 2005;447:996–9.

105. Patrizi A, Savoia F, Negosanti F, Posar A, Santucci M, Neri I. Telogen effluvium caused by magnesium valproate and lamotrigine. Acta Derm Venereol 2005;85(1):77–8.

106. Rasgon NL, Altshuler LL, Fairbanks L, Elman S, Bitran J, Labarca R, Saad M, Kupka R, Nolen WA, Frye MA, Suppes T, McElroy SL, Keck PE, Leverich G, Grunze H, Walden J, Post R, Mintz J. Reproductive function and risk for PCOS in women treated for bipolar disorder. Bipolar Disord 2005;7(3):246–59.

107. Eriksson K, Viinikainen K, Monkkonen A, Aikia M, Nieminen P, Heinonen S, Kalviainen R. Children exposed to valproate in utero—population based evaluation of risks and confounding factors for long-term neurocognitive development. Epilepsy Res 2005;65:189–200.

108. Schorry EK, Oppenheimer SG, Saal HM. Valproate embryopathy: clinical and cognitive profile in 5 siblings. Am J Med Genet 2005;133:202–6.

109. Miller BP, Perry W, Moutier CY, Robinson SK, Feifel D. Rapid oral loading of extended release divalproex in patients with acute mania. Gen Hosp Psychiatry 2005;27(3):218–21.

110. Peters CAN, Pohlmann-Eden B. Intravenous valproate as an innovative therapy in seizure emergency situations including status epilepticus—experience in 102 adult patients. Seizure 2005;14(3):164–9.

111. Reiter PD, Nickisch J, Merritt G. Efficacy and tolerability of intravenous valproic acid in acute adolescent migraine. Headache 2005;45:899–903.

112. Eyer F, Felgenhauer N, Gempel K, Steimer W, Gerbitz K-D, Zilker T. Acute valproate poisoning: pharmacokinetics, alteration in fatty acid metabolism, and changes during therapy. J Clin Psychopharmacol 2005;25:376–80.

113. Ikeda H, Murakami T, Takano M, Usui T, Kihira K. Pharmacokinetic interaction on valproic acid and recurrence of epileptic seizures during chemotherapy in an epileptic patient. Br J Clin Pharmacol 2005;59:593–7.

114. Ragueneau-Majlessi I, Levy RH, Brodie M, Smith D, Shah J, Grund JS. Lack of pharmacokinetic interactions between steady-state zonisamide and valproic acid in patients with epilepsy. Clin Pharmacokinet 2005;44:517–23.

115. Coves-Orts FJ, Borras-Blasco J, Navarro-Ruiz A, Murcia-Lopez A, Palacios-Ortega F. Acute seizures due to a probable interaction between valproic acid and meropenem. Ann Pharmacother 2005;39:533–7.

116. Herzog AG, Farina EL, Blum AS. Serum valproate levels with oral contraceptive use. Epilepsia 2005;46:970–1.

117. Fleming J, Chetty M. Psychotropic drug interactions with valproate. Clin Neuropharmacol 2005;28:96–101.

118. LoVecchio F, Shriki J, Samaddar R. L-carnitine was safely administered in the setting of valproate toxicity. Am J Emerg Med 2005;23(3):321–2.

119. Camilleri C, Albertson T, Offerman S. Fatal cerebral edema after moderate valproic acid overdose. Ann Emerg Med 2005;45:337–8.

120. Tseng YL, Lan MY, Lai SL, Huang FC, Tsai JJ. Vigabatrin-attributable visual field defects in patients with intractable partial epilepsy. Acta Neurol Taiwan 2006;15(4):244–50.

121. Sorri I, Herrgard E, Viinikainen K, Paakkonen A, Heinonen S, Kalviäinen R. Ophthalmologic and neurologic findings in two children exposed to vigabatrin in utero. Epilepsy Res 2005;65(1–2):117–20.

122. Scaioli V, Franceschetti S, Binelli S, Casazza M, Villani F, Granata T, Balestrini MR,

Curzi S, Agazzi P, Avanzino G. Serial electro-physiological studies of the visual pathway in patients treated with vigabatrin. Int Congr Ser 2005;1278:41–4.

123. Hammoudi DS, Lee SSF, Madison A, Mirabella G, Buncic JR, Logan WJ, Snead OC, Westall CA. Reduced visual function associated with infantile spasms in children on vigabatrin therapy. Investig Ophthalmol Vis Sci 2005;46:514–20.

124. Brodie MJ, Duncan R, Vespignani H, Solyom A, Bitenskyy V, Lucas C. Dose-dependent safety and efficacy of zonisamide: a randomized, double-blind, placebo-controlled study in patients with refractory partial seizures. Epilepsia 2005;46:31–41.

125. Chadwick DW, Marson AG. Zonisamide add-on for drug-resistant partial epilepsy. Cochrane Database Syst Rev 2005;19(4).

126. Wilfong A, Schultz R. Zonisamide for absence seizures. Epilepsy Res 2005;64(1–29):31–4.

127. Go T. Effect of antiepileptic drug polytherapy on crystalluria. Pediatr Neurol 2005;32(2):113–5.

128. Santos CS, Brotherton T. Use of zonisamide in pediatric patients. Pediatr Neurol 2005;33(1):12–4.

129. Wilfong AA. Zonisamide monotherapy for epilepsy in children and young adults. Pediatr Neurol 2005;32(2):77–80.

130. Yanagaki S, Oguni H, Yoshii K, Hayashi K, Imai K, Funatsuka M, Osawa M. Zonisamide for West syndrome: a comparison of clinical responses among different titration rate. Brain Develop 2005;27(4):286–90.

131. Bookheimer S, Schrader LM, Rausch R, Sankar R, Engel Jr J. Reduced anesthetization during the intracarotid amobarbital (Wada) testing patients taking carbonic anhydrase-inhibiting medications. Epilepsia 2005;46:236–43.

132. Griffith SG, Dai Y. Effect of zonisamide on the pharmacokinetics and pharmacodynamics of a combination ethinylestradiol–norethindrone oral contraceptive in healthy women. Clin Ther 2005;26(12):2056–65.

A.H. Ghodse and S. Galea

8 Opioid analgesics and narcotic antagonists

℞ **Routes of administration of opioids**

The usefulness and adverse effects of different routes of administration of opioids have been discussed in several articles.

Oral *Oral administration is the method most often used because it is non-invasive, convenient and easy to titrate. In chronic pain oral opioid formulations that provide longer durations of effect are preferred, because they provide more stable pain control, better tolerability, and increased convenience, patient options, and flexibility.*

Modified-release oxymorphone is a new oral tablet formulation aimed to provide a 12-hour dosing interval. In a prospective, open, sequential crossover pilot study patients with cancer with moderate or severe pain, using either modified-release morphine or oxycodone, were safely switched to modified-release oxymorphone at a lower equivalent dosage with no reduction in pain relief or increase in adverse effects (1^c). This study was a pilot study with a small sample size. Further studies are required for more robust findings.

In another study oral and rectal tramadol were compared (2^c). The two routes were equally effective in pain relief and were associated with similar adverse events. However, both patients and physicians preferred the oral route. Nevertheless, rectal administration of tramadol can be safe, reliable, and non-invasive for patients who cannot take oral tramadol.

Sublingual *The combination of naloxone and buprenorphine has been used sublingually with the aim of reducing the abuse potential of buprenorphine. When crushed and injected, naloxone will act as an opioid receptor antagonist. This combination when administered parenterally to non-physically dependent individuals attenuated (but did not block) the effects of buprenorphine (3^R).*

Intramuscular and subcutaneous *The intramuscular and subcutaneous routes are most often used in postoperative analgesia (4^R). The limitations are: discomfort due to repeated injections; large interpersonal variation in dosage requirements; peaks and troughs in blood concentrations with inconsistent pain relief and incidence of adverse effects; and delayed response times from staff in delivering the analgesic (4^R).*

In patients undergoing posterior lumbar interbody fusion, continuous epidural morphine was compared with continuous subcutaneous morphine as pre-emptive analgesia (5^c). There were no differences in analgesic effects. However, there were more adverse effects with epidural morphine, despite the fact that subcutaneous doses of morphine were about three times higher. In addition, preoperative epidural catheterization was difficult without seeing the dura mater. Thus, continuous epidural morphine was not suitable for pre-emptive analgesia; continuous subcutaneous morphine was the preferred option because of technical ease and fewer complications.

Patient-controlled analgesia *Patient-controlled analgesia (PCA), intravenously, subcutaneously, intramuscularly, epidurally, or transdermally, is the method that patients prefer (6^R). It gives them increased autonomy, greater control, reduced anxiety, "better pain relief",*

Side Effects of Drugs, Annual 30
J.K. Aronson (Editor)
ISSN: 0378-6080
DOI: 10.1016/S0378-6080(08)00008-1

and "not worrying about receiving too much drug" (4^R, 6^R, 7^M). The technique's effectiveness depends on appropriate patient alertness, education, and motivation. Methods that require a pump have some disadvantages—well trained nursing staff are required and pumps can be cumbersome, limiting patient mobility. Potentially life-threatening adverse events can occur through errors in programming (8^A).

- A 51-year-old man was given postoperative piritramide by perfusor pump. He was found dead a few hours later. Autopsy, histopathology, and toxicology suggested piritramide overdose. Recent servicing of the perfusor pump had resulted in a change in settings from mg/hour to ml/hour. Consequently, he had received 1.5 times the intended dose of piritramide.

Despite its limitations the technique has the advantage of reducing peaks and troughs and is superior to ordinary intramuscular administration. Recent technology has seen the development of a fentanyl–PCA transdermal patch. This is a needle-free patch that delivers fentanyl on demand through a low-intensity direct electric current, transferring ionizable drug transdermally into the systemic circulation. It is programmed to deliver fixed doses over 10 minutes, to a total of 80 doses or over a total period of 24 hours. This system overcomes the various limitations of PCA outlined above. It reduces programming errors, is non-invasive, does not require patient motivation, and is not attached to a pump, facilitating early mobility and recovery (6^R). It is easy to use and produces adequate pain relief. It is also well-tolerated, the most common adverse effect being nausea. It is less sedating and disorientating than intravenous PCA morphine and may therefore be more suitable for elderly patients (6^R).

Intrathecal   The intrathecal route of administration is effective but has the potential for an increased frequency of adverse effects. Pruritus is the most frequent adverse effect of intrathecal morphine. Concern has also been raised about the possible association of pruritus with re-activation of herpes labialis virus type II. Reactivation of oral Herpes simplex infection has been explored in patients receiving intrathecal morphine and intravenous morphine (9^c). More patients had reactivation of Herpes simplex with intrathecal morphine than with intravenous morphine (19 versus 8). There was

also a significantly higher incidence of pruritus with intrathecal morphine. These results suggest that there is a cause-and-effect relation between pruritus and herpes re-activation.

Other adverse effects associated with intrathecal morphine include nausea and vomiting, urinary retention, and early or delayed respiratory depression.

In a comparison of intrathecal morphine and remifentanil in patients undergoing off-pump coronary surgery opioid-related cardiac effects were similar; intrathecal morphine did not produce central neuroaxial hematoma or post-spinal tap headache (10^c).

Intrathecal lipid-soluble agents, such as fentanyl and sufentanil, do not predispose to nausea and vomiting, but do predispose to dose-related pruritus (4^R). In a comparison of intrathecal fentanyl and systemic hydromorphone (1 mg intramuscularly + 1 mg intravenously) in nulliparous women in spontaneous labor, intrathecal administration was associated with less nausea and vomiting than systemic administration (11^{Cr}).

In a comparison of sufentanil 7.5 micrograms intrathecally and 7.5 micrograms intravenously, intrathecal sufentanil had superior analgesic efficacy (12^C). There was pruritus in significantly more patients with intrathecal sufentanil (5 versus 0). Peripheral oxygen desaturation was only observed with intravenous sufentanil (n = 6).

Intrathecal nalbuphine for elective cesarean delivery is associated with fewer adverse effects than other opioids (such as morphine) (4^R).

Long-term intrathecal administration of pethidine may be associated with toxicity, owing to accumulation of its metabolite, norpethidine. This was explored in a study in 10 patients with neuropathic cancer pain, who had not responded sufficiently to recommended regimens (13^c). There were high plasma concentrations of pethidine and norpethidine in three subjects; however, norpethidine concentrations were still below the concentration reported to induce nervous system toxicity, i.e. under 500 ng/ml, and no patient had evidence of nervous system toxicity. One patient developed a tremor and twitches on day 7; however, these were unlikely to be due to nervous system excitability because they resolved spontaneously in 3 hours and further administration of pethidine was not accompanied by further excitation.

Epidural   *The epidural route tends to provide high-quality analgesia and is rational in patients with a short life expectancy when systemic treatment of chronic pain has failed. Fentanyl and morphine are the most common opioids given in this way. Some limitations of this route include: risk of infection; spinal hematoma; reduced mobility due to cumbersome equipment (4^R). Adverse effects are not infrequent but do not tend to be severe or life-threatening.*

All forms of epidural analgesia (both continuous epidural infusion and patient-controlled infusion) provide superior analgesia compared with patient-controlled intravenous analgesia (7^M, 14^C). Continuous infusion epidural analgesia is superior to patient-controlled epidural analgesia; patients on continuous epidural infusion have a lower incidence of pruritus but higher incidences of nausea, vomiting, and motor block (7^M).

In comparisons of lipophilic and hydrophilic opioids, the latter are associated with higher pain scores (7^M). The epidural method is the preferred route by patients undergoing cesarean section, because often the anesthetic procedure itself is epidural.

Lipid-encapsulated morphine (DepoDur™) has the advantage of sustained release and prolonged analgesia when given epidurally (4^R). In a comparison of DepoDur™ (5, 10, 15, 20, or 25 mg) and standard epidural morphine a single-dose of DepoDur™ was well tolerated; 97% of patients rated adverse events (nausea, vomiting, pruritus, and hypotension) as mild to moderate (15^C). Fewer of the patients who received DepoDur™ (87%) required intravenous fentanyl for breakthrough pain than those who received standard epidural morphine (98%). All doses of DepoDur™ were well tolerated and the adverse effects profile was acceptable and predictable. However, further studies are required to determine the optimum dosage and safety in different patient populations.

A similar study of DepoDur™ up to 48 hours after elective cesarean section showed that DepoDur™ was well tolerated, with mild to moderate adverse events, and was as beneficial as standard morphine (16^C).

In a study of a low-volume continuous infusion mix (9 ml of bupivacaine 0.5%, clonidine 150 micrograms, and diamorphine over 30 hours) in 65 patients, pain relief improved as did adverse effects, such as drowsiness, confusion, hallucinations, and constipation. Serious adverse reactions were infrequent. More common adverse events were related to the route of administration, such as superficial infections (11%), deep infections (2.1%), paresthesia (4.3%), and line migration/dislocation (32%) (17^c).

The use of epidural buprenorphine to treat cancer pain is associated with early respiratory depression (18^R).

Rectal   *Transdermal fentanyl patches typically contain large amounts of fentanyl, thus giving the potential for abuse and toxicity. Fentanyl toxicity has been reported after rectal insertion of fentanyl patches (19^{Ar}).*

- *A 41-year-old man became comatose after inserting three fentanyl patches (100 µg/hour) into his rectum. He was given naloxone 6 mg without a response. The patches were removed digitally and he recovered 1 hour later.*

This report shows the importance of being aware of the toxic potential of patches. Increased absorption by the rectal mucosa and the relatively high rectal temperature facilitate rapid release and high fentanyl concentrations. The authors pointed out that the low price of the patches could result in more cases of accidental, abusive, or intentional fentanyl toxicity.

Musculoskeletal   Opioid use results in *reduced bone mineral density*, probably mediated by suppression of endogenous production of sex hormones. In a large sample of the US population opioid users had a reduced bone mineral density compared with non-users, when adjusting for all co-variates (20^C). This effect was more evident in long-term users. Owing to lack of data on testosterone and estradiol, the investigators could not prove causality.

A report of bilateral femoral neck stress fractures in a heroin addict has highlighted the importance of early identification of osteopenia (21^A).

Drug–drug interactions   Analgesic agents are commonly used in combination, with the aim of benefiting from their additive or synergistic effect on analgesia and from the potential to reduce the prevalence of adverse effects due to lower dosage regimens. There has been a systematic review of opioid-related adverse events in studies of opioid-sparing postoperative pain treatment with *COX-2 inhibitors* (rofecoxib, celecoxib, parecoxib, and valdecoxib) (22[M]). The opioids were hydrocodone, fentanyl, hydromorphone, morphine, tramadol, and pethidine. The results did not support the opinion that opioid-sparing is associated with a reduced frequency of adverse events. Vomiting was significantly reduced in only three of the 18 trials. There was also no evidence to support a reduced risk of other opioid-related adverse events, except for dizziness.

OPIOID RECEPTOR AGONISTS

Dextromethorphan   *(SED-15, 1088; SEDA-27, 88; SEDA-28, 106; SEDA-29, 105)*

Dextromethorphan is a non-competitive antagonist at N-methyl-D-aspartate (NMDA) receptors. It is antitussive and has antihyperalgesic effects. In 25 volunteers intravenous dextromethorphan 0.5 mg/kg significantly reduced areas of established hyperalgesia after tissue injury by 39% and prevented the development of further hyperalgesia (23[c]). There was large inter-subject variability in the timing of this effect, with an average duration of 2 hours in relation to peak serum concentration. Most of the volunteers ($n = 22$) reported adverse events, such as mild to moderate *dizziness* and *drowsiness*. However, attention should be paid to the potential for dextromethorphan to cause phencyclidine-like effects and its potential as a drug of abuse.

Susceptibility factors   When dextromethorphan hydrobromide 80 mg orally (equivalent to 62 mg of dextromethorphan base) was given to 419 healthy subjects, adverse events were experienced by 17%, most being mild (24[C]). Dextromethorphan is metabolized by CYP2D6 in the liver to its active metabolite dextrorphan (SEDA-29, 105). *Body mass index, weight, female sex, increased CYP2D6 and CYP3A4 metabolic ratios*, and *CYP2D6 poor metabolizer phenotypes* were significantly associated with adverse events, but CYP2D6 extensive metabolizers were not protected against adverse

events. Adverse events were more closely associated with CYP2D6 activity than with the CYP2D6 phenotype. There was no association between the μ opioid (OP$_3$, MOR) receptor and the occurrence of adverse events, possibly because dextromethorphan is a weak opioid agonist, binding to sigma rather than μ opioid receptors (24[C]).

Drug formulations   A fixed-dose combination of dextromethorphan 30 mg and quinidine 30 mg has been developed and is undergoing Phase II and Phase III trials in the treatment of emotional lability, neuropathic pain, chronic cough, and weaning drug-dependent patients from opioid analgesics and antidepressants. The usefulness of the combination results from the ability of quinidine to sustain therapeutic concentrations of dextromethorphan over a 12-hour dosing schedule by inhibiting oxidative first-pass metabolism of dextromethorphan, and hence reducing dosage requirements to only 2.5–5% of the usual dose. The combination significantly improved emotional lability in different patient populations, for example those with multiple sclerosis and amyotrophic lateral sclerosis, and was well tolerated (25[c]). The most commonly reported adverse events were *nausea, constipation, diarrhea, dry mouth, fatigue, dizziness, insomnia, headache, upper respiratory tract infection*, and *somnolence*. In most cases the adverse events were mild to moderate. Of those with diabetic neuropathy 24% withdrew because of adverse events from the combination drug compared with 6% of those taking dextromethorphan alone and 8% of those taking quinidine alone.

Dextropropoxyphene   *(SED-15, 1092; SEDA-27, 89)*

Drug overdose   Self-poisoning with co-proxamol (dextropropoxyphene hydrochloride 32.5 mg+paracetamol 325 mg) is a common method of self-poisoning in the UK; it accounts for 5% of all cases and is the second most commonly used drug in cases of self-poisoning (26[C], 27[r]). When it was marketed in the UK about 1.7 million people received 7.5 million prescriptions annually (27[r]). In a multicenter study based on an examination of coroners' reports in 2000–1, death resulted from respiratory depression and/or cardiac effects (26^C). There were 123 deaths from co-proxamol poisoning, of which 42% were in those aged 55 years or more, possibly because of increased prescribing in older age groups, increased vulnerability to toxicity, and higher degrees of suicidal intent. Alcohol was consumed in 59% of cases and most of these were young people with low degrees of suicide intent. About half had a history of self-harm and one-third were in contact with psychiatric services. Co-proxamol has been withdrawn in the UK.

Diamorphine (heroin) *(SED-15, 1096; SEDA-27, 89; SEDA-28, 106; SEDA-29, 106)*

Respiratory In a retrospective study of the case notes of patients who had been admitted to hospital with acute attacks of *asthma*, there was a high prevalence of heroin use—15% had used only heroin and another 16% had used both heroin and cocaine (28^c). Heroin users had been intubated more often than non-drug users (17 versus 2.3%). Similarly, more heroin users were admitted to ICU than non-users (21 versus 12%). However, they did not spend more time receiving mechanical ventilation or being in hospital. These findings suggest that heroin induced some degree of bronchoconstriction and respiratory depression, which worsened the initial presentation of asthma.

Nervous system Two cases of possible *toxic leukoencephalopathy* following probable inhalation of heroin vapor have been reported (29^A).

- A 55-year-old man developed confusion, behavioral change, aggression, poor attention, disorientation in time, and impaired short-term memory. He had full ocular movements with no nystagmus, brisk deep tendon reflexes, and bilateral extensor plantar responses. He became progressively drowsy with myoclonic jerks and died 2 weeks later.
- A 36-year-old man with a history of substance abuse became unresponsive, with his eyes in mid-position gaze, with pinpoint pupils, brisk deep tendon reflexes, and bilateral extensor plantar responses. On day 9 he spontaneously opened his

eyes. However, he died 1 month later with persistent pyrexia from methicillin resistant *Staphylococcus aureus*.

Neuroimaging and neuropathology in both cases showed diffuse symmetrical degeneration of white matter, with sparing of subcortical U fibers, cerebellum, and brain stem. Toxicology was negative, but was done some time after the report of substance use. In these case reports heroin use could not be confirmed. Although the findings suggested the possibility of heroin toxicity due to inhalation, sparing of the cerebellum and brain stem, frontal predominance of degeneration, and the more prominent axonal involvement are not typical of heroin toxicity, throwing speculation on an unidentified impurity.

Drug abuse The prevalence of heroin as a drug of abuse has been reviewed (30^R). There are over 1 million heroin addicts in the USA. The lifetime prevalence among those aged 12–25 years continues to increase gradually.

Drug contamination Atypical reactions after the use of heroin have been attributed to contamination with *clenbuterol* (31^A).

- Four patients, aged 21–43 years, all developed chest pain, palpitation, and shortness of breath after inhaling heroin. They had tachycardias, low blood pressure, hypokalemia, and hyperglycemia.

In all the cases the heroin had been adulterated with veterinary clenbuterol.

Fentanyl *(SED-15, 1346; SEDA-27, 90; SEDA-28, 108; SEDA-29, 106)*

Observational studies In 31 patients undergoing transurethral resection of the prostate fentanyl ($n = 15$) or saline ($n = 16$) was added to ropivacaine for subarachnoid block; the only significant adverse effect was *pruritus* (32^C).

Transdermal fentanyl 25 micrograms/hour has been assessed in 22 patients with painful oral mucositis induced by high-dose chemotherapy after stem cell transplantation (33^c). Three had severe *dizziness*, severe *vomiting*, and extensive *rashes*. These patients were subsequently withdrawn from the analysis. Mild *nausea* (in 32%) and *dizziness* (in 11%) were the two most common adverse events. There was no respiratory depression, constipation, or withdrawal symptoms.

Respiratory   The respiratory effects of fentanyl have been demonstrated in 21 volunteers who were given a high-dose infusion (34[c]). Four of them developed *apnea* shortly after the infusion, thought to be due to rapid crossing of the blood–brain barrier and rapid depression of respiratory neurons.

A method of estimating analgesic fentanyl requirements after surgery, while avoiding respiratory depression, has been evaluated prospectively (35[c]). The method was based on a fentanyl challenge before surgery. The patients required only very small adjustments to the settings that were based on estimates from the challenge. There was no evidence of respiratory depression.

The incidence of fentanyl-induced *cough* has been studied in patients undergoing surgery (36[C]). Fentanyl (100 micrograms for those weighing 40–69 kg; 150 micrograms for those weighing 70–90 kg) was given intravenously at three different rates, over 2, 15, or 30 seconds. A longer injection time resulted in a reduced incidence of cough. Light smoking was associated with a reduced incidence of cough.

Endocrine   *Hypothalamic–pituitary–adrenal (HPA) axis suppression* has been attributed to chronic administration of opioids (37[A]).

- A 64-year-old man with chronic sciatic pain had been taking transdermal fentanyl 200 micrograms/hour for 2 years. He developed back pain, miosis, somnolence, and a blood pressure of 70/40 mmHg. Adrenocortical insufficiency was diagnosed, but the cause was unclear, and he was given hydrocortisone 25 mg/day. After poor compliance with hydrocortisone he again presented in adrenal crisis. On re-stabilization, opiate-induced suppression of the HPA axis was suspected. On gradual reduction of the dose of fentanyl, HPA axis function improved markedly.

Gastrointestinal   Fentanyl and remifentanil have been compared in patients undergoing plastic surgery, anesthetized with propofol (38[C]). There was a higher incidence of postoperative *nausea and vomiting* in those who received fentanyl. Despite this, patient satisfaction was the same in the two groups.

In a comparison of transdermal fentanyl (*n* = 299) and modified-release oral morphine (*n* = 298) in patients with chronic low back pain, transdermal fentanyl was associated with significantly less constipation (31 versus 48%); a smaller proportion of those who received transdermal fentanyl needed to use laxatives (39[C]). In both groups, the most common adverse events leading to treatment withdrawal were *nausea, vomiting*, and *constipation*.

Drug abuse   Abuse of fentanyl-containing analgesics is increasing. In the USA, reports of fentanyl abuse increased to over 6000% (1506 cases) from 1995 to 2002 (29[R]).

Breast feeding   The method by which infants were fed at discharge from hospital has been studied in a random sample of 425 healthy primiparae who delivered healthy singleton babies at term (40[c]). The main determinants of bottle feeding were: maternal age (OR = 0.90, 95% CI = 0.85, 0.95); occupation (OR = 0.63, 95% CI = 0.40, 0.99 for each category, unemployed, manual, non-manual); antenatal feeding intentions (OR = 0.12, 95% CI = 0.08, 0.19 for each category, bottle feeding, undecided, breast-feeding); cesarean section (OR = 0.25, 95% CI = 0.13, 0.47, cesarean or vaginal delivery); and the dose of fentanyl administered intrapartum (OR = 1.004, 95% CI = 1.000, 1.008). The authors suggested that intrapartum fentanyl, particularly at higher doses, may impede the establishment of breast feeding by impairing suckling.

Susceptibility factors

Age   In children aged 2–16 years with chronic malignant and non-malignant pain, the adverse effects of transdermal fentanyl were those of a potent opioid, with no specific risks in this group of patients (41[C]).

Levo-α-acetylmethadol (LAAM)

Cardiovascular   Levo-α-acetylmethadol has been removed from the market throughout the European Union and in the USA production has ceased because of a report of 10 cases of *prolongation of the QT interval* (29[R]).

Drug–drug interactions   Levo-α-acetylmethadol is metabolized by CYP3A4 N-demethylation and CYP3A-mediated inactivation. Hence, patients who take CYP3A inducers (for example *rifampicin*) are susceptible to increased metabolism, reduced plasma concentrations, and withdrawal symptoms. Those taking CYP3A inhibitors (for example *troleandomycin*) are susceptible to reduced metabolism, increased plasma concentrations, and toxicity (42[E]).

Methadone   *(SED-15, 2270; SEDA-27, 91; SEDA-28, 47; SEDA, 107)*

Observational studies   Methadone 16 mg/day was effective in 29 patients with restless legs syndrome that had not responded to dopamine receptor agonists (43[c]). Most ($n = 17$) were still taking methadone at follow-up and reported a 75% reduction in symptoms. Of 27 patients, 17 reported at least one adverse event while taking methadone, including *constipation* ($n = 11$), *fatigue* ($n = 2$), and *insomnia, sedation, rash, reduced libido, confusion*, and *hypertension* (one each). Five patients stopped treatment because of adverse events.

Cardiovascular   Recent reports have implicated methadone in potentially fatal cardiac effects (SEDA-27, 91; SEDA-29, 107). Methadone-related *torsade de pointes* has been reported in a patient with chronic bone and vaso-occlusive pain due to sickle cell disease (44[Ar]).

- A 40-year-old man with sickle cell disease, hypertension, congestive heart failure, and a past history of cocaine and marihuana abuse, was given a large dose of oral methadone 560 mg/day, following hydromorphone 170 mg intravenously and by PCA for progressive back and leg pain. On day 2, he developed asymptomatic bradycardia and QT_c prolongation (454–522 msec). On day 3, he developed profuse sweating and non-sustained polymorphous ventricular tachycardia consistent with torsade de pointes. He had hypokalemia and hypocalcaemia. Echocardiography showed normal bilateral ventricular function, mild pulmonary hypertension, and trivial four-valve regurgitation. Methadone was replaced by modified-release morphine and a continuous epidural infusion of hydromorphone + bupivacaine. Daily electrocardiography showed a heart rate of 50–69/minute, a QT_c interval of 375–463 msec, and no further dysrhythmias.

This case highlights the importance of very careful monitoring especially when prescribing such large doses of methadone. The effects of methadone on cardiac function are potentially fatal.

Another report has highlighted the potential risks of combining prodysrhythmic drugs on cardiovascular function (45[Ar]).

- A 39-year-old man had recurrent episodes of sinus tachycardia at 115/minute, with no other abnormalities. He was taking methadone 120 mg/day for opioid dependency and doxepin 100 mg/day for anxiety, and was given metoprolol 50 mg/day. During the next few weeks he had episodes of recurrent syncope with sinus bradycardia (47/minute) and prolongation of the QT interval (542 ms). The QT interval and heart rate normalized after withdrawal of all treatment.

In this case it is likely that the myocardial repolarization potential of methadone and doxepin may have been influenced or triggered by bradycardia induced by metoprolol. This shows the importance of cardiac monitoring in patients receiving combination therapy with potential adverse cardiac effects. Patients with co-morbidities are at high risk.

The association between methadone treatment and *QT_c interval prolongation*, QRS widening, and bradycardia has been explored prospectively in 160 patients with at least a 1-year history of opioid misuse (46[C]). The QT_c interval increased significantly from baseline at 6 months ($n = 149$) and 12 months ($n = 108$). The QRS duration and heart rate did not change. There were no cases of torsade de pointes, cardiac dysrhythmias, syncope, or sudden death. There was a positive correlation between methadone concentration and the QT_c interval.

Psychiatric   The combinations of methadone + carbamazepine and buprenorphine + carbamazepine have been compared in the treatment of mood disturbances during the detoxification of 26 patients with co-morbidities (47[c]). The buprenorphine combination had more of an effect. More patients taking the methadone combination dropped out of the study (58 versus 36%). However, both regimens were considered safe and without unexpected adverse effects. The results of this study need to be interpreted with caution because of the small sample size.

Immunologic The immunotoxic potential of methadone has been studied in rats that were given methadone 20 or 40 mg/kg/day for 6 weeks (48[ER]). The higher dose increased serum IgG concentrations but had no effect on functioning of the immune system. This suggests that methadone is not associated with immunotoxicity, even at dosages that were very high compared with usual clinical doses. The author advised caution in extrapolating animal data to humans.

Pregnancy and fetotoxicity In a randomized controlled trial in 18 pregnant women in the second trimester, a change from short-acting morphine to methadone or buprenorphine was explored (49[c]). The transition was accomplished without any adverse events in mother or fetus and with minimal withdrawal discomfort.

In 42 methadone-maintained women methadone had profound effects on fetal neurobehavioral functioning, implying a disruption of or threat to fetal neural development (50[C]). At peak concentrations the fetuses had slower heart rates, less heart rate variability, fewer heart rate accelerations, reduced duration of movements, reduced motor activity, and a lower degree of coupling between fetal movement and fetal heart rate. The long-term effects of such daily changes in the fetus are not known. There were very few effects on maternal physiology.

Morphine   *(SED-15, 2386; SEDA-27, 92; SEDA-28, 109; SEDA-29, 107)*

Comparative studies Opioids are often combined with other analgesics to reduce the need for larger doses of opioids, which is often accompanied by a reduction in adverse effects. In a study of the effect of adding ketamine and nefopam to morphine for postoperative analgesia, ketamine ($n = 22$) caused more intense sedation and nefopam ($n = 22$) more *tachycardia* and profuse *sweating* than morphine ($n = 21$); other adverse effects did not differ (51[c]).

Drug combination studies

Morphine + droperidol A morphine-sparing effect is produced when droperidol is given in combination with morphine (52[C]). However,

the combination therapy is also associated with a greater frequency of postoperative *nausea and vomiting*.

Morphine + gabapentin Gabapentin and morphine are often used for neuropathic pain. In 57 patients the combination of gabapentin and morphine was more effective in managing pain than either tablet alone (53[C]). At the maximum tolerated dose, the gabapentin + morphine combination gave a similar frequency of adverse effects as either drug alone. However, there was an increased frequency of *dry mouth* compared with morphine alone and an increased frequency of *constipation* compared with gabapentin.

Morphine + ketamine In an observational study in more than 1000 patients of the combination of morphine + ketamine the combination was safe but was associated with frequent treatable adverse effects (54[C]). Therapy had to be withdrawn in 72 patients because of adverse effects. The most common reasons were *nausea, vivid dreams or hallucinations*, and *pruritus*. *Respiratory depression* and *sedation* not responding to naloxone occurred in three patients (two of whom had undiagnosed renal insufficiency, resulting in reduced elimination of morphine-6-glucuronide, the active metabolite of morphine). A substantial proportion experienced *vivid dreams* and/or *hallucinations* (6.2%), not unpleasant dreams (3.3%), and unpleasant dreams (0.8%). Two patients had *confusion* (one had brain metastases and another had a history of alcohol abuse) and one patient had an *anxiety attack*. Pain was still not adequately controlled in one-third of patients. Thus, although the combination therapy was overall beneficial, adverse effects were frequent. In another study intravenous ketamine 20 ng/ml or more enhanced morphine analgesia without causing intolerable adverse effects (55[c]).

Morphine + ketorolac In a study of the combination of ketorolac + morphine as intravenous PCA for postoperative ileus after colorectal resection, the combination resulted in 29% less morphine consumption and a reduction in the duration of recovery of bowel movement and ambulation (56[C]). Opioid-induced adverse effects were similar with morphine and morphine + ketorolac. In another study of pain relief after anterior cruciate ligament reconstruction, the combination of ketorolac + morphine was associated with morphine sparing, and patient satisfaction was similar in the two groups (57[c]).

Morphine + physostigmine The addition of physostigmine to morphine postoperatively enhances opioid analgesia. In adults undergoing open lower abdominal surgery who were randomly assigned to either morphine-based patient-controlled analgesia ($n = 25$) or morphine-based patient-controlled analgesia+a continuous infusion of physostigmine ($n = 25$), those who received the combination had an enhanced analgesic response and required significantly less morphine (58[C]). Physostigmine has antinociceptive properties, attenuates the production of proinflammatory cytokines (IL-1β) that reduce pain, attenuates morphine-induced respiratory depression, antagonizes the depressant effect of morphine on the apneic threshold, reverses postoperative somnolence and loss of consciousness through enhancing cholinergic muscarinic transmission, and reduces the postoperative anticholinergic syndrome, which is characterized by agitation, restlessness, disorientation, and respiratory depression. Physostigmine increased *nausea and vomiting*, especially in the early postoperative period, and the authors suggested that aggressive antiemetic treatment be added to the physostigmine+morphine regimen.

Psychological In a double-blind, crossover, randomized, placebo-controlled study of the acute effects of immediate-release morphine on everyday cognitive functioning in 14 patients who were also taking modified-release opioids, immediate-release morphine on top of modified-release morphine produced discrete *impairment of cognitive functioning* (59[c]). Both immediate and delayed memory recall were affected. Impairment in delayed recall was more pronounced. Retrograde amnesia suggested that morphine produces additional difficulties in retrieval of information. Simple tracking tasks were enhanced in the morphine group; however, more demanding tasks and set shifting were impaired. There was no effect on backwards digit span. These findings suggest that morphine produces discrete impairment that is likely to affect quality of life.

Gastrointestinal In a study of intrathecal morphine 50 micrograms after postpartum bilateral tubal ligation, those who received morphine had significantly more *vomiting* than the controls (21 versus 3.5%) (60[c]).

Skin *Pruritus* is a well known adverse effect of opioids. In a randomized study of the effects of ondansetron and dolasetron, given 30 minutes before anesthesia, to prevent pruritus induced by morphine (61[c]). One theory of the cause of morphine-induced pruritus is direct stimulation of 5-HT$_3$ receptors, at which ondansetron and dolasetron are antagonists. The results support this hypothesis, because the frequency of pruritus in the first 8 hours after the operation was reduced by 48% by ondansetron and 70% by dolasetron. Pruritus was still present in a significant number of patients (34% of the ondansetron group and 20% of the dolasetron group), suggesting that several mechanisms are involved in morphine-induced pruritus. The study was methodologically sound but lacked statistical power owing to a small sample size.

Immunologic The immunotoxic potential of morphine 25 or 50 mg/kg/day has been explored in a 6-week study in rats (48[ER]). Morphine had no effect on serum immunoglobulin concentrations, the antibody response to sheep erythrocytes, or host resistance to *Listeria monocytogenes*. However, it was associated with an increase in muscle larvae count after *T spiralis* infection. These findings suggest that morphine has a marginal effect on the immune system. However, these results cannot be extrapolated to effects in humans except with caution.

Death In 57 039 patients with non-ST segment elevation acute coronary syndromes—the CRUSADE study (Can Rapid Risk Stratification of Unstable Angina Patients Suppress Adverse Outcomes With Early Implementation of the ACC/AHA Guidelines)—patients taking morphine had a higher risk of death (62[C], 63[r]). These findings were consistent even when baseline characteristics and concomitant use of glyceryl trinitrate were accounted for.

Drug abuse Abuse of morphine-containing analgesics reported by emergency departments in the USA increased to 116% (2775 cases) from 1995 to 2002 (29[R]).

Susceptibility factors

Sex   In a study of sex differences in the experience of pain in 4317 patients (54% men), the women had more postoperative pain and required a higher dosage of morphine (+11%) than the men in the immediate postoperative period; these differences disappeared in elderly patients (64[C]).

Drug dosage regimens   Three different dosage regimens for epidural morphine have been compared in a double-blind study in women undergoing postpartum tubal ligation (65[C]). The patients were randomized to receive epidural saline and epidural morphine 2, 3, or 4 mg after epidural anesthesia with lidocaine. Postoperatively they received oral ibuprofen every 6 hours and paracetamol 325 mg + hydrocodone 10 mg on request. Pain was better controlled by epidural morphine. Those who received morphine had opioid-related adverse effects, namely, nausea, vomiting, and pruritus. Those who received morphine 4 mg required treatment for nausea, vomiting, and pruritus more often than those who received 2 mg, without analgesic benefit. Thus, morphine 2 mg caused the least "analgesic burden" and is probably the ideal regimen in women undergoing postpartum tubal ligation. There was no respiratory depression. The study did not explore options of smaller dosage regimens and may have lacked power to detect analgesic benefits between the various regimens.

In 45 children aged 1–15 years undergoing hip orthopedic surgery with 0.25% bupivacaine, three dosage regimens of morphine 11.2, 15, or 20 micrograms/kg were used for caudal or epidural administration that would produce at least 8 hours of postoperative analgesia (66[c]). The adverse effects of morphine were dose-related: 11.2 micrograms/kg produced the lowest frequency of *sleeping* and *vomiting*. However, the frequency of vomiting was unacceptably high: almost 50% of children given the lowest dose of morphine had vomiting. This high frequency was unlikely to have been due to the adverse effects of morphine alone, and the authors suggested possible contributory factors, such as the administration of oxygen via a facemask with gastric distension and prolonged preoperative fasting. Morphine was not associated with urinary retention or pruritus.

Oxycodone   *(SED-15, 2651; SEDA-27, 93; SEDA-28, 110; SEDA-29, 108)*

Drug abuse   In 2002 an estimated 1.9 million people were using oxycodone illicitly in the USA; emergency room reports of oxycodone abuse increased to 560% (22 397 cases) from 1995 to 2002 (29[R]).

Papaverine

Cardiovascular   A study in neonates has confirmed the hypothesis that continuous infusion of papaverine-containing solutions in peripheral arterial catheters reduces the catheter failure rate and increases the functional duration of the catheter (67[c]). There was no difference in the incidence of intraventricular hemorrhage and no evidence of hepatotoxicity.

Sexual function   Intracavernous injection of papaverine for erectile impotence is invasive and is generally associated with *pain, anxiety*, and *priapism*. Vardenafil, on the other hand, is used orally with a lower risk of priapism. In 24 men, vardenafil was compared with papaverine and was as effective and safer (68[c]). There was prolonged erection requiring pharmacological detumescence in three of those given papaverine.

Pethidine (meperidine)   *(SED-15, 2791; SEDA-27, 94; SEDA-28, 111; SEDA-29, 108)*

Gastrointestinal   Non-steroidal anti-inflammatory drugs have been compared with opioids in the treatment of acute renal colic in a meta-analysis of 20 studies (69[M]). Seven different opioids were studied. In most of the studies there was a higher incidence of adverse events in patients who took opioids. Pooled analysis showed significantly more *vomiting* in those who took opioids, particularly pethidine. No serious adverse events were reported and adverse event rates did not vary with dosage.

Pregnancy and fetotoxicity   In 407 women in labor with dystocia, pethidine, contrary to the belief that it has oxytocic properties, did not reduce the duration of labor and was not useful in the management of first-stage dystocia (70[Cr]). More of those who received pethidine than the controls required augmentation of labor with oxytocic agents. Also more women in the pethidine group had *nausea, vomiting*, and *dizziness*. The fetuses that had been exposed to pethidine were more likely to have an Apgar score under 7 at 1 minute, had an umbilical cord blood pH under 7.10, and were more likely to be admitted to the neonatal intensive care unit.

Lactation   Pethidine is not often used in postcesarean analgesia because its active metabolite, norpethidine, can accumulate in breast milk, resulting in reduced scores on neonatal behavior assessment scales (4[R]).

Pholcodine

Immunologic   *Hypersensitivity* has been attributed to pholcodine (71[A]).

- A 33-year-old woman developed facial angioedema 8 hours after taking Respilène®syrup (which contains pholcodine, domperidone, tixocortol, and bacitracin). The symptoms resolved with an intravenous glucocorticoid. An intradermal test was positive for pholcodine but negative for domperidone, tixocortol, and bacitracin. Open oral challenge with pholcodine 20 mg was positive.

This is believed to have been the first report of allergy to pholcodine.

Remifentanil   *(SED-15, 3030; SEDA-27, 94; SEDA-28, 111; SEDA-29, 109)*

Observational studies   Remifentanil 0.054 micrograms/kg/minute for postoperative pain after cardiac surgery produced adequate analgesia in 73% of tracheally extubated patients without causing respiratory compromise (72[c], 73[c]). However, the investigators suggested careful monitoring by trained personnel (72[c]).

In infants and children undergoing cardiac surgery, spinal anesthetic blockade with remifentanil significantly reduced postoperative pain and reduced the requirement for fentanyl without significant adverse effects (73[c]).

Cardiovascular   Remifentanil can cause *bradycardia* and *hypotension*. In 40 children, cardiac effects were monitored after the administration of remifentanil with or without atropine (74[c]). Remifentanil reduced blood pressure, heart rate, and cardiac index, even when atropine was added (75[c]). Glycopyrrolate 6 micrograms/kg prevented the bradycardia caused by remifentanil + sevoflurane anesthesia for cardiac catheterization in children with congenital heart disease (76[C]). Remifentanil attenuated the rapid rise in systolic blood pressure after electroconvulsive therapy. This sympathetic response can be harmful to patients who already have cardiac problems. Thus the cardiac effects of remifentanil may be beneficial in patients with compromised cardiac function.

Respiratory   In 11 volunteers remifentanil 0.035 micrograms/kg/minute *reduced normoxic and hypoxic ventilation* (77[c]). In children who were breathing spontaneously and receiving inhalational anesthesia, large variations in dosages of remifentanil (0.053–0.3 micrograms/kg/minute) werc well tolerated (78[c]). A dose of 0.05 micrograms/kg/minute allowed spontaneous respiration in over 90% of children and 0.3 micrograms/kg/minute prevented spontaneous respiration in 90%. Although this study provided useful information on the respiratory effects of increasing infusion rates of remifentanil in children, it had several limitations, including not comparing respiratory parameters with blood concentrations.

Nervous system   Intraoperative administration of large doses of remifentanil produces postoperative peri-incisional *hyperalgesia*. In a randomized study 75 patients undergoing major abdominal surgery were given one of two doses of remifentanil (0.05 and 0.4 micrograms/kg/minute) or remifentanil + ketamine (remifentanil 0.4 micrograms/kg/minute; ketamine 0.5 mg/kg after induction, 5 micrograms/kg/minute intraoperatively up to skin closure, and 2 micrograms/kg/minute for 48 hours thereafter) (79[C]). High-dose remifentanil was associated with hyperalgesia. The addition of ketamine prevented this, implying involvement of NMDA receptors. There were similar results in a smaller study in patients undergoing major abdominal surgery, in which high-dose remifentanil added to epidural anesthesia resulted in acute opioid tolerance and hyperalgesia immediately after surgery (80[C]).

Gastrointestinal Remifentanil produced less postoperative *nausea and vomiting* than fentanyl in a prospective, randomized, double-blind study in patients anesthetized with propofol undergoing plastic surgery (38[C]). The incidence of nausea and vomiting 2–12 hours postoperatively was less if remifentanil was used intraoperatively rather than fentanyl. The need for antiemetic rescue drugs was also less with remifentanil. Known susceptibility factors for postoperative nausea and vomiting were accounted for through exclusion criteria. The patients who received remifentanil also required less postoperative opioid analgesia. Despite these benefits, the degree of patient satisfaction was the same in the two groups.

Pregnancy and fetotoxicity In 20 women in labor remifentanil gave better analgesia than nitrous oxide (81[C]). The adverse effects were similar in the two groups, with some exceptions—sedation was more profound with remifentanil and two subjects reported slight itching. The effects on the fetus were similar in the two groups, including reduced beat-to-beat variability in fetal heart rate. The neonates did not suffer from depression; however, there were withdrawals in the remifentanil group because of a requirement for respiratory support or fetal compromise.

Remifentanil has been compared with diazepam during fetoscopic surgery in 54 women in the second trimester, who were randomly assigned to either incremental doses of diazepam or a continuous infusion of remifentanil after combined spinal epidural anesthesia (82[C]). Remifentanil produced adequate maternal sedation, with mild clinically irrelevant respiratory depression and faster and more pronounced fetal immobilization, resulting in better surgical conditions. No respiratory depression was observed with diazepam and sedation was more pronounced.

Susceptibility factors

Age Remifentanil and remifentanil + midazolam provided safe and effective analgesia for bone marrow aspiration in 80 children aged 5–16 years of age (83[C]). There were no cases of deep sedation, hypotension, bradycardia, hypoxemia, or respiratory depression.

Drug–drug interactions The addition of *neostigmine* after anesthesia with propofol + remifentanil alters the state of anesthesia and may enhance recovery (84[C]).

The effects of two doses of remifentanil by intravenous infusion (7.5 micrograms/kg/hour, $n = 15$, and 30 micrograms/kg/hour, $n = 15$) have been compared with the effects of equal volumes of saline ($n = 15$) before induction of anesthesia with *propofol* (85[C]). Remifentanil significantly reduced propofol requirements and accelerated its hypnotic effects.

In 21 children, mean age 6.5 years, with lymphoblastic leukemia or lymphoma undergoing intrathecal chemotherapy, the combination of propofol and remifentanil achieved earlier recovery (86[C]). Similarly, in 20 children, the addition of remifentanil resulted in reduced propofol consumption and faster emergence times, as measured by the composite auditory evoked potential index.

For intracranial surgery, the combination of propofol + remifentanil produced fewer hypotensive events than the combination of sevoflurane + remifentanil (87[C]).

Tramadol   *(SED-15, 3469; SEDA-27, 96; SEDA-28, 112; SEDA-29, 110)*

Comparative studies In a comparison of intramuscular tramadol and intramuscular diclofenac sodium in acute migraine, the two treatments were equally effective (88[C]). The adverse effects profiles were also similar and were not considered to be severe. Nausea and vomiting were not associated with tramadol.

In a comparison of tramadol + midazolam and electro-acupuncture in relieving pain during shockwave lithotripsy, electro-acupuncture was more effective (89[C]). There were no adverse effects of electro-acupuncture, but tramadol + midazolam caused mild *orthostatic hypotension* and *dizziness*.

Cardiovascular *Pericarditis* has been attributed to tramadol (90[A]).

- An 88-year-old man took tramadol and 2 days later developed precordial chest pressure radiating to the scapula and increasing with inspiration and movement. His blood pressure was 75/45 mmHg

and his heart rate 60/minute. There was a soft pericardial rub, mild cardiomegaly, diffuse ST segment
elevation and PR interval shortening, normal left
ventricular systolic function, and no wall motion
abnormalities or effusion on echocardiography.

The temporal relation between the development
of acute pericarditis and the resolution of symptoms on withdrawal of tramadol suggested a
causal link.

Immunologic   Tramadol has been associated
with *angioedema*, a rare but a potentially life
threatening adverse effect (91[A]).

- A 52-year-old lady developed swelling of the
  tongue, peripheral sensory loss, difficulty in standing, and swelling below both eyes after taking
  tramadol 50 mg bd. Her symptoms resolved on
  withdrawal.
- A 36-year-old woman developed swelling of the
  tongue, difficulty swallowing, intense pruritus,
  sweating, hallucinations, vertigo, and, loss of sensory perception over the mouth and cheeks after
  taking tramadol.
- An 83-year-old woman with a history of heart
  failure, paroxysmal atrial fibrillation, chronic obstructive airways disease, and angina was given
  tramadol 50 mg tds and 5 days later developed
  swelling of the throat due to edema of the oral
  mucous membrane, uvula, tongue, and supraglot-
  tis. Tramadol was withdrawn and she was treated
  with cortisone, antihistamines, and adrenaline by
  inhalation.
- A 79-year-old man with a history of myocardial
  infarctions, anemia, heart failure, and angina, was
  given tramadol for back pain. After 17 days he developed respiratory distress and a swollen tongue.
  He was treated with cortisone and adrenaline, and
  tramadol and ramipril were withdrawn.
- A 61-year-old woman was given tramadol 50
  mg/day for sciatic pain and 2 hours later developed respiratory distress and difficulty opening her
  mouth. Anti-allergy treatment was given and tramadol was withdrawn.
- A 55-year-old man with a history of hypertension
  and chronic bronchitis was given tramadol 50–
  100 mg 2–3 times daily and 5 days later developed
  swelling of the tongue and edema of the oral cavity. Betamethasone and adrenaline were given and
  tramadol and enalapril were withdrawn.

Four of these patients were taking concomitant ACE inhibitors, which can also cause
angioedema (SEDA-29, 207). Whether an interaction of tramadol and ACE inhibitors increases
the risk of angioedema is not known.

PARTIAL OPIOID RECEPTOR AGONISTS

Buprenorphine   *(SED-15, 571; SEDA-27, 97; SEDA-28, 112; SEDA-29, 111)*

Placebo-controlled studies   In a randomized
controlled trial the safety of buprenorphine
for detoxification from opiates was highlighted
(92[C]). There were no withdrawals because of
treatment-related adverse events.

Respiratory   Buprenorphine showed a ceiling
effect in its ability to cause *respiratory depression* in both rats and humans (34[Ec]). There was
a non-linear dose-response relation, due to partial μ (OP₃, MOR) receptor agonism, between
buprenorphine and respiratory effect.

Psychiatric   In a comparison of buprenorphine and methadone in alleviating mood disturbances in conjunction with carbamazepine in
30 patients buprenorphine was associated with
better mood stabilization and short-term relief
of depressive symptoms than methadone; both
treatments were safe and without unexpected
adverse effects (47[c]).

Gastrointestinal   Buprenorphine has a low
incidence of *constipation* compared with other
opioids (18[R]).

Liver   Buprenorphine can cause *increased
liver enzymes* at normal doses and at high doses
can cause *hepatitis* (18[R]).

Sexual function   Buprenorphine causes less
sexual dysfunction than other opioids (18[R]).

Immunologic   There is some evidence of *immune system stimulation* by buprenorphine at
toxic concentrations (48[ER]). However, these results are based on experimental studies in rats
and are unlikely to be relevant to humans.

Infection risk   Soft tissue infections due to
Gamella morbillorum have been reported in patients who had received buprenorphine (93[A]).

- A 38-year-old male drug user with hepatitis C developed fever, pain, erythema, and areas of necrosis at the site of intravenous administration of
  buprenorphine. *Gamella morbillorum* was identified and he was treated with amoxicillin and
  gentamicin.

- A 39-year-old male drug user developed fever and a subcutaneous abscess at the site of intravenous administration of buprenorphine. *Gamella morbillorum* was grown from pus cultures. He was treated with co-amoxiclav and gentamicin followed by amoxicillin.

Although cutaneous infections are frequent in drug addicts, they are not usually due to *Gamella morbillorum*. However, contamination by *Gamella morbillorum*, which forms part of the normal flora of the mouth, is possible because addicts often use saliva to convert solid forms of drugs into solutions for intravenous administration.

Death   Buprenorphine-related deaths have been reviewed (94[R]). Between 1980 and 2002 43 deaths were identified in which buprenorphine was mentioned either in the death certificate or in the coroner's report. In most cases other drugs (often benzodiazepines) and alcohol had also been used, suggesting that the risk of death increased when buprenorphine was used in combination with other drugs. In seven cases, buprenorphine only was detected, questioning its high safety profile.

Pregnancy   In a randomized controlled study, 18 pregnant women in the second trimester were switched from short-acting morphine to buprenorphine without difficulty and minimal withdrawal effects to either mother or fetus (49[c]).

Lactation   Buprenorphine passes into breast milk in concentrations similar to those in maternal plasma. However, exposure tends to be minimal, with no reported cases of neonatal abstinence symptoms after cessation of breast feeding (3[R]).

Susceptibility factors

Renal impairment   The long-term use of buprenorphine by patients with renal impairment could result in accumulation of metabolites (norbuprenorphine) in the plasma, although this may not be clinically significant (3[R]).

Liver disease   Patients with hepatitis treated with buprenorphine should have liver enzymes monitored (3[R]). HIV-positive patients taking drug therapy are susceptible to increased concentrations of buprenorphine because of drug interactions (3[R], 95[R]).

Drug interactions   Buprenorphine is mainly metabolized by CYP3A4. Concomitant use of medications that induce CYP3A4 (for example *rifampicin, phenytoin*) or inhibit it (for example *fluoxetine, cimetidine, saquinavir*) may increase or inhibit buprenorphine metabolism and caution should be taken when buprenorphine is given with such drugs (3[R], 29[R]).

Nalbuphine   *(SED-15, 2416; SEDA-29, 111)*

Cardiovascular   The effects of nalbuphine 5 mg on the cardiovascular and subjective effects of cocaine have been studied in a randomized controlled trial in seven patients (96[C]). The combination of nalbuphine and cocaine was safe and did not have synergistic effects on heart rate and blood pressure or subjective effects. Nalbuphine was safe and well tolerated and its acute administration moderately attenuated the abuse-related effects of cocaine.

OPIOID RECEPTOR ANTAGONISTS

Nalmefene   *(SED-15, 2420; SEDA-29, 111)*

Reproductive system   The hypothesis that endogenous opioids have a role in the premenstrual dysphoric disorder has been explored in 22 subjects, who received either placebo or nalmefene during the follicular phase and the rest of their cycles (97[c]). Of those who received nalmefene, one complained of *insomnia* throughout the study. Withdrawal was required in one of those who took nalmefene but none of those who took placebo. Nalmefene did not beneficially affect the symptoms of premenstrual dysphoric disorder.

Naloxone   *(SED-15, 2421; SEDA-27, 97; SEDA-28, 113)*

Placebo-controlled studies   The effects of naloxone 0.25 micrograms/kg on the adverse effects of intravenous morphine have been explored in a double-blind, randomized, placebo-controlled trial in 131 patients in pain (98[C]). Naloxone failed to improve nausea, pruritus, and vomiting and failed to reduce the need for rescue antiemetics. Naloxone did not affect pain reduction.

In a postoperative placebo-controlled study in 46 children and adolescents, average age 14 years, naloxone 0.25 micrograms/kg significantly reduced the incidence and severity of opioid-induced adverse effects (pruritus and nausea), without affecting opioid-induced analgesia (99[c]).

Naltrexone   *(SED-15, 2423; SEDA-27, 97; SEDA-28, 113; SEDA-29, 112)*

Drug dependence   The use of naltrexone as constraint therapy in addicted physicians has been reviewed (29[R]). Drug-free retention rates were less than 20%, suggesting that naltrexone was not very effective.

Susceptibility factors   The safety and effectiveness of naltrexone in alcohol-dependent populations with co-morbid axis 1 disorders has been explored in a 12-week multicenter randomized study (100[C]). The results suggested that naltrexone can be used safely in this group of individuals. Naltrexone was associated with more reported nervousness and restlessness than disulfiram or placebo. Other adverse effects, including after-taste, blurred vision, confusion, constipation, drowsiness, dry mouth, loss of appetite, nausea, and tremor, were more likely to be experienced by subjects taking any

Table 1. *Frequency of adverse effects of naltrexone (101[C])*

Adverse event	Dose	Frequency (n)
Nausea	190 mg	25% (53)
	380 mg	33% (68)
Headache	190 mg	16% (33)
	380 mg	22% (45)
Fatigue	190 mg	16% (34)
	380 mg	20% (41)
Discontinuation because of adverse events	Placebo	6.7% (14)
	190 mg	6.7% (14)
	380 mg	14% (29)

medication, i.e. naltrexone (*n* = 59), disulfiram (*n* = 66), naltrexone+disulfiram (*n* = 65), than subjects taking placebo (*n* = 64). The combination of naltrexone+disulfiram was associated with significantly more abdominal pain, nausea, vomiting, numb limbs, pins and needles, irregular heartbeat, restlessness, and higher degrees of depression and general distress, than those taking either medication alone.

Drug formulations   Parenteral modified-release naltrexone in two doses (190 and 380 mg) together with low-intensity psychosocial intervention has been studied in a randomized placebo-controlled trial in 627 individuals with alcohol dependence (101[C]). There were few adverse events, the most common being *nausea* (mostly mild or moderate and during only in the first month of treatment), *headache*, and *fatigue* (Table 1). There was no hepatotoxicity. Other adverse events included *insomnia, vomiting, reduced appetite, diarrhea, dizziness, nasopharyngitis, upper respiratory tract infection,* and *pain at the injection site*.

References

1. Sloan P, Slatkin N, Ahdieh H. Effectiveness and safety of oral extended-release Oxymorphone for the treatment of cancer pain: a pilot study. Supportive Care Cancer 2005;13(1):57–65.

2. Mercadante S, Arcuri E, Fusco F, Tirelli W, Villari P, Bussolino C, Campa T, De Conno F, Ripamonti C. Randomized double-blind, double-dummy crossover clinical trial of oral tramadol

A. Del Favero

9

Anti-inflammatory and antipyretic analgesics and drugs used in gout

Strategies to reduce upper gastrointestinal tract damage caused by non-steroidal anti-inflammatory drugs (NSAIDs)

NSAID-induced gastrointestinal damage is an important cause of hospital admissions and deaths world wide. It has been responsible every year for about 7000 deaths in the USA and 1000 in the elderly population in the UK (1^R, 2^R). Other estimates suggest that the number of cases of bleeding ulcers attributable to NSAIDs in the UK is about 2400. It is therefore not surprising that guidelines have been produced to assist clinicians in choosing the most appropriate preventive strategies in patients with varying degrees of gastrointestinal risk (3^R, 4^R). Clinical trials have also been carried out to explore possible preventive strategies. Several theoretical options are available in clinical practice, but the best preventive choice depends on a careful consideration of several factors, such as: the intrinsic gastrotoxic potential of the NSAID used; the treatment regimen adopted, with particular attention to dose and duration of therapy; the characteristics of the individual subject, i.e. the identification of high-risk patients; and the availability and appropriate use of the most efficacious pharmacological prophylactic regimen.

1. Choosing the least toxic NSAID in the first step on the way to choosing the best prophylaxis

There is a consistent body of evidence that traditional NSAIDs are not all the same with respect to gastrointestinal toxicity (SEDA-18, 99; Table 1) (5^C, 6^C), and the clinical and epidemiological relevance of this fact should not be ignored (2^R, 7^R, 8^R). In fact, if one takes in account epidemiological data on the frequency of bleeding ulcers and deaths attributable to NSAIDs as well as the relative risks associated with different NSAIDs, substitution of ibuprofen (which has the least gastrointestinal toxicity at a dose of 2.4 g/day) for all other NSAIDs would reduce the number of such events in the UK from 2431 to 695 annually. Substituting ibuprofen (or another "safe" NSAID) at a lower dose of 1200 g/day would be likely to reduce events nearly to zero. Similarly, substitution of ibuprofen 1.2 g/day, or another relatively safe NSAID, would be likely to reduce events nearly to zero. These estimates should be interpreted with cau-

Table 1. Odds ratios (and 95% CI) for gastrointestinal adverse effects of NSAIDs (SEDA-18, 99)

	Odds ratio for gastrointestinal bleeding and perforation (95% CI) (5^c)	Odds ratio for acute gastrointestinal bleeding (95% CI) (6^c)
Ibuprofen	2.9 (1.8, 5.0)	2.0 (1.4, 2.8)
Diclofenac	3.9 (2.3, 6.5)	4.2 (2.6, 6.8)
Naproxen	3.1 (1.7, 5.9)	9.1 (5.5, 15)
Indometacin	6.3 (3.3, 12)	11.3 (6.3, 20)
Ketoprofen	5.4 (2.6, 11)	23.7 (7.6, 74)
Piroxicam	18 (8.2, 40)	14 (7.1, 26)
Azapropazone	23 (6.9, 80)	32 (10.3, 97)
Overall	4.7 (3.8, 5.7)	4.5 (3.6, 5.6)
Low dose	2.6 (1.8, 3.8)	2.5 (1.7, 3.8)
Intermediate dose	–	4.5 (3.3, 6.0)
High dose	7.0 (5.2, 9.6)	8.6 (5.8, 13)

Side Effects of Drugs, Annual 30
J.K. Aronson (Editor)
ISSN: 0378-6080
DOI: 10.1016/S0378-6080(08)00009-3

tion, as the overall incidence of bleeding ulcers may be inaccurate, and reduced efficacy at a lower dose, albeit accompanied by better tolerability, may affect the benefit to harm balance.

Similar data are obtained for patients taking low-dose aspirin. The total number of excess cases attributable to aspirin in the UK is 753 annually. If prophylactic aspirin was prescribed solely at a dose of 75 mg/day, the safest efficacious dose for cardiovascular prophylaxis, the number of cases would fall to 445 annually, and the number of related deaths from 87 to 51.

On the basis of these data it is likely that an appropriate clinical strategy could prevent many episodes of peptic ulcer bleeding by selecting the least toxic NSAIDs at the lowest effective doses and using them only in patients who do not respond to simple analgesics.

2. Identification of patients at high risk of complicated ulcers

Epidemiological data show that about 50% of patients who regularly take NSAIDs have gastric erosions and 15–30% have endoscopic ulcers. However, the clinical relevance of these manifestations varies greatly, and the incidence of clinically significant gastrointestinal events caused by NSAIDs is much lower. In fact, upper gastrointestinal events may occur in 3.0–4.5% of patients taking NSAIDs, and serious complicated events (upper gastrointestinal bleeding and perforation) develop in about 1.5% (7^R, 8^R).

There have been several studies of the factors that increase the risk of serious gastrointestinal complications and of methods to reduce the risk. Advanced age (over 65 years) has been consistently found to be a primary risk factor for gastrointestinal toxicity; the risk increases linearly with age and remains constant over an extended period of observation. Other risk factors that have been identified in multiple studies are higher doses of NSAIDs, including the use of two or more NSAIDs; a history of ulceration or gastrointestinal bleeding; concomitant use of some drugs, such as glucocorticoids and anticoagulants, and consumption of alcohol. Concomitant disease should also be considered (9^R). Not all of these possible risk factors have the same quality of evidence, as many of them have been based on univariate analyses and have not considered the interactions among multiple factors and co-existing conditions.

However, these risk factors should be carefully considered when choosing to start a NSAID.

3. Eradication of Helicobacter pylori

Eradication of Helicobacter pylori has previously been reviewed (SEDA 27, 105), but it merits further attention.

Many patients who have had upper gastrointestinal bleeding have to continue to take low-dose aspirin (under 325 mg/day) for cardiovascular prophylaxis or other NSAIDs for musculoskeletal pain. It is uncertain whether infection with Helicobacter pylori is a susceptibility factor for bleeding in such patients. Nor is it known whether eradicating the infection would substantially reduce the risk of bleeding ulcers, and thus obviate the need for acid suppression. New information can be derived from a randomized study of omeprazole or eradication therapy in patients with a history of upper gastrointestinal bleeding who were infected with Helicobacter pylori and who were taking low-dose aspirin or other NSAIDs (10^C). Among patients with Helicobacter pylori infection and a history of upper gastrointestinal bleeding who were taking low-dose aspirin, eradication was equivalent to treatment with omeprazole in preventing recurrent bleeding. However, omeprazole was superior to eradication in preventing recurrent bleeding in patients who were taking other NSAIDs, such as naproxen, and by implication other non-aspirin NSAIDs.

In light of the increasing use of aspirin for cardiovascular prophylaxis, these findings suggest that patients who are at risk of bleeding from ulcers should be tested for Helicobacter pylori infection and treated if necessary.

The role of gastric acid suppression with a proton pump inhibitor (lansoprazole) in preventing the recurrence of ulcer complications after eradication of Helicobacter pylori in patients taking long-term low-dose aspirin has been further better defined in another randomized study, in which patients with healed ulcers in whom Helicobacter pylori had been eradicated were randomized for 12 months to aspirin 100 mg + either lansoprazole 30 mg or placebo (11^C). Those who took lansoprazole were significantly less likely to have recurrent ulcer complications while taking low-dose aspirin, compared with those in whom only eradication was used.

4. COX-2 selective inhibitors in preventing upper gastrointestinal bleeding

There is a consistent body of evidence that concurrent therapy with non-selective NSAIDs and a proton pump inhibitor can reduce the risk of ulceration or ulcer complications (12^C, 13^C, 14^C), and this approach is therefore recommended for prophylaxis in patients at high risk for ulcer complications. COX-2 selective inhibitors (coxibs) were developed with the goal of delivering effective pain relief without causing the serious gastrointestinal adverse effects (mainly complicated ulcers) linked to the non-selective NSAIDs (SEDA-25, 126). Unfortunately the claims of better gastrointestinal safety of coxibs relative to traditional NSAIDs were open to criticism (SEDA-29, 116). Most of the data on gastric safety profile of coxibs came from a study (CLASS) that failed to demonstrate a significant reduction in ulcer complications in patients taking celecoxib compared with patients taking non-selective NSAIDs. However, the coxibs were widely adopted, both in clinical practice and official guidelines (4^R). Moreover, more recent data have linked coxibs with serious cardiovascular, renal, and cutaneous adverse reactions, prompting regulatory authorities to withdraw some compounds from the market.

There have been two studies of the efficacy of selective COX-2 inhibitors with respect to co-therapy with proton pump inhibitors and NSAIDs.

The aim of the first study was to assess whether celecoxib is similar to diclofenac plus omeprazole in reducing the risk of recurrent ulcer bleeding in high-risk patients. Patients who used NSAIDs for arthritis and who developed ulcer bleeding were randomly assigned to either celecoxib 200 mg bd or diclofenac 75 mg bd + omeprazole 20 mg/day for 6 months (15^C). The therapeutic and point was recurrent ulcer bleeding. The probability of recurrent bleeding during 6 months was 4.9% (CI = 3.1, 6.7) in patients taking celecoxib and 6.4% (4.3, 8.4) in those taking diclofenac + omeprazole, a non-significant difference. In the second trial eligible patients were randomly assigned to celecoxib 200 mg/day or naproxen 250 mg tds + lansoprazole 30 mg/day (16^C). The primary therapeutic end point was recurrent ulcer complications. During a median follow-up of 24 weeks 3.7% (CI = 0, 7.3%) of those who took celecoxib compared with 6.3% (1.6, 16%) of those who took lansoprazole developed recurrent ulcer complications. Celecoxib was therefore as effective as lansoprazole co-therapy in preventing recurrences of ulcer complications in subjects with a history of NSAID-related complicated peptic ulcers.

The results of these studies should be interpreted with caution, for two reasons.

Firstly, in both studies a significant proportion (4–6%) of patients still had recurrent ulcer complications over the period of follow-up, showing that neither prophylactic regimen was completely protective in high-risk patients. In view of these data an important question is whether the addition of a proton pump inhibitor to celecoxib (or other COX-2 inhibitors) will further reduce upper gastrointestinal events. The problem awaits the results of further studies.

Secondly, there was an unexpectedly high rate of renal adverse effects, including acute renal insufficiency, in both studies. Careful monitoring of patients taking proton pump inhibitors + NSAIDs or celecoxib is wise.

Conclusions   What are the practical implications of these data? To reduce the substantial risk of ulcer-related bleeding and perforation associated with all NSAIDs we must take into account all possible strategies that might prevent complications in as many patients as possible. Too many patients continue to take NSAIDs when simple analgesics, such as paracetamol, would provide the same benefit with less toxicity and cost. Moreover, when an NSAID is needed, the least toxic compound should be selected on the basis of available data. Finally, because of the substantial increase in risk from low-dose to high-dose NSAID therapy, it is wise, whenever possible, to start treatment with low dosages.

Individual risk factors must lead clinicians to choose the best prophylaxis. However, the gastrointestinal advantage of a combination of a traditional NSAID with a proton pump inhibitor should not be interpreted without careful consideration of competing risks from the cardiovascular perspective. For NSAIDs with competing cardiovascular and gastrointestinal risks, the trade off between reducing gastrointestinal adverse events must be weighed against concerns about cardiovascular adverse effects.

These simple guidelines, if followed, would provide a realistic strategy for preventing many complications related to the use of NSAID.

Urinary tract   Prostaglandins play an important role in genitourinary function, as they provoke contraction of the detrusor muscle. Relaxation of the detrusor muscle by inhibition of prostaglandin synthesis by NSAIDs could therefore result in *acute urinary retention*. In a population-based case-control study of 536 men each matched with up to 10 controls ($n = 5348$ in all) from a source population of 72 114, the risk of acute urinary retention in current users of NSAIDs was twice that in non-users (CI = 1.23, 3.31) (17[C]). The highest risk (adjusted OR = 3.3; CI = 1.2, 9.2) was in those who had recently started using NSAIDs and in those using high doses.

Drug–drug interactions   In a population-based study in Finland of co-prescription of NSAIDs and other drugs that may potentiate their gastrointestinal toxicity, combining NSAIDs with *corticosteroids, anticoagulants,* or *selective serotonin reuptake inhibitors* (SSRIs) increased the risk of upper gastrointestinal haemorrhage by 15, 15, and 13 times respectively (18[c]).

The Australian Adverse Drug Reactions Advisory Committee (ADRAC) and the New Zealand Pharmacovigilance Centre have received and published case reports of raised International Normalized Ratios (INR) and hemorrhage when celecoxib and rofecoxib were given to patients stabilized on *warfarin*. Small increases in INR have also been reported with valdecoxib (19[c], 20[c], 21[c], 22[c]). This possible interaction could be mediated by several mechanisms. Firstly, many NSAIDs are substrates for CYP2C9 and may interfere with the oxidative metabolism of S-warfarin, thereby increasing the hypoprothrombinemic response. Secondly, the non-selective NSAIDs may significantly inhibit COX-1 generated thromboxane A_2, impairing platelet aggregation, impairing hemostasis if bleeding occurs. Thirdly, NSAIDs can cause gastric damage and further increase the risk of gastrointestinal bleeding in patients taking warfarin. Differences in the risk of gastrointestinal toxicity may be relevant when evaluating the risk of the interaction in an individual.

Despite the clinical and epidemiological importance of the problem, there is little information on the comparative safety of coxibs and NSAIDs in patients taking warfarin. A nested case-control study has provided some information about the risk of upper gastrointestinal hemorrhage in patients taking warfarin and a non-selective NSAID or a COX-2 inhibitor (23[C]). The patients had had an upper gastrointestinal hemorrhage while taking warfarin. After adjusting for potential confounders, patients taking warfarin were more likely to have been taking celecoxib (OR = 1.7; CI = 1.2, 3.6), rofecoxib (OR = 2.4; CI = 1.7, 3.6), or a non-selective NSAID (OR = 1.9; CI = 1.4, 3.7) relative to controls. These findings suggest that the risk of upper gastrointestinal hemorrhage is equally increased in warfarin users taking either a coxib or a traditional NSAID. If there is co-prescription, careful monitoring of the INR is mandatory and gastric protection wise.

INDIVIDUAL DRUGS AND CLASSES

Acetylsalicylic acid (aspirin) and related compounds   *(SED-15, 15; SEDA-27, 109; SEDA-28, 123; SEDA-29, 124)*

Gastrointestinal   The incidence of upper *gastrointestinal haemorrhage* has been reported to be similar in patients taking either 75 or 325 mg of aspirin per day (24[C], 25[C]). This confirms the previous finding of a large meta-regression analysis (26[C]).

Enteric-coated aspirin has been associated with *gastroduodenal ulcer formation*; the enteric coating has been shown to be toxic to the bowel and it is postulated that it is also toxic to the stomach (27[C]).

Urinary tract   Studies of the association between the long-term use of aspirin or other NSAIDs and *end-stage renal disease* have given conflicting results (SEDA-26, 111). In order to examine this association, a case-control study was carried out in 583 patients with end-stage renal disease and 1190 controls (28[C]). Long-term use of any analgesic was associated with an overall non-significant odds ratio of 1.22 (CI = 0.89, 1.66). For specific groups of drugs the risks were:

- aspirin 1.56 (1.05, 2.30);
- paracetamol 0.80 (0.39, 1.63);
- pyrazolones 1.03 (0.60, 1.76);
- other NSAIDs 0.94 (0.57, 1.56).

There was thus a small increased risk of end-stage renal disease associated with aspirin, which was related to the cumulative dose and duration of use; it was particularly high among the subset of patients with vascular nephropathy as underlying disease.

These results suggest that long-term use of non-aspirin analgesics and NSAIDs is not associated with an increased risk of end-stage renal disease but that long-term use of aspirin is associated with a small increase in the risk of end-stage renal disease. However, these results should be taken with caution since they have arisen from a subgroup analysis, and should be confirmed by other studies.

Management of adverse drug reactions De-sensitization was attempted in 16 patients with acute coronary artery disease and a history of aspirin hypersensitivity (of whom three had a history of angioedema) in a protocol that lasted a few hours (29[c]). None received pretreatment with antihistamines or glucocorticoids, and beta-blockers were withheld. The first seven received eight oral doses of aspirin, starting at 1 mg and doubling each 30 minutes; the next nine patients underwent a shorter version using five doses (5, 10, 20, 40, and 75 mg). The patients were monitored in the coronary care unit; blood pressure, pulse, and peak expiratory flow were measured every 30 minutes, and cutaneous, naso-ocular, and pulmonary reactions were monitored closely until 3 hours after the procedure. Immediate tolerance was obtained in 14 patients, all of whom continued treatment uneventfully. One patient developed angioedema 3 hours after the procedure, which resolved immediately with a glucocorticoid and adrenaline. The patient was rechallenged successfully 2 days later and continued to take aspirin. Another patient, who had had a severe recent attack of asthma, developed nasal swelling and shortness of breath 1 hour after the last dose; although the symptoms resolved rapidly with inhaled salbutamol, rechallenge was not attempted. In 11 patients who then underwent coronary stenting aspirin + clopidogrel was given for 9–12 months; four were treated

with aspirin alone. There were no major adverse cardiac events or new revascularization during a median follow-up of 14 months (range 1–35).

ANILINE DERIVATIVES   (SED-15, 2679; SEDA-27, 110; SEDA-28, 125)

Paracetamol and the risk of asthma   R

The prevalence of asthma has risen worldwide in recent years, but the reason for this increase is unclear. A number of hypotheses have been formulated, and among them attention has been paid to epidemiological and pathophysiological evidence underlying the hypothesis that paracetamol may be a risk factor for asthma (30[R]).

The first study to suggest a link between asthma and paracetamol was one using data from the International Study of Asthma and Allergies in Childhood of the European Community Respiratory Health Survey (ECHRIS) (31[C]). There was a positive correlation between paracetamol sales and asthma symptoms. For each gram increase in per capita paracetamol sales in 1994–5 the prevalence of wheeze increased by 0.52% among 13- to 14-year-old subjects in this study. Similarly, wheezing rose by 0.26% per gram increase among young adults.

While ecological findings such as these are helpful for the description of group-level (in this case country-level) patterns of association, inferences about individuals cannot be made. However, an association between paracetamol and asthma at the individual level has been seen in a large case-control study (32[C]). After controlling for potential confounding factors, the odds ratio (OR) for asthma, compared with newer users of paracetamol was 1.06 (CI = 0.77, 1.45) in infrequent users (less than monthly), 1.22 (CI = 0.87, 1.77) in monthly users, 1.79 (CI = 1.21, 2.65) in weekly users, and 2.38 (CI = 1.22, 4.64) in daily users. The effect was much stronger for severe asthma (OR = 8.2; CI = 2.8, 23). However, the study had limitations, such as selection bias, and did not take into account factors such as respiratory tract infections. Furthermore, the cross-sectional design of the study makes it unclear whether the use of paracetamol contributed to asthma or vice versa (33[C]).

Further evidence came from the Nurses' Health Study, a prospective cohort study of 121 200 women (34[C]). The objective was to examine the relation between paracetamol use and new-onset asthma. During 352 719 person-years of follow-up, 346 participants reported a new diagnosis of asthma. Increasing frequency of paracetamol use was positively associated with newly diagnosed asthma. The multivariate rate ratio for asthma for participants who took paracetamol for more than 14 days/month was 1.65 (CI = 1.11, 2.39) compared with non-users. The positive association were not affected by the use of aspirin. In a multivariate analysis aspirin was inversely related to newly diagnosed asthma. There was no association with NSAIDs. However, these results cannot be generalized, as the study was conducted in an older, female, and predominantly white population not representative of the general population.

A more recent study using data from the US-based Third National Health and Nutrition Examination Survey has provided further evidence that use of paracetamol is associated with asthma in a dose-related way (adjusted OR = 1.20; CI = 1.12, 1.28) (35[C]). Increased use of paracetamol was also dose-dependently associated with COPD.

In a well conducted, double-blind, randomized study aimed at determining the safety of ibuprofen in children with febrile illnesses, there was a significant association between increased out-patient visits for asthma and use of paracetamol (36[C]). However, the lack of a placebo group in this study made it unclear whether ibuprofen reduced the risk of asthma, paracetamol increased the risk, or a combination of the two.

Finally, there have been multiple case reports and case series of respiratory symptoms and acute reductions in respiratory function indexes after ingestion of paracetamol among both aspirin-sensitive and aspirin tolerant patients (30[C]). Plausible mechanisms that explain the association of paracetamol with asthma include depletion of pulmonary glutathione and thereby a reduced capability of the host to mitigate oxidative stress produced by reactive oxygen species.

COX-2 SELECTIVE INHIBITORS
(SEDA-27, 111; SEDA-28, 128; SEDA-29, 116)

Celecoxib

Urinary tract   As more experience accumulates it appears that celecoxib has the same adverse renal effects as other NSAIDs. *Minimal-change disease with interstitial nephritis* and *nephritic syndrome* have been described in two elderly patients taking celecoxib (37[A], 38[A]). However, it has been claimed that celecoxib is less nephrotoxic than conventional NSAIDs, from the results of a double-blind, randomized, placebo-controlled comparison of the effect of celecoxib, 200 mg every 12 hours to a total of 5 doses, on renal function with that of naproxen 500 mg every 12 hours to a total of 5 doses, in 28 patients with cirrhosis and ascites (39[C]). There was a significant reduction in glomerular filtration rate and renal plasma flow in the patients who took naproxen but not in the other two groups. This suggests that short-term celecoxib does not impair renal function in patients with decompensated cirrhosis. However, further studies are needed before concluding that celecoxib is safer than other NSAIDs in such patients.

Parecoxib

Respiratory   Non-selective NSAIDs are more likely to precipitate *bronchconstriction* than COX-2 inhibitors (SEDA-26, 119). However, there has been a recent report of two patients who developed severe, life-threatening bronchospasm soon after receiving parenteral parecoxib (40[A]). Both had a history of mild asthma. This suggests that COX-2 inhibitors are not without risk and should be used with great caution, especially in patients with asthma.

Rofecoxib

Sensory systems   Visual impairment associated with rofecoxib and other coxibs may be more frequent than has previously been thought and may be under-recognised (SEDA-28, 129). There have been three reports of *central retinal vein occlusion* after starting rofecoxib or after a dosage increase (41[A]).

- A 72-year-old woman took rofecoxib 25 mg/day for rheumatoid arthritis for 6 months. She then increased the dose to 50 mg/day and 3 days later she had sudden deterioration of vision in her right eye due to central retinal vein occlusion.
- A 69-year-old woman had severe deterioration of vision in her right eye 24 hours after starting to take rofecoxib 25 mg/day for osteoarthritis. Ophthalmic examination showed severe intraretinal hemorrhage and retinal vein occlusion.
- A 47-year-old man started to take rofecoxib for hip pain. A week later he had temporary blotches in his right eye. He stopped treatment but started rofecoxib again 1 month later, after which his vision progressively deteriorated. Ophthalmic examination showed central retinal vein occlusion.

All three patients stopped taking rofecoxib. About 1 year later visual acuity in the first two had improved.

Mouth There have been three reports of *oral lesions* attributed to rofecoxib (42[A]).

- A 72-year-old woman, who had taken rofecoxib 50 mg/day for rheumatoid arthritis for 4 weeks, developed atrophic erosive lesions on her right buccal mucosa. Rofecoxib was withdrawn and within 15 days the lesions had resolved. Six months later she again took rofecoxib and the same mucosal lesions appeared at the same site. Rofecoxib was again withdrawn and the buccal lesions resolved. There was no recurrence 8 months later.
- An 83-year-old woman, who had taken rofecoxib 50 mg/day for osteoarthritis for 6 weeks developed erosive lesions on the left side of her tongue and floor of her mouth. Rofecoxib was withdrawn and the lesions resolved completely within 10 days. There was no recurrence 1 year later.
- A 67-year-old woman, who had taken rofecoxib 25 mg/day for osteoarthritis for 16 months, developed severe erosive oral lesions with pseudomembranes. Topical triamcinolone was ineffective. Rofecoxib was replaced by meloxicam and 2 weeks later her symptoms had eased markedly.

Gastrointestinal Contrasting data on the safety of rofecoxib in patients with pre-existing primary *inflammatory bowel disease* have been reported. In one study in 32 patients rofecoxib did not exacerbate inflammatory bowel disease (SEDA 28, 132), but in isolated cases inhibition of COX-2 in the large bowel worsened inflammatory bowel disease, as has again been reported in three patients exposed to

rofecoxib—two patients developed inflammatory bowel disease de novo and one had exacerbation of pre-existing disease (43[A]).

- A 42-year-old man developed abdominal pain and diarrhea with 15 loose bowel movements per day after taking rofecoxib 25 mg/day for 3 days. Rofecoxib was withdrawn but over the next few weeks his symptoms improved only partially. Colonoscopy showed focal shallow ulceration with adherent exudate. Biopsy showed active colitis with a focal erosion involving the transverse colon. Colonoscopy at 4 months showed resolution of the inflammatory changes, but a biopsy still showed patchy active ileitis with focal erosions in the transverse colon. Normal bowel function gradually returned and the abdominal pain resolved.
- A 65-year-old woman developed a change in bowel habit and rectal bleeding after taking aspirin for 5 days, ibuprofen for 2 days, and then rofecoxib (dosage not stated) for 10 days. While taking rofecoxib she developed loose bowel movements with small amounts of bright red blood. Rofecoxib was withdrawn and her symptoms resolved completely. Colonoscopy after 12 days showed segmental inflammatory changes with serpiginous ulceration. Biopsy showed active colitis with erosions, cryptitis, and crypt abscesses.
- A 52-year-old man with a 14-month history of inflammatory bowel disease, currently in remission, took rofecoxib 50 mg/day for 5 days and developed abdominal cramp and loose stools with bright red blood. Colonoscopy showed focal ulceration of the cecum and descending colon. Biopsy showed patchy acute cryptitis and active colitis with ulceration. Rofecoxib was withdrawn and his symptoms resolved.

These observations suggest that extreme caution should be taken when prescribing rofecoxib for patients with inflammatory bowel disease. Furthermore, patients who develop symptoms of diarrhea and abdominal pain should be monitored carefully for possible inflammatory bowel disease.

Skin A 63-year-old woman developed *Stevens–Johnson syndrome* while taking rofecoxib for arthralgia. Despite early withdrawal she developed serious corneal and conjunctival complications (44[A]).

Immunologic Rofecoxib has been implicated in a case of combined *interstitial nephritis and acute hepatitis* (45[A]).

- A 62-year-old man who had taken rofecoxib for 6 months, developed malaise, anorexia, weight loss, pruritus, jaundice, and upper quadrant abdominal discomfort. His liver function tests were abnormal:

serum bilirubin 240 μmol/l (reference range <20), γ-glutamyl transferase 98 units/l (<60), alkaline phosphatase 218 units/l (<150). A liver biopsy was consistent with drug-induced hepatic damage. He was treated with ursodeoxycholic acid, but his cholestasis deteriorated. Over the next few days his renal function also worsened (serum creatinine 540 μmol/l) and urinalysis showed heavy proteinuria. He needed hemodialysis for 6 weeks. A renal biopsy was consistent with drug-induced acute interstitial nephritis and acute tubular necrosis. He was given a glucocorticoid and his renal and liver function recovered after 3 months.

Isolated severe acute cholestatic and cytolytic hepatitis has previously been attributed to rofecoxib (46[A]).

Valdecoxib

Cardiovascular   Despite claims from the results of a meta-analysis conducted by its manufacturer that valdecoxib appears to be associated with significantly fewer adverse gastrointestinal events that non-selective NSAIDs (47[M]), its marketing authorization has been suspended in many countries because of an increased risk of serious cardiovascular outcomes (48[C]) found in two randomized placebo-controlled trials in high-risk patients (SEDA-29, 122).

Urinary tract   Acute *anuric renal insufficiency* has been described with NSAIDs and can also occur with coxibs (SEDA-26, 125).

• A 31-year-old woman with pyelonephritis developed acute anuric renal insufficiency while taking valdecoxib for back pain and needed hemodialysis (49[A]). No susceptibility factor for acute renal insufficiency was identified.

Skin   Various serious skin reactions to valdecoxib have been described in publications and/or reported to drug control agencies (SEDA-29, 122), including *exanthematous skin eruptions, purpura*, and systemic *allergic contact dermatitis* (50[A], 51[A], 52[A]).

Musculoskeletal   Exacerbation of pre-existing *carpal tunnel syndrome* has been attributed to valdecoxib (53[A]).

• A 40-year old patient had worsening of carpal tunnel syndrome after a single dose of valdecoxib 40 mg for a knee contusion. Valdecoxib was switched to ibuprofen and within 12 hours the symptoms resolved.

Valdecoxib-associated edema may have aggravated pre-existing carpal tunnel syndrome

---

OXICAMS   *(SEDA-15, 2555; SEDA-27, 116; SEDA-28, 128; SEDA-29, 125)*

Lornoxicam

Gastrointestinal   Multiple small hemispheric polyps, associated with luminal narrowing, were found in the gastric antrum of a 74-year-old man who had taken lornoxicam (54[A]). The polyps consisted of granulation tissue and immature regenerative epithelium. The authors suggested that in the hypoacidic conditions induced by nizatidine, inflammatory polyps could have arisen through rapid and excessive regeneration after gastric mucosal injury due to the NSAID. However, there was no evidence in this case of a cause-and-effect relation.

PYRAZOLONE DERIVATIVES

Dipyrone   *(SEDA-27, 111)*

Hematologic   Dipyrone is associated with an increased risk of *agranulocytosis* (SEDA-27, 111). In a case-control study in patients identified from a large database designed for the surveillance of blood dyscrasias, during 78.73 million person-years follow-up there were 396 confirmed cases of agranulocytosis, 177 of which were analysed, with 586 matched controls (55[C]). In the week before agranulocytosis developed, 30 cases (17%) and 9 controls (1.5%) had been exposed to dipyrone (adjusted RR = 26; CI = 8.4, 79). Among exposed patients there was a trend towards an increased risk of agranulocytosis, with increased duration of exposure. However, the risk disappeared 10 days after the last dose of dipyrone.

The balance of benefit and harm for dipyrone is controversial. One must remember that it is often associated with severe anaphylactic reactions, especially when it is infused intravenously for analgesia (56[A]).

DRUGS USED IN THE TREATMENT OF GOUT

Colchicine   *(SEDA-15, 883; SEDA-28, 133; SEDA-29, 125)*

Prescribers have been reminded by New Zealand's Medsafe Pharmacovigilance Team of the revised dosage advice for colchicine, which is now second-line therapy for acute gout, because of the risk of serious adverse effects (57[S], 58[S]). Colchicine is very toxic in overdose, and deaths have occurred. The use of high doses in acute gout is not appropriate, especially in patients who are elderly, have impaired renal or hepatic function, or weigh less than 50 kg. Medsafe has advised that:

- colchicine should be considered a second-line treatment for acute gout, when NSAIDs are contraindicated, inefficacious, or poorly tolerated;
- the dosage interval should be increased to 6 hours;
- the maximum daily dose in the first 24 hours should be 2.5 mg;
- the maximum cumulative dose over 4 days should not exceed 6 or 3 mg in elderly people;
- colchicine is contraindicated in severe renal or hepatic impairment and the dose should be reduced in patients with less severe impairment.

In addition, continued dosing until adverse gastrointestinal events occur "is no longer considered safe or appropriate". Medsafe has urged prescribers to write clear dosage advice on the prescription, to inform patients of the revised dosage advice, to stress how important it is not to exceed the maximum doses, to warn patients of the symptoms of colchicine toxicity, and to advise them to stop taking the drug immediately and see a doctor if symptoms such as nausea, vomiting, and diarrhea occur.

Susceptibility factors

Renal disease   There have been single case reports of severe colchicine-induced myopathy in which impaired renal function caused insufficient elimination of colchicine (59[A]).

Drug–drug interactions   Drug interactions with colchicine may occur more often than has previously been thought (SEDA-28, 133).

Clarithromycin   Concomitant treatment with clarithromycin can increase the risk of fatal colchicine toxicity. In a retrospective case-control study of 116 patients who took clarithromycin and colchicine, nine of the 88 patients who took the two drugs concomitantly died, compared with only one of the 28 patients who took the two drugs sequentially (60[C]). Multivariate analysis of the 88 patients showed that longer overlapping therapy, baseline renal function impairment, and pancytopenia were independently associated with death. This study had several limitations but it cannot be dismissed, as further reports have been published that document severe adverse reactions after co-administration of colchicine with clarithromycin (61[A], 62[A]).

- A 68-year-old man with acute gouty arthritis and a community-acquired pneumonia was given colchicine 0.5 mg every 6 hours and clarithromycin 500 mg tds. On day 5 the dose of colchicine was reduced to 0.5 mg every 8 hours because of diarrhea. On day 11 both drugs were withdrawn and the next day he developed a paralytic ileus, recurrence of fever, hypotension, pancytopenia, and acute renal and hepatic insufficiency. He died on day 13 and post-mortem examination showed agranulocytosis and massive hepatic necrosis.
- A 55-year-old woman with acute gout and pneumonia was given colchicine 0.5 mg tds and clarithromycin 250 mg bd. After five doses of colchicine and three of clarithromycin she developed severe leukopenia and thrombocytopenia. Bone marrow biopsy showed marked hypocellularity. She developed a febrile neutropenia and died after 12 days.
- A 71-year-old man taking colchicine 1.5 mg/day for Familial Mediterranean Fever was given clarithromycin, amoxicillin and omeprazole for 7 days for *Helicobacter pylori* eradication. After 3 days he developed fever, abdominal pain, and bloody diarrhea, and after 8 days pancytopenia, dehydration, and metabolic acidosis. The dosage of colchicine was reduced to 0.5 mg/day. He was rehydrated and recovered fully. The previous dosage of colchicine was gradually reinstituted without adverse effects.

Statins Concomitant treatment with statins can cause myopathy or rhabdomyolysis.

- A 70-year-old man, who had taken fluvastatin for 2 years for dyslipidemia, developed rhabdomyolysis and acute renal insufficiency 10 days after starting to take colchicine 1.5 mg/day (63[A]). He had raised creatine kinase and aspartate transaminase activities, and serum myoglobin and creatinine concentrations. Colchicine and fluvastatin were withdrawn and his gout was treated with intra-articular glucocorticoid injections. The laboratory findings normalized over about 10 days. Fluvastatin was subsequently restarted without problems and 2 months later his renal function was normal.
- A 65-year-old woman, who was taking pravastatin 20 mg/day and losartan, diuretics, and aspirin for ischemic heart disease, was given colchicine 1.5 mg/day for gout, and 20 days later developed symmetrical proximal muscle weakness in the legs with reduced tendon reflexes and electromyography consistent with muscle disease (64[A]). She had raised creatine kinase, aspartate transaminase, and lactate dehydrogenase activities. Blood urea nitrogen and serum creatinine concentrations were

slightly raised. Colchicine and pravastatin were withdrawn and within 7 days her clinical and laboratory findings normalized. She had another attack of gout 12 days later and was given colchicine 1.0 mg/day without adverse effects.

There have also been single case reports of rhabdomyolysis with simvastatin, atorvastatin, and possibly gemfibrozil (SEDA-28, 133). The combination of colchicine with other potentially myotoxic drugs, such as gemfibrozil and other statins, has clinical relevance, as these classes of drugs are often co-prescribed in patients with renal insufficiency.

Colchicine and most of the statins are biotransformed in the liver, primarily by CYP3A4, which may explain the increased risk of myopathy during concurrent therapy. However, pravastatin and fluvastatin are not primarily metabolized by cytochrome P450 isoenzymes (65[E]) and in such cases the interaction may be mediated by P glycoprotein.

References

1. Roth SH, Fries JF, Abadi IA, Hubscer O, Mintz G, Samara AM. Prophylaxis of non-steroidal anti-inflammatory drug gastropathy: a clinical opinion. J Rheumatol 1991;18:956–8.
2. Langman MJ. Ulcer complications associated with anti-inflammatory drug use. What is the extent of the disease burden? Pharmacoepidemiol Drug Saf 2001;10:13–9.
3. Dubois RW, Melmed GY, Henning JM, Bernal M. Risk of upper gastrointestinal injury and events in patients treated with cyclooxygenase (COX)-1/COX-2 nonsteroidal anti-inflammatory drugs (NSAIDs), COX-2 selective NSAIDs, and gastroprotective cotherapy: an appraisal of the literature. Clin Rheumatol 2004;10:178–89.
4. Schnitzer TJ. Update on guidelines for the treatment of chronic musculoskeletal pain. Clin Rheumatol 2006;25:S22–9.
5. Langman MJ, Weil J, Wainwright P, Lawson DH, Rawlins MD, Logan RF, Murphy M, Vessey MP, Colin-Jones DG. Risks of bleeding peptic ulcer associated with individual non-steroidal anti-inflammatory drugs. Lancet 1994;343:1075–8.
6. Garcìa Rodrìguez LA, Ruigòmez A. Secondary prevention of upper gastrointestinal bleeding associated with maintenance acid-suppressing treatment in patients with peptic ulcer bleed. Epidemiology 1999;10:228–32.
7. Laine L. Approaches to nonsteroidal anti-inflammatory drug use in the high-risk patient. Gastroenterology 2001;120:594–606.
8. Langman M. Population impact of strategies designed to reduce peptic ulcer risks associated with NSAID use. Int J Clin Pract Suppl 2003;135:38–42.
9. Wolfe MM, Lichtenstein DR, Singh G. Gastrointestinal toxicity of nonsteroidal anti-inflammatory drugs. N Engl J Med 1999;340:1888–99.
10. Chan FK, Chung SC, Suen BY, Lee YT, Leung WK, Leung VK, Wu JC, Lau JY, Hui Y, Lai MS, Chan HL, Sung JJ. Preventing recurrent upper gastrointestinal bleeding in patients with Helicobacter pylori infection who are taking low-dose aspirin or naproxen. N Engl J Med 2001;344:967–73.
11. Lai KC, Lam SK, Chu KM, Wong BC, Hui WM, HUWH, Lau GK, Wong WM, Yuen MF, Chan AO, Lai CL, Wong J. Lansoprazole for the prevention of recurrences of ulcer complications from long-term low-dose aspirin use. N Engl J Med 2002;346:2033–8.
12. Graham DY, Agrawal NM, Campbell DR, Haber MM, Collis C, Lukasik NL, Huang B, NSAID-Associated Gastric Ulcer Prevention Study Group. Ulcer prevention in long-term

users of nonsteroidal anti-inflammatory drugs: results of a double-blind, randomized, multicenter, active-and placebo-controlled study of misoprostol vs lansoprazole. Arch Intern Med 2002;162:169–75.

13. Silverstein FE, Graham Dy, Senior JR, Davies HW, Struthers BJ, Bittman RM, Geis GS. Misoprostol redices serious gastrointestinal complications in patients with rheumatoid arthritis receiving nonsteroidal anti-inflammatory drugs. A randomized, double-blind, placebo-controlled trial. Ann Intern Med 1995;123:241–9.

14. Garcia Rodriguez LA, Ruigomez A. Secondary prevention of upper gastrointestinal bleeding associated with maintenance acid-suppressing treatment in patients with peptic ulcer bleed. Epidemiology 1999;10:228–32.

15. Chan FK, Hung LC, Suen BY, Wu JC, Lee KC, Leung VK, Hui AJ, To KF, Leung WK, Wong VW, Chung SC, Sung JJ. Celecoxib versus diclofenac and omeprazole in reducing the risk of recurrent ulcer bleeding in patients with arthritis. N Engl J Med 2002;347:2104–10.

16. Lai KC, Chu KM, Hui WM, Wong BC, Hu WH, Wong WM, Chan AO, Wong J, Lam SK. Celecoxib compared with lansoprazole and naproxen to prevent gastrointestinal ulcer complications. Am J Med 2005;118:1271–8.

17. Verhamme KM, Dieleman JP, Van Wijk MA, van der Lei J, Bosch JL, Stricker BH, Sturkenboom MC. Nonsteroidal anti-inflammatory drugs and increased risk of acute urinary retention. Arch Intern Med 2005;165:1547–51.

18. Helin-Salmivaara A, Huupponen R, Virtanen A, Lammela J, Klaukka T. Frequent prescribing of drugs with potential gastrointestinal toxicity among continuous users of non-steroidal anti-inflammatory drugs. Eur J Clin Pharmacol 2005;61:425–31.

19. Adverse Drug Reactions Advisory Committee (ADRAC). Interaction of celecoxib and warfarin. Adv Drug React Bull 2001;20:2.

20. Med Safe Editorial Team. Interaction between COX-2 inhibitors and warfarin. Prescriber Update 2001;22:16–8.

21. Adverse Drug Reactions Advisory Committee (ADRAC). Interaction of rofecoxib and warfarin. Adv Drug React Bull 2002;21:3.

22. Savage R. Cyclo-oxygenase-2 inhibitors: when should they be used in the elderly? Drugs Aging 2005;22:185–200.

23. Battistella M, Mamdami MM, Juurlink DN, Rabeneck L, Laupacis A. Risk of upper gastrointestinal hemorrage in warfarin users treated with nonselective NSAIDs or COX-2 inhibitors. Arch Intern Med 2005;24:158–60.

24. Fisher M, Knappertz V. Comments in response to "Analysis of risk of bleeding complications after different doses of aspirin in 192,036 patients enrolled in 31 randomised controlled trials". Am J Cardiol 2005;96(10):1467.

25. Laine L, McQuaid K. Bleeding complications related to aspirin dose. Am J Cardiol 2005;96(7):1035–6.

26. Derry S, Loke YK. Risk of gastrointestinal haemorrhage with long term use of aspirin: meta-analysis. BMJ 2000;321(7270):1183–7.

27. Graham D, Chan F. Endoscopic ulcers with low-dose aspirin and reality testing. Gastroenterology 2005;128(3):807.

28. Ibáñez L, Morlans M, Vidal X, Martínez MJ, Laporte J-R. Case-control study of regular analgesic and nonsteroidal anti-inflammatory use and end-stage renal disease. Kidney Int 2005;67:2393–8.

29. Silberman S, Neukirch-Stoop C, Steg PG. Rapid desensitization procedure for patients with aspirin hypersensitivity undergoing coronary stenting. Am J Cardiol 2005;95(4):509–10.

30. Eneli I, Sadri K, Camargo Jr C, Barr RG. Acetaminophen and the risk of asthma: the epidemiologic and pathophysiologic evidence. Chest 2005;127:604–12.

31. Newson RB, Shaheen SO, Chinn S, Burney PG. Paracetamol sales and atopic disease in children and adults: an ecological analysis. Eur Respir J 2000;16:817–23.

32. Shaheen SO, Sterne JA, Songhurst CE, Burney PG. Frequent paracetamol use and asthma in adults. Thorax 2000;55:266–70.

33. Shaheen SO, Newson RB, Sherriff A, Henderson AJ, Heron JE, Burney PG, Golding J, ALSPAC Study Team. Paracetamol use in pregnancy and wheezing in early childhood. Thorax 2002;57:958–63.

34. Barr RG, Wentowsky CC, Curhan GC, Somers SC, Stampfer MJ, Schwarts J, Speizer FE, Camargo CA. Prospective study of acetaminophen use and newly diagnosed asthma among women. Am J Respir Crit Care Med 2004;169:836–41.

35. McKeever TM, Lewis SA, Smit HA, Burney P, Britton JR, Cassano PA. The association of acetaminophen, aspirin, and ibuprofen with respiratory disease and lung function. Am J Respir Crit Care Med 2005;171:966–71.

36. Lesko SM, Mitchell AA. The safety of acetaminophen and ibuprofen among children younger than two years old. Pediatrics 1999;104:39.

37. Almansori M, Kovithavongs T, Qarni MU. Cyclooxygenase-2 inhibitor-associated minimal-change disease. Clin Nephrol 2005;63:381–4.

38. Sirvent AE, Enriquez R, Amoros F, Reyes A. Nephrotic syndrome associated with celecoxib. Nefrologia 2005;25:81–2.

39. Clària J, Kent JD, Lòpez-Parra M, Escolar G, Ruiz-Del-Arbol L, Ginès P, Jimènez W, Vucelic B, Arroyo V. Effects of celecoxib and naproxen on renal function in nonazotemic patients with cirrhosis and ascites. Hepatology 2005;42:579–87.

40. Looney Y, O'Shea A, O'Dwyer R. Severe bronchospasm after parenteral parecoxib: cyclooxygenase-2 inhibitors: not the answer yet. Anesthesiology 2005;102:473–5.

41. Meyer CH, Schmidt JC, Rodrigues EB, Mennel S. Risk of retinal vein occlusions in patients treated with rofecoxib (Vioxx). Ophthalmologica 2005;219:243–7.

42. Bagàan JV, Thongprasom K, Scully C. Adverse oral reactions associated with the COX-2 inhibitor rofecoxib. Oral Dis 2004;10:401–3.

43. Wilcox GM, Mattia AR. Rofecoxib and inflammatory bowel disease: clinical and pathologic observations. J Clin Gastroenterol 2005;39:142–3.

44. Goldberg D, Panigrahi D, Barazi M, Abelson M, Butrus S. A case of rofecoxib-associated Stevens–Johnson syndrome with corneal and conjunctival changes. Cornea 2004;23:736–7.

45. Haider M, Gain E, Khadem G, Pilmore H, Yun K, Jayasinghe N, Walker R. Simultaneous presentation of rofecoxib-induced acute hepatitis and acute interstitial nephritis. Intern Med J 2005;35:370–2.

46. Ouar S, Bellaïche G, Belloc J, Tordjman G, Ley G, Slama JL. Severe acute cholestatic and cytolytic hepatitis induced by rofecoxib. Gastroenterol Clin Biol 2005;29:471–2.

47. Eisen GM, Goldstein JL, Hanna DB, Rublee DA. Meta-analysis: upper gastrointestinal tolerability of valdecoxib, a cyclooxygenase-2-specific inhibitor, compared with nonspecific nonsteroidal anti-inflammatory drugs among patients with osteoarthritis and rheumatoid arthritis. Aliment Pharmacol Ther 2005;21:591–8.

48. Ray A, Griffin MR, Stein CM. Cardiovascular toxicity of valdecoxib. N Engl J Med 2004;351:2767.

49. Muhlfeld AS, Gloege J. Cox-2 inhibitors induced anuric renal failure in a previously healthy young woman. Clin Nephrol 2005;63:221–4.

50. Talhari C, Lauceviciute U, Enderlein E, Ruzicka T, Homey B. Cox-2-selective inhibitor valdecoxib induces severe allergic skin reactions. J Allergy Clin Immunol 2005;115:1089–90.

51. Knowles SR, Phillips EJ, Wong G, Shera NH. Serious dermatologic reaction associated with valdecoxib: report of two cases. J Am Acad Dermatol 2004;51:1028–9.

52. Jaeger C, Jappe U. Valdecoxib. Valdecoxib-induced systemic contact dermatitis confirmed by positive patch test. Contact Dermatitis 2005;52:47–8.

53. Ruppen W, Schüpfer GK. Exacerbation of carpal tunnel syndrome under treatment with valdecoxib. Anesth Analg 2005;100:1215–6.

54. Hizawa K, Takeya T, Yao T, Yamamoto H, Aomi H, Nakahara T, Matsumoto T, Iida M. Gastric inflammatory polyposis after long term intermittent use of nonsteroidal anti-inflammatory drugs and histamine 2 receptor antagonists. Endoscopy 2005;37:685.

55. Ibàñèz L, Vidal X, Ballarìn E, Laporte JR. Population-based drug-induced agranulocytosis. Arch Intern Med 2005;165:869–74.

56. Eckle T, Ghanayim N, Trick M, Unerti K, Eltzsching HK. Intraoperative metamizol as cause for acute anaphylactic collapse. Eur J Anaesthesiol 2005;22:810–2.

57. Anonymous. Colchicine. Toxic in overdose: reminder. WHO Newslett 2006;4:5–6.

58. Australian Adverse Drug Reactions Advisory Committee, Medsafe Pharmacovigilace Team. Colchicine–safe use is critical. Prescriber Update 2006;27(1):2.

59. Wilbur K, Makowsky M. Colchicine myotoxicity: case reports and literature review. Pharmacotherapy 2004;24:1784–92.

60. Hung IF, Wu AK, Cheng VC, Tang BS, To KW, Yeung CK, Woo PC, Lau SK, Cheung BM, Yuen KY. Fatal interaction between clarithromycin and colchicine in patients with renal insufficiency: a retrospective study. Clin Infect Dis 2005;41:291–300.

61. Cheng VCC, Ho PL, Yuen KY. Two probable cases of serious drug interaction between clarithromycin and colchicine. South Med J 2005;98:811–3.

62. Rollot F, Pajot O, Chauvelot-Moachon L, Nazal EM, Kélaïdi C, Blache P. Acute colchicines intoxication during clarithromycin administration. Ann Pharmacother 2004;38:2074–7.

63. Atasoyu EM, Evrenkaya TR, Solmazgul E. Possible colchicine rhabdomyolysis in a fluvastatin-treated patient. Ann Pharmacother 2005;39:1368–9.

64. Alayli G, Cengiz K, Cantürk F, Durmus D, Akyol Y, Menekse EB. Acute myopathy in a patient with concomitant use of pravastatin and colchicine. Ann Pharmacother 2005;39:1358–61.

65. Hsu WC, Chen WH, Chang MT, Chiu HC. Colchicine-induced acute myopathy in a patient with concomitant use of simvastatin. Clin Neuropharmacol 2002;25:266–8.

I.D. Welters and M. Leuwer

10 General anesthetics and therapeutic gases

ANESTHETIC VAPORS (SEDA-27, 119; SEDA-28, 139; SEDA-29, 129)

HALOGENATED VAPORS

Comparative studies   In a systematic review of 25 published, randomized controlled comparisons of sevoflurane (746 patients) and desflurane (752 patients) there was no significant difference in the rates of postoperative *nausea and vomiting* (1[M]).

Endocrine   The effects of anesthesia for more than 10 hours with either isoflurane or sevoflurane on *hormone secretion* have been studied in 20 patients (2[c]). Adrenaline and noradrenaline concentrations increased continuously during and after surgery in the isoflurane group whereas they increased only after surgery in the sevoflurane group; both concentrations were higher in the isoflurane group during anesthesia. Cortisol increased continuously but adrenocorticotropic hormone increased only during surgery. Antidiuretic hormone increased during surgery and the isoflurane group had significantly higher values than the sevoflurane group. Glucose increased both during and after surgery but insulin increased only after surgery; glucagon fell during surgery in both groups.

Metabolism   The effects of anesthesia with sevoflurane (0.5, 1.0, and 1.5 MAC) and isoflurane (0.5, 1.0, and 1.5 MAC) on *glucose tolerance* have been studied in a randomized study in 30 patients (3[C]). The insulinogenic index

(change in concentration of immunoreactive insulin/change in glucose concentration), the acute insulin response, and the rates of glucose disappearance were significantly lower in all anesthesia groups than in the control group. However, there were no differences among the six anesthesia groups.

Desflurane   (SED-15, 1072)

Cardiovascular   *Cardiac arrest* due to desflurane toxicity has been attributed to accidental delivery of a high concentration of desflurane due to vaporizer malfunction (4[A]).

- A healthy 36-year-old woman underwent anesthesia maintained with desflurane, which was delivered at 3.5% using a Tec 6 Plus Vaporizer (Datex Ohmeda, Steeton, England) via a partially closed circuit with a low flow of fresh gases (1 l/minute). Five minutes after induction, she developed hypoxia and bradycardia, rapidly followed by cardiac arrest with asystole. She was resuscitated and a chest x-ray showed pulmonary edema.

Examination of the memory of the halogenated anesthetic monitor (Viridia 24 C; Hewlett Packard, Boeblingen, Germany) showed a progressive increase in end-expiratory desflurane concentration up to 23%. There was an internal crack in the control dial, which normally regulates the control valve, but the damage did not limit the rotation of the control valve, which remained uncontrolled. The authors thought that this defect had been responsible for massive administration of desflurane in the inhalation circuit. Cardiac arrest was probably due to the negative inotropic effect of desflurane.

Duchenne's muscular dystrophy can be associated with cardiac arrest during anesthesia, and this has been reported in a 16-year-old boy who was anesthetized with desflurane (5[A]).

Side Effects of Drugs, Annual 30
J.K. Aronson (Editor)
ISSN: 0378-6080
DOI: 10.1016/S0378-6080(08)00010-X

Respiratory   The effects of 6 or 12% desflurane and 1.8 or 3.6% sevoflurane, which have markedly different pungencies, on *airway reactivity* have been tested in 60 patients breathing equivalent concentrations through a laryngeal mask airway (6[c]). Compared with sevoflurane, desflurane titration to 12% increased heart rate, increased mean arterial blood pressure, and initiated frequent coughing (53 versus 0%) and body movements (47 versus 0%). During emergence, there was a two-fold greater incidence of coughing and a five-fold increase in breath holding with desflurane.

Liver   All halogenated anesthetics can cause *acute liver damage*, and this has been reported in an 81-year-old woman after general anesthesia with desflurane (7[A]).

Body temperature   Halogenated anesthetics can cause *malignant hyperthermia* (SED-15, 1496), and another case has been reported with desflurane (8[A]).

Genotoxicity   The effects of desflurane on the frequency of *sister chromatid exchange* has been studied in peripheral blood lymphocytes of 15 women during and after anesthesia maintained with desflurane 5–6% in an oxygen/air mixture (9[E]). The numbers of sister chromatid exchanges per cell at 60 and 120 minutes were significantly higher than the numbers before anesthesia. In addition, the numbers of sister chromatid exchange per cell on the 1st, 3rd, and 7th postoperative days were significantly higher than preoperatively, but there was no difference by the 12th postoperative day. The authors concluded that desflurane may be capable of causing genetic damage. This view has been supported by the results of an in vitro study of the effect of desflurane on peripheral blood lymphocytes, in which both halothane and desflurane increased DNA migration in a concentration-related manner (10[E]).

Isoflurane   *(SED-15, 1921)*

Cardiovascular   Isoflurane can cause marked *hypertension* during induction of anesthesia. Of 26 patients who were anesthetized with 0.5% isoflurane in oxygen, increased to 4% in

2 minutes, nine had increases in systolic blood pressure by more than 10 mmHg (mean 26) (11[c]). Tracheal intubation markedly increased the blood pressure in all patients, but there was a negative correlation between the isoflurane-induced increase and that induced by intubation. Tracheal intubation produced a larger increase in blood pressure in the isoflurane-induced hypertensive patients.

Psychological   *Memory function* and its relation to depth of hypnotic state has been prospectively evaluated in anesthetized and non-anesthetized subjects, using the Bispectral Index during general anesthesia and an auditory word stem completion test and process dissociation procedure after anesthesia (12[C]). Isoflurane was used in 47 patients and propofol in one. There was evidence of memory for words presented during light anesthesia (Bispectral Index score 61–80) and adequate anesthesia (score 41–60) but not during deep anesthesia (score 21–40). The process dissociation procedure showed a significant implicit memory contribution but not reliable explicit memory contribution. Memory performance was better in non-anesthetized subjects than in anesthetized patients, with a higher contribution from explicit memory and a comparable contribution from implicit memory. The authors concluded that during general anesthesia for elective surgery, implicit memory persists, even in adequate hypnotic states, to a comparable degree as in non-anesthetized subjects.

Sevoflurane   *(SED-15, 3123; SEDA-28, 139; SEDA-29, 129)*

Observational studies   In 640 infants aged 1 day to 12 months, who were given sevoflurane in high concentrations for sedation during MRI examination, the only adverse events were one case of *vomiting*, eight of *minor hypoxia*, and two of *severe hypoxia* (13[c]).

Cardiovascular   *Prolongation of the QT interval* is associated with torsade de pointes, susceptibility to which arises from increased transmural dispersion of repolarization across the myocardial wall, which can be measured electrocardiographically as the time interval between the peak and end of the T wave. Several anesthetic drugs prolong the QT interval, but their effect on transmural dispersion of repolarization is unknown. The effects of propofol and sevoflurane on the corrected QT (QT_c) and transmural dispersion of repolarization have been investigated in 50 unpremedicated children aged 1–16 years (14[c]). Sevoflurane significantly prolonged the preoperative QT_c; propofol did not. Neither anesthetic had any significant effect on the preoperative transmural dispersion of repolarization.

Respiratory The incidence and duration of *apnea* during sevoflurane anesthesia has been studied in 131 women who were given increasing concentrations of sevoflurane from 1 to 8% ($n = 42$), decremental–incremental concentrations from 8 to 4% and then from 4 to 8% ($n = 36$), or fixed concentrations of 8% ($n = 53$) (15[C]). Although apnea occurred in all groups, it was more frequent and more pronounced in the fixed-dose group.

Nervous system A 3-year-old child had *tonic convulsions* after inhaling 3.9% sevoflurane for 45 minutes associated with moderate hyperventilation; he was later discovered to have epileptiform activity on electroencephalography (16[A]).

Two types of *tonic–clonic movement disorders* during sevoflurane anesthesia have been described (17[R]):

- agitation during early induction shortly after the loss of the eyelash reflex, characterized by discoordinate movements of the arms and legs, often followed by hypertonia and respiratory obstruction, both of which resolve with deepening of anesthesia;
- localized or generalized tonic–clonic movements during deep anesthesia at the end of induction and persisting at that level of anesthesia.

During sevoflurane anesthesia electroencephalography shows a brief increase in beta activity, which occurs at around the time when the eyelash reflex is lost (30–60 seconds after beginning induction); this is rapidly followed by sudden slowing to <2 Hz delta activity maximal at the end of the second minute of induction, and then acceleration to delta predominance (2–4 Hz) until the pupils are constricted and central. The bispectral index monitor also shows a higher index number at concentric pupils than during the middle of induction, when slowing down is maximal. Some subjects have episodes of burst suppression with deeper anesthesia (higher end-tidal sevoflurane and longer duration of anesthesia). Epileptiform activity also occurs. Spikes occur first, usually during delta oscillations (spike-wave). They may be simple or complex or periodic, leading to periods of epileptiform discharges or frank seizures. Generally, major discharges or frank seizure activity occur during deep anesthesia and are occasionally accompanied by tonic–clonic movements. Susceptibility factors include pre-existing epilepsy, febrile convulsions, and intracranial pathology.

The authors of this review made the following recommendations:

- benzodiazepine premedication, such as midazolam in children, might be useful;
- nitrous oxide might have a minimal protective effect;
- narcotic analgesics might be useful, but their protective qualities have not yet been documented.

The use of sevoflurane in children is complicated by a high incidence of *postanesthetic agitation*, probably due to residual sevoflurane during washout. It is not related to the speed of emergence (18[c]). Nitrous oxide has been used to mitigate this in 20 children, by continued administration after the end of sevoflurane anesthesia (19[c]). The end-tidal concentrations of sevoflurane at awakening were significantly lower in those who had been given nitrous oxide than in the control group and postanesthetic agitation was significantly less.

The effect of clonidine 2 micrograms/kg on the risk of sevoflurane-induced postanesthetic agitation has been quantified in 169 children (20[c]). Clonidine significantly reduced pain and discomfort scores, reduced the overall incidence of agitation by 57%, and reduced the incidence of severe agitation by 67%. The relative risks of agitation and severe agitation were 0.43 (95% CI = 0.24, 0.78) and 0.32 (0.09, 1.17) respectively.

Liver   Severe *hepatotoxicity* occurred after anesthesia with sevoflurane in a child with pre-existing mild renal dysfunction (21[A]).

Trichloroethylene   *(SED-15, 3488; SEDA-28, 140; SEDA-29, 130)*

Trichloroethylene is not used as an inhalational anesthetic, but still has industrial uses.

Immunologic   In 35 workers who had been exposed to environmental trichloroethylene there were significant *increases in serum inter-leukin-2 and interferon-gamma concentrations* and a *reduction in interleukin-4 concentrations* compared with 30 control workers (22[C]).

Teratogenicity   Reviewers of the industrial uses of trichloroethylene have concluded that there is no evidence that it is teratogenic (23[M], 24[M]).

Drug overdose   Overdosage with trichloro-ethylene has been reported (25[A]).

- A man in his 40s drank an unknown amount of trichloroethylene in a suicide attempt. He became comatose, with acute respiratory failure, hypotension, sinus tachycardia, and severe diarrhea. He was mechanically ventilated and on day 4 developed ventricular bigeminy. His serum creatine kinase and lactate dehydrogenase activities were persistently raised. He died with complete heart block after 24 days.

A muscle biopsy in this case showed evidence of muscle damage, with large lipid droplets compressed the myofilaments, degenerating mitochondria, and markedly reduced succinate and NAD cytochrome c reductase activities.

OTHER VAPORS

Nitrous oxide   *(SED-15, 2550; SEDA-27, 120; SEDA-28, 140; SEDA-29, 131)*

Nervous system   *Myelopathy* associated with nitric oxide anesthesia typically occurs in individuals who have been discovered postoperatively to be B_{12} deficient, and another case has

been reported in a 24-year-old man who used nitric oxide for recreational purposes (26[A]).

A patient who developed a diffuse myelopathy after receiving nitrous oxide on two occasions within 8 weeks had hyperhomocysteinemia and low concentrations of vitamin B_{12}, and had a polymorphism in the 5,10-methylenetetrahydrofolate reductase (MTHFR) gene associated with the thermolabile isoform of the enzyme (27[A]). The authors suggested that this explained the myelopathy. Treatment with folic acid and vitamin B_{12} caused the neurological symptoms to improve.

Subacute combined degeneration of the cord occurred 4 weeks after prolonged exposure to nitrous oxide in a man with diabetes who had hyperhomocysteinemia and vitamin B_{12} deficiency (28[A]).

Drug–device interactions   Nitrous oxide is 34 times more soluble than nitrogen in enclosed body cavity gas spaces, and it enters such spaces rapidly, causing expansion and a rise in pressure. It can therefore cause pneumothorax, air embolism, or pneumocephalus. Nitrous oxide also diffuses into the cuff of endotracheal tubes and can cause a marked increase in cuff pressure. In a 27-year-old woman with placenta percreta at 37 weeks gestation who required elective cesarean hysterectomy, internal iliac artery occlusion balloons ruptured during nitrous oxide anesthesia (29[A]).

INTRAVENOUS AGENTS: NON-BARBITURATE ANESTHETICS

Etomidate   *(SED-15, 1302; SEDA-27, 121)*

Nervous system   *Myoclonic movements* and *pain on injection* are common during induction of anesthesia with etomidate. In a double-blind study in 100 patients in whom anesthesia was induced with etomidate, ketamine 0.2 mg/kg, ketamine 0.5 mg/kg, magnesium sulfate 2.48 mmol, or isotonic saline were used to prevent myoclonic muscle movements. Of the 25 patients who received magnesium sulfate, 19 did not have myoclonic movements after the administration of etomidate; ketamine did not reduce the incidence of myoclonic movements (30^c).

Endocrine   Etomidate inhibits adrenal function resulting in *reduced steroidogenesis* after administration of both single boluses and maintenance infusions (31^c). In a prospective cohort study of 62 critically ill patients who were mechanically ventilated for more than 24 hours, about half developed adrenal insufficiency on the day after intubation. Administration of a single intravenous dose of etomidate 0.2–0.4 mg/kg for intubation led to a 12-fold increased risk of adrenal insufficiency (32^c). Etomidate should therefore be avoided as an induction agent in critically illness, in particular in patients with septic shock, among whom the incidence of adrenal insufficiency is high (33^R, 34^R, 35^R).

Ketamine   *(SED-15, 1964; SEDA-27, 120; SEDA-28, 141; SEDA-29, 131)*

Ketamine is a non-competitive antagonist at the phencyclidine site of the N-methyl-d-aspartate (NMDA) receptor for glutamate. However, its effects are also mediated by interactions with many others receptors. It was introduced as early as the 1960s, and is not generally used today as a general anesthetic, because of its adverse psychological effects, including *delirium, disturbed dreaming, motor adverse effects*, and *emergence reactions* in about 12% of patients. In the last decade, ketamine has increasingly been used in subanesthetic doses for the treatment of acute and chronic pain

Placebo-controlled studies   The effect of low-dose intravenous ketamine in combination with continuous femoral nerve block on postoperative pain and rehabilitation after total knee arthroplasty has been evaluated in a randomized placebo-controlled study (36^C). Those who received ketamine required significantly less morphine. No patients reported sedation, hallucinations, nightmares, or diplopia, and there were no differences in the incidence of nausea and vomiting between the two groups.

Systematic reviews   In a systematic review perioperative subanesthetic doses of ketamine reduced rescue analgesic requirements, pain intensity, or both in 27 of 37 clinical trials (2240 participants) (37^M, 38^M). Ketamine reduced both 24-hour PCA morphine consumption and postoperative nausea and vomiting. Adverse effects were mild or absent.

Nervous system   Ketamine has long been regarded as contraindicated in patients with, or at risk of, neurological damage. However, this view has recently been revised, with emphasis that there is evidence that ketamine does not increase intracranial pressure when used under conditions of controlled ventilation, co-administration of a gamma-aminobutyric acid (GABA) receptor agonist, and without nitrous oxide (39^R). Based on clinical, laboratory, and experimental results, ketamine may be safely used in patients with neurological damage. Ketamine may have neuroprotective effects, and S(+)-ketamine additional neuroregenerative effects, even when administered after the onset of a cerebral insult. Ketamine's hemodynamic effects may also improve cerebral perfusion and thereby influence outcome.

Psychological   The effects of ketamine 50 or 100 ng/ml on *memory* have been investigated in a double-blind, placebo-controlled, randomized, within-subject study in 12 healthy volunteers (40^C). Deleterious effects of ketamine on episodic memory were primarily attributable to its effects on encoding, rather than retrieval. The authors suggested that the effects they observed were similar to the memory deficits seen in schizophrenia and thus provide some support for the ketamine model of the disease.

Drug abuse   The illegal use of ketamine as a recreational drug is rapidly growing (41^R). It is sold as a liquid or powder that can be injected, ingested, or added to materials for smoking. Its psychedelic effects usually dissipate within 1 hour, and repeated use is therefore common. Its acute pharmacological effects include *tachycardia, increased blood pressure, impaired memory and cognitive function*, and *visual alterations*. High doses can cause *out-of-body or near-death experiences*. Its toxic effects include *hyperexcitability, severe agitation*, and *paranoid psychoses. Hyperthermia,* *seizures, rhabdomyolysis,* and *transient respiratory depression* can occur. Physical dependence has not been reported.

Dopamine D_1 receptor availability has been assessed using positron emission tomography and the selective D_1 receptor radioligand $[^{11}C]$-NNC 112 $((+)$-5-(7-benzofuranyl)-8-chloro-7-hydroxy-3-methyl-2,3,4,5-tetrahydro-1H-3-benzazepine) in 14 chronic recreational users of ketamine and matched healthy subjects (42^c). Dorsolateral prefrontal cortex D_1 receptor availability was significantly up-regulated in chronic ketamine, confirming similar observations in animals. Prefrontal dopamine neurotransmission is important for working memory and executive functions.

Drug overdose   Chronic homicidal ketamine poisoning has been reported in a 34-year-old married woman with no previous medical history, who died in her own home (43^A). She had been chronically poisoned by her husband over about 1 year. There was cardiac muscle fibrosis and hyaline degeneration of the small cardiac arteries.

Propofol   *(SED-15, 2945; SEDA-27, 121; SEDA-28, 142; SEDA-29, 132)*

Cardiovascular   In a double-blind, randomized, placebo-controlled study of the effects of ephedrine 70 micrograms/kg and ketamine 0.5 mg/kg in 75 patients, both drugs attenuated *hypotension* caused by propofol (44^C).

Nervous system   *Myoclonic movements* during induction of propofol anesthesia have been described in a 1-year-old boy undergoing adenotonsillectomy (45^A). Anesthetic maintenance, emergence, and neurological outcome were uneventful. Similar symptoms have been reported during emergence of a 14-year-old boy after propofol anesthesia for suturing of an upper limb laceration (46^A). Although the pathophysiological mechanisms are not known, it has been proposed that the seizure activity that occurs is subcortical in origin, as it is not related to electroencephalographic changes (47^C). Seizure activity has also been reported in a 78-year-old man who was given propofol and

had no subsequent evidence of epileptic activity (48^A).

Hallucinations have been attributed to propofol in a 70-year-old man (49^A).

Metabolism

Propofol infusion syndrome   A constellation of clinical symptoms including rhabdomyolysis, metabolic acidosis, cardiac dysrhythmias, cardiovascular collapse, and death associated with long-term administration of propofol has been termed the propofol infusion syndrome (SEDA-29, 132). Although it was initially recognized in children, the propofol infusion syndrome is now known to occur in both children (50^C, 51^C) and adults (52^A).

Three fatal cases of propofol infusion syndrome in adults have been reported (53^A):

- a 27-year-old woman who developed a metabolic acidosis, hypotension, and bradycardia;
- a 64-year-old man who developed a metabolic acidosis, hypotension, and rhabdomyolysis;
- a 24-year-old woman who developed hypotension, metabolic acidosis, and bradydysrhythmias.

Propofol infusion syndrome may present with one component only, such as lactic acidosis (52^A) or rhabdomyolysis (54^A). Initially, it was thought to result from cumulative toxicity, with reports after high-dose infusion as well as after prolonged administration of lower doses. However, recent reports suggest that it can occur even after short-term use and low-dose administration (55^A). It has been suggested that patients who are susceptible to metabolic acidosis or rhabdomyolysis after propofol administration may have subclinical forms of mitochondrial diseases that affect either the respiratory chain complex or fatty acid oxidation (56^r). In order to minimize the development of propofol infusion syndrome as a potentially lethal complication, a maximum dose of 3 mg/kg/hour has been recommended for sedation in intensive care patients.

Hypertriglyceridemia   The frequency and severity of hypertriglyceridemia and pancreatitis have been studied in 159 adults in intensive care who were given propofol for 24 hours or longer (57^c). There was hypertriglyceridemia in 29 (18%), of whom six had a serum triglyceride concentration of 11 mmol/l or more;

the median maximum serum triglyceride concentration was 8.0 (range 4.6–20) mmol/l. At the time when hypertriglyceridemia was detected, the median infusion rate of propofol was 50 (range 5–110) micrograms/kg/minute. The median time from the start of propofol therapy to identification of hypertriglyceridemia was 54 (range 14–319) hours. *Pancreatitis* developed in three of the 29 patients with hypertriglyceridemia.

Pancreas   (*See also Metabolism above.*) A 12-year-old girl developed acute *pancreatitis* within hours after exposure to a single dose of propofol (58[A]). In the context of two cases of pancreatitis due to propofol in young patients with Cushing's syndrome, it has been suggested that such patients may be at increased risk (59[A]).

Musculoskeletal   A *metabolic myopathy* has been described in a patient who received propofol (60[A]).

- During administration of propofol 3 mg/kg/hour, a 40-year-old man developed a fever of 41 °C, resistant to diclofenac and physical cooling. Propofol was replaced by midazolam. His urine darkened and his urinary output fell and eventually ceased completely. His serum creatine kinase activity was 708 nmol/1 and his serum myoglobin concentration 4625 nmol/1. His serum creatinine rose from 130 to 480 µmol/1 during the next 12 hours and he developed hyperkalemia (5.9 mmol/1) and a metabolic acidosis. Histological examination of skeletal muscle showed vacuole formation and cytochrome oxidase-negative fibers. Biochemical examination of the muscle fibers showed an increased free carnitine concentration and NADH-CoQ-oxidoreductase activity.

Drug formulations   The problems of formulating propofol have been reviewed (61[R]). It was originally formulated in Cremophor EL, which was later replaced by 10% soybean oil because of non-IgE-mediated anaphylactic reactions. However, such formulations can cause injection pain, sepsis, and hyperlipidemia and this has led to the development of propofol emulsions with altered propofol and lipid contents, the addition of different excipients to emulsions for antimicrobial activity, and non-emulsion formulations including cyclodextrin and polymeric micelle formulations. In addition, propofol prodrugs have been evaluated.

For a discussion of the effects of different formulations of propofol on injection pain see the special review below.

A lipid-free solution of propofol avoids bacterial contamination but is associated with a high incidence of thrombophlebitis (62[C]).

Drug interactions   It has been suggested that seizures in a 48-year-old man who was given intravenous propofol were potentiated by concurrent therapy with baclofen (63[A]).

Prevention of pain due to propofol injection   ℞

The most common adverse effect of propofol is pain on injection. It is particularly the case when propofol is injected into the small veins on the back of the hand, compared with the forearm or antecubital fossa. The incidence is 25–74%; in one series of 18 patients, mean age 46 years, to whom propofol was given into a vein in the back of the hand over 30 seconds, pain was reported in 10 cases (64[C]).

Many strategies to prevent propofol-induced pain have been tried. It may be reduced by rapid injection (65[C]). In 100 patients anesthesia was induced with propofol injected in a sterile ground-glass syringe at a rate of 10 ml over 10–15 seconds; only 16% complained of pain; of the 24 patients aged under 50 years, 33% complained of pain (66[c]).

Warming propofol to 37 °C has no effect on the incidence of pain (67[C], 68[C]).

Mechanism   *The mechanism of propofol-induced pain is not known, but it is probably related to the concentration of aqueous propofol at the site of injection (see drug formulations below). Other proposed mechanisms involve the generation of bradykinin, although there are conflicting results (69[C], 70[C]), and pH, since the addition of lidocaine reduces the pH of propofol solution (71[C]).*

Lidocaine   *Lidocaine is the most extensively studied treatment for propofol-induced pain (72[C], 73[C]) and is usually used as a comparator for other compounds. It should be given about half a minute before the propofol or mixed with the propofol immediately before administration.*

In a double-blind, randomized study in 310 patients undergoing anesthesia three doses of lidocaine were compared, 0.1, 0.2, and 0.4 mg/kg; the lowest dose significantly reduced the incidence of pain and there was no improvement when the dose was increased (74^C).

In 183 patients aged 15–65 years who were given propofol into a vein on the back of the hand, lidocaine was added to the solution before injection in concentrations of 0.05, 0.10, 0.15, and 0.20% and compared with saline in the same concentrations (75^C). Severe pain in those given lidocaine occurred in 11–30% compared with 35–67% in those given saline, and overall the incidence of pain was reduced significantly by lidocaine. However, there was no benefit in using lidocaine in a concentration above 0.05%, although in another study a 0.1% strength was optimal (76^C).

Intravenous lidocaine + prilocaine in 70 patients aged 19–65 years, given either separately or together, reduced the amount of pain produced by propofol (77^c).

Topical anesthesia using 60% lidocaine tape also reduces the incidence of propofol-induced pain (78^c, 79^c), but in a double-blind, randomized, placebo-controlled study in 90 patients, topical 5% lidocaine + prilocaine cream (Emla) was not effective, whereas the addition of lidocaine to propofol was (80^c). However, Emla was applied for only 1 hour before the administration of propofol, and there is evidence that longer exposure is required; in 65 propofol anesthetics in 28 children during lumbar puncture and/or bone marrow aspiration, application of Emla 4 hours before propofol was effective (81^c).

Alfentanil   *In 22 patients the pain caused by propofol was modified by a bolus intravenous dose of alfentanil 1 mg (82^c).*

Dexamethasone   *In a randomized, placebo-controlled, double-blind study in 70 patients, 18–60 years of age, intravenous dexamethasone 0.15 mg/kg up to a maximum of 8 mg reduced the incidence of propofol injection pain significantly when it was given 1 minute before propofol (83^C). However, it was associated with perineal itching and pain in some cases.*

Dexmedetomidine   *In a randomized, placebo-controlled comparison of the α_2-adrenoceptor agonist dexmedetomidine 0.25 micrograms/kg and lidocaine 0.5 mg/kg in 90 patients, both drugs reduced pain from propofol (84^C).*

Glyceryl trinitrate   *Glyceryl trinitrate ointment applied to the back of the hand reduced the incidence of propofol-induced pain in a placebo-controlled study in 60 women (85^c). There was no pain in 18 of 30 women who were pretreated with glyceryl trinitrate compared with 10 of 30 women who were pretreated with placebo. There was moderate or severe pain in 11 of those treated with placebo compared with only one of those who were treated with glyceryl trinitrate. The pain occurred 10 seconds or more after the start of injection in more than half the subjects, and in more than half the patients the site at which the pain was felt was above the injection site. No patient had a headache or postural hypotension.*

5HT$_3$ receptor antagonists   *In a double-blind, randomized, placebo-controlled study in 150 patients, intravenous granisetron 2 mg was as effective as intravenous lidocaine 40 mg with 120 seconds of venous occlusion at preventing propofol-induced pain and significantly better than placebo (86^C).*

In a double-blind, randomized, placebo-controlled study in 80 patients, ondansetron reduced propofol-induced pain (87^C).

Ketamine   *In a placebo-controlled study in 100 women, pretreatment with intravenous ketamine 10 mg reduced the incidence of propofol-induced injection pain from 84 to 26% of patients (88^C).*

Metoclopramide   *In a randomized, double-blind, placebo-controlled study in 90 patients, the addition of metoclopramide improved the analgesic effect of lidocaine in patients given intravenous propofol (89^C). However, in another study metoclopramide was less effective than lidocaine (90^C).*

Nafamostat   *In a double-blind, randomized, placebo-controlled study in 213 patients, nafamostat mesilate 0.02 mg/kg significantly reduced propofol-induced pain (91^C). Nafamostat is an inhibitor of bradykinin generation* from kallikrein, and in another study the same authors found increased bradykinin concentrations after injection of the lipid solvent of propofol, an effect that was attenuated by nafamostat (69^C). They suggested that the effect of bradykinin on the injected vein increases contact between aqueous propofol and the free nerve endings of the vessel.

Nitrous oxide   In a randomized, double-blind study in 90 patients, 50% nitrous oxide in oxygen + lidocaine 40 mg mixed in 1% propofol 20 ml was compared with 50% nitrous oxide in oxygen without lidocaine and 50% oxygen in air + lidocaine (92^C). The combination of 50% nitrous oxide + lidocaine was the most effective treatment. A similar result was found in a randomized, double-blind study in 102 adults (93^C).

NSAIDs   In 250 patients intravenous flurbiprofen 50 mg immediately before propofol injection completely abolished injection pain and was more effective than lidocaine; when flurbiprofen was given 1 minute before propofol injection it was less effective (94^C).
    In a randomized, double-blind study in 180 patients pretreatment with intravenous ketorolac 15 mg and 30 mg reduced propofol-induced pain (95^C). A lower dose of ketorolac 10 mg with venous occlusion for 120 seconds achieved the same effect. However, in another study in 22 patients, ketorolac 30 mg given before propofol had no effect (77^c).

Ondansetron   Ondansetron and tramadol have been compared in 100 patients being given propofol in a randomized, double-blind study (96^C). Tramadol 50 mg intravenously was as effective as ondansetron 4 mg intravenously with 15 seconds of venous occlusion at preventing propofol injection pain. However, there was significantly less nausea and vomiting in those given ondansetron.

Remifentanil   In 225 patients aged 19–73 years, remifentanil 0.25 or 1 micrograms/kg immediately before propofol, remifentanil 0.25 micrograms/kg 1 minute before propofol, and pethidine (meperidine) 40 mg immediately before propofol were compared with saline; remifentanil 1 micrograms/kg provided the most effective pain relief (97^C).

The effects of remifentanil on the incidence and severity of pain after propofol injection have been compared with those of lidocaine in a double-blind, randomized, placebo-controlled study in 155 patients (98^C). Pretreatment with intravenous remifentanil infusion 0.25 micrograms/kg/minute significantly reduced the pain after propofol injection. Lidocaine 40 mg achieved the same effect.

Thiopental   In 90 women aged 15–34 years who were given propofol into a vein in the back of the hand, co-induction with thiopental reduced the severity of the pain but not its frequency (99^C). However, lidocaine reduced both the severity (to a greater extent than thiopental) and the frequency.

Tramadol   Tramadol was less effective than lidocaine in preventing propofol-induced pain (100^C), but equivalent to ondansetron (96^C).

Effect of formulation   The effect of altering the lipid emulsion carrier in propofol formulations on pain after injection has been evaluated in several studies. In particular, a modified lipid emulsion of propofol containing a mixture of medium-chain and long-chain triglycerides (MCT/LCT; Propofol-Lipuro) has been compared with the usual formulation (LCT; Diprivan), which contains long-chain triglycerides only.
    In two prospective randomized studies in 222 and 80 patients respectively MCT/LCT propofol was equivalent to LCT propofol with lidocaine pretreatment (101^C, 102^C). Lidocaine before MCT/LCT propofol conferred an additional advantage.
    In 130 adults randomly assigned to a propofol emulsion containing medium-chain triglycerides or a lipid-free formulation, the latter caused more pain on injection (103^C).
    A medium-chain/long-chain triglyceride emulsion has been evaluated in a randomized, double-blind, crossover comparison with a long-chain triglyceride emulsion in subanesthetic doses In a comparison of MCT/LCT propofol and LCT propofol in 60 healthy subjects there was significantly less pain with MCT/LCT (104^c). However, when MCT/LCT was given first there was no significant difference. The authors concluded that MCT/LCT propofol is associated with less injection pain

than LCT propofol and also seems to attenuate subsequent injection pain of LCT propofol when administered first. The mechanism is unknown, but they suggested that it might be related to a reduction in the concentration of propofol in the aqueous phase.

In 80 adults the maximal intensity of pro-pofol-induced local pain was significantly lower after MCT/LCT propofol than after LCT propofol (105[A]).

In a randomized, double-blind comparison of MCT/LCT propofol and LCT propofol in 194 patients, the former produced a significantly lower incidence of moderate injection pain (11 versus 26%) (106[c]). Similar results were reported in 200 adults in whom the mechanism of the pain was also sought; bradykinin concentrations were the same after the two types of formulations and the authors concluded that the pain was probably due to propofol in the aqueous phase (70[C]).

In a randomized double-blind comparison of MCT/LCT propofol and LCT propofol + lidocaine in 83 children undergoing day case surgery, the former was associated with significantly less pain (107[C]).

In 75 patients the addition of lidocaine to MCT/LCT propofol further reduced the incidence of pain (108[C]).

Another strategy has been to alter the amount of lipid in the emulsion. A lipid formulation ("Ampofor") that contains 50% less soybean oil and egg lecithin (5 and 0.6% respectively) has been compared with the most commonly available propofol formulations in two randomized studies in 63 and 60 patients respectively (109[C], 110[C]). Ampofor was associated with an increased incidence of pain on injection.

Conclusions   Propofol-induced pain has been reviewed (111[R]). The authors reached the following conclusions:

- guaranteed pain-free propofol injection is not possible;
- single preventive interventions are not as effective as combinations of different measures;
- the application of a venous tourniquet improves the pain-reducing effect of drugs such as lidocaine;
- a propofol MCT/LCT emulsion should be used;

- for general anesthesia opioids or ketamine can be used and for sedation a subanesthetic dose of thiopental;
- for children Emla cream (lidocaine + prilocaine) is suitable, because it reduces the pain of both propofol injection and venous cannulation [it should be applied for several hours before the administration of propofol].

INTRAVENOUS AGENTS: BARBITURATE ANESTHETICS

Thiopental sodium   (SED-15, 3395; SEDA-27, 121)

Electrolyte balance   There has been a previous report of severe *hyperkalemia* following hypokalemia related to prolonged thiopental coma (112[A]) and a second report has now appeared (60[A]).

- A 35-year-old woman with a history of tonic–clonic seizures gave birth to a healthy child at term, but 2 weeks later developed tonic–clonic seizures refractory to combined antiepileptic drug therapy. She was mechanically ventilated and was sedated with midazolam, sufentanil, and thiopental (2–3 mg/kg/hour) for 84 hours, controlled by burst suppression on continuous electroencephalographic monitoring. After 2 days she developed symptoms of puerperal sepsis and underwent hysterectomy. During thiopental coma, she developed mild hypokalemia, which was treated with potassium 2–5 mmol/hour. The potassium infusion was stopped several hours before hysterectomy. Renal function was not compromised. A few hours later she developed a ventricular tachycardia, associated with a serum potassium concentration of 7.1 mmol/l. Despite treatment with insulin, glucose, calcium, and immediate hemofiltration, the hyperkalemia persisted, and she became asystolic and died.

It is unclear whether the rise in serum potassium in this case was related to rhabdomyolysis or some other effect. However, hypokalemia has previously been described after barbiturate coma, with hyperkalemia after withdrawal; hyperkalemia in such cases may therefore be a rebound effect.

Multiorgan failure   A syndrome with striking similarities to propofol infusion syndrome has been reported in association with thiopental (113[A]).

- A 59-year-old man with a history of epileptic convulsions developed status epilepticus. Intravenous midazolam was ineffective and he was mechanically ventilated and given high-dose thiopental with continuous electroencephalographic monitoring. After 3 days he developed a fever, severe hemodynamic instability, and multiorgan dysfunction. He was given inotropic drugs in high doses, low-dose glucocorticoids, and renal replacement therapy. After 5 days, thiopental and midazolam were withdrawn. He died after 2 weeks with persistent cardiac failure, severe rhabdomyolysis, renal insufficiency, metabolic acidosis, and fulminant hepatic failure.

The clinical symptoms that led to this patient's death mimicked propofol infusion syndrome. The authors hypothesized that total suppression of cerebral activity by any sedative drug could lead to physiological compromise and development of a lethal syndrome resembling the propofol infusion syndrome. As observed in propofol infusion syndrome, which is usually associated with high-dose propofol infusion, very high dosages of thiopental were used as a sedative anticonvulsant regimen in this patient. Although rhabdomyolysis and renal insufficiency have been described as complications of status epilepticus (114[A]), a toxic drug-related cellular effect in susceptible patients, possibly involving mitochondrial pathways, could provide an alternative explanation.

References

1. Macario A, Dexter F, Lubarsky D. Meta-analysis of trials comparing postoperative recovery after anesthesia with sevoflurane or desflurane. Am J Health Syst Pharm 2005;62(1):63–8.
2. Nishiyama T, Yamashita K, Yokoyama T. Stress hormone changes in general anesthesia of long duration: isoflurane-nitrous oxide vs sevoflurane-nitrous oxide anesthesia. J Clin Anesth 2005;17(8):586–91.
3. Tanaka T, Nabatame H, Tanifuji Y. Insulin secretion and glucose utilization are impaired under general anesthesia with sevoflurane as well as isoflurane in a concentration-independent manner. J Anesth 2005;19(4):277–81.
4. Geffroy JC, Gentili ME, Le Pollès R, Triclot P. Massive inhalation of desflurane due to vaporizer dysfunction. Anesthesiology 2005;103(5):1096–8.
5. Smelt WL. Cardiac arrest during desflurane anaesthesia in a patient with Duchenne's muscular dystrophy. Acta Anaesthesiol Scand 2005;49(2):267–9.
6. Arain SR, Shankar H, Ebert TJ. Desflurane enhances reactivity during the use of the laryngeal mask airway. Anesthesiology 2005;103(3):495–9.
7. Tung D, Yoshida EM, Wang CS, Steinbrecher UP. Severe desflurane hepatotoxicity after colon surgery in an elderly patient. Can J Anaesth 2005;52(2):133–6.
8. Uskova AA, Matusic BP, Brandom BW. Desflurane, malignant hyperthermia, and release of compartment syndrome. Anesth Analg 2005;100(5):1357–60.
9. Akin A, Ugur F, Ozkul Y, Esmaoglu A, Gunes I, Ergul H. Desflurane anaesthesia increases sister chromatid exchanges in human lymphocytes. Acta Anaesthesiol Scand 2005;49(10):1559–61.
10. Karpiński TM, Kostrzewska-Poczekaj M, Stachecki I, Mikstacki A, Szyfter K. Genotoxicity of the volatile anaesthetic desflurane in human lymphocytes in vitro, established by comet assay. J Appl Genet 2005;46(3):319–24.
11. Kobayashi Y. Pressor responses to inhalation of isoflurane during induction of anesthesia and subsequent tracheal intubation. Masui 2005;54(8):869–74.
12. Iselin-Chaves IA, Willems SJ, Jermann FC, Forster A, Adam SR, Van der Linden M. Investigation of implicit memory during isoflurane anaesthesia for elective surgery using the process dissociation procedure. Anesthesiology 2005;103(5):925–33.
13. De Sanctis Briggs V. Magnetic resonance imaging under sedation in newborns and infants: a study of 640 cases using sevoflurane. Paediatr Anaesth 2005;15(1):9–15.
14. Whyte SD, Booker PD, Buckley DG. The effects of propofol and sevoflurane on the QT interval and transmural dispersion of repolarization in children. Anesth Analg 2005;100(1):71–7.
15. Pancaro C, Giovannoni S, Toscano A, Peduto VA. Apnea during induction of anesthesia

with sevoflurane is related to its mode of administration. Can J Anaesth 2005;52(6):591–4.

16. Boutin F, Bonnet A, Cros AM. Survenue d'une crise épileptiforme avec le sévoflurane chez un enfant. Ann Fr Anesth Reanim 2005;24(5):559–60.

17. Constant I, Seeman R, Murat I. Sevoflurane and epileptiform EEG changes. Paediatr Anaesth 2005;15(4):266–74.

18. Oh AY, Seo KS, Kim SD, Kim CS, Kim HS. Delayed emergence process does not result in a lower incidence of emergence agitation after sevoflurane anesthesia in children. Acta Anaesthesiol Scand 2005;49(3):297–9.

19. Shibata S, Shigeomi S, Sato W, Enzan K. Nitrous oxide administration during washout of sevoflurane improves postanesthetic agitation in children. J Anesth 2005;19(2):160–3.

20. Tesoro S, Mezzetti D, Marchesini L, Peduto VA. Clonidine treatment for agitation in children after sevoflurane anesthesia. Anesth Analg. 2005;101(6):1619–22.

21. Jang Y, Kim I. Severe hepatotoxicity after sevoflurane anesthesia in a child with mild renal dysfunction. Paediatr Anaesth 2005;15(12):1140–4.

22. Iavicoli I, Marinaccio A, Carelli G. Effects of occupational trichloroethylene exposure on cytokine levels in workers. J Occup Environ Med 2005;47(5):453–7.

23. Hardin BD, Kelman BJ, Brent RL. Trichloroethylene and dichloroethylene: a critical review of teratogenicity. Birth Defects Res A Clin Mol Teratol 2005;73(12):931–55.

24. Watson RE, Jacobson CF, Williams AL, Howard WB, DeSesso JM. Trichloroethylene-contaminated drinking water and congenital heart defects: a critical analysis of the literature. Reprod Toxicol 2006;21(2):117–47.

25. Vattemi G, Tonin P, Filosto M, Rizzuto N, Tomelleri G, Perbellini L, Iacovelli W, Petrucci N. Human skeletal muscle as a target organ of trichloroethylene toxicity. JAMA 2005;294(5):554–6.

26. Waters MF, Kang GA, Mazziotta JC, DeGiorgio CM. Nitrous oxide inhalation as a cause of cervical myelopathy. Acta Neurol Scand 2005;112(4):270–2.

27. Lacassie HJ, Nazar C, Yonish B, Sandoval P, Muir HA, Mellado P. Reversible nitrous oxide myelopathy and a polymorphism in the gene encoding 5,10-methylenetetrahydrofolate reductase. Br J Anaesth 2006;96(2):222–5.

28. Ahn SC, Brown AW. Cobalamin deficiency and subacute combined degeneration after nitrous oxide anesthesia: a case report. Arch Phys Med Rehabil 2005;86(1):150–3.

29. Kuczkowski KM, Eisenmann UB. Nitrous oxide as a cause of internal iliac artery occlusion balloon rupture. Ann Fr Anesth Reanim 2005;24(5):564.

30. Guler A, Satilmis T, Akinci SB, Celebioglu B, Kanbak M. Magnesium sulfate pretreatment reduces myoclonus after etomidate. Anesth Analg 2005;101(3):705–9.

31. Wagner RL, White PF, Kan PB, Rosenthal MH, Feldman D. Inhibition of adrenal steroidogenesis by the anesthetic etomidate. N Engl J Med 1984;310:1415–21.

32. Malerba G, Romano-Girard F, Cravoisy A, Dousset B, Nace L, Lévy B, Bollaert PE. Risk factors of relative adrenocortical deficiency in intensive care patients needing mechanical ventilation. Intensive Care Med 2005;31:388–92.

33. Jackson WL Jr.. Should we use etomidate as an induction agent for endotracheal intubation in patients with septic shock? A critical appraisal. Chest 2005;127:1031–8.

34. Annane D. ICU physicians should abandon the use of etomidate! Intensive Care Med 2005;31:325–6.

35. Morris C, McAllister C. Etomidate for emergency anaesthesia; mad, bad and dangerous to know? Anaesthesia 2005;60(8):737–40.

36. Adam F, Chauvin M, Du MB, Langlois M, Sessler DI, Fletcher D. Small-dose ketamine infusion improves postoperative analgesia and rehabilitation after total knee arthroplasty. Anesth Analg 2005;100:475–80.

37. Bell RF, Dahl JB, Moore RA, Kalso E. Perioperative ketamine for acute post-operative pain: a quantitative and qualitative systematic review (Cochrane review). Acta Anaesthesiol Scand 2005;49:1405–28.

38. Bell RF, Dahl JB, Moore RA, Kalso E. Perioperative ketamine for acute postoperative pain. Cochrane Database Syst Rev 2006:CD004603.

39. Himmelseher S, Durieux ME. Revising a dogma: ketamine for patients with neurological injury? Anesth Analg 2005;101:524–34.

40. Honey GD, Honey RA, Sharar SR, Turner DC, Pomarol-Clotet E, Kumaran D, Simons JS, Hu X, Rugg MD, Bullmore ET, Fletcher PC. Impairment of specific episodic memory processes by sub-psychotic doses of ketamine: the effects of levels of processing at encoding and of the subsequent retrieval task. Psychopharmacology (Berl) 2005;181(3):445–57.

41. Ricaurte GA, McCann UD. Recognition and management of complications of new recreational drug use. Lancet 2005;365(9477):2137–45.

42. Narendran R, Frankle WG, Keefe R, Gil R, Martinez D, Slifstein M, Kegeles LS, Talbot PS, Huang Y, Hwang DR, Khenissi L, Cooper TB, Laruelle M, Abi-Dargham A. Altered prefrontal dopaminergic function in chronic recreational ketamine users. Am J Psychiatry 2005;162(12):2352–9.

43. Tao Y, Chen XP, Qin ZH. A fatal chronic ketamine poisoning. J Forensic Sci 2005;50(1):173–6.

44. Ozkoçak I, Altunkaya H, Ozer Y, Ayoğlu H, Demirel CB, Ciçek E. Comparison of ephedrine and ketamine in prevention of injection pain and hypotension due to propofol induction. Eur J Anaesthesiol 2005;22(1):44–8.

45. Nimmaanrat S. Myoclonic movements following induction of anesthesia with propofol: a case report. J Med Assoc Thai 2005;88:1955–7.

46. Saravanakumar K, Venkatesh P, Bromley P. Delayed onset refractory dystonic movements following propofol anesthesia. Paediatr Anaesth 2005;15:597–601.

47. Borgeat A, Dessibourg C, Popovic V, Meier D, Blanchard M, Schwander D. Propofol and spontaneous movements: an EEG study. Anesthesiology 1991;74:24–7.

48. Hickey KS, Martin DF, Chuidian FX. Propofol-induced seizure-like phenomena. J Emerg Med 2005;29(4):447–9.

49. Venkatesh KH, Chandramouli BA. Postoperative hallucinations following propofol infusion in a neurosurgical patient: a diagnostic dilemma. J Neurosurg Anesthesiol 2005;17(3):176–7.

50. Martin PH, Murthy BV, Petros AJ. Metabolic, biochemical and haemodynamic effects of infusion of propofol for long-term sedation of children undergoing intensive care. Br J Anaesth 1997;79:276–9.

51. Hansen TG. Propofol infusion syndrome in children. Ugeskr Laeger 2005;167(39):3672–5.

52. Liolios A, Guerit JM, Scholtes JL, Raftopoulos C, Hantson P. Propofol infusion syndrome associated with short-term large-dose infusion during surgical anesthesia in an adult. Anesth Analg 2005;100:1804–6.

53. Kumar MA, Urrutia VC, Thomas CE, Abou-Khaled KJ, Schwartzman RJ. The syndrome of irreversible acidosis after prolonged propofol infusion. Neurocrit Care 2005;3(3):257–9.

54. Betrosian AP, Papanikoleou M, Frantzeskaki F, Diakalis C, Georgiadis G. Myoglobinemia and propofol infusion. Acta Anaesthesiol Scand 2005;49:720.

55. Haase R, Sauer H, Eichler G. Lactic acidosis following short-term propofol infusion may be an early warning of propofol infusion syndrome. J Neurosurg Anesthesiol 2005;17:122–3.

56. Farag E, Deboer G, Cohen BH, Niezgoda J. Metabolic acidosis due to propofol infusion. Anesthesiology 2005;102:697–8.

57. Devlin JW, Lau AK, Tanios MA. Propofol-associated hypertriglyceridemia and pancreatitis in the intensive care unit: an analysis of frequency and risk factors. Pharmacotherapy 2005;25(10):1348–52.

58. Gottschling S, Larsen R, Meyer S, Graf N, Reinhard H. Acute pancreatitis induced by short-term propofol administration. Paediatr Anaesth 2005;15(11):1006–8.

59. Priya G, Bhagat H, Pandia MP, Chaturvedi A, Seth A, Goswami R. Can propofol precipitate pancreatitis in patients with Cushing's syndrome? Acta Anaesthesiol Scand 2005;49(9):1381–3.

60. Machata AM, Gonano C, Birsan T, Zimpfer M, Spiss CK. Rare but dangerous adverse effects of propofol and thiopental in intensive care. J Trauma 2005;58:643–5.

61. Baker MT, Naguib M. Propofol: the challenges of formulation. Anesthesiology 2005;103(4):860–76.

62. Paul M, Dueck M, Kampe S, Fruendt H, Kasper SM. Pharmacological characteristics and side effects of a new galenic formulation of propofol without soyabean oil. Anaesthesia 2003;58:1056–62.

63. Manikandan S, Sinha PK, Neema PK, Rathod RC. Severe seizures during propofol induction in a patient with syringomyelia receiving baclofen. Anesth Analg 2005;100(5):1468–9.

64. Sear JW, Jewkes C, Wanigasekera V. Hemodynamic effects during induction, laryngoscopy, and intubation with eltanolone (5β-pregnanolone) or propofol. A study in ASA I and II patients. J Clin Anesth 1995;7:126–31.

65. Shimizu T, Inomata S, Kihara S, Toyooka H, Brimacombe JR. Rapid injection reduces pain on injection with propofol. Eur J Anaesthesiol 2005;22(5):394–6.

66. Lomax D. Propofol injection pain. Anaesth Intensive Care 1994;22:500–1.

67. Ozturk E, Izdes S, Babacan A, Kaya K. Temperature of propofol does not reduce the incidence of injection pain. Anesthesiology 1998;89:1041.

68. Uda R, Kadono N, Otsuka M, Shimizu S, Mori H, Ozturk E, Izdes S, Babacan A, Kaya K. Strict temperature control has no effect on injection pain with propofol. Anesthesiology 1999;91:591–2.

69. Nakane M, Iwama H. A potential mechanism of propofol-induced pain on injection based on studies using nafamostat mesilate. Br J Anaesth 1999;83:397–404.

70. Ohmizo H, Obara S, Iwama H. Mechanism of injection pain with long and long-medium chain triglyceride emulsive propofol. Can J Anaesth 2005;52(6):595–9.

71. Eriksson M, Englesson S, Niklasson F, Hartvig P. Effect of lignocaine and pH on propofol-induced pain. Br J Anaesth 1997;78(5):502–6.

72. Scott RP, Saunders DA, Norman J. Propofol: clinical strategies for preventing the pain of injection. Anaesthesia 1988;43(6):492–4.

73. King SY, Davis FM, Wells JE, Murchison DJ, Pryor PJ. Lidocaine for the prevention of pain due to injection of propofol. Anesth Analg 1992;74(2):246–9.

74. Gehan G, Karoubi P, Quinet F, Leroy A, Rathat C, Pourriat JL. Optimal dose of lignocaine for preventing pain on injection of propofol. Br J Anaesth 1991;66(3):324–6.

75. Tham CS, Khoo ST. Modulating effects of lignocaine on propofol. Anaesth Intensive Care 1995;23:154–7.

76. Ho C-M, Tsou M-Y, Sun M-S, Chu C-C, Lee T-Y. The optimal effective concentration of lidocaine to reduce pain on injection of propofol. J Clin Anesth 1999;11:296–300.

77. Eriksson M. Prilocaine reduces injection pain caused by propofol. Acta Anaesthesiol Scand 1995;39:210–3.

78. Uda R, Ohtsuka M, Doi Y, Inamori K, Kunimasa K, Ohnaka M, Minami T, Akatsuka M,

Mori H. Sixty percent lidocaine tape alleviates pain on injection of propofol after diminishing venipuncture pain. Masui 1998;47(7):843–7.

79. Yokota S, Komatsu T, Komura Y, Nishiwaki K, Kimura T, Hosoda R, Shimada Y. Pretreatment with topical 60% lidocaine tape reduces pain on injection of propofol. Anesth Analg 1997;85(3):672–4.

80. McCluskey A, Currer BA, Sayeed I. The efficacy of 5% lidocaine-prilocaine (EMLA) cream on pain during intravenous injection of propofol. Anesth Analg 2003;97(3):713–4.

81. Von Heijne M, Bredlöv B, Söderhäll S, Olsson GL. Propofol or propofol–alfentanil anesthesia for painful procedures in the pediatric oncology ward. Paediatr Anaesth 2004;14(8):670–5.

82. Fletcher JE, Seavell CR, Bowen DJ. Pretreatment with alfentanil reduces pain caused by propofol. Br J Anaesth 1994;72:342–4.

83. Singh M, Mohta M, Sethi AK, Tyagi A. Efficacy of dexamethasone pretreatment for alleviation of propofol injection pain. Eur J Anaesthesiol 2005;22(11):888–90.

84. Turan A, Memis D, Kaya G, Karamanlioglu B. The prevention of pain from injection of propofol by dexmedetomidine and comparison with lidocaine. Can J Anaesth 2005;52(5):548–9.

85. Wilkinson D, Anderson M, Gauntlett IS. Pain on injection of propofol. Modification by nitroglycerin. Anesth Analg 1993;77:1139–42.

86. Dubey PK, Prasad SS. Pain on injection with propofol: the effect of granisetron pretreatment. Clin J Pain 2003;19:121–4.

87. Ambesh SP, Dubey PK, Sinha PK. Ondansetron pretreatment to alleviate pain on propofol injection: a randomized, controlled, double-blinded study. Anesth Analg 1999;89:197–9.

88. Tan CH, Onsiong MK, Kua SW. The effect of ketamine pretreatment on propofol injection pain in 100 women. Anaesthesia 1998;53:296–307.

89. Fujii Y, Nakayama M. A lidocaine/metoclopramide combination decreases pain on injection of propofol. Can J Anaesth 2005;52(5):474–7.

90. Mok MS, Pang W-W, Hwang M-H. The analgesic effect of tramadol, metoclopramide, meperidine and lidocaine in ameliorating propofol injection pain: a comparative study. J Anaesthesiol Clin Pharmacol 1999;15:37–42.

91. Iwama H, Nakane M, Ohmori S, Kaneko T, Kato M, Watanabe K, Okuaki A. Nafamostat mesilate, a kallikrein inhibitor, prevents pain on injection with propofol. Br J Anaesth 1998;81(6):963–4.

92. Sinha PK, Neema PK, Rathod RC. Effect of nitrous oxide in reducing pain of propofol injection in adult patients. Anaesth Intensive Care 2005;33(2):235–8.

93. Niazi A, Galvin E, Elsaigh I, Wahid Z, Harmon D, Leonard I. A combination of lidocaine and nitrous oxide in oxygen is more effective in preventing pain on propofol injection

than either treatment alone. Eur J Anaesthesiol 2005;22(4):299–302.

94. Nishiyama T. How to decrease pain at rapid injection of propofol: effectiveness of flurbiprofen. J Anesth 2005;19(4):273–6.

95. Huang YW, Buerkle H, Lee TH, Lu CY, Lin CR, Lin SH, Chou AK, Muhammad R, Yang LC. Effect of pre-treatment with ketorolac on propofol injection pain. Acta Anaesthesiol Scand 2002;46:1021–4.

96. Memis D, Turan A, Karamanlioglu B, Kaya G, Pamukcu Z. The prevention of propofol injection pain by tramadol or ondansetron. Eur J Anaesthesiol 2002;19:47–51.

97. Basaranoglu G, Erden V, Delatioglu H, Saitoglu L. Reduction of pain on injection of propofol using meperidine and remifentanil. Eur J Anaesthesiol 2005;22(11):890–2.

98. Roehm KD, Piper SN, Maleck WH, Boldt J. Prevention of propofol-induced injection pain by remifentanil: a placebo-controlled comparison with lidocaine. Anaesthesia 2003;58:165–70.

99. Haugen RD, Vaghadia H, Waters T, Merrick PM. Thiopentone pretreatment for propofol injection pain in ambulatory patients. Can J Anaesth 1995;42:1108–12.

100. Pang W-W, Huang P-Y, Chang D-P, Huang M-H. The peripheral analgesic effect of tramadol in reducing propofol injection pain: a comparison with lidocaine. Reg Anesth Pain Med 1999;24:246–9.

101. Adam S, von Bommel J, Pelka M, Dirckx M, Jonsson D, Klein J. Propofol-induced injection pain: comparison of a modified propofol emulsion to standard propofol with premixed lidocaine. Anesth Analg 2004;99:1076–9.

102. Kunitz O, Losing R, Schulz-Stubner S, Haaf-von-Below S, Rossaint R, Kuhlen R. Propofol-LCT versus propofol MCT/LCT with or without lidocaine – a comparison on pain on injection. Anaesthesiol Intensivmed Notfallmed Schmerzther 2004;39:10–4.

103. Dubey PK, Kumar A. Pain on injection of lipid-free propofol and propofol emulsion containing medium-chain triglyceride: a comparative study. Anesth Analg 2005;101(4):1060–2.

104. Sun NC, Wong AY, Irwin MG. A comparison of pain on intravenous injection between two preparations of propofol. Anesth Analg 2005;101(3):675–8.

105. Liljeroth E, Akeson J. Less local pain on intravenous infusion of a new propofol emulsion. Acta Anaesthesiol Scand 2005;49(2):248–51.

106. Nagao N, Uchida T, Nakazawa K, Makita K. Medium-/long-chain triglyceride emulsion reduced severity of pain during propofol injection. Can J Anaesth 2005;52(6):660–1.

107. Nyman Y, von Hofsten K, Georgiadi A, Eksborg S, Lönnqvist PA. Propofol injection pain in children: a prospective randomized double-blind trial of a new propofol formulation versus propofol with added lidocaine. Br J Anaesth 2005;95(2):222–5.

108. Yew WS, Chong SY, Tan KH, Goh MH. The effects of intravenous lidocaine on pain during injection of medium- and long-chain triglyceride propofol emulsions. Anesth Analg 2005;100(6):1693–5.

109. Song D, Hamza MA, White PF, Byerly SI, Jones SB, Macaluso AD. Comparison of a lower-lipid propofol emulsion with the standard emulsion for sedation during monitored anesthesia care. Anesthesiology 2004;100:1072–5.

110. Song D, Hamza MA, White PF, Klein K, Recart A, Khodaparasat O. The pharmacodynamic effects of a lower-lipid emulsion of propofol: a comparison with the standard propofol emulsion. Anesth Analg 2004;98:687–91.

111. Auerswald K, Pfeiffer F, Behrends K, Burkhardt U, Olthoff D. Injektionsschmerzen nach Propofolgabe. Anaesthesiol Intensivmed Notfallmed Schmerzther 2005;40(5):259–66.

112. Schaefer M, Link J, Hannemann L, Rudolph KH. Excessive hypokalemia and hyperkalemia following head injury. Intensive Care Med 1995;21:235–7.

113. Enting D, Ligtenberg JJ, Aarts LP, Zijlstra JG. Total suppression of cerebral activity by thiopental mimicking propofol infusion syndrome: a fatal common pathway? Anesth Analg 2005;100:1864–5.

114. Guven M, Oymak O, Utas C, Emeklioglu S. Rhabdomyolysis and acute renal failure due to status epilepticus. Clin Nephrol 1998;50:204.

Stephan A. Schug and Alagirisamy Raajkumar

11

Local anesthetics

EFFECTS RELATED TO MODES OF USE   *(SED-15, 2121; SEDA-27, 124; SEDA-28, 145; SEDA-29, 135)*

Airway anesthesia

Respiratory   *Laryngospasm* can occur after airway anesthesia by local anesthetic spray.

- A 54-year-old patient scheduled for flexible fiber-optic bronchoscopy, following a lung transplantation 18 months before, had intravenous induction with propofol (1[A]). The vocal cords and vocal folds adducted immediately after a rapid injection of 2 ml of 2% lidocaine via a bronchoscope injection port. Ventilation ceased and the end-tidal carbon dioxide concentration fell to zero. There was spontaneous recovery after 40 seconds and ventilation resumed.

Laryngospasm is a serious event that results in partial or complete upper airway obstruction. The authors postulated that direct application of a drug on the vocal cords has the potential to induce laryngospasm, although this has never been described before in clinical practice.

Caudal, epidural, and spinal anesthesia

Caudal anesthesia

Susceptibility factors

Children   Caudal anesthesia is a common regional technique in children. Both ropivacaine and bupivacaine are widely used in regional

anesthesia. Unlike in adults, there are conflicting pharmacokinetic data in children.

In a randomized study of the unbound plasma concentrations of bupivacaine and ropivacaine for caudal block, 38 children were randomized to 0.5 ml/kg of bupivacaine or ropivacaine 0.25% (2[c]). After bupivacaine the unbound concentrations were 47 and 24 ng/ml at 1 and 2 hours respectively. After ropivacaine the corresponding unbound concentrations were 61 and 50 ng/ml. The differences between the groups were statistically significant. These concentrations are far below the toxic concentrations quoted in the literature for bupivacaine (unbound plasma concentrations >250 ng/ml) and ropivacaine (>150–600 ng/ml).

Epidural anesthesia

Respiratory   *Hiccups* that last longer than 48 hours are referred to as persistent hiccups, and those lasting more than 2 months are considered intractable. Persistent or intractable hiccups can lead to fatigue, sleep disturbances, dehydration, and even wound dehiscence in the perioperative period.

- A 65-year-old man received a series of three epidural injections, each with 11 ml of a mixture of 0.08% bupivacaine and triamcinolone 80 mg, in an anesthesia pain clinic for evaluation and treatment of lumbar spinal stenosis (3[A]). After the first two injections he developed leg weakness, which resolved after about 4 hours. After the third injection he developed mild urinary retention, which resolved without consequence 6 hours later. All three injections were associated with hiccups after about 1 hour and persisting for 5–7 days. He received two further epidural injections of a glucocorticoid in isotonic saline and did not develop hiccups. All the procedures were 8 weeks apart. A year later, after an epidural injection for a total knee replacement he developed hiccups, which resolved 9 days later.

Side Effects of Drugs, Annual 30
J.K. Aronson (Editor)
ISSN: 0378-6080
DOI: 10.1016/S0378-6080(08)00011-1

There are many causes of hiccups. They are most commonly gastrointestinal in origin, such as gastric distention or gastro-esophageal reflux disease. Metabolic derangements and drugs are also frequently implicated. Two cases of hiccups after thoracic epidural injections of glucocorticoids have previously been reported, but in this case a glucocorticoid injection without bupivacaine did not lead to hiccups.

Skin Delayed-type *hypersensitivity* to epidural ropivacaine has been described.

- A 74-year-old man with postherpetic neuralgia and no history of drug allergies developed a purpuric rash and widespread blotchy erythema on his legs, trunks, and arms following continuous epidural blockade with ropivacaine 0.2% without preservatives (up to 96 ml/day) (4[A]). He had normal white cell and platelet counts and a slight eosinophilia (640 × 10[6]/l). The epidural infusion and other drugs (amitriptyline, alprazolam, and laxoprofen) were withheld and the eruptions completely resolved within 7 days. Intradermal ropivacaine 0.2% produced erythema (maximum size 23 mm × 13 mm) at 8–72 hours. Histology showed perivascular infiltrates of lymphocytes and eosinophils in the dermis. Patch testing with amitriptyline, alprazolam, and loxoprofen induced no eruptions, and neither did restarting the drugs.

This report led to a correspondence questioning the duration of the infusion and also possible cumulative toxicity of ropivacaine (5[r]).

Spinal (intrathecal) anesthesia

Cardiovascular Intra-operative *hypotension* is common and potentially dangerous in elderly patients undergoing spinal anesthesia for repair of hip fractures. Combining an intrathecal opioid with a local anesthetic allows a reduction in the dose of local anesthetic and causes less sympathetic block and hypotension, while still maintaining adequate anesthesia.

In a double-blind, randomized comparison in 40 patients of glucose-free bupivacaine 9.0 mg and fentanyl 20 micrograms with glucose-free bupivacaine 11.0 mg alone, the incidence and frequency of hypotension was reduced by the addition of fentanyl (6[c]). Similarly, falls in systolic, diastolic, and mean blood pressures were all less. However, there were four failed blocks in those given fentanyl compared with one in those given bupivacaine alone.

Nervous system The incidence of *transient neurological symptoms* with lidocaine compared with other local anesthetics has been the subject of a systematic review of 14 randomized, controlled trials in 1347 patients, 117 of whom developed transient neurological symptoms (7[M]). Of the 117, 94 developed the symptoms after the use of lidocaine (out of 674 patients treated with lidocaine). The clinical picture was typically bilateral pain in the buttocks, thighs, and legs, which started within 24 hours after the initiation of spinal anesthesia and after complete recovery from spinal anesthesia. The pain varied in intensity from mild to severe (visual analogue scale score 2–9.5), and most patients complained of mild to moderate pain. A non-steroidal anti-inflammatory drug was the treatment of choice and a few patients were given opioids as well. In most cases the pain disappeared by the second day and the maximum duration was 5 days; only one patient had symptoms for 10 days. None had any neurological symptoms. The relative risk of transient neurological symptoms after spinal anesthesia with lidocaine was 4.35 (95% CI = 1.98, 9.54) and therefore significantly higher than with other local anesthetics (bupivacaine, prilocaine, procaine, and mepivacaine). This increased risk must be weighed against the benefit of rapid, short-acting anesthesia when considering whether to use lidocaine for ambulatory anesthesia.

As early ambulation after spinal anesthesia has been described as a risk factor for transient neurological symptoms, the effects of ambulation after subarachnoid lidocaine have been subjected to a randomized, double-blind study in 60 patients, comparing early ambulation with 6 hours recumbent position postoperatively (8[C]). There was no significant difference between the groups in the incidence of transient neurological symptoms (23 versus 27%). In all patients the symptoms resolved spontaneously. The authors proposed that there is no correlation between the time of ambulation and the incidence of transient neurological symptoms.

While lidocaine is primarily regarded as the agent causing transient neurological symptoms, mepivacaine has also infrequently been implicated (9[C]). In a prospective single-center study of 1273 patients who received spinal or combined spinal–epidural anesthesia with plain mepivacaine 1.5% for ambulatory surgery, transient neurological symptoms occurred in 78 patients (6.4%) (10^C). None of the 372 combined spinal–epidural anesthetics was inadequate for surgery, but 14 of 838 spinal anesthetics (1.7%) were inadequate. The mean age of patients who developed transient neurological symptoms was 48 years, older than that of patients without symptoms, 41 years. Transient neurological symptoms were not influenced by sex or intraoperative position. None of the patients had permanent neurological sequelae. The authors concluded that spinal anesthesia with mepivacaine is associated with a high success rate and infrequent transient neurological symptoms, making it likely to be a safe and effective technique for ambulatory patients.

In contrast to transient neurological symptoms with no permanent neurological deficits, rare cases of neurological consequences after spinal anesthesia continue to be reported. In one case persistent cauda equina syndrome occurred after uneventful spinal anesthesia.

• A 72-year-old man of ASA status 1 had spinal anesthesia with hyperbaric bupivacaine 0.5% for an inguinal hernia repair, and anesthesia and surgery were uneventful (11^A). However, the next morning he had difficulty in defecating and complained of impaired ambulation and urinary retention, which required bladder catheterization. He had impaired sensation to pinprick in both L5 dermatomes, in the perineal region, and over the left calf, with reduced reflexes, gait changes, and sleep disturbances. Cauda equina syndrome was diagnosed.

The authors concluded that bupivacaine neurotoxicity had occurred, in view of the absence of any other identifiable cause for the neurological deficit. One previous case of persistent cauda equina syndrome after a single intrathecal dose of hyperbaric bupivacaine has been reported (12^A). This was attributed to maldistribution of local anesthetic due to spinal stenosis by adhesions secondary to meningitis. Local anesthetic neurotoxicity is believed to occur mainly in the cauda equina, because the sacral root sheaths are substantially longer (and larger for S1) than neighboring lumbar roots, are devoid of protective sheaths, and given their dorsal position in the thecal sac (in particular L5, S1, and S2), are more exposed to pooling of a hyperbaric anesthetic.

Unusually *prolonged spinal anesthesia* has also been reported.

• A 67-year-old man with significant peripheral arterial disease scheduled for femoropopliteal bypass surgery had an uneventful spinal injection with hyperbaric bupivacaine 15 mg (13^A). A sensory level was recorded bilaterally at T10. Nine hours later there was complete motor blockade and no sensory level regression. A CT scan with contrast was negative. About 24 hours later there was sensory regression to L1-L2 and complete spontaneous recovery from sensory and motor blockade occurred at 29 hours. There was no permanent neurological deficit or pain.

Negative radiology and complete resolution of symptoms ruled out spinal hematoma in this case. The authors assumed caudal maldistribution of hyperbaric solution hypothetically related to a low volume of CSF, reduced elimination from the subarachnoid space secondary to atherosclerosis, or an unknown cause, although transient spinal artery syndrome could not be ruled out.

Dental anesthesia

Sensory systems   *Visual disturbances* after dental extraction under local anesthesia are uncommon, but do happen.

• A 73-year-old man with a history of infective endocarditis was admitted for multiple dental extractions and received prilocaine 144 mg after aspiration (14^A). Within 2 minutes he reported that he could not see in his left eye. Fundoscopy showed diffusely obstructed retinal vessels, with multiple segmented clear fluid emboli and an incomplete cherry-red spot. There was no evidence of choroidal abscess or central nervous system signs of recent thromboembolism. Anterior chamber ocular paracentesis with ocular massage was attempted without improvement. Five days later his visual acuity remained at light perception only. Two months later his vision was unchanged.

The authors noted that this is a rare event and proposed causative mechanisms: intra-arterial injection causing retrograde flow in an abnormal anatomy or injection through vascular abnormalities from previous trauma or inflammation. It was difficult to implicate endocarditis, in the absence of calcific or platelet fibrin emboli. They concluded that delivery of local anesthetic must be done with aspiration before and care during injection. This will possibly prevent intravascular injection.

Infiltration anesthesia

Cardiovascular   *Hemodynamic changes* due to additives in local anesthetics have been described. Local anesthetics containing adrenaline are routinely used in functional endoscopic sinus surgery (FESS) for achieving hemostasis. In a prospective double-blind study of the hemodynamic effects of infiltration with lidocaine + 1:200,000 adrenaline 76 patients were randomly allocated to three groups (15^c). Group I received 2% lidocaine 2 ml with adrenaline, group II received saline 2 ml with adrenaline, and group III received saline 2 ml without adrenaline. Adrenaline, with and without lidocaine, caused significant hemodynamic changes compared with saline. The changes lasted no more than 4 minutes. The authors concluded that the changes were due to the effects of adrenaline on β_2 adrenoceptors.

Nervous system   *Spinal cord infarction* is an extremely rare but catastrophic complication of paravertebral injection.

- A 66-year-old man with a painful cervical spine received a paravertebral cervical infiltration of lidocaine + cortisone at C5-6 (16^A). He developed respiratory failure 2.5 hours later and was successfully resuscitated. However, he developed a tetraplegia with full consciousness and was ventilation for the next 2 months, when he died. An MRI scan confirmed an ischemic lesion of the upper anterior cervical myelin. Neuropathology confirmed anterior infarction of the cervical myelin at C2/C3, with obstruction of the anterior spinal artery by an epithelialized fibrocartilaginous embolus.

It was not possible to conclude with absolute certainty, for legal purposes, that the cervical infiltration had caused the fibrocartilaginous embolism. However, the authors suggested that without any other relevant evidence anatomically or at post-mortem, there was a strong suggestion that puncture of an intervertebral fibrous disc and subsequent transportation of the material into an arterial lumen by the cannula caused the ultimately fatal outcome.

Facial paralysis can be the consequence of local anesthetic administration in the laryngeal area.

- A 4-year-old boy was given a peritonsillar infiltration of bupivacaine hydrochloride 0.5%, in a volume of 2–3 ml per tonsil, and both tonsils were removed uneventfully (17^A). A few minutes later, he developed right-sided peripheral facial paralysis, which worsened over the next hour. There was neither laceration nor bleeding. The facial paralysis improved slowly and completely resolved after 8 hours.

The authors assumed that the paralysis had been caused by a direct effect of the local anesthetic agent on the facial nerve.

Sensory systems   Tumescent anesthesia is a form of protracted infiltration anesthesia using large volumes of diluted local anesthetics. It is used for liposuction, which has become the most frequently performed cosmetic procedure in the world. In eight consecutive patients of ASA grade I, plasma concentrations and objective/subjective symptoms over 20 hours after tumescent anesthesia with lidocaine 35 mg/kg (3 liters of a buffered solution of 0.08% lidocaine with adrenaline) at an average rate of 116 ml/minute were noted (18^c). Peak plasma concentration of 2.3 µg/ml of lidocaine occurred after 5–17 hours. There was no correlation between peak concentrations and dose per kg or total amount of lidocaine infiltrated. One patient had tinnitus after 14 hours at a plasma concentration of 3.3 µg/ml. The authors suggested that even though no fluid overload or toxic symptoms occurred in this small group of patients, there is still a risk of toxicity in association with peak concentrations of lidocaine that may occur after discharge.

Interpleural anesthesia

Respiratory   Unilateral *bronchospasm* after interpleural block with bupivacaine has been described.

- A 55-year-old man received an interpleural block with 20 ml of bupivacaine 0.5% + adrenaline 100 µg (1:200000) after a test dose and 45 minutes later there was a fall in SpO$_2$ from 98 to 93% accompanied by a rise in respiratory rate to 30/minute and mild respiratory distress (19^A). On auscultation there were expiratory wheezes on the right side and normal breath sounds on the left. The unilateral bronchospasm resolved spontaneously, coinciding with a three-segment regression of analgesia to T4.

Anesthetic techniques that can cause bronchospasm in non-asthmatic patients include:

interscalene brachial plexus block, interpleural block, spinal and general anesthesia, and intercostal nerve block. Bronchospasm can be initiated by any technique that interrupts sympathetic innervation in the lungs but spares the parasympathetic.

Intravenous regional anesthesia

Bier's block, because of its ease of administration, rapid onset, and recovery, continues to be widely used.

Skin An unexplained skin reaction to intravenous regional anesthesia has been described.

- A 41-year-old man was given 40 ml of lidocaine 0.5% for intravenous regional anesthesia for release of a trigger finger (20[A]). He developed a uniform, circumferential, reddish brown and in places purple discoloration of the forearm below the tourniquet. Ultrasound and Doppler sonography ruled out a hematoma, a collection, or circulatory predicament. After 8 days the rash disappeared completely.

The authors observed that although this did not need any particular treatment, it caused undue psychological trauma and inconvenience to the patient.

Obstetric anesthesia

Fetotoxicity Two cases of neonatal intoxication resulting from the administration of a local anesthetic to the mother for episiotomy during labor, initially diagnosed as perinatal asphyxia, have been reported (21[A]).

- Within minutes of vaginal birth, two full-term neonates developed signs of central nervous and cardiovascular system toxicity, including hypertonia, convulsions, apnea, bradycardia, and hypotension. In neither case was there evidence of fetal distress, and fetal monitoring was normal. The first mother had received lidocaine (2.5%) + prilocaine (2.5%) cream and the second 10 ml of mepivacaine solution 2%. Blood samples from both babies at 2 hours showed high concentrations of the respective local anesthetics. In both cases neurodevelopment at 12 months was normal.

The authors suggested that "unexplained perinatal asphyxia" could be ruled out by finding high concentrations of local anesthetic in the blood, urine, and cerebrospinal fluid. Therefore, if neonatal intoxication is suspected, an early urine specimen for toxicology screening is the cheapest and easiest way to secure the diagnosis.

Ocular anesthesia

Sensory systems *A conjunctival cyst and orbital cellulitis* have been described after sub-Tenon's block.

- A 68-year-old man received a sub-Tenon's block for cataract surgery (22[A]). During a routine follow up for glaucoma, a conjunctival cyst was noticed adjacent to the carbuncle of the right eye at the site of the sub-Tenon's injection. The cyst had apparently developed over the previous 4–6 months and was about 8 mm in diameter, transparent, and multiloculated. Although conspicuous, the cyst did not cause discomfort.

Sub-Tenon's block has become a popular anesthetic technique for cataract surgery because of its safety, faster onset of anesthetic effect, and patient preference. Inclusion cyst formation as a complication is a late event and has not previously been reported. While without consequences in this case, raised lesions of the eyeball, such as cysts, if close to the limbus, can prevent uniform coating of the cornea by tears, resulting in focal dryness and eventually thinning of the cornea. The authors proposed that simple and meticulous technique, including perpendicular positioning of the scissors, smaller snips, gentle holding of the conjunctival edges, and teasing the edges of inversion if present, will help to avoid this potential complication.

Two cases of *orbital swelling* after sub-Tenon's anesthesia have been reported (23[A]).

- Two patients presented with proptosis and chemosis after the third post-operative day. Computed tomography showed non-specific inflammation of the orbital soft tissues. They were treated with oral glucocorticoids and antibiotics, and the inflammation subsided within 4 weeks. Both patients had otherwise uneventful cataract surgery, were apyrexial, and were generally well.

Possible explanations for these episodes were infection, reactions to povidone-iodine or local anesthetic, or trauma due to the sub-Tenon's cannula.

Topical anesthesia

Nervous system   *Seizures* after the application of local anesthetic gel for urological catheterization have been reported (24[A]).

- A 40-year-old man received a spinal anesthetic with 3 ml of hyperbaric bupivacaine 0.5%. A gel containing lidocaine 2% (40 ml) was used for cystoscopy to aid bladder catheterization. He developed circumoral tingling followed by a generalized tonic–clonic seizure and was given a barbiturate and diazepam. The serum lidocaine concentration was 20 µg/ml (in the high toxic range) and fell to 12 µg/ml after 12 hours.

Absorption across the urethral mucosa would be expected to be rapid, because of the rich vascular supply, and that peak plasma concentrations would be higher by this route because of the absence of hepatic first-pass removal. In this case, the dose of lidocaine was high. The authors suggested that a gel without a local anesthetic should be used when the patient is given some form of regional anesthesia for catheterization.

Sensory systems   Permanent *anosmia* after topical nasal anesthesia with lidocaine 4% has been described.

- A 62-year-old man had fiberoptic endoscopy with lidocaine 4% spray and 10 minutes later complained of anosmia (25[A]). Computed tomography ruled out tumor, infection, and obstruction.

The authors postulated, in the absence of other obvious causes, that lidocaine had caused mitochondrial dysfunction, with activation of apoptotic pathways. They concluded that endoscopic topical local anesthesia should be done with the subject sitting and the head upwards to reduce contact of the anesthetic with the olfactory cleft.

Skin   Different types of *topical reactions* have been reported after the use of EMLA cream (a eutectic mixture of prilocaine 2.5% and lidocaine 2.5%).

- A 9-year-old boy with beta thalassemia major, who required subcutaneous infusions of deferoxamine 5 times a week, had been having EMLA cream applied to the injection sites and later developed an eczematous rash at these sites (26[A]). Initial patch testing 4 months later elicited a positive response to EMLA cream. Subsequent testing confirmed a positive test to prilocaine. Lidocaine and related anesthetics gave negative results. He continued further treatment with tetracaine 4% cream with no problems, and an allergic contact dermatitis was diagnosed.
- A 2-year-old Caucasian boy developed purpuric reactions at the sites of application of EMLA cream, used for curettage of molluscum contagiosum (27[A]). He had no other symptoms, but had a family history of atopy and had had mild atopic dermatitis since the age of 6 months. He was not treated and the purpura healed without sequelae in about 2 weeks.
- A 5-year-old girl with acute lymphoblastic leukemia developed a purpuric rash at sites where EMLA cream had been used to obtain local anesthesia before lumbar puncture (27[A]). Her routine hematological tests showed thrombocytopenia with a platelet count of 38×10^9/l. The lesion was asymptomatic and completely resolved without treatment in about 2 weeks.

Patch tests were not performed in the second and third cases, but allergic contact dermatitis does not present with purpuric lesions. The mechanisms of action of local anesthetics, including a direct action on voltage-gated sodium channels, a direct effect on the membrane lipid matrix with subsequent structural alterations, and a direct effect on lipid-protein interfaces, all support a potential hypothesis of a direct toxic effect of EMLA cream on the blood vessels. The authors reported other factors that may be involved in the pathogenesis of such a condition, including atopic dermatitis, predisposition in children, prematurity, trauma, and thrombocytopenia.

Localized *angioedema* has been described subsequent to the use of EMLA.

- A 46-year-old man with idiopathic genital pain syndrome was given EMLA cream (28[A]). After using it for 2 weeks, he complained of swelling of the glans penis associated with mild itching and edema. A patch test with EMLA cream, half diluted with white soft paraffin, lidocaine 2%, and cream base, gave a positive reaction to lidocaine + prilocaine and not to lidocaine alone. The symptoms resolved with topical glucocorticoids.

The diagnosis was contact angioedema secondary to contact allergy to prilocaine.

Death   A fatal reaction to topical use of a mixed local anesthetic gel has been described (29[A]).

- A 22-year-old college student died after applying a topical gel containing lidocaine 10%, tetracaine 10%, and phenylephrine. She had seizures in her car and although the conclusion was death due to high dose of lidocaine, questions were raised about the relevance of tetracaine, which is better absorbed.

The author highlighted the variable doses of local anesthetics in compounded products, their easy availability as non-prescription items, and the unnecessary use of higher doses when alternatives with appropriate doses are available (30[r]).

INDIVIDUAL COMPOUNDS

Articaine   *(SED-15, 348)*

Immunologic   An *immediate skin reaction* has been reported after the use of articaine.

- A 51-year-old woman developed immediate erythema and edema of the lips, face, and eyelids without any other symptoms after subcutaneous administration of a combination of articaine and adrenaline (31[A]). The reaction resolved with a glucocorticoid in 2 days. Skin prick tests with local anesthetics (lidocaine, bupivacaine, mepivacaine, articaine) were negative except for articaine.

The results suggested that there is no cross-reactivity between articaine and other amide local anesthetics. A difference in the chemical structure between articaine, being a tiofen, and the other amide local anesthetics, which have a phenyl-methylated ring, is a possible explanation.

Metabolism   Articaine has been implicated in an episode of *weakness of the limb muscles*, *fatigue*, and *anorexia* in a patient with a rare respiratory chain disorder due to a genetic defect in mitochondrial DNA (Kearns–Sayre Syndrome).

- A 28-year-old woman with Kearns–Sayre Syndrome, previously exposed multiple times to lidocaine, underwent planned tooth extraction after injection of articaine 1.5 ml (60 mg) with adrenaline (0.009 mg) (32[A]). Within 5 minutes she complained of a feeling of heat, fatigue, weakness, and a desire to sleep. She was unable to walk or stand and had frequent urination. At 20 hours after the injection she had diffuse weakness, reduced tendon and absent patellar reflexes, and subclonic Achilles tendon reflexes. She recovered fully 48 hours after the injection.

The authors assumed a direct mitochondrial toxic effect of articaine, although this was disputed by others in correspondence (33[r]).

Benzocaine   *(SED-15, 427; SEDA-28, 150)*

Cardiovascular   An 11-month-old child consumed about 2 ml of a benzocaine anesthetic gel 20% accidentally (34[A]). He developed a *tachycardia* (200/minute) which resolved over 24 hours. The author explained that although the cardiotoxicity of benzocaine is milder than that of other local anesthetics, it can cause life-threatening effects and so pediatricians should counsel parents about the potential hazard of anesthetic teething gels; formulations that contain benzocaine should be in a childproof container.

Hematologic   *Methemoglobinemia* is a well-known adverse effect of benzocaine (SED-15, 427). The FDA has issued a Public Health Advisory warning to highlight the fact that the use of benzocaine sprays in the mouth and throat has occasionally been linked with methemoglobinemia (35[S]). The agency has also advised that the Veterans Health Administration has announced its decision to cease using benzocaine spray for local numbing of the mouth and throat mucous membranes for minor surgical procedures or tube insertion. It has further warned that methemoglobinemia has occurred when benzocaine spray was used for a longer duration or more often than recommended. The agency has suggested the following points for consideration when using benzocaine in the mouth or throat:

- Patients with breathing problems, or who smoke, are at greater risk of methemoglobinemia.
- The use of products with different active ingredients (for example lidocaine) may be beneficial in patients who are more likely to

develop methemoglobinemia, such as children aged less than 4 months and older patients with certain inborn defects.

- Patients should receive the minimum dosage required to reduce the risk of methemoglobinemia.
- Patients who receive benzocaine should be carefully monitored for methemoglobinemia.
- Blood analysis for methemoglobinemia should be done using co-oximetry.
- A change in the color of the blood to chocolate-brown may be a danger sign.
- Patients with suspected methemoglobinemia should be promptly treated.

Methemoglobinemia followed the use of topical benzocaine for transesophageal echocardiography in three cases and fiberoptic intubation in one case (36[A], 37[A], 38[A]). All the patients were successfully treated with methylthioninium chloride (methylene blue) 1–2 mg/kg. Another case occurred with use of benzocaine to treat throat ache after intubation (39[A]).

In a cohort study of this problem, two out of more than 1000 gastric bypass patients who underwent endoscopy developed methemoglobinemia (40[c]). In both cases benzocaine spray 20% had been used and the patients developed cyanosis, dyspnea, and tachycardia within 7 and 13 minutes. The methemoglobin concentrations were 19 and 36%. Both were resuscitated successfully with methylthioninium chloride and one with added ascorbic acid 1 g orally. The authors suggested that benzocaine spray should be limited and pointed out that pulse oximetry underestimates the degree of hypoxia. Prompt diagnosis and treatment with methylthioninium chloride can be life-saving. In subsequent correspondence others acknowledged the difficulty in determining the dose in a spray and suggest nebulized lidocaine as an alternative (41[r]).

Two other cases of methemoglobinemia in morbidly obese patients who underwent bariatric surgery have been reported (42[A]). Blood gas analysis was the only clue that led to the diagnosis in both these patients, in whom pulmonary compromise would have otherwise been blamed on obesity. Both recovered well with methylthioninium chloride.

Bupivacaine *(SED-15, 568; SEDA-27, 131; SEDA-28, 150)*

In a randomized controlled study after total knee arthroplasty in 14 patients the effects of a continuous infusion of intra-articular bupivacaine were examined (43[C]). The patients were randomized to three groups who received 4 ml/hour of isotonic saline, bupivacaine 0.25%, and bupivacaine 0.5%. Opioid-sparing effects and patient satisfaction were the primary observations, and serum bupivacaine was also measured in two patients who received bupivacaine 0.5%. The study was halted because of a serum bupivacaine concentration of 1.2 μg/ml in one of these patients, close to presumed toxic concentrations.

Cardiovascular   The longer-acting, more lipophilic agents, such as bupivacaine, can cause cardiovascular toxicity at serum concentrations that are not much greater than those required to cause nervous system toxicity.

- A 65-year-old man had 15 ml of plain bupivacaine 0.5% infiltrated before a planned radiofrequency ablation of a lumbar sympathetic ganglion (44[A]). He immediately developed respiratory arrest with bradycardia and hypotension (54/40 mmHg). Asystolic cardiac arrest was treated successfully but he subsequently developed pulmonary edema after a hypotensive episode. Angiography showed left anterior descending artery ischemia and his electrocardiographic T waves normalized 7 months later.

The authors report this case as bupivacaine-induced *cardiovascular collapse* with several novel features. Firstly, it developed after the administration of a relatively low dose of bupivacaine, less than 1.1 mg/kg. Secondly, the presentation was that of mixed cardiogenic and vasomotor shock. Finally, he developed an unexplained delayed cardiographic finding of symmetrically inverted anterior T waves. The authors thought that drug–drug interactions may also have contributed; since he was taking amitriptyline and carbamazepine, each of which is potentially cardiotoxic and may have lowered the threshold for bupivacaine toxicity.

Levobupivacaine   (SED-15, 2037)

Drug overdose   Successful resuscitation after accidental intravenous infusion of levobupivacaine has again been described.

- A 63-year-old man with localized prostate cancer scheduled for brachytherapy received an infusion of levobupivacaine 100 ml (125 mg) instead of an antibiotic after intravenous induction (45[A]). He developed severe hypotension and bradycardia without a recordable blood pressure and was treated with boluses of adrenaline. Later he developed a supraventricular tachycardia, nodal rhythm, and ST changes. He was extubated uneventfully and his postoperative electrocardiogram and troponin were normal. The arterial levobupivacaine concentrations were 1.74 µg/ml after 40 minutes of infusion, 0.81 µg/ml at 100 minutes, and 0.61 µg/ml at 160 minutes.

The packaging of the intended antibiotic and L-bupivacaine were similar. This illustrates the value of having clearly identifiable packaging and color coding of giving sets and pumps.

Lidocaine   (SED-15, 2051; SEDA-26, 146; SEDA-27, 133; SEDA-28, 152)

Nervous system   Two cases of toxicity associated with excessive lidocaine concentrations during low-dose treatment in terminally ill patients have been reported (46[A]).

- An 82-year-old woman with mucinous adenocarcinoma received intravenous lidocaine 300 mg/day for neuropathic pain. Her renal function and liver function were normal. After 2 days her pain was controlled, but 1 week later she developed severe somnolence. Her serum lidocaine concentration was 8.4 µg/ml. The symptoms were attributed to lidocaine, which was withdrawn. She improved the next day and was given an intravenous infusion of lidocaine 100 mg/day and achieved adequate pain control without any adverse effects.
- A 70-year-old woman with ovarian cancer was given a neurolytic mesenteric plexus block, NSAIDs, transdermal fentanyl 75 micrograms/hour, and intravenous morphine 80 mg/day. On day 100 intravenous lidocaine 200 mg/day was added for new neuropathic pain in the legs secondary to progressive intrapelvic tumor. One week later she became somnolent. Her serum lidocaine concentration was 8.4 µg/ml. Her renal and liver tests were normal. Lidocaine was withdrawn and 2 days later the somnolence disappeared without an increase in pain.

The authors suggested that measuring lidocaine concentrations helps to avoid toxicity in terminally ill patients, who seem to tolerate much lower daily doses.

Immunologic   The predictability of allergy to local anesthetics still remains elusive, owing to its rarity. *Hypersensitivity* due to local anesthetics and its additives continues to be reported.

- A 63-year-old man without any known allergies developed pruritus, generalized urticaria, and dyspnea and collapsed after application of topical lidocaine gel in a dental clinic (47[A]). After treatment a prick test, performed with various agents and components, turned positive for guar gum, which is included as a gelling agent in lidocaine gel. Total serum immunoglobulin E (IgE) was raised to 99.0 Ku/l but specific IgE to guar gum was negative.

This case highlights the importance of meticulous investigation and testing of all components of local anesthetics. The authors suggested that a possible explanation of the negative guar-specific IgE could have been a varying degree of contamination in guar products not detected by commercial highly purified assays.

Mepivacaine   (SED-15, 2256)

Skin   *Allergic skin reactions* to amide local anesthetics are uncommon and little is known about cross-reactivity among these drugs. Two cases of cross-reactivity of mepivacaine with ropivacaine and lidocaine have been reported.

- A 35-year-old woman with no previous history of allergy developed urticaria on her face, neck, and legs 15 minutes after receiving mepivacaine for extirpation of a nevus (48[A]). She was treated with an oral antihistamine, and the rash completely resolved in 1 hour. Prick and intradermal tests with undiluted mepivacaine 1% were negative. A single-blind, placebo-controlled, subcutaneous challenge test and an intradermal test with mepivacaine were positive. A latex-prick test was negative. In order to evaluate cross-reactivity among different amides, prick and intradermal tests were carried out with undiluted lidocaine 1%, bupivacaine 0.5%, and ropivacaine 1%. The tests were negative with lidocaine and bupivacaine, but positive with ropivacaine. An intradermal test with ropivacaine was also positive.

- A 54-year-old woman with no history of atopy or allergy developed a maculopapular rash and pruritus in the injection area 2 days after surgery (49[A]). The skin lesions resolved in 7 days without treatment. Skin prick and intradermal tests for cross-reactivity to various dilutions of lidocaine, mepivacaine, bupivacaine, and articaine were performed. Patch tests at 2 and 4 days with lidocaine and mepivacaine were positive.

Amide local anesthetics rarely cause allergic reactions. Formerly, cross-reactivity among them was considered non-existent, but these cases demonstrate that that is not necessarily so.

Ropivacaine   *(SED-15, 3078; SEDA-27, 134; SEDA-28, 152)*

Cardiovascular   The cases reported this year support the suggestion that ropivacaine-induced *cardiac toxicity* is not nearly as troublesome as bupivacaine toxicity (50[r]).

Successful resuscitation after systemic ropivacaine toxicity during peripheral nerve block has been described.

- A 15-year-old girl was given 18 ml of ropivacaine 0.75% to the sciatic nerve after negative aspiration, and developed convulsions, immediately followed by ventricular fibrillation (51[A]). Oxygen was delivered by face mask and she received two DC shocks of 200 J. The convulsions stopped and sinus rhythm returned. Postoperatively, there was no evidence of sciatic block. She did not remember the episode and was discharged the next day.

The authors emphasized the importance of electrocardiographic monitoring during nerve block for early identification of complications, the effectiveness of appropriate resuscitation measures in ropivacaine toxicity, and the potential usefulness of low-dose adrenaline in the test dose to detect inadvertent intravascular injection.

Nervous system   A *generalized tonic–clonic seizure* after epidural injection of ropivacaine has been described.

- A 48-year-old woman scheduled for abdominal total hysterectomy had an uneventful lumbar epidural insertion for postoperative pain relief (52[A]). She was asymptomatic after a test dose of 2 ml of lidocaine 1%. To begin epidural anesthesia, ropivacaine 1% was injected epidurally at a rate of about 12 ml/minute. She became confused and had a classical tonic–clonic seizure after injection of 8 ml of ropivacaine. The convulsions ceased with intravenous midazolam 5 mg. Aspiration was negative for blood before the catheter was removed.

The arterial plasma concentration of ropivacaine 2 minutes after the start of the seizure was 1.5 µg/ml. Although tachycardia occurred at this time, the effect on the cardiovascular system was minimal. The authors repeated the suggestion that adding adrenaline to the test dose could have predicted intravascular injection.

Tetracaine   *(SED-15, 3327)*

Skin   A *severe skin reaction* to tetracaine has been reported.

- A 71-year-old man developed severe contact dermatitis in the groin area after transurethral resection of prostate, during which a probe lubricated with an ointment containing tetracaine was used (53[A]). Biopsy and patch testing showed a positive reaction to tetracaine. The dermatitis resolved with topical glucocorticoids and antihistamines.

References

1. Riley RH, Musk MT. Laryngospasm induced by topical application of lignocaine. Anaesth Intensive Care 2005;33(2):278.
2. Bozkurt P, Arslan I, Bakan M, Cansever MS. Free plasma levels of bupivacaine and ropivacaine when used for caudal block in children. Eur J Anaesthesiol 2005;22(8):640–1.
3. McAllister RK, McDavid AJ, Meyer TA, Bittenbinder TM. Recurrent persistent hiccups after epidural steroid injection and analgesia with

bupivacaine. Anesth Analg 2005;100(6):1834–6.

4. Ban M, Hattori M. Delayed hypersensitivity due to epidural block with ropivacaine. BMJ 2005;330(7485):229.

5. Wildsmith JA. Delayed hypersensitivity due to epidural block with ropivacaine: report raises several issues. BMJ 2005;330(7497):966 [author reply].

6. Martyr JW, Stannard KJ, Gillespie G. Spinal-induced hypotension in elderly patients with hip fracture. A comparison of glucose-free bupivacaine with glucose-free bupivacaine and fentanyl. Anaesth Intensive Care 2005;33(1):64–8.

7. Zaric D, Christiansen C, Pace NL, Punjasawadwong Y. Transient neurologic symptoms after spinal anesthesia with lidocaine versus other local anesthetics: a systematic review of randomized, controlled trials. Anesth Analg 2005;100(6):1811–6.

8. Cramer BG, Stienstra R, Dahan A, Arbous MS, Veering BT, Van Kleef JW. Transient neurological symptoms with subarachnoid lidocaine: effect of early mobilization. Eur J Anaesthesiol 2005;22(1):35–9.

9. Zaric D, Christiansen C, Pace NL, Punjasawadwong Y. Transient neurologic symptoms (TNS) following spinal anaesthesia with lidocaine versus other local anaesthetics. Cochrane Database Syst Rev 2003(2):CD003006.

10. YaDeau JT, Liguori GA, Zayas VM. The incidence of transient neurologic symptoms after spinal anesthesia with mepivacaine. Anesth Analg 2005;101(3):661–5.

11. Chabbouh T, Lentschener C, Zuber M, Jude N, Delaitre B, Ozier Y. Persistent cauda equina syndrome with no identifiable facilitating condition after an uneventful single spinal administration of 0.5% hyperbaric bupivacaine. Anesth Analg 2005;101(6):1847–8.

12. Kubina P, Gupta A, Oscarsson A, Axelsson K, Bengtsson M. Two cases of cauda equina syndrome following spinal–epidural anesthesia. Reg Anesth 1997;22(5):447–50.

13. Zeidan A, Samii K. A case of unusually prolonged hyperbaric spinal anesthesia. Acta Anaesthesiol Scand 2005;49(6):885.

14. Rishiraj B, Epstein JB, Fine D, Nabi S, Wade NK. Permanent vision loss in one eye following administration of local anesthesia for a dental extraction. Int J Oral Maxillofac Surg 2005;34(2):220–3.

15. Yang JJ, Wang QP, Wang TY, Sun J, Wang ZY, Zuo D, Xu JG. Marked hypotension induced by adrenaline contained in local anesthetic. Laryngoscope 2005;115(2):348–52.

16. Meyer HJ, Monticelli F, Kiesslich J. Fatal embolism of the anterior spinal artery after local cervical analgetic infiltration. Forensic Sci Int 2005;149(2–3):115–9.

17. Shlizerman L, Ashkenazi D. Peripheral facial nerve paralysis after peritonsillar infiltration of bupivacaine: a case report. Am J Otolaryngol 2005;26(6):406–7.

18. Nordstrom H, Stange K. Plasma lidocaine levels and risks after liposuction with tumescent anaesthesia. Acta Anaesthesiol Scand 2005;49(10):1487–90.

19. Sudhakar S, Kundra P, Madhurima S, Ravishankar M. Unilateral bronchospasm following interpleural analgesia with bupivacaine. Acta Anaesthesiol Scand 2005;49(1):104–5.

20. Ansari MM, Abraham A. Unusual discoloration of forearm with Bier's block using 0.5% lidocaine. Anesth Analg 2005;100(6):1866–7.

21. Pignotti MS, Indolfi G, Ciuti R, Donzelli G. Perinatal asphyxia and inadvertent neonatal intoxication from local anaesthetics given to the mother during labour. BMJ 2005;330(7481):34–5.

22. Vishwanath MR, Jain A. Conjunctival inclusion cyst following sub-Tenon's local anaesthetic injection. Br J Anaesth 2005;95(6):825–6.

23. Mukherji S, Esakowitz L. Orbital inflammation after sub-Tenon's anesthesia. J Cataract Refract Surg 2005;31(11):2221–3.

24. Priya V, Dalal K, Sareen R. Convulsions with intraurethral instillation of lignocaine. Acta Anaesthesiol Scand 2005;49(1):124.

25. Salvinelli F, Casale M, Hardy JF, D'Ascanio L, Agro F. Permanent anosmia after topical nasal anaesthesia with lidocaine 4%. Br J Anaesth 2005;95(6):838–9.

26. Ismail F, Goldsmith PC. Emla cream-induced allergic contact dermatitis in a child with thalassaemia major. Contact Dermatitis 2005;52(2):111.

27. Neri I, Savoia F, Guareschi E, Medri M, Patrizi A. Purpura after application of EMLA cream in two children. Pediatr Dermatol 2005;22(6):566–8.

28. Ajith C, Somesh G, Kumar B. Iatrogenic swollen penis. Sex Transm Infect 2005;81(1):15–6.

29. Perrin JH. Hazard of compounded anesthetic gel. Am J Health Syst Pharm 2005;62(14):1445–6.

30. Young D. Student's death sparks concerns about compounded preparations. Am J Health Syst Pharm 2005;62(5):450–2.

31. El-Qutob D, Morales C, Pelaez A. Allergic reaction caused by articaine. Allergol Immunopathol (Madr) 2005;33(2):115–6.

32. Finsterer J, Haberler C, Schmiedel J. Deterioration of Kearns–Sayre syndrome following articaine administration for local anesthesia. Clin Neuropharmacol 2005;28(3):148–9.

33. Stehr SN, Oertel R, Schindler C, Hubler M. Re: deterioration of Kearns–Sayre syndrome following articaine administration for local anesthesia. Clin Neuropharmacol 2005;28(5):253.

34. Calello DP, Muller AA, Henretig FM, Osterhoudt KC. Benzocaine: not dangerous enough? Pediatrics 2005;115(5):1452.

35. Anonymous. Benzocaine. Mouth and throat use linked with methaemoglobinaemia. WHO Newslett 2006;2:4.

36. Hegedus F, Herb K. Benzocaine-induced methemoglobinemia. Anesth Prog 2005;52(4):136–9.

37. Alonso GF. A wild reaction to a topical anesthetic. RN 2005;68(10):57–60.

38. Birchem SK. Benzocaine-induced methemoglobinemia during transesophageal echocardiography. J Am Osteopath Assoc 2005;105(8):381–4.

39. LeClaire AC, Mullett TW, Jahania MS, Flynn JD. Methemoglobinemia secondary to topical benzocaine use in a lung transplant patient. Ann Pharmacother 2005;39(2):373–6.

40. Srikanth MS, Kahlstrom R, Oh KH, Fox SR, Fox ER, Fox KM. Topical benzocaine (Hurricaine) induced methemoglobinemia during endoscopic procedures in gastric bypass patients. Obes Surg 2005;15(4):584–90.

41. Wong DH, Wilson SE. Avoiding topical anesthesia-induced methemoglobinemia. Obes Surg 2005;15(7):1088.

42. Carrodeguas L, Szomstein S, Jacobs J, Arias F, Antozzi P, Soto F, Zundel N, Whipple O, Simpfendorfer C, Gordon R, Villares A, Rosenthal RJ. Topical anesthesia-induced methemoglobinemia in bariatric surgery patients. Obes Surg 2005;15(2):282–5.

43. Hoeft MA, Rathmell JP, Dayton MR, Lee P, Howe JG, Incavo SJ, Lawlis JF. Continuous, intra-articular infusion of bupivacaine after total-knee arthroplasty may lead to potentially toxic serum levels of local anesthetic. Reg Anesth Pain Med 2005;30(4):414–5.

44. Levsky ME, Miller MA. Cardiovascular collapse from low dose bupivacaine. Can J Clin Pharmacol 2005;12(3):e240–5.

45. Salomaki TE, Laurila PA, Ville J. Successful resuscitation after cardiovascular collapse following accidental intravenous infusion of levobupivacaine during general anesthesia. Anesthesiology 2005;103(5):1095–6.

46. Tei Y, Morita T, Shishido H, Inoue S. Lidocaine intoxication at very small doses in terminally ill cancer patients. J Pain Symptom Manage 2005;30(1):6–7.

47. Roesch A, Haegele T, Vogt T, Babilas P, Landthaler M, Szeimies RM. Severe contact urticaria to guar gum included as gelling agent in a local anaesthetic. Contact Dermatitis 2005;52(6):307–8.

48. Prieto A, Herrero T, Rubio M, Tornero P, Baeza ML, Velloso A, Perez C, De Barrio M. Urticaria due to mepivacaine with tolerance to lidocaine and bupivacaine. Allergy 2005;60(2):261–2.

49. Sanchez-Morillas L, Martinez JJ, Martos MR, Gomez-Tembleque P, Andres ER. Delayed-type hypersensitivity to mepivacaine with cross-reaction to lidocaine. Contact Dermatitis 2005;53(6):352–3.

50. Finucane BT. Ropivacaine cardiac toxicity—not as troublesome as bupivacaine. Can J Anaesth 2005;52(5):449–53.

51. Gielen M, Slappendel R, Jack N. Successful defibrillation immediately after the intravascular injection of ropivacaine. Can J Anaesth 2005;52(5):490–2.

52. Iwama H. A case of normal ropivacaine concentration causing grand mal seizure after epidural injection. Eur J Anaesthesiol 2005;22(4):322–3.

53. Huerta Brogeras M, Aviles JA, Gonzalez-Carrascosa M, de la Cueva P, Suarez R, Lazaro P. Dermatitis sistemica de contacto por tetracainas. Allergol Immunopathol (Madr) 2005;33(2):112–4.

O. Zuzan and M. Leuwer

12 Neuromuscular blocking agents and skeletal muscle relaxants

DEPOLARIZING NEUROMUSCULAR BLOCKING AGENTS *(SED-15, 2489; SEDA-28, 155)*

Suxamethonium

Musculoskeletal   Generalized *muscle pain* after the use of suxamethonium is well recognized and common. Various interventions for prevention of this myalgia have been studied and have been subjected to meta-analysis (1[M]). Small doses of non-depolarizing neuromuscular blocking agents (precurarization), sodium channel blockers (local anesthetics such as lidocaine), and non-steroidal anti-inflammatory drugs were effective, with numbers-needed-to-treat (NNT$_B$) of 2.5–6. Precurarization, however, was associated with adverse effects such as blurred vision (NNT$_H$ = 3), diplopia (NNT$_H$ = 5), heavy eyelids (NNT$_H$ = 2), weakness (NNT$_H$ = 4), difficulty in breathing (NNT$_H$ = 26), difficulty in swallowing (NNT$_H$ = 7), and a lower voice (NNT$_H$ = 6). The authors concluded that precurarization should only be used cautiously. In response to this publication, a correspondent highlighted the fact that the incidence of these adverse effects was dose-related and that the published doses used for precurarization studies had increased significantly over the last 20 years (2[r]). This correspondent, a well-known expert in the field, suggested that precurarization with a non-depolarizing blocking agent is both safe and effective, provided that the dose does not exceed 10% of the ED95. We agree with this, but should also like to endorse the following statement: "Clinicians should be aware of

this risk when using precurarization. To maximize patients' safety, close monitoring for precurarization-related side effects is strongly recommended" (3[r]). It should also be noted that the incidence of myalgia in this meta-analysis was still rather high despite precurarization, at 21–38%. Because of their methods, the authors could not assess the impact of combining different interventions. An incidence of 5% has been reported for the combined use of atracurium (0.05 mg/kg) and lidocaine (1.5 mg/kg) for pre-treatment followed by suxamethonium 1.5 mg/kg (4[c]). Similarly, the combination of a small dose of d-tubocurarine with lidocaine 1.5 mg/kg was more effective than either drug alone (5[c]). All this could be summarized in a protocol for rapid-sequence intubation of the airway:

1. Preoxygenate for at least 2 minutes.
2. Give a small dose (no more than $0.1 \times$ ED95) of a non-depolarizing muscle relaxant.
3. Give lidocaine 1.5 mg/kg 90 seconds after the non-depolarizing muscle relaxant.
4. Give an induction agent no later than 120 seconds after the non-depolarizing muscle relaxant, followed by suxamethonium 1.5 mg/kg.
5. Intubate no earlier than 50 seconds after suxamethonium.

SKELETAL MUSCLE RELAXANTS

Baclofen *(SED-15, 408; SEDA-27, 141; SEDA-28, 157)*

The adverse effects of baclofen in the treatment of gastroesophageal reflux have been reviewed (6[R]). The most common adverse effects

Side Effects of Drugs, Annual 30
J.K. Aronson (Editor)
ISSN: 0378-6080
DOI: 10.1016/S0378-6080(08)00012-3

were *somnolence, dizziness, nausea, vomiting,* and *seizures.*

Susceptibility factors

Epilepsy   Baclofen is used to treat spasticity in children with cerebral palsy. These children often have epilepsy as well. The effect of baclofen on the frequency of seizures may therefore be relevant. It has been suggested that baclofen may increase seizure frequency and have pro-convulsive properties (SEDA-27, 141) (7[A], 8[A], 9[A]). In the largest study so far, the seizure frequency in 150 children with cerebral palsy before and after the institution of intrathecal baclofen therapy was recorded (10[c]). The prevalence of epilepsy before the intervention was 60/150 (40%). Eight of those 60 children had a reduced seizure frequency after intrathecal baclofen was started; in four of those eight no more seizures occurred and antiepileptic treatment was withdrawn. On the other hand, two of 60 children had an increased frequency of seizures. In addition, one child developed new-onset seizures after intrathecal baclofen was started. The authors concluded that baclofen does not aggravate seizure activity in epileptic patients. Indeed, their results support the use of intrathecal baclofen to treat spasticity in patients with cerebral palsy and seizures. To what extent this can be extrapolated to other conditions, for example in patients with spasticity after trauma, who might also have post-traumatic epilepsy, is currently not clear.

Drug overdose   Seizures have previously been reported in cases of baclofen overdose (11[A]). In a review of cases presenting to an Australian toxicology service there were 23 cases in which baclofen intoxication was involved (12[c]). In eight of these, baclofen was the only agent involved, and seizures occurred in four. Therefore, although it is a potent nervous system depressant, baclofen can have proconvulsive effects, especially in overdose. Other symptoms associated with overdose were miosis or mydriasis, depressed level of consciousness or coma, absent or depressed reflexes, hypertension, and bradycardia or tachycardia.

Botulinum toxins   *(SED-15, 551;*
SEDA-27, 161; SEDA-28, 168; SEDA-29, 156)

Botulinum toxins A and B are used for the treatment of facial rhytides (for example, lateral orbital wrinkles, lower eyelid wrinkles, and labial lines), by producing weakness or paralysis of the associated muscles, and in the treatment of hyperhidrosis. Complications such as *temporary bruising, discomfort, incomplete muscle paralysis*, and *headache* can occur. Fortunately, adverse effects and undesirable sequelae after injection are temporary. Several extensive reviews have covered these complications and their management (13[R], 14[R], 15[R]).

Systematic reviews   In a review of four publications reporting adverse events after local injection of botulinum toxin into the lower urinary tract the reported adverse effects included *generalized muscle weakness, arm weakness, hyposthenia with reduced supralesional muscle force, vision disturbances*, and *fever* (16[M]). All the adverse effects were self-limiting and lasted 2 weeks to 2 months after injection.

Observational studies   In a review of all adverse events after therapeutic and cosmetic use reported to the FDA during the 13.5 years since botulinum A toxin was first licensed, there were 1437 reports—406 after therapeutic use (217 serious and 189 non-serious) and 1031 after cosmetic use (36 serious and 995 non-serious) (17[c]). The adverse events occurred predominantly in women, median age 50 years. Over a single year the proportion of reports classified as serious was 33-fold higher for therapeutic than for cosmetic cases. The 217 serious adverse events reported in therapeutic cases included all 28 reported deaths; six deaths were attributed to *respiratory arrest*, five to *myocardial infarction*, three to *strokes*, two to *pulmonary embolism*, two to *pneumonia*, five to other causes, and five to unknown causes. Of the 36 serious events after cosmetic use of botulinum toxin, 30 were included as possible complications in the FDA-approved label; the other six may not have been related to the drug. *Seizures* were reported in 17 patients; 15 of these had either a history of seizures or a condition that increase their risk of seizures (for example a history of cerebral infarction).

Other serious adverse events included *dyspha-gia* (n = 26), *muscle weakness* (13), *allergic reactions* (13), *flu-like syndromes* (10), *injection site trauma* (9), *dysrhythmias* (9), and *myocardial infarction* (6). Among the 995 cosmetic cases associated with non-serious events, the most common were lack of effect (63%), *injection site reactions* (19%), and *ptosis* (11%).

While this review revealed very interesting information about the adverse effects of botulinum toxin, it did not allow the incidence of such effects to be estimated. The survey covered 1989–2003, but the cosmetic use of botulinum toxin was only approved by the FDA in 2002. On the other hand, the estimated number of cosmetic uses over those 2 years in the USA was impressive (1 123 510 injections in 2002 and 2 891 390 injections in 2003) (18[c]). Of course, botulinum toxin was also used for cosmetic purposes, even before FDA approval.

Adverse events have been studied in 327 patients (202 women, 125 men) who received 1043 injections of botulinum A toxin for cervical dystonia (n = 58), blepharospasm (n = 31), hemifacial spasm (n = 39), spasticity due to cerebral palsy (n = 96), chronic anal fissure (n = 96), or esophageal achalasia (n = 7) (19[c]). The following adverse events were observed in those with cervical dystonias: *dysphagia* (27% of patients and 7% of sessions), *weakness of the neck muscles* (6.7 and 1.3%), *pain during swallowing* (5.1 and 1%), and a *flu-like syndrome* (3.4 and 0.7%); the dysphagia appeared 8.2 days after injection and lasted 15 days on average. In patients with blepharospasm there were *unilateral ptosis* (22 and 6.3%), *bilateral ptosis* (3 and 1.9%), and *hematomas* (3 and 0.6%), and in hemifacial spasm *excessive weakness resulting in asymmetry of the face*, either mild (28 and 20%) or moderate (46 and 27%). In spasticity due to cerebral palsy there was *excessive weakness of the legs*, which lasted 14 days on average (6.2 and 1.9%), *pain* (5.2 and 1.6%), and a *flu-like syndrome* (4.1 and 1.3%). In chronic anal fissure there were *mild incontinence of flatus and feces* (9 and 5%), *hematomas* (5%), a *flu-like syndrome* (3%), *inflammation of external anal varices* (2%), and *epididymitis* (1%). In esophageal achalasia, *chest pain* in six patients (on the day of injection and for 2–4 days) and *esophageal reflux* in two (4–8 weeks after the injection, lasting 2–3 weeks). The adverse

effects were transient, mostly local, and completely reversible.

Nervous system   In a double-blind, randomized, placebo-controlled trial in 60 patients with lateral epicondylitis a single injection of botulinum toxin type A significantly reduced pain (20[C]). However, there was mild *paresis of the fingers* at 4 weeks in four patients who received botulinum and in none of those who received placebo; 10 patients who received botulinum and six who received placebo had weak finger extension on the same side as the injection.

Sensory systems   *Parasympathetic dysfunction of the visual system* occurred in three patients after injection of botulinum toxin type B at remote sites (21[A]).

Skin   An unusual case of a *generalized rash* starting 30 hours after an injection of botulinum toxin A to treat blepharospasm has been reported (22[A]).

A man who received botulinum A toxin injections every 3 months for 18 months for left-sided oromandibular dystonia developed left-sided madarosis and facial alopecia (23[A]).

Musculoskeletal   *Myofascial necrosis* has been attributed to botulinum toxin (24[A]).

- 36-year-old woman with multiple sclerosis was given electromyographically guided botulinum toxin (total dose 400 IU) into the medial hamstrings and adductor muscles in both legs. Two months she presented with a foul-smelling, painless, necrotic lesion measuring 2–3 cm in diameter in the groin skin crease overlying the adductor compartment of both thighs with no surrounding erythema. A large amount of foul-smelling pus, necrosed skin, and underlying adductor muscles was debrided. No organisms were grown.

The authors suggested that the necrosis might have been linked to excessive paralysis caused by the toxin, but they could not explain the underlying mechanism. Previous reports of botulinum-induced local paralysis did not mention necrosis. Previously, muscle fiber necrosis has only been noted in animal experiments (25[E]). If excessive paralysis of the adductor muscles was the precipitating event, the patient should have noticed a significant change in muscle tone, but that was not mentioned. Also, negative cultures do not rule out infectious causes. Despite these uncertainties, the authors concluded that all patients who receive injections of botulinum toxin should be warned of this effect. For the time being we do not think there is enough evidence to back up this conclusion. This case report does not justify the assumption that extensive myofascial necrosis is a direct adverse effect of botulinum toxin. However, patients who receive deep intramuscular injections still need to be warned of infectious complications, which include abscess formation and soft tissue infections.

Immunologic   In a long-term study of 45 patients (mean age 69 years, 32 women) who had received injection of botulinum toxin repeatedly for at least 12 years (mean 16 years), there were 20 adverse events in 16 patients after their initial visit and 11 adverse events in 10 patients at their most recent injection visit (26[c]). In four of 22 non-responsive patients *blocking antibodies* were confirmed by the mouse protection assay. Of the antibody-negative patients, 16 again became responsive after dosage adjustments and two remained non-responders.

Drug tolerance   Secondary non-responsiveness can occur in patients who are given repeated injections of botulinum toxin type A, especially for focal dystonias and spasticity. Botulinum toxin type B has been used as an alternative but has been disappointing. Of 36 patients with cervical dystonia resistant to type A toxin, only 13 had a reasonable response to type B; the other 23 patients had either no response or a poor response, or had unacceptable adverse effects and stopped treatment (27[c]). A few patients with blepharospasm, hemifacial spasm, or foot dystonia also had disappointing responses. Of 20 patients with spasticity, seven had some response to type B without unacceptable adverse effects.

Resistance to botulinum toxin type B has also been described in those with and without prior resistance to botulinum toxin type A (28[c]). Of 24 patients with cervical dystonias treated with botulinum toxin type B for up to 64 months, mean treatment dose 14 828 (range 2500–28 000) units, eight became secondarily resistant, and four were primary non-responders, possibly because of the severity and nature of their disease.

Susceptibility factors

Genetic   Patients with diseases that affect the neuromuscular junction, such as myasthenia gravis or Lambert–Eaton syndrome can develop systemic muscle weakness, even with low doses of botulinum toxin; they should therefore not be treated with botulinum toxin. Patients with mitochondrial cytopathies seem to be hypersensitive to the effects of botulinum toxin and have an increased risk of adverse reactions, as has been reported in two siblings with mitochondrial myopathy (29[c]).

- A 30-year-old man with complex II and III deficiency of the mitochondrial respiratory chain had unspecified intellectual and movement disorders going back to infancy, was wheelchair bound, and could only speak single words or simple phrases, but had good comprehension and memory and normal sphincter function. He received two injections of botulinum toxin (Dysport 120 mU in each parotid gland for excessive drooling and 100 mU into the right tibialis anterior muscle and 200 mU into the right tibialis posterior muscle for right foot inturning). There were no adverse effects. About 2 months later he received Dysport 120 mU into each parotid gland and 60 mU into each submandibular gland, 300 mU into the right tibialis anterior muscle, and 100 mU into the right tibialis posterior muscle. Ten days later he developed swallowing difficulties which resolved within 2 months.
- The second patient was the first patient's 32-year-old sister, who had a very similar clinical picture. She received Dysport 120 mU into each parotid gland, and 50 mU into each submandibular gland. She developed fluctuating dysphagia, which lasted 2 months.

The authors quoted one previous report of remote symptoms after botulinum toxin in a patient with mitochondrial myopathy (30[R]). They suggested that neuromuscular junction defects might have resulted in the exacerbated response to botulinum toxin and concluded that botulinum toxin should be avoided in patients with mitochondrial cytopathies.

Management of adverse reactions   Prevention of the adverse effects of botulinum toxin has been reviewed (31[R]). The correct injection technique is essential, since most unwanted effects are caused by incorrect technique. The most common adverse effects are pain and hematoma. In the periocular region, lid and brow ptosis are important. Pain and bruising can also occur in the upper and lower face and at extrafacial sites. The most important methods of avoiding most unwanted adverse effects are the proper techniques of dilution, storage, and injection, and careful exclusion of patients with contraindications. Pain and bruising can be prevented by cooling the skin before and after injection. Upper lid ptosis can be partly

corrected using apraclonidine or phenylephrine eye-drops.

Apraclonidine, an α_2 adrenoceptor agonist that causes Muller's muscles to contract, quickly raising the upper eyelid by 1–3 mm, has been used to treat ptosis secondary to the use of botulinum toxin (32^A).

References

1. Schreiber JU, Lysakowski C, Fuchs-Buder T, Tramer MR. Prevention of succinylcholine-induced fasciculation and myalgia: a meta-analysis of randomized trials. Anesthesiology 2005;103:877–84.
2. Donati F. Dose inflation when using precurarization. Anesthesiology 2006;105:222–3.
3. Schreiber J, Fuchs-Buder T, Lysakowski C, Tramer M. Dose inflation when using precurarization. Anesthesiology 2006;105:223 [authors' reply].
4. Raman SK, San WM. Fasciculations, myalgia and biochemical changes following succinylcholine with atracurium and lidocaine pretreatment. Can J Anaesth 1997;44:498–502.
5. Melnick B, Chalasani J, Uy NT, Phitayakorn P, Mallett SV, Rudy TE. Decreasing post-succinylcholine myalgia in outpatients. Can J Anaesth 1987;34:238–41.
6. Cappell MS. Clinical presentation, diagnosis and management of gastroesophageal reflux disease. Med Clin N Am 2005;89:243–91.
7. Hansel DE, Hansel CR, Shindle MK, Reinhardt EM, Madden L, Levey EB, Johnston MV, Hoon Jr AH. Oral baclofen in cerebral palsy: possible seizure potentiation? Pediatr Neurol 2003;29:203–6.
8. Kofler M, Kronenberg MF, Rifici C, Saltuari L, Bauer G. Epileptic seizures associated with intrathecal baclofen application. Neurology 1994;44:25–7.
9. Zak R, Solomon G, Petito F, Labar D. Baclofen-induced generalized nonconvulsive status epilepticus. Ann Neurol 1994;36:113–4.
10. Buonaguro V, Scelsa B, Curci D, Monforte S, Iuorno T, Motta F. Epilepsy and intrathecal baclofen therapy in children with cerebral palsy. Pediatr Neurol 2005;33:110–3.
11. Perry HE, Wright RO, Shannon MW, Woolf AD. Baclofen overdose: drug experimentation in a group of adolescents. Pediatrics 1998;101:1045–8.
12. Leung NY, Whyte IM, Isbister GK. Baclofen overdose: defining the spectrum of toxicity. Emerg Med Australas 2006;18:77–82.
13. Carruthers A, Carruthers J. Botulinum toxin type A. J Am Acad Dermatol 2005;53:284–90.
14. Vartanian AJ, Dayan SH. Complications of botulinum toxin A use in facial rejuvenation. Facial Plast Surg Clin North Am 2005;13:1–10.
15. Wollina U, Konrad H. Managing adverse events associated with botulinum toxin type A. A focus on cosmetic procedures. Am J Clin Dermatol 2005;6:141–50.
16. De Laet K, Wyndaele JJ. Adverse events after botulinum A toxin injection for neurogenic voiding disorders. Spinal Cord 2005;43(7):397–9.
17. Coté TR, Mohan AK, Polder JA, Walton MK, Braun MM. Botulinum toxin type A injections: adverse events reported to the US Food and Drug Administration in therapeutic and cosmetic cases. J Am Acad Dermatol 2005;53:407–15.
18. American Society of Plastic Surgeons. 2000/2001/2002/2003 National Plastic Surgery Statistics. Available at http://www.plasticsurgery.org/media/statistics/2003Statistics.cfm [accessed October 2007].
19. Sławek J, Madalinski MH, Maciag-Tymecka I, Duzynski W. Frequency of side effects after botulinum toxin A injections in neurology, rehabilitation and gastroenterology. Pol Merkur Lekarski 2005;18(105):298–302.
20. Wong SM, Hui AC, Tong PY, Poon DW, Yu E, Wong LK. Treatment of lateral epicondylitis with botulinum toxin: a randomized, double-blind, placebo-controlled trial. Ann Intern Med 2005;143(11):793–7.
21. Dubow J, Kim A, Leikin J, Cumpston K, Bryant S, Rezak M. Visual system side effects caused by parasympathetic dysfunction after botulinum toxin type B injections. Mov Disord 2005;20(7):877–80.
22. Mezaki T, Sakai R. Botulinum toxin and skin reaction. Mov Disord 2005;20:770.
23. Kowing D. Madarosis and facial alopecia presumed secondary to botulinum a toxin injections. Optom Vis Sci 2005;82(7):579–82.
24. Agaba AE, Mahmoud S, Esmail H, Sutton J, Bertalot JC, Jibani MM. Extensive myofascial necrosis: a delayed complication of botulinum

toxin therapy. Eur J Intern Med 2005;16(8):603–5.

25. Kim HS, Hwang JH, Jeong ST, Lee YT, Lee PK, Suh YL, Shim JS. Effect of muscle activity and botulinum toxin dilution volume on muscle paralysis. Dev Med Child Neurol 2003;45:200–6.

26. Mejia NI, Vuong KD, Jankovic J. Long-term botulinum toxin efficacy, safety, and immunogenicity. Mov Disord 2005;20(5):592–7.

27. Barnes MP, Best D, Kidd L, Roberts B, Stark S, Weeks P, Whitaker J. The use of botulinum toxin type-B in the treatment of patients who have become unresponsive to botulinum toxin type-A—initial experiences. Eur J Neurol 2005;12(12):947–55.

28. Berman B, Seeberger L, Kumar R. Long-term safety, efficacy, dosing, and development of resistance with botulinum toxin type B in cervical dystonia. Mov Disord 2005;20(2):233–7.

29. Gioltzoglou T, Cordivari C, Lee PJ, Hanna MG, Lees AJ. Problems with botulinum toxin treatment in mitochondrial cytopathy: case report and review of the literature. J Neurol Neurosurg Psychiatry 2005;76(11):1594–6.

30. Muller-Vahl KR, Kolbe H, Egensperger R, Dengler R. Mitochondriopathy, blepharospasm, and treatment with botulinum toxin. Muscle Nerve 2000;23:647–8.

31. Wollina U, Konrad H. Managing adverse events associated with botulinum toxin type A: a focus on cosmetic procedures. Am J Clin Dermatol 2005;6(3):141–50.

32. Scheinfeld N. The use of apraclonidine eyedrops to treat ptosis after the administration of botulinum toxin to the upper face. Dermatol Online J 2005;11(1):9.

Michael Schachter

13 Drugs that affect autonomic functions or the extrapyramidal system

This year has seen relatively few significant additions to the literature concerning the adverse effects of anti-Parkinsonian drugs and a rather more equal spread of reports in other areas. However, this chapter includes a special review of a very intriguing adverse effect of the use of dopamine receptor agonists, the apparent link with pathological gambling. The literature on this topic has grown very considerably in the last couple of years, particularly because of interest in the possible light it may shed on the neuropsychology of addictive behaviors.

DRUGS THAT STIMULATE BOTH ALPHA- AND BETA-ADRENOCEPTORS
(SEDA-27, 145; SEDA-28, 160; SEDA-29, 148)

Adrenaline (epinephrine) (SED-15, 41; SEDA-29, 148)

Cardiovascular It is somewhat surprising to see cellular phones cited as a cause of acute poisoning, but just that has been suggested in a report from New York (1[A]).

- An 18-year-old man with septic shock was given an infusion of adrenaline at an initial rate of 0.15 micrograms/kg/minute. During the following 9 hours his systolic blood pressure varied from 92 to 105 mmHg and the infusion rate was 0.1–0.2 micrograms/kg/minute. He then complained of a sudden headache and chest and abdominal pain. His blood pressure was 250/188 mmHg with a pulse of 198/minute. He developed pulmonary edema and raised cardiac enzymes. It was noted that the infusion bag was much emptier than it should have been—he had acutely received 10.5 mg of adrenaline more than had been intended.

Just before this episode a member of the family had received a call on a cellular phone. Subsequent testing by hospital engineers showed that the proximity of the phone during a call could have triggered the pump to run at nearly 1 litre/hour. Most hospitals, certainly in the UK, ask visitors to switch off their phones when entering clinical areas, although the need for this has been questioned (2[r], 3[r]). It is possible that this problem varies with the type and make of equipment, but this report suggests that it needs careful examination.

Inhaled adrenaline is available as an over-the-counter medication in at least some parts of the USA. In one case the use of inhaled adrenaline resulted in a stroke secondary to presumed hypertension (4[A]).

> **DoTS classification:**
> *Reaction*: Hypertension due to adrenaline
> *Dose-relation*: Toxic
> *Time-course*: Time-independent
> *Susceptibility factors*: ?Age

- A 73-year-old man in North Carolina developed acute confusion, fluent aphasia, and vomiting. He had no lateralizing motor signs other than slight right arm weakness, although both plantar responses were extensor. The blood pressure was 160/81 mmHg. A CT scan of the brain

Side Effects of Drugs, Annual 30
J.K. Aronson (Editor)
ISSN: 0378-6080
DOI: 10.1016/S0378-6080(08)00013-5

showed a left thalamic hemorrhage. It emerged that he was using large doses of inhaled adrenaline (0.22 mg/puff) as self-medication for chronic obstructive pulmonary disease. The maximum recommended dose was 2 puffs every 3 hours on not more than 2 days of the week, and this had clearly been exceeded by a large margin. He made an almost complete recovery, with slight residual weakness, and stopped using inhaled adrenaline.

Presumably the cause of the cerebral hemorrhage in this case was an acute episode of hypertension.

Noradrenaline (norepinephrine)
(SED-15, 2582)

Cardiovascular   *Dynamic left ventricular outflow tract obstruction* associated with catecholamine therapy in a patient *without* evidence of hypertrophic cardiomyopathy has been reported, possibly for the first time (5[A]).

- A 31-year-old man developed acute pancreatitis with hypovolemia and shock. Apart from large volumes of fluid and colloid, he was given dopamine 20 micrograms/kg/minute and noradrenaline 0.1 micrograms/kg/minute. After initial improvement he became severely hypotensive, with a blood pressure of 65/40 mmHg, a pulse of 134/minute, and a new loud systolic murmur at the left sternal edge. Echocardiography showed severe left ventricular outflow obstruction with a maximal pressure gradient of 106 mmHg. There was rapid hemodynamic improvement after the withdrawal of catecholamines and he survived, with type 1 diabetes and several pancreatic pseudocysts.

The authors pointed out that this problem can occur in the presence of catecholamine therapy and hypovolemia even in patients with an entirely normal heart, and that early diagnosis and correct management is vital.

Ephedra and ephedrine   *(SED-15, 1221; SEDA-29, 148)*

Nervous system   Metabolife 356, which is marketed as an aid to weight loss, contains ma huang (ephedrine 12 mg), guaraná extract (caffeine 40 mg), chromium picolinate, and various herbs and vitamins.

DoTS classification:
Reaction: Vasospasm due to ephedrine
Dose-relation: Toxic
Time-course: Time-independent
Susceptibility factors: Unknown

- A 20-year-old, otherwise healthy woman had symptoms of a transient ischemic attack less than 30 minutes after taking four tablets of Metabolife 356 (6[A]). She had also taken 6–15 tablets/day during the 3 days before in an attempt to lose weight. Two-point discrimination was reduced over the whole of the left side, but there were no other neurological abnormalities and her blood pressure was 134/84 mmHg. Her symptoms resolved within 4 hours. Rechallenge was not attempted.

Cerebral vasospasm was presumably the main mechanism in this case, but the authors noted reports of hemorrhagic as well as ischemic stroke associated with ephedrine-containing formulations. The manufacturer of this product has removed all ephedra-containing products, including Metabolife 356, from the market. However, the authors commented that although many ephedra-containing formulations are no longer available over the counter, they can be easily bought on the Internet.

Liver   There has been a further report of *fulminant hepatic failure* requiring liver transplantation after the use of *Ephedra sinica* or Ma huang, a traditional Chinese remedy that contains ephedrine-type alkaloids (7[A]).

Pseudoephedrine   *(SED-15, 1221; SEDA-29, 149)*

Cardiovascular   In a meta-analysis of 24 studies involving 1285 subjects the authors concluded that in healthy individuals pseudoephedrine significantly *increased heart rate* (2.83/minute; CI = 2.0, 3.6) and *increased systolic blood pressure* (0.99 mmHg; 95% CI = 0.08, 1.9), with no effect on diastolic pressure (8[M]). In patients with controlled hypertension there was an increase of similar magnitude in systolic blood pressure (1.2 mmHg; CI = 0.56, 1.84). Higher doses and immediate-release formulations were associated with greater increases in blood pressure, although it was difficult to be certain what the average dose was in these studies; from the data presented it was usually 60 mg once or twice daily. The authors reported isolated cases of much greater rises in blood pressure (up to 20 mmHg systolic) but again it was difficult to determine the doses used. They concluded that immediate-release formulations had a greater effect than modified-release formulations, and that a dose-response relation could be discerned. Evidently many cases of pseudoephedrine-related cardiovascular effects involved higher doses than have been used in formal studies or are recommended by manufacturers. There appeared to be a smaller effect in women than in men. Shorter duration of use was associated with greater increases in systolic and diastolic blood pressures. There were no clinically significant adverse outcomes. However, a rare adverse event may not be seen with such a small sample size.

Coronary vasospasm has been attributed to pseudoephedrine (9[A]).

• A previously healthy 32-year-old man from Nigeria developed substernal chest pain at rest associated with nausea and sweating 45 minutes after taking two tablets of an over-the-counter cold remedy containing pseudoephedrine 30 mg and paracetamol 500 mg per tablet. He recalled a similar but less severe episode 1 week earlier after taking the same medication. There was no relevant past medical history or family history of coronary artery disease. An electrocardiogram showed ST elevation in the inferolateral leads and the plasma creatine kinase activity and troponin I concentration were both raised. Coronary angiography showed normal arteries.

The authors concluded that this episode had been caused by coronary vasospasm initiated by pseudoephedrine and warned of the dangers of this type of medication, even in otherwise healthy individuals. The temporal association between ingestion of pseudoephedrine and the myocardial infarction suggested a causal relation. The absence of coronary artery disease at catheterization combined with the cardiac magnetic resonance imaging findings were consistent with an acute myocardial infarction caused by vasospasm due to pseudoephedrine.

Hypertensive strokes have been attributed to pseudoephedrine in 22 patients (10[cr]). The effects of pseudoephedrine may be important when considered on a population basis, given its widespread use as decongestants. Although

marked rises in blood pressure were uncommon, there were rises above 140/90 mmHg in nearly 3% of the patients. The benefit to harm balance should therefore be evaluated carefully before pseudoephedrine is used in individual patients most at risk of rises in blood pressure and heart rate.

Skin Toxic epidermal necrolysis has been reported in a patient taking pseudoephedrine (11[A]).

> ***DoTS classification:***
> *Reaction*: Toxic epidermal necrolysis due to pseudoephedrine
> *Dose-relation*: Hypersusceptibility
> *Time-course*: First-dose
> *Susceptibility factors*: Unknown

• A 57-year-old woman developed a pruritic generalized maculopapular rash with occasional target lesions 8 days after taking two doses of pseudoephedrine, 240 mg in total. She also had oropharyngeal ulceration. Over the next week she developed bullae covering about 15% of the body, which subsided over the next 2 weeks with supportive therapy. Biopsy was consistent with toxic epidermal necrolysis. Three years later she took a single dose of a compound medication containing pseudoephedrine and developed a rash 12 hours later. This was successfully treated with glucocorticoids, topical and systemic.

DRUGS THAT PREDOMINANTLY STIMULATE ALPHA₁-ADRENOCEPTORS
(SEDA-27, 147; SEDA-28, 161; SEDA-29, 150)

Phenylephrine   *(SED-15, 2808; SEDA-27, 147)*

Cardiovascular *Cardiographic U waves* have been reported to have been caused by phenylephrine (12[A]).

• A 71-year-old woman suddenly developed global aphasia. She was hypertensive and a heavy smoker and had previously undergone left carotid endarterectomy. There were multiple ischemic areas in the brain on the left side and total occlusion of the common, internal, and external carotid arteries on that side. Perhaps surprisingly, it was thought that hypoperfusion of the language areas of the cortex could be overcome by increasing the arterial pressure. This was done by an intravenous infusion of phenylephrine up to a dose of 180 micrograms/minute, which produced a blood pressure of 220/100 mmHg. Unfortunately, this did not produce any clinical improvement but positive U waves developed in the chest leads of the electrocardiogram; these disappeared after the infusion was discontinued.

The authors noted that while U waves are usually considered to be pathological and may reflect a tendency to the development of ventricular dysrhythmias, particularly torsade de pointes, the mechanisms by which they are formed are still conjectural. In any case, this approach to therapy does not appear very promising.

Phenylpropanolamine   *(SED-15, 2811; SEDA-29, 150)*

Drug overdose   It is several years since phenylpropanolamine was withdrawn from sale in many countries, but it seems that these do not include Japan, where a case of overdose has been reported.

- A 22-year-old Japanese woman took an unquantified overdose of an over-the-counter formulation containing phenylpropanolamine (13[A]). She was admitted to hospital 6 hours later, when she appeared to be well. Her blood pressure was 108/62 mmHg with a heart rate of 125/minute in sinus rhythm. However, she had clinical and radiological signs of pulmonary edema, with an ejection fraction of only 20%. Creatine kinase activity was raised and reached a peak 18 hours after admission. During this time hemoperfusion was carried out in order to reduce very high plasma concentrations of phenylpropanolamine. After initial deterioration she made a full recovery and was clinically and radiologically normal by the 9th day after admission, by which time the ejection fraction was 70%. Coronary angiography was entirely normal. She was entirely well 1 year later.

The authors commented that phenylpropanolamine-induced myocardial damage has been reported only eight times before this episode and was less severe in all those cases. The precise mechanism of damage is uncertain but may include direct catecholamine-induced cytotoxicity, coronary vasoconstriction, or a combination of the two.

DRUGS THAT STIMULATE BETA$_1$-ADRENOCEPTORS   *(SEDA-27, 147; SEDA-29, 150)*

Dobutamine   *(SED-15, 1169; SEDA-29, 150)*

Cardiovascular   Dobutamine is very commonly used in stress echocardiography. One well-recognised complication is *non-sustained ventricular tachycardia*. The prognostic implications have been considered in 1266 consecutive patients, of whom 65 (5.1%) had this dysrhythmia (14[C]). After 3 years of follow-up there was no significant difference in all-cause mortality between patients who had ventricular tachycardia and those who did not (22 versus 17%). However, further analysis showed that patients who had (i) non-sustained ventricular tachycardia, (ii) no evidence of inducible ischemia, and (iii) a moderately reduced ejection fraction (0.35–0.45) did have significantly reduced survival. On the other hand, as the authors pointed out, this was a retrospective study with post hoc subgroup analysis, and the results should be confirmed by a prospective study. Even allowing for this, these results support earlier findings that this type of dysrhythmia when induced by dobutamine does not in itself indicate significantly increased risk.

As mentioned above, catecholamines can cause *midventricular obstruction*, and a similar effect has been described during dobutamine stress echocardiography (15[A]).

- A 73-year-old woman with chest pain had ST segment elevation on the electrocardiogram and raised creatine kinase activity and troponin concentrations. However, coronary angiography showed no significant obstructive lesions. She was given intravenous glyceryl trinitrate, with resolution of both the chest pain and the electrocardiographic changes. Stress echocardiography with dobutamine 10 micrograms/kg/minute was carried out 5 days later. This led to severe midventricular obstruction (a pressure gradient of 150 mmHg) and mitral regurgitation, with marked pulmonary hypertension. There was no pulmonary edema or cardiogenic shock, and she recovered fully after being given propranolol.

The authors commented that sympathetic stimulation may play a crucial role in this syndrome, whether it occurs spontaneously or after sympathomimetic drug administration.

DRUGS THAT STIMULATE DOPAMINE RECEPTORS

(SEDA-27, 148; SEDA-28, 162; SEDA-29, 151)

Levodopa and dopamine receptor agonists

Nervous system   The susceptibility factors for levodopa-induced peak dose *dyskinesias* have been examined in 215 consecutive patients with Parkinson's disease, of whom nearly half (105) had peak dose dyskinesias (16^C). Independent clinical predictors included female sex, early onset of Parkinson's disease, longer duration of treatment, and a higher dosage of levodopa, in other words greater overall exposure to the drug. This is in keeping with the results of previous studies. However, the investigators in this case also examined the effect of a polymorphism of the D2 receptor gene (DRD2 CA_n−STR) and found that in men only the presence of the 13,14+ genotype was strongly protective. The risk of peak dose dyskinesias was in fact three times greater in women than in men, and this over-rode the potential protective effect of this genotype. Although the authors emphasized the preliminary nature of their findings, they suggested that these considerations might be helpful in making therapeutic choices.

℞ *Pathological gambling and dopamine receptor agonists*

> **DoTS classification:**
> *Reaction*: Pathological gambling due to dopamine receptor agonists (particularly pramipexole)
> *Dose-relation*: Collateral
> *Time-course*: Intermediate
> *Susceptibility factors*: Genetic (dopamine D_1 receptor gene allele DRD1–800 T/C); age (younger age of onset of Parkinson's disease); sex (male); combined therapy with levodopa

It has become increasingly clear over the last decade that the non-motor disturbances that are associated with Parkinson's disease and its treatment are far more complex than was previously recognized. One of these abnormalities is pathological gambling. Although the increasing availability of opportunities for gambling, for instance online, has probably led to a general increase of such cases, it is now clear that there is a specific problem with drugs used to treat Parkinson's disease.

Prevalence   It is possible that the disease itself increases the likelihood of pathological gambling, but few patients are now left without drug treatment, so it is difficult to assess the true drug-free prevalence. Neurologists in several countries have attempted to assess the prevalence of this compulsive behavior in treated patients with Parkinson's disease.

In an Italian sample of 98 patients, 6.1% displayed pathological gambling, compared with 0.25% in age-matched controls (17^c): estimates in the general population in several countries all suggest rates of 1% at most.

In a larger study in Glasgow the prevalence was estimated at 4.4% overall but 8% for those taking dopamine receptor agonists, since all affected patients were taking these drugs (18^C).

In 297 patients in Toronto it was estimated that the lifetime prevalence of pathological gambling was 3.4%, with a figure of 7.2% for those taking dopamine receptor agonists (19^C). There were no cases among patients taking levodopa monotherapy.

Case series   A multidisciplinary team from the Mayo Clinic described 11 patients with idiopathic Parkinson's disease who developed pathological gambling (although the total number of patients in that clinic was not stated) (20^c). All were taking a dopamine receptor agonist at standard doses, eight of them in combination with levodopa. In most cases the abnormal behavior occurred within 3 months of starting dopamine receptor agonist therapy. The authors commented that nine of their patients were taking the dopamine receptor agonist pramipexole, and at the time that their article was published this was true of 10 out of 17 published cases.

In a more recent survey of published cases of pathological gambling in Parkinson's disease 28 case series were identified, including a total of 177 patients (21^M). There was a male preponderance (76%), a mean age at diagnosis of 57 years (range 30–78 years), and a mean disease duration of 7.8 years (range 2–22 years). In some but not all series the presence of other psychopathologies, particularly depression, was noted but the data were too incomplete to allow estimates of prevalence. Probably the most striking finding was that all but three of the patients were taking dopamine receptor agonists, although only in 17 cases as monotherapy. Pramipexole was the most commonly prescribed dopamine receptor agonist (in 44% of patients) and the mean dose was higher than that recommended for this drug (4.6 against 3.3 mg/day). This excess was not seen with the other synthetic dopamine receptor agonist, ropinirole, or in the approximately 30% of subjects who were taking an ergot-derived dopamine receptor agonist. Overall there was a trend towards an increased risk associated with pramipexole but this did not reach statistical significance.

In a series of 21 patients from the previously cited group in Toronto, published at the same time and therefore not included in this analysis, all the affected individuals were taking adjunctive dopamine receptor agonist therapy and none either levodopa or dopamine receptor agonist monotherapy (22[c]). There were very few patients in the latter group or in the control group of Parkinsonian patients without pathological gambling. The patients with compulsive gambling were younger at the time of onset of Parkinson's disease, had higher novelty seeking scores (by a ratio of nearly two to one), and had a higher incidence of a personal or family history of alcohol abuse (nearly 60% compared with 19% in the control group).

Mechanisms   Although a detailed discussion of the mechanisms of this adverse effect and its relevance to basic neuroscience and practical therapeutics is beyond the scope of this review, several researchers have concluded that in some susceptible individuals, possibly with premorbid psychological problems, dopamine receptor agonists may activate exaggerated novelty-seeking and risk-taking behaviors (21[C], 23[C], 24[c], 25[r]). Hypersexuality has long been recognized in this context (23[C]). Although it has been tempting to regard this as specifically linked to dopamine D_3 receptor stimulation, as seen with pramipexole, it has already been

noted that this is made more difficult to interpret because of the tendency to use higher doses of the drug than are generally recommended, reducing selectivity for D_3 receptors.

- A 63-year-old man developed pathological gambling after bilateral subthalamic stimulation was added to pharmacotherapy, including pergolide 3 mg/day (26[A]). The abnormal behavior ceased when pergolide was withdrawn, but the precise location of the stimulus was also changed, so a cause-and-effect relation was not certain.

In striking contrast another report, from Genoa, described two men aged 43 and 51 years who developed pathological gambling while taking levodopa combined respectively with pramipexole and bromocriptine (27[A]). Both underwent subthalamic stimulation for relief of motor symptoms and both improved sufficiently in this respect to allow rapid withdrawal of dopaminergic drugs. The gambling behavior ceased entirely, but it is very difficult to ascertain whether this was a direct consequence of the brain stimulation or of the withdrawal of dopamine receptor agonists.

Susceptibility factors   In a Brazilian study of pathological gambling in 70 discordant sib pairs, none of whom had Parkinson's disease, all the pathological gamblers were male, while of the matched non-gambling sibs only 37 were male (28[C]). The only positive association with the abnormal behavior was with the dopamine D_1 receptor gene allele DRD1–800 T/C.

Metabolism   There has been interest in the possible effect of anti-Parkinsonian drug therapy to *increase plasma homocysteine concentrations* and ultimately the risk of vascular disease (although this is currently controversial, given the lack of success of recent interventional trials), and possibly also of progressive cognitive impairment. The effects of catechol-O-methyl transferase (COMT) inhibitors on plasma concentrations of homocysteine and of folic acid and vitamin B_{12}, co-factors in homocysteine metabolism, have been studied in 26 patients with Parkinson's disease taking levodopa, 20 taking levodopa plus a COMT inhibitor, and 32 age-matched controls not suffering from Parkinson's disease (29[c]). Homocysteine concentrations were raised in both groups of Parkinsonian patients, but the effect was less marked in patients taking COMT inhibitors as well as levodopa (18 versus 14 µmol/l; 10 µmol/l in the controls). Plasma folate concentrations were lowest in the patients who took levodopa only but were actually highest in those also taking COMT inhibitors (5.8 versus 8.8 µmol/l; 7.5 µmol/l in the controls). Vitamin B_{12} concentrations were similar in the three groups. The difference in homocysteine concentrations was attributable to the presence of the COMT inhibitor rather than to individual folate concentrations. This is the first time this effect has been described and the authors speculated that it may be due to enzyme inhibition, leading to a reduced supply of S-adenosylhomocysteine, which is then converted to homocysteine. The practical implications are uncertain and designing clinical studies to follow up on this observation may prove quite difficult.

Serosae   It will come as no surprise that reports of *fibrotic reactions* to ergot-derived dopamine receptor agonists continue to appear. Indeed, regulatory authorities in many countries have modified their prescribing recommendations because of such reactions, especially those affecting heart valves. Sometimes these problems occur only after years of treatment.

> *DoTS classification*:
> *Reaction*: Fibrotic reactions due to ergot-derived dopamine receptor agonists
> *Dose-relation*: Collateral
> *Time-course*: Late
> *Susceptibility factors*: Unknown

• A man whose Parkinson's disease started at the age of 55 was treated initially with bromocriptine and then with levodopa (30[A]). Six years later pergolide 1.5 mg/day was added. After 11 years of this therapy he developed a cough and shortness of breath. A CT scan of the chest showed pleural plaques, which on biopsy proved to be fibrosis with a mild inflammatory component. Pergolide was withdrawn and replaced by the synthetic dopamine receptor agonist pramipexole. His pulmonary symptoms resolved completely, as did the radiological signs, and he was well 2 years later, although with possibly some deterioration in the control of his Parkinson's disease.

This report reinforces the relative safety of the newer synthetic dopamine receptor agonists, if possibly at the expense of somewhat lower efficacy. It also shows that fibrotic reactions can take several years to appear. The authors speculated that the metabolic disposition of the drug may change with increased accumulation, but it is not clear what might have triggered such a change in this patient.

ERGOT DERIVATIVES   *(SED-15, 1230; SEDA-27, 224; SEDA-28, 151)*

Although the use of non-dopamine receptor agonist ergot derivatives has declined, serious adverse effects are still reported.

Methylergonovine

Cardiovascular   *Fatal cardiac arrest* has been reported in a woman with hypertension who was given methylergonovine after termination of pregnancy (31[A]).

• A 38-year-old Taiwanese woman, with a history of hypertension treated with verapamil and valsartan, was given intravenous methylergonovine 0.2 mg and intramuscular oxytocin 10 IU after termination of pregnancy at 5 weeks of gestation. Five minutes later she complained of chest pain and then had a cardiac arrest. Attempted resuscitation was unsuccessful.

The authors acknowledged that methylergonovine should have been avoided in this case, and in any case is best given intramuscularly. They also noted that six of the seven published cases of ergot alkaloid-induced post-partum myocardial infarction occurred in Asians, suggesting increased susceptibility.

Methysergide   *(SED-15, 2316)*

Skin   *Scleroderma-like skin changes* have been attributed to long-term methysergide treatment (32[A]).

• A 63-year-old woman developed inflammatory edema of the legs and feet after taking methysergide 1.65 mg/day for migraine for over 10 years. It emerged that she had been taking. There were scleroderma-like changes in the legs and on the dorsa of the feet. Investigations for auto-immune disease were all negative. Biopsy showed fibrosis with some perivascular lymphocytic in-filtrate. A CT scan showed peri-aortic fibrosis without evidence of compression, which is a well-known adverse effect of methysergide. Methy-sergide was withheld and betamethasone ointment was prescribed "but not applied". However, there was some improvement after 2 weeks; the edema and erythema resolved completely within 2 months and the induration had partially regressed at that time, leaving hyperpigmentation. There was no change in the peri-aortic fibrosis.

Although fibrotic reactions to methysergide have been known for many years this appears to be the first description of scleroderma-like skin changes such as these.

DRUGS THAT AFFECT THE CHOLINERGIC SYSTEM
(SEDA-27, 152; SEDA-28, 165; SEDA-29, 153)

Anticholinergic drugs   *(SED-15, 264; SEDA-29, 153)*

Nervous system   Antimuscarinic drugs that are used in management of bladder hyperac-tivity and incontinence are designed to have a very limited effect on the nervous system. However, there is no absolute guarantee of this, as has been shown by a subanalysis of data from the OPERA (Overactive Bladder: Perfor-mance of Extended Release Agents) study, in which modified-release tolterodine 4 mg/day and modified-release oxybutynin 10 mg/day over 12 weeks were compared in 790 women with overactive bladders (33[C]). The incidence of nervous system adverse effects was similar in the two groups (8 and 9%). *Dizziness* was the most common (2.5 and 3.8%) but *somno-lence* was also relatively frequent with oxybu-tynin (2.3 versus 1.0%). All these effects were rated as mild to moderate by the patients, and only six individuals taking oxybutynin and two taking tolterodine cited adverse effects as the reason for withdrawing. This supports the view that oxybutynin is more lipophilic than toltero-dine and therefore better able to penetrate the brain.

Sensory systems   Of 52 Turkish women aged 22–60 years with urodynamically demonstrated bladder overactivity and no history of eye dis-ease, 28 were given tolterodine 2 mg bd and 24 oxybutynin 5 mg tds (34[c]). Best corrected visual acuity did not change significantly with either drug. Oxybutynin, but not tolterodine, significantly *reduced accommodation ampli-tude. Pupil diameter was significantly larger* in dim light with tolterodine while there was no change with oxybutynin. Perhaps unexpectedly, neither drug affected the pupillary response to bright light. Both drugs *reduced tear secretion* but neither caused significant rises in intraoc-ular pressure. Overall therefore there seems to be a slight advantage for tolterodine in terms of ocular adverse effects, although both drugs will exacerbate any pre-existing symptoms of dry eyes.

Psychological   The effects of oxybutynin on cognitive function have been studied in 25 chil-dren (aged 5–17 years, 14 girls) with daytime enuresis (35[c]). Ten were treated with behavior modification and 15 with behavior modifica-tion plus oxybutynin 7.5–20 mg/day, depend-ing on body weight. Patient allocation was not random but according to parental choice. Neu-ropsychological testing was done at baseline (after 4 weeks of behavior modification) and at the end of the treatment period. There was no cognitive impairment in the oxybutynin-treated children, but surprisingly baseline function was lower in those who were allocated to oxybu-tynin. This may have introduced selection bias, making it difficult to interpret any possible drug effect.

Electrolyte balance   *Hyponatremia* has been attributed to tolterodine (36[A]).

- A 78-year-old woman who was taking chlorpro-mazine, temazepam, trimipramine, and tolterodine developed increasing confusion and urinary in-continence. She had a urinary tract infection, a hemoglobin of 9.1 g/dl, a plasma creatinine of 139 µmol/l, and a plasma sodium concentration of 133 mmol/l. She was treated with norfloxacin but developed antibiotic-associated diarrhea and her plasma sodium fell to 125 mmol/l. However, this did not improve after resolution of the diarrhea or after withdrawal of all drugs other than tolterodine. When this too was withdrawn the plasma sodium rose to 135 mmol/l and on rechallenge fell again, this time even lower to 117 mmol/l.

This is the first published report of hyponatremia due to tolterodine. The mechanism is
unclear, but the authors speculated that it might
have been due to increased antidiuretic hormone, in the same way as fluoxetine, which it
resembles structurally. This would imply that
this effect is independent of antimuscarinic activity, since this property is very much attenuated in the case of fluoxetine.

Drug–drug interactions   A possible interaction of oxybutynin with *carbamazepine* has
been reported (37[A]).

- A 37-year-old woman with incomplete tetraplegia due to cervical spondylosis had taken carbamazepine 1000 mg/day for neuropathic pain
  for 2 years and was also taking baclofen and

dantrolene 125 mg/day to alleviate spasticity and
fluvoxamine 100 mg/day for depression. Oxybutynin 5 mg bd was added because of bladder
hyperactivity, and 2 weeks later she became dizzy,
unsteady, and confused, with bilateral nystagmus.
The plasma carbamazepine concentration was
16 µg/ml, the upper limit of the usual target range
being 12 µg/ml. All the drugs were withdrawn and
she returned to her previous state. However, because her symptoms also recurred all the drugs
except fluvoxamine were restarted, but with a
lower dose of carbamazepine 600 mg/day. Within
1 day the plasma carbamazepine concentration had
risen from 9.2 to 29 µg/ml. Carbamazepine was
replaced by sodium valproate, with good efficacy
and no problems.

The authors suggested that oxybutynin or dantrolene or both may inhibit the metabolism of
carbamazepine.

References

1. Hahn I-H, Schnadower D, Dakin RJ, Nelson LS. Cellular phone interference as a cause
   of acute epinephrine poisoning. Ann Emerg Med
   2005;46:298–9.
2. Myerson SG, Mitchell ARJ. Mobile phones in
   hospitals. BMJ 2003;326:460–1.
3. Derbyshire SWG, Burgess A. Use of mobile
   phones in hospitals. BMJ 2006;333:767–8.
4. Cartwright MS, Reynolds PS. Intracerebral hemorrhage associated with over-the-counter inhaled
   epinephrine. Cerebrovasc Dis 2005;19:415–6.
5. Auer J, Berent R, Weber T, Lamm G, Eber B.
   Catecholamine therapy inducing dynamic left
   ventricular outflow tract obstruction. Int J Cardiol
   2005;101:325–8.
6. Lo Vecchio F, Sawyers B, Eckholdt PA. Transient ischemic attack associated with Metabolife
   356 use. Am J Emerg Med 2005;23:199–200.
7. Skoulidis F, Alexander GJ, Davies SE. Ma
   huang associated acute liver failure requiring
   liver transplantation. Eur J Gastroenterol Hepatol
   2005;17(5):581–4.
8. Salerno SM, Jackson JL, Berbano EP. Effect
   of oral pseudoephedrine on blood pressure and
   heart rate. A meta-analysis. Arch Intern Med
   2005;165:1686–94.
9. Manini AF, Kabrehl C, Thomsen TW. Acute myocardial infarction after over-the-counter use of
   pseudoephedrine. Ann Emerg Med 2005;45:213–
   6.
10. Cantu C, Arauz A, Murillo-Bonilla LM,
    Lopez M, Barinagarrementeria F. Stroke as-
    sociated with sympathomimetics contained in

over-the-counter cough and cold drugs. Stroke
2003;34:1667–72.
11. Nagge JJ, Knowles SR, Juurlink DN, Shear NH.
    Pseudoephedrine-induced toxic epidermal necro-
    lysis. Arch Dermatol 2005;141:907–8.
12. Hefer D, Bukharovich I, Nasrallah EJ, Plot-
    nikov A. Prominent positive U waves appear-
    ing with high-dose intravenous phenylephrine.
    J Electrocardiol 2005;38:378–82.
13. Nozoe M, Namera A, Kohriyama K, Take-
    moto M. Over-the-counter medication and acute
    life-threatening myocardial damage. Int J Cardiol
    2005;102:545–7.
14. Cox DE, Farmer LD, Hoyle JR, Wells GL. Prog-
    nostic significance on nonsustained ventricular
    tachycardia during dobutamine stress echocar-
    diography. Am J Cardiol 2005;96:1293–8.
15. Previtali M, Repetto A, Scuteri L. Dobutamine
    induced severe midventricular obstruction and
    mitral regurgitation in left ventricular apical bal-
    looning syndrome. Heart 2005;91:353–5.
16. Zappia M, Annesi G, Nicoletti G, Arabia G,
    Annesi F, Messina D, Pugliese P, Spadafora P,
    Tarantino P, Carrideo S, Civitelli D, De
    Marco EV, Ciro-Candiano IC, Gambardella A,
    Quattrone A. Sex differences in clinical and ge-
    netic determinants of levodopa peak-dose dysk-
    inesias in Parkinson disease. An exploratory
    study. Arch Neurol 2005;62:601–5.
17. Avanzi M, Baratti M, Cabrini S, Uber E,
    Brighetti G, Bonfà F. Prevalence of pathologi-
    cal gambling in patients with Parkinson's disease.
    Mov Disord 2006;12:2068–72.

18. Grosset KA, Macphee G, Pal G, Stewart D, Watt A, Davie J, Grosset DG. Problematic gambling on dopamine agonists: not such a rarity. Mov Disord 2006;21:2206–8.
19. Voon V, Hassan K, Zurowski M, Duff-Canning S, de Souza M, Fox S, Lang AE, Miyasaki J. Prospective prevalence of pathologic gambling and medication association in Parkinson disease. Neurology 2006;66:1750–2.
20. Dodd ML, Klos KJ, Bower JH, Geda YE, Josephs KA, Ahlskog JE. Pathological gambling caused by drugs used to treat Parkinson disease. Arch Neurol 2005;62:1377–81.
21. Gallagher DA, O'Sullivan SS, Evans AH, Lees AJ, Schrag A. Pathological gambling in Parkinson's disease: risk factors and differences from dopamine dysregulation. Mov Disord [epublication ahead of print].
22. Voon V, Thomsen T, Miyasaki JM, de Souza M, Shafro A, Fox SH, Duff-Canning S, Lang AE, Zurowski M. Factors associated with dopaminergic drug-related pathological gambling in Parkinson disease. Arch Neurol 2007;64:212–6.
23. Weintraub D, Siderwowf AD, Potenza MN, Goveas J, Morales KH, Duda JE, Moberg PJ, Stern MB. Association of dopamine agonist use with impulse control disorders in Parkinson disease. Arch Neurol 2006;63:969–73.
24. Gschwandtner U, Aston J, Renaud S, Fuhr P. Pathologic gambling in patients with Parkinson's disease. Clin Neuropharmacol 2001;24:170–2.
25. Stocchi F. Pathological gambling in Parkinson's disease. Lancet Neurol 2005;4:590–2.
26. Smeding HMM, Goudriaan AE, Foncke EMJ, Schuurman PR, Speelman JD, Schmand B. Pathological gambling after bilateral subthalamic stimulation in Parkinson disease. J Neurol Neurosurg Psychiatry 2007;78:517–9.
27. Bandini F, Primavera A, Pizzorno M, Cocito L. Using STN DBS and medication reduction as a strategy to treat pathological gambling in Parkinson's disease. Parkinsonism Relat Disord 2007;13:369–71.
28. da Silva Lobo DS, Vallada HP, Knight J, Martins SS, Tavares H, Gentil V, Kennedy JL. Dopamine genes and pathological gambling in discordant sib-pairs. J Gambl Stud 2007 [epublication ahead of print].
29. Lamberti P, Zoccolella S, Iliceto G, Armenise E, Fraddosio A, de Mari M, Livrea P. Effects of levodopa and COMT inhibitors on plasma homocysteine in Parkinson's disease patients. Mov Disord 2005;20:69–72.
30. Tintner R, Manian P, Gauthier P, Jankovic J. Pleuropulmonary fibrosis after long-term treatment with the dopamine agonist pergolide for Parkinson disease. Arch Neurol 2005;62:1290–5.
31. Lin Y-H, Seow K-M, Hwang J-L, Chen H-H. Myocardial infarction and mortality caused by methylergonovine. Acta Obstet Gynecol Scand 2005;84:1022.
32. Kluger N, Girad C, Bessis D, Guillot B. Methysergide-induced scleroderma-like changes in the legs. Br J Dermatol 2005;153:224–5.
33. Chu FM, Dmochowski RR, Lama DJ, Anderson RU, Sand PK. Extended-release formulations of oxybutynin and tolterodine exhibit similar central nervous system tolerability profiles: a subanalysis of data from the OPERA trial. Am J Obstet Gynecol 2005;192:1849–55.
34. Altan-Yaycioglu R, Yaycioglu O, Aydin Akova Y, Guvel S, Ozkardes H. Ocular side-effects of tolterodine and oxybutynin, a single-blind prospective randomized trial. Br J Clin Pharmacol 2005;59:588–92.
35. Sommer BR, O'Hara R, Askari N, Kraemer HC, Kennedy WA. The effect of oxybutynin treatment on cognition in children with diurnal incontinence. J Urol 2005;173:2125–7.
36. Juss JK, Radhamma AKJ, Forsyth DR. Tolterodine-induced hyponatraemia. Age Ageing 2005;34:524–5.
37. Vander T, Odi H, Bluvstein V, Ronen J, Catz A. Carbamazepine toxicity following oxybutynin and dantrolene administration: a case report. Spinal Cord 2005;43:252–5.

A.E. Goossens and J.K. Aronson

14 Dermatological drugs, topical agents, and cosmetics

COSMETICS

Reviews of the 7th Amendment to the Cosmetics Directive (2003/15/EC) have been published ([1R], [2R]). The Directive foresees the phasing out of animal experiments by 2009, by introducing bans on animal testing of cosmetics and on the marketing in the EU of cosmetics tested on animals. For toxicity studies relevant to humans the ban would apply by 2013, with a possible postponement in case of technical difficulties in the development of alternative methods. The Directive also requires an immediate marketing ban if alternative methods have already been validated by the European Centre for the Validation of Alternative Methods and adopted by the Community.

The safety of various ingredients of cosmetics, including tert-butyl alcohol, polyacrylamide and acrylamide residues, and a wide variety of antioxidants have been reviewed on the basis of animal toxicology ([3ER], [4ER], [5ER]).

Observational studies   The prevalence and characteristic of adverse cosmetic events have been studied using a questionnaire supplied by ten community pharmacies to 4373 customers in Naples ([6c]). There were 2716 female and 812 male respondents, of whom 98.5% reported using cosmetics. There were 1507 adverse cosmetic events; 848 customers had had at least one adverse cosmetic events and 18% reported more than one event. There was a significantly higher prevalence of adverse cosmetic events in women (27 versus 17% in men). In 95.9% the event affected the skin and 4.1% were systemic.

Among cutaneous reactions, *burning* and *itching* were the most prominent and accounted for 36 and 33% respectively. The most frequently reported systemic event was *headache* (40%) followed by *nausea* (24%). The authors concluded that there is a sizeable problem and they advocated a system to report, collect, and evaluate adverse cosmetic events.

Skin   The role of contact allergy in *rosacea* has been investigated in a retrospective study of the results of patch tests in 361 of 76697 patients with rosacea ([7c]). There were positive reactions to nickel (II) sulfate in 9.3%, fragrance mix in 8.8%, thimerosal in 6.9%, *Myroxylon pereirae* resin in 5.9%, potassium dichromate in 4.6%, and propolis in 2.8%. Patients with rosacea had a significantly higher risk of contact allergy to propolis and contact allergy to nickel was significantly less frequent. Only 2/329 patients were positive to neomycin sulfate and 1/100 to gentamicin sulfate. Of 118 patients tested with their own products, three were tested to metronidazole, and one had a positive reaction.

Immunologic   Products brought in by 5911 patients were subjected to 34082 single patch tests and assigned to 1 of 26 categories, based on the EU Classification Annex I to 76/768/EEC ([8c]). The leave-on products most commonly tested were creams, emulsions, lotions, gels, and oils for the skin (3621 tested, 312 positive). The rinse-off products most commonly tested were bath and shower preparations (1333 tested, 71 positive). Positive reactions to the fragrance mix, *Myroxylon pereirae* resin, methyldibromoglutaronitrile, (chloro-)methylisothiazolinone, 2-bromo-2-nitropropane-1,3-diole and other ingredients of cosmetics and toiletries were more common than in product-negative patients.

Side Effects of Drugs, Annual 30
J.K. Aronson (Editor)
ISSN: 0378-6080
DOI: 10.1016/S0378-6080(08)00014-7

In patch tests with a cosmetic and fragrance series in 50 patients of both sexes with clinically suspected cosmetic dermatitis for more than 1 year, most of whom were young adults aged 10–29 years, 33 reacted to one or more allergens (9[c]). Fragrance components were most commonly implicated (in 52%) followed by preservatives (39%), paraphenylenediamine (21%), and cetrimide and tertiary butyl hydroquinone (12% each).

Infection risk   In an assessment of the risk of transmission of the BSE prion in cosmetics, the FDA has concluded that cosmetics that contain proteins derived from bovine sources might be sources of exposure and that the preferred way of preventing such transmission by cosmetics would be by avoiding the use of high-risk cattle-derived protein in their manufacture (10[c]). The FDA has therefore prohibited the use of certain cattle materials in cosmetics and human foods, including the brain, skull, trigeminal ganglia, spinal cord, parts of the vertebral column and the transverse processes of the thoracic and lumbar vertebrae, tonsils, and distal ileum.

Gold

Immunologic   Of 49 respondents to a questionnaire that was sent to 102 gold-allergic patients, all but one were women (11[c]). Most of the patients reported that their dermatitis had improved after patch testing, but most had avoided other allergens as well as gold. The authors concluded that avoidance of gold earrings did not appear to benefit patients with earlobe dermatitis, but that total avoidance of gold jewelry on the hands and wrists did seem to benefit a subgroup of patients with facial and eyelid dermatitis who wore powder, eye shadow, or foundation on affected areas.

Hair dyes

The Cosmetic Ingredient Review (CIR) program was established in 1976 by the Cosmetics, Toiletry, and Fragrance Association, with the support of the Food and Drug Administration

(FDA) and the Consumer Federation of America (CFA). The safety of cosmetics has been reviewed by the CIR, with particular emphasis on hair dyes (12[R]).

Respiratory   The causes of *occupational asthma* over 8 year have been studied in 47 hairdressers, mean age 25 (range 17–52) years, using responses to specific inhalation (13[c]). In 24 patients with asthma it was attributed to persulfate salts in 21, permanent hair dyes in two, and latex in one. In 13 of these 24 patients with occupational rhinitis, it was due to persulfate salts in 11 and to paraphenylenediamine in two. Patients with persulfate-induced asthma had a long period of exposure to bleaching agents and a long latent period between the start of exposure and the onset of symptoms.

Immunologic   An interview-based study in a representative random sample ($n = 4000$) of the Danish population showed that allergic skin reactions to hair dyes was more common than expected from patch-test studies (14[c]). In all, 18% of the male respondents and 75% of the female respondents had at some point dyed their hair, the median age at first exposure being 16 years. Adverse skin reactions to hair dyes compatible with allergic reactions were reported in 5.3% of individuals who had ever used a hair dye. Of these, only 16% had been in contact with health-care services after the reaction.

Direct oxidative DNA damage and production of tumor necrosis factor alfa have been studied in 19 hairdressers with contact dermatitis of the hands who had been exposed to irritants and allergens, mainly hair dyes; 14 had allergic contact dermatitis and five had irritant contact dermatitis (15[c]). The serum concentrations of TNF alfa in those with allergic contact dermatitis were significantly higher than in controls; the effect increased with increasing exposure. There was significant exposure-related DNA damage in those with irritant contact dermatitis.

Genotoxicity/mutagenicity/carcinogenicity
The members of a biopharmaceutical drug development services contract research organization, Covance Laboratories Ltd, have reviewed the guidelines of the European Scientific Committee on Cosmetics and Non-Food Products (SCCNFP) for testing hair dyes for genotoxic/

mutagenic/carcinogenic potential (16^{SR}). They have pointed out that the battery of six in vitro tests recommended in those guidelines differs substantially from the batteries of two or three in vitro tests recommended in other guidelines and suggested that potential genotoxic activity may effectively be determined by the use of a limited number of well-validated test systems that are capable of detecting induced gene mutations and structural and numerical chromosomal change, and that increasing the number of in vitro assays would merely reduce increase the number of false positives. They recommended the use of three assays, the bacterial gene mutation assay, the mammalian cell gene mutation assay (preferably the mouse lymphoma tk assay), and the in vitro micronucleus assay, combined with metabolic activation systems optimized for the individual chemical types. One could comment, however, that it a high rate of false positives in such testing would be preferable to a high rate of false negatives. Problems in testing include the fact that new compounds are formed on the scalp by reaction between the chemicals in hair dyes and that one component could mask the genotoxicity of another.

Tumorigenicity   The possible association between the personal use of hair dyes and *non-Hodgkin's lymphoma, leukemia, multiple myeloma*, and *Hodgkin's disease* has been investigated in a case-control study in 2737 patients and 1779 controls (17^{C}). Among women, there was no association between ever using hair dyes and the risk of lymphopoietic malignancies. For permanent hair dyes, there was a slightly but non-significantly increased risk of lymphocytic leukemia (OR = 1.3; 95% CI = 0.8, 2.2) and of follicular subtypes of non-Hodgkin's lymphoma (OR = 1.3; 95% CI = 0.8, 2.0). Women who used black hair dye colors were at an increased risk of leukemia (OR = 1.9; 95% CI = 1.0, 3.4), in particular chronic lymphocytic leukemia (OR = 3.0; 95% CI = 1.1, 7.5).

In a case-control study of 112 white women with *gliomas* and 215 controls there was a 1.7-fold increased risk of glioma among women who had ever used hair coloring products (95% CI = 1.0, 2.9; n = 62), and a 2.4-fold risk among those who had used permanent hair coloring products (OR = 2.4; 95% CI = 1.3, 4.5; n = 39) (18^{C}). For women with the most

aggressive form of glioma, glioblastoma multiforme, the risk increased with duration of exposure to 4.9 (95% CI = 1.6, 15.7; n = 10) after 21 or more years of permanent hair coloring use. The risk was higher with earlier age at first use. There was no association with non-permanent (sometimes called temporary or semi-permanent) hair coloring products.

Teratogenicity   The relation between maternal hair dye use in pregnancy and the risk of *neuroblastoma* in their offspring has been studied in 538 mothers of children with neuroblastoma and 504 controls (19^{C}). The use of any hair dye in the month before and/or during pregnancy was associated with a moderately increased risk of neuroblastoma (adjusted OR = 1.6; 95% CI = 1.2, 2.2). Temporary hair dyes (OR = 2.0, CI = 1.1, 3.7) were more strongly associated with neuroblastoma than permanent hair dyes (OR = 1.4, CI = 1.0, 2.0). It is not known whether or how the risk is affected by the color and chemical composition of the dye and the method of application.

Aminophenols

Immunologic   *Allergic contact dermatitis* due to paraphenylenediamine after tattooing with black henna has been reviewed (20^{R}).

Paraphenylenediamine (PPD) is the most common screening agent used to diagnose allergic contact dermatitis from oxidative hair dyes. However, testing with this allergen does not pick up all cases. Contact allergy to two frequently used hair dye chemicals has been described: 3-nitro-para-hydroxyethylaminophenol for the first time and 4-amino-3-nitrophenol for the second time (21^{A}).

- A 50-year-old woman developed severe scalp dermatitis and vesicular hand eczema for the first time in her life. She had a +? reaction to paraphenylenediamine and to her own hair collected at day 3 after exposure to the hair dye that had elicited the reaction. Open exposure to the product (often advised on the packaging of such products) was negative both before and after the allergic reaction to the product.

This adverse reaction could only be explained by patch testing with the individual hair dye product ingredients and the positive reactions to the dyes present.

Work is currently going on to establish a new screening patch-test series for hair-dye allergy.

Sodium stearoyl lactylate

Immunologic   Contact allergy to sodium stearoyl lactylate, an emulsifier commonly used in food (E481), has been reported as the cause of dermatitis, because of its presence in a cosmetic cream (22[A]).

Nail cosmetics

The adverse effects of nail cosmetics have been reviewed (23[R]). Nail cosmetics are of three types: (1) coatings that harden on evaporation; (2) coatings that polymerize; and (3) stick-on nail dressings (synthetic covers). The adverse effects of the two first types consist of both local reactions and distant contact dermatitis. Nail enamels especially cause *ectopic contact dermatitis*, while polymerizing coatings and synthetic covers are more likely to cause *local reactions*, which can be severe. Systemic adverse effects and infections can also occur.

Corticosteroids, topical

Immunologic   Corticosteroids not infrequently cause *contact allergy*. In most cases the reaction is eczematous, but occasionally other types of skin reactions occur. A generalized exanthematous reaction with pustulosis (AGEP), a drug eruption that is in most cases caused by systemic medication, has been reported in association with topical application of a glucocorticoid (24[A]).

Colophony   *(SEDA-29, 156)*

Colophony (rosin) derives from pine resin, tall oil, and stump extracts (25[R]). It is used in its native or chemically modified forms, hydrogenated, disproportionated, esterified, polymerized, as salts, or reacted with maleic anhydride or formaldehyde. It is used in the sizing of paper and paperboard, to make waxes and varnishes, for coating the strings of bows used to play stringed musical instruments, and in permanent color markers. Exposure can occur by contact with adhesive tapes, soaps, coatings on price labels, eye shadow, periodontal and surgical dressings, furniture polish, glues, musician's rosin, printing inks, printing paper surfaces, rubber, and plastics. The main sensitizing components are abietic acid and abitol (a mixture of hydroabietyl alcohols).

Respiratory   Some workers exposed to colophony during soldering can develop *occupational asthma*. Serum obtained from seven exposed symptomatic individuals, some with a likely diagnosis of occupational asthma, 10 exposed asymptomatic individuals, and 11 unexposed individuals was tested for specific IgE antibodies against a protein extract produced following in vitro challenge of mono-mac-6 cells with colophony extract (26[c]). The serum from exposed symptomatic individuals showed increased binding of specific IgE antibodies to a range of colophony-cell protein conjugates compared with both the exposed asymptomatic and the non-exposed control populations. The authors concluded that they were able to assess sensitization to colophony by detecting specific IgE in colophony-exposed workers with a likely diagnosis of occupational asthma.

Immunologic   *Contact dermatitis* from colophony is common. Of 250 Iranian patients with a diagnosis of contact dermatitis and/or atopic dermatitis 126 (50%) had at least one positive patch test reaction and 23 (9.2%) had more than two positive reactions to a range of allergens (27[c]). Colophony caused reactions in 13 cases (5.2%) and was the fifth most common allergen.

Minoxidil   *(SED-15, 2354; SEDA-27, 217; SEDA-29, 215)*

Immunologic   Allergic *contact dermatitis* has been reported in a 72-year-old woman during treatment with topical minoxidil for alopecia (28[A]).

PHOTOTHERAPY AND PHOTOCHEMOTHERAPY

(SED-15, 2823; SEDA-28, 171; SEDA-29, 158)

Aminolevulinic acid

Nervous system   Photodynamic therapy with topical 5-aminolevulinic acid generally causes few adverse effects, which are mild and transient, such as *itching, stinging* or *burning pain* (29[c]), and slight to moderate *edema* and *erythema* (30[c]), although *pain* during illumination can be problematic, for example in psoriasis (31[c]). The pain occasionally persists for up to 24 hours and rarely for several days. The mechanism may be related to GABA receptors, by which ALA is transported into peripheral nerve endings, resulting in fiber stimulation (32[R]). Cooling by fanning or water spray directed at the treatment site is effective. Topical anesthesia with local anesthetics is not, but cold-air anesthesia can help.

A severe, acute, predominantly *motor polyneuropathy*, with signs of autonomic involvement, and skin changes followed aminolevulinic acid administration in an 82-year-old man (33[A]). There were changes in heme metabolism and the authors interpreted this as a rare response to aminolevulinic resembling an acute attack of hepatic porphyria with neurological features.

Skin   *Photocontact urticaria* has been attributed to topical aminolevulinic acid in a patient with unilesional mycosis fungoides (34[A]). In a photopatch test black light and visible light irradiation after topical aminolevulinic acid provoked an urticarial reaction in the uninvolved skin, suggesting an allergic reaction.

PUVA

Tumorigenicity   There is an increased incidence of *skin cancer* in Caucasians who have been treated with psoralen plus ultraviolet A

therapy. However, in 4294 Japanese patients who had been exposed to long-term PUVA therapy in Korea, Thailand, Egypt, and Tunisia, with a follow-up period of at least 5 years, the risk of non-melanoma skin cancer relative to general dermatology out-patients was 0.86 (CI = 0.36, 1.35) (35[c]).

UVB

Tumorigenicity   UVB phototherapy is commonly used to treat psoriasis and other skin diseases. The risk of skin cancer associated with UVB phototherapy has been surveyed in a systematic review of 11 prospective and retrospective studies in about 3400 patients published from 1966 to June 2002 (36[M]). Other than the most recent Finnish study, none showed an increased risk of *skin cancer*. In one of the studies there was an increased rate of *genital tumors* associated with UVB phototherapy.

The incidence of skin cancer in 1380 adults in a long-term study of PUVA has been investigated in relation to UVB exposure (37[c]). High UVB exposure (at least 300 treatments) was associated with a modest but significant increase in the risk of squamous cell carcinoma (adjusted incidence rate ratio = 1.37, 95% CI = 1.03, 1.83) and basal cell carcinoma (adjusted IRR = 1.45, 95% CI = 1.07, 1.96). Among patients with under 100 PUVA treatments, high exposure to UVB was significantly associated with a risk of squamous cell carcinoma (adjusted IRR = 2.75, 95% CI = 1.11, 6.84) and basal cell carcinoma (adjusted IRR = 3.00, 95% CI = 1.30, 6.91) on body sites typically exposed to UVB but not on chronically sun-exposed sites, which are typically covered during therapy.

SUNSCREENS

Drometrizole trisiloxane

Immunologic   Allergic *contact dermatitis* from drometrizole trisiloxane, a chemical UVA and UVB sunscreen agent used in cosmetic products, has been reported, with concomitant sensitivities to other sunscreens (38[A]). Allergic reactions to drometrizole trisiloxane seem to be rare, but this could be due to lack of appropriate testing.

VITAMIN A (RETINOIDS)

(SED-15, 3653; SEDA-27, 159; SEDA-28, 171; SEDA-29, 158; for vitamin A carotenoids see Chapter 34)

Teratogenicity   Although the teratogenicity of oral retinoids is well known, it is not clear what the risks are with topical retinoids (adapalene and tretinoin). Although the results of two flawed epidemiological studies were reassuring, new cases of birth defects were subsequently reported in children exposed in utero to topical tretinoin. However, the epidemiological data are still scant and unconvincing, neither confirming the risk nor ruling it out completely. It has been suggested that it is best to avoid topical retinoids altogether in early pregnancy (39[R]).

Acitretin

Ear, nose, throat   *Dysphonia* has been attributed to acitretin (40[A]).

- A 36-year-old woman, who had taken acitretin 20 mg/day for palmoplantar keratoderma for about 3 months, complained of dysphonia. She had bilateral vocal fold edema and congestion, consistent with vocal abuse. Reduction of the dose of acitretin to 10 mg/day did not produce and the acitretin was withdrawn. Within 5 days, her voice recovered spontaneously. Acitretin was reintroduced and 8 days later she was dysphonic. When the acitretin was withdrawn the dysphonia resolved.

Sensory systems   Sudden bilateral symmetrical *sensorineural hearing loss* has been attributed to oral acitretin (41[A]).

Gastrointestinal   *Rectal bleeding* has been attributed to acitretin in a patient with discoid lupus erythematosus (42[A]).

Skin   *Pseudoporphyria*, with erosions and crusts on the backs of the hands and millium cysts, has been attributed to acitretin used to prevent cutaneous malignancies (43[A]). The acitretin was not withdrawn and the skins symptoms varied in severity, worsening in the summer.

Musculoskeletal   Retinoids can rarely cause *hyperostosis* when they are used in high dosages and over long periods. In one case exuberant enthesitis occurred in a 60-year-old man with psoriatic arthropathy who had taken acitretin 25 mg/day for 10 years (44[A]).

Adapalene

See tazarotene.

Isotretinoin

Ear, nose, throat   *Hoarseness*, possibly caused by excess granulomatous tissue formation over nodules on the vocal cords, has been reported in a patient taking isotretinoin (45[A]).

- A 38-year-old woman with papulopustular acne took isotretinoin 30 mg/day (0.6 mg/kg) for 3 weeks and noticed mild hoarseness, which gradually worsened. After 5 months, isotretinoin was withdrawn; 2 weeks later the hoarseness started to improve and it disappeared completely after 6 weeks. As the woman was a teacher, vocal abuse could have been the origin of this adverse event.

Psychiatric   The possible association of isotretinoin with *depression, suicidal ideation*, and *attempted suicide* is still controversial. A series of cases suggesting an association between exposure to isotretinoin and *manic psychosis* has been reported (46[c]). Five young adults developed manic psychosis during 1 year in association with isotretinoin treatment, resulting in suicidality and progression to long-standing psychosis. Associated risk factors were a family and personal history of psychiatric morbidity. The cases were drawn from 500 soldiers who had been evaluated in a military specialist dermatology clinic for severe acne.

Skin   An acquired *port wine stain* has been reported in a patient taking isotretinoin (47[A]).

- An 18-year-old man with severe comedonal and pustular acne took isotretinoin 40 mg/day for 6 months and 6 weeks after the end of the course of treatment developed a large erythematous telangiectatic area on his left cheek and upper lip, consistent with an acquired port stain.

The mechanism by which isotretinoin could cause this adverse effect is not clear, but increased skin dryness might have been the main pathological change.

Tazarotene

Tazarotene has been included in a review of treatments for psoriasis, including adalimumab, efalizumab, and infliximab, alefacept and etanercept, and pimecrolimus (48[R]).

Skin   Tazarotene cream 0.05 and 0.1% and adapalene 0.1% cream and gel have been compared in 26 subjects (49[c]). They were applied under occlusive dressings at randomized sites on the upper back for about 24 hours 4 times a week and for 72 hours once a week for 3 weeks. In all, 16 subjects stopped using one or more of the test products because of severe irritation scores; all but one of these were at sites treated with tazarotene. The mean 21-day cumulative irritancy scores for adapalene 0.1% cream and gel were significantly lower than those for tazarotene cream 0.05 and 0.1% and not higher than with the control product.

Tretinoin (all-trans retinoic acid, ATRA)

Placebo-controlled studies   There has been a 2-year placebo-controlled study of the efficacy and safety of tretinoin emollient cream 0.05% in 204 subjects with photodamaged facial skin, including histopathological assessment of safety and an analysis of markers of collagen deposition (50[c]). Tretinoin produced significantly greater improvement than placebo in the signs of photodamage (fine and coarse wrinkling, mottled hyperpigmentation, lentigines, and sallowness), the overall severity of photodamage, and the investigators' global assessment of response. Histological evaluation showed no increase in keratinocytic or melanocytic atypia, dermal elastosis, or untoward effects on the stratum corneum compared with placebo. Immunohistochemistry showed a significant increase relative to placebo in facial procollagen 1C terminal, a marker for procollagen synthesis, at month 12.

VITAMIN D ANALOGUES, TOPICAL

Calcipotriol   *(SED-15, 594; SEDA-28, 169; SEDA-29, 156; for oral vitamin D analogues see Chapter 34)*

Skin   In three patients with psoriasis calcipotriol ointment resulted in severe *eczematous eruptions*, which resolved after withdrawal of calcipotriol and topical application of a glucocorticoid. Patch tests showed a strong reaction to calcipotriol; there was no cross-reactivity to other vitamin D3 analogues, tacalcitol and calcitriol (51[c]).

Exacerbation of pustular psoriasis has been attributed to calcipotriol (52[A]).

- A 55-year-old Japanese man with generalized pustular psoriasis controlled by oral etretinate, oral ciclosporin, and topical beclometasone dipropionate was given calcipotriol ointment (Dovonex®; 50 µg/g) instead of the steroid, and 2 weeks later became feverish, with numerous pustules on most of the body, a white blood cell count of 10.8×10^9/l, and a CRP concentration of 263 mg/l, consistent with exacerbation of pustular psoriasis. The lesions were controlled within 2 weeks by withdrawing calcipotriol, restarting topical 0.025% beclometasone dipropionate ointment, and increasing the dose of oral ciclosporin to 5 mg/kg/day. During remission, 2 months later, calcipotriol ointment again caused exacerbation of the pustular psoriasis.

Nails   In 24 patients (19 women and 5 men) with nail psoriasis calcipotriol ointment (50 µg/g), 14 patients improved significantly after 3 months and two were completely free of nail lesions after 5 months (53[c]). There were adverse reactions in two patients: *periungual irritation and inflammation* in one, *irritation, pruritus, and oozing* in the other; these patients withdrew from the study.

Tacalcitol

The efficacy and safety of tacalcitol have been reviewed (54[R]). The adverse effects are uncommon and generally mild, and include *local irritation* and *pruriginous or burning sensations*.

References

1. Manou I, Eskes C, de Silva O, Renner G, Zuang V. Safety data requirements for the purposes of the Cosmetics Directive. Altern Lab Anim 2005;33(Suppl 1):21–6.
2. Ruet Rossignol M. The 7th Amendment to the Cosmetics Directive. Altern Lab Anim 2005;33(Suppl 1):19–20.
3. Chen M. Amended final report of the safety assessment of t-butyl alcohol as used in cosmetics. Int J Toxicol 2005;24(Suppl 2):1–20.
4. Anonymous. Amended final report on the safety assessment of polyacrylamide and acrylamide residues in cosmetics. Int J Toxicol 2005;24(Suppl 2):21–50.
5. Elmore AR. Final report of the safety assessment of L-ascorbic acid, calcium ascorbate, magnesium ascorbate, magnesium ascorbyl phosphate, sodium ascorbate, and sodium ascorbyl phosphate as used in cosmetics. Int J Toxicol 2005;24(Suppl 2):51–111.
6. Di Giovanni C, Arcoraci V, Gambardella L, Sautebin L. Cosmetovigilance survey: are cosmetics considered safe by consumers? Pharmacol Res 2006;53(1):16–21.
7. Jappe U, Schnuch A, Uter W. Rosacea and contact allergy to cosmetics and topical medicaments—retrospective analysis of multicentre surveillance data 1995–2002. Contact Dermatitis 2005;52(2):96–101.
8. Uter W, Balzer C, Geier J, Frosch PJ, Schnuch A. Patch testing with patients' own cosmetics and toiletries—results of the IVDK*, 1998–2002. Contact Dermatitis 2005;53(4):226–33.
9. Tomar J, Jain VK, Aggarwal K, Dayal S, Gupta S. Contact allergies to cosmetics: testing with 52 cosmetic ingredients and personal products. J Dermatol 2005;32(12):951–5.
10. Epstein HA. Risk assessment of variant Creutzfeldt–Jakob disease in cosmetics. Skinmed 2005;4(6):377–8.
11. Nedorost S, Wagman A. Positive patch-test reactions to gold: patients' perception of relevance and the role of titanium dioxide in cosmetics. Dermatitis 2005;16(2):67–70.
12. Bergfeld WF, Belsito DV, Marks Jr JG, Andersen FA. Safety of ingredients used in cosmetics. J Am Acad Dermatol 2005;52(1):125–32; Erratum: J Am Acad Dermatol 2005;53(1):137.
13. Moscato G, Pignatti P, Yacoub MR, Romano C, Spezia S, Perfetti L. Occupational asthma and occupational rhinitis in hairdressers. Chest 2005;128(5):3590–8.
14. Sösted H, Hesse U, Menné T, Andersen KE, Johansen JD. Contact dermatitis to hair dyes in a Danish adult population: an interview-based study. Br J Dermatol 2005;153:132–5.
15. Cavallo D, Ursini CL, Setini A, Chianese C, Cristaudo A, Iavicoli S. DNA damage and TNFalpha cytokine production in hairdressers with contact dermatitis. Contact Dermatitis 2005;53(3):125–9.
16. Kirkland DJ, Henderson L, Marzin D, Muller L, Parry JM, Speit G, Tweats DJ, Williams GM. Testing strategies in mutagenicity and genetic toxicology: an appraisal of the guidelines of the European Scientific Committee for Cosmetics and Non-Food Products for the evaluation of hair dyes. Mutat Res 5 2005;88(2):88–105.
17. Miligi L, Costantini AS, Benvenuti A, Veraldi A, Tumino R, Ramazzotti V, Vindigni C, Amadori D, Fontana A, Rodella S, Stagnaro E, Crosignani P, Vineis P. Personal use of hair dyes and hematolymphopoietic malignancies. Arch Environ Occup Health 2005;60(5):249–56.
18. Heineman EF, Ward MH, McComb RD, Weisenburger DD, Zahm SH. Hair dyes and risk of glioma among Nebraska women. Cancer Causes Control 2005;16(7):857–64.
19. McCall EE, Olshan AF, Daniels JL. Maternal hair dye use and risk of neuroblastoma in offspring. Cancer Causes Control 2005;16(6):743–8.
20. Arranz Sanchez DM, Corral de la Calle M, Vidaurrazaga Diaz de Arcaya C, de Lucas Laguna R, Diaz Diaz R. Risks of black henna tattoos. An Pediatr (Barc) 2005;63(5):448–52.
21. Sösted H, Menné T. Allergy to 3-nitro-p-hydroxyethylaminophenol and 4-amino-3-nitrophenol in a hair dye. Contact Dermatitis 2005;52:317–9.
22. Jensen CD, Andersen K. Allergic contact dermatitis from sodium stearoyl lactylate, an emulsifier commonly used in food products. Contact Dermatitis 2005;53:116.
23. Baran R, Andre J. Side effects of nail cosmetics. J Cosmet Dermatol 2005;4(3):204–9.
24. Mur EC, González-Carrascosa Ballesteros M, Fernández RS, Marco CB. Generalized exanthematous reaction with pustulosis induced by topical corticosteroids. Contact Dermatitis 2005;52:114–5.
25. Hausen BM, Kuhlwein A, Schulz KH. Colophony allergy. A contribution to the origin, chemistry, and uses of colophony and modified colophony products, 1. Derm Beruf Umwelt. 1982;30(4):107–15.
26. Elms J, Fishwick D, Robinson E, Burge S, Huggins V, Barber C, Williams N, Curran A. Specific IgE to colophony? Occup Med (Lond) 2005;55(3):234–7.
27. Kashani MN, Gorouhi F, Behnia F, Nazemi MJ, Dowlati Y, Firooz A. Allergic contact dermatitis in Iran. Contact Dermatitis 2005;52(3):154–8.
28. Hagemann T, Schlutter-Bohmer B, Allam JP, Bieber T, Novak N. Positive lymphocyte transformation test in a patient with allergic contact dermatitis of the scalp after short-term use of topical minoxidil solution. Contact Dermatitis 2005;53(1):53–5.
29. Radakovic-Fijan S, Blecha-Thalhammer U, Schleyer V, Szeimies RM, Zwingers T, Honigsmann H, Tanew A. Topical aminolaevulinic acid-based photodynamic therapy as a treatment

option for psoriasis? Results of a randomized, observer-blinded study. Br J Dermatol
2005;152(2):279–83.

30. Alster TS, Tanzi EL, Welsh EC. Photorejuvena-
tion of facial skin with topical 20% 5-amino-
levulinic acid and intense pulsed light treatment:
a split-face comparison study. J Drugs Dermatol
2005;4(1):35–8.

31. Fransson J, Ros AM. Clinical and immunohistochemical evaluation of psoriatic plaques treated
with topical 5-aminolaevulinic acid photodynamic therapy. Photodermatol Photoimmunol
Photomed 2005;21(6):326–32.

32. Wennberg AM. Pain, pain relief and other practical issues in photodynamic therapy. Australas J
Dermatol 2005;46(Suppl):S3–4.

33. Sylantiev C, Schoenfeld N, Mamet R, Grooz-
man GB, Drory VE. Acute neuropathy mimicking porphyria induced by aminolevulinic acid
during photodynamic therapy. Muscle Nerve
2005;31(3):390–3.

34. Yokoyama S, Nakano H, Nishizawa A,
Kaneko T, Harada K, Hanada K. A case of
photocontact urticaria induced by photodynamic
therapy with topical 5-aminolaevulinic acid.
J Dermatol 2005;32(10):843–7.

35. Murase JE, Lee EE, Koo J. Effect of ethnicity on
the risk of developing nonmelanoma skin cancer
following long-term PUVA therapy. Int J Dermatol 2005;44(12):1016–21.

36. Lee E, Koo J, Berger T. UVB phototherapy and
skin cancer risk: a review of the literature. Int J
Dermatol 2005;44(5):355–60.

37. Lim JL, Stern RS. High levels of ultraviolet B
exposure increase the risk of non-melanoma skin
cancer in psoralen and ultraviolet A-treated patients. J Invest Dermatol 2005;124(3):505–13.

38. Hughes TM, Martin JA, Lewis VJ, Stone NM.
Allergic contact dermatitis to drometrizole
trisiloxane in a sunscreen with concomitant sensitivities to other sun screens. Contact Dermatitis
2005;52:226–7.

39. Anonymous. Topical retinoids during pregnancy
(continued). Prescrire Int 2005;14(77):100–1.

40. Petitpain N, Pouaha J, Cosserat F, Gambier N,
Truchetet F, Cuny JF. Recurrent dysphonia and
acitretin. J Voice 2006;20(4):642–3.

41. Mahasitthiwat V. A woman with sudden bilateral sensorineural hearing loss after treatment psoriasis with acitretin. J Med Assoc Thai
2005;88(Suppl 1):S79–81.

42. Fairhurst DA, Clark SM. Rectal bleeding following acitretin therapy for discoid lupus erythematosus. Dermatology 2005;211(4):385.

43. Martin Ezquerra G, Sola Casas M, Herrera
Acosta E, Umbert Millet P. Pseudoporhyria
secondary to acitretin. J Am Acad Dermatol
2005;53(1):169–71.

44. Fairhurst DA, Clark SM. Rectal bleeding following acitretin therapy for discoid lupus erythematosus. Dermatology 2005;211(4):385.

45. Busso CIM, Serrano RL. Hoarseness during
isotretinoin therapy. J Am Acad Dermatol
2005;52:168.

46. Barak YAC, Wohl YBC, Greenberg YA,
Dayan YBB, Friedman TB, Shoval GA, Kno-
bler HAD. Affective psychosis following Ac-
cutane (isotretinoin) treatment. Int Clin Psychopharmacol 2005;20:39–41.

47. Hoque S, Holden C. Acquired port wine stain
following oral isotretinoin. Clin Exp Dermatol
2005;30:587–8.

48. Saini R, Tutrone WD, Weinberg JM. Advances in
therapy for psoriasis: an overview of infliximab,
etanercept, efalizumab, alefacept, adalimumab,
tazarotene, and pimecrolimus. Curr Pharm Design 2005;11:273–80.

49. Dosik JS, Homer K, Arsonnaud S. Cumulative irritation potential of adapalene 0.1% cream and
gel compared with tazarotene cream 0.05 and
0.1%. Cutis 2005;75(5):289–93.

50. Kang S, Bergfeld W, Gottlieb AB, Hickman J,
Humeniuk J, Kempers S, Lebwohl M, Lowe N,
McMichael A, Milbauer J, Phillips T, Powers J,
Rodriguez D, Savin R, Shavin J, Sherer D, Sil-
vis N, Weinstein R, Weiss J, Hammerberg C,
Fisher GJ, Nighland M, Grossman R, Nyirady J.
Long-term efficacy and safety of tretinoin emollient cream 0.05% in the treatment of photodamaged facial skin: a two-year, randomized,
placebo-controlled trial. Am J Clin Dermatol
2005;6:245–53.

51. Foti C, Carnimeo L, Bonamonte D, Conserva A,
Casulli C, Angelini G. Tolerance to calcitriol
and tacalcitol in three patients with allergic contact dermatitis to calcipotriol. J Drugs Dermatol
2005;4(6):756–9.

52. Tamiya H, Fukai K, Moriwaki K, Ishii M.
Generalized pustular psoriasis precipitated by
topical calcipotriol ointment. Int J Dermatol
2005;44(9):791–2.

53. Zakeri M, Valikhani M, Mortazavi H, Barze-
gari M. Topical calcipotriol therapy in nail psoriasis: a study of 24 cases. Dermatol Online J
2005;11(3):5.

54. Leone G, Pacifico A. Profile of clinical efficacy
and safety of topical tacalcitol. Acta Biomed
2005;76(1):13–9.

Garry M. Walsh

15 Antihistamines (H_1 receptor antagonists)

The adverse effects of antihistamines, including drug–drug interactions in elderly atopic patients, in whom co-morbidities and polypharmacy are common, have again been reviewed ([1R]).

Cetirizine *(SED-15, 702; SEDA-27, 166; SEDA-28, 178; SEDA-29, 161)*

Drug–drug interactions In 17 men, of whom 16 completed the study, cetirizine did not significantly alter the pharmacokinetics of the HIV-1 protease inhibitor *ritonavir*, also a potent inhibitor of cytochrome P450 isozymes ([2c]). However, this study was conducted in healthy subjects rather than in patients infected with HIV-1.

Desloratadine *(SED-15, 1074; SEDA-27, 167; SEDA-28, 179; SEDA-29, 162)*

Biliary tract *Biliary colic* has been attributed to desloratadine ([3A]).

- A 41-year-old Peruvian woman took desloratadine 5 mg/day for 1 month for recurrent rhinitis and had an episode of biliary colic, with acute abdominal pain in the right upper quadrant, abdominal distension, nausea, and vomiting. Desloratadine was withdrawn and she recovered within 10 days, having only received analgesia.

Although this adverse event appeared to have occurred as a consequence of taking desloratadine, this was not confirmed by a subsequent drug challenge.

Susceptibility factors

Children Desloratadine is available for use in children as a syrup, and in a non-randomized uncontrolled study it was effective and well tolerated in 49 children aged 6–12 years with pollen-induced rhinitis ([4c]). In all, 22 adverse events were reported in 13 children; of these, one case of insomnia and one of diarrhea were considered possibly related to treatment.

Renal and hepatic disease No specific precautions appear to be required with respect to the administration of desloratadine in renal or hepatic insufficiency; nor have clinically relevant racial or sex variations in its disposition been noted ([5R], [6R]).

Diphenhydramine *(SED-15, 1134; SEDA-27, 167; SEDA-28, 179; SEDA-29, 163)*

Drug overdose Diphenhydramine overdose can cause central nervous system, anticholinergic, and cardiovascular effects. In addition to inhibition of cardiac fast sodium channels, higher concentrations of the drug also inhibit potassium channels, which can result in QT interval prolongation.

- A 40-year-old woman took 25 tablets of Tylenol-PM (McNeil Pharmaceutical, Raritan, NJ, USA), an over-the-counter combination of diphenhydramine 25 mg and paracetamol 500 mg ([7A]). She was intubated and a 12-lead electrocardiogram showed a sinus tachycardia with a markedly prolonged QT interval (QT_c 588 ms). Ventricular

Side Effects of Drugs, Annual 30
J.K. Aronson (Editor)
ISSN: 0378-6080
DOI: 10.1016/S0378-6080(08)00015-9

repolarization on the electrocardiogram was abnormal, with broad biphasic T waves, which were more apparent in the mid-precordial leads. Torsade de pointes was absent. By day 2, the QT interval and T waves were normal. She recovered fully.

Paracetamol does not prolong the QT interval or affect cardiac repolarization. The authors concluded that the tachycardia caused by the anticholinergic and hypotensive effects of diphenhydramine may have protected against torsade de pointes. They further suggested that it may be practical to avoid bradycardia in the acute phase of diphenhydramine toxicity.

- A 17-year-old man was found unconscious next to a bottle of diphenhydramine, which had contained up to 40 tablets of 50 mg each (8[A]). He had a tachycardia of 150/minute, a tachypnea of 32/minute, a metabolic acidosis, with a pH of 7.21, and an unspecified number of seizures. Electrocardiography showed right bundle branch block and QT interval prolongation at 522 ms. He was treated with intravenous benzodiazepines to suppress seizures and with physostigmine 0.5 ml (concentration not stated). He was then able to speak and the metabolic and cardiovascular parameters all improved and reverted to normal, though the time scale was unclear.

The authors noted that although the clinical features of diphenhydramine toxicity are well described, electrocardiographic changes have not been reported extensively. They emphasized that diphenhydramine overdose can occasionally cause prolongation of the QT interval. Although torsade de pointes has been described with diphenhydramine overdose it did not occur here. Presumably the cardiovascular toxicity of diphenhydramine is partly related to its anticholinergic activity, similar to that seen with tricyclic antidepressants. However, other antihistamines without anticholinergic effects have been implicated in QT prolongation and torsade de pointes (SEDA-26, 180; SEDA-27, 165). Furthermore, the dramatic response to physostigmine, a cholinesterase inhibitor, in this case is very interesting, in view of the controversy associated with its use in poisoning.

- A 36-year-old woman became agitated and confused, with uncoordinated limb movements and opsoclonus (9[A]). Toxicology screening was positive only for diphenhydramine, and it subsequently emerged that she had taken 40 tablets of 50 mg strength. She was treated with clonazepam 3 mg/day and by the third day all her neurological symptoms had disappeared.

Whether the outcome in this case was due to the clonazepam or merely due to elimination of the drug was not clear. Opsoclonus has not previously been described with diphenhydramine toxicity but has occurred with amitriptyline. The authors pointed out this parallel and suggested that an anticholinergic effect on brainstem neurons involved in the control of eye movements was neurophysiologically plausible.

- A 39-year-old man took an overdose of diphenhydramine and became unconscious and hypotensive. His electrocardiogram showed changes suggestive of the Brugada syndrome (10[A]). However, normalization of the electrocardiogram as he recovered and a negative flecainide test ruled out Brugada syndrome.

Fexofenadine   *(SED-15, 1357; SEDA-27, 168; SEDA-28, 179)*

Fexofenadine is a substrate of P glycoprotein and organic anion transporting polypeptides. In 12 healthy men a single oral dose of fexofenadine 120 mg was followed by 6-day courses of verapamil 240 mg/day (an inhibitor of P glycoprotein), cimetidine 800 mg/day (an inhibitor of organic cation transporters), or probenecid 2000 mg/day (an inhibitor of organic anion transporting polypeptides) (11[c]). Verapamil significantly increased the peak plasma fexofenadine concentration 2.9 times (95% CI = 2.4, 4.0) and the AUC 2.5 times (CI = 2.0, 3.0). Cimetidine did not affect the plasma concentrations of fexofenadine but reduced its renal clearance to 61% (CI = 50, 98). Probenecid increased the AUC of fexofenadine 1.5 times (CI = 1.1, 2.4) and reduced its renal clearance to 27% (CI = 20, 58). These results suggest that verapamil increases exposure to fexofenadine, probably because of an increase in systemic availability by inhibition of P glycoprotein, and that probenecid slightly increases exposure to fexofenadine by inhibiting its renal clearance.

Levocetirizine   *(SED-15, 2038; SEDA-27, 169; SEDA-28, 180; SEDA-29, 163)*

Levocetirizine is the single R-isomer of the racemic mixture cetirizine dihydrochloride, which undergoes minimal hepatic metabolism. Compared with cetirizine levocetirizine has twice the affinity for H$_1$ histamine receptors, has an improved pharmacokinetic profile, and appears to be safe and effective for the treatment of allergic diseases, including chronic urticaria and allergic rhinitis (12[R], 13[R]).

Skin   *Fixed drug eruptions* are the most frequent types of adverse cutaneous drug reactions with tetracyclines, sulfonamides, sulfones, penicillins, pyrazolones, barbiturates, and phenolphthalein, which are also among the most frequent culprits. A number of first-generation antihistamines, such as cyclizine lactate, diphenhydramine hydrochloride, phenothiazines, dimenhydrinate, and hydroxyzine, can cause fixed drug eruptions.

- A 52-year-old man took levocetirizine for urticaria and developed a solitary well-circumscribed hyperpigmented macule on the volar aspect of his right forearm (14[A]). A provisional diagnosis of a fixed drug eruption from levocetirizine was made and subsequently confirmed based on the clinical findings and a positive drug re-challenge test.
- A 33-year-old woman developed an intense generalized pruritic urticarial eruption without angioedema about 90 minutes after taking cetirizine 10 mg for relapsing generalized urticaria (15[A]). Following a symptom-free interval of 2 weeks, skin prick tests with cetirizine, levocetirizine, loratadine, and desloratadine were negative. A subsequent placebo-controlled single-blind oral provocation test with cetirizine 10 mg provoked no adverse reaction. However, within 90 minutes of an oral challenge performed the next day with cetirizine 20 mg, lentil-sized wheals and pruritus developed, beginning at the forearms and spreading over the whole body. In contrast, a placebo produced no reaction. Two days later oral challenge with two doses of levocetirizine 5 mg resulted in the same reaction as seen after cetirizine. A later oral provocation test with loratadine had no effect.

It is important to note that the adverse effects in this individual were only seen when twice the recommended dose of either cetirizine or levocetirizine was given orally. Multilocalized fixed drug eruption and localized as well as generalized urticaria have been reported for the parent drug cetirizine (SEDA 26, 27). Levocetirizine is an enantomer of cetirizine and they have the same piperazinic ring, which may act as an immunogen, giving rise to the adverse cutaneous reactions reported in a few individuals. The authors pointed out that although such reactions are rare it is essential to recognize urticarial adverse reactions caused by H$_1$ receptor antagonists, since this adverse effect may mimic the underlying disease that led the patient to take the drug.

- A 34-year-old man developed a fixed drug eruption after taking levocetirizine 5 mg/day for a recurrent urticarial rash (16[A]). The morning after the first night-time dose he felt a tingling and burning sensation over his lower lip and the tip of his tongue. Mild swelling, erythema, light brown pigmentation, erosion, and crusting followed over the next few hours. A similar lesion developed over the glans penis. There was no other drug history during this time. A year before he had had similar lesions after taking a single dose of cetirizine 10 mg, which he had been avoiding since then. There were superficial, crusted lesions of a fixed drug eruption on the lower lip and the glans penis, and these subsided with topical betamethasone 0.05% cream in about 3 days. Separate oral re-challenge tests 2 weeks later with cetirizine and levocetirizine produced similar lesions. He was advised to avoid both drugs in the future.

Owing to their rarity, fixed drug eruptions from antihistamines can be difficult to detect, as in many cases they can mimic the underlying disease for which the drug was prescribed.

Susceptibility factors

Children   Levocetirizine appears to be safe and effective in children (17[R]). For example, the effect of levocetirizine has been assessed in a double-blind, randomized, placebo-controlled 6-week study in 177 children with seasonal allergic rhinitis (18[C]). Compared with placebo levocetirizine was effective in relieving symptoms and it conferred significant improvements in quality of life. Adverse effects were no different from placebo and no subject in the levocetirizine arm withdrew from the study.

References

1. Hansen J, Klimek L, Hormann K. Pharmacological management of allergic rhinitis in the elderly: safety issues with oral antihistamines. Drugs Aging 2005;22:28996.
2. Peytavin G, Gautran C, Otoul C, Cremieux AC, Moulaert B, Delatour F, Melac M, Strolin-Benedetti M, Farinotti R. Evaluation of pharmacokinetic interaction between cetirizine and ritonavir, an HIV-1 protease inhibitor, in healthy male volunteers. Eur J Clin Pharmacol 2005;61:267–73.
3. Perez R, Rodrigo L, Perez R, de Francisco R. Acute cholestasis related to desloratidine. World J Gastroenterol 2005;11(21):3647–8.
4. Rossi GA, Tosca MA, Passalacqua G, Bianchi B, Le Grazie C, Canonica GW. Evidence of desloratadine syrup efficacy and tolerability in children with pollen-induced allergic rhinitis. Allergy 2005;60:416–7.
5. DeBuske LM. Review of desloratadine for the treatment of allergic rhinitis, chronic idiopathic urticaria and allergic inflammatory disorders. Expert Opin Pharmacother 2005;6:2511–23.
6. Berger WE. The safety and efficacy of desloratadine for the management of allergic disease. Drug Saf 2005;28:1101–18.
7. Sype JW, Khan IA. Prolonged QT interval with markedly abnormal ventricular repolarization in diphenhydramine overdose. Int J Cardiol 2005;99:333–5.
8. Thakur AC, Aslam AK, Aslam AF, Vasavada BC, Sacchi TJ, Khan IA. QT interval prolongation in diphenhydramine toxicity. Int J Cardiol 2005;98:341–3.
9. Hermann DM, Bassetti CL. Reversible opsoclonus after diphenhydramine misuse. Eur Neurol 2005;53:46–7.
10. Lopez-Barbeito B, Lluis M, Delgado V, Jimenez S, Diaz-Infante E, Nogue-Xarau S, Brugada J. Diphenhydramine overdose and Brugada sign. Pacing Clin Electrophysiol 2005;28:730–2.
11. Yasui-Furukori N, Uno T, Sugawara K, Tateishi T. Different effects of three transporting inhibitors, verapamil, cimetidine, and probenecid, on fexofenadine pharmacokinetics. Clin Pharmacol Ther 2005;77(1):17–23.
12. Walsh GM. Levocetirizine—an update. Curr Medicinal Chem 2006;13:2711–5.
13. Holgate S, Powell R, Jenkins M, Ali O. A treatment for allergic rhinitis: a view on the role of levocetirizine. Curr Med Res Opin 2005;21:1096–9.
14. Guptha SD, Prabhakar SM, Sacchidanand S. Fixed drug eruption due to levocetirizine. Indian J Dermatol Venereol Leprol 2005;71:361–2.
15. Kränke B, Mayr-Kanhäuser S. Urticarial reaction to the antihistamine levocetirizine dihydrochloride. Dermatology 2005;210:246–7.
16. Mahajan VK, Lal Sharma N, Sharma VC. Fixed drug eruption: a novel side-effect of levocetirizine. Int J Dermatol 2005;44:796–8.
17. Simons FER, Simons KJ. Levocetirizine: pharmacokinetics and pharmacodynamics in children age 6 to 11 years. J Allergy Clinical Immunol 2005;116:335–61.
18. de Blic J, Wahn U, Billard E, Alt R, Pujazon MC. Levocetirizine in children: evidenced efficacy and safety in a 6-week randomized seasonal allergic rhinitis trial. Pediatr Allergy Immunol 2005;16:267–75.

Markus Joerger, Katharina Hartmann, and Max Kuhn

16 Drugs acting on the respiratory tract

INHALED GLUCOCORTICOIDS

(SED-15, 958; SEDA-27, 174; SEDA-28, 184, SEDA-29, 168)

Systemic availability of inhaled glucocorticoids in adults Determination of growth hormone secretion has been reported to be a potential alternative to adrenal function testing to assess the systemic availability of inhaled glucocorticoids, according to a double-blind, placebo-controlled crossover study (1^C). There was a dose-related increase in growth hormone secretion over the dose-range of 100–1000 micrograms of inhaled beclomethasone dipropionate in eight healthy volunteers.

Local and cutaneous adverse effects of inhaled glucocorticoids Local adverse effects (hoarseness, dysphonia, oral candidiasis) and cutaneous adverse effects (bruising) of inhaled glucocorticoids were reviewed in SEDA-29 (p. 168). The long-term safety of budesonide has been confirmed in a randomized, placebo-controlled, double-blind study in 7221 adults and children with asthma (aged 5–66 years) using inhaled budesonide 400 micrograms/day (adolescents and adults ≥11 years) or 200 micrograms/day (children <11 years) for 3 years in mild persistent asthma (2^C). *Oral candidiasis* was more common with budesonide (1.2%) than with placebo (0.5%), as were *dysphonia* (1.4 versus 1.0%), *throat irritation* (1.0 versus 0.7%), and *bruising* (0.4 versus 0.2%).

Side Effects of Drugs, Annual 30
J.K. Aronson (Editor)
ISSN: 0378-6080
DOI: 10.1016/S0378-6080(08)00016-0

Budesonide

Pregnancy Pregnancy outcomes after exposure to inhaled glucocorticoids were reviewed in SEDA-28 (p. 186). Evidence-based guidelines have since stressed the importance of inhaled glucocorticoids as first-line therapy in controlling asthma during pregnancy, with preference given to budesonide. Data from clinical and epidemiological studies up to January 2005 have been reviewed (3^C) and have confirmed previous assessments.

Budesonide is the only inhaled corticosteroid to be given a category B pregnancy rating by the US Food and Drug Administration, based on observational data from the Swedish Medical Birth Registry. In a double-blind, randomized, placebo-controlled trial 2473 women aged 15–50 years used once-daily budesonide (400 micrograms) or placebo via a dry powder inhaler for 3 years in addition to their usual asthma medication (4^C). This trial was followed by a 2-year open study in 319 pregnancies, of which 313 were analysed. Healthy children were delivered in 81 and 77% of all pregnancies in the budesonide and placebo groups respectively. Of the 196 pregnancies reported by participants taking budesonide, 23 (12%) had miscarriages, three (2%) had congenital malformations, and 12 (6%) had other outcomes. Of the 117 pregnancies reported in the placebo group, 11 (9%) had miscarriages, four (3%) had congenital malformations, and 12 (10%) had other outcomes. Thus, treatment with low-dose inhaled budesonide does not seem to affect the outcome of pregnancy.

Fetotoxicity Retrospective epidemiological studies (5^c, 6^c, 7^c, 8^c) and a randomized, placebo-controlled trial (9^C) have shown no clinically or statistically significant effects on fetal outcomes among more than 6600 infants

193

whose mothers were exposed to inhaled budesonide during pregnancy. Rates of stillbirths, multiple births, and congenital malformations were not increased.

℞ *Susceptibility factors for the adverse effects of budesonide in children and very young children*

The systemic availability of nebulized budesonide has been assessed in 10 young children aged 3–6 years, comparing drug pharmacokinetics after intravenous infusion of budesonide 125 micrograms and inhalation of budesonide 1 mg from a Pari[TM] nebulizer (10[c]). Of the nominal dose 6% (corresponding to 26% of the dose administered after accounting for drug that was not inhaled) reached the systemic circulation, which is about half the systemic availability in healthy adults using the same nebulizer (11[c]). Lung deposition was estimated to be 18% of the administered dose, which is markedly lower than the 58% found in adults. Deposition in the oropharynx was estimated to be 82% of the administered dose in young children compared with 42% in adults, which indicates a very different deposition pattern in young children. Mean clearance was estimated to be around 30 ml/minute/kg, which is about 50% higher than in healthy adults. The low systemic availability in combination with a higher clearance corrected for body weight means that young children can be treated with the same doses of nebulized budesonide as adults, without an increased risk of unwanted systemic effects.

Systemic availability has been similarly assessed from inhalation of single dose of budesonide 800 micrograms via Turbuhaler[TM] in 15 children aged 8–14 years, and compared with a single dose of fluticasone propionate 750 micrograms via Diskus[TM] (12[c]). Mean lung deposition was 31% for budesonide via Turbuhaler[TM] and 8% for fluticasone propionate via Diskus[TM]. Pulmonary deposition was four times higher via Turbuhaler[TM] than via Diskus[TM]. The increased lung deposition and systemic availability of budesonide when given by Turbuhaler[TM] may be due to the smaller particle sizes that it generates. Overall, the results of deposition studies in children are similar to those in adults (13[c]).

Endocrine   Adrenal function was suppressed by high-dose inhaled budesonide (400–900 micrograms/m^2/day) in a dose-related manner in 19 children aged 5–12 years (14[c]). Baseline assessments showed significantly less adrenal suppression with budesonide than beclomethasone at comparable doses. In a subsequent randomized, double-blind, placebo-controlled study in 404 asthmatic children aged 6–18 years, inhaled budesonide at a daily dose of up to 800 micrograms for 12 weeks was associated with adrenal suppression in 12%, but adrenal suppression was not clinically apparent in any of the children (15[c]). In a case-control study, 21% of asthmatic children using therapeutic doses of budesonide had signs and symptoms of adrenal suppression (16[c]), but these were not clinically important. Current data suggest individual idiosyncratic sensitivity of some children to inhaled glucocorticoids: eight cases of symptomatic adrenal insufficiency have been identified with therapeutic doses of budesonide (17[c]).

Musculoskeletal   Long-term budesonide safety data on growth rate are contradictory. In one study there was no growth reduction in 216 children aged 3–11 years using budesonide 400 micrograms/day over up to 6 years, compared with control patients using standard antiasthmatic treatment without glucocorticoids (18[c]). A small case-control study showed a growth rate reduction of 0.44 cm/year in a subgroup of male adolescents using budesonide 600 micrograms/day (19[c]). However, asthma-associated pubertal delay and subsequent growth delay was probably a significant bias in this study, as control subjects were free of asthmatic symptoms. In very young children (<3 years of age), more than 6 months of treatment with nebulized budesonide 1 mg/day did not result in reduced growth velocity compared with individual pre-study measurements (20[c]).

Growth velocity was further assessed using pooled data from three randomized, placebo-controlled studies (21[C], 22[C], 23[C]) in a total of 1018 asthmatic children aged 6 months to 8 years (24[R], 25[R]). The children used budesonide inhalation suspension at doses of 0.25, 0.5, or 1.0 mg either daily (26[C]), twice daily (23[C]), or variations thereof (21[C]), or placebo. Mean growth velocity was similar with budesonide (6.64 cm/year) and conventional treatment (6.45 cm/year). However, there was a small but statistically significant reduction in growth velocity in the budesonide group in one study (0.8 cm/year) (16[C]). This may be explained by the fact that the use of oral or inhaled glucocorticoids during the enrolment and/or study period was restricted in this study and not in the two other studies. In another study there was an initial small transient reduction in growth velocity in 1041 children aged 5–12 years, which generally occurred within the first year of treatment with budesonide 200 micrograms twice daily (26[C]). However, long-term data on final adult height suggest that children and adolescents who use inhaled budesonide in a mean daily dose of 412 micrograms ultimately achieve their adult target height (27[C]).

Additional data from a large randomized, placebo-controlled, double-blind study have confirmed budesonide-associated initial growth reduction with later compensation. In this study, 1000 children aged 5–10 years who used inhaled budesonide 200 micrograms/day for 3 years had a mean growth reduction of 1.34 cm over 3 years compared with the placebo group (28[C]). The reduction was greatest in the first year of treatment (0.58 cm) and fell during years two and three (0.43 and 0.33 cm respectively).

Data on the correlation of adrenal function with growth velocity are very limited. In a small non-randomized study there was no correlation between adrenal suppression as assessed by low-dose tetracosactide stimulation and growth deceleration in 72 asthmatic children aged 4–16 years using long-term budesonide (22[c]). There was a positive correlation between severity of asthma, assessed by FEV_1, and height, confirming the known relation between the severity of pulmonary symptoms and the degree of growth retardation.

In conclusion, while data on final adult height are reassuring (28[C], 29[C]), evidence is still insufficient as to whether long-term budesonide treatment in childhood allows children to attain their full genetic growth potential. The interpretation of growth studies is often complicated by confounding variables, including inadequate evaluation of pubertal status, inadequate control groups, lack of titration according to asthma severity, and baseline differences in age, height, and oral glucocorticoid exposure between cases and controls. Peak bone density attained during childhood may be a critical determinant of the risk of fracture in adulthood. The effects of long-term inhaled budesonide on bone mineral density have been measured in 157 asthmatic children age 5–16 years in a case-control study, by dual energy photon absorptiometry (DEXA scans) (27[C]). After treatment with budesonide at a mean daily dose of 504 micrograms for 3–6 years there were no measurable differences in bone mineral density, total bone calcium, or body composition (total fat tissue and lean body weight). There was no correlation between any of these parameters and the duration of treatment or the cumulative or current dose of budesonide.

Long-term effects   The short-term and long-term safety of budesonide in children is of paramount interest as it potentially affects growth, metabolic function (adrenals) and sensory function (the eyes). However, long-term safety data of budesonide in very young children are limited. In an open study, 198 asthmatic children aged 8 years or younger were treated with adjusted doses of budesonide inhalation suspension (initial daily doses of 0.5 mg for patients under 4 years and 1.0 mg for older children) (30[c]). There were treatment-related adverse effects in 8.6%. Oral candidiasis was the most frequent drug-related adverse event, in 2.5%. There were no cases of cataract. Adverse effects did not increase with increasing duration of treatment. Overall, this study gives evidence of a favorable long-term safety-profile of budesonide in young children. However, adrenal function and growth rate were not assessed.

In a case-control study in asthmatic children cutaneous and ocular adverse effects were specifically assessed during treatment over 3–6 years with budesonide, mean daily dose of 504 micrograms (157 cases and 111 age-matched controls) (31[c]). Budesonide was not associated with posterior subcapsular cataract, bruises, hoarseness, or other noticeable voice changes. These data suggest a beneficial long-term safety profile of budesonide at therapeutic doses in children.

Drug formulations   The lung disposition of budesonide has been studied by pharmacokinetic evaluation after a single dose of 1000 micrograms, after the use of administered from two budesonide DPIs (Giona™ Easyhaler™ and Pulmicort™ Turbuhaler™) in an open, randomized, crossover study in 33 healthy volunteers (32[c]). The two devices delivered equivalent doses of budesonide to the lungs.

℞ Ciclesonide

Ciclesonide, a non-halogenated glucocorticoid, is converted locally in the airways to an active metabolite, desisobutyrylciclesonide, which has a 100-fold greater relative glucocorticoid receptor binding affinity than ciclesonide itself (33[R]). The pharmacokinetic–pharmacodynamic profile of inhaled ciclesonide suggests a reduced potential for adverse systemic effects.

Ciclesonide is formulated in a hydrofluoroalkane-propelled MDI, and a daily dosing schedule of 160 micrograms was as active and safe in asthmatic patients as fluticasone propionate 88 micrograms twice daily (34[C]) or budesonide 200 micrograms twice daily (35[C]).

Mean intrapulmonary deposition of inhaled ciclesonide is 52%, while mean oropharyngeal deposition is 38% (36[r], 37[r]). Oropharyngeal deposition of desisobutyrylciclesonide was more than one order of magnitude lower than that of budesonide when ciclesonide was administered in a dose of 800 micrograms in healthy volunteers (38[r]). Low oropharyngeal deposition of ciclesonide and low conversion of ciclesonide to desisobutyrylciclesonide in the oropharynx (39[c], 40[c]) result in reduced local adverse effects.

Placebo-controlled studies   In a double-blind, placebo-controlled study, 1031 children with persistent asthma used ciclesonide 40, 80, or 160 micrograms daily for 12 weeks (41[C]). Oral candidiasis was reported in 0.4% and hoarseness in 0.1% of those who used ciclesonide. In a double-blind, randomized, placebo-controlled study, 531 patients with moderate to severe asthma used ciclesonide 160 or 320 micrograms twice daily or fluticasone propionate 440 micrograms twice daily for 12 weeks (42[C]). The frequency of local adverse effects was similar with ciclesonide and placebo, but significantly higher with fluticasone. The low frequency of local adverse effects with ciclesonide was confirmed in a meta-analysis in 6846 patients enrolled in ciclesonide clinical trials (43[M]).

Metabolism   The effect of ciclesonide on adrenal function has been analysed in 164 asthmatic adults in a double-blind, randomized, placebo-controlled study (44[C]). The patients used ciclesonide 320 micrograms once daily, ciclesonide 320 micrograms twice daily, or fluticasone propionate 440 micrograms twice daily for 12 weeks. Adrenal function was significantly suppressed by fluticasone propionate but not by ciclesonide. Oral candidiasis was reported in 2.4% of patients on ciclesonide versus 22% of patients on fluticasone propionate. Even high daily doses of ciclesonide up to 1280 micrograms did not suppress adrenal function, as measured by 24-hour urinary cortisol excretion (45[c]). This is in accordance with other studies in asthmatic subjects, in which serum or 24-hour urinary cortisol concentrations were unchanged by ciclesonide (46[c], 47[c], 48[c], 49[c], 50[c], 51[c], 52[c]).

A pharmacokinetic–pharmacodynamic modelling analysis pooled data from 635 adult and children using ciclesonide in daily doses of 40–2880 micrograms to study the effect of ciclesonide on endogenous cortisol release (53[C]). Using an E_{max} model, less than 1% of all observed desisobutyrylciclesonide concentrations were higher than the EC_{50} for cortisol suppression, indicating negligible changes in cortisol concentrations at therapeutically relevant doses. Systemic availability was estimated to be about 50% in patients with impaired liver function, compared with healthy individuals, but this was unlikely to be clinically significant.

In general, ciclesonide in daily doses of up to 640 micrograms can be considered to be safe with respect to adrenal function. Its long-term safety profile is similarly advantageous, and administration in daily doses up to 1280 micrograms over 52 weeks was not associated with systemic or local adverse effects in patients with persistent asthma (54[c]).

Short-term lower-leg growth rate and adrenal function was assessed in 24 children aged 6–12 years using increasing doses of ciclesonide (40, 80, and 160 micrograms) in a randomized, double-blind, placebo-controlled, crossover study (55[c]). Ciclesonide had no effect on lower-leg growth rate or adrenal function.

Fluticasone propionate

Susceptibility factors

Age   Current evidence for the safety of inhaled glucocorticoids in very young children (<4 years of age) is limited. In a double-blind, controlled multicenter study, 160 children aged 1–4 years were randomized to either fluticasone propionate 100 micrograms or placebo twice daily, both administered by MDI and Babyhaler™ for 12 weeks (56[C]). There was a significant 20% reduction in corrected urinary cortisol excretion after treatment with fluticasone group compared with placebo. The relevance of adrenal suppression is unclear, as it is unlikely that there would be clinical sequelae during this short treatment period.

Fluticasone propionate has been compared with montelukast in two randomized, double-blind studies. In the first study, 495 asthmatic children 6 to 14 years of age received montelukast 5 mg once daily or fluticasone 100 μg twice daily for one year (57[C]). Both treatments were well tolerated. Adrenal function was not assessed, but the one-year overall growth rate was lower with fluticasone than with montelukast (5.81 versus 6.18 cm/year). In the second study, 342 children aged 6–12 years used fluticasone propionate inhalation powder 50 micrograms twice daily or chewable montelukast 5 mg once daily for 12 weeks (58[C]). The mean ratios of end-point to baseline 12-hour urinary cortisol excretion rates were similar in small subsets of the groups (fluticasone propionate $n = 14$, montelukast $n = 15$). However, mean adjusted growth rates were similar between treatment groups in a previous randomized, open study in 625 children aged 1–3, using fluticasone propionate 100 micrograms twice daily or sodium cromoglicate 5 mg four times daily for 1 year (59[C]). Very young children might be less sensitive to the same daily dose of inhaled fluticasone propionate with respect to growth rate and compared with older children.

Drug formulations   The systemic effects of two formulations of fluticasone (DPI and MDI) in adults given for 1 week or 6 weeks have been studied by pooling data from two studies (60[C]). The patients in one study ($n = 33$) used fluticasone 800 micrograms/day given by DPI (Rotadisk™ Diskhaler™) or fluticasone 704 micrograms/day given by MDI with OptiChamber™ for 1 week; the patients in the other study ($n = 9$) used fluticasone 704 micrograms/day by MDI with OptiChamber™ for 6 weeks. Plasma drug concentrations were higher and accompanied by adrenal suppression with MDI than with DPI. This might be because MDIs generate smaller particle sizes, which result in increased systemic availability.

Mometasone furoate   ℞

Comparative studies   *Mometasone furoate 400 micrograms once daily has been compared with budesonide 400 micrograms once daily, both administered by DPI, in 262 patients with moderate asthma in a double-blind, randomized, placebo-controlled study (61[C]). There were treatment-related adverse effects in 8% with mometasone and placebo and in 9% with budesonide. The most common were headache and pharyngitis (both 4% or less). There was oral candidiasis in one patient using mometasone furoate.*

In another randomized, open, parallel-group study, mometasone furoate 400 micrograms once daily via DPI was compared with fluticasone propionate 250 micrograms twice daily via MDI in 167 asthmatic adults and adolescents (62[C]). Two subjects in each group developed mild-to-moderate oral candidiasis.

Mometasone furoate 400 micrograms once daily via MDI has been compared with beclomethasone dipropionate twice daily via hydrofluoroalkane or chlorofluorocarbon MDIs, given over 2 weeks in a randomized, parallel-group study (63[C]). The mean reduction in 24-hour serum cortisol $AUC_{0-2\,4}$ was significantly less with mometasone furoate (−9%) than with either beclomethasone dipropionate formulation (−23 and −24%). These data do not support negligible systemic availability or a lower potential for systemic adverse effects of mometasone furoate compared with fluticasone propionate, but suggest that adrenal suppression is less for mometasone furoate compared with beclomethasone dipropionate at therapeutic doses.

Metabolism   Adrenal suppression with DPI formulations of mometasone furoate and fluticasone propionate has been studied in 21 asthmatic patients in a randomized crossover study (64^C). Every 2 weeks the patients used consecutive doubling incremental doses of either mometasone furoate via Twisthaler^{TM} (400, 800, and 1600 micrograms/day) or fluticasone propionate via Accuhaler^{TM} (500, 1000, and 2000 micrograms/day). There was significant suppression of adrenal function with both mometasone furoate and fluticasone propionate at high and medium doses.

Drug dosage regimens   Various schedules of mometasone furoate (200 micrograms or 400 micrograms once daily, 200 micrograms twice daily) have been assessed in a double-blind, placebo-controlled study in 400 asthmatic patients (65^C). The only treatment-related adverse event that occurred at an incidence of 5% or more was oral candidiasis (6%). The incidence of treatment-related pharyngitis was under 2%.

In a similar randomized, placebo-controlled study in 268 asthmatic patients, mometasone furoate 400 micrograms once daily and 200 micrograms twice daily were compared (66^C). The most common treatment-related adverse event was oral candidiasis, which occurred in 3% of patients using 400 micrograms once daily and in 2% using 200 micrograms twice daily. Dysphonia was reported in 3% of the patients using 400 micrograms once daily and pharyngitis in 2%.

BETA$_2$-ADRENOCEPTOR AGONISTS   *(SED-15, 448; SEDA-27, 179; SEDA-28, 188; SEDA-29, 171)*

R.   *Respiratory adverse effects of long-acting beta$_2$-adrenoceptor agonists*

The long-acting beta$_2$-adrenoceptor agonists salmeterol and formoterol have proven therapeutic activity in asthmatic patients who remain symptomatic despite treatment with inhaled glucocorticoids (67^C). However, the US Food and Drug Administration (FDA) has issued a public health advisory notice alerting health care professionals and patients to the fact that these medicines may increase the chance of episodes of severe asthma and death when those episodes occur (68^S, 69^r). The announcement followed a July 2005 meeting of an FDA advisory committee on this topic. Accordingly, current FDA guidelines recommend that salmeterol or formoterol should only be added to inhaled glucocorticoids if asthma is insufficiently controlled by the latter. Furthermore, salmeterol and formoterol should be withdrawn only after consulting the treating physician, and they should not be used for the treatment of exacerbations of acute asthma. In the UK, concern about increased rates of severe illness and asthma-related deaths associated with these agents prompted researchers to undertake a large randomized, double-blind comparison of salmeterol 50 micrograms twice daily and salbutamol 200 micrograms four times daily, supplementing usual antiasthmatic treatment in 25 180 patients (70^C). Patients who used salmeterol were three times more likely to die from asthma during the trial than those who used salbutamol (12 of 16 787 patients versus two of 8393). Overall, asthma-associated deaths were very infrequent, and the study was not designed to test the hypothesis that salmeterol increased the risk of death. Moreover, the fact that a significantly higher proportion of patients in the salbutamol group than in the salmeterol group (3.8 versus 2.9%) were withdrawn might have biased the study.

In a further large study (the Salmeterol Multicenter Asthma Research Trial, SMART), 26 355 asthmatic patients were randomized to either salmeterol or placebo for 28 weeks in addition to their usual therapy (71^C). The primary study endpoint was the occurrence of respiratory-related deaths or life-threatening experiences (expressed as necessitating intubation and mechanical ventilation). Many patients withdrew from the study: 2959 (22%) in the salmeterol group and 3143 (24%) in the placebo group. Similar numbers of subjects in the two groups had severe potentially treatment-related adverse effects (143 and 134 patients in the salmeterol and placebo groups respectively). Respiratory-related deaths or life-threatening experiences were similar in the two groups, but respiratory-related deaths alone as well as asthma-related deaths were more frequent in the salmeterol group than in the placebo group (respectively: $RR = 2.16$; 95% $CI = 1.06, 4.41$; $RR = 4.4$; 95% $CI = 1.3, 15.3$). Respiratory-related and asthma-related deaths were more frequent in the salmeterol group in African–Americans ($n = 4685$), but were balanced between the groups in Caucasians ($n = 18\,642$). A possible explanation is more severe asthma in African–Americans, with less use of inhaled glucocorticoids at baseline (38%) compared with Caucasians (49%). In patients who used baseline glucocorticoids, the incidence of respiratory-related and asthma-related deaths was not increased. The low rate of baseline corticosteroid treatment is a major shortcoming of this study.

Studies similar to SMART are not available for formoterol. However, pooled data from placebo-controlled registration studies have shown an increased incidence of serious asthma-related events in 3768 patients taking formoterol compared with 1863 patients taking placebo (3.9 versus 0.9 events per 100 treatment years) (68^S). There were similar rates among patients who were using inhaled glucocorticoids concomitantly and those who were not. There was one asthma-related death among 5907 patients taking formoterol, and no asthma-related deaths in 1238 patients taking salbutamol in the analysis of all pooled controlled and uncontrolled asthma studies.

In conclusion, current data suggest an increased risk of asthma-related serious adverse effects, including asthma-related deaths in patients taking long-term ($\geqslant 6$ months) salmeterol or formoterol. There is uncertainty about the susceptibility factors that predispose patients to respiratory-related and asthma-related serious adverse effects when using salmeterol or formoterol, but current data suggest that genetics, ethnicity, and baseline corticosteroid treatment are important co-variates. The results of the SMART study in particular suggest that patients who use insufficient baseline corticosteroid treatment are at increased risk of an asthma-related death when using salmeterol.

Genetic susceptibility factors that affect the use of long-acting beta$_2$-adrenoceptor agonists

Safety data on the interrelation between beta$_2$-adrenoceptor genotypes and salbutamol treatment were reviewed in SEDA-29 (p. 173). There are several beta$_2$-adrenoceptor polymorphisms that appear to alter the behavior of the receptor after exposure to an agonist (72^R). These include the polymorphisms Arg–Gly 16 and Glu–Gln 27. The Gly 16 receptor variant down-regulates after agonist administration to a greater extent and is associated with increased airway reactivity, while the Glu 27 variant appears to protect against down-regulation and is associated with less airway reactivity. Homozygous Gly 16 was significantly more susceptible to bronchodilator tolerance in a small group of asthmatic patients (46%) than homozygous Arg 16 (8%) after administration of formoterol 24 micrograms twice daily for 4 weeks (73^c). It was suggested that the effect of Gly 16 dominates any putative protective effects of Glu 27.

In a six placebo-controlled randomized studies, in which asthmatic patients took formoterol or salmeterol for 1–2 weeks, the primary end point was either methacholine or adenosine monophosphate provocative dose/dilution causing a 20% fall in FEV_1 from baseline (PD_{20} and PC_{20} respectively) (74^M). Bronchoprotection was measured after the first and last dose of formoterol or salmeterol. Homozygous or heterozygous Arg 16 polymorphism correlated significantly with increased bronchoprotective subsensitivity compared with homozygous Gly 16 after the last dose. Bronchoprotective subsensitivity was greater with formoterol than with salmeterol for all genotypes, especially for the Arg 16 receptor variant. The results of this analysis, showing increased bronchoprotective subsensitivity with Gly 16, are apparently contrary to those of previous in vitro and in vivo studies, perhaps owing to the artificial increase in bronchomotor tone with methacholine/AMP bronchial challenge. However, the results are in line with those of previous long-term studies, in which asthmatic patients with homozygous Arg 16 taking regular salbutamol had worse outcomes than patients not homozygous for Arg 16 $(75^C, 76^C)$.

The effect of Arg 16/Gly 16 on bronchodilator response to salmeterol and the potential effect of concurrent treatment with inhaled glucocorticoids has been assessed in a retrospective analysis of two randomized, double-blind, placebo-controlled studies (77^M). In both studies, salmeterol-treated patients homozygous for Arg 16 did not benefit from the treatment *compared with patients homozygous for Gly 16, independent of the additional use of inhaled glucocorticoids. Overall, current data suggest that there is a subset of corticosteroid-treated asthmatics with increased susceptibility to bronchodilator tolerance to long-acting beta$_2$-adrenoceptor agonists used regularly, and preliminary study results suggest that formoterol may have greater bronchoprotective subsensitivity than salmeterol, probably as a consequence of the fact that formoterol is a full beta$_2$-adrenoceptor agonist while salmeterol is a partial agonist.*

Cardiovascular   Beta$_1$- and beta$_2$-adrenoceptors co-exist in the heart, in a ratio of about 3:1 (78[R]), and the cardiac effects of beta$_2$-adrenoceptor agonists are a consequence of direct activation of cardiac beta$_2$-adrenoceptors. There has been an extended meta-analysis of the cardiovascular effects of various beta$_2$-adrenoceptor agonists in randomized, placebo-controlled trials in patients with asthma or chronic obstructive pulmonary disease (COPD), including 13 single-dose trials ($n = 232$) and 20 trials of longer durations ($n = 6623$) (79[M]). At the start of treatment heart rate rose and potassium concentrations fell compared with placebo. In trials lasting from 3 days to 1 year, beta$_2$-adrenoceptor agonists significantly increased the *risk of a cardiovascular event* (RR = 2.54; 95% CI = 1.59, 4.05) compared with placebo. In most cases the event was *sinus tachycardia*. The relative risk of a cardiovascular event other than sinus tachycardia (ventricular tachycardia, atrial fibrillation, syncope, congestive heart failure, myocardial infarction, cardiac arrest, and sudden death) was not significantly increased (RR = 1.66; 95% CI = 0.76, 3.6).

A standard dose of nebulized salbutamol 5 mg significantly enhanced atrioventricular nodal conduction and reduced atrioventricular nodal, atrial, and ventricular refractoriness, in addition to its positive chronotropic effect, in adults patients with asthma or COPD (80[c]). Although dysrhythmias were not reported in this study, these effects could contribute to the generation of spontaneous dysrhythmias.

Tolerance to the hemodynamic effects of regularly inhaled salbutamol has been studied in 10 asthmatic patients and 10 matched healthy controls in a randomized, placebo-controlled,

double-blind, crossover study (81[c]). Asthmatic adults using intermittent beta$_2$-adrenoceptor agonists had a greater cardiovascular response to sympathetic stimulation by isometric exercise, but also an attenuated hemodynamic response (tachycardia, hypertonia, increased cardiac index) to acute inhalation of salbutamol 200 micrograms, suggesting hemodynamic tolerance. It is unclear if these findings represent a group effect of beta$_2$-adrenoceptor agonists or apply to salbutamol only.

Susceptibility factors

Age   In a small group of children with severe acute asthma who took fenoterol 0.5 mg/kg/dose (in total up to 15 mg) over 1 hour, there was significant tachycardia, and additional electrocardiographic changes compatible with myocardial ischemia in six of them (82[c]).

Formoterol   *(SED-15, 1443; SEDA-27, 179; SEDA-28, 188; SEDA-29, 171)*

Drug formulations   Systemic availability, as determined by serum potassium, was similar after a cumulative dose of formoterol 96 micrograms delivered via Easyhaler™ or via Aerolizer™ in 32 asthmatic patients (83[c]). The occurrence of adverse events was dose-related, the most common events being *tremor, hypokalemia, headache*, and *bouts of palpitation*; all occurred with similar frequency after both formoterol formulations. QT$_c$ intervals over 450 ms were seen only after cumulative doses of 48 and 96 micrograms, but one patient had an atrial dysrhythmia after a cumulative dose of formoterol 96 micrograms via Easyhaler™.

In a second study, the safety profile of cumulative doses of formoterol up to 96 micrograms delivered via the HFA-134a-propelled MDI device Modulite™ was comparable with that of formoterol via Foradil™ Aerolizer™ (84[c]). There were no relevant cardiac dysrhythmias during 24-hour electrocardiography in this study.

In a placebo-controlled comparison of formoterol via Modulite™, Foradil™, or Aerolizer™, at single dose of 12 micrograms in 49 patients with moderate to severe stable asthma there were no significant changes in blood pressure, heart rate, QT_c interval, or serum potassium in the two active treatment groups, but blood glucose rose significantly (85[c]).

In 500 patients with moderate to severe asthma there was similar tolerability of formoterol 12 micrograms twice daily over 12 weeks delivered via the MDI device Modulite[TM] or via the Foradil[TM] Aerolizer[TM] (86[c]).

In a multicenter, double-blind, randomized study in patients with persistent asthma, formoterol 10 micrograms delivered twice daily via the new DPI device Certihaler[TM] and compared with salbutamol 180 micrograms four times daily or placebo resulted in no clinically relevant changes in laboratory tests, vital signs, physical examination, or unexpected adverse effects (87[c]).

Drug dosage regimens   The safety of high-dose formoterol, total daily dose 108 micrograms (88[c]) and 96 micrograms (89[c]), has been assessed in two randomized, double-blind, crossover studies, compared with or high-dose salbutamol (total daily dose 1800 and 2400 micrograms respectively). In both studies, high-dose formoterol and salbutamol resulted in pronounced but clinically insignificant hypokalemia, hyperglycemia, and minimal increases in mean QT_c interval. However, the number of patients in both studies was small ($n = 16$ and $n = 17$ respectively), and the studies took no account of the idiosyncratic nature of individual increased cardiac susceptibility.

Levosalbutamol (levalbuterol)

(SEDA-28, 189, SEDA-29, 172)

Levosalbutamol is the R-enantiomer of racemic salbutamol (albuterol). A dose of 0.63 mg of levosalbutamol is considered to be equipotent to salbutamol 2.5 mg (90[c]). So far, the data on a potential negative impact of the S-enantiomer (S-salbutamol) on drug safety are controversial.

In a retrospective observational review of the admission data of 736 emergency department patients over 9 months, there were fewer admissions in patients who used nebulized levosalbutamol 1.25 mg compared with those who used racemic salbutamol 2.5 mg in addition to standard antiasthmatic treatment (91[c]). Other outcome variables were not analysed.

Susceptibility factors

Age   The safety of levosalbutamol has been assessed in 211 children aged 2–5 years in a randomized, double-blind study (92[C]). They received either levosalbutamol (0.31 or 0.63 mg regardless of body weight), racemic salbutamol (1.25 for children under 15 kg, 2.5 mg for children over 15 kg), or placebo over 3 weeks. Levosalbutamol was generally well tolerated. Racemic salbutamol and levosalbutamol 0.63 mg, but not levosalbutamol 0.31 mg or placebo, significantly increased ventricular rate. There were no significant QT_c interval changes in any treatment group. All the groups experienced hypokalemia and hyperglycemia 30–60 minutes after the last dose.

In another study, levosalbutamol 1.25 mg (up to six nebulizations) was compared with combined racemic salbutamol 5 mg + ipratropium bromide 0.25 mg (up to three nebulizations) in 140 patients aged 6–18 years with acute asthma (93[C]). The median increase in heart rate was greater with salbutamol + ipratropium bromide group than with levosalbutamol. Other safety outcomes, including nervousness, nausea/vomiting, palpitation, or headache were similar in the groups. Besides causing less tachycardia, levosalbutamol provided no advantage over combined salbutamol+ipratropium.

Salbutamol (albuterol)   *(SED-15, 3093; SEDA-27, 179, SEDA-28, 189, SEDA-29, 172)*

Metabolism   *Lactic acidosis* can occur in adults with acute severe asthma, but there is some controversy about its significance. In a prospective study, lactic acidosis was assessed in 18 adults who presented to an emergency department with acute severe asthma and were treated with high doses of salbutamol 400 micrograms at 10-minute intervals over 2 hours (94[c]). At the end of treatment, mean plasma lactate concentrations were significantly higher than at baseline. Higher plasma lactate concentrations after salbutamol treatment correlated with a shorter duration of asthma attack before presentation, higher pre-treatment heart rate, lower pre-treatment SpO_2, higher pre-treatment PCO_2, and lower pre-treatment serum potassium concentration. Therefore, the hyperadrenergic state before salbutamol treatment predisposes patients to lactic acidosis. Lactic acidosis probably results from combined endogenous adrenergic stimulation and the use of $beta_2$-adrenoceptor agonists, resulting in increased conversion of pyruvate to lactate.

The effect of nebulized salbutamol 2.5 mg on blood glucose concentration has been assessed in a double-blind, placebo-controlled study in 19 patients with insulin-dependent diabetes (9 of whom had cystic fibrosis-related diabetes) (95[c]). There were no significant differences in blood glucose concentrations at baseline or changes during treatment in the two treatment groups.

Salmeterol   *(SED-15, 3099; SEDA-28, 190)*

Drug combinations

Combined salmeterol and fluticasone propionate   In a randomized, double-blind, parallel-group study in 282 adults with asthma there was a similar overall frequency of adverse effects in patients who used combined salmeterol 50 micrograms + fluticasone propionate 250 micrograms twice daily via Diskus[TM] inhaler for 12 months, compared with monotherapy with either salmeterol or fluticasone propionate alone (96[C]). However, candidiasis and hoarseness/dysphonia were more frequent in those who used salmeterol + fluticasone propionate (6 and 11% respectively) compared with salmeterol (2 and 1% respectively) or fluticasone propionate (0 and 9% respectively). The absence of candidiasis with fluticasone propionate group raises some doubts about the accuracy of the safety assessments, as safety was not the primary study end point. Despite obvious synergistic therapeutic effects between salmeterol and fluticasone propionate, concerns about the development of tolerance to the bronchoprotective effect of salmeterol remain.

In a single-blind, crossover study in nine asthmatic patients, tolerance to the protective effect on allergen challenge of a single dose of salmeterol + fluticasone (50/250 micrograms) was compared with the effect of salmeterol + fluticasone (50/250 micrograms) twice daily for 1 week (97[c]). The results suggested minimal tolerance to the protective effect, as 80% of patients were still protected against an allergen challenge (protection index ⩾80%). Simultaneous administration of salmeterol + fluticasone propionate seems to induce less tolerance than monotherapy with a $beta_2$-adrenoceptor agonist. However, tolerance to the bronchoprotective effect of salmeterol against allergen challenge may not be homogeneously distributed in the asthmatic population.

Another controversy is fixed-dose versus adjustable maintenance dosing with combination antiasthmatic drug treatment. Fixed-dose salmeterol + fluticasone propionate 50/250 micrograms twice daily has been compared with adjustable-dose formoterol + budesonide (starting dose 6/200 micrograms twice daily) (98[C]). While the incidence of asthma exacerbations was significantly lower in the fixed-dose group, drug-related adverse effects were similar (6.3% in the fixed-dose group versus 5.9% in the adjustable-dose group). Probably a minimum daily amount of maintenance therapy is necessary to prevent asthma exacerbations in adults.

In 270 Chinese patients, a DPI formulation of salmeterol + fluticasone propionate (Seretide[TM] Diskus[TM]) 50/250 micrograms twice daily did not differ from a hydrofluoroalkane MDI formulation, consisting of the same combination and daily dose (99[C]). Overall safety was similar in the two groups, but voice alterations were more frequent with the DPI (2.9%) than the MDI (0%). Candidiasis was not reported in either group.

In 203 asthmatic children aged 4 to 11 years, twice-daily salmeterol + fluticasone propionate 50/100 micrograms has been compared with twice-daily fluticasone propionate 100 micrograms for 12 weeks in a randomized, double-blind study (100[C]). The most common drug-related adverse effects with salmeterol + fluticasone propionate and fluticasone group included headache (<1 and 4%), oral or pharyngeal candidiasis (4 and 0%), throat irritation (3 and 2%), dizziness (2 and <1%), and mood disorders (<1 and 2%). There were no signs of impaired adrenal function.

ANTICHOLINERGIC DRUGS

(SED-15, 264; SEDA-27, 179; SEDA-28, 190; SEDA-29, 174)

Tiotropium bromide   *(SED-15, 3433; SEDA-27, 180; SEDA-28, 190; SEDA-29, 174)*

Comparative studies   In a randomized, double-blind comparative study there were fewer serious adverse effects in 653 patients with COPD using tiotropium 18 micrograms daily compared with patients using salmeterol 50 micrograms twice daily over 12 weeks (2.4 versus 5.5% respectively) (101[C]). The most common adverse event related to tiotropium was a *dry mouth*, which occurred more often in patients using tiotropium than in those using salmeterol (4.9 versus 1.2% respectively).

In a second randomized, double-blind, crossover comparison of tiotropium 18 micrograms daily, formoterol 12 micrograms twice daily, or both treatments combined over 6 weeks in 71 patients with COPD seven patients withdrew owing to adverse events that were not classified as study-drug related (102[C]). Safety assessments, including blood pressure and pulse rate, electrocardiography, and laboratory safety screening (blood chemistry, hematology, and urine analysis), showed no differences between treatment periods. These results suggest that the combination of tiotropium with formoterol in the tested doses is more effective than either treatment alone at comparable tolerability.

Cardiovascular   Electrocardiographic and 24-hour Holter monitoring in 196 patients with COPD at baseline and after 8 and 12 weeks of treatment with tiotropium 18 micrograms daily was performed in a randomized, double-blind, placebo-controlled study (103[C]). Tiotropium was not associated with changes in heart rate, heart rhythm, QT interval, or conduction.

LEUKOTRIENE MODIFIERS

(SED-15, 2025; SEDA-27, 177; SEDA-28, 191; SEDA-29, 174)

Immunologic   Montelukast has been reported to be associated with systemic eosinophilia

and small vessel vasculitis or *Churg–Strauss syndrome* (reviewed in SEDA-27, 177). In a retrospective analysis of 20 cases of Churg–Strauss syndrome between 1995 and 2003, eight were associated with pranlukast; the onset was at 1–6 months after the start of pranlukast treatment (104[c]). Five of the eight patients with pranlukast-associated Churg–Strauss syndrome had taken low doses of oral or inhaled glucocorticoids without withdrawal before the onset of the syndrome, while three had not taken prior glucocorticoids. The patients with pranlukast-related Churg–Strauss syndrome had significantly higher blood eosinophil counts, higher neurological disability scores, and poor responses to glucocorticoids, compared with patients with Churg–Strauss syndrome not associated with pranlukast. However, initial disease activity was not different between the two groups. A possible explanation of pranlukast-associated Churg–Strauss syndrome in patients without prior exposure to oral or inhaled glucocorticoids may be an imbalance in activity between leukotriene B4 (LTB4) and cysteinyl leukotriene receptors, resulting in modification of chemoattraction of eosinophils and neutrophils. Patients taking pranlukast therefore have to be monitored carefully for at least 6 months after the start of treatment. This must also be considered for patients whose corticosteroid dose has not been reduced while on pranlukast, and also patients taking montelukast or zafirlukast.

Montelukast   *(SED-15, 2384; SEDA-27, 179; SEDA-28, 192, SEDA-29, 175)*

Immunologic   A *leukocytoclastic vasculitis* has been associated with montelukast in a young man (105[A]).

- A 20-year-old man with allergic rhinitis developed colicky abdominal pain and recurrent vomiting from subacute obstructive ileus. Two days later, he developed arthralgia and purpura over the arms and legs. Laboratory tests showed an acute inflammatory reaction with eosinophilia and positive antineutrophilic cytoplasmic antibodies. Endoscopy confirmed suspected ulcerative gastroenteritis and intestinal ulcers and skin lesions showed leukocytoclastic vasculitis. He recovered quickly after withdrawal of montelukast and introduction of oral prednisolone.

Susceptibility factors

Age   Montelukast 4 mg oral granules daily for 6 weeks has been assessed in children aged 6–24 months in a randomized, double-blind, placebo-controlled study (106[C]). The incidence of drug-related adverse effects was similar in the two groups, and there were no clinically important differences between treatment groups in clinical or laboratory adverse effects.

References

1. Bertoldo F, Olivieri M, Franchina G, De Blasio F, Lo Cascio V. Inhaled beclomethasone dipropionate acutely stimulates dose-dependent growth hormone secretion in healthy subjects. Chest 2005;128:902–5.
2. Sheffer AL, Silverman M, Woolcock AJ, Diaz PV, Lindberg B, Lindmark B. Long-term safety of once-daily budesonide in patients with early-onset mild persistent asthma: results of the Inhaled Steroid Treatment as Regular Therapy in Early Asthma (START) study. Ann Allergy Asthma Immunol 2005;94:48–54.
3. Gluck PA, Gluck JC. A review of pregnancy outcomes after exposure to orally inhaled or intranasal budesonide. Curr Med Res Opin 2005;21:1075–84.
4. Silverman M, Sheffer A, Diaz PV, Lindmark B, Radner F, Broddene M, de Verdier MG, Pedersen S, Pauwels RA, START Investigators Group. Outcome of pregnancy in a randomized controlled study of patients with asthma exposed to budesonide. Ann Allergy Asthma Immunol 2005;95(6):566–70.
5. Kallen B, Rydhstroem H, Aberg A. Congenital malformations after the use of inhaled budesonide in early pregnancy. Obstet Gynecol 1999;93:392–5.
6. Kallen BA, Otterblad OP. Maternal drug use in early pregnancy and infant cardiovascular defect. Reprod Toxicol 2003;17:255–61.
7. Namazy J, Schatz M, Long L, Lipkowitz M, Lillie MA, Voss M, Deitz RJ, Petitti D. Use of inhaled steroids by pregnant asthmatic women does not reduce intrauterine growth. J Allergy Clin Immunol 2004;113:427–32.
8. Norjavaara E, de Verdier MG. Normal pregnancy outcomes in a population-based study including 2,968 pregnant women exposed to budesonide. J Allergy Clin Immunol 2003;111:736–42.
9. Silverman M, Sheffer A, Diaz PV, Lindmark B, Radner F, Broddene M, de Verdier MG, Pedersen S, Pauwels RA. Outcome of pregnancy in a randomized controlled study of patients with asthma exposed to budesonide. Ann Allergy Asthma Immunol 2005;95(6):566–70.
10. Agertoft L, Andersen A, Weibull E, Pedersen S. Systemic availability and pharmacokinetics of nebulised budesonide in preschool children. Arch Dis Child 1999;80:241–7.
11. Dahlström K, Larsson P. Lung deposition and systemic availability of budesonide inhaled as nebulised suspension from different nebulisers. J Aerosol Med 1995;8:79.
12. Agertoft L, Pedersen S. Lung deposition and systemic availability of fluticasone Diskus and budesonide Turbuhaler in children. Am J Respir Crit Care Med 2003;168:779–82.
13. Thorsson L, Edsbacker S, Kallen A, Lofdahl CG. Pharmacokinetics and systemic activity of fluticasone via Diskus and pMDI, and of budesonide via Turbuhaler. Br J Clin Pharmacol 2001;52:529–38.
14. Yiallouros PK, Milner AD, Conway E, Honour JW. Adrenal function and high dose inhaled corticosteroids for asthma. Arch Dis Child 1997;76:405–10.
15. Shapiro G, Bronsky EA, LaForce CF, Mendelson L, Pearlman D, Schwartz RH, Szefler SJ. Dose-related efficacy of budesonide administered via a dry powder inhaler in the treatment of children with moderate to severe persistent asthma. J Pediatr 1998;132:976–82.
16. Priftis KN, Papadimitriou A, Gatsopoulou E, Yiallouros PK, Fretzayas A, Nicolaidou P. The effect of inhaled budesonide on adrenal and growth suppression in asthmatic children. Eur Respir J 2006;27:316–20.
17. Patel L, Wales JK, Kibirige MS, Massarano AA, Couriel JM, Clayton PE. Symptomatic adrenal insufficiency during inhaled corticosteroid treatment. Arch Dis Child 2001;85:330–4.
18. Agertoft L, Pedersen S. Effects of long-term treatment with an inhaled corticosteroid on growth and pulmonary function in asthmatic children. Respir Med 1994;88:373–81.
19. Merkus PJ, Essen-Zandvliet EE, Duiverman EJ, van Houwelingen HC, Kerrebijn KF, Quanjer PH. Long-term effect of inhaled corticosteroids on growth rate in adolescents with asthma. Pediatrics 1993;91:1121–6.
20. Reid A, Murphy C, Steen HJ, McGovern V, Shields MD. Linear growth of very young asthmatic children treated with high-dose nebulized budesonide. Acta Paediatr 1996;85:421–4.

21. Baker JW, Mellon M, Wald J, Welch M, Cruz-Rivera M, Walton-Bowen K. A multiple-dosing, placebo-controlled study of budesonide inhalation suspension given once or twice daily for treatment of persistent asthma in young children and infants. Pediatrics 1999;103:414–21.

22. Kemp JP, Skoner DP, Szefler SJ, Walton-Bowen K, Cruz-Rivera M, Smith JA. Once-daily budesonide inhalation suspension for the treatment of persistent asthma in infants and young children. Ann Allergy Asthma Immunol 1999;83:231–9.

23. Shapiro G, Mendelson L, Kraemer MJ, Cruz-Rivera M, Walton-Bowen K, Smith JA. Efficacy and safety of budesonide inhalation suspension (Pulmicort Respules) in young children with inhaled steroid-dependent, persistent asthma. J Allergy Clin Immunol 1998;102:789–96.

24. Scott MB, Skoner DP. Short-term and long-term safety of budesonide inhalation suspension in infants and young children with persistent asthma. J Allergy Clin Immunol 1999;104:200–9.

25. Skoner DP, Szefler SJ, Welch M, Walton-Bowen K, Cruz-Rivera M, Smith JA. Longitudinal growth in infants and young children treated with budesonide inhalation suspension for persistent asthma. J Allergy Clin Immunol 2000;105:259–68.

26. The Childhood Asthma Management Program Research Group. Long-term effects of budesonide or nedocromil in children with asthma. N Engl J Med 2000;343:1054–63.

27. Agertoft L, Pedersen S. Effect of long-term treatment with inhaled budesonide on adult height in children with asthma. N Engl J Med 2000;343:1064–9.

28. Pauwels RA, Pedersen S, Busse WW, Tan WC, Chen YZ, Ohlsson SV, Ullman A, Lamm CJ, O'Byrne PM. Early intervention with budesonide in mild persistent asthma: a randomised, double-blind trial. Lancet 2003;361:1071–6.

29. Agertoft L, Pedersen S. Bone mineral density in children with asthma receiving long-term treatment with inhaled budesonide. Am J Respir Crit Care Med 1998;157:178–83.

30. Agertoft L, Larsen FE, Pedersen S. Posterior subcapsular cataracts, bruises and hoarseness in children with asthma receiving long-term treatment with inhaled budesonide. Eur Respir J 1998;12:130–5.

31. Leflein JG, Baker JW, Eigen H, Lyzell E, McDermott L. Safety features of budesonide inhalation suspension in the long-term treatment of asthma in young children. Adv Ther 2005;22:198–207.

32. Lahelma S, Kirjavainen M, Kela M, Herttuainen J, Vahteristo M, Silvasti M, Ranki-Pesonen M. Equivalent lung deposition of budesonide in vivo: a comparison of dry powder inhalers using a pharmacokinetic method. Br J Clin Pharmacol 2005;59:167–73.

33. Christie P. Ciclesonide: a novel inhaled corticosteroid for asthma. Drugs Today (Barc) 2004;40:569–76.

34. Buhl R, Vinkler I, Magyar P, Gyori Z, Rybacki C, Middle MV, Escher A, Engelstatter R. Comparable efficacy of ciclesonide once daily versus fluticasone propionate twice daily in asthma. Pulm Pharmacol Ther 2006;19(6):404–12.

35. Niphadkar P, Jagannath K, Joshi JM, Awad N, Boss H, Hellbardt S, Gadgil DA. Comparison of the efficacy of ciclesonide 160 mug QD and budesonide 200 mug BID in adults with persistent asthma: a phase III, randomized, double-dummy, open-label study. Clin Ther 2005;27:1752–63.

36. Bethke TD, Boudreau RJ, Hasselquist BE High lung deposition fo ciclesonide in 2D- and 3D-imaging. In: 12th annual congress of the European Respiratory Society (ERS), vol. 30. September 14–18, Stockholm, Sweden. 2002, p. S38.

37. Drollmann A, Hasselquist BE, Boudreau RJ Ciclesonide shows high lung deposition in 2D and 3D-imaging. In: 98th international conference of the American Thoracic Society (ATS). May 17–22, Atlanta. 2002, p. 165.

38. Nave R, Zech K, Bethke TD. Lower oropharyngeal deposition of inhaled ciclesonide via hydrofluoroalkane metered-dose inhaler compared with budesonide via chlorofluorocarbon metered-dose inhaler in healthy subjects. Eur J Clin Pharmacol 2005;61:203–8.

39. Nave R, Bethke TD, van Marle SP, Zech K. Pharmacokinetics of [14C]ciclesonide after oral and intravenous administration to healthy subjects. Clin Pharmacokinet 2004;43:479–86.

40. Richter K, Kanniess F, Biberger C, Nave R, Magnussen H. Comparison of the oropharyngeal deposition of inhaled ciclesonide and fluticasone propionate in patients with asthma. J Clin Pharmacol 2005;45:146–52.

41. Gelfand E, Boguniewicz M, Weinstein S, Bernstein C, Lloyd M, Zhang P, Williams J, Banerji D, Hamedani P. Ciclesonide, administered once daily, has a low incidence of oropharyngeal adverse events in pediatric asthma patients. J Allergy Clin Immunol 2005;115(2):213.

42. Bernstein JA, Nonan MJ, Rim C, Fish J, Kundu S, Williams J, Banerji DD, Hamedani P. Ciclesonide has minimal oropharyngeal side effects in the treatment of patients with moderate-to-severe asthma. J Allergy Clin Immunol 2004;113(2):113.

43. Engelstätter R, Banerji D, Steinijans VW Low incidence of oropharyngeal adverse events in asthma patients treated with ciclesonide: results from a pooled analysis. In: 100th international conference of the American Thoracic Society (ATS). May 21–26, Orlando, Florida. 2004.

44. Lipworth BJ, Kaliner MA, LaForce CF, Baker JW, Kaiser HB, Amin D, Kundu S, Williams JE, Engelstaetter R, Banerji DD. Effect of ciclesonide and fluticasone on hypothalamic–pituitary–adrenal axis function in adults with mild-to-moderate persistent

asthma. Ann Allergy Asthma Immunol 2005;94:465–72.

45. Szefler SJ, Rohatagi S, Williams JE, Lloyd M, Kundu S, Banerji D. Ciclesonide, a novel inhaled steroid, does not affect hypothalamic–pituitary–adrenal axis function in patients with moderate-to-severe persistent asthma. Chest 2005;128(3):1104–14.

46. Derom E, Van DV, Marissens S, Engelstatter R, Vincken W, Pauwels R. Effects of inhaled ciclesonide and fluticasone propionate on cortisol secretion and airway responsiveness to adenosine 5'monophosphate in asthmatic patients. Pulm Pharmacol Ther 2005;18:328–36.

47. Langdon CG, Adler M, Mehra S, Alexander M, Drollmann A. Once-daily ciclesonide 80 or 320 microg for 12 weeks is safe and effective in patients with persistent asthma. Respir Med 2005;99:1275–85.

48. Pearlman DS, Berger WE, Kerwin E, LaForce C, Kundu S, Banerji D. Once-daily ciclesonide improves lung function and is well tolerated by patients with mild-to-moderate persistent asthma. J Allergy Clin Immunol 2005;116:1206–12.

49. Postma DS, Sevette C, Martinat Y, Schlosser N, Aumann J, Kafe H. Treatment of asthma by the inhaled corticosteroid ciclesonide given either in the morning or evening. Eur Respir J 2001;17:1083–8.

50. Szefler S, Rohatagi S, Williams J, Lloyd M, Kundu S, Banerji D. Ciclesonide, a novel inhaled steroid, does not affect hypothalamic–pituitary–adrenal axis function in patients with moderate-to-severe persistent asthma. Chest 2005;128:1104–14.

51. Weinbrenner A, Huneke D, Zschiesche M, Engel G, Timmer W, Steinijans VW, Bethke T, Wurst W, Drollmann A, Kaatz HJ, Siegmund W. Circadian rhythm of serum cortisol after repeated inhalation of the new topical steroid ciclesonide. J Clin Endocrinol Metab 2002;87:2160–3.

52. Lee DK, Fardon TC, Bates CE, Haggart K, McFarlane LC, Lipworth BJ. Airway and systemic effects of hydrofluoroalkane formulations of high-dose ciclesonide and fluticasone in moderate persistent asthma. Chest 2005;127:851–60.

53. Rohatagi S, Krishnaswami S, Pfister M, Sahasranaman S. Model-based covariate pharmacokinetic analysis and lack of cortisol suppression by the new inhaled corticosteroid ciclesonide using a novel cortisol release model. Am J Ther 2005;12:385–97.

54. Chapman KR, Boulet LP, D'Urzo AD Long-term administration of ciclesonide is safe and well tolerated in patients with persistent asthma. In: 4th triennial World Asthma Meeting (WAM). February 16–19, Bangkok, Thailand. 2004, p. 61.

55. Agertoft L, Pedersen S. Short-term lower-leg growth rate and urine cortisol excretion in children treated with ciclesonide. J Allergy Clin Immunol 2005;115:940–5.

56. Carlsen KC, Stick S, Kamin W, Cirule I, Hughes S, Wixon C. The efficacy and safety of fluticasone propionate in very young children with persistent asthma symptoms. Respir Med 2005;99:1393–402.

57. Garcia Garcia ML, Wahn U, Gilles L, Swern A, Tozzi CA, Polos P. Montelukast, compared with fluticasone, for control of asthma among 6- to 14-year-old patients with mild asthma: the MOSAIC study. Pediatrics 2005;116:360–9.

58. Ostrom NK, Decotiis BA, Lincourt WR, Edwards LD, Hanson KM, Carranza Jr R, Crim C. Comparative efficacy and safety of low-dose fluticasone propionate and montelukast in children with persistent asthma. J Pediatr 2005;147:213–20.

59. Bisgaard H, Allen D, Milanowski J, Kalev I, Willits L, Davies P. Twelve-month safety and efficacy of inhaled fluticasone propionate in children aged 1 to 3 years with recurrent wheezing. Pediatrics 2004;113:e87–94.

60. Whelan GJ, Blumer JL, Martin RJ, Szefler SJ. Fluticasone propionate plasma concentration and systemic effect: effect of delivery device and duration of administration. J Allergy Clin Immunol 2005;116:525–30.

61. Corren J, Berkowitz R, Murray JJ, Prenner B. Comparison of once-daily mometasone furoate versus once-daily budesonide in patients with moderate persistent asthma. Int J Clin Pract 2003;57:567–72.

62. Wardlaw A, Larivee P, Eller J, Cockcroft DW, Ghaly L, Harris AG. Efficacy and safety of mometasone furoate dry powder inhaler vs fluticasone propionate metered-dose inhaler in asthma subjects previously using fluticasone propionate. Ann Allergy Asthma Immunol 2004;93:49–55.

63. Chrousos GP, Ghaly L, Shedden A, Iezzoni DG, Harris AG. Effects of mometasone furoate dry powder inhaler and beclomethasone dipropionate hydrofluoroalkane and chlorofluorocarbon on the hypothalamic–pituitary–adrenal axis in asthmatic subjects. Chest 2005;128:70–7.

64. Fardon TC, Lee DK, Haggart K, McFarlane LC, Lipworth BJ. Adrenal suppression with dry powder formulations of fluticasone propionate and mometasone furoate. Am J Respir Crit Care Med 2004;170:960–6.

65. D'Urzo A, Karpel JP, Busse WW, Boulet LP, Monahan ME, Lutsky B, Staudinger H. Efficacy and safety of mometasone furoate administered once-daily in the evening in patients with persistent asthma dependent on inhaled corticosteroids. Curr Med Res Opin 2005;21:1281–9.

66. Karpel JP, Busse WW, Noonan MJ, Monahan ME, Lutsky B, Staudinger H. Effects of mometasone furoate given once daily in the evening on lung function and symptom control in persistent asthma. Ann Pharmacother 2005;39:1977–83.

67. Greening AP, Ind PW, Northfield M, Shaw G. Added salmeterol versus higher-dose corticosteroid in asthma patients with symptoms on existing inhaled corticosteroid. Allen &

Hanburys Limited UK Study Group. Lancet 1994;344:219–24.

68. Food and Drug Administration. Pulmonary-Allergy Drugs Advisory Committee, June 13, 2005. Briefing information. www.fda.gov/ohrms/dockets/ac/05/briefing/2005-4148% 20index%20with%20disclaimer-13.htm [last visited April 12, 2007].

69. Martinez FD. Safety of long-acting beta-agonists—an urgent need to clear the air. N Engl J Med 2005;353:2637–9.

70. Castle W, Fuller R, Hall J, Palmer J. Serevent nationwide surveillance study: comparison of salmeterol with salbutamol in asthmatic patients who require regular bronchodilator treatment. BMJ 1993;306:1034–7.

71. Perera BJ. Salmeterol multicentre asthma research trial (SMART): interim analysis shows increased risk of asthma related deaths. Ceylon Med J 2003;48:99.

72. Johnson M. The beta-adrenoceptor. Am J Respir Crit Care Med 1998;158:S146–53.

73. Tan S, Hall IP, Dewar J, Dow E, Lipworth B. Association between beta 2-adrenoceptor polymorphism and susceptibility to bronchodilator desensitisation in moderately severe stable asthmatics. Lancet 1997;350:995–9.

74. Lee DK, Currie GP, Hall IP, Lima JJ, Lipworth BJ. The arginine-16 beta2-adrenoceptor polymorphism predisposes to bronchoprotective subsensitivity in patients treated with formoterol and salmeterol. Br J Clin Pharmacol 2004;57:68–75.

75. Israel E, Drazen JM, Liggett SB, Boushey HA, Cherniack RM, Chinchilli VM, Cooper DM, Fahy JV, Fish JE, Ford JG, Kraft M, Kunselman S, Lazarus SC, Lemanske RF, Martin RJ, McLean DE, Peters SP, Silverman EK, Sorkness CA, Szefler SJ, Weiss ST, Yandava CN. The effect of polymorphisms of the beta(2)-adrenergic receptor on the response to regular use of albuterol in asthma. Am J Respir Crit Care Med 2000;162:75–80.

76. Taylor DR, Drazen JM, Herbison GP, Yandava CN, Hancox RJ, Town GI. Asthma exacerbations during long term beta agonist use: influence of beta(2) adrenoceptor polymorphism. Thorax 2000;55:762–7.

77. Wechsler ME, Lehman E, Lazarus SC, Lemanske Jr RF, Boushey HA, Deykin A, Fahy JV, Sorkness CA, Chinchilli VM, Craig TJ, Dimango E, Kraft M, Leone F, Martin RJ, Peters SP, Szefler SJ, Liu W, Israel E. Beta-adrenergic receptor polymorphisms and response to salmeterol. Am J Respir Crit Care Med 2006;173:519–26.

78. Bristow MR. Beta-adrenergic receptor blockade in chronic heart failure. Circulation 2000;101:558–69.

79. Salpeter SR, Ormiston TM, Salpeter EE. Cardiovascular effects of beta-agonists in patients with asthma and COPD: a meta-analysis. Chest 2004;125:2309–21.

80. Kallergis EM, Manios EG, Kanoupakis EM, Schiza SE, Mavrakis HE, Klapsinos NK, Vardas PE. Acute electrophysiologic effects of inhaled salbutamol in humans. Chest 2005;127:2057–63.

81. Waring WS, Leigh RB. Haemodynamic responses to salbutamol and isometric exercise are altered in young adults with mild asthma. Eur J Clin Pharmacol 2005;61:9–14.

82. Zanoni LZ, Palhares DB, Consolo LC. Myocardial ischemia induced by nebulized fenoterol for severe childhood asthma. Indian Pediatr 2005;42:1013–8.

83. Randell J, Saarinen A, Walamies M, Vahteristo M, Silvasti M, Lahelma S. Safety of formoterol after cumulative dosing via Easyhaler and Aerolizer. Respir Med 2005;99:1485–93.

84. Molimard M, Guenole E, Duvauchelle T, Vicaut E, Lefrancois G. A randomized, double-blind, double-dummy, safety crossover trial comparing cumulative doses up to 96 microg of formoterol delivered via an HFA-134a-propelled pMDI vs. same cumulative doses of formoterol DPI and placebo in asthmatic patients. Respiration 2005;72(Suppl 1):28–34.

85. Bousquet J, Huchon G, Leclerc V, Vicaut E, Lefrancois G. A randomized, double-blind, double-dummy, single-dose, efficacy crossover trial comparing formoterol-HFA (pMDI) versus formoterol-DPI (Aerolizer) and placebo (pMDI or Aerolizer) in asthmatic patients. Respiration 2005;72(Suppl 1):6–12.

86. Dusser D, Vicaut E, Lefrancois G. Double-blind, double-dummy, multinational, multicenter, parallel-group design clinical trial of clinical non-inferiority of formoterol 12 microg/unit dose in a b.i.d. regimen administered via an HFA-propellant-pMDI or a dry powder inhaler in a 12-week treatment period of moderate to severe stable persistent asthma in adult patients. Respiration 2005;72(Suppl 1):20–7.

87. LaForce C, Prenner BM, Andriano K, Lavecchia C, Yegen U. Efficacy and safety of formoterol delivered via a new multidose dry powder inhaler (Certihaler) in adolescents and adults with persistent asthma. J Asthma 2005;42:101–6.

88. Kruse M, Rosenkranz B, Dobson C, Ayre G, Horowitz A. Safety and tolerability of high-dose formoterol (Aerolizer) and salbutamol (pMDI) in patients with mild/moderate, persistent asthma. Pulm Pharmacol Ther 2005;18:229–34.

89. Rosenkranz B, Rouzier R, Kruse M, Dobson C, Ayre G, Horowitz A, Fitoussi S. Safety and tolerability of high-dose formoterol (via Aerolizer®) and salbutamol in patients with chronic obstructive pulmonary disease. Respir Med 2006;100(4):666–72.

90. Handley DA, Tinkelman D, Noonan M, Rollins TE, Snider ME, Caron J. Dose-response evaluation of levalbuterol versus racemic albuterol in patients with asthma. J Asthma 2000;37:319–27.

91. Schreck DM, Babin S. Comparison of racemic albuterol and levalbuterol in the treatment of acute asthma in the ED. Am J Emerg Med 2005;23:842–7.

92. Skoner DP, Greos LS, Kim KT, Roach JM, Parsey M, Baumgartner RA. Evaluation of the safety and efficacy of levalbuterol in 2–5-year-old patients with asthma. Pediatr Pulmonol 2005;40:477–86.

93. Ralston ME, Euwema MS, Knecht KR, Ziolkowski TJ, Coakley TA, Cline SM. Comparison of levalbuterol and racemic albuterol combined with ipratropium bromide in acute pediatric asthma: a randomized controlled trial. J Emerg Med 2005;29:29–35.

94. Rodrigo GJ, Rodrigo C. Elevated plasma lactate level associated with high dose inhaled albuterol therapy in acute severe asthma. Emerg Med J 2005;22:404–8.

95. Konig P, Goldstein D, Poehlmann M, Rife D, Ge B, Hewett J. Effect of nebulized albuterol on blood glucose in patients with diabetes mellitus with and without cystic fibrosis. Pediatr Pulmonol 2005;40:105–8.

96. Lundback B, Ronmark E, Lindberg A, Jonsson AC, Larsson LG, Petavy F, James M. Control of mild to moderate asthma over 1-year with the combination of salmeterol and fluticasone propionate. Respir Med 2006;100:2–10.

97. Paggiaro PL, Giannini D, Di Franco A, Bacci E, Dente FL, Vagaggini B, Tonelli M, Zingoni M. Minimal tolerance to the bronchoprotective effect of inhaled salmeterol/fluticasone combination on allergene challenge. Pulm Pharmacol Ther 2006;19(6):425–9.

98. FitzGerald JM, Boulet LP, Follows RM. The CONCEPT trial: a 1-year, multicenter, randomized, double-blind, double-dummy comparison of a stable dosing regimen of salmeterol/fluticasone propionate with an adjustable maintenance dosing regimen of formoterol/budesonide in adults with persistent asthma. Clin Ther 2005;27:393–406.

99. You-Ning L, Humphries M, Du X, Wang L, Jiang J. Efficacy and safety of salmeterol/fluticasone propionate delivered via a hydrofluoroalkane metered dose inhaler in Chinese patients with moderate asthma poorly controlled with inhaled corticosteroids. Int J Clin Pract 2005;59:754–9.

100. Malone R, LaForce C, Nimmagadda S, Schoaf L, House K, Ellsworth A, Dorinsky P. The safety of twice-daily treatment with fluticasone propionate and salmeterol in pediatric patients with persistent asthma. Ann Allergy Asthma Immunol 2005;95:66–71.

101. Briggs Jr DD, Covelli H, Lapidus R, Bhattycharya S, Kesten S, Cassino C. Improved daytime spirometric efficacy of tiotropium compared with salmeterol in patients with COPD. Pulm Pharmacol Ther 2005;18:397–404.

102. van Noord JA, Aumann JL, Janssens E, Smeets JJ, Verhaert J, Disse B, Mueller A, Cornelissen PJ. Comparison of tiotropium once daily, formoterol twice daily and both combined once daily in patients with COPD. Eur Respir J 2005;26:214–22.

103. Covelli H, Bhattacharya S, Cassino C, Conoscenti C, Kesten S. Absence of electrocardiographic findings and improved function with once-daily tiotropium in patients with chronic obstructive pulmonary disease. Pharmacotherapy 2005;25:1708–18.

104. Shimbo J, Onodera O, Tanaka K, Tsuji S. Churg–Strauss syndrome and the leukotriene receptor antagonist pranlukast. Clin Rheumatol 2005;24:661–2.

105. Khanna S, Uniyal B, Kumar D, Vij J. Henoch–Schonlein purpura probably due to montelukast presenting as subacute intestinal obstruction. Indian J Gastroenterol 2005;24:86.

106. van Adelsberg J, Moy J, Wei LX, Tozzi CA, Knorr B, Reiss TF. Safety, tolerability, and exploratory efficacy of montelukast in 6- to 24-month-old patients with asthma. Curr Med Res Opin 2005;21:971–9.

J.K. Aronson

17 Positive inotropic drugs and drugs used in dysrhythmias

CARDIAC GLYCOSIDES (SED-15, 648; SEDA-27, 185; SEDA-28, 196; SEDA-29, 182)

Cardiovascular Any type of cardiac dysrhythmia can occur in digitalis intoxication, and further examples have been reported:

- *bidirectional ventricular tachycardia* in an 86-year-old woman with renal insufficiency whose serum digoxin concentration was 13 ng/ml (digoxin dose 250 micrograms/day) (1[A]); the tachycardia resolved after 6 days, when the digoxin concentration fell to 1.6 ng/ml.
- a *broad complex tachycardia* due to hyperkalemia and mild digoxin toxicity in a 78-year-old woman (2[A]);
- *asystolic cardiac arrest* 1 week after surgical repair of a congenital heart anomaly in a 12-week-old girl (3[A]).

Hematologic Cardiac glycosides inhibit Na/K-ATPase, causing changes in intracellular calcium concentration. Increased intracellular calcium is a key event in *platelet activation*, and there is evidence that cardiac glycosides activate platelets in vitro, albeit in high concentrations (4[E], 5[E]). Platelet and endothelial functions have been studied in 30 patients with non-valvular atrial fibrillation, 16 of whom were taking digoxin (mean plasma digoxin concentration 1.2 nmol/l) (6[c]). Digoxin significantly increased platelet CD62P expression and platelet–leukocyte conjugates and markedly increased EMP62E and EMP31, markers of

endothelial activation. After adjusting for potential confounders (including age, congestive heart failure, coronary artery disease, ejection fraction, antiplatelet drugs, beta-blockers, and calcium channel blockers), the differences persisted. The authors concluded that if digitalis activates endothelial cells and platelets it could predispose to thrombosis and vascular events. However, there is no evidence that that happens clinically.

Death The only prospective randomized trial of the use of digoxin in patients with congestive heart failure, the Digitalis Investigation Group (DIG) study, showed that there were no beneficial effects on mortality (SEDA-20, 173). However, a post hoc re-analysis of the data from that study suggested that mortality might be increased in patients with higher plasma digoxin concentrations (SEDA-27, 185). If this were true, it would suggest that lower digoxin concentrations (0.5–0.8 ng/ml) would be associated with a reduced death rate and this has again been hypothesized (7[H]).

Evidence that that is in fact so has come from another retrospective analysis of the Digitalis Investigation Group (DIG) study, in which continuous multivariable analysis showed a significant linear relation between serum digoxin concentration and mortality, with no effect of sex (8[c]). The hazard ratios (HR) for mortality varied with serum concentration, with reduced mortality at serum concentrations of 0.5–0.9 ng/ml (HR = 0.81; 95% CI = 0.71, 0.92) and increased mortality at concentrations of 1.2–2.0 ng/ml (HR = 1.21; CI = 1.05, 1.40). However, digoxin reduced the risk of hospitalization at all serum concentrations.

Gastrointestinal Digitalis can rarely cause ischemic colitis and a case of *necrotic enterocolitis* might have been related to digoxin

Side Effects of Drugs, Annual 30
J.K. Aronson (Editor)
ISSN: 0378-6080
DOI: 10.1016/S0378-6080(08)00017-2

toxicity in a neonate (9[A]). However, the authors did not highlight this in their report, but instead emphasized that digitalis intoxication in neonates may present with vomiting and no cardiac signs of toxicity.

Susceptibility factors

Sex   Post-hoc analysis of the results of the DIG study suggested that digoxin may adversely affect survival in women but not in men (SEDA-27, 185). Among patients with left ventricular dysfunction enrolled in the Studies of Left Ventricular Dysfunction (SOLVD) with left ventricular ejection fractions of 0.35 and below, there was no interaction between sex and digitalis treatment in respect of survival, and there was no significant difference in the hazard ratios for men and women taking digitalis with respect to all-cause mortality, cardiovascular mortality, heart failure mortality, or dysrhythmic death with worsening heart failure (10[c]). The authors concluded that there was no evidence of a difference between men and women in the effect of digitalis on survival. This has been confirmed by a reanalysis of the data from the Digitalis Investigation Group (DIG) study (8[c]).

Drug overdose   A fatal case of poisoning involving verapamil, metoprolol, and digoxin has been reported (11[A]).

- A 39-year-old man was found dead in his room with empty packets of prescribed drugs nearby. The blood concentrations of verapamil, norverapamil, metoprolol and digoxin were 9.2, 3.0, 3.6 µg/ml, and 3.2 ng/ml respectively.

This was a complicated case of overdose. There is a pharmacodynamic interaction of beta-blockers with verapamil (SED-15, 603) and verapamil may have inhibited the metabolism of metoprolol via CYP2D6 (12[E]); verapamil also inhibits the clearance of digoxin (SED-15, 604). Based on the results of an autopsy and toxicological examination, death was attributed to cardiac failure, hypotension, and bradycardia due to combined overdose of verapamil, metoprolol, and digoxin.

Digoxin-specific Fab antibody fragments have been used to treat oleander intoxication in a 7-year-old child (13[Ar]) and a 44-year-old man (14[A]).

Drug–drug interactions

Clarithromycin   The macrolide antimicrobial drugs can reportedly interact with digoxin by at least two mechanisms: by reducing its metabolism in the gut before absorption (by inhibiting the growth of the bacterium *Eubacterium glenum*) and by inhibiting P glycoprotein. However, there have been conflicting reports that clarithromycin can either reduce or increase the renal clearance of digoxin (SEDA-27, 186; SEDA-28, 198). In six men with end-stage renal disease clarithromycin increased serum digoxin concentrations by 1.8–4.0 times (15[A]). In three cases the increase occurred within 12 days and in the other three at 53–190 days. The authors attributed the increase in serum digoxin to inhibition by clarithromycin of P glycoprotein in the intestine and/or bile capillaries rather than the kidneys, since renal function was dramatically impaired and four of the patients were anuric.

Exenatide   In an open study exenatide had little effect on the steady-state pharmacokinetics of digoxin in 21 healthy men (16[C]). A small fall in $C_{ss.max}$ and a small prolongation of $t_{ss.max}$ were thought to be of no clinical importance.

Hypericum perforatum (St John's wort)   There are conflicting reports about a possible interaction of *Hypericum perforatum* with digoxin.

The effect of an extract of *Hypericum perforatum* (St John's wort) on the pharmacokinetics of digoxin have been investigated in 25 subjects in a single-blind, parallel, placebo-controlled study (17[C]). St John's wort had no effect on the pharmacokinetics of digoxin after a single dose but after 10 days there was a 25% reduction in the steady-state AUC of digoxin and reductions in $C_{ss.max}$ (33%) and $C_{ss.min}$ (26%). The authors suggested that the mechanism might be induction of P glycoprotein.

In another randomized, placebo-controlled, parallel-group study in 96 healthy volunteers a 7-day loading phase with digoxin was followed by 14 days of co-medication with placebo or one of 10 St John's wort products varying in dose and type of formulation (18[C]). The high-dose hyperforin-rich extract LI 160 reduced the steady-state AUC of digoxin by 25% (95% CI = 21, 28), the $C_{ss.max}$ by 37% (32, 42), and the $C_{ss.min}$ by 19% (11, 27). Co-medication with hypericum powder 4 g with comparable hyper-forin content resulted in reductions in digoxin AUC by 27% (16, 37), $C_{ss.max}$ by 38% (18, 48), and $C_{ss.min}$ by 19% (10, 27). Hypericum powder 2 g with half the hyperforin content reduced AUC by 18% (14, 22), $C_{ss.max}$ by 21% (2, 40), and $C_{ss.min}$ by 13% (5, 21). The authors concluded that the interaction of St John's wort with digoxin correlates with the dose of hyperforin.

In contrast, in a randomized, placebo-controlled study of a low-dose extract of *Hypericum*, hyperforin had no effect on the steady-state AUC of digoxin (19[C]).

- An 80-year-old man taking long-term digoxin started to take St John's wort herbal tea 2 l/day and later developed digoxin poisoning, with a nodal bradycardia at 36/minute and bigeminy (20[A]).

This was not a convincing report.

It is likely that St John's wort has a small effect on the pharmacokinetics of digoxin, since the transport of digoxin in the gut and kidneys is partly mediated by P glycoprotein, which is induced by St John's wort. However, different formulations of St John's wort are likely to have different effects and it is not clear whether any interaction has clinical significance.

Lasofoxifene In 12 healthy postmenopausal women lasofoxifene had no effect on the steady-state pharmacokinetics of digoxin (21[C]).

Selective serotonin reuptake inhibitors There is in vitro evidence that some selective serotonin reuptake inhibitors (SSRIs) inhibit P glycoprotein, which is responsible for active transport of digoxin in the gut and kidneys. In a nested case–control study of patients aged 66 years or older, hospital admissions for digoxin toxicity were related to SSRI therapy in the previous 30 days (22[C]). Among 245 305 patients taking digoxin there were 3144 cases of digoxin toxicity. After adjusting for potential confounders, there was an increased risk of digoxin toxicity after the start of therapy with paroxetine (OR = 2.8; 95% CI = 1.6, 4.7), fluoxetine (OR = 2.9; CI = 1.5, 5.4), sertraline (OR = 3.0; CI = 1.9, 4.7), and fluvoxamine (OR = 3.0; CI = 1.5, 5.7). However, there was also an increased risk with tricyclic antidepressants (OR = 1.5; 95% CI = 1.0,

2.4) and benzodiazepines (OR = 2.1; 95% CI = 1.7, 2.5), drug classes that have no known pharmacokinetic interaction with digoxin and do not inhibit P glycoprotein. There were no statistical differences in the risks of digoxin toxicity among any of the agents tested. The authors therefore suggested that SSRIs do not increase the risk of digoxin toxicity and that inhibition of P glycoprotein by sertraline and paroxetine is unlikely to be of major clinical significance.

Interference with diagnostic tests In one case *Eleutheroccus senticosus* (Siberian ginseng) increased the serum concentration of digoxin (23[A]), probably because ginseng can give false readings in digoxin radioimmunoassay rather than by an in vivo interaction. This effect varies from formulation to formulation and from assay to assay (24[E], 25[E]).

Therapeutic doses of cardiac glycosides increase serum concentrations of A and B natriuretic peptides (ANP and BNP) (26[c], 27[c]). There has now been a report of a large *increase in BNP* in a patient with digitalis toxicity (28[A]).

- A 78-year-old woman with congestive heart failure developed nausea, increasing dyspnea on exertion, and leg edema. Her heart rate was 50/minute and her respiratory rate 30/minute. An electrocardiogram showed sinus bradycardia with left bundle-branch block. The serum potassium concentration was 7.0 mmol/l, the serum creatinine was 221 mol/l, and she had a compensated metabolic acidosis. The serum digoxin concentration was 4.2 ng/ml. The serum concentration of B natriuretic peptide (BNP) was greater than 1300 pg/ml (the upper limit of the assay).

Monitoring drug therapy In a patient with digoxin toxicity the plasma digoxin concentration measured with a microparticle enzyme immunoassay (MEIA/AxSYM) gave consistently lower results than other methods, enzyme multiplied immunoassay (EMIT/Cobas), fluorescence polarization immunoassay (FPIA/FLx), and liquid chromatography–electrospray–mass spectrometry (29[A]). The source of the negative interference was not discovered.

OTHER POSITIVE INOTROPIC DRUGS   (SED-15, 2822; SEDA-27, 188; SEDA-28, 199; SEDA-29, 183)

Milrinone   (SED-15, 2346; SEDA-27, 188; SEDA-28, 199; SEDA-29, 183)

Systematic reviews   The role of intravenous inotropic agents with vasodilator properties (so-called inodilators) in the management of acute heart failure syndromes has been reviewed (30[M]). Randomized controlled trials of the currently available medications, dobutamine, dopamine, and milrinone, have failed to show benefits and the results suggest that acute, intermittent, or continuous intravenous use of such drugs may increase morbidity and mortality. Their use should be restricted to patients who are hypotensive as a result of low cardiac output despite a high left ventricular filling pressure.

Hematologic   In a historically controlled trial in 24 children with severe pulmonary edema induced by enterovirus 71 (EV71) in southern Taiwan the mortality was lower in those who were given milrinone (36 versus 92%) (31[c]). There were significant *reductions in white blood cell count* (10.8 versus 19.5×10^9/l) *and platelet count* (257 versus 400×10^9/l).

DRUGS USED IN DYSRHYTHMIAS

Cardiovascular   Prolongation of the QT_c interval, resulting from inhibition of the human ether-a-go-go related gene (HERG) potassium channels by antidysrhythmic drugs, can cause serious ventricular dysrhythmias and sudden death. In 284 426 patients with suspected adverse reactions to drugs that are known to inhibit HERG channels reported to the International Drug Monitoring Program of the World Health Organization (WHO-UMC) up to the first quarter of 2003, 5591 cases (cardiac arrest, sudden death, torsade de pointes, ventricular fibrillation, and ventricular tachycardia) were compared with 278 835 non-cases (32[S]). HERG inhibitory activity was defined as the effective

Table 1. *HERG inhibitory activities of antidysrhythmic drugs and the frequencies of dysrhythmias (32[S])*

Drug	Log HERG inhibitory activity	Cases	Non-cases	Cases/total (%)
Amiodarone	−3.3	271	10 467	2.52
Cibenzoline	−1.4	13	214	5.73
Bepridil	−1.3	59	125	32.07
Procainamide	−0.8	101	2652	3.67
Flecainide	−0.7	332	1894	14.92
Disopyramide	−0.4	110	1843	5.63
Dofetilide	−0.4	68	676	9.14
Propafenone	−0.3	97	1146	7.80
Aprindine	0.0	1	164	0.61
Quinidine	1.0	181	3399	5.06
Ibutilide	1.1	154	27	85.08

therapeutic unbound plasma concentration divided by the HERG IC_{50} value of the suspected drug. There was a significant association between HERG inhibitory activity and the risk of serious ventricular dysrhythmias and sudden death (Table 1). The antidysrhythmic drugs that least followed the predicted pattern were amiodarone, bepridil, flecainide, ibutilide, and sotalol, for which the odds were higher than expected, and aprindine, for which the odds were lower than expected.

ADENOSINE RECEPTOR AGONISTS   (SED-15, 36; SEDA-27, 189; SEDA-28, 203; SEDA-29, 185)

Adenosine and analogues

Comparative studies   The effects of abciximab or intracoronary adenosine distal to the occlusion on immediate angiographic results and 6-month left ventricular remodelling have been studied in 90 patients undergoing primary angioplasty with coronary stenting (33[c]). Abciximab enhanced myocardial reperfusion, with a reduced incidence of 6-month left ventricular remodelling. In contrast, adenosine improved angiographic results but did not prevent left ventricular remodelling. Adverse events were not reported.

Cardiovascular   *Sinus arrest* during adenosine stress testing has been reviewed in the context of three cases in liver transplant recipients with graft failure (34[AR]). The authors concluded that patients with orthotopic liver transplants have an increased risk of sinus arrest from adenosine. They attributed this to stimulation of adenosine A_1 receptors in the sinoatrial node, activating an outward potassium current, and resulting in a direct negative chronotropic effect.

Adenosine is contraindicated in patients with accessory conduction pathways, but it is not always possible to detect this contraindication.

- A previously healthy 35-year-old man was given adenosine 6 mg for a narrow-complex tachycardia at 217/minute (35[A]). The rhythm suddenly changed to wide QRS atrial fibrillation at an average ventricular rate of 250/minute and transient higher rates over 300/minute, degenerating into ventricular fibrillation after a few minutes. DC shock 200 J resulted in sinus rhythm. An accessory pathway was subsequently diagnosed.

Adenosine receptor agonists

To date, four subtypes of adenosine receptor have been described: A_1, A_{2A}, A_{2B}, and A_3 (34[AR]). Stimulation of specific cell-surface A_1 receptors shortens the duration, depresses the amplitude, and reduces the rate of rise of the action potential in the atrioventricular node, slowing conduction; this is the mechanism by which adenosine terminates re-entrant supraventricular tachycardias. In myocardial perfusion imaging adenosine causes coronary vasodilatation by stimulating A_{2A} receptors in vascular endothelium and smooth muscle cells. Stimulation of A_{2B} receptors in mast cells causes bronchospasm in susceptible individuals. Stimulation of A_3 receptors reduces the degree of apoptosis resulting from ischemia reperfusion injury in the heart, although most of the cardioprotective effects of adenosine are thought to be mediated by A_1 receptors.

A high proportion of patients experience transient adverse effects after the administration of adenosine (SED-15, 36); selective agonists developed for clinical use might be safer and would be longer acting. Over a dozen selective agonists are now in clinical trials: A_1 agonists

for cardiac dysrhythmias and neuropathic pain; A_{2A} agonists for myocardial perfusion imaging and as anti-inflammatory agents (36[R]); A_{2B} agonists for treatment of cardiac ischemia; and A_3 agonists for rheumatoid arthritis and colorectal cancer (37[R]). Apadenoson, binodenoson, and regadenoson are new selective adenosine A_{2A} receptor agonists (38[R]).

Binodenoson and adenosine have been compared in a multicenter, randomized, single-blind, two-arm crossover study in 226 patients who underwent two single photon emission computed tomographic (SPECT) imaging studies (39[C]). There were fewer adverse events, specifically *chest pain, dyspnea*, and *flushing*, with any dose of binodenoson than with adenosine, and the adverse effects were less severe. There were no cases of atrioventricular block with binodenoson compared with seven cases among 226 patients who were given adenosine.

Regadenoson has been studied in 36 patients as a pharmacological stress agent for detecting reversible myocardial hypoperfusion combined with single-photon emission computed tomography (SPECT) (40[c]). The reported adverse events (frequencies in parentheses) were *chest pain* (33), *flushing* (31), *dyspnea* (31), *headache* (25), *dizziness* (19), *abdominal pain* (11), *hypesthesia* (8), and *palpitation* (6).

Ajmaline and derivatives
(SED-15, 45)

Cardiovascular   Class I antidysrhythmic drugs can precipitate *Brugada syndrome* in susceptible individuals by sodium channel blockade. Ajmaline challenge was positive in 48 of 103 patients (41[c]). J wave elevation in −2V2 and a reduced T wave amplitude in V3 at baseline were independent predictors of a positive response.

Amiodarone   *(SED-15, 148; SEDA-27, 189; SEDA-28, 205; SEDA-29, 185)*

Comparative studies   In a double-blind, placebo-controlled trial 665 patients who were taking anticoagulants and had persistent atrial fibrillation were randomized to amiodarone

($n = 267$), sotalol ($n = 261$), or placebo ($n = 137$) for 1.0–4.5 years (42^C). Amiodarone and sotalol were equally effective in producing cardioversion to sinus rhythm (27 and 24% versus placebo 0.8%), but the effect of amiodarone lasted significantly longer (487, 74, and 6 days according to intention to treat, and 809, 209, and 13 days according to treatment received). There were no significant differences in the rates of adverse events, except *minor bleeding*, which was significantly more common with amiodarone than sotalol or placebo (8.33 versus 6.37 and 6.71 per 100 patient-years). The rates of major bleeding were 2.07, 3.10, and 3.97 per 100 patient-years; of minor strokes 1.19, 0.68, and 0.96; and of major strokes 0.87, 2.03, and 0.95. There were two cases of non-fatal adverse pulmonary effects with amiodarone and one with placebo. There was one case of non-fatal torsade de pointes with sotalol.

Cardiovascular   *Atrial flutter with 1:1 conduction* is very rare in patients taking class III antidysrhythmic drugs (SEDA-27, 190), but another case has been reported, with prolongation of the flutter cycle and infra-Hissian block (43^A).

Of six patients with *torsade de pointes* taking chronic amiodarone, five were women, three were taking drugs that inhibit CYP3A4 (loratadine or trazodone), three had hypokalemia, and four had reduced left ventricular function (44^c).

Respiratory   *Lung damage* due to amiodarone can occur within days or weeks of the start of therapy, and death can occur. The prognosis is worse in those with pre-existing lung damage and the incidence can be reduced by using lower loading and maintenance doses. The speed with which amiodarone-induced lung damage can occur has been illustrated by the case of a 75-year-old man who received a total dose of amiodarone of only 1500 mg and developed dyspnea, tachypnea, and hypoxemia, with diffuse crackles over both lungs, multiple bilateral acinar pattern infiltrates without Kerley B lines or peribronchial cuffing on the chest X ray, and diffuse ground glass opacities associated with smooth interlobular thickening, more prominent in the lower lung zones, and intralobular interstitial thickening in subpleural regions on a high-resolution chest CT scan;

there were foamy macrophages in the bronchoalveolar lavage fluid (45^{Ar}).

Of 613 Chinese patients taking amiodarone 200 mg/day 12 (1.9%) had amiodarone-induced lung damage; nine were men (46^c). Their mean age was 77 years. The average duration of therapy was 14 (range 1–27) months. Three patients developed the complication within 4 months of starting the medication. Eight developed their complications at 12–24 months. Two died of respiratory failure.

- A 73-year-old man who had taken amiodarone 200 mg/day, 5 days a week, for 15 years was given a glucocorticoid for suspected giant cell arteritis (47^c). The glucocorticoid was suddenly withdrawn 2 weeks later, and 10 days later he developed dyspnea and fever and rapidly developed acute respiratory failure. Post-mortem findings were consistent with amiodarone-induced acute interstitial pneumonitis, with mild fibrosis and numerous intra-alveolar foamy macrophages.

The authors hypothesized that the glucocorticoid had masked amiodarone-associated lung damage.

Nervous system   *Ataxia* is an occasional adverse effect of amiodarone (48^A).

- An 84-year-old woman with hypertrophic obstructive cardiomyopathy and paroxysmal atrial fibrillation developed a progressively debilitating ataxia, which abated over 4 months after withdrawal of amiodarone. Despite the long half-life of amiodarone, her symptoms began to improve after several days, and she was walking without assistance within 1 week.

Sensory systems   Morphological changes in the cornea caused by amiodarone (*vortex keratopathy* or *cornea verticillata*) have been evaluated by in vivo slit scanning confocal microscopy in 49 eyes of 25 patients taking amiodarone and 26 eyes of 13 age- and sex-matched healthy controls (49^c). The mean dosage of amiodarone was 224 mg/day and the mean duration of treatment was 21 months. There were deposits in all but eight eyes of the patients who took amiodarone, and they were detected as early as 2 months after the start of treatment. Deposition correlated significantly with the duration of treatment and therefore the cumulative dose. The deposits were seen in the basal lamina in all eyes and in the superficial epithelium, anterior stroma, mid-stroma, and subepithelial nerves in eyes with grades 2–4 keratopathy. There were also abnormalities in anterior stromal keratocytes, subepithelial and stromal nerves, and endothelium. The authors suggested that confocal microscopy will prove to be useful in early diagnosis and in understanding the pathophysiology of amiodarone keratopathy.

Unilateral amiodarone vortex keratopathy in an 87-year-old woman was explained by the presence of corneal dysplasia in the unaffected eye, which did not allow amiodarone to bind to corneal lipid (50[A]).

Optic neuropathy in patients on amiodarone has been reviewed (51[R]) and an unusual case reported in which bilateral inferior field loss progressed to upper and lower field loss bilaterally despite withdrawal of the amiodarone (52[Ar]).

Endocrine   There are two types of amiodarone-induced *hyperthyroidism*: type 1 occurs in subjects with underlying thyroid disease and type 2 is a form of destructive thyroiditis; the former is rare. Thyroid function tests were measured before and after treatment of amiodarone-induced hyperthyroidism ($n = 12$) and the response to combined antithyroid and glucocorticoid treatment ($n = 11$) was recorded (53[c]). One patient had type 1 hyperthyroidism, nine had type 2, and two probably had a mixed form. Six patients had diffuse hypoechoic goiters. The median time to euthyroidism (defined as a normal free T3 concentration) with a thionamide + prednisolone (starting dose 20–75 mg/day) was 2 (interquartile range 1.0–2.7) months. Thionamide treatment was stopped after a median duration of 5.7 (4.2–8.7) months and glucocorticoids were completely withdrawn after 6.7 (5.5–8.7) months.

Thyroid hormone-producing thyroid carcinoma is an uncommon cause of thyrotoxicosis. Precipitation of thyrotoxicosis by iodine-containing compounds in patients with thyroid carcinoma is rare, but has been attributed to amiodarone in a 77-year-old man with extensive hepatic metastases from a well-differentiated thyroid carcinoma (54[A]).

Treatment of amiodarone-induced hyperthyroidism is difficult (SED-15, 158).

- A 40 year-old patient with severe amiodarone-induced hyperthyroidism after heart transplantation did not respond to high doses of antithyroid

drugs combined with glucocorticoids (55[A]). A low dose of lithium carbonate resulted in normalization of thyroid function.

Liver   *Acute hepatic damage* after intravenous amiodarone can be fatal. Three cases of acute hepatocellular injury after intravenous amiodarone in critically ill patients have been described and another 25 published cases and six cases reported to the Swiss Pharmacovigilance Center (Swissmedic) discussed (56[Ar]). The authors suggested that acute liver damage after intravenous amiodarone may have been caused by the solubilizing excipient polysorbate 80. However, ischemic hepatitis due to hemodynamic changes could not be ruled out (57[r]).

Liver damage can occur very quickly after the start of amiodarone therapy (58[A]).

- A 54-year-old man with 70% burns developed atrial fibrillation and was given intravenous amiodarone 150 mg followed by 1 mg/minute and then 0.5 mg/minute overlapped with oral doses of 400 mg tds (total dose 6.2 g). Liver function tests had been normal, but after 5 days the aspartate transaminase and alanine transaminase activities rose to 739 and 1303 units/l respectively. Amiodarone was withdrawn and the transaminase activities fell immediately.

Although amiodarone can cause liver damage, it usually takes the form of a hepatitis associated with phospholipid deposition; *hepatic cirrhosis* is uncommon (SEDA-28, 208; SEDA-29, 186).

- A 63-year-old man developed ascites after taking amiodarone 200 mg/day for 23 months (59[Ar]). A liver biopsy showed grade 3 chronic hepatitis and micronodular cirrhosis. The presence of striking microvesicular steatosis on light microscopy and lysosomal inclusion bodies on electron microscopy suggested amiodarone-induced hepatotoxicity.
- An 85-year-old man took amiodarone for 7 years (total dose 528 g) (60[A]). He had hepatomegaly and mild elevations of serum transaminases. Liver biopsy showed cirrhosis, and electron microscopy showed numerous lysosomes with electron-dense, whorled, lamellar inclusions characteristic of a secondary phospholipidosis. Initially, withdrawal of amiodarone led to a slight improvement, but his general condition deteriorated and he died from complications of pneumonia and renal insufficiency.

Skin   The adverse effects of amiodarone on the skin usually resolve within 2 years of drug withdrawal. However, in a 67-year-old woman who developed both *phototoxicity* and a *slate-grey discoloration* while taking amiodarone, the dyspigmentation gradually resolved after withdrawal but the phototoxicity persisted for more than 17 years (61[A]). The authors offered four possible explanations: continuing phototoxicity due to persistence of amiodarone or its metabolites in the skin, which seems unlikely; persistent postinflammatory cutaneous hypersensitivity; transfer to a photoallergic mechanism; conversion to light-exacerbated seborrheic dermatitis.

Musculoskeletal   Two patients with atrial fibrillation had acute devastating *low back pain* a few minutes after the start of intravenous loading with amiodarone (62[A]).

Immunologic   *Angioedema* has only been reported once in a patient taking amiodarone (SEDA-25, 216). Two more cases have now been reported (63[A]).

Oral formulations of amiodarone contain iodine, about 10% of which is released into the circulatory system and may increase the risks of *hypersensitivity reactions* in iodine-sensitive patients. Reactions to iodinated contrast media are usually due to their high osmolar or ionic content. Although amiodarone has a high content of iodine, there is no known association between amiodarone and reactions to contrast media. Three patients who were allergic to iodine were given amiodarone for chemical cardioversion of dysrhythmias (64[c]). There were no anaphylactic or anaphylactoid reactions. However, the authors suggested that in patients with true iodine hypersensitivity there is a possibility of such reactions.

Susceptibility factors

Lung disease   In the Atrial Fibrillation Follow-up Investigation of Rhythm Management (AFFIRM) study, pre-existing lung disease was present in 591 of 4060 patients and was associated with a higher risk of pulmonary death and a higher risk of amiodarone-associated pulmonary toxicity (65[C]). At 4 years amiodarone-induced pulmonary toxicity had occurred in 52 of 1468 patients (3.5%) and was present in more patients with pre-existing pulmonary disease (14 of 238 patients, 5.9%) than in those without (38 of 1230 patients, 3.1%). However, the use

of amiodarone in the presence of pre-existing pulmonary disease did not increase the rates of pulmonary deaths or all-cause mortality. The authors concluded that cautious use of amiodarone to treat atrial fibrillation is acceptable in elderly patients, even if there is pre-existing pulmonary disease.

Drug–drug interactions   Amiodarone toxicity has been attributed to impaired metabolism by *metronidazole* (66[C]).

- A 71-year-old Caucasian woman was given metronidazole 500 mg tds for antibiotic-associated pseudomembranous colitis. The QT_c interval was 440 ms. After 3 days she developed atrial fibrillation and was given intravenous amiodarone as a 450 mg bolus followed by 900 mg/day. Conversion to sinus rhythm occurred 2 days later and the QT_c interval was prolonged to 625 ms. Later she developed sustained polymorphic torsade de pointes. Metronidazole and amiodarone were immediately withdrawn, and over the next 6 days the QT_c interval gradually normalized.

Diagnosis of adverse drug reactions   Krebs von den Lungen-6 (KL-6), a sialylated carbohydrate antigen, has previously been recognized as a serum marker for diffuse interstitial lung disease (SED-15, 154). There has been a report of another patient, a 69-year-old woman, with lung damage due to amiodarone who had increased blood concentrations of KL-6 (67[A]).

Aprindine   *(SED-15, 330; SEDA-27, 194)*

Hematologic   In a case-control study, 177 cases of *agranulocytosis* were compared with 586 sex-, age-, and hospital-matched control subjects with regard to previous use of medicines (68[C]). The annual incidence of community-acquired agranulocytosis was 3.46 per million, and it increased with age. The fatality rate was 7.0% and the mortality rate was 0.24 per million. The following drugs were most strongly associated with a risk of agranulocytosis:

- ticlopidine hydrochloride (OR = 103; 95% CI = 13, 837);
- calcium dobesilate (78; 4.5, 1346);
- antithyroid drugs (53; 5.8, 478);

- dipyrone (metamizole sodium and metamizole magnesium) (26; 8.4, 179);
- spironolactone (20; 2.3, 176).

Aprindine was among other drugs associated with a significant risk. However, the size of the risk was not stated.

Cibenzoline *(SED-15, 740; SEDA-27, 195)*

Cardiovascular Cibenzoline has been reported to have unmasked *Brugada syndrome* in a 61-year-old woman (69[A]). Ajmaline reproduced the effect. The authors concluded that cibenzoline should probably be avoided in patients with Brugada syndrome.

Disopyramide *(SED-15, 1145; SEDA-27, 195; SEDA-28, 209)*

Observational studies Because of its negative inotropic effect, disopyramide reduces the left ventricular outflow gradient and improves symptoms in patients with hypertrophic obstructive cardiomyopathy. However, its long-term effects have not been well studied. In 118 patients who took disopyramide (mean dose 432 mg/day for a mean of 3.1 years) and 373 who did not, all-cause annual cardiac death rates (1.4 versus 2.6% per year) and sudden death rates (1.0 versus 1.8% per year) did not differ significantly, although there was a tendency for disopyramide to reduce mortality (70[C]). The authors concluded that disopyramide is not prodysrhythmic in hypertrophic obstructive cardiomyopathy. The main adverse effects of disopyramide were attributable to its *anticholinergic effects*—dry mouth and prostatism, which required drug withdrawal in 7% of the patients.

Dofetilide *(SED-15, 1173; SEDA-27, 195; SEDA-28, 209; SEDA-29, 187)*

Cardiovascular Dofetilide can cause *torsade de pointes* (SED-15, 1175). It occurs in 0.8–3.3% of patients and most episodes occur within 3 days of the start of therapy (71[Ar]). Two unusual variants of ventricular dysrhythmias have been reported in patients taking dofetilide—non-sustained runs of monomorphic ventricular tachycardia shortly after the first dose of dofetilide, confirmed by rechallenge, and torsade de pointes that followed isolated ventricular extra beats during an exercise test in a patient without baseline QT interval prolongation but with significant QT interval prolongation after the postectopic pause (72[A]).

Flecainide *(SED-15, 1370; SEDA-27, 195; SEDA-28, 209; SEDA-29, 188)*

Cardiovascular Sodium channel blockers have been used to improve muscle strength and relaxation in myotonic dystrophy. However, myotonic dystrophy is associated with cardiac abnormalities and 30% of deaths are attributable to cardiac causes, mainly dysrhythmias. A 41-year-old woman with myotonic dystrophy developed a *ventricular tachycardia* while talking flecainide (73[A]). When flecainide was withdrawn ventricular tachycardia could not be induced. The authors recommended careful cardiac assessment, risk stratification, and consideration of high-risk patients for electrophysiological studies, especially if considering use of a class I antidysrhythmic drug.

Nervous system Another case of flecainide-associated *neuropathy* has been reported (74[A]).

Susceptibility factors

Genetic Among 40 patients taking flecainide or propafenone adverse effects were more frequent in poor CYP2D6 metabolizers (21%) than in extensive metabolizers (4.8%) (75[c]). Only the poor metabolizers had adverse effects that required drug withdrawal.

Monitoring therapy The usual target range for plasma flecainide concentrations is 200–1000 ng/ml (76[c]). The relation between plasma flecainide concentration and its effect on atrial fibrillatory rate has been studied in 10 patients during acute and maintenance therapy of persistent lone atrial fibrillation (77[c]). Flecainide was given as a single oral bolus of 300 mg followed by 200–400 mg/day for 5 days. The initial bolus resulted in plasma concentrations of 288–629 ng/ml; day 5 plasma concentrations were lower in those taking a dosage of 200 mg/day than in those taking higher doses (mean 508 versus 974 ng/ml). The fibrillatory rate was reduced after the initial bolus but remained stable thereafter and was independent of flecainide plasma concentration. There was significant prolongation of the QRS duration but no change in RR or QT_c interval and no correlation between plasma flecainide concentration and QRS duration. Presumably plasma flecainide concentrations do not well reflect concentrations in the heart.

In a double-blind, randomized, placebo-controlled study of the effects of flecainide in six men with congenital long QT syndrome with the DeltaKPQ gene deletion, the lowest dose of flecainide associated with at least a 40 ms reduction in the QT_c interval was determined in an initial open, dose-ranging investigation using one-quarter or half of the recommended maximal antidysrhythmic dose; QT_c interval reduction was achieved with a dose of 1.5 mg/kg/day in four subjects and with 3.0 mg/kg/day in two (78[c]). They were then randomized to four 6-month alternating periods of flecainide and placebo. Average QT_c intervals during placebo and flecainide were 534 ms and 503 ms respectively, with an adjusted reduction in QT_c interval of −27 ms (95% CI = −37, −17 at a mean flecainide blood concentration of 110 ng/ml.

Drug–drug interactions   In a double-blind, placebo-controlled, randomized, three-way, crossover study, *fluvoxamine* (a CYP1A2 inhibitor) 100 mg/day reduced the clearance of intravenous lidocaine by 41% and prolonged its half-life from 2.6 to 3.5 hours (80[c]). During co-administration of fluvoxamine + *erythromycin* (a CYP3A4 inhibitor) 500 mg tds, lidocaine clearance was reduced by 53% compared with placebo and 21% compared with fluvoxamine alone and the half-life was further prolonged to 4.3 hours. The apparent volume of distribution of lidocaine was not affected. The half-life of monoethylglycinexylidide, an active metabolite of lidocaine, was significantly prolonged by both fluvoxamine alone and the combination of fluvoxamine + erythromycin. The authors concluded that the minor effect of inhibitors of CYP3A4 on the pharmacokinetics of lidocaine can be explained by compensatory metabolism by CYP1A2.

Mexiletine   *(SED-15, 2329; SEDA-27, 197)*

Immunologic   A drug-induced *hypersensitivity syndrome* occurred in a 66-year-old man taking mexiletine (81[A]). Withdrawal of the mexiletine and glucocorticoid treatment led to temporary improvement, but tapering the glucocorticoid dose twice led to recrudescence, during which there were raised antibody titers against HHV-6 and cytomegalovirus and viral DNA in the blood, suggesting that these two viruses may have been involved in the recrudescence.

Lidocaine (lignocaine)   *(SED-15, 2051; SEDA-27, 196; SEDA-28, 210; SEDA-29, 188)*

Sensory systems   The efficacy of intravenous lidocaine 100 mg over 5 minutes in treatment-resistant pruritus in chronic cholestatic liver disease has been studied in a placebo-controlled study 18 patients (79[c]). There were no severe adverse events. Five patients who were given lidocaine had mild *tinnitus*, associated in two cases with *lingual paresthesia* during infusion.

Propafenone   *(SED-15, 2939; SEDA-27, 197; SEDA-28, 211)*

Cardiovascular   Propafenone and ibutilide have been compared in 40 patients with atrial flutter (82[c]). Ibutilide was superior to propafenone for treating atrial flutter (90 versus 30%) and the respective mean conversion times were 11 and 35 minutes. *Bradycardia* (2/20) and *hypotension* (4/20) were more common adverse effects with propafenone.

Skin   *Acute generalized exanthematous pustulosis* has been attributed to propafenone in an 85-year-old man (83[A]). The mechanism of this type of eruption is thought to be via the preferential production of IL-8 by T cells after the drug binds to the cells and elicits a CD4 and CD8 immune reaction.

Procainamide   *(SED-15, 2923;*
SEDA-27, 197; SEDA-28, 210)

Hematologic   *Pure red cell aplasia* has previously been attributed to procainamide, but it was not clear whether it was due to drug-induced lupus-like syndrome (SED-15, 2924). Another case has been reported in a 63-year-old man (84[A]).

Drug–drug interactions   In a randomized, crossover drug interaction study in 10 healthy adults, *levofloxacin* reduced the renal clearances and prolonged the half-lives of both procainamide and N-acetylprocainamide; *ciprofloxacin* reduced the renal clearances of procainamide and N-acetylprocainamide only slightly (85[C]).

Quinidine and derivatives   *(SED-15, 2997; SEDA-28, 212; SEDA-29, 189)*

Cardiovascular   Intravenous quinidine has been used to study the susceptibility to *QT interval prolongation* in 14 relatives of patients who had safely tolerated chronic therapy with a QT interval-prolonging drug (controls) and 12 relatives of patients who had developed acquired long QT syndrome (86[c]). The interval from the peak to the end of the T wave, an index of transmural dispersion of repolarization, was significantly prolonged (from 63 to 83 ms) by quinidine in the relatives of those with acquired long QT syndrome but not in control relatives (from 66 to 71 ms). The time from the peak to the end of the T wave as a fraction of the QT interval was similar in the two groups at baseline but was longer in the relatives of those with acquired long QT syndrome after quinidine. The authors concluded that first-degree relatives of patients with acquired long QT syndrome have greater drug-induced prolongation of terminal repolarization than control relatives, supporting a genetic predisposition to acquired long QT syndrome.

Quinidine syncope has again been reported, in a 46-year-old woman, associated with bradycardia and torsade de pointes due to *prolongation of the QT interval* (660 ms); it responded to intravenous sodium bicarbonate and pacing (87[A]).

References

1. Grimard C, De Labriolle A, Charbonnier B, Babuty D. Bidirectional ventricular tachycardia resulting from digoxin toxicity. J Cardiovasc Electrophysiol 2005;16(7):807–8.

2. Goranitou G, Stavrianaki D, Babalis D. Wide QRS tachycardia caused by severe hyperkalaemia and digoxin intoxication. Acta Cardiol 2005;60(4):437–41.

3. Eyal D, Molczan KA, Carroll LS. Digoxin toxicity: pediatric survival after asystolic arrest. Clin Toxicol (Phila) 2005;43(1):51–4.

4. Prodouz KN, Poindexter BJ, Fratantoni JC. Ouabain affects platelet reactivity as measured in vitro. Thromb Res 1987;46:337–46.

5. Andersson TL, Vinge E. Effects of ouabain on ^{86}Rb-uptake, ^{3}H-5-HT-uptake and aggregation by 5-HT and ADP in human platelets. Pharmacol Toxicol 1988;62:172–6.

6. Chirinos JA, Castrellon A, Zambrano JP, Jimenez JJ, Jy W, Horstman LL, Willens HJ, Castellanos A, Myerburg RJ, Ahn YS. Digoxin use is associated with increased platelet and endothelial cell activation in patients with nonvalvular atrial fibrillation. Heart Rhythm 2005;2(5):525–9.

7. Wang L, Song S. Digoxin may reduce the mortality rates in patients with congestive heart failure. Med Hypotheses 2005;64(1):124–6.

8. Adams Jr KF, Patterson JH, Gattis WA, O'Connor CM, Lee CR, Schwartz TA, Gheorghiade M. Relationship of serum digoxin concentration to mortality and morbidity in women in the Digitalis Investigation Group trial a retrospective analysis. J Am Coll Cardiol 2005;46:497–504.

9. Nybo M, Damkier P. Gastrointestinal symptoms as an important sign in premature newborns with severely increased S-digoxin. Basic Clin Pharmacol Toxicol 2005;96(6):465–8.

10. Domanski M, Fleg J, Bristow M, Knox S. The effect of gender on outcome in digitalis-treated heart failure patients. J Card Fail 2005;11(2):83–6.

11. Kinoshita H, Taniguchi T, Nishiguchi M, Ouchi H, Minami T, Utsumi T, Motomura H, Tsuda T, Ohta T, Aoki S, Komeda M, Kamamoto T, Kubota A, Fuke C, Arao T, Miyazaki T, Hishida S. An autopsy case of combined drug intoxication involving verapamil, metoprolol and digoxin. Forensic Sci Int 2003;133:107–12.

12. Ma B, Prueksaritanont T, Lin JH. Drug interactions with calcium channel blockers: possible involvement of metabolite-intermediate complexation with CYP3A. Drug Metab Dispos 2000;28(2):125–30.

13. Camphausen C, Haas NA, Mattke AC. Successful treatment of oleander intoxication (cardiac glycosides) with digoxin-specific Fab antibody fragments in a 7-year-old child: case report and review of literature. Z Kardiol 2005;94(12):817–23.

14. Bourgeois B, Incagnoli P, Hanna J, Tirard V. Traitement par anticorps antidigitalique d'une intoxication volontaire par laurier rose. Ann Fr Anesth Reanim 2005;24(6):640–2.

15. Hirata S, Izumi S, Furukubo T, Ota M, Fujita M, Yamakawa T, Hasegawa I, Ohtani H, Sawada Y. Interactions between clarithromycin and digoxin in patients with end-stage renal disease. Int J Clin Pharmacol Ther 2005;43(1):30–6.

16. Kothare PA, Soon DK, Linnebjerg H, Park S, Chan C, Yeo A, Lim M, Mace KF, Wise SD. Effect of exenatide on the steady-state pharmacokinetics of digoxin. J Clin Pharmacol 2005;45(9):1032–7.

17. Johne A, Brockmöller J, Bauer S, Maurer A, Langheinrich M, Roots I. Pharmacokinetic interaction of digoxin with an herbal extract from St John's wort (Hypericum perforatum). Clin Pharmacol Ther 1999;66(4):338–45.

18. Mueller SC, Uehleke B, Woehling H, Petzsch M, Majcher-Peszynska J, Hehl EM, Sievers H, Frank B, Riethling AK, Drewelow B. Effect of St John's wort dose and preparations on the pharmacokinetics of digoxin. Clin Pharmacol Ther 2004;75(6):546–57.

19. Arold G, Donath F, Maurer A, Diefenbach K, Bauer S, Henneicke-von Zepelin HH, Friede M, Roots I. No relevant interaction with alprazolam, caffeine, tolbutamide, and digoxin by treatment with a low-hyperforin St John's wort extract. Planta Med 2005;71(4):331–7.

20. Andelić S. Bigeminy—the result of interaction between digoxin and St. John's wort. Vojnosanit Pregl 2003;60(3):361–4.

21. Roman D, Bramson C, Ouellet D, Randinitis E, Gardner M. Effect of lasofoxifene on the pharmacokinetics of digoxin in healthy postmenopausal women. J Clin Pharmacol 2005;45(12):1407–12.

22. Juurlink DN, Mamdani MM, Kopp A, Herrmann N, Laupacis A. A population-based assessment of the potential interaction between serotonin-specific reuptake inhibitors and digoxin. Br J Clin Pharmacol 2005;59(1):102–7.

23. McRae S. Elevated serum digoxin levels in a patient taking digoxin and Siberian ginseng. CMAJ 1996;155(3):293–5.

24. Dasgupta A, Wu S, Actor J, Olsen M, Wells A, Datta P. Effect of Asian and Siberian ginseng on serum digoxin measurement by five digoxin immunoassays. Significant variation in digoxin-like immunoreactivity among commercial ginsengs. Am J Clin Pathol 2003;119(2):298–303.

25. Dasgupta A, Reyes MA. Effect of Brazilian, Indian, Siberian, Asian, and North American ginseng on serum digoxin measurement by immunoassays and binding of digoxin-like immunoreactive components of ginseng with Fab fragment of antidigoxin antibody (Digibind). Am J Clin Pathol 2005;124(2):229–36.

26. Kobusiak-Prokopowicz M, Swidnicka-Szuszkowska B, Mysiak A. Effect of digoxin on ANP, BNP, and cGMP in patients with chronic congestive heart failure. Pol Arch Med Wew 2001;105(6):475–82.

27. Tsutamoto T, Wada A, Maeda K, Hisanaga T, Fukai D, Maeda Y, Ohnishi M, Mabuchi N, Kinoshita M. Digitalis increases brain natriuretic peptide in patients with severe congestive heart failure. Am Heart J 1997;134(5 Pt 1):910–6.

28. Heinrich K, Prendergast HM, Erickson T. Chronic digoxin toxicity and significantly elevated BNP levels in the presence of mild heart failure. Am J Emerg Med 2005;23(4):561–2.

29. Tribut O, Gaulier JM, Allain H, Bentué-Ferrer D. Major discrepancy between digoxin immunoassay results in a context of acute overdose: a case report. Clin Chim Acta 2005;354(1–2):201–3.

30. Bayram M, De Luca L, Massie MB, Gheorghiade M. Reassessment of dobutamine, dopamine, and milrinone in the management of acute heart failure syndromes. Am J Cardiol 2005;96(6A):47G–58G.

31. Wang SM, Lei HY, Huang MC, Wu JM, Chen CT, Wang JN, Wang JR, Liu CC. Therapeutic efficacy of milrinone in the management of enterovirus 71-induced pulmonary edema. Pediatr Pulmonol 2005;39(3):219–23.

32. De Bruin ML, Pettersson M, Meyboom RH, Hoes AW, Leufkens HG. Anti-HERG activity and the risk of drug-induced arrhythmias and sudden death. Eur Heart J 2005;26(6):590–7.

33. Petronio AS, De Carlo M, Ciabatti N, Amoroso G, Limbruno U, Palagi C, Di Bello V, Romano MF, Mariani M. Left ventricular remodeling after primary coronary angioplasty in

patients treated with abciximab or intracoronary adenosine. Am Heart J 2005;150(5):1015.

34. Giedd KN, Bokhari S, Daniele TP, Johnson LL. Sinus arrest during adenosine stress testing in liver transplant recipients with graft failure: three case reports and a review of the literature. J Nucl Cardiol 2005;12(6):696–702.

35. Copetti R, Proclemer A, Paolo Pillinini P, Chizzola G. Life-threatening proarrhythmia in a patient with orthodromic atrioventricular tachycardia treated with low-dose adenosine. J Cardiovasc Electrophysiol 2005;16(1):106.

36. Lappas CM, Sullivan GW, Linden J. Adenosine A$_{2A}$ agonists in development for the treatment of inflammation. Expert Opin Investig Drugs 2005;14(7):797–806.

37. Gao ZG, Jacobson KA. Emerging adenosine receptor agonists. Expert Opin Emerg Drugs 2007;12(3):479–92.

38. Miller DD. Impact of selective adenosine A$_{2A}$ receptor agonists on cardiac imaging: feeling the lightning, waiting on the thunder. J Am Coll Cardiol 2005;46(11):2076–8.

39. Udelson JE, Heller GV, Wackers FJ, Chai A, Hinchman D, Coleman PS, Dilsizian V, DiCarli M, Hachamovitch R, Johnson JR, Barrett RJ, Gibbons RJ. Randomized, controlled dose-ranging study of the selective adenosine A$_{2A}$ receptor agonist binodenoson for pharmacological stress as an adjunct to myocardial perfusion imaging. Circulation 2004;109(4):457–64.

40. Hendel RC, Bateman TM, Cerqueira MD, Iskandrian AE, Leppo JA, Blackburn B, Mahmarian JJ. Initial clinical experience with regadenoson, a novel selective A$_{2A}$ agonist for pharmacologic stress single-photon emission computed tomography myocardial perfusion imaging. J Am Coll Cardiol 2005;46(11):2069–75.

41. Hermida JS, Denjoy I, Jarry G, Jandaud S, Bertrand C, Delonca J. Electrocardiographic predictors of Brugada type response during Na channel blockade challenge. Europace 2005;7(5):447–53.

42. Singh BN, Singh SN, Reda DJ, Tang XC, Lopez B, Harris CL, Fletcher RD, Sharma SC, Atwood JE, Jacobson AK, Lewis Jr HD, Raisch DW, Ezekowitz MD, Sotalol Amiodarone Atrial Fibrillation Efficacy Trial (SAFE-T) Investigators. Amiodarone versus sotalol for atrial fibrillation. N Engl J Med 2005;352(18):1861–72.

43. Perdrix-Andujar L, Paziaud O, Ricard G, Diebold B, Le Heuzey JY. 1/1 nodo-ventricular conduction atrial flutter with amiodarone. Arch Mal Coeur Vaiss 2005;98(3):259–62.

44. Antonelli D, Atar S, Freedberg NA, Rosenfeld T. Torsade de pointes in patients on chronic amiodarone treatment: contributing factors and drug interactions. Isr Med Assoc J 2005;7(3):163–5.

45. Skroubis G, Galiatsou E, Metafratzi Z, Karahaliou A, Kitsakos A, Nakos G. Amiodarone-induced acute lung toxicity in an ICU setting. Acta Anaesthesiol Scand 2005;49(4):569–71. Erratum: Acta Anaesthesiol Scand 2005;49(6):886.

46. Fung RC, Chan WK, Chu CM, Yue CS. Low dose amiodarone-induced lung injury. Int J Cardiol 2006;113(1):144–5.

47. Charles PE, Doise JM, Quenot JP, Muller G, Aube H, Baudouin N, Piard F, Besancenot JF, Blettery B. Amiodarone-related acute respiratory distress syndrome following sudden withdrawal of steroids. Respiration 2006;73(2):248–9.

48. Krauser DG, Segal AZ, Kligfield P. Severe ataxia caused by amiodarone. Am J Cardiol 2005;96(10):1463–4.

49. Uçakhan OO, Kanpolat A, Yilmaz N. In vivo confocal microscopy of megalocornea with central mosaic dystrophy. Clin Experiment Ophthalmol 2005;33(1):102–5.

50. Chilov MN, Moshegov CN, Booth F. Unilateral amiodarone keratopathy. Clin Experiment Ophthalmol 2005;33(6):666–8.

51. Murphy MA, Murphy JF. Amiodarone and optic neuropathy: the heart of the matter. J Neuroophthalmol 2005;25(3):232–6.

52. Clement CI, Myers P, Tan KP. Bilateral optic neuropathy due to amiodarone with recurrence. Clin Experiment Ophthalmol 2005;33(2):222–5.

53. Dietlein M, Schicha H. Amiodarone-induced thyrotoxicosis due to destructive thyroiditis: therapeutic recommendations. Exp Clin Endocrinol Diabetes 2005;113(3):145–51.

54. Mackie GC, Shulkin BL. Amiodarone-induced hyperthyroidism in a patient with functioning papillary carcinoma of the thyroid and extensive hepatic metastases. Thyroid 2005;15(12):1337–40.

55. Boeving A, Cubas ER, Santos CM, Carvalho GA, Graf H. Use of lithium carbonate for the treatment of amiodarone-induced thyrotoxicosis. Arq Bras Endocrinol Metabol 2005;49(6):991–5.

56. Rätz Bravo AE, Drewe J, Schlienger RG, Krähenbühl S, Pargger H, Ummenhofer W. Hepatotoxicity during rapid intravenous loading with amiodarone: description of three cases and review of the literature. Crit Care Med 2005;33(1):128–34.

57. Guglin M. Intravenous amiodarone: offender or bystander? Crit Care Med 2005;33(1):245–6.

58. Maker AV, Orgill DP. Rapid acute amiodarone-induced hepatotoxicity in a burn patient. J Burn Care Rehabil 2005;26(4):341–3.

59. Puli SR, Fraley MA, Puli V, Kuperman AB, Alpert MA. Hepatic cirrhosis caused by low-dose oral amiodarone therapy. Am J Med Sci 2005;330(5):257–61.

60. Oikawa H, Maesawa C, Sato R, Oikawa K, Yamada H, Oriso S, Ono S, Yashima-Abo A, Kotani K, Suzuki K, Masuda T. Liver cirrhosis induced by long-term administration of a daily low dose of amiodarone: a case report. World J Gastroenterol 2005;11(34):5394–7.

61. Yones SS, O'Donoghue NB, Palmer RA, Menagé Hdu P, Hawk JL. Persistent severe amiodarone-induced photosensitivity. Clin Exp Dermatol 2005;30(5):500–2.

62. Korantzopoulos P, Pappa E, Karanikis P, Kountouris E, Dimitroula V, Siogas K. Acute low back pain during intravenous administration of

amiodarone: a report of two cases. Int J Cardiol 2005;98(2):355–7.

63. Lahiri K, Malakar S, Sarma N. Amiodarone-induced angioedema: report of two cases. Indian J Dermatol Venereol Leprol 2005;71(1):46–7.

64. Brouse SD, Phillips SM. Amiodarone use in patients with documented allergy to iodine-containing compounds. Pharmacotherapy 2005;25(3):429–34.

65. Olshansky B, Sami M, Rubin A, Kostis J, Shorofsky S, Slee A, Greene HL, NHLBI AFFIRM Investigators. Use of amiodarone for atrial fibrillation in patients with preexisting pulmonary disease in the AFFIRM study. Am J Cardiol 2005;95(3):404–5.

66. Kounas SP, Letsas KP, Sideris A, Efraimidis M, Kardaras F. QT interval prolongation and torsades de pointes due to a coadministration of metronidazole and amiodarone. Pacing Clin Electrophysiol 2005;28(5):472–3.

67. Bernal Morell E, Hernández Madrid A, Marín Marín I, Rodríguez Pena R, González Gordaliza MC, Moro C. Multiple pulmonary nodules and amiodarone. KL-6 as a new diagnostic tool. Rev Esp Cardiol 2005;58(4):447–9.

68. Ibáñez L, Vidal X, Ballarín E, Laporte JR. Population-based drug-induced agranulocytosis. Arch Intern Med 2005;165(8):869–74.

69. Sarkozy A, Caenepeel A, Geelen P, Peytchev P, de Zutter M, Brugada P. Cibenzoline induced Brugada ECG pattern. Europace 2005;7(6):537–9.

70. Sherrid MV, Barac I, McKenna WJ, Elliott PM, Dickie S, Chojnowska L, Casey S, Maron BJ. Multicenter study of the efficacy and safety of disopyramide in obstructive hypertrophic cardiomyopathy. J Am Coll Cardiol 2005;45(8):1251–8.

71. Nagra BS, Ledley GS, Kantharia BK. Marked QT prolongation and torsades de pointes secondary to acute ischemia in an elderly man taking dofetilide for atrial fibrillation: a cautionary tale. J Cardiovasc Pharmacol Ther 2005;10(3):191–5.

72. Reiffel JA. Atypical proarrhythmia with dofetilide: monomorphic VT and exercise-induced torsade de pointes. Pacing Clin Electrophysiol 2005;28(8):877–9.

73. Gorog DA, Russell G, Casian A, Peters NS. A cautionary tale. The risks of flecainide treatment for myotonic dystrophy. J Clin Neuromuscular Dis 2005;7:25–8.

74. Malesker MA, Sojka SG, Fagan NL. Flecainide-induced neuropathy. Ann Pharmacother 2005;39(9):1580.

75. Martínez-Sellés M, Castillo I, Montenegro P, Martín ML, Almendral J, Sanjurjo M. Pharmacogenetic study of the response to flecainide and propafenone in patients with atrial fibrillation. Rev Esp Cardiol 2005;58(6):745–8.

76. Breindahl T. Therapeutic drug monitoring of flecainide in serum using high-performance liquid chromatography and electrospray mass spectrometry. J Chromatogr B Biomed Sci Appl 2000;746(2):249–54.

77. Husser D, Binias KH, Stridh M, Sornmo L, Olsson SB, Molling J, Geller C, Klein HU, Bollmann A. Pilot study: noninvasive monitoring of oral flecainide's effects on atrial electrophysiology during persistent human atrial fibrillation using the surface electrocardiogram. Ann Noninvasive Electrocardiol 2005;10(2):206–10.

78. Moss AJ, Windle JR, Hall WJ, Zareba W, Robinson JL, McNitt S, Severski P, Rosero S, Daubert JP, Qi M, Cieciorka M, Manalan AS. Safety and efficacy of flecainide in subjects with long QT-3 syndrome (DeltaKPQ mutation): a randomized, double-blind, placebo-controlled clinical trial. Ann Noninvasive Electrocardiol 2005;10(4 Suppl):59–66.

79. Villamil AG, Bandi JC, Galdame OA, Gerona S, Gadano AC. Efficacy of lidocaine in the treatment of pruritus in patients with chronic cholestatic liver diseases. Am J Med 2005;118(10):1160–3.

80. Olkkola KT, Isohanni MH, Hamunen K, Neuvonen PJ. The effect of erythromycin and fluvoxamine on the pharmacokinetics of intravenous lidocaine. Anesth Analg 2005;100(5):1352–6.

81. Sekiguchi A, Kashiwagi T, Ishida-Yamamoto A, Takahashi H, Hashimoto Y, Kimura H, Tohyama M, Hashimoto K, Iizuka H. Drug-induced hypersensitivity syndrome due to mexiletine associated with human herpes virus 6 and cytomegalovirus reactivation. J Dermatol 2005;32(4):278–81.

82. Sun JL, Guo JH, Zhang N, Zhang HC, Zhang P. Clinical comparison of ibutilide and propafenone for converting atrial flutter. Cardiovasc Drugs Ther 2005;19(1):57–64.

83. Huang YM, Lee WR, Hu CH, Cheng KL. Propafenone-induced acute generalized exanthematous pustulosis. Int J Dermatol 2005;44(3):256–7.

84. Pasha SF, Pruthi RK. Procainamide-induced pure red cell aplasia. Int J Cardiol 2006;110(1):125–6.

85. Bauer LA, Black DJ, Lill JS, Garrison J, Raisys VA, Hooton TM. Levofloxacin and ciprofloxacin decrease procainamide and N-acetylprocainamide renal clearances. Antimicrob Agents Chemother 2005;49(4):1649–51.

86. Kannankeril PJ, Roden DM, Norris KJ, Whalen SP, George Jr AL, Murray KT. Genetic susceptibility to acquired long QT syndrome: pharmacologic challenge in first-degree relatives. Heart Rhythm 2005;2(2):134–40.

87. Tsai CL. Quinidine cardiotoxicity. J Emerg Med 2005;28(4):463–5.

A.P. Maggioni, M.G. Franzosi, and R. Latini

18   Beta-adrenoceptor antagonists and antianginal drugs

BETA-ADRENOCEPTOR ANTAGONISTS (SED-15, 452; SEDA-27, 203; SEDA-28, 217; SEDA-29, 194)

Cardiovascular   Carvedilol has been evaluated in patients with heart failure (1[C]). In more than 50% of the patients given carvedilol the dosage could be titrated up to the maximum (50 mg/day). The major reason for missing the target dose was *hypotension* followed by bradycardia. Carvedilol had to be withdrawn in 21/316 patients (6.6%), in 14 (4.4%) for cardiovascular reasons: six with *worsening heart failure*, five with *hypotension*, two with *syncope*, and one with *bradycardia*. The most frequent non-cardiovascular reason for withdrawal was *chronic obstructive pulmonary disease*. Age did not influence tolerability: the rate of discontinuation was similar in patients aged 70 years or older and in younger patients. These data have confirmed in a real clinical context what controlled studies have shown, that carvedilol is generally well tolerated and that the maximum target dose can be reached in a relevant number of patients irrespective of age and severity of heart failure.

In an unusual case of Munchausen's syndrome, a female general practitioner repeatedly took high doses of beta-blockers in order to simulate symptomatic *sick sinus syndrome* (2[A]).

Respiratory   In a randomized controlled clinical trial in 21 otherwise healthy individuals with high-pressure primary open-angle glaucoma, six of 11 who used topical timolol 0.5% for 3 years had subclinical *increases in bronchial reactivity* not completely reversible in three cases on withdrawal of the beta-blocker (3[c]).

Nervous system   *Delirium* has been attributed to metoprolol (4[A]).

- A 53-year-old man with a history of alcohol abuse suffered personality changes and multiple hallucinogenic episodes for 2 years, attributed to dementia probably caused by alcohol abuse. He also taking acenocoumerol, atorvastatin, quinapril, and metoprolol 50 mg bd for atrial flutter. Metoprolol, which had been started 2 years before, was withdrawn. Within 24 hours the delirium had disappeared completely and the liver enzymes fell.

Gastrointestinal   Propranolol can rarely cause *mesenteric ischemia* (5[A]).

- A 59-year-old white man with hyperthyroidism was given propylthiouracil 100 mg tds and propranolol 20 mg bd. The next day, he developed increased abdominal pain and bloody diarrhea. Angiography showed superior mesenteric artery occlusion. Antegrade aorta-mesenteric bypass surgery was performed for revascularization.

Propranolol can reduce splanchnic blood flow by reducing cardiac output and selectively inhibiting vasodilatory receptors in the splanchnic circulation.

Urinary tract   The lower urinary tract *symptoms of benign prostatic hyperplasia* in a 60-year-old man worsened antihypertensive treatment with bisoprolol (6[A]). Withdrawal resulted in relief whereas and rechallenge caused repeated deterioration.

Skin   Various drugs can cause a lupus-like syndrome. Beta-adrenoceptor antagonists have been implicated only infrequently and there have been no cases of *subacute cutaneous lupus erythematosus* associated with the use of

Side Effects of Drugs, Annual 30
J.K. Aronson (Editor)
ISSN: 0378-6080
DOI: 10.1016/S0378-6080(08)00018-4

beta-adrenoceptor antagonists. Subacute cutaneous lupus erythematosus has been attributed to acebutolol (7[A]).

- A 57-year-old woman with hypertension developed a cutaneous eruption taking acebutolol for 1 month. She had no history of photosensitivity, photodermatosis, or immunological diseases. A complete blood cell count, liver and kidney tests, rheumatoid factor, and complement fractions were all within the reference ranges. There was a positive titer of antinuclear antibodies. A biopsy specimen showed atrophy of the epidermis. A positive lupus band test was found at direct immunofluorescence. Acebutolol was withdrawn, and she was given chloroquine sulfate associated with photoprotection. The cutaneous eruption resolved progressively. After 4 months the skin lesions had completely cleared. A Seroly test was negative for antihistone antibodies.

While several cases of subacute cutaneous lupus erythematosus have been described with other antihypertensive agents, such as captopril, calcium channel blockers, and hydrochlorothiazide, this seems to have been the first case described in a patient taking a beta-adrenoceptor antagonist. This case and its evolution suggest a link between acebutolol therapy and the onset of a lupus-like syndrome, whose pathogenesis is unclear.

Toxic epidermal necrolysis occurred 1 week after the combined use of dorzolamide, timolol, and latanoprost eyedrops in an otherwise healthy 60-year-old woman; the authors attributed it to the combination of timolol and dorzolamide (8[A]).

Sexual function *Erectile dysfunction* is common in men with hypertension, particularly in those who take beta-adrenoceptor antagonists. New-generation beta-blockers, such as nebivolol, seem to cause less sexual dysfunction, probably because they increase the release of nitric oxide. In a randomized, single-blind, multicenter trial, 131 patients with a new diagnosis of hypertension, without prior erectile dysfunction, were randomized to either atenolol or atenolol plus chlorthalidone or nebivolol (9[C]). Over 12 weeks the patients who were allocated to nebivolol did not have any change in the number of satisfactory episodes of sexual intercourse, while those who took atenolol or atenolol plus chlorthalidone had a significant reduction from baseline. Given a similar effect in reducing blood pressure, nebivolol seems to maintain a more active sexual life in hypertensive men than atenolol. Increased release of nitric oxide due to nebivolol may counteract the detrimental effect of beta-adrenoceptor antagonists on sexual activity.

Peyronie's disease has been attributed to long-term therapy with timolol eye drops 0.25% bd in a 74-year-old man who had used it for 22 years; the conditon improved when he stopped using timolol (10[A]). This seems to have been the first report of this condition in a patient using beta-blocker eye drops.

Immunologic The authors of a brief review of the risk of *anaphylaxis* with beta-blockers have concluded that the risk is not increased (11[r]).

Drug formulations Timolol hydrogel eyedrops 0.1% have been compared with timolol aqueous solution 0.5% in a randomized, double-blind, crossover study in 24 healthy subjects (12[c]). The aqueous solution had about 10 times more systemic availability than the hydrogel. There was no difference between the two formulations in efficacy in reducing intraocular pressure, but the mean peak heart rate during exercise was reduced by 19/minute by the aqueous solution and by only 5/minute by the hydrogel.

Drug overdose The management of self-poisoning with beta-blockers has again been reviewed (13[R]). In one case an overdose of propranolol unmasked *Brugada syndrome* (14[A]).

- A 24-year-old healthy man took propranolol 2.28 g. After gastric lavage, electrolytes, cardiac enzymes, chest X-ray, and echocardiography were normal, but an electrocardiogram showed the typical coved pattern of Brugada syndrome. An ajmaline test confirmed Brugada syndrome.

The electrocardiographic effects in this case may have been due to the membrane stabilizing effect of high concentration of propranolol and/or inhibition of calcium channels.

NITRATES, ORGANIC   (SED-15, 2529; SEDA-27, 204; SEDA-28, 218; SEDA-29, 195)

Glyceryl trinitrate (nitroglycerin)

Cardiovascular   Of 118 patients (66 men and 52 women) with chest pain (mean age 63 years) 30 patients had normal coronary arteries or minimal or non-obstructive coronary artery disease and 88 had obstructive lesions defined as luminal narrowing greater than 50% in any one or more of the left or right coronary arteries or their major branches (15[c]). Glyceryl trinitrate produced variable relief of chest pain within 10 minutes in all cases. Significant *headache* occurred in 36% and the patients with normal or minimally diseased coronary arteries had a greater risk of significant headache than those with obstructive lesions (73 versus 23%).

Respiratory   Episodes of severe *oxygen desaturation* occurred in a 43-year-old man with obesity, hypertension, and diabetes mellitus after intravenous administration of glyceryl trinitrate on two occasions, which the authors attributed to inhibition of hypoxic pulmonary vasoconstriction (16[A]).

Nervous system   In a patient with *migraine* triggered on two separate occasions by glyceryl trinitrate positron emission tomography showed activation in the primary visual area of the occipital cortex during the aura (17[A]).

Management of adverse reactions   Abrupt cessation of intravenous glyceryl trinitrate after infusion for more than 24 hours often causes *rebound vasoconstriction*; this can be prevented by the use of oral isosorbide dinitrate (18[A]).

Molsidomine   (SED-15, 2371)

Drug formulations   A new form of molsidomine, a prolonged-release tablet containing 16 mg for once-a-day administration has been evaluated in 533 patients (19[C]). Blood pressure and heart rate, electrocardiographic findings, and blood parameters were not affected by molsidomine. Drug-related adverse events occurred

in respectively 4.7, 5.4, and 6.9% of patients allocated to placebo, molsidomine 8 mg, and molsidomine 16 mg. The difference was not statistically significant. The most commonly reported events were headache and hypotension; the latter was significantly associated with molsidomine 16 mg, although the hypotension episodes were reported as being non-serious.

CALCIUM CHANNEL BLOCKERS   (SED-15, 598; SEDA-27, 224; SEDA-28, 218; SEDA-29, 195)

Drug overdose   The management of self-poisoning with calcium channel blockers has again been reviewed (13[R]).

- A 43-year old man took amlodipine 560 mg and failed to respond to fluid resuscitation, calcium salts, glucagon, and noradrenaline/adrenaline inotropic support (20[A]). However, intravenous metaraminol 2 mg followed by 83 micrograms/minute produced an improvement in his blood pressure, cardiac output, and urine output.
- A 65-year-old man with aortic stenosis died after mistakenly taking six tablets of modified-release diltiazem SR 360 mg (21[A]). He developed symptoms of toxicity within 7 hours and died after 17 hours. The diltiazem concentration in an antemortem blood sample 11.5 hours after ingestion was 2.9 μg/ml and in a postmortem sample of central blood 6 μg/ml.

Amlodipine   (SED-15, 175; SEDA-27, 205; SEDA-28, 219; SEDA-29, 195)

Nails   *Longitudinal melanonychia* is tan, brown, or black longitudinal streaking in the nail plate due to increased melanin deposition and *Hutchinson's sign* is periungual pigmentation. In a 75-year-old Indian man longitudinal melanonychia and periungual pigmentation affecting several fingernails and toenails were attributed to amlodipine, which he had taken for 2 years for hypertension (22[A]).

Fluid balance   Calcium channel blockers often cause peripheral *edema*, usually limited to the lower legs; periocular and perioral edema are less common. Occasionally edema can be more severe, and a case of anasarca has been reported in a 77-year-old woman with essential hypertension taking amlodipine 10 mg/day (23[A]).

Diltiazem   *(SED-15, 1126; SEDA-27, 205; SEDA-28, 219; SEDA-29, 196)*

Mouth   *Gingival enlargement* has been studied in 46 patients taking diltiazem ($n = 32$) or verapamil ($n = 14$) compared with 49 cardiovascular controls who had never taken them (24[c]). There was more gingival enlargement in the patients taking diltiazem compared with controls: 31% as assessed by the vertical gingival overgrowth index and in 50% as assessed by the horizontal Miranda & Brunet index. The corresponding figures for verapamil were 21 and 36% (not different from controls). The risk of gingival enlargement (odds ratio) associated with diltiazem therapy, adjusted for gingival index values, was 3.5 (1.0–12) the vertical gingival overgrowth index and 6.2 (1.9, 20) for the horizontal Miranda & Brunet index. Verapamil had no significant effect.

Gastrointestinal   *Intestinal pseudo-obstruction* has been attributed to diltiazem (25[A]).

- A 74-year-old man with acute myelogenous leukemia and neutropenia was given five doses of intravenous diltiazem 5 mg every 5–10 minutes plus amiodarone for atrial fibrillation, followed by diltiazem 30 mg orally qds and a continuous infusion of amiodarone. Amiodarone was withdrawn after 1 day because of an adverse effect and the dose of diltiazem was increased to 120 mg qds orally by day 14. On day 15, he developed increasing abdominal distention with hyperactive bowel sounds. An abdominal X-ray showed multiple dilated loops in the small and large bowel and diltiazem was withdrawn, after which he recovered.

Medications rarely cause intestinal pseudo-obstruction, but calcium channel blockers cause smooth muscle relaxation, which was probably the causative mechanism in this case.

Skin   Skin reactions to calcium channel blockers have been reviewed in the light of a report of three reactions to diltiazem, which causes skin reactions more often than other calcium channel blockers (26[A]).

- A 54-year-old man developed a generalized erythema-multiforme-like reaction followed by erythrodermia and exfoliative dermatitis after taking diltiazem for 6–7 days.
- An 80-year-old woman had a pruritic exanthematous eruption on her trunk 10 days after taking diltiazem, which evolved to generalized erythrodermia and superficial desquamation; it gradually improved in 10–12 days after withdrawal.
- A 79-year-old man developed erythema and pruritus initially on the back, and then affecting the thorax, limbs, and face after taking diltiazem for 3 days. Diltiazem was withdrawn and the skin improved, but verapamil was started 3 days later and the skin worsened again.

The authors carried out skin tests with different calcium channel blockers. Diltiazem was positive in all three patients; nifedipine was positive in patient 2 and verapamil in patient 3.

Felodipine   *(SEDA-29, 197; SEDA-29, 197)*

Mouth   Felodipine-associated *gingival enlargement* has been reported in a patient with type 2 diabetes (27[A]). The changes resolved after withdrawal of felodipine and control of the diabetes, and there were further improvements after scaling and root planing and instruction about oral hygiene. The histological features, elongated rete pegs, fibrous hyperplasia, a low-grade chronic inflammatory infiltrate, predominantly consisting of lymphocytes, and collagen bundle groups randomly distributed, were similar to those present in other cases of drug-associated gingival enlargement.

Lercanidipine   *(SED-15, 2024; SEDA-28, 219; SEDA-29, 197)*

Susceptibility factors

Renal disease   Dihydropyridine calcium channel blockers often cause adverse effects that necessitate withdrawal, particularly in more fragile patients, such as those with renal dysfunction. Lercanidipine has been assessed in a multicenter trial in 203 hypertensive patients with chronic renal insufficiency (28[C]). None had achieved a target blood pressure (systolic pressure >130 mmHg or diastolic blood pressure

>90 mmHg) despite treatment with a blocker of the renin-angiotensin system, either an ACE inhibitor or an angiotensin receptor blocker. Lercanidipine was added in a dosage of 10 mg/day for 6 months. In all, 43/203 patients (21%) withdrew from the study for several reasons, poor adherence and uncontrolled blood pressure being the most frequent. In three of these 43 the reason was possibly related to lercanidipine: erectile dysfunction in one, urinary incontinence in one, and dry mouth and eosinophilia in one. Biochemical values did not change significantly during treatment, with the exception of (a) creatinine clearance, which improved significantly after 6 months; (b) proteinuria, which improved significantly, and (c) cholesterol and trygliceride concentrations, which were significantly lower at the end of the treatment period.

Nicardipine   *(SED-15, 2502; SEDA-27, 206; SEDA-29, 197)*

Cardiovascular   A 38-year-old parturient developed *acute pulmonary edema* more than 48 hours after tocolytic treatment with nicardipine and salbutamol at 30 weeks gestation (29[A]). The authors discussed the question of whether a second tocolytic should be used after a first has failed.

Nifedipine   *(SED-15, 2516; SEDA-27, 206; SEDA-28, 220; SEDA-29, 198)*

Cardiovascular   Rapid blood pressure reduction is not recommended in severe hypertension in older people because of adverse effects related to impaired cerebral autoregulation, although sublingual nifedipine is still used in children, in whom the cerebral circulation is more robust. *Ventricular dysrhythmias* have been described in a teenager who was given nifedipine 10 mg sublingually for symptomatic, severe hypertension (blood pressure 180/120) (30[A]). Within minutes she complained of palpitation and had a tachycardia of 100/minute with ventricular bigeminy and later ventricular extra beats. The authors suggested that reflex sympathetic activation following an abrupt drop in blood pressure

may have caused the dysrhythmias, because of raised catecholamine concentrations, and that it may be more appropriate to treat severe hypertension in young people with intravenous antihypertensive agents that can be titrated to produce controlled reductions in blood pressure.

Gastrointestinal   Retention of modified-release capsules can cause *bezoar* formation. In a patient with a enteric stricture, modified-release capsules of nifedipine caused *recurrent small bowel obstruction* (31[A]).

Pregnancy   Severe *hypotension followed by fetal death* has been reported after the administration of nifedipine as a tocolytic (32[A]).

- A 23-year-old woman of African origin went into preterm labor and was given tocolytic therapy with atosiban. The uterine contractions continued and indometacin was added until the contractions ceased after 24 hours. After 48 hours the atosiban was withdrawn and 5 hours later the uterine contractions started again. She was given oral nifedipine 10 mg but after the second dose the blood pressure fell to 73/30 mmHg. Ultrasound examination showed severe fetal bradycardia soon followed by death. Tocolytic therapy was withdrawn and a colloid infusion started. After 6 hours the blood pressure was again normal.

The authors concluded that care should be taken when administering nifedipine as a tocolytic in pregnancy. They did not deny that nifedipine is generally safe and effective in these circumstances, but others disagreed that nifedipine had caused severe hypotension in this case: "In our 15 years of personal experience with nifedipine for the management of preterm labour, we have never seen such severe hypotension in a previously normotensive 'euvolemic' patient" (33[r]). They pointed out that the half-life of nifedipine is only 1.3 hours and that its adverse effects are generally mild and transient side. They cited several meta-analyses that have shown that nifedipine is associated with better neonatal outcomes and fewer adverse maternal outcomes than other tocolytic agents, especially beta-adrenoceptor agonists.

However, other authors described another case of severe hypotension, in a 24-year-old woman in her third pregnancy who had suspected preterm labour at 26 weeks of gestation and was given nifedipine tocolysis, 30 mg orally followed by two doses of 20 mg, after which she complained of severe headache, visual disturbances, flushing, dizziness, palpitation, nausea, and vomiting; her pulse rate was 120/minute and her blood pressure 80/40 mmHg (34[A]). She required circulatory resuscitation using intravenous infusions of crystalloids and colloids, and her blood pressure returned to normal over the next 30 minutes. There was no evidence of fetal compromise during these events.

Furthermore, there is no doubt that severe hypotension can happen in these cases. Of 73 consultant obstetricians in the United Kingdom who replied to a survey, 53% used nifedipine as their first-line tocolytic and 40% used atosiban (35[c]). Of these, 17 reported maternal hypotension of sufficient severity to cause fetal compromise necessitating cesarean section with nifedipine, compared with four with ritodrine and two with atosiban.

Others have pointed out that conclusions from meta-analyses that favor the use of nifedipine as a tocolytic agent are not supported by close examination of the data, since the tocolytic actions have been studied primarily in normal pregnancies (36[r]). They have suggested that care should be taken in giving nifedipine when the maternal cardiovascular condition is compromised, such as in intrauterine infection, twin pregnancy, maternal hypertension, and cardiac disease, because of the risks of life-threatening pulmonary edema and/or cardiac failure, in which baroreceptor-mediated increases in sympathetic tone may not balance the cardiac depressant activity of nifedipine.

Drug–drug interactions   Severe hypotension with reduced systemic vascular resistance occurred in a patient taking nifedipine and *clarithromycin* (37[A]).

- A 77-year-old ex-smoker with a history of type 2 diabetes and hypertension took modified-release nifedipine 60 mg tds, doxazosin 8 mg tds, captopril 25 mg tds, metformin 850 mg tds, and aspirin 300 mg/day. Clarithromycin 500 mg tds was added for a presumed chest infection. Two days later he developed shock, heart block, and multi-organ failure, with reduced systemic vascular resistence, compatible with septic shock secondary to a respiratory infection. However, no causative micro-organisms were identified and the leukocyte

count was normal. The antihypertensive agents were withdrawn and noradrenaline was given. He recovered.

The authors suggested that extreme hypotension had occurred secondary to a fall in systemic vascular resistence, because of excessive hypotension, due to an interaction of nifedipine with clarithromycin. The time course supported this hypothesis.

Verapamil   *(SED-15, 3618; SEDA-27, 207; SEDA-28, 220; SEDA-29, 199)*

Endocrine   Marked *hyperprolactinemia* has been attributed to verapamil in a 42-year-old woman who may have been hypersusceptible to this action of verapamil (38[AR]).

Mouth   Four patients with cluster headache developed *gingival enlargement* after taking verapamil. In two it was treated by optimizing oral hygiene and dental plaque control (39[AR]). In the other one it was also necessary to reduce the dose of verapamil, and in one the verapamil had to be withdrawn to reverse the gingival enlargement.

Skin   Subacute *cutaneous lupus erythematosus* has been attributed in a single case to verapamil (40[A]).

Drug overdose   The management of verapamil overdose has been reviewed in the context of a case report (41[AR]).

- A 29-year-old woman took an overdose of sotalol 4.8 g and verapamil 3.6 g and had cardiovascular collapse (42[A]). After 4 hours of normothermic cardiopulmonary resuscitation extracorporeal heart lung assist was established. Vasoactive drugs were withheld after 2 days. She recovered after 5 days, after experiencing several complications (intestinal bleeding, transient nerve paralysis, and renal insufficiency due to rhabdomyolysis).

Drug–drug interactions   Verapamil has a marked negative inotropic effect and can cause refractory cardiogenic shock, particularly when it is used in combination with a *beta-blocker*, as combination that is generally to be avoided (43[AR]).

Verapamil toxicity has been attributed to inhibition of verapamil metabolism by *telithromycin* (44^{AR}).

- A 76-year-old white woman taking verapamil 180 mg/day for hypertension took telithromycin 800 mg/day for 2 days for acute sinusitis and became short of breath, weak, profoundly hypotensive and bradycardic, with a systolic blood pressure of 50–60 mmHg and a heart rate of 30/minute. She recovered after drug withdrawal and supportive measures.

Telithromycin is a substrate of CYP3A4 and presumably inhibited the metabolism of verapamil.

References

1. Nul D, Zambrano C, Diaz A, Ferrante D, Varini S, Soifer S, Grancelli H, Doval H, Grupo de Estudio de la Sobrevida en la Insuficiencia Cardiaca en Argentina. Impact of a standardized titration protocol with carvedilol in heart failure: safety, tolerability, and efficacy—a report from the GESICA Registry. Cardiovasc Drugs Ther 2005;19:125–34.
2. Steinwender C, Hofmann R, Kypta A, Leisch F. Recurrent symptomatic bradycardia due to secret ingestion of beta-blockers—a rare manifestation of cardiac Munchhausen syndrome. Wien Klin Wochenschr 2005;117(18):647–50.
3. Gandolfi SA, Chetta A, Cimino L, Mora P, Sangermani C, Tardini MG. Bronchial reactivity in healthy individuals undergoing long-term topical treatment with beta-blockers. Arch Ophthalmol 2005;123(1):35–8.
4. van der Vleuten PA, van den Brink E, Schoonderwoerd BA, van den Berg F, Tio RA, Zijlstra F. Delirant beeld, toegeschreven aan het gebruik van metoprolol. Ned Tijdschr Geneeskd 2005;149(39):2183–6.
5. Köksal AS, Usküdar O, Köklü S, Yüksel O, Beyazit Y, Sahin B. Propranolol-exacerbated mesenteric ischemia in a patient with hyperthyroidism. Ann Pharmacother 2005;39(3):559–62.
6. Sein Anand J, Chodorowski Z, Hajduk A. Repeated intensification of lower urinary tract symptoms in the patient with benign prostatic hyperplasia during bisoprolol treatment. Przegl Lek 2005;62(6):522–3.
7. Fenniche S, Dhaoui A, Ben Ammar F, Benmously R, Marrak H, Mokhtar I. Acebutolol-induced subacute cutaneous lupus erythematosus. Skin Pharmacol Physiol 2005;18:230–3.
8. Flórez A, Rosón E, Conde A, González B, García-Doval I, de la Torre C, Cruces M. Toxic epidermal necrolysis secondary to timolol, dorzolamide, and latanoprost eyedrops. J Am Acad Dermatol 2005;53(5):909–11.
9. Boydak B, Nalbantgil S, Fici F, Nalbantgil I, Zoghi M, Ozerkan F, Tengiz I, Ercan E, Yilmaz H, Yoket U, Onder R. A randomised comparison of the effects of nebivolol and atenolol with and without chlorthalidone on the sexual function of hypertensive men. Clin Drug Invest 2005;25(6):409–16.
10. Ross JJ, Rahman I, Walters RF. Peyronie's disease following long-term use of topical timolol. Eye 2006;20(8):974–6.
11. Miller MM, Miller MM. Beta-blockers and anaphylaxis: are the risks overstated? J Allergy Clin Immunol 2005;116(4):931–3.
12. Uusitalo H, Nino J, Tahvanainen K, Turjanmaa V, Ropo A, Tuominen J, Kahonen M. Efficacy and systemic side-effects of topical 0.5% timolol aqueous solution and 0.1% timolol hydrogel. Acta Ophthalmol Scand 2005;83(6):723–8.
13. Ojetti V, Migneco A, Bononi F, De Lorenzo A, Gentiloni Silveri N. Calcium channel blockers, beta-blockers and digitalis poisoning: management in the emergency room. Eur Rev Med Pharmacol Sci 2005;9(4):241–6.
14. Aouate P, Clerc J, Viard P, Seoud J. Propranolol intoxication revealing a Brugada syndrome. J Cardiovasc Electrophysiol 2005;16(3):348–51.
15. Hsi DH, Roshandel A, Singh N, Szombathy T, Meszaros ZS. Headache response to glyceryl trinitrate in patients with and without obstructive coronary artery disease. Heart 2005;91(9):1164–6.
16. Karaaslan P, Dönmez A, Arslan G. Severe hypoxaemia following intravenous nitroglycerine administration in an obese patient: case report. Eur J Anaesthesiol 2005;22(12):957–8.
17. Afridi S, Kaube H, Goadsby PJ. Occipital activation in glyceryl trinitrate induced migraine with visual aura. J Neurol Neurosurg Psychiatry 2005;76(8):1158–60.
18. Kelly EA, Ahmed RM, Horowitz JD. Withdrawal of intravenous glyceryl trinitrate: absence of rebound phenomena with transition to oral isosorbide dinitrate. Clin Exp Pharmacol Physiol 2005;32(4):269–72.
19. Messin R, Opolski G, Fenyvesi T, Carreer-Bruhwyler F, Dubois C, Famaey JP, Géczy J. Efficacy and safety of molsidomine once-a-day in patients with stable angina pectoris. Int J Cardiol 2005;98:79–89.

20. Wood DM, Wright KD, Jones AL, Dargan PI. Metaraminol (Aramine) in the management of a significant amlodipine overdose. Hum Exp Toxicol 2005;24(7):377–81.
21. Cantrell FL, Williams SR. Fatal unintentional overdose of diltiazem with antemortem and postmortem values. Clin Toxicol (Phila) 2005;43(6):587–8.
22. Sladden MJ, Mortimer NJ, Osborne JE. Longitudinal melanonychia and pseudo-Hutchinson sign associated with amlodipine. Br J Dermatol 2005;153(1):219–20.
23. Sener D, Halil M, Yavuz BB, Cankurtaran M, Ariogul S. Anasarca edema with amlodipine treatment. Ann Pharmacother 2005;39(4):761–3.
24. Miranda J, Brunet L, Roset P, Berini L, Farre M, Mendieta C. Prevalence and risk of gingival overgrowth in patients treated with diltiazem or verapamil. J Clin Periodontol. 2005;32(3):294–8.
25. Young RP, Wu H. Intestinal pseudo-obstruction caused by diltiazem in a neutropenic patient. Ann Pharmacother 2005;39(10):1749–51.
26. Gonzalo Garijo MA, Pérez Calderón R, de Argila Fernández-Durán D, Rangel Mayoral JF. Cutaneous reactions due to diltiazem and cross reactivity with other calcium channel blockers. Allergol Immunopathol (Madr) 2005;33(4):238–40.
27. Fay AA, Satheesh K, Gapski R. Felodipine-influenced gingival enlargement in an uncontrolled type 2 diabetic patient. J Periodontol 2005;76(7):1217.
28. Robles NR, Ocon J, Gomez CF, Manjon M, Pastor L, Herrera J, Villatoro J, Calls J, Torrijos J, Rodríguez VI, Rodriguez MM, Mendez ML, Morey A, Martinez FI, Marco J, Liebana A, Rincon B, Tornero F. Lercanidipine in patients with chronic renal failure: the ZAFRA Study. Renal Failure 2005;1:73–80.
29. Chapuis C, Menthonnex E, Debaty G, Koch FX, Rancurel E, Menthonnex P, Pons JC. Oedème aigu du poumon au decours d'une tocolyse par nicardipine et salbutamol lors d'une menace d'accouchement prématuré sur grossesse gémellaire. J Gynecol Obstet Biol Reprod (Paris) 2005;34(5):493–6.
30. Castaneda MP, Walsh CA, Woroniecki RP, Del Rio M, Flynn JT. Ventricular arrhythmia following short-acting nifedipine administration. Pediatr Nephrol 2005;20(7):1000–2.
31. Yeen WC, Willis IH. Retention of extended release nifedipine capsules in a patient with enteric stricture causing recurrent small bowel obstruction. South Med J 2005;98(8):839–42.
32. van Veen AJ, Pelinck MJ, van Pampus MG, Erwich JJ. Severe hypotension and fetal death due to tocolysis with nifedipine. BJOG 2005;112(4):509–10.
33. Papatsonis DN, Carbonne B, Dekker GA, Flenady V, King JF. Severe hypotension and fetal death due to tocolysis with nifedipine. BJOG 2005;112(11):1582–3.
34. Kandysamy V, Thomson AJ. Severe hypotension and fetal death due to tocolysis with nifedipine. BJOG 2005;112(11):1583–4.
35. Johnson KA, Mason GC. Severe hypotension and fetal death due to tocolysis with nifedipine. BJOG 2005;112(11):1583.
36. van Geijn HP, Lenglet JE, Bolte AC. Nifedipine trials: effectiveness and safety aspects. BJOG 2005;112(Suppl 1):79–83.
37. Gerònimo-Pardo M, Cuartero-del-Pozo AB, Jimènez-Vizuete JM, Cortinas-Sàez M, Peyrò-Garcia R. Clarithromycin-nifedipine interaction as possible cause of vasodilatory shock. Ann Pharmacother 2005;39:538–42.
38. Krysiak R, Okopieh B, Herman ZS. Hiperprolaktynemia spowodowana przez werapamil. Opis przypadku. Arch Med Wewn 2005;113(2):155–8.
39. Matharu MS, van Vliet JA, Ferrari MD, Goadsby PJ. Verapamil induced gingival enlargement in cluster headache. J Neurol Neurosurg Psychiatry 2005;76(1):124–7.
40. Kurtis B, Larson MJ, Hoang MP, Cohen JB. Case report: verapamil-induced subacute cutaneous lupus erythematosus. J Drugs Dermatol 2005;4(4):506–8.
41. Morales MG, Guerrero SG, Garcia GR, Villalobos SJ, Camarena AG, Aguirre SJ, Martinez SJ. Intoxicacion grave con verapamilo. Arch Cardiol Mex 2005;75(Suppl 3):S3-100–5.
42. Rygnestad T, Moen S, Wahba A, Lien S, Ingul CB, Schrader H, Knapstad SE. Severe poisoning with sotalol and verapamil. Recovery after 4 h of normothermic CPR followed by extra corporeal heart lung assist. Acta Anaesthesiol Scand 2005;49(9):1378–80.
43. Nanda U, Ashish A, Why HJ. Modified release verapamil induced cardiogenic shock. Emerg Med J 2005;22(11):832–3.
44. Reed M, Wall GC, Shah NP, Heun JM, Hicklin GA. Verapamil toxicity resulting from a probable interaction with telithromycin. Ann Pharmacother 2005;39(2):357–60.

R. Verhaeghe and P. Verhamme

19   Drugs acting on the cerebral and peripheral circulations

DRUGS USED IN THE TREATMENT OF ARTERIAL DISORDERS OF THE BRAIN AND LIMBS

Cilostazol   *(SED-15, 773; SEDA-27, 209; SEDA-29, 202)*

Drug–drug interactions   The phosphodiesterase inhibitor cilostazol has antiplatelet properties in addition to an action on vascular smooth muscle and was therefore initially thought to be unsafe in combination with other commonly used antiplatelet drugs, such as aspirin or clopidogrel. However, in a crossover study in 21 patients with peripheral disease cilostazol did not significantly increase bleeding time, nor further prolong it when it was added to any regimen containing *aspirin* or *clopidogrel* (1[C]). Thus, cilostazol is not expected to increase the risk of adverse bleeding effects when combined with aspirin or clopidogrel.

Ginkgo biloba (Ginkgoaceae)

See Chapter 48.

Pentoxifylline   *(SED-15, 2779; SEDA-27, 210)*

Skin   Acute *urticaria* triggered by pentoxifylline and confirmed by skin tests and oral rechallenge has been reported in a 60-year-old man (2[A]).

DRUGS USED IN THE TREATMENT OF VENOUS DISORDERS

Drugs used for venous disease, in Mediterranean countries often called phlebotonics, are in general poorly evaluated. The authors of a Cochrane review have concluded that these drugs have minor effects on edema, but this is of uncertain clinical significance (3[M]).

Calcium dobesilate   *(SED-15, 610; SEDA-29, 202)*

Hematologic   In a recent overview calcium dobesilate ranked second in a list of drugs associated with *agranulocytosis* (4[R]). Nevertheless, in a previous review it was estimated that the incidence is very low (less than one in a million) and lower than in the general population (SEDA-29, 202).

DRUGS USED IN THE TREATMENT OF MIGRAINE

Triptans   *(SED-15, 3525; SEDA-27, 210; SEDA-29, 203)*

Cardiovascular   *Vasoconstriction* leading to organ ischemia is the most feared adverse effect of triptans. It can occur in very young people with presumed normal blood vessels (5[A]).

Side Effects of Drugs, Annual 30
J.K. Aronson (Editor)
ISSN: 0378-6080
DOI: 10.1016/S0378-6080(08)00019-6

• A 16-year-old boy developed chest pain which started 20 minutes after he took a first intranasal dose of sumatriptan for cluster headache. A diagnosis of non Q wave myocardial infarction was made on the basis of ST segment changes and increased cardiac enzymes. Angiography showed normal coronary arteries.

Nervous system   *Serotonin syndrome* has been reported in a 65-year-old woman taking sumatriptan and paroxetine (6[A]). The authors argued that the combined use of a presynaptic serotonin reuptake inhibitor with a postsynaptic serotonin receptor agonist may have facilitated the occurrence of the serotonin syndrome. However, the two drugs can also both cause the serotonin syndrome when taken separately (7[r]).

OTHER PERIPHERAL VASODILATORS

Inhibitors of phosphodiesterase type V   *(SED-15, 3133; SEDA-27, 210; SEDA-28, 224; SEDA-29, 203)*

Reviews of inhibitors of phosphodiesterase type V repeatedly stress the overall good tolerance of this class of drugs (8[R], 9[R], 10[R]). The most common complaints are *headache, facial flushing, nasal congestion*, and *dyspepsia*. *Prolonged erection* and *priapism* are rare. There is a risk of hypotension when the triptans are combined with *nitrates*.

Cardiovascular   *Prolongation of the QT_c interval* has been reported but usually without serious dysrhythmias, although ventricular tachycardia has been reported after sildenafil (SED-15, 3133).

• A healthy 50-year-old man took vardenafil 10 mg and 15 minutes later developed persistent palpitation lasting 2 hours (11[A]). He had atrial fibrillation and no structural heart disease. The dysrhythmia converted spontaneously to sinus rhythm 4 hours later.

The authors suggested that hypotension induced by vardenafil had led to a reflex tachycardia.

Sensory systems   *Non-arteritic anterior ischemic optic neuropathy* (NAION) is the most common acquired optic neuropathy after the age of 50 and has repeatedly been connected to inhibitors of phosphodiesterase type V, most often sildenafil. Case reports are being published in ever increasing numbers, but they do not clarify the problem. In a recent review the weak points in the possible connection between inhibitors of phosphodiesterase type V and NAION have been emphasized (12[R]).

Liver   *Acute hepatitis* has been reported in association with sildenafil (SEDA-28, 224). There have now been further reports in two men, aged 49 and 56 years, without apparent risk factors for liver disease (13[A], 14[A]). The evidence in favor of a link between acute liver disease and sildenafil is largely circumstantial but corresponds to accepted criteria for drug-induced hepatitis.

• Fatal variceal rupture occurred in a 41-year-old man with alcoholic liver cirrhosis and portal hypertension 3–4 hours after he took an unknown dose of sildenafil (15[A]).

The authors hypothesized that sildenafil caused vasodilatation and increased splanchnic blood flow, thereby augmenting intravariceal pressure. He also had a high blood concentration of ethanol, another vasodilator.

Skin   *Rashes* have been attributed to sildenafil.

• A 57-year-old man developed lichenoid lesions on the upper half of the body (16[A]). Biopsy showed degeneration of keratinocytes and a dense lymphohistioid infiltrate arranged in a lichenoid pattern. He had been taken sildenafil irregularly. The eruption resolved within 3 weeks of withdrawal of sildenafil and recurred after rechallenge a few weeks later.
• A 67-year-old man developed toxic epidermal necrolysis, having during the previous 48 hours taken sildenafil between 300 and 400 mg (partly as a commercially available drug and partly in a Chinese aphrodisiac herbal medicine) (17[A]). He had also been taking eight different medicines for diabetes, hypertension, hyperlipidemia, heart failure, gout, and osteoarthritis. The serum concentration of tumor necrosis factor was initially raised. He was given infliximab and recovered.

References

1. Comerota AJ. Effect on platelet function of cilostazol, clopidogrel, and aspirin, each alone or in combination. Atheroscler Suppl 2005;6:13–9.
2. Gonzales-Mahave I, Del Pozo MD, Blasco A, Lobera T, Venturini M. Urticaria due to pentoxyfylline. Allergy 2005;60:705.
3. Martinez MJ, Bonfill X, Moreno RM, Vargas E, Capella D. Phlebotonics for venous insufficiency. Cochrane Database Syst Rev 2005;3:CD003229.
4. Ibanez L, Vidal X, Ballarin E, Laporte JR. Population-based drug-induced agranulocytosis. Arch Intern Med 2005;165:869–74.
5. Erbilen E, Ozhan H, Akdemir R, Yazici M. A case of myocardial infarction with sumatriptan use. Pediatr Cardiol 2005;26:464–6.
6. Hendrix Y, van Zagten MS. Serotonin syndrome as a result of concomitant use of paroxetine and sumatriptan. Ned Tijdschr Geneeskd 2005;149:1654.
7. Mathew NT, Tietjen GE, Lucker C. Serotonin syndrome complicating migraine pharmacotherapy. Cephalalgia 1996;16:323–7.
8. Rashid A. The efficacy and safety of PDE5 inhibitors. Clin Cornerstone 2005;7:47–56.
9. Reffelmann T, Kloner RA. Pharmacotherapy of erectile dysfunction: focus on cardiovascular safety. Expert Opin Drug Saf. 2005;4:531–40.
10. Carson 3rd CC. Cardiac safety in clinical trials of phosphodiesterase 5 inhibitors. Am J Cardiol 2005;96:37M–41M.
11. Veloso HH, de Paola AAV. Atrial fibrillation after vardenafil therapy. Emerg Med J 2005;22:823.
12. Tomsak R. PDE5 inhibitors and permanent visual loss. Int J Impot Res 2005;17:547–9.
13. Balian A, Touati F, Huguenin B, Prevot S, Perlemuter G, Naveau S, Chaput JC. Probable sildenafil induced acute hepatitis in a patient with no other risk factors. Gastroenterol Biol Clin 2005;29:89.
14. Daghfous R, El Aidli S, Zaiem A, Loueslati MH, Belkahia C. Sildenafil-associated hepatotoxicity. Am J Gastroenterol 2005;100(8):1895–6.
15. Finley DS, Lugo B, Ridgway J, Teng W, Imagawa D. Fatal variceal rupture after sildenafil use: report of a case. Curr Surg 2005;62:55–6.
16. Antiga E, Melani L, Cardinali C, Giomi B, Caproni M, Francalanci S, Fabbri P. A case of lichenoid drug eruption associated with sildenafil citratus. J Dermatol 2005;32:972–5.
17. Al-Shouli S, Abouchala N, Bogusz MJ, Al Tufail M, Thestrup-Pedersen K. Toxic epidermal necrolysis associated with high intake of sildenafil and is response to infliximab. Acta Derm Venereol 2005;85:534–5.

Jamie J. Coleman and Una Martin

20 Antihypertensive drugs

Monitoring therapy The publication of clear and explicit guidance on monitoring therapy in order to maximize efficacy and minimize adverse drug reactions is rare. The publication of practical recommendations for the use of ACE inhibitors, beta-blockers, aldosterone antagonists, and angiotensin receptor antagonists in heart failure may also be helpful in the safer administration of these drugs in hypertension ([1S]). These guidelines provide advice about how these drugs should be used safely, including what advice should be given to the patient and what monitoring needs to be undertaken. Of equal value are the recommendations about the actions to be taken if problems occur, for example what to do in the event of electrolyte imbalance or renal dysfunction in patients taking ACE inhibitors.

ANGIOTENSIN CONVERTING ENZYME INHIBITORS *(SED-15, 226; SEDA-27, 213; SEDA-28, 227; SEDA-29, 207)*

Respiratory *Cough* was reported as an adverse effect of ACE inhibitors in the mid-1980s. It can be distressing and inconvenient, leading to withdrawal of therapy. Certain susceptibility factors are clearly recognized (for example non-smoking and female sex), but racial group can also affect the incidence. HOPE TIPS was a prospective study of patients with high cardiovascular risk, in which the practicability and tolerability of ramipril titration was tested in 1881 patients ([2C]). Cough occurred in 14% over a period of up to 3 months, and 4% discontinued ramipril as a result. The author of an accompanying editorial ([3r]) pointed out that the true incidence of ramipril-induced cough had conceivably been overestimated in the study, owing to the large proportions of patients with type 2 diabetes (52%) and non-smokers (80%) and the high doses used. The authors suggested that cough was not necessarily more common in Asian patients (79% of the patients in this study), although within this broad category the differential susceptibility to cough may be quite large, and the editorial examined this; on the balance of evidence, Chinese patients (and perhaps some other racial groups in Asian countries) probably develop cough more commonly with ACE inhibitors than Caucasian patients do.

Autacoids

Angioedema Angiotensin converting enzyme inhibitors commonly cause angioedema, probably by an effect on bradykinin (SEDA-29, 207). In a large, double-blind, randomized comparison of enalapril maleate and omapatrilat, angioedema occurred in 86 (0.86%) of 12 557 patients who were randomized to enalapril ([4C]).

The characteristics of treated hypertensive patients in the Antihypertensive and Lipid-Lowering treatment to prevent Heart Attack Trial (ALLHAT) who developed angioedema have been published ([5C]). There were 42 418 participants, of whom 53 developed angioedema; 70% were assigned to the ACE inhibitor lisinopril. Susceptibility factors included, as expected, black ethnicity (55%), but unusually there was a male preponderance (60%). The timing of the adverse effect fitted with the known variable time-course: three cases (6%) within 1 day of randomization, 22% within the first week, 34% within the first month, and 68% within the first year.

Five cases of angioedema in association with various ACE inhibitors have been reported ([6A]). The patients were taking lisinopril, trandalopril, or ramipril, and all presented with increasing breathlessness and/or dysphagia associated

Side Effects of Drugs, Annual 30
J.K. Aronson (Editor)
ISSN: 0378-6080
DOI: 10.1016/S0378-6080(08)00020-2

with significant tongue edema. There was significant airway obstruction in all cases, requiring either tracheostomy or intubation. Withdrawal of the ACE inhibitor and standard supportive care, including glucocorticoids, antihistamines, and adrenaline in two cases, led to resolution of the angioedema.

Orolingual angioedema has been attributed to benazepril after recombinant tissue plasminogen activator (rtPA) treatment for acute stroke (7[A]).

- A 58-year-old man taking amlodipine and benazepril received intravenous rtPA for an acute left middle cerebral artery territory stroke. He developed orolingual angioedema 5 minutes later. There was no airway compromise or hemodynamic instability to suggest an anaphylactic reaction. He was treated with dexamethasone and an antihistamine. The angioedema resolved completely over the next 48 hours, as did his neurological deficits.

Lisinopril-associated angioedema has been reported in a patient undergoing maxillofacial surgery (8[A]).

Small bowel angioedema has been attributed to perindopril (9[A]).

Angioedema occurred in a 57-year-old man who had taken trandolapril for 2 days, not having occurred while he took ramipril for 3 years (10[A]). The authors suggested that this implied that angioedema is not a class effect of ACE inhibitors. However, the association could have been coincidental.

The Australian Adverse Reactions Advisory Committee has issued a warning in its bulletin about the continued reporting of angioedema due to ACE inhibitors (11[SA]). Of over 7000 reports of angioedema since 1970, 13% had been attributable to ACE inhibitors. In some cases angioedema occurred episodically with long symptom-free intervals.

- An elderly woman, who had been taking ramipril for 1 year without adverse effects, had several episodes of unilateral swelling of the face, lips, jaw line, and cheek, each lasting 2–3 days over 4 months.

Drug–drug interactions *Aprotinin*, a proteolytic enzyme inhibitor acting on plasmin and kallidinogenase (kallikrein), is hypothesized to contribute significantly to a reduction in glomerular perfusion pressure when it is used in combination with ACE inhibitors. In a retrospective investigation of this combination in adults undergoing coronary artery bypass surgery, the combination of preoperative ACE inhibition and intraoperative aprotinin was associated with a significant increase in the incidence of acute renal insufficiency (OR = 2.9; 95% CI = 1.4, 5.8) (12[c]). The authors concluded that this combination should be avoided in cardiac surgery.

Cilazapril   *(SED-15, 773)*

Cardiovascular Refractory *hypotension* occurred when the long-acting ACE inhibitor cilazapril was used in a patient undergoing spinal surgery (13[A]).

- A 76-year-old woman, who had taken cilazapril 2.5 mg/day for 5 years for hypertension, underwent back surgery. On the morning of the procedure she took her usual dose of cilazapril, and 10 minutes after induction of anesthesia her blood pressure fell to 60/40 mmHg. She was successfully treated with ephedrine and fluid boluses. However, about 1 hour later her blood pressure fell to 60/30 mmHg when she was placed in the prone position. She was given ephedrine and fluids, with no effect on blood pressure. After a dopamine infusion her systolic blood pressure stabilized at 80–100 mmHg. Cilazapril was withdrawn. On the third postoperative day her blood pressure progressively increased, and she was weaned from the vasopressor. By the end of that day her blood pressure was 185/65 mmHg and cilazapril was restarted.

Urinary tract *Uremia* has been reported in association with cilazapril (14[A]).

- A 72-year-old man had taken captopril, cilazapril, and enalapril for heart disorders and developed uremia in the context of progressive symptoms of renal impairment and dehydration, presenting with renal insufficiency and hyperkalemia. The plasma potassium concentration normalized after hemodialysis but the creatinine concentration remained high and the eventual outcome was not clearly stated.

The association with cilazapril was relatively weak in this case.

Enalapril   *(SED-15, 1210; SEDA-26, 235; SEDA-28, 227; SEDA-29, 210)*

Endocrine The *syndrome of inappropriate antidiuretic hormone secretion* has been reported in association with enalapril (15[A]).

Electrolyte imbalance   The management of *hyperkalemia* caused by inhibitors of the renin–angiotensin–aldosterone system has previously been reviewed (16[R]). Volume depletion is a risk factor for the development of both renal impairment and subsequent hyperkalemia, because of the effects of ACE inhibitors on the renal vasculature. A further case of life-threatening hyperkalemia has been reported in a woman who developed a severe diarrheal illness on a background of widespread vascular disease, for which she was taking enalapril, bisoprolol, bumetanide, and isosorbide mononitrate (17[A]).

Pancreas   *Pancreatitis* has been reported in a 74-year-old woman with chronic renal insufficiency on hemodialysis taking enalapril (18[A]).

Urinary tract   Because of concerns over the adverse effects of prostaglandin synthesis inhibitors (for example non-steroidal anti-inflammatory drugs) in patients taking ACE inhibitors for heart failure, a human experimental study has been undertaken in 14 elderly healthy subjects, who were randomized to oral diclofenac or placebo with either no pre-treatment or after the administration of bendroflumethiazide and enalapril to activate the renin–angiotensin system (19[E]). Diclofenac caused significant *reductions in urine flow, the excretion rates of electrolytes, osmolality clearance, and free water clearance*, although all of these were further reduced by pre-treatment with a diuretic and an ACE inhibitor. The authors deduced that in elderly patients with congestive cardiac failure, NSAIDs can counteract the beneficial effects of ACE inhibitors.

Fetotoxicity   The use of ACE inhibitors in pregnancy can have serious effects on the fetus. A further case of fatal *neonatal renal insufficiency* associated with maternal enalapril use during the third trimester has been reported (20[A]).

- A woman with pregnancy-induced hypertension took enalapril 5 mg/day for 21 days before delivery, in addition to other antihypertensive drugs. The use of enalapril was temporally associated with oligohydramnios. The neonate had intrauterine growth retardation, hydrops, and oliguric renal insufficiency, which did not respond to furosemide, peritoneal dialysis, and exchange transfusion. Autopsy showed macroscopically and microscopically normal kidneys.

Drug–drug interactions   An interaction of *sirolimus* with ramipril, causing tongue edema, has previously been described after renal transplantation (SEDA-29, 209). There have been two further cases in renal graft patients, both of whom developed acute severe allergic reactions (21[A]).

- A 54-year-old woman was given sirolimus to allow tacrolimus withdrawal 26 months after a renal transplant when she had also been taking enalapril for 2 months for difficult blood pressure control. Nine days later she developed an urticarial erythematous skin lesion with localized non-pitting edema on the face, neck, and upper thorax.
- A 61-year-old man developed non-pitting facial edema after ramipril was added to an immunosuppressive regimen.

In neither case was rechallenge performed.

Imidapril   *(SED-15, 1718)*

Skin   There has been a report of atenolol-induced lupus erythematosus followed 4 years later by imidapril-induced *pemphigus foliaceus* (22[A]). The patient had HLA type DR4, which the authors surmised to be a predisposing factor to these two rare drug-induced immune-mediated dermatoses.

- A 67-year-old woman developed photo-distributed telangiectatic erythema together with periungual erythema and ragged posterior cuticles; this was attributed to atenolol, which she had taken for 1 year. She had a positive antinuclear antibody titer (1:160, homogeneous pattern), anti-dsDNA antibodies 125 IU (0–30), and antihistone antibodies 44 IU (0–5), which confirmed drug-induced lupus erythematosus. The photosensitive erythema improved and her autoantibodies returned to normal 3 months after atenolol was withdrawn. Four years later she developed crusted plaques and erosions over her upper back, arms, and scalp. Her medication included imidapril, which she had taken for 2.5 years, and thyroxine. The clinical presentation and skin histology and immunofluorescence were consistent with pemphigus foliaceus, which was thought to be drug-induced. Imidapril was withdrawn and she was given prednisolone 30 mg/day and hydroxychloroquine 200 mg bd. Within 4 months the pemphigus improved significantly.

Serosae   An unusual case of *eosinophilic pleurisy* has been described in association with imidapril (23[A]). Eosinophilic lung diseases have been rarely reported and only with some ACE inhibitors (for example captopril and perindopril); this is the first reported case with imidapril. The authors made no formal assessment of the probability that this was drug-induced. Rechallenge was not attempted, but the result of dechallenge was dramatic, and improvements in both diagnostic imaging and laboratory findings made the association probable.

Lisinopril   *(SED-15, 2071; SEDA-27, 213; SEDA-28, 228; SEDA-29, 210)*

Pancreas   *Pancreatitis* has been reported in a patient taking lisinopril and atorvastatin (24[A]). The relative contributions of each drug were not explored.

Drug–drug interactions   *Lithium* toxicity occurred in a patient who took concomitant lisinopril (25[A]).

- A 46-year-old man with a schizoaffective disorder took increasing doses of lithium for breakthrough hypomanic symptoms, in addition to neuropsychotherapies and antihypertensive drugs. Initially he had been taking atenolol and fosinopril; however, the latter was replaced by lisinopril because of supply shortage. A month after substitution, and from a stable lithium concentration and stable renal function, he developed symptoms of lithium toxicity, confirmed by serum lithium concentration measurement. Withdrawal of therapy and supportive measures resolved the problem.

Perindopril   *(SED-15, 2782)*

The effects of perindopril on the renin–angiotensin system and its adverse effects have been reviewed (26[R]).

Respiratory   Perindopril has previously been reported to cause *pulmonary eosinophilia*. Various types of drug-induced eosinophilic lung diseases have been described, varying from mild, simple pulmonary eosinophilia-like syndrome to fulminant, acute eosinophilic pneumonia-like syndromes. A further case of pulmonary eosinophilia-like syndrome has been reported, with symptoms occurring 5 weeks after the introduction of perindopril for hypertension (27[A]). No rechallenge was performed, but multiple investigations to exclude other causes and the temporal association were fairly convincing for drug-induced pulmonary eosinophilia.

Pancreas   ACE inhibitors have often been implicated in *pancreatitis*, although few cases have occurred in association with perindopril. A case of probable perindopril-induced pancreatitis has been reported (28[A]).

Quinapril   *(SED-15, 2996; SEDA-29, 211)*

Skin   *Pemphigus vulgaris* and *pemphigus foliaceus* have both been attributed to ACE inhibitors, including quinapril.

- A 54-year-old man developed a skin reaction 2 months after starting to take quinapril, with skin biopsy findings of IgG and complement fragment C3 deposits, consistent with drug-induced pemphigus (29[A]).

Ramipril   *(SED-15, 3022; SEDA-27, 214; SEDA-28, 228; SEDA-29, 211)*

Electrolyte balance   *Hyperkalemia* is a concern when ACE inhibitors are co-administered with potassium-sparing diuretics, such as triamterene or amiloride, or aldosterone antagonists, such as spironolactone. Both classes of agents are increasingly being used, in both heart failure and hypertension. A 59-year-old patient with both of these diagnoses was given ramipril 5 mg/day, hydrochlorothiazide 12.5 mg/day, and spironolactone 25 mg/day and developed acute renal impairment and severe hyperkalemia (9.3 mmol/l) (30[A]).

Hematologic   *Neutropenia* and *agranulocytosis* have both rarely been attributed to ACE inhibitors.

- Ramipril-induced agranulocytosis has been reported in a 55-year-old man with hypertensive chronic renal insufficiency (31[A]). He was also taking metoprolol, clonidine, furosemide, simvastatin, aspirin, and amlodipine, but was given ramipril 4 days before developing weakness and a neutropenic fever. A bone marrow biopsy showed moderate hypocellularity. An in vitro lymphocyte cytotoxicity assay was performed with furosemide and ramipril; there was a cytotoxic response to ramipril.

Salivary glands *Sialadenitis* has been reported with ACE inhibitors, although the mechanism is unclear and probably multifactorial. The primary pathogenesis is reduced salivary volume and/or flow rate. Disruption in salivary secretion at the cellular level can affect volumes, while flow rates can be affected by spasm or edema in the salivary ducts.

- An adult woman developed recurrent, painless, unilateral parotid gland swelling, which was initially thought to be recurrent sialadenitis (32[A]). However, her symptoms resolved on withdrawal of ramipril. The clue to the diagnosis came from the fact that after multiple episodes of localized, pre-auricular gland swelling, she developed swelling that extended anteriorly to her nasal-labial crease, which became indistinct. This was considered to be a sign of angioedema and the ACE inhibitor was withdrawn. There was no recurrence.

It was presumed that the angioedema was the cause of the gland swelling, due to obstruction of the salivary gland ducts.

Serosae *Polyserositis* is an unusual adverse drug reaction.

- A 63-year-old man developed bilateral pleural effusions and a substantial pericardial effusion (33[A]). He had taken nitrendipine, ramipril, hydrochlorothiazide, and carvedilol for 10 years. After withdrawal of these drugs and treatment of his condition, ramipril alone was restarted. Within 1 week the symptoms and effusions recurred.

A subsequent positive lymphocyte transformation test facilitated the probable diagnosis of an adverse drug reaction to ramipril.

Temocapril *(SED-15, 3313; SEDA-29, 211)*

Cardiovascular A 72-year-old woman developed exercise-related *syncope* during treatment with amlodipine and temocapril for hypertension (34[A]).

ANGIOTENSIN II RECEPTOR ANTAGONISTS *(SED-15, 223; SEDA-27, 214; SEDA-28, 229; SEDA-29, 211)*

Angioedema due to angiotensin II receptor antagonists †

DoTS classification:
Reaction: Angioedema due to angiotensin II receptor antagonists
Dose-relation: ?Collateral
Time-course: Time-independent
Susceptibility factors: Previous angioedema with an ACE inhibitor

The introduction of the angiotensin II receptor antagonists has provided a new tool for inhibition of the renin–angiotensin system (Figure 1), and these drugs are used extensively in the treatment of hypertension and heart failure, in diabetic nephropathy, and after myocardial infarction. They are purported to be as efficacious as the ACE inhibitors, owing to downstream receptor antagonism, and were also originally thought to cause fewer adverse effects, such as cough (35[R]). More recently it has become clear that some of the common adverse effects of ACE inhibitors also occur with angiotensin II receptor antagonists. In particular, angioedema has been reported both with initial therapy and when substituting treatment in patients who have had ACE inhibitor-induced angioedema.

Angioedema is a self-limiting, but potentially fatal condition caused by non-pitting edema affecting the skin and mucous membranes, including the upper respiratory and intestinal epithelial linings. Angioedema due to ACE inhibitors (36[R]) was reviewed in SEDA-29 (p. 207), covering the general features of presentation, incidence, causative mechanisms, and management. Here we review angioedema due to angiotensin II receptor antagonists.

Mechanisms Angioedema may be bradykinin-mediated or dependent on mast cell degranulation or other mechanisms (37[R]). It is thought that ACE inhibitors induce angioedema by increasing the availability of bradykinin, due to reduced enzymatic degradation (38[R]) (see Figure 1). Angiotensin II receptor antagonists

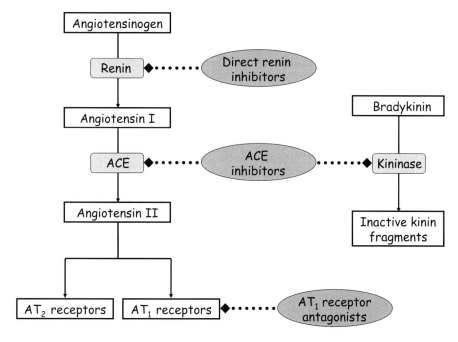

Fig. 1. Renin angiotensin system and drug targets.

theoretically do not affect bradykinin, so they should be appropriate substitutes in patients with ACE inhibitor-associated angioedema. However, there have been several reports of angioedema associated with angiotensin II receptor antagonists, and it has been suggested that they cause it by potentiating the effects of bradykinin (39[R]).

The antihypertensive effects of angiotensin II receptor antagonists are thought to be secondary to inhibition of the binding of angiotensin II to AT_1 receptors, which are the receptors responsible for most of the deleterious effects of angiotensin II, including increased blood pressure due to vasoconstriction and salt retention due to aldosterone synthesis. However, there is increasing evidence that unopposed activation of AT_2 receptors by angiotensin II during therapy with angiotensin II receptor antagonists can produce vasodilatation and increased vascular permeability through mechanisms that involve nitric oxide release and potentiation of the effects of bradykinin (39[R]).

Under normal circumstances the angiotensin II receptor antagonists have a low affinity for AT_2 receptors compared with AT_1 receptors. Antagonism of AT_1 receptors causes a

transient rise in angiotensin II concentrations, which may increase AT_2 receptor expression and activity (40[A]). In animals angiotensin II receptor antagonists increase aortic and renal bradykinin concentrations, perhaps secondary to increased stimulation of AT_2 receptors (41[E], 42[E]). They may therefore precipitate angioedema by causing increased AT_2 receptor activity, leading to increased tissue bradykinin concentrations (43[A]). Although these increased concentrations may not be detectable in the serum, in the tissues they may cause angioedema (40[A]). However, increased serum bradykinin concentrations can sometimes be detected; in one study losartan increased the serum bradykinin concentration two-fold in hypertensive humans (44[c]).

Other mechanisms have been proposed by which angiotensin II receptor antagonists could increase bradykinin, including inhibition of neutral endopeptidase, an enzyme involved in the breakdown of bradykinin (44[A]); there was reduced neutral endopeptidase activity in homogenates of isolated heart components in rats that had been treated with angiotensin II receptor antagonists (45[E]). It has also been proposed that increased plasma angiotensin II concentra-

tions caused by angiotensin II receptor antagonists can cause negative feedback inhibition of ACE activity (46[A]). Finally, an abnormality of degradation of an active metabolite of bradykinin, des-arginine(9)-bradykinin may be involved (47[E]). All of these factors would favor the development of angioedema.

Incidence *Angioedema has been reported with losartan (48[r], 49[A], 50[A], 51[A], 52[A], 54[A], 55[A], 56[A]), valsartan (40[A], 46[A], 53[A], 57[A]), candesartan (58[A]), irbesartan (59[A]), olmesartan (43[A]), and telmisartan (60[A]). The incidence of angioedema associated with the use of ACE inhibitors is 0.1–1% (39[R], 61[R], 62[c]), whereas the incidence of angioedema due to angiotensin II receptor antagonists is reported to be 0.1–0.4% (63[C]).*

Dose-relation *There is little information about the relation to dose of this adverse effect. In one case valsartan-induced angioedema occurred when the dose of valsartan was increased from 160 to 320 mg/day (40[A]). The patient taking the lower dose for 2 years and the symptoms of lip and tongue swelling occurred within 2 hours of taking the higher dose; once the dose was reduced to 160 mg/day no further episodes of angioedema occurred.*

Time course *The time of onset varies with angiotensin II receptor antagonists, ranging from hours to years. For example, losartan has been associated with angioedema from within 30 minutes after administration to 3 years after starting therapy.*

Susceptibility factors *There is evidence that angioedema due to angiotensin II receptor antagonists is more likely in patients who have had angioedema while taking ACE inhibitors (62[c], 64[r]). In one series, 32% of patients reported to have angioedema with angiotensin II receptor antagonists had had a prior episode of angioedema attributable to an ACE inhibitor (48[R]). It has also been reported that almost half of those who have angioedema due to an angiotensin II receptor antagonist have also had it with an ACE inhibitor (65[A]). Despite this, angioedema due to angiotensin II receptor antagonists has also been reported to occur in*

patients not previously exposed to an ACE inhibitor and in patients who have previously received an ACE inhibitor without developing angioedema (46[A]). There is no information about other factors that increase susceptibility.

Conclusions *Although angioedema due to angiotensin II receptor antagonists is uncommon, caution is advised when they are prescribed, particularly if there is a history of ACE inhibitor-associated angioedema.*

Cardiovascular Angiotensin II receptor blockers have provoked concerns about the risk of *myocardial infarction*. The use of this class as an alternative to ACE inhibitors for all indications has been suggested, but an incomplete analysis of some of the evidence led to a provocative suggestion that angiotensin II receptor antagonists confer a risk of harm (66[r]). However, several meta-analyses have been performed to examine the association between angiotensin II receptor antagonists and the risk of myocardial infarction in a variety of clinical trial settings; there was no significant increase in the risk (67[M], 68[M]).

Fetotoxicity Angiotensin II receptor antagonists can cause a wide variety of fetotoxic effects, including *oligohydramnios, fetal growth retardation*, and *pulmonary hypoplasia*, abnormalities that are similar to those seen with ACE inhibitors. The available evidence has been reviewed, with the conclusion that pharmacological suppression of the fetal renin–angiotensin system through AT_1 receptor blockade disrupts fetal vascular perfusion and renal function, and that angiotensin II receptor antagonists should be withdrawn as soon as pregnancy is recognized (69[R]). Furthermore, there has been a report of a child born with *renal impairment* after anhydramnios due to maternal exposure to valsartan and hydrochlorothiazide during the first 28 weeks of pregnancy (70[A]).

• A hypertensive woman taking valsartan 80 mg/day, hydrochlorothiazide 12.5 mg/day, prazosin 10 mg/day, lysine acetylsalicylate 100 mg/day, and levothyroxine 250 micrograms/day became pregnant. At 28 weeks anhydramnios associated with high β_2-microglobulin concentrations in fetal cord blood was observed. On withdrawal of valsartan, fetal renal prognosis improved. At the age of 2.5 years the child had mild chronic renal insufficiency. Growth parameters were within the expected range, and there was no evidence of developmental delay.

In this case the Naranjo probability scale suggested that the child's renal impairment was probably related to valsartan.

Candesartan   *(SED-15, 612; SEDA-28, 229; SEDA-29, 211)*

Electrolyte balance   As angiotensin II receptor antagonists are often used for similar indications or substituted for ACE inhibitor therapy, the combination of an angiotensin II receptor antagonist with spironolactone will become more commonly used in treating cardiovascular and renal disease. Severe *hyperkalemia*, due to a combination of candesartan and spironolactone, has been described in a patient with hypertensive nephrosclerosis and only mild renal impairment (71[A]). The authors reasonably advised that close monitoring of serum potassium should be mandatory during combination therapy, in order to prevent hyperkalemia. They also suggested that the transtubular potassium gradient and fractional excretion of potassium should be assessed before starting therapy to identify high-risk patients, and that a thiazide or loop diuretic be co-administered in order to reduce the risk of hyperkalemia; however, neither of these strategies has clear evidence to support it.

Biliary tract   Prolonged severe *cholestasis* induced by candesartan cilexetil improved after extracorporeal albumin dialysis (72[A]).

Pancreas   A 75-year-old hypertensive man taking long-term candesartan cilexetil died after developing fulminant *pancreatitis*, complicated by acute renal insufficiency, respiratory insufficiency, and septic shock (73[A]).

Eprosartan   *(SED-15, 1229)*

The use of eprosartan in hypertension has been reviewed (74[R]).

Irbesartan   *(SED-15, 1908; SEDA-28, 229; SEDA-29, 212)*

Sensory systems   Acute bilateral *angle closure glaucoma* is often due to an adverse drug reaction in patients who are predisposed by having narrowed angles in the anterior chambers of the eye. This has been reported with a wide variety of agents, including adrenergic agents, antidepressants, sulpha drugs, and ACE inhibitors.

- A 42-year-old woman gradually developed a severe, pulsatile, temporal headache, with nausea, blurred vision, and red eyes 2 weeks after starting to take a combination of irbesartan and hydrochlorothiazide for hypertension (75[A]). She was also taking gabapentin and pantoprazole. She had severe bilateral intraocular hypertension and was given topical antiglaucoma treatment. The next day she had laser iridotomy, and her symptoms resolved.

The authors suggested that the timing made a drug-induced cause probable, although they did not specifically discuss the possible contribution of irbesartan. There have been several reports of angle closure glaucoma with hydrochlorothiazide, but only one with angiotensin II receptor antagonists. It is likely that the combination antihypertensive treatment was responsible, but unclear which of the agents (or both) was causative.

Liver   There have been a few reports of *hepatitis* in association with irbesartan.

- A 69-year-old man developed autoimmune cholestatic hepatitis while taking irbesartan for essential hypertension (76[A]).
- A 51-year-old woman developed acute hepatitis while taking irbesartan (77[A]).

Pancreas   An elderly patient developed pancreatitis soon after starting to take irbesartan 300 mg/day (78[A]). The Naranjo criteria suggested a probable drug-induced event.

Drug–drug interactions   *Lithium* toxicity developed in a 74-year-old woman with bipolar disorder, type 2 diabetes mellitus, hypertension, and ischemic heart disease (79[A]). She was taking several potentially causative drugs, including two diuretics, an ACE inhibitor, and irbesartan, which had been started several weeks before. The authors suggested that the addition of the angiotensin II receptor antagonist may have contributed to lithium intoxication. Since ACE inhibitors enhance tubular reabsorption of lithium they proposed that the mechanism of this interaction is probably similar.

Losartan   *(SED-15, 2168)*

The clinical pharmacokinetics of losartan have been reviewed (80[R]).

Observational studies   Losartan 2.5–100 mg has been studied in 175 hypertensive children aged 6–16 years (81[c]). There were non-severe adverse events in 14; *headache* was the most common. In a comparison of losartan and nebivolol, headache was a common symptom in patients taking losartan; there were no serious adverse events (82[c]).

Electrolyte balance   Severe *hyperkalemia* (8.4 mmol/l), which required hemodialysis, occurred in an 84-year-old woman taking losartan 50 mg/day and spironolactone 25 mg/day for hypertension and severe mitral insufficiency (83[A]).

Metal metabolism   Zinc, magnesium, and nitric oxide have been studied in a prospective observational study in patients with hypertension taking losartan alone and in combination with hydrochlorothiazide (84[c]). Losartan caused *zinc deficiency* with increased urinary zinc excretion, an effect that was exacerbated by co-administration of hydrochlorothiazide. There were no effects on magnesium or nitric oxide. Zinc deficiency can aggravate hypertension and is also reported to be responsible for some adverse drug effects, such as dysgeusia.

Hematologic   Losartan has been used after renal transplantation to control both blood pressure and post-transplant *erythrocytosis*. The interaction between the renin–angiotensin system and erythropoietic mechanisms is complex, and after transplantation ACE inhibition can cause anemia without erythrocytosis. In a prospective controlled study renal transplant patients taking losartan had a significant fall in hemoglobin concentration compared with controls (85[c]). This suggested that losartan can

have an effect beyond its antihypertensive efficacy.

Telmisartan   *(SED-15, 3311; SEDA-28, 229; SEDA-29, 212)*

Susceptibility factors

Renal disease   Telmisartan has been studied in patients with varying severity of chronic kidney disease in a non-randomized study (86[c]). It was an effective antihypertensive with few adverse effects.

Valsartan   *(SED-15, 3593; SEDA-29, 213)*

Respiratory   *Pneumonitis* has been reported in association with valsartan (87[A]).

• A 70-year-old man with dyspnea had diffuse pulmonary infiltrates on chest X-ray and ground-glass changes and non-segmental consolidation on CT imaging. He had been taking the Chinese herbal drug saiko-ka-ryukotsu-borei-to and valsartan for about 3 months, and drug-induced pneumonitis was suspected. The drugs were withdrawn and oral prednisolone given. He improved symptomatically.

DIRECT RENIN INHIBITORS

Direct renin inhibitors—a new class of antihypertensive drugs but the same adverse effects?

The development of novel antihypertensive agents is important, as the number of patients with hypertension continues to burgeon throughout the world. Identifying novel targets is an important prelude to developing appropriate leads, but the identification of the target for the latest class of antihypertensive agents, direct renin inhibitors, is not new. The idea of blocking renin at the proximal step of the renin–angiotensin–aldosterone pathway was proposed several decades ago. However, early attempts at producing renin inhibitors were thwarted by difficulties in achieving either adequate systemic availability or acceptable blood pressure lowering activity. Previous peptide-like molecules were successful when given parenterally, but had little activity when given orally (88^R).

It was the advent of computational molecular modelling that made the non-peptide renin inhibitors a reality. Aliskiren is a novel compound that was developed by the use of X-ray crystallography of the active site of renin and subsequent computational modelling. Its non-peptide structure overcame some of the difficulties of previous attempts at producing renin inhibitors, although it still has some interesting pharmacokinetic properties. It is the first in class of the orally active, non-peptide, direct renin inhibitors for the treatment of hypertension to go into phase III trials. Here we outline current knowledge about the clinical effects and safety of this new drug.

Mechanism of action   The renin–angiotensin system plays a central role in hypertension, mediating its effects through the peptide hormone angiotensin II, which increases arterial tone, stimulates aldosterone release, activates sympathetic neurotransmission, and promotes renal sodium reabsorption. Overactivation of the renin–angiotensin system therefore contributes to hypertension and its associated end-organ damage. The system can be inhibited at various points: ACE inhibitors reduce the conversion of angiotensin I to angiotensin II and angiotensin II receptor blockers antagonize the interaction of angiotensin II with the type-1 angiotensin II (AT_1) receptor (Figure 1). However, both of these classes of agent interfere with the normal feedback mechanism to the juxtaglomerular apparatus in the kidneys and thus lead to a reactive rise in plasma renin activity, which can partially counteract their effects. Optimal blockade of the renin–angiotensin–aldosterone system should therefore be achievable by blocking the proximal step in the conversion of angiotensinogen to angiotensin I by directly inhibiting the action of renin, thus attenuating the reactive rise in plasma renin activity.

In healthy volunteers aliskiren produces dose-dependent reductions in plasma renin activity and angiotensin I and angiotensin II concentrations (89^c), which translates into effective blood pressure lowering.

Pharmacokinetics   The systemic availability of aliskiren is limited, less than 3% of the parent compound being absorbed (88^R). Its half-life is in the region of 40 hours, which allows effective once-daily dosing; steady-state plasma concentrations are achieved after 5–8 days (90^c). Aliskiren has little clinically significant interaction with cytochrome P450 liver enzymes and no significant hepatic metabolism. Mild to severe hepatic impairment had no significant effect on the single-dose pharmacokinetics of aliskiren (91^c). The main route of elimination is biliary excretion and consequent fecal elimination. Renal clearance plays a minor role, about 1% being excreted in the urine. Aliskiren is a substrate for P glycoprotein and co-administration of other drugs that interfere with P glycoprotein could theoretically alter exposure to aliskiren (92^c). In elderly patients (65 years and over) there were only modest increases in drug exposure (92^c).

Clinical studies   The largest clinical studies to date with aliskiren have investigated the use of doses of up to 600 mg/day and have shown effective blood pressure lowering in patients with hypertension. In an 8-week study in 652 patients, aliskiren (150, 300, and 600 mg) was compared with placebo and irbesartan (93^C). Aliskiren 150 mg was as effective as irbesartan 150 mg, while higher doses lowered mean sitting diastolic blood pressure significantly more. The incidences of adverse events were comparable with aliskiren, irbesartan, and placebo.

In an 8-week placebo-controlled study in 672 hypertensive patients, aliskiren 150–600 mg/day was significantly superior to placebo in lowering mean sitting systolic and diastolic blood pressures at all doses; maximal or near-maximal reductions were achieved by week 4 (94^C). In a subgroup of patients evaluated with ambulatory blood pressure monitoring, the blood pressure lowering effect was sustained throughout the 24-hour dosing interval. There are many more clinical studies in progress or soon to be published.

Combination therapy   The favorable effect of aliskiren on plasma renin activity implies that combination treatment with antihypertensive agents that otherwise increase renin activity should be beneficial. Aliskiren has been investigated in open studies in combination with hydrochlorothiazide, ramipril, and irbesartan (95^c). Plasma renin activity did not increase compared with baseline, which suggests that combination therapy can achieve increased renin–angiotensin system suppression and improved blood pressure control.

In a comparison of aliskiren and ramipril, alone or in combination, the incidence of cough with aliskiren was lower than with ramipril, but the incidence with the combination was, surprisingly, lower still (90^c). Combination treatment with calcium channel blockers may also reduce the incidence of edema seen with agents such as amlodipine and provide an advantage to this combination. In a comparison of the combined use of aliskiren and valsartan against both agents alone or placebo in 1979 patients with hypertension the combination produced significantly greater reductions in blood pressure than either agent alone (96^R).

Adverse effects   The adverse effects of renin inhibitors compared with other renin–angiotensin blockers have been reviewed (97^R). The renin inhibitors should lack the effects of ACE inhibitors that are mediated through the accumulation of substance P, bradykinin, and other peptides, such as dry cough and angioedema. Aliskiren has been purported in trials to have "placebo-like" tolerability and a safety profile equivalent to that of angiotensin receptor antagonists (98^R). The most common adverse effects reported in the trials to date have been headache, diarrhea, and dizziness, all at low incidence rates. It has been suggested that gastrointestinal tolerability of aliskiren is dose-limiting above doses of 300 mg/day (99^R). Long-term adverse effects have not been studied, as trials reported to date have been principally short-term, with trials lasting up to 12 months in the more recent larger phase III studies.

Electrolyte balance and renal function   One would expect aliskiren to have the same effects on electrolytes and renal function as those seen with angiotensin receptor antagonists or ACE inhibitors. Hyperkalemia and rises in creatinine have not been described in many of the early-phase trials published to date, most of which have reported that clinical laboratory values remained normal. However, combination therapy in the aliskiren/valsartan trial was associated with laboratory abnormalities—there were higher serum potassium concentrations and clinically relevant increases in serum creatinine in patients who took the combination (96^R). In an accompanying commentary it was pointed out that in the absence of trials with hard end-point data, the routine use of combinations of agents with dual inhibition of the renin–angiotensin system may expose patients to hyperkalemia and renal insufficiency, and this strategy is unlikely to become routine in conditions such as hypertension (100^r).

Pregnancy   The reproductive effects of renin inhibitors have not been reported, although it is likely that aliskiren will be contraindicated in pregnant women and those who are planning a pregnancy, as are ACE inhibitors and angiotensin receptor antagonists, because of concerns about potential teratogenic effects.

Susceptibility factors

Age   Aliskiren has not been evaluated in children, and this is therefore a contraindication pending clinical trials or further experience in younger subjects.

Renal impairment   As with other inhibitors of the renin–angiotensin system, aliskiren is contraindicated in patients with bilateral renal artery stenosis or renal artery stenosis in a single functioning kidney.

Biliary disease   As the excretion of aliskiren depends on hepatobiliary routes, care should be taken in patients with biliary abnormalities.

Drug–drug interactions   Some of the most important potential drug interactions with aliskiren have been investigated in trials. There were no significant changes in drug exposure when it was combined with amlodipine, atenolol, celecoxib, cimetidine, hydrochlorothiazide, lovastatin, ramipril, or valsartan (101^c, 102^c), or in single-dose studies with warfarin (103^c).

Conclusions   Further development of renin inhibitors will continue in the near future to produce other agents with different receptor affinities and binding kinetics. There are also some important questions to be answered, such as whether long-term use of renin inhibitors *will provide adequate end-organ protection, in terms of reducing diabetic proteinuria and left ventricular hypertrophy, and produce beneficial effects on arterial compliance. Further studies will also be needed to determine long-term safety and tolerability, both as monotherapy and in combination with other agents.*

ENDOTHELIN RECEPTOR ANTAGONISTS   *(SED-15, 1215; SEDA-27, 214; SEDA-29, 213)*

Several endothelin receptor antagonists are in clinical use or currently in trials in the treatment of idiopathic pulmonary hypertension or pulmonary artery hypertension secondary to connective tissue disorders. Some agents block both endothelin A (ET_A) receptors and endothelin B (ET_B) receptors (bosentan); others block ET_A only (sitaxsentan and ambrisentan). They antagonize the effect of the powerful vasoconstrictor and smooth muscle mitogen hormone endothelin-1. Theoretically, the selective ET_A receptor antagonists should inhibit the vasoconstrictor effects of ET_A stimulation while preserving the natural vasodilator responses that are mediated through ET_B receptors. All of the endothelin receptor antagonists have adverse effects typical of vasodilatory agents, including *headache, nasal congestion, dizziness*, and *peripheral edema*.

Ambrisentan

Ambrisentan has been investigated in a double-blind, dose-ranging study in 64 patients with pulmonary hypertension, either idiopathic or secondary (to collagen vascular disease, anorexigen use, or human immunodeficiency infection), over 12 weeks for dose ranging followed by a 12-week open extension phase (104[c]). There were improvements in most of the outcome variables, including exercise capacity and cardiopulmonary hemodynamics. Adverse events reflected those common to the endothelin receptor antagonist class (see above), but two patients developed *raised serum transaminase activities*, one of whom required treatment withdrawal. Raised liver enzymes have previ-

ously been seen with bosentan (SEDA-29, 213) and other drugs in this class; the incidence of abnormalities between the difference agents requires further clarification.

Bosentan   *(SED-15, 549; SEDA-27, 214; SEDA-29, 213)*

The risk management strategies and post-marketing surveillance plans in place in the USA and Europe have been described in a paper that also briefly describes the potential *hepatotoxicity* and *teratogenicity* of bosentan (105[R]).

Sitaxsentan   *(SEDA-29, 213)*

The selective ET_A receptor antagonist sitaxsentan has been reviewed (106[R]).

DRUGS THAT ACT ON THE SYMPATHETIC NERVOUS SYSTEM   *(SEDA-27, 216; SEDA-28, 230; SEDA-29, 214)*

PRESYNAPTIC ALPHA-ADRENOCEPTOR AGONISTS

Clonidine   *(SED-15, 817; SEDA-27, 216; SEDA-28, 230; SEDA-29, 214)*

The mechanism of action of clonidine is attributed to its central action as an alpha₂ adrenoceptor agonist, although this assumption may not explain all of its antihypertensive actions. In an experimental study of the hemodynamic response to clonidine in 28 young healthy men, the hemodynamic response suggested that the hypotensive action of clonidine is caused by both an immediate reduction in peripheral vascular resistance and a prolonged reduction in cardiac output (107[c]). The study also showed that central blood pressure was reduced more than peripheral blood pressure, according to pulse wave velocity indices.

Nervous system   Anecdotal reports have shown that clonidine can induce *epileptic activity*. In 22 patients with chronic, medically intractable, localization-related epilepsy, magnetoencephalography was used to investigate whether oral clonidine can aid localization of spike or sharp-wave activity as well as to gain knowledge about whether clonidine is epileptogenic (108[c]). Oral clonidine-induced magnetoencephalographic activity was superior to sleep deprivation, and therefore may be an aid to localization as well as showing epileptogenic activity.

Drug overdose   In a prospective evaluation of clonidine overdose in children, all of the clinical effects occurred rapidly after ingestion, but all of the patients recovered fully with observation and supportive therapy (109[c]). The authors suggested that direct medical evaluation should be undertaken for all children aged 4 years or younger who have taken an unintentional overdose of at least 0.1 mg, in children 5–8 years of age who have taken at least 0.2 mg, and in children older than 8 years of age who have taken at least 0.4 mg; and that observation for 4 hours may be sufficient to detect patients who will develop severe adverse effects.

POSTSYNAPTIC α-ADRENOCEPTOR ANTAGONISTS   *(SEDA-27, 216; SEDA-29, 214)*

Current guidelines on the use of postsynaptic α-adrenoceptor antagonists have been reviewed (110[R]).

Drug–drug interactions   Postsynaptic α-adrenoceptor antagonists are used both in hypertension and for urological conditions, and can cause orthostatic hypotension due to vasodilatation. This adverse effect can be potentiated

considerably if they are co-administered with *inhibitors of phosphodiesterase type V* for the treatment of erectile dysfunction (111[R]).

Alfuzosin   *(SED-15, 74; SEDA-29, 214)*

In a systematic review, 11 trials of alfuzosin in 3901 men were analysed (112[M]). Alfuzosin was safe and well tolerated. Most of the reported adverse events, such as *dizziness* and *syncope*, were related to its vasodilatory action.

Doxazosin   *(SED-15, 1188; SEDA-27, 217; SEDA-29, 214)*

Drug overdose   Acute intoxication with doxazosin has been reported (113[A]).

- A 19-year-old girl took doxazosin 60 mg and developed drowsiness, hypotension, and tachycardia. She was given supportive therapy, including activated charcoal to reduce gastrointestinal absorption, and her hypotension resolved with crystalloid infusion. She survived and was discharged after 48 hours.

Tamsulosin   *(SED-15, 3303; SEDA-29, 214)*

Sensory systems   The *intraoperative floppy iris syndrome* (IFIS) has been reported in current or recent users of α-adrenoceptor antagonists undergoing phacoemulsification cataract surgery, as reported by the manufacturers of Flomax®, a formulation of tamsulosin hydrochloride (114[S]). The company stated that no definitive causal relation has been established, but it has changed its product information to warn patients to tell their surgeons if they are taking tamsulosin, who may need to alter their surgical technique to minimize the risk of IFIS. A retrospective and prospective study has substantiated this association (115[c]).

Drug overdose Overdosage of tamsulosin has been reported (116[A]).

- A 78-year-old woman took an unintentional overdose of tamsulosin 2 mg, mistaking it for herbal tablets. On the next day she developed headache and dizziness and had hypotension, orthostatic hypotension, and bradycardia. She recovered rapidly after supportive care.

Overdose with α-adrenoceptor antagonists usually causes hypotension, often accompanied by reflex tachycardia or bradycardia, as in this case. The mechanism of the bradycardia is unclear.

IMIDAZOLINE RECEPTOR ANTAGONISTS

Moxonidine   *(SED-15, 2395; SEDA-29, 214)*

Moxonidine has been used as add-on therapy in elderly patients with resistant hypertension (117[c]). The results suggested that moxonidine is efficacious and well tolerated in patients who are already taking two or more antihypertensive agents.

References

1. McMurray J, Cohen-Solal A, Dietz R, Eichhorn E, Erhardt L, Hobbs FD, Krum H, Maggioni A, McKelvie RS, Pina IL, Soler-Soler J, Swedberg K. Practical recommendations for the use of ACE inhibitors, beta-blockers, aldosterone antagonists and angiotensin receptor blockers in heart failure: putting guidelines into practice. Eur J Heart Fail 2005;7(5):710–21.
2. Sharpe N, International HOPE TIPS Investigators. The HOPE TIPS: the HOPE study translated into practices. Cardiovasc Drugs Ther 2005;19(3):197–201.
3. Nicholls MG, Gilchrist NL. Cough with ACE inhibitors: a bigger problem in some racial groups? Cardiovasc Drugs Ther 2005;19(3):173–5.
4. Kostis JB, Kim HJ, Rusnak J, Casale T, Kaplan A, Corren J, Levy E. Incidence and characteristics of angioedema associated with enalapril. Arch Intern Med 2005;165(14):1637–42.
5. Piller L, Ford C, Davis B, Nwachuku C, Black H, Oparil S, Gappy S, Retta T, Probstfield J. Angioedema in the antihypertensive and lipid-lowering treatment to prevent heart attack trial (ALLHAT). Am J Hypertens 2005;18(5 Suppl):92A.
6. Rai MR, Amen F, Idrees F. Angiotensin-converting enzyme inhibitor related angioedema and the anaesthetist. Anaesthesia 2004;59(3):283–9.
7. Rafii MS, Koenig M, Ziai WC. Orolingual angioedema associated with ACE inhibitor use after rtPA treatment of acute stroke. Neurology 2005;65(12):1906.
8. O'Ryan F, Poor DB, Hattori M. Intraoperative angioedema induced by angiotensin-converting enzyme inhibitors: overview and case report. J Oral Maxillofac Surg 2005;63(4):551–6.
9. Salloum H, Locher C, Chenard A, Bigorie B, Beroud P, Gatineau-Sailliant G, Glikmanas M. Angiœdème intestinal après prise de perindopril. Gastroenterol Clin Biol 2005;29(11):1180–1.
10. Karagiannis A, Pyrpasopoulou A, Tziomalos K, Florentin M, Athyros V. Angioedema may not be a class side-effect of the angiotensin-converting-enzyme inhibitors. Q J Med 2005;99:197–8.
11. Adverse Drug Reactions Advisory Committee (ADRAC). Angioedema—still a problem with ACE inhibitors. Aust Adv Drug React Bull 2005;24(2):7.
12. Kincaid EH, Ashburn DA, Hoyle JR, Reichert MG, Hammon JW, Kon ND. Does the combination of aprotinin and angiotensin-converting enzyme inhibitor cause renal failure after cardiac surgery? Ann Thorac Surg 2005;80(4):1388–93.
13. Akinci SB, Ayhan B, Kanbak M, Aypar U. Refractory hypotension in a patient chronically treated with a long acting angiotensin-converting enzyme inhibitor. Anaesth Intensive Care 2004;32(5):722–3.
14. Fomin VV, Taronishvili OI, Shvetsov MIu, Shilov EM, Moiseev SV, Kushnir VV, Sorokin IuD. Progressive azotemia provoked by ACE inhibitor in renal ischemia. Ter Arkh 2004;76(9):66–70.
15. Fernandez Fernandez FJ, De la Fuente AJ, Vazquez TL, Perez FS. Síndrome de secre-

ción inadecuada de hormona antidiurética causado por enalapril. Med Clin (Barc) 2004;123(4):159.

16. Palmer BF. Managing hyperkalemia caused by inhibitors of the renin–angiotensin–aldosterone system. N Engl J Med 2004;351(6):585–92.

17. McGuigan J, Robertson S, Isles C. Life threatening hyperkalaemia with diarrhoea during ACE inhibition. Emerg Med J 2005;22(2):154–5.

18. Kishino T, Nakamura K, Mori H, Yamaguchi Y, Takahashi S, Ishida H, Saito S, Watanabe T. Acute pancreatitis during haemodialysis. Nephrol Dial Transplant 2005;20(9):2012–3.

19. Juhlin T, Bjorkman S, Hoglund P. Cyclooxygenase inhibition causes marked impairment of renal function in elderly subjects treated with diuretics and ACE-inhibitors. Eur J Heart Fail 2005;7(6):1049–56.

20. Murki S, Kumar P, Dutta S, Narang A. Fatal neonatal renal failure due to maternal enalapril ingestion. J Matern Fetal Neonatal Med 2005;17(3):235–7.

21. Burdese M, Rossetti M, Guarena C, Consiglio V, Mezza E, Soragna G, Gai M, Segoloni GP, Piccoli GB. Sirolimus and ACE-inhibitors: a note of caution. Transplantation 2005;79(2):251–2.

22. Ah-Weng A, Natarajan S. A case report of drug-induced pemphigus foliaceus preceded by a history of drug-induced lupus erythematosus. J Am Acad Dermatol 2005;52(3 Suppl 1):42.

23. Yoshida H, Hasegawa R, Hayashi H, Irie Y. Imidapril-induced eosinophilic pleurisy. Case report and review of the literature. Respiration 2005;72(4):423–6.

24. Kanbay M, Sekuk H, Yilmaz U, Gur G, Boyacioglu S. Acute pancreatitis associated with combined lisinopril and atorvastatin therapy. Dig Dis 2005;23(1):92–4.

25. Meyer JM, Dollarhide A, Tuan IL. Lithium toxicity after switch from fosinopril to lisinopril. Int Clin Psychopharmacol 2005;20(2):115–8.

26. Ferrari R, Pasanisi G, Notarstefano P, Campo G, Gardini E, Ceconi C. Specific properties and effect of perindopril in controlling the renin–angiotensin system. Am J Hypertens 2005;18(9 Pt 2):142S–54S.

27. Rochford AP, Smith PR, Khan SJ, Pearson AJ. Perindopril and pulmonary eosinophilic syndrome. J R Soc Med 2005;98(4):163–5.

28. Famularo G, Minisola G, Nicotra GC, De SC. Idiosyncratic pancreatitis associated with perindopril. JOP 2005;6(6):605–7.

29. Centre de Pharmacovigilance. Angiotensin-converting enzyme inhibitors and pemphigus. Folia Pharmacother 2005;32(1):9.

30. Nurnberger J, Daul A, Philipp T. Patient mit schwerer Hyperkaliämie—ein Notfall nach RALES. Dtsch Med Wochenschr 2005;130(36):2008–11.

31. Horowitz N, Molnar M, Levy Y, Pollack S. Ramipril-induced agranulocytosis confirmed by a lymphocyte cytotoxicity test. Am J Med Sci 2005;329(1):52–3.

32. Moss JR, Zanation AM, Shores CG. ACE inhibitor associated recurrent intermittent parotid gland swelling. Otolaryngol Head Neck Surg 2005;133(6):992–4.

33. Brunkhorst FM, Bloos F, Klein R. Ramipril induced polyserositis with pericardial tamponade and pleural effusion. Int J Cardiol 2005;102(2):355–6.

34. Ogimoto A, Mizobuchi T, Shigematsu Y, Hara Y, Ohtsuka T, Fukuoka T, Okura T, Higaki J. Exercise-related syncope induced by vasodilator therapy in an elderly hypertensive patient. J Am Geriatr Soc 2005;53(2):351–2.

35. Pylypchuk GB. ACE inhibitor-versus angiotensin II blocker-induced cough and angioedema. Ann Pharmacother 1998;32(10):1060–6.

36. Agostoni A, Cicardi M. Drug-induced angioedema without urticaria. Drug Saf 2001;24(8):599–606.

37. Kaplan AP, Greaves MW. Angioedema. J Am Acad Dermatol 2005;53(3):373–88.

38. Vleeming W, van Amsterdam JG, Stricker BH, de Wildt DJ. ACE inhibitor-induced angioedema. Incidence, prevention and management. Drug Saf 1998;18(3):171–88.

39. Howes LG, Tran D. Can angiotensin receptor antagonists be used safely in patients with previous ACE inhibitor-induced angioedema? Drug Saf 2002;25(2):73–6.

40. Irons BK, Kumar A. Valsartan-induced angioedema. Ann Pharmacother 2003;37(7–8):1024–7.

41. Siragy HM, de GM, El-Kersh M, Carey RM. Angiotensin-converting enzyme inhibition potentiates angiotensin II type 1 receptor effects on renal bradykinin and cGMP. Hypertension 2001;38(2):183–6.

42. Gohlke P, Pees C, Unger T. AT2 receptor stimulation increases aortic cyclic GMP in SHRSP by a kinin-dependent mechanism. Hypertension 1998;31(1 Pt 2):349–55.

43. Nykamp D, Winter EE. Olmesartan medoxomil-induced angioedema. Ann Pharmacother 2007;41(3):518–20.

44. Campbell DJ, Krum H, Esler MD. Losartan increases bradykinin levels in hypertensive humans. Circulation 2005;111(3):315–20.

45. Walther T, Siems WE, Hauke D, Spillmann F, Dendorfer A, Krause W, Schultheiss HP, Tschöpe C. AT1 receptor blockade increases cardiac bradykinin via neutral endopeptidase after induction of myocardial infarction in rats. FASEB J 2002;16(10):1237–41.

46. Arakawa M, Murata Y, Rikimaru Y, Sasaki Y. Drug-induced isolated visceral angioneurotic edema. Intern Med 2005;44(9):975–8.

47. Molinaro G, Cugno M, Perez M, Lepage Y, Gervais N, Agostoni A, Adam A. Angiotensin-converting enzyme inhibitor-associated angioedema is characterized by a slower degradation of des-arginine(9)-bradykinin. J Pharmacol Exp Ther 2002;303(1):232–7.

48. Warner KK, Visconti JA, Tschampel MM. Angiotensin II receptor blockers in patients with

ACE inhibitor-induced angioedema. Ann Pharmacother 2000;34(4):526–8.

49. van Rijnsoever EW, Kwee-Zuiderwijk WJ, Feenstra J. Angioneurotic edema attributed to the use of losartan. Arch Intern Med 1998;158(18):2063–5.

50. Acker CG, Greenberg A. Angioedema induced by the angiotensin II blocker losartan. N Engl J Med 1995;333(23):1572.

51. Boxer M. Accupril- and Cozaar-induced angioedema in the same patient. J Allergy Clin Immunol 1996;98(2):471.

52. Sharma PK, Yium JJ. Angioedema associated with angiotensin II receptor antagonist losartan. South Med J 1997;90(5):552–3.

53. Frye CB, Pettigrew TJ. Angioedema and photosensitive rash induced by valsartan. Pharmacotherapy 1998;18(4):866–8.

54. Rivera JO. Losartan-induced angioedema. Ann Pharmacother 1999;33(9):933–5.

55. Cha YJ, Pearson VE. Angioedema due to losartan. Ann Pharmacother 1999;33(9):936–8.

56. Chiu AG, Krowiak EJ, Deeb ZE. Angioedema associated with angiotensin II receptor antagonists: challenging our knowledge of angioedema and its etiology. Laryngoscope 2001;111(10):1729–31.

57. Tojo A, Onozato ML, Fujita T. Repeated subileus due to angioedema during renin–angiotensin system blockade. Am J Med Sci 2006;332(1):36–8.

58. Lo KS. Angioedema associated with candesartan. Pharmacotherapy 2002;22(9):1176–9.

59. Nielsen EW. Hypotensive shock and angiooedema from angiotensin II receptor blocker: a class effect in spite of tripled tryptase values. J Intern Med 2005;258(4):385–7.

60. Borazan A, Ustun H, Yilmaz A. Angioedema induced by angiotensin II blocker telmisartan. Allergy 2003;58(5):454.

61. Israili ZH, Hall WD. Cough and angioneurotic edema associated with angiotensin-converting enzyme inhibitor therapy. A review of the literature and pathophysiology. Ann Intern Med 1992;117(3):234–42.

62. Cicardi M, Zingale LC, Bergamaschini L, Agostoni A. Angioedema associated with angiotensin-converting enzyme inhibitor use: outcome after switching to a different treatment. Arch Intern Med 2004;164(8):910–3.

63. Dickstein K, Kjekshus J. Effects of losartan and captopril on mortality and morbidity in high-risk patients after acute myocardial infarction: the OPTIMAAL randomised trial. Optimal Trial in Myocardial Infarction with Angiotensin II Antagonist Losartan. Lancet 2002;360(9335):752–60.

64. Fuchs SA, Meyboom RH, van Puijenbroek EP, Guchelaar HJ. Use of angiotensin receptor antagonists in patients with ACE inhibitor induced angioedema. Pharm World Sci 2004;26(4):191–2.

65. Abdi R, Dong VM, Lee CJ, Ntoso KA. Angiotensin II receptor blocker-associated angioedema: on the heels of ACE inhibitor angioedema. Pharmacotherapy 2002;22(9):1173–5.

66. Verma S, Strauss M. Angiotensin receptor blockers and myocardial infarction. BMJ 2004;329(7477):1248–9.

67. McDonald MA, Simpson SH, Ezekowitz JA, Gyenes G, Tsuyuki RT. Angiotensin receptor blockers and risk of myocardial infarction: systematic review. BMJ 2005;331(7521):873.

68. Volpe M, Mancia G, Trimarco B. Angiotensin II receptor blockers and myocardial infarction: deeds and misdeeds. J Hypertens 2005;23(12):2113–8.

69. Alwan S, Polifka JE, Friedman JM. Angiotensin II receptor antagonist treatment during pregnancy. Birth Defects Res A Clin Mol Teratol 2005;73(2):123–30.

70. Bos-Thompson MA, Hillaire-Buys D, Muller F, Dechaud H, Mazurier E, Boulot P, Morin D. Fetal toxic effects of angiotensin II receptor antagonists: case report and follow-up after birth. Ann Pharmacother 2005;39(1):157–61.

71. Fujii H, Nakahama H, Yoshihara F, Nakamura S, Inenaga T, Kawano Y. Life-threatening hyperkalemia during a combined therapy with the angiotensin receptor blocker candesartan and spironolactone. Kobe J Med Sci 2005;51(1–2):1–6.

72. Sturm N, Hilleret MN, Dreyfus T, Barnoud D, Leroy V, Zarski JP. Hépatite sévère et prolongée secondaire à la prise de candesartan cilexitil (Atacand®) améliorée par le système MARS. Gastroenterol Clin Biol 2005;29(12):1299–301.

73. Gill CJ, Jennings AE, Newton JB, Schwartz DE. Fatal acute pancreatitis in a patient chronically treated with candesartan. J Pharm Tech 2005;21(2):79–82.

74. Robins GW, Scott LJ. Eprosartan: a review of its use in the management of hypertension. Drugs 2005;65(16):2355–77.

75. Rahim SA, Sahlas DJ, Shadowitz S. Blinded by pressure and pain. Lancet 2005;365(9478):2244.

76. Annicchiarico BE, Siciliano M. Could irbesartan trigger autoimmune cholestatic hepatitis? Eur J Gastroenterol Hepatol 2005;17(2):247–8.

77. Peron JM, Robic MA, Bureau C, Vinel JP. Hépatite aiguë cytolytique du a la prise d'irbesartan (Aprovel): à propos d'un cas. Gastroenterol Clin Biol 2005;29(6–7):747–8.

78. Famularo G, Minisola G, Nicotra GC, De SC. Acute pancreatitis associated with irbesartan therapy. Pancreas 2005;31(3):294–5.

79. Spinewine A, Schoevaerdts D, Mwenge GB, Swine C, Dive A. Drug-induced lithium intoxication: a case report. J Am Geriatr Soc 2005;53(2):360–1.

80. Sica DA, Gehr TW, Ghosh S. Clinical pharmacokinetics of losartan. Clin Pharmacokinet 2005;44(8):797–814.

81. Shahinfar S, Cano F, Soffer BA, Ahmed T, Santoro EP, Zhang Z, Gleim G, Miller K, Vogt B, Blumer J, Briazgounov I. A double-blind, dose-response study of losartan in hypertensive chil-

dren. Am J Hypertens 2005;18(2 Pt 1):183–90. Erratum: Am J Hypertens 2006;19(6):658.

82. Van Bortel LM, Bulpitt CJ, Fici F. Quality of life and antihypertensive effect with nebivolol and losartan. Am J Hypertens 2005;18(8):1060–6.

83. Kauffmann R, Orozco R, Venegas JC. Hiperkalemia grave asociada a drogas que actúan sobre el sistema renina, angiotensina, aldosterona: Un problema que requiere atención. Caso clínico. Rev Med Chil 2005;133(8):947–52.

84. Koren-Michowitz M, Dishy V, Zaidenstein R, Yona O, Berman S, Weissgarten J, Golik A. The effect of losartan and losartan/hydrochlorothiazide fixed-combination on magnesium, zinc, and nitric oxide metabolism in hypertensive patients: a prospective open-label study. Am J Hypertens 2005;18(3):358–63.

85. Ersoy A, Kahvecioglu S, Ersoy C, Cift A, Dilek K. Anemia due to losartan in hypertensive renal transplant recipients without posttransplant erythrocytosis. Transplant Proc 2005;37(5):2148–50.

86. Sharma AM, Hollander A, Koster J. Telmisartan in patients with mild/moderate hypertension and chronic kidney disease. Clin Nephrol 2005;63(4):250–7.

87. Tokunaga T. A case of drug-induced pneumonitis associated with Chinese herbal drugs and valsartan. Nihon Kokyuki Gakkai Zasshi 2005;43(7):406–11.

88. Staessen JA, Li Y, Richart T. Oral renin inhibitors. Lancet 2006;368(9545):1449–56.

89. Nussberger J, Wuerzner G, Jensen C, Brunner HR. Angiotensin II suppression in humans by the orally active renin inhibitor aliskiren (SPP100): comparison with enalapril. Hypertension 2002;39(1):E1–8.

90. Schmieder RE. Aliskiren: a clinical profile. J Renin Angiotensin Aldosterone Syst 2006;7(Suppl 2):S16–20.

91. Vaidyanathan S, Warren V, Yeh C, Bizot MN, Dieterich HA, Dole WP. Pharmacokinetics, safety, and tolerability of the oral renin inhibitor aliskiren in patients with hepatic impairment. J Clin Pharmacol 2007;47(2):192–200.

92. Vaidyanathan S, Reynolds C, Yeh CM, Bizot MN, Dieterich HA, Howard D, Dole WP. Pharmacokinetics, safety, and tolerability of the novel oral direct renin inhibitor aliskiren in elderly healthy subjects. J Clin Pharmacol 2007;47(4):453–60.

93. Gradman AH, Schmieder RE, Lins RL, Nussberger J, Chiang Y, Bedigian MP. Aliskiren, a novel orally effective renin inhibitor, provides dose-dependent antihypertensive efficacy and placebo-like tolerability in hypertensive patients. Circulation 2005;111(8):1012–8.

94. Oh BH, Mitchell J, Herron JR, Chung J, Khan M, Keefe DL. Aliskiren, an oral renin inhibitor, provides dose-dependent efficacy and sustained 24-hour blood pressure control in patients with hypertension. J Am Coll Cardiol 2007;49(11):1157–63.

95. O'Brien E, Barton J, Nussberger J, Mulcahy D, Jensen C, Dicker P, Stanton A. Aliskiren reduces blood pressure and suppresses plasma renin activity in combination with a thiazide diuretic, an angiotensin-converting enzyme inhibitor, or an angiotensin receptor blocker. Hypertension 2007;49(2):276–84.

96. Oparil S, Yarows SA, Patel S, Zhang J, Satlin A. Efficacy and safety of combined use of aliskiren in patients with hypertension: a randomised double-blind trial. Lancet 2007;370:221–9.

97. Cheng H, Harris RC. Potential side effects of renin inhibitors—mechanisms based on comparison with other renin–angiotensin blockers. Expert Opin Drug Saf 2006;5(5):631–41.

98. Van Tassell BW, Munger MA. Aliskiren for renin inhibition: a new class of antihypertensives. Ann Pharmacother 2007;41(3):456–64.

99. Krum H, Gilbert RE. Novel therapies blocking the renin–angiotensin–aldosterone system in the management of hypertension and related disorders. J Hypertens 2007;25(1):25–35.

100. Birkenhäger WH, Staessen JA. Dual inhibition of the renin system by aliskiren and valsartan. Lancet 2007;370:195–6.

101. Dieterle W, Corynen S, Vaidyanathan S, Mann J. Pharmacokinetic interactions of the oral renin inhibitor aliskiren with lovastatin, atenolol, celecoxib and cimetidine. Int J Clin Pharmacol Ther 2005;43(11):527–35.

102. Vaidyanathan S, Valencia J, Kemp C, Zhao C, Yeh CM, Bizot MN, Denouel J, Dieterich HA, Dole WP. Lack of pharmacokinetic interactions of aliskiren, a novel direct renin inhibitor for the treatment of hypertension, with the antihypertensives amlodipine, valsartan, hydrochlorothiazide (HCTZ) and ramipril in healthy volunteers. Int J Clin Pract 2006;60(11):1343–56.

103. Dieterle W, Corynen S, Mann J. Effect of the oral renin inhibitor aliskiren on the pharmacokinetics and pharmacodynamics of a single dose of warfarin in healthy subjects. Br J Clin Pharmacol 2004;58(4):433–6.

104. Galié N, Badesch D, Oudiz R, Simonneau G, McGoon MD, Keogh AM, Frost AE, Zwicke D, Naeije R, Shapiro S, Olschewski H, Rubin LJ. Ambrisentan therapy for pulmonary arterial hypertension. J Am Coll Cardiol 2005 Aug 2;46(3):529–35.

105. Segal ES, Valette C, Oster L, Bouley L, Edfjall C, Herrmann P, Raineri M, Kempff M, Beacham S, van Lierop C. Risk management strategies in the postmarketing period: safety experience with the US and European bosentan surveillance programmes. Drug Saf 2005;28(11):971–80.

106. Widlitz AC, Barst RJ, Horn EM. Sitaxsentan: a novel endothelin-A receptor antagonist for pulmonary arterial hypertension. Exp Rev Cardiovasc Ther 2005;3(6):985–91.

107. Mitchell A, Buhrmann S, Opazo Saez A, Rushentsova U, Schafers RF, Philipp T, Nurnberger J. Clonidine lowers blood pressure by reducing vascular resistance and cardiac output

in young, healthy males. Cardiovasc Drugs Ther 2005;19(1):49–55.

108. Kettenmann B, Feichtinger M, Tilz C, Kaltenhauser M, Hummel C, Stefan H. Comparison of clonidine to sleep deprivation in the potential to induce spike or sharp-wave activity. Clin Neurophysiol 2005;116(4):905–12.

109. Spiller HA, Klein-Schwartz W, Colvin JM, Villalobos D, Johnson PB, Anderson DL. Toxic clonidine ingestion in children. J Pediatr 2005;146(2):263–6.

110. Sica DA. Alpha1-adrenergic blockers: current usage considerations. J Clin Hypertens (Greenwich) 2005;7(12):757–62.

111. Kloner RA. Pharmacology and drug interaction effects of the phosphodiesterase 5 inhibitors: focus on alpha-blocker interactions. Am J Cardiol 2005;96(12B):42M–6M.

112. MacDonald R, Wilt TJ. Alfuzosin for treatment of lower urinary tract symptoms compatible with benign prostatic hyperplasia: a systematic review of efficacy and adverse effects. Urology 2005;66(4):780–8.

113. Satar S, Sebe A, Avci A, Yesilagac H, Gokel Y. Acute intoxication with doxazosin. Hum Exp Toxicol 2005 Jun;24(6):337–9.

114. Boehringer Ingelheim. Important safety information on Intraoperative Floppy Iris Syndrome (IFIS). 14 Oct 2005; http://hc-sc.gc.ca/dhp-mps/medeff/advisories-avis/prof/2005/flomax_hpc-cps_e.html.

115. Chang DF, Campbell JR. Intraoperative floppy iris syndrome associated with tamsulosin. J Cataract Refract Surg 2005;31(4):664–73.

116. Anand JS, Chodorowski Z, Wisniewski M. Acute intoxication with tamsulosin hydrochloride. Clin Toxicol (Phila) 2005;43(4):311.

117. Martin U, Hill C, O'Mahoney D. Use of moxonidine in elderly patients with resistant hypertension. J Clin Pharm Ther 2005;30(5):433–7.

Domenic A. Sica

21

Diuretics

Sensory systems In 1077 patients with intraocular pressures of 22–29 mmHg, normal visual fields, and normal optic discs, who were followed every 6 months for 5 years in the European Glaucoma Prevention Study, a multivariate analysis showed that the use of diuretics (HR = 2.41, 95% CI = 1.12, 5.19) was one of several factors associated with the development of *open-angle glaucoma* (1^C). Systemic hypertension was not associated with the conversion to open-angle glaucoma. Information concerning the use of any medications was obtained at baseline and every 6 months throughout the study. However, particular classes of diuretics were not separately cited. This contributory effect of diuretics may be explained by the play of chance alone or by as yet unknown detrimental effects of diuretics on the retinal ganglion cells. A possible reduction in ocular perfusion pressure induced by a diuretic-related reduction in systemic pressure may be an additional mechanism. In this study, diuretics were more often used in combination with other antihypertensive drugs, particularly in the patients who developed open-angle glaucoma. Blood pressure readings were not obtained during the study, and so it could not be determined whether there was hypotension.

℞ *Hypersensitivity reactions to sulfonamide derivatives*

In patients who are allergic to antimicrobial sulfonamides a decision has to be made as to whether other sulfonamide derivatives can be given safely.

Side Effects of Drugs, Annual 30
J.K. Aronson (Editor)
ISSN: 0378-6080
DOI: 10.1016/S0378-6080(08)00021-4

Sulfonamide structures *Sulfonamides are characterized by a sulfur dioxide (SO$_2$) moiety and a nitrogen (N) moiety directly linked to a benzene ring (Figure 1). Many classes of drugs contain this chemical structure, including antimicrobial sulfonamides (for example sulfamethoxazole), carbonic anhydrase inhibitors (for example acetazolamide), thiazide, thiazide-like, and loop diuretics (for example hydrochlorothiazide, chlorthalidone, furosemide, bumetanide), sulfonylureas (for example glibenclamide, glipizide), uricosuric drugs (for example probenecid), sulfasalazine, selective serotonin receptor agonists (for example sumatriptan), and the selective cyclooxygenase COX-2 inhibitor celecoxib.*

However, there are several structural differences among these classes. A major difference between sulfonamide antimicrobial drugs and other sulfonamide-containing compounds is the presence of an arylamine group (NH$_2$) at the N4 position. It has been hypothesized that only sulfonamides that contain the N4 primary amine are implicated in allergic reactions. This primary arylamine is oxidized to a highly reactive hydroxylamine intermediate, which is further oxidized to a highly immunogenic nitroso metabolite with a high affinity for cysteine residues on proteins. Non-antimicrobial sulfonamides are thought to be less immunogenic because they lack the N4 primary amine.

Case reports

- *A 57-year-old woman with decompensated heart failure and a history of allergy to co-trimoxazole (rash and pancreatitis) was given ethacrynic acid instead of a sulfonamide diuretic (2^A). However, owing to a shortage of oral ethacrynic acid she went without diuretic therapy and developed acute decompensated heart failure. She was given intravenous furosemide 40 mg bd and 5 weeks later developed nausea, vomiting, and abdominal pain and raised serum amylase and lipase activities. Intravenous furosemide was withdrawn and 2 days later the abdominal symptoms resolved. Because of worsening pulmonary edema, she was given*

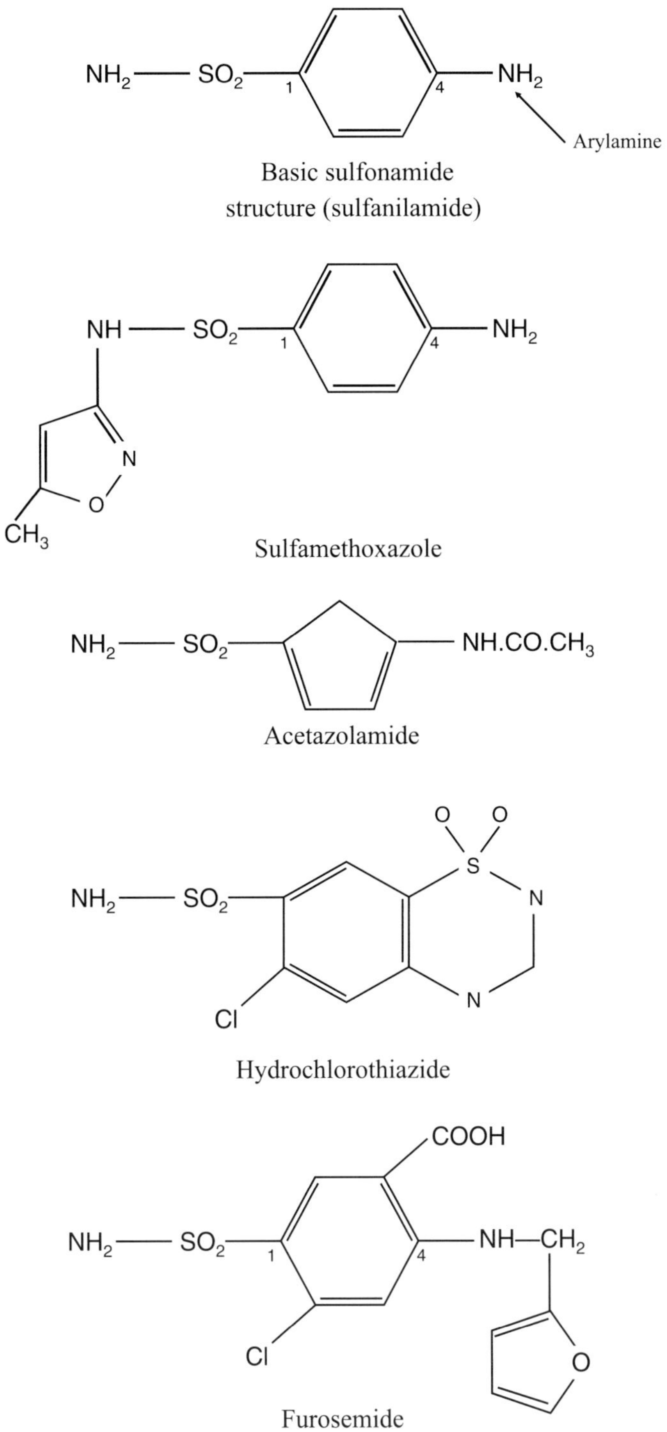

Fig. 1. Chemical structures of sulfonamide antimicrobial drugs containing an arylamine group (NH_2) at the N4 position and non-antimicrobial sulfonamides absent an arylamine group at this position.

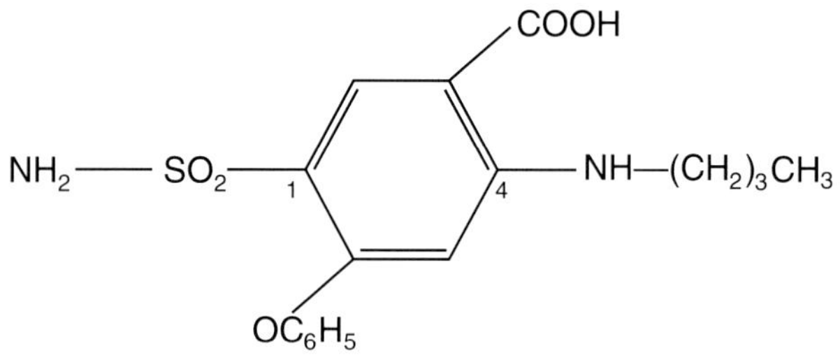

COOH

NH$_2$—SO$_2$—[1]——[4]—NH—(CH$_2$)$_3$CH$_3$

OC$_6$H$_5$

Bumetanide

Fig. 1. (*continued*)

intravenous bumetanide and within 24 hours developed myalgias. After 3 days bumetanide was withdrawn and intravenous torsemide begun. Four days later she developed severe abdominal pain similar to prior episodes, and laboratory and imaging studies were consistent with a diagnosis of pancreatitis. Torsemide was withdrawn and her symptoms resolved quickly. Intravenous ethacrynic acid was started with no further complications.

- *An 82-year-old woman, who had a history of angioedema with co-trimoxazole, developed angioedema, severe dysphagia, dyspnea, and a rash after taking valsartan and hydrochlorothiazide for 4 months (3^A). She was given subcutaneous adrenaline and intravenous antihistamines and glucocorticoids. The angioedema resolved in under 24 hours, and she was discharged with instructions to continue her regular medications, with the exception of valsartan. After 12 weeks she had another episode of angioedema, dyspnea, dysphagia, and rash. Hydrochlorothiazide was withdrawn but was later restarted. Within 2 days she developed mild swelling of the face and lips. Hydrochlorothiazide was permanently withdrawn.*

In the second patient the similarity between the allergic reactions that occurred during treatment with hydrochlorothiazide and co-trimoxazole suggested true cross-reactivity.

Formal studies   There have been very few studies of the incidence of cross-reactivity between antimicrobial sulfonamides and other sulfonamide derivatives. In a retrospective cohort study, of 969 patients who had an allergic reaction to an antimicrobial sulfonamide, 96 (9.9%; adjusted OR = 2.8; 95% CI = 2.1, 3.7) had an allergic reaction to a non-antimicrobial sulfonamide (4^c). Of 19 257 who had no allergic reaction to an antimicrobial sulfonamide, 315 (1.6%) had an allergic reaction to a non-antimicrobial sulfonamide (adjusted OR = 2.8; 95% CI = 2.1, 3.7). However, the risk of an

allergic reaction was even greater with a penicillin among patients with a prior hypersensitivity reaction to an antimicrobial sulfonamide, compared with patients with no such history (adjusted OR = 3.9; 95% CI = 3.5, 4.3). Finally, the risk of an allergic reaction with a non-antimicrobial sulfonamide was lower among patients with a history of hypersensitivity to an antimicrobial sulfonamide than among those with a history of hypersensitivity to a penicillin (adjusted OR = 0.6; 95% CI = 0.5, 0.8).

Thus, although a history of an allergic reaction to antimicrobial sulfonamides marks a heightened risk on exposure to non-antimicrobial sulfonamides, this risk is not exclusive to antimicrobial sulfonamides. In point of fact, patients with a history of hypersensitivity to an antimicrobial sulfonamide are at even greater risk of a reaction to a penicillin than to a non-antimicrobial sulfonamide.

Prescribers should appreciate that patients with a history of allergic reactions to antimicrobial sulfonamides may be at increased risk of all drug-induced adverse events of a seeming allergic nature.

CARBONIC ANHYDRASE INHIBITORS   (*SED-15, 643; SEDA-27, 220; SEDA-28, 233; SEDA-29, 220*)

Acetazolamide

Nervous system   Acetazolamide is used to reduce the frequency of attacks of ataxia in patients with episodic ataxia type 2. However, the metabolic acidosis that acetazolamide causes can result in nervous system complications (5[A]).

- A 49-year-old man with episodic ataxia type 2 responded to acetazolamide 250 mg qds. However, during an attack of ataxia he developed gaze-evoked nystagmus, positional nystagmus, dysarthria, and aggravated gait ataxia; he was also excessively drowsy and unable to speak unless subjected to painful stimuli. Imaging studies and laboratory data were normal, except for hyperammonemia (1.58 mg/l, reference range 0.08–0.48 mg/l) and a compensated metabolic acidosis. Acetazolamide was continued, but 3 days later the ammonia concentration increased to 6.6 mg/l, with worsening of the ataxia and dysarthria. Acetazolamide was withdrawn, and within 10 days his symptoms had almost completely resolved and the serum ammonia concentration had fallen to 1.22 mg/l.

This is the first report of *ataxia* secondary to acetazolamide-induced hyperammonemia in a patient with episodic ataxia type 2. Acetazolamide increases the renal production of NH_3, and the consequent metabolic acidosis can cause hyperammonemia. Acetazolamide should therefore be used cautiously in patients with a history of hepatic or renal disease (conditions that predispose to hyperammonemia).

Metabolic acidosis due to acetazolamide causes increased minute ventilation, which can cause *increased intracranial pressure* and result in neurological complications (6[A]).

- A 19-year-old woman with postoperative bilateral raised intracranial pressure was given intravenous acetazolamide 500 mg followed by 250 mg every 6 hours. After 3 days she developed a metabolic acidosis (serum HCO_3 18 mmol/l), which was attributed to acetazolamide. The metabolic acidosis progressed over the next 3 days (HCO_3 15 mmol/l) with appropriate hypocapnia (P_aCO_2 3.2–3.6 kPa). After 6 days she became agitated, and a propofol infusion was begun, but her mechanical respiratory rate was not increased to maintain her prior hypocapnia. After 5 hours her P_aCO_2 was 4.7 kPa and her arterial pH was 7.26. She developed extreme hypertension and a tachycardia. A CT scan of the brain showed cerebral edema, brain stem herniation, and bilateral watershed infarcts. At post mortem there were multiple fat emboli in the brain and lungs.

The use of acetazolamide in the presence of unrecognized cerebral edema due to fat embolism, with sudden normalization of brain CO_2, as occurred in this patient when her previous state of hypocapnia was no longer sustained by ventilatory effort, resulted in cerebral acidosis, vasodilatation, and a further increase in intracranial pressure. This proved catastrophic and led to brainstem herniation and brain death. Acetazolamide should be avoided if at all possible in patients with bony and traumatic brain injuries, particularly during weaning from mechanical ventilation, since it can precipitate coning in patients with raised intracranial pressure.

Sensory systems   Acetazolamide-induced *transient myopia and angle closure glaucoma* can occur in patients without glaucoma (7[A]).

- A 66-year-old man with chronic open-angle glaucoma underwent routine left cataract surgery and intraocular lens implantation. He was given oral acetazolamide 250 mg the evening before and immediately after surgery and 3 hours later developed severe left eye pain. He had corneal edema, a uniformly shallow anterior chamber, and an intraocular pressure of 52 mmHg. The right eye showed circumcorneal congestion, corneal edema, and an intraocular pressure of 40 mmHg. He was treated with intravenous mannitol, oral acetazolamide, intraocular timolol, ofloxacin, and dexamethasone. After 24 hours the corneal edema and shallow anterior chamber persisted, with an intraocular pressure of 32 mmHg in each eye. Acetazolamide was withdrawn. Ultrasound showed bilateral choroidal effusions and intravenous dexamethasone was begun. On day 5, all ocular signs had resolved and the intraocular pressure was 18 mmHg bilaterally.

Angle closure glaucoma has been reported as an adverse effect of acetazolamide. It has been suggested that this relates to an induced forward shift of the crystalline lens in addition to ciliary body edema. Although glucocorticoids have been reported to cause choroidal effusions, an exaggeration of this phenomenon by the combination of a glucocorticoid and acetazolamide has not been previously reported.

Electrolyte balance   Children with heart disease often require high-dose diuretic therapy, which can lead to hypochloremic metabolic alkalosis. There are limited data on the safety of acetazolamide in the treatment of hypochloremic metabolic alkalosis in children. In 28 patients, median age 2 (range 0.3–20) months who took acetazolamide 5 mg/kg for 3 days, there were no adverse events (8[c]). There was no significant difference in any electrolyte concentration, except for serum HCO_3, which fell from 36 to 31 mmol/l, and serum chloride, which rose from 91 to 95 mmol/l. There was no change in urine output. Acetazolamide appears to be safe in very young patients when given for 3 consecutive days.

Skin   Carbonic anhydrase inhibitors can rarely cause *Stevens–Johnson syndrome* (9[A]).

- A 62-year-old man with cerebrovascular disease underwent regional cerebrovascular reactivity to intravenous acetazolamide 1000 mg using single-photon emission computed tomography with [^{123}I] N-isopropyl-para-iodoamfetamine 0.45 mg. Three days later he developed erythematous eruptions of varying sizes on his back, which then spread over his entire body. The presumptive diagnosis was Stevens–Johnson syndrome and he was given a glucocorticoid. The skin and mucous lesions became bullous or erosive, ruptured spontaneously, and dried with crusting. He gradually improved over 21 days. Lymphocyte transformation tests were positive with acetazolamide.

All previous cases have occurred in patients taking oral acetazolamide for glaucoma and have been limited to Japanese or Indian patients or patients of Japanese descent, as was the case here.

Brinzolamide

Acid-base balance   Topical brinzolamide can be systemically absorbed and could cause systemic adverse effects. In one case it was reported to have caused a *metabolic acidosis* (10[A]).

- A 66-year-old man with glaucoma was given brinzolamide twice daily to only one eye in addition to topical latanoprost. After 3 months he reported having stopped using brinzolamide because of lethargy and a bad taste in the mouth. He also reported that a silver chain worn around his neck had turned black within 2 days of starting brinzolamide and again soon after it had been cleaned. Electrolyte and acid-base status were not assessed.

Although a metabolic acidosis could occur with topical brinzolamide if sufficient drug were systemically absorbed, a change in the color of a silver chain worn around the neck is hardly an adequate basis for a diagnosis of a metabolic acidosis.

Dorzolamide

Sensory systems   *Anosmia* has been attributed to topical dorzolamide (11[A])

- A 49-year-old man with glaucoma was given 2% dorzolamide in addition to timolol. After 1 month he developed reduced smell and after 2 months anosmia. Dorzolamide was withdrawn and latanoprost substituted. His sense of smell returned to normal within 20 days. Rechallenge with several different glaucoma medications resulted in recurrence of the anosmia whenever dorzolamide was used.

Carbonic anhydrase exists in multiple forms in the nasal mucosa, where its inhibition may have resulted in anosmia. However, the absence of previous reports of anosmia with dorzolamide suggests a patient-specific isoenzyme variability/susceptibility to carbonic anhydrase inhibition.

Skin   *Allergic contact dermatitis* has been attributed to topical dorzolamide (12[A]).

- An 80-year-old woman developed conjunctival inflammation and a severe eczematous rash affecting the eyelids and cheeks within 1 week of switching from latanoprost + benzalkonium chloride to Cosopt® (dorzolamide hydrochloride 2% + timolol maleate 0.5% + benzalkonium chloride). Cosopt® was withdrawn and the dermatitis was treated with topical glucocorticoids and emollients, with rapid resolution. Subsequent patch testing was positive with pure dorzolamide 40% and timolol 10%, with no reactions to product excipients or benzalkonium chloride.

Contact dermatitis to two separate topical agents, timolol and dorzolamide, is decidedly uncommon. Patch testing, albeit at higher drug concentrations, showed sensitivity to both compounds.

THIAZIDE AND THIAZIDE-LIKE DIURETICS   *(SED-15, 3375; SEDA-27, 220; SEDA-28, 233; SEDA-29, 221)*

Mineral balance   *Hypercalcemia* associated with thiazide diuretics is probably due to reduced urine calcium excretion. However, the incidence of thiazide diuretic-associated hypercalcemia has not been reported. In a study that included 72 patients with thiazide diuretic-associated hypercalcemia (68 women and 4 men; mean age 64 years), the overall age and sex-adjusted incidence was 7.7 per 100 000 (95% CI = 5.9, 9.5), with an increase in incidence after 1996, peaking at 16 per 100 000 (95% CI = 8.3, 24) in 1998 (13[c]). The highest rate was in women aged 70–79 years (55/100 000). Thiazide diuretic-associated hypercalcemia was typically discovered several years (mean 6.0) after the start of therapy. The mean highest serum calcium was 2.7 (range 2.54–2.88) mmol/l and the serum parathyroid hormone concentration (obtained in 53 patients) was 4.8 pmol/l (reference range 1.0–5.2). In 21 of 33 patients who stopped taking the thiazide diuretic there was persistent hypercalcemia, and 18 were subsequently found to have primary hyperparathyroidism. The observed sex discrepancy in these studies suggests that postmenopausal women are predisposed to hypercalcemia with thiazide diuretics and/or that women more often take thiazides for the treatment of hypertension. This phenomenon tends to be mild, asymptomatic, and non-progressive; it calls for establishing whether primary hyperparathyroidism is present.

Chlorthalidone

Sensory systems   Chlorthalidone has been associated with acute *myopia* (14[A]).

• A 30-year-old man with hypertension developed visual blurring after taking chlortalidone 12.5 mg/day for 4 days in addition to atenolol. Visual acuity was 20/120 in both eyes and slit-lamp biomicroscopy showed retinal striae radiating from the fovea. B-scan ultrasonography showed shallow peripheral serous choroidal detachment. The blood pressure was 140/100, hematological and renal function tests and serum electrolytes were within the reference ranges, and a CT scan of the head was normal. Atenolol and chlorthalidone were withdrawn and 5 days later his visual acuity had returned to 20/20. Fundoscopy showed disappearance of the retinal striae at the macula and resolution of the peripheral choroidal effusion.

The exact mechanism whereby chlorthalidone caused acute myopia in this case was unclear, but the authors suggested that it could have been due to ciliary body effusion, peripheral uveal effusion, ciliary spasm, and lens swelling.

Hydrochlorothiazide

Sensory systems   Bilateral *angle closure glaucoma* has been reported with hydrochlorothiazide (15[A]).

• A 70-year-old woman with hypertension developed bilateral worsening vision over 1 day. She had started to take hydrochlorothiazide 1 month before. Visual acuity was substantially impaired and intraocular pressures were about 40 mmHg bilaterally. Slit lamp examination showed bilateral shallow anterior chambers with anterior bowing of the iris and a centered posterior chamber intraocular lens. She was given dorzolamide, timolol, brimonidine, and prednisolone acetate and by the next day the intraocular pressures were ≈15 mmHg, although the anterior chambers remained shallow. Anterior choroidal effusions were suspected and the hydrochlorothiazide was withdrawn. After 3 days later the best-corrected vision was substantially improved, deep anterior chambers were present bilaterally, and the intraocular pressures were 12 mmHg.

Hydrochlorothiazide has only been associated with bilateral secondary angle closure once before. The proposed mechanism involves an idiosyncratic reaction in the uvea, with expansion of the extracellular tissues of the ciliary body and choroid. Presumably in cases in which there is mild expansion of the ciliary body and choroid there might only be a period of transient myopia. If uveal expansion is unrelenting there is appositional closure of the angle to such a degree that the intraocular pressure cannot equilibrate to normal. It is unclear whether there is cross-reactivity amongst various sulfonamide derivatives for this ocular complication.

Pancreas   Fatal *necrotizing pancreatitis* has been reported in a patient taking hydrochlorothiazide (16[A]).

• A 49-year-old man with hypertension, who had taken hydrochlorothiazide 12.5 mg/day and lisinopril 10 mg/day for 1 year, developed severe diffuse abdominal pain and vomiting. The diagnosis was pancreatic inflammation and necrosis. Other causes of pancreatitis, including hypertriglyceridemia, hypercalcemia, HIV infection, alcohol, and trauma, were excluded. Despite aggressive treatment he developed multi-organ failure and refractory shock and died shortly thereafter.

Thiazide-induced necrotizing pancreatitis is very rare, only three cases having previously been reported. The exact mechanism is incompletely understood and the susceptibility factors are not known. The intensity varies and can range from mild to life-threatening.

Indapamide

Cardiovascular   Indapamide has been associated with *QT interval prolongation* and *torsade de pointes* independent of electrolyte changes (17[A]).

- A 42-year-old woman with systemic lupus erythematosus and hypertension developed palpitation and near syncope. Her medications included prednisolone 5 mg/day and indapamide 2.5 mg/day. A baseline electrocardiogram showed sinus rhythm, several episodes of non-sustained ventricular tachycardia, and a QT_c interval of 510 ms. Serum potassium, magnesium, and free calcium concentrations were all normal. Despite withdrawal of indapamide and prednisolone, torsade de pointes occurred and degenerated into ventricular fibrillation. Over the next two days the QT_c interval gradually shortened to 430 ms. Coronary angiography did not show any significant stenotic lesions.

Several non-antidysrhythmic drugs, including diuretics, prolong cardiac repolarization, predisposing to torsade de pointes. Diuretic-induced hypokalemia can exacerbate this effect. However, indapamide blocks the slow component of the delayed inward rectifier potassium current, leading to excessive lengthening of cardiac repolarization and thereby a predisposition to torsade de pointes. Indapamide should therefore be used with caution in patients who are at risk of torsade de pointes, especially when the patient is also taking drugs that block the rapid component of the delayed inward rectifier potassium current. Such drugs include class III antidysrhythmic drugs, macrolide antibiotics, antipsychotic drugs, and antihistamines.

LOOP DIURETICS   *(SED-15, 567, 1454; SEDA-27, 220; SEDA-28, 233; SEDA-29, 222)*

Sensory systems

Ear   Sensorineural hearing loss is an important adverse outcome in survivors of neonatal intensive care illnesses, particularly those with persistent pulmonary hypertension of the new-

born. The relations between ototoxic drugs and 4-year sensorineural hearing loss have been assessed in a prospective, longitudinal outcome study in near-term and term survivors of severe neonatal respiratory failure who were enrolled in the Canadian arm of the Neonatal Inhaled Nitric Oxide Study (18[C]). A combination of loop diuretic use for more than 14 days and an average dose of neuromuscular blocker greater than 0.96 mg/kg/day contributed to sensorineural hearing loss among survivors (OR = 5.2; 95% CI = 1.6, 17). Cumulative dose and duration of diuretic use and overlap of diuretic use with neuromuscular blockers, aminoglycosides, and vancomycin were individually linked to sensorineural hearing loss. These studies implicate loop diuretics and neuromuscular blockers individually and possibly synergistically in sensorineural hearing loss.

Mineral balance   Loop diuretics can affect bone by *increasing urine calcium excretion* and *modifying the diurnal rhythm of parathyroid hormone*. In a double-blind, randomized study 87 otherwise healthy postmenopausal women with osteopenia were randomized to bumetanide 2 mg/day or placebo for 1 year (19[C]). Calcium (800 mg/day) and vitamin D (10 micrograms/day) were administered throughout the study. Compared with placebo, urine calcium and plasma parathyroid hormone concentrations rose by 17 and 9% respectively. Bone mineral density fell by 2% at the hip (95% CI = 0.7, 3.2%) and ultradistal forearm. Six months after completion of bumetanide therapy between-group differences in bone mineral density were no longer statistically significant. The negative effect of bumetanide on bone metabolism and density was probably mitigated in these studies by calcium and vitamin D.

Musculoskeletal   Although loop diuretics increase renal calcium excretion, there have been variable results in studies of their effects on the risk of fractures. In a case–control study of the risk of fracture in 44 001 patients who had taken a loop diuretic in the preceding 5 years and 194 111 age- and sex-matched controls, "ever" use of a loop diuretic was associated with a crude 51% increased risk of any fracture (OR = 1.51; 95% CI = 1.48, 155) and a 72% increased risk of hip fracture (OR = 1.72; 95% CI = 1.64, 181) (20[C]). After adjustment for potential confounders, the risk reduction was only slightly increased for any fracture (OR = 1.04) and for hip fracture (OR = 1.16). With an increased average daily dose the estimates increased in former users but fell in current users. Furosemide was associated with higher risk estimates than bumetanide. This study does not provide a definitive answer to the risk of fractures with loop diuretics but suggests that particular caution should be taken.

Death   In 1354 patients (76% men, mean age 53 years) with advanced systolic heart failure (mean ejection fraction 24%) four groups were identified according to daily furosemide equivalent dosages: 0–40, 41–80, 81–160, and over 160 mg/day (21[C]). The four groups were comparable as regards sex, body mass index, a history of hypertension, ischemic etiology of heart failure, and use of spironolactone. The highest dose was associated with lower hemoglobin and serum sodium concentrations and higher blood urea nitrogen and serum creatinine concentrations. There was reduced survival with increased diuretic dosage at 2 years: 83, 81, 68, and 53%. Diuretic dosage was an independent predictor of mortality at 1 year and 2 years, even with co-variate adjustment for multiple potentially confounding variables. Kaplan–Meier survival estimate curves showed persistence of the prognostic value of diuretic dosage in men/women, patients with and without coronary artery disease, and those with a serum creatinine above or below 133 µmol/l. The association of larger doses of loop diuretics with poorer outcomes has been demonstrated in a number of retrospective analyses. However, this study differed, in that it showed a stepwise, dose-dependent effect of loop diuretics on mortality. Propensity matching was not performed in these studies and so it is not known whether the relation between loop diuretic dosage and increased mortality is causative.

ALDOSTERONE RECEPTOR ANTAGONISTS

Eplerenone   *(SED-15, 1227; SEDA-27, 231; SEDA-28, 235)*

Susceptibility factors

Renal disease   In 64 subjects mild, moderate, or severe renal impairment had no effect on the

pharmacokinetics of a single dose of eplerenone 100 mg followed by 100 mg/day on days 3–8 (22[c]). Hemodialysis removed about 10% of the dose.

Spironolactone   *(SED-15, 3176; SEDA-27, 231; SEDA-28, 235; SEDA-29, 222)*

Electrolyte balance   In 3995 patients for whom spironolactone was prescribed in a single teaching hospital and two community hospitals, *hyperkalemia* was identified in 419 (10.5%); the median age of all the patients was 65 years and the median daily dose was 25 mg (23[c]).

One would expect the risk of hyperkalemia in patients taking spironolactone to be increased by concomitant therapy with an ACE inhibitor or an angiotensin receptor antagonist (24[A], 25[A]). However, this effect may be mitigated by the addition of a potassium-wasting diuretic, as exemplified by a retrospective study of 259 patients with chronic heart failure who were taking spironolactone (25 mg/day, n = 210, or 50 mg/day, n = 49) plus furosemide 40 mg/day, plus either an ACE inhibitor or an angiotensin receptor antagonist, and 251 who were taking the same drugs without spironolactone (26[c]). The serum potassium concentration was raised only in those who were taking spironolactone, regardless of other potassium-sparing therapy (enalapril maleate 5 mg/day, losartan potassium 50 mg/day, or candesartan cilexetil 8 mg/day).

Endocrine   In an open study in 35 women with acne, mean age 21 years, spironolactone 100 mg/day on 16 days each month for 3 months had no effect on serum total testosterone concentrations but *reduced serum dehydroepiandrosterone sulfate concentrations* (27[c]).

Breasts   In a man with chronic heart failure and *gynecomastia* attributed to spironolactone there was bilaterally increased uptake of ^{67}Ga citrate and ^{18}F FDG in the breast tissues (28[A]).

Susceptibility factors

Children   In 100 children (average age 21 months, weight 9.5 kg), 62 of whom had heart disease, 29 had chronic lung disease, and 9 had other conditions, spironolactone 1.7–2.0 mg/kg/day plus a potassium-wasting diuretic was associated with hyperkalemia initially, but hypokalemia was more frequent during long-term use (29[c]).

Elderly patients In a retrospective survey of 64 patients aged over 75 years, there was hyperkalemia (over 5.5 mmol/l) in 36% and severe hyperkalemia (over 6.0 mmol/l) in 11% (30[c]). The incidence of severe renal insufficiency was 11% and 38% of the patients had a more than 50% rise in creatinine concentration. Three deaths were thought to be drug related. Only severe intercurrent illness predicted the adverse outcomes. In contrast to the results of other studies, age, baseline creatinine, creatinine clearance, ACE inhibitor dose, NYHA class, diabetes mellitus, intensity of monitoring, co-morbidity, and number of co-medications were not predictive. These results suggest that elderly patients are more susceptible to hyperkalemia and renal insufficiency when taking spironolactone.

OSMOTIC DIURETICS

Mannitol *(SED-15, 2203; SEDA-29, 222)*

Electrolyte balance Intraoperative *hyperkalemia* and cardiac toxicity have been reported during intraoperative infusion of mannitol.

- A 31-year old woman received two 40 g doses of intravenous mannitol over about 45 minutes during a right frontal craniotomy and debulking of a recurrent astrocytoma (31[A]). About 15 minutes later she developed peaked T waves on the electrocardiogram in conjunction with a plasma potassium concentration of 6.1 mmol/l. Serum potassium was lowered and the electrocardiographic changes resolved.
- A 41-year old man received 200 g of 20% intravenous mannitol during elective craniotomy for clipping of a left middle cerebral artery aneurysm (32[A]). After about 40 minutes, about 120 g having been infused, his electrocardiogram showed peaked T waves and a prolonged QRS duration. Despite withdrawal of mannitol the electrocardiogram deteriorated into a sine-wave ventricular tachycardia and soon afterwards coarse ventricular fibrillation. The serum potassium concentration was 7.5 mmol/l and the serum sodium 116 mmol/l. The serum potassium was reduced to 3.9 mmol/l and sinus rhythm was eventually restored.

These cases illustrate that hypertonic mannitol, when rapidly infused, can prompt extracellular shifts of potassium. Under these circumstances, when the plasma potassium concentration increases rapidly, hyperkalemic cardiotoxicity can occur. Accordingly, plasma potassium concentration should be monitored whenever significant quantities of mannitol (80 grams or more) are given rapidly (in under 1 hour).

References

1. Miglior S, Torri V, Zeyen T, Pfeiffer N, Vaz JC, Adamsons I, EGPS Group. Intercurrent factors associated with the development of open-angle glaucoma in the European Glaucoma Prevention Study. Am J Ophthalmol 2007;144:266–75.
2. Juang P, Page II RL, Zolty R. Probable loop diuretic-induced pancreatitis in a sulfonamide-allergic patient. Ann Pharmacother 2006;40:128–34.
3. Ruscin JM, Page RL, Scott J. Hydrochlorothiazide-induced angioedema in a patient allergic to sulfonamide antibiotics: evidence from a case report and a review of the literature. Am J Geriatr Pharmacother 2006;4:325–9.
4. Strom BL, Schinnar R, Apter AJ, Margolis DJ, Lautenbach E, Hennessy S, Bilker WB, Pettitt D. Absence of cross-reactivity between sulfonamide antibiotics and sulfonamide nonantibiotics. N Engl J Med 2003;349:1628–35.
5. Kim JM, Ryu WS, Hwang YH, Kim JS. Aggravation of ataxia due to acetazolamide induced hyperammonaemia in episodic ataxia. J Neurol Neurosurg Psychiatry 2007;78:771–2.
6. Walshe CM, Cooper JD, Kossmann T, Hayes I, Iles L. Cerebral fat embolism syndrome causing brain death after long-bone fractures and acetazolamdie therapy. Crit Care Resusc 2007;9:184–6.

7. Parthasarathi S, Myint K, Singh G, Mon S, Sadasivam P, Dhillon B. Bilateral acetazolamide-induced choroidal effusion following cataract surgery. Eye 2007;21:870–2.

8. Moffett BS, Moffett TI, Dickerson HA. Acetazolamide therapy for hypochloremic metabolic alkalosis in pediatric patients with heart disease. Am J Ther 2007;14:331–5.

9. Ogasawara K, Tomitsuka N, Kobayashi M, Komoribayashi N, Fukuda T, Saitoh H, Inoue T, Ogawa A. Stevens–Johnson syndrome associated with intravenous acetazolamide administration for evaluation of cerebrovascular reactivity. Neurol Med Chir 2006;46:161–3.

10. Menon GJ, Vernon SA. Topical brinzolamide and metabolic acidosis. Br J Ophthalmol 2006;90:247–8.

11. Turgut B, Türkçüoğlu P, Güler M, Akyol N, Celiker U, Demir T. Anosmia as an adverse effect of dorzolamide. Acta Ophthalmol Scand 2007;85:228–9.

12. Kalavala M, Statham BN. Allergic contact dermatitis from timolol and dorzolamide eye drops. Contact Dermatitis 2006;54:345.

13. Wermers RA, Kearns AE, Jenkins GD, Melton LJ. Incidence and clinical spectrum of thiazide-associated hypercalcemia. Am J Med 2007;120:e9–15.

14. Mahesh G, Giridhar A, Saikumar SJ, Fegde S. Drug-induced myopia following chlorthalidone treatment. Indian J Ophthalmol 2007;55:386–8.

15. Lee GC, Tam CP, Danesh-Meyer HV, Myers JS, Katz LJ. Bilateral angle closure glaucoma induced by sulphonamide-derived medications. Clin Experiment Ophthalmol 2007;35:55–8.

16. Bedrossian S, Vahid B. A case of fatal necrotizing pancreatitis: complication of hydrochlorothiazide and lisinopril therapy. Dig Dis Sci 2007;52:558–60.

17. Letsas KP, Alexanian IP, Pappas LK, Kounas SP, Efremidis M, Sideris A, Kardaras F. QT interval prolongation and torsade de pointes associated with indapamide. Int J Cardiol 2006;112:373–4.

18. Robertson CM, Tyebkhan JM, Peliowski A, Etches PC, Cheung PY. Ototoxic drugs and sensorineural hearing loss following severe neonatal respiratory failure. Acta Paediatrica 2006;95:214–23.

19. Rejnmark L, Vestergaard P, Heickendorff L, Andreasen F, Mosekilde L. Loop diuretics increase bone turnover and decrease BMD in osteopenic postmenopausal women: results from a randomized controlled study with bumetanide. J Bone Min Res 2006;21:163–70.

20. Rejnmark L, Vestergaard P, Mosekilde L. Fracture risk in patients treated with loop diuretics. J Intern Med 2006;259:117–24.

21. Eshaghian S, Horwich TB, Fonarow GC. Relation of loop diuretic dose to mortality in advanced heart failure. Am J Cardiol 2006;97:1759–64.

22. Ravis WR, Reid S, Sica DA, Tolbert DS. Pharmacokinetics of eplerenone after single and multiple dosing in subjects with and without renal impairment. J Clin Pharmacol 2005;45(7):810–21.

23. Huang C, Noirot LA, Reichley RM, Bouselli DA, Dunagan WC, Bailey TC. Automatic detection of spironolactone-related adverse drug events. AMIA Annu Symp Proc 2005;989.

24. Fujii H, Nakahama H, Yoshihara F, Nakamura S, Inenaga T, Kawano Y. Life-threatening hyperkalemia during a combined therapy with the angiotensin receptor blocker candesartan and spironolactone. Kobe J Med Sci 2005;51(1–2):1–6.

25. Kauffmann R, Orozco R, Venegas JC. Severe hyperkalemia associated to the use of losartan and spironolactone: case report. Rev Med Chil 2005;133(8):947–52.

26. Saito M, Takada M, Hirooka K, Isobe F, Yasumura Y. Serum concentration of potassium in chronic heart failure patients administered spironolactone plus furosemide and either enalapril maleate, losartan potassium or candesartan cilexetil. J Clin Pharm Ther 2005;30(6):603–10.

27. Yemisci A, Gorgulu A, Piskin S. Effects and side-effects of spironolactone therapy in women with acne. J Eur Acad Dermatol Venereol 2005;19(2):163–6.

28. Fukuchi K, Sasaki H, Yokoya T, Noguchi T, Goto Y, Hayashida K, Ishida Y. Ga-67 citrate and F-18 FDG uptake in spironolactone-induced gynecomastia. Clin Nucl Med 2005;30(2):105–6.

29. Buck ML. Clinical experience with spironolactone in pediatrics. Ann Pharmacother 2005;39(5):823–8.

30. Dinsdale C, Wani M, Steward J, O'Mahony MS. Tolerability of spironolactone as adjunctive treatment for heart failure in patients over 75 years of age. Age Ageing 2005;34(4):395–8.

31. Hassan ZU, Kruer JJ, Fuhrman TM. Electrolyte changes during craniotomy caused by administration of hypertonic mannitol. J Clin Anesth 2007;19:307–9.

32. Flynn BC. Hyperkalemia cardiac arrest with hypertonic mannitol infusion: the strong ion difference revisited. Anesth Analg 2007;104:225–6.

Gijsbert B. van der Voet and J.A. Centeno

22 Metals

Aluminium *(SED-15, 97; SEDA-27, 224; SEDA-28, 244; SEDA-29, 225)*

Aluminium compounds are used as phosphate binders and as adjuvants in vaccines. Aluminium is also part of dental and medical implant material such as glass ionomer cement. Because of aluminium's known adverse effects, aluminium-based phosphate binders (aluminium hydroxide) have gradually lost their place in the treatment of hyperphosphatemia (1[R]) especially in patients with renal insufficiency. Calcium and magnesium salts and a synthetic polyallamine hydrochloride have been more often used. Recently lanthanum carbonate has also been introduced as a phosphate binder and it is effective in short-term treatment; however, caution is required, keeping in mind the lessons learned from aluminium (2[R]).

Neuromuscular function Current evidence suggests that aluminium from adjuvants in vaccines can persist at the site of injection for years. However, its relation to *macrophagic myofasciitis* is controversial (3[R]), as has been illustrated by the following case report.

- A 32-year-old man had intermittently raised serum creatine kinase activity (78 U/l in April 2003, 484 U/l in July 2003, and 8846 U/l in August 2003; reference range <196 U/l), with normal troponin concentrations (4[A]). He had no neuromuscular symptoms. He had been given inactivated hepatitis A vaccine (Havrix) and poliomyelitis vaccine in March 2000 and a booster inoculation for hepatitis A in February 2001. He had no evidence of muscle weakness or wasting and no fasciculation, and the rest of the neurological examination and needle electromyography was normal. In a deltoid muscle biopsy the interstitial connective tissue contained a dense infiltrate of large

macrophages. Electron microscopy showed spiculated structures within these macrophages. An EDAX X-ray detector showed an aluminium peak from the aggregates. There was no correlation between macrophage myofasciitis and the clinical signs and symptoms in this patient.

Skin In 19 children *pruritic nodules* occurred at the injection site after immunization with aluminium hydroxide-adsorbed DTaP/polio + Hib (Infanrix, Pentavac) and persisted for many years (5[c]). The nodules were often aggravated during upper respiratory tract infections and local skin alterations. The median time between immunization and the onset of symptoms was 1 month. Epicutaneous tests for aluminium were positive in all 16 children who were tested, indicating delayed hypersensitivity to aluminium. This condition is not common but is important to recognize, as the child and the family can suffer considerably. Subsequent immunization with aluminium-adsorbed vaccines can aggravate the symptoms. Aluminium-containing skin products, such as antiperspirants, can cause contact dermatitis, while nodules can be mistaken for tumors. Even though the incidence of itchy nodules and aluminium allergy after the administration of Infanrix, Pentavac, and other aluminium-adsorbed vaccines is probably low, research to replace aluminium adjuvants would be appropriate.

Susceptibility factors Although the toxicity of aluminium in end-stage renal insufficiency is well known and apparently under control, a recent report has suggested that *infection* might lead to raised plasma aluminium and neurotoxicity (6[Ac]).

- A 67-year-old man with end-stage renal insufficiency secondary to diabetic nephropathy had been treated with hemodialysis for 15 years and had taken aluminium hydroxide 1 g tds for 5 years. He developed a pyrexia of 37.8 °C because of a cellulitis at the dialysis catheter exit site. There was no hemodynamic compromise, but he was encephalopathic with reduced consciousness, impaired cognition, and agitation. The C-reactive protein was

Side Effects of Drugs, Annual 30
J.K. Aronson (Editor)
ISSN: 0378-6080
DOI: 10.1016/S0378-6080(08)00022-6

121 mg/l. Although an exit-site swab grew *Staphylococcus aureus*, blood cultures were persistently negative. The dialysis catheter was removed and he was given intravenous flucloxacillin 500 mg qds. The plasma aluminium concentration was very high (25 µmol/l). Subsequent estimations showed a return to the basal concentration (<1 µmol/l), with neurological recovery by day 7.

In the same study, five patients on hemodialysis with bacteremia, not taking aluminium hydroxide had no appreciable rise in plasma aluminium concentration (mean 1.3, range 0.6–2.0 µmol/l). This case suggests that aluminium toxicity may be under-diagnosed and raises questions about the frequency of aluminium monitoring and the effects of acute septic episodes. The authors suggested that infection can cause the release of tissue aluminium, leading to acutely increased plasma aluminium concentrations and signs of neurotoxicity.

Antimony *(SED-15, 316; SEDA-27, 224; SEDA-28, 244; SEDA-29, 226)*

Antimonials, especially the pentavalent compounds, remain important in the treatment of various forms of leishmaniasis (visceral, cutaneous, and mucosal) (7[R], 8[R]).

Cardiovascular Cardiac adverse effects of antimony compounds, such as *prolongation of the QT interval* and *ventricular tachycardia*, are still often observed.

- A 12-year-old girl was referred to hospital with recurrent syncopal attacks for 4 days, each lasting 10–15 minutes (9[A]). She had seven such episodes. She had completed a course of sodium stibogluconate 20 mg/kg/day for 30 days for visceral leishmaniasis 5 days before. She had frequent runs of sustained polymorphous ventricular tachycardia (torsade de pointes) with a prolonged QT_c interval (460 ms). Lidocaine was temporarily beneficial and hypokalemia (3.3 mmol/l) was managed by intravenous potassium. Recurrent ventricular tachycardia with giddiness was aborted by synchronized cardioversion (0.5 J/kg), as was a later episode of ventricular fibrillation. She recovered slowly, with episodes of sustained ventricular tachycardia, each requiring cardioversion, over the next 2 days. Her QT_c interval eventually shortened to 350 ms.

Arsenic *(SED-15, 339; SEDA-27, 225; SEDA-28, 245; SEDA-29, 227)*

The efficacy of arsenic trioxide in cancer (10[R], 11[R]), especially hematological malignancies such as acute promyelocytic anemia (12[R], 13[R]), is still being explored. Arsenic trioxide belongs to a new category of anticancer agents, which target mitochondria. Cardiotoxicity is a frequent adverse effect. Arsenic is often found in herbal medicines of Asian origin (14[R]).

Respiratory *Acute lung injury* has been reported in a patient who received arsenic trioxide (15[A]).

- A 68-year-old man with pancytopenia due to myelodysplastic syndrome was given arsenic trioxide and 8 weeks later developed a chronic non-productive cough, weight loss, and dyspnea on exertion. He had bilateral crackles over the lower two-thirds of the lungs, mild pitting edema in both legs, and multiple petechiae diffusely scattered over the skin. Lung function tests showed a restrictive pattern with an FEV_1 of 1.85 l (60% of predicted), FVC 2.34 l (59% of predicted), FEV_1/FVC of 79%, total lung capacity of 4.15 l (66% of predicted), and 93% predicted diffusion capacity of carbon monoxide. A chest CT scan showed dense parenchymal consolidation throughout both lungs, with bilateral pleural effusions. There was mosaic perfusion, suggesting air trapping, and areas of ground glass opacity. He was transfused with platelets and packed erythrocytes and given a broad-spectrum antibiotic. Bronchoscopy showed normal central airways and no evidence of alveolar hemorrhage. Bronchoalveolar lavage yielded no infectious organisms. He was given high-dose intravenous dexamethasone and rapidly improved. Later, another dose of arsenic trioxide produced the same clinical syndrome, which again responded to a corticosteroid.

Fluid balance *Fluid retention* has been reported during therapy with arsenic trioxide (16[A]).

- A 78-year-old man with acute promyelocytic anemia developed systemic edema and a pleural effusion during therapy with arsenic trioxide. He had neither cardiac nor renal insufficiency. Dexamethasone was not effective. The fluid retention disappeared after withdrawal of arsenic trioxide but recurred when it was readministered. Its appearance was not related to the number of leucocytes in the peripheral blood.

The clinical features suggested that the fluid retention in this case was different from that caused by acute promyelocytic leukemia differentiation syndrome and was probably an adverse effect of arsenic trioxide.

Bismuth   *(SED-15, 518; SEDA-27, 225; SEDA-28, 245; SEDA-29, 227)*

Bismuth compounds (colloidal bismuth subcitrate, bismuth subsalicylate) are used for a host of gastrointestinal complaints, and bismuth-based quadruple therapy is still the second-line treatment of choice in the eradication of *Helicobacter pylori* (17[R]). Bismuth compounds continue to be used after tonsillectomy for hemostasis and also in dental medicine.

Bismacine, also known as chromacine, is an injectable product that has been used to treat Lyme disease. It is not a pharmaceutical, is not approved for anything, including Lyme disease, and contains high amounts of bismuth, which is not approved for use by injection. The US FDA has warned consumers and health-care providers against using bismacine, after investigating one report of death and several reports of injuries (18[S]). One person died, one was hospitalized, and others had serious adverse events after receiving bismacine. The possible effects of bismuth poisoning include *renal insufficiency* and *cardiovascular collapse*.

Urinary tract   *Acute renal insufficiency* is an infrequent adverse effect of colloidal bismuth citrate overdose but continues to occur (19[A]).

- A 16-year-old girl developed nausea, vomiting, and facial paresthesia 10 days after taking 60 tablets (18 g) of colloidal bismuth subcitrate (De-Nol) in a suicide attempt. She had undergone gastric lavage 6 hours later and had received intravenous fluids. However, for the next 9 days she had continued to vomit 3 or 4 times a day. Her blood urea nitrogen was 37 mmol/l, serum creatinine 1759 µmol/l, and her serum electrolytes and liver enzymes were normal. Creatinine clearance was 8.8 ml/minute/1.73 m^2, fractionated sodium excretion 6.6%, renal failure index 9.2%, and tubular phosphate reabsorption 63%. Abdominal ultrasonography showed slightly large kidneys bilaterally and slightly increased echogenicity in the renal parenchyma. Electrocardiography and echocardiography were normal. The serum bismuth concentration 2 days after admission was 495 µg/l. She was given intravenous fluids, hemodialysis, first on alternate days and then twice weekly, and oral penicillamine 20 mg/kg/day. The

serum blood urea nitrogen and creatinine concentrations fell gradually over about 1 month and hemodialysis was discontinued. After seven weeks her renal function had returned to normal and her serum bismuth concentration had fallen to almost one-half.

Chromium   *(SED-15, 737; SEDA-27, 226; SEDA-28, 246; SEDA-29, 228)*

Chromium supplements continue to be used in performance enhancement and may also have a beneficial role in the treatment of diabetes (20[R], 21[R]). Chromium, often combined with cobalt, is used in medical implant materials.

Cardiovascular   In a recent study the importance of chromium supplementation on specific cardiac measurements during diabetes was reported (22[C]). *Prolongation of the QT$_c$ interval* was a powerful predictor of total mortality, cardiac death, and stroke in patients with type 2 diabetes mellitus. Experimental and clinical studies suggested that chromium supplementation improves insulin sensitivity, lowers plasma insulin concentrations, and improves glucose homeostasis.

The potential effects of chromium supplementation on QT$_c$ interval duration in patients with type 2 diabetes have been studied in 60 patients randomly assigned to chromium picolinate 1000 micrograms/day for 3 months and placebo for 3 months in either order. Baseline QT$_c$ interval was similar in the two groups (422 versus 425 milliseconds), it was shorter after 3 months in those who took chromium picolinate first (406 versus 431 milliseconds). In the next 3 months, the QT$_c$ interval shortened in those who took chromium picolinate second and did not alter in the others, resulting in comparable QT$_c$ intervals at the end of the study (414 versus 409 milliseconds). Apart from body mass index (31.4 kg/m^2 in patients with QT$_c$ shortening versus 28.7 kg/m^2 in those without), no clinical or laboratory variables predicted QT$_c$ interval shortening.

Cobalt   *(SED-15, 847; SEDA-24, 255)*

Skin   See under *Nickel*.

Musculoskeletal   Cobalt–chromium alloys are used as implant devices. *Fatigue fractures* of the cemented cobalt–chromium stem in 10 patients after total hip arthroplasty have been reviewed (23[AR]). The average age at the time of surgery was 54 (range 34–70) years and the average body mass index was 29 (range 20–38) kg/m^2. The time *in situ* of the prosthesis at the time of fracture averaged 8 (range 4–12) years. Obesity, undersizing, varus positioning, retroversion, and loss of medial calcar support have all been associated with an increased risk of this complication. Five patients had a body mass index of 25–29 and three had a BMI of 30 or greater. There was loss of medial calcar support in 7 patients in whom intermediate follow-up radiographs were taken before the fracture occurred; as proximal medial bone support is lost, the stem must withstand all the cyclic loads that are applied to the hip, eventually leading to fatigue failure and fracture.

Copper   *(SED-15, 901; SEDA-27, 226; SEDA-28, 246; SEDA-29, 228)*

The roles of copper in Wilson's disease and neurodegenerative disease have been reviewed (24[R], 25[R]).

Gallium   *(SED-15, 1477; SEDA-27, 227; SEDA-28, 246; SEDA-29, 228)*

Gallium nitrate is used as an antitumor agent. Gallium-67 is used as a radio-imaging agent for cancer detection. Gallium-68 labelled peptides are now being used increasingly in imaging (26[R]). Gallium-based dental alloys are being increasingly used in dental medicine.

Gold and gold salts   *(SED-15, 1520; SEDA-27, 227; SEDA-28, 246; SEDA-29, 228)*

The traditional disease-modifying antirheumatic drugs have been compared with modern biological drugs, such as TNF-alfa blockers (27[R]). The author concluded that conventional compounds, such as gold salts, continue to maintain their place in the treatment of rheumatoid arthritis.

Observational studies   Of 49 respondents to a questionnaire that was sent to 102 gold-allergic patients, all but one were women (28[c]). Most of them reported that their dermatitis had improved after patch testing, but most had avoided other allergens as well as gold. The authors concluded that avoidance of gold earrings did not appear to benefit patients with earlobe dermatitis, but that total avoidance of gold jewelry on the hands and wrists did seem to benefit a subgroup of patients with facial and eyelid dermatitis who wore powder, eye shadow, or foundation on affected areas.

Comparative studies   Of 120 patients with rheumatoid arthritis who switched from aurothioglucose to aurothiomalate after the former was withdrawn from the Dutch market because of insufficient quality of the raw material at the end of 2001, 19 reported an adverse drug reaction with aurothiomalate that they had not previously experienced with aurothioglucose (29[C]). The most common adverse effects were *pruritus, dermatitis/stomatitis, and chrysiasis/hyperpigmentation*. There were 29 withdrawals within 12 months because of lack of efficacy ($n = 17$), adverse drug reactions ($n = 8$), or remission ($n = 3$). Kaplan–Meier plots showed a survival rate with aurothiomalate of 79% after 12 months. There were no statistically significant differences in disease activity indicators during follow-up visits compared with baseline.

Iron salts   *(SED-15, 1911; SEDA-27, 227; SEDA-28, 247; SEDA-29, 229)*

Iron deficiency has recently been reviewed (30[R]), as have adverse drug events associated with parenteral iron (31[R], 32[R]). These reviews have suggested that there are increased risks associated with iron dextran, especially *hypersensitivity reactions*, while non-dextran supplements appear to be safer.

Immunologic   *Acute hypersensitivity reactions* have been attributed to sodium ferric gluconate in a woman with anemia (33[A]).

• A 38-year-old woman with persistent anemia that
failed to respond to oral iron was given parenteral ferric gluconate 125 mg intravenously over
10 minutes. She tolerated this dose well, with
no immediate reaction. However, about 1 hour
after the end of the ferric gluconate infusion
she felt dizzy and nauseated and had a swollen
tongue. These effects abated without intervention. One week later, she had a second course
of parenteral iron, preceded by intravenous dexamethasone 10 mg, intravenous diphenhydramine
25 mg, and oral prochlorperazine 10 mg. Before
treatment her blood pressure was 132/65 mmHg
and her heart rate 65/minute. She was given ferric gluconate in the same dose, but to be infused
over 30 minutes. About halfway through the infusion, she developed epigastric pain, nausea, and
swelling of her lips and tongue. Her blood pressure fell to 90/50 mmHg. The iron infusion was
immediately discontinued and she was given intravenous diphenhydramine 25 mg, dexamethasone
10 mg, cimetidine 300 mg, morphine 1 mg for
epigastric pain, and fluids 250 ml/hour, and oxygen 2 1/minute by nasal cannula. The redness
and swelling of her lips and tongue subsided
within minutes and her blood pressure rose to
90/62 mmHg.

An *anaphylactoid reaction* to sodium ferric
gluconate has been reported during pregnancy
(34[A]).

• A 24-year-old woman at 38 weeks' gestation was
given intravenous sodium ferric gluconate complex for iron deficiency anemia. Shortly after the
start of the infusion her tongue started to swell.
She was given diphenhydramine 50 mg and the
sodium ferric gluconate was continued. Her blood
pressure then fell suddenly and she developed severe angioedema of the eyes, lips, and oral mucosa.
The infusion was stopped. Her blood pressure was
70/30 mmHg, the heart rate 110 beats/minute, and
the SpO_2 100%. The fetal heart was monitored
throughout treatment, resuscitation, and stabilization, and was normal. She was given several doses
of adrenaline 50 micrograms, ranitidine 50 mg, and
dexamethasone 10 mg, with 2 liters of crystalloid.
She delivered a healthy child 1 week later.

Magnesium salts   *(SED-15, 2196; SEDA-28, 248)*

Magnesium sulfate is used in the treatment of
pre-eclampsia and to arrest preterm labor (35[R]);
other magnesium salts are used as laxatives.

Cardiovascular   In a retrospective, case-control study in 150 women treated for preterm

labor with magnesium sulfate, the susceptibility
factors for pulmonary edema included greater
magnesium sulfate and intravenous fluid infusion rates, use of a less concentrated solution
of magnesium sulfate, infection, multiple ges-
tations, concomitant tocolytics, large positive
net fluid balances, and maternal transport (36[R]).
The mean latency period to diagnosis was 1.96
days. Six percent of patients had recurrence if
magnesium sulfate tocolysis was continued.

Hematologic   The effects of magnesium sulfate on cord blood neutrophil functional activity
has been studied in 30 preterm neonates, 10
of whom had been exposed to maternal tocolysis with magnesium sulfate perterm, 10
of whose mothers had not received tocolysis,
and 10 term infants (37[c]). Neutrophil functional activity in the cord blood of the preterm
neonates was significantly lower than in term
neonates. Alterations in neutrophil chemotaxis,
random motility, and chemiluminescence were
more noticeable in neonates with intrapartum
exposure to magnesium sulfate than in preterm
infants whose mothers had received no tocolysis. Furthermore, the reduction in neutrophil
functional activity correlated with maternal
serum magnesium concentrations.

Musculoskeletal   Tocolysis with magnesium
sulfate can affect calcium homeostasis and
cause *osteoporosis*. A woman in her mid thir-
ties was given intravenous magnesium sulfate
for 101 days (loading dose 2 g, infused over
30 minutes, followed by a maintenance dose of
1 g/hour); after delivery she developed osteoporosis, leading to significant morbidity (38[AR]).

Magnesium causes hypocalcemia and hypercalciuria by several mechanisms. It is taken
up by bone, displacing calcium; in the kidneys
magnesium ions compete with calcium for reabsorption in the loop of Henle; and magnesium
suppresses parathyroid hormone secretion.

Because of the risk of osteoporosis during
prolonged intravenous administration of magnesium sulfate, the authors made the following
recommendations:

• alternatives to prolonged infusion of magnesium sulfate in the treatment of preterm labor
should be considered;
• for early prevention and treatment of possible
osteoporosis, the diagnosis must be thought
of and established as early as possible;

- radiography in the third trimester is not feasible, but bone mineral density screening of the heels by ultrasonography can be performed;
- if patients have magnesium sulfate tocolysis and bed rest for more than 2 months, they should have the bone density screening by ultrasonography, especially before their first attempt to get out of bed;
- specific stresses on the bones, which might lead to fractures, must be avoided—protected and progressively increased weight bearing and, in some instances, adjusted analgesics and physical therapy for pain control are recommended;
- lactation should be discouraged, because it could be associated with a negative calcium balance and marked bone loss;
- calcium and vitamin D supplementation can be prescribed during tocolysis—the daily calcium requirement should be increased to higher than the recommended dietary allowance in single pregnancy (1200 mg/day) to meet maternal needs in pregnancies that require prolonged magnesium sulfate tocolysis and continuous bed rest;
- because women are not exposed to sunlight during tocolysis, vitamin D 400 IU/day, should be given;
- in severe cases, antiresorptive drugs given postpartum may help in restoring bone mineral density, but controlled trials are needed to confirm this.

Management of adverse drug reactions The effect of nifedipine on magnesium-induced adverse effects has been studied in a retrospective chart review of 377 women who were given intravenous magnesium sulfate for pre-eclampsia 162 received magnesium sulfate and contemporaneous nifedipine and 215 controls received magnesium sulfate and either another antihypertensive ($n = 32$) or no antihypertensive ($n = 183$) (39[c]). The cases had more severe pre-eclampsia and a longer infusion of magnesium sulfate. However, they had no excess of neuromuscular weakness (53%) compared with controls who received antihypertensive medication (53%), or controls who received no antihypertensive medication (45); nor were there other serious magnesium-related effects. Those who received magnesium had less neuromuscular blockade than controls who received antihypertensive medication (OR = 0.04; 95%

CI = 0.002, 0.80) and less maternal hypotension than those who received no antihypertensive medication (41 versus 53%). The authors concluded that nifedipine does not alter the risk of serious magnesium-related effects.

Manganese   *(SED-15, 2200; SEDA-27, 229; SEDA-28, 248; SEDA-29, 230)*

Manganese compounds are used as mineral supplements and as contrast agents in radiodiagnostics.

Nervous system *Parkinsonism* has been reported in a patient taking manganese-containing supplements (40[A]).

- A 62-year-old Japanese man, who had been managed on maintenance hemodialysis therapy for chronic renal insufficiency caused by diabetic nephropathy, developed progressive worsening of gait, dysarthria, slowing of actions, and impaired handwriting. He had a mask-like face, flexed posture, minimal cogwheel rigidity, tremor of the hands, and disturbance of fine finger movements. He walked with short steps. His handwriting was micrographic. An MRI scan of the brain showed symmetrical abnormalities in the bilateral basal ganglia, with low-intensity areas on T1-weighted images and high-intensity areas on T2-weighted images and flair images. The serum manganese concentration was 8 μg/l, and the CSF concentration 2 μg/l. The serum manganese concentration in hemodialysis is generally reported to be low (mean 2 μg/l) compared with that in the healthy population (6.1 μg/l). Although the reference range for the manganese concentration in the CSF has not been reported in patients on hemodialysis, the CSF concentration in this patient was high compared with that in healthy subjects (0.88 μg/l) and patients with Parkinson disease (1.20 μg/l). A 4-hour hemodialysis session did not change his serum manganese concentration, and the manganese concentration in the dialysate was below the limit of detection. He had been taking several health supplements for as long as 4 years, including *Chlorella* extract (12 g/day), taro extract (2.5 g/day), and *Umbelliferae* powder (4 g/day). His daily intake of manganese was calculated from the listed content to be 0.02 mg for taro extract and 0.5 mg for *Umbelliferae* powder. The *Chlorella* extract contained manganese 139 μg/g of, a daily oral intake of 1.7 mg. Thus, his total daily manganese intake was 2.22 mg. The supplements were withdrawn and he was given levodopa, without improvement. EDTA also was tried intravenously, 1 g bd for 10 days; the manganese concentration in the CSF increased six-fold and 2 weeks later an MRI scan showed dramatic improvement. During the next 4 months his symptoms gradually improved, and his gait, handwriting, speech, and rigidity became almost normal.

Although a definitive diagnosis of manganese-induced parkinsonism can be made only by confirmation of manganese accumulation in the brain, the diagnosis was presumed in this patient from his symptoms, high serum and CSF manganese concentrations, and bilateral MRI scan abnormalities in the basal ganglia.

Mercury and mercurial salts

(SED-15, 2259; SEDA-27, 229; SEDA-28, 248; SEDA-29, 230)

The adverse effects of mercury-containing dental amalgams continue to be debated (41[R]). Mercury is also commonly found in herbal medicines of Asian origin (14[R]).

The use of thiomersal (an ethylmercury preservative) in vaccines still gives reason for concern (42[R]) especially its purported role in *autism* (43[R]). Several affluent countries are moving to eliminate it from vaccines as a precautionary measure. However, the WHO has advocated continued use of thiomersal-containing vaccines in developing countries because of their effectiveness, safety, low cost, wide availability, and logistical suitability in such countries.

In a major review of the risk of adverse effects of vaccines that contain thiomersal, the authors supported the WHO position, concluding that the benefit to harm balance is favorable, and that these vaccines should continue to be used, especially in developing countries, until thiomersal-free substitutes become practical and affordable (44[R]).

Gastrointestinal   The use of heavy metals, such as mercury, in folk remedies to treat abdominal pain is relatively common in certain Hispanic communities (45[A]).

- A 4-month-old Mexican–American boy with a 4-week history of abdominal colic developed a fever and irritability. There was tenderness over McBurney's point, and a plain abdominal X-ray showed a metallic density in the right lower quadrant, presumably within the appendix. The child had received elemental mercury for abdominal pain for 4–6 weeks. The blood mercury concentration was 31 µg/l. Positional maneuvers and whole bowel irrigation with polyethylene glycol were unsuccessfully used in an attempt to empty the mercury from the appendix. Persistent fever and irritability eventually necessitated appendicectomy.

Immunologic   A generalized reaction to thiomersal in an influenza vaccine has been reported (46[A]).

- A 39-year-old white woman developed pruritus and a rash on all four limbs 8 hours after influenza immunization in the right deltoid muscle. She initially had pruritus on the right arm, which spread to the left arm, both legs, and the upper chest. She had received influenza vaccine each year for the past 6 years without adverse effects. However, she had had a rash on her eyelids 10 years before from a thiomersal-containing contact lens solution. She had an erythematous, maculopapular eruption on all four limbs and the torso. The rash spread to her buttocks and persisted for 2 weeks, after which she was given a 5-day course of oral prednisone and an antihistamine. The rash resolved after 4 days. Patch testing 4 weeks later was positive only with thiomersal.

Nickel   *(SED-15, 2502; SEDA-27, 229; SEDA-28, 249; SEDA-29, 230)*

Skin   Of 250 Iranian patients with a diagnosis of contact dermatitis and/or atopic dermatitis 126 (50%) had at least one positive patch test reaction and 23 (9.2%) had more than two positive reactions (47[c]). The five most common allergens were nickel sulfate 70 (28%), cobalt chloride 32 (13%), para-tertiarybutyl phenol formaldehyde resin 20 (8.0%), potassium dichromate 13 (5.2%), and colophony 13 (5.2%). Contact allergy to nickel sulfate was significantly more common in women and in patients under 40 years of age, probably because of more exposure.

Immunologic   *Pericarditis* has been attributed to hypersensitivity to the nickel in an Amplatzer occluder device, which contains nitinol, an alloy that is composed of 55% nickel and 45% titanium (48[A]).

- A 38-year-old man with a history of migraine had an ischemic stroke, which was attributed to paradoxical embolism through a patent foramen ovale. A 35 mm Amplatzer patent foramen ovale occluder device was inserted percutaneously without complications. Several days later he complained of intermittent episodes of substernal chest pressure and tingling in the left arm. The pain progressed to severe left scapular discomfort, exacerbated by inspiration and movement. His migraines became more frequent and he had more visual auras without headache. CT angiography showed a small pericardial effusion. He was given prednisone 40 mg/day for pericarditis. Allergy patch testing showed a positive reaction to nickel, consistent with a type IV hypersensitivity reaction.

Contact dermatitis has been attributed to nickel in a peripheral intravenous catheter (49[A]). The catheter (OPTIVA, Medex, Johnson and Johnson Medical and Vascular Access) was made of polyurethane and was latex free, but the eyelet was made of brass (30%) and nickel plated (70%).

- A 37-year-old woman had several recurrent episodes of itchy macular exanthems each time she had an infusion of glucose for several hours. She had a history of allergic contact dermatitis to nickel, confirmed by a highly positive patch test to nickel sulfate. She was given a glucose infusion for 4 hours under medical supervision thorugh a peripheral intravenous catheter, OPTIVA 20G with OCRILON polyurethane (Medex, Johnson & Johnson Medical and Vascular Access, Arlington, TX, USA). One hour later she developed an itchy, macular, slightly swollen rash, predominantly in the flexural folds, which abated after 2 days of loratidine therapy. There was no reaction at the infusion site on the forearm.
- A 33-year-old woman had recurrent episodes of an itchy rash, which appeared 10 hours after three surgical operations for a malignant pulmonary tumour and ovarian metastases and after an injection of an iodine-containing contrast medium for a chest scan. The rash consisted of dark-red maculopapular lesions predominantly localized in the periumbilical area and in the folds, with no lesions at the infusion site on the forearm. After an infusion via a central venous polyurethane catheterization set (Arrow, Arrow International, Reading, PA, USA) instead of a peripheral catheter there was no recurrence. She had a past history of severe allergic contact dermatitis to nickel, confirmed by highly positive patch tests to nickel sulfate.

Selenium   *(SED-15, 3119; SEDA-27, 230; SEDA-28, 250; SEDA-29, 231)*

Selenium compounds are being increasingly used in cancer prevention (50[R], 51[R]). Attention has been focussed on the speciation of human selenium compounds (52[R]). No new adverse effects of selenium have been reported.

Silver salts and derivatives
(SED-15, 3140; SEDA-27, 230; SEDA-28, 250; SEDA-29, 231)

Silver-based compounds continue to be used as antimicrobial agents in wound healing (53[R], 54[R]). The general view is that silver can be a useful tool in treating infected wounds, but that its effectiveness depends on the form of silver used. Silver-alloy coated catheters reduce catheter-associated urinary tract infections (55[R]).

Urinary tract   Prolonged topical application of silver sulphadiazine cream was associated with *acute renal insufficiency* (56[A]).

- A 61-year-old woman with rheumatoid arthritis, Sjögren's syndrome, and scleroderma was given prednisone 1 mg/kg/day and topical silver sulfadiazine cream 200 g/day for extensive pyoderma gangrenosum on the legs. After 3 weeks she developed pulmonary edema, oliguria, and altered consciousness. She had a leukopenia (1.1×10^9/l), renal insufficiency (serum creatinine 316 μmol/l), and moderate proteinuria; ultrasonography of the kidneys was normal. The blood silver concentration was 1818 nmol/l (reference range <92 nmol/l) and the urine concentration was 1381 nmol/l (reference range <9 nmol/l). Sulfadiazine was undetectable in the blood. All the signs abated after withdrawal of silver sulfadiazine and several sessions of hemodialysis.

Silver-induced renal toxicity was most likely in this case, and this was supported by the high concentrations of silver in blood and urine and the improvement on withdrawal of the topical cream, without change in oral treatment. The absence of erythrocytes and crystals in the urine and the absence of sulfadiazine in the blood did not support sulphonamide-induced renal toxicity.

Skin   Cases of *argyria* continue to be reported with existing allopathic silver-based medicines and especially with colloidal silver solutions that are recommended in various types of complementary and alternative medicine (57[A]).

- A 58-year-old white man treated a presumed kidney infection with a home-made colloidal silver solution. He had brewed the colloidal silver solution using a 38 000-V generator, 100% pure silver coins, and distilled water. He had drunk 8 oz of this solution every hour from 0800 to 2000 h for 4 days. About 4 weeks later he noticed a bluish staining of the oral mucosa with progressive involvement of his face, trunk, and limbs. He had striking, diffuse blue-gray discoloration of the skin, most prominent on the sun-exposed areas of his forearms, hands, face, neck, and V of the chest. The lunulae, sclerae, and conjunctiva were also involved. There were spotty blue-gray macules on the oral mucosa of the soft palate. Histological examination of a punch biopsy from the forearm showed fine, minute, round, brown-black granules deposited primarily in the basement membrane of the eccrine glands. The particles were also found to a lesser extent in the fibrous sheath around the pilosebaceous units, erector pili muscles, arteriolar walls, and dermal elastic fibers.

Titanium   *(SED-15, 3434; SEDA-27, 230; SEDA-28, 250; SEDA-29, 231)*

Titanium is widely used in medical and dental implant materials (58[R]). Nickel–titanium alloys are often used and allergic reactions are often related to the nickel and not the titanium (59[E]).

Zinc   *(SED-15, 3717; SEDA-27, 230; SEDA-28, 251; SEDA-29, 232)*

Metal metabolism   Zinc supplementation can cause *acquired copper deficiency* and incidentally lead to both hematological symptoms and neuromuscular symptoms (60[A]).

• A 53-year-old woman developed a mild motor and sensory polyneuropathy, including some demyelinating features, with altered gait and spasticity of the legs. Her white blood cell count was $2.6 \times 10^9/l$. The serum copper concentration was markedly low at 70 µg/l (reference range 70–155), as was the serum ceruloplasmin concentration (21 mg/l; reference range 229–431). Serum zinc was raised at 2.28 mg/l (reference range 0.66–1.10). She had taken zinc capsules for a year or more for sinusitis, each containing 50 mg of elemental zinc in the form of zinc gluconate. The recommended dose was 15 mg/day, but she had taken 4–8 capsules daily and would increase the dose according to the severity of her symptoms, taking up to 400 mg/day. The zinc was withdrawn. She received one dose of intravenous copper chloride and oral copper sulfate supplementation (2.0 mg/day elemental copper). A bone marrow biopsy 12 days later was normocellular. Her copper concentration, white blood cell count, and mean corpuscular volume normalized after 3 months of treatment. There was significant but incomplete improvement in her gait and spasticity at 6 months. There was also some improvement in her nerve conduction studies.

Acknowledgement

This manuscript has been reviewed in accordance with the policy of the US Armed Forces Institute of Pathology and the Department of Defense, and approved for publication. Approval does not signify that the contents necessarily reflect the views and policies of the Department of the Army or the Department of Defense, nor does the mention of trade names or commercial products constitute endorsement or recommendation for use.

References

1. Schucker JJ, Ward KE. Hyperphosphatemia and phosphate binders. Am J Health System Pharm 2005;62:2355–61.

2. Canavese C, Mereu C, Nordio M, Sabbioni E, Aime S. Blast from the past: the aluminum's ghost on the lanthanum salts. Curr Med Chem 2005;12:1631–6.

3. Siegrist CA. Vaccine adjuvants and macrophagic myofasciitis. Arch Pediatr 2005;12:96–101.

4. Shingde M, Hughes J, Boadle R, Wills EJ, Pamphlett R. Macrophagic myofasciitis associated with vaccine-derived aluminium. Med J Aust 2005;183:145–6.

5. Grau MV, Baron JA, Barry EL, Sandler RS, Haile RW, Mandel JS, Cole BF. Nineteen cases of persistent pruritic nodules and contact allergy to aluminium after injection of commonly used aluminium-absorbed vaccines. Eur J Pediatr 2005;164:2353–8.

6. Fenwick S, Roberts EA, Mahesh BS, Roberts NB. In end-stage renal failure, does infection lead to elevated plasma aluminium and

neurotoxicity? Implications for monitoring. Ann Clin Biochem 2005;42(Pt 2):149–52.

7. Murray HW, Berman JD, Davies CR, Saravia NG. Advances in leishmaniasis. Lancet 2005;366:1561–77.

8. Berman J. Clinical status of agents being developed for leishmaniasis. Expert Opin Investig Drugs 2005;14:1337–46.

9. Baranwal AK, Mandal RN, Singh R, Singhi SC. Sodium stibogluconate and polymorphic ventricular tachycardia. Indian J Pediatr 2005;72:269–71.

10. Gazzitt Y, Akay C. Arsenic trioxide: an anticancer missile with multiple warheads. Hematology 2005;10:205–13.

11. Hu J, Fang J, Dong Y, Chen SJ, Chen Z. Arsenic in cancer therapy. Anticancer Drugs 2005;16:119–27.

12. Amadori S, Fenaux P, Ludwig H, O'Dwyer M, Sanz M. Use of arsenic trioxide in haematological malignancies: insight into the clinical development of a novel agent. Curr Med Res Opin 2005;21:403–11.

13. Douer D, Tallman MS. Arsenic trioxide: new clinical experience with an old medication in hematologic malignancies. J Clin Oncol 2005;23:2396–410.

14. Lynch E, Braithwaite R. A review of the clinical and toxicological aspects of "traditional" (herbal) medicines adulterated with heavy metals. Expert Opin Drug Saf 2005;4:769–78.

15. Hassaballa HA, Lateef OB, Silver MR, Balk RA. Acute lung injury induced by arsenic trioxide in a patient with refractory myelodysplastic syndrome. J Crit Care 2005;20:111–3.

16. Arai A, Kitano A, Kurosu T, Yamamoto K, Miki T, Murakami N, Miura O. Fluid retention during arsenic trioxide treatment in acute promyelocytic leukemia. Am J Hematol 2005;79:247–8.

17. McLoughlin RM, O'Morain CA, O'Connor HJ. Eradication of *Helicobacter pylori*: recent advances in treatment. Fundam Clin Pharmacol 2005;19:421–7.

18. Anonymous. Bismacine. Warning against use. WHO Newslett 2006;5:3.

19. Cengiz N, Uslu Y, Gok F, Anarat A. Acute renal failure after overdose of colloidal bismuth subcitrate. Pediatr Nephrol 2005;20:1355–8.

20. Guerrero-Romero F, Rodriguez-Moran M. Complementary therapies for diabetes: the case for chromium, magnesium, and antioxidants. Arch Med Res 2005;36:250–7.

21. McCarty MF. Nutraceutical resources for diabetes prevention—an update. Med Hypotheses 2005;64:151–8.

22. Vrtovec M, Vrtovec B, Briski A, Kocijancic A, Anderson RA, Radovancevic B. Chromium supplementation shortens QTc interval duration in patients with type 2 diabetes mellitus. Am Heart J 2005;149:632–6.

23. Della Valle AG, Becksac B, Anderson J, Wright T, Nestor B, Pellici PM. Late fatigue fracture of a modern cemented forged cobalt chrome stem for total hip arthroplasty: a report of 10 cases. J Arthroplasty 2005;20:1084–8.

24. Kitzberger R, Madl C, Ferenci O. Wilson disease. Metab Brain Dis 2005;20:295–302.

25. Cerpa W, Vareia-Nallar L, Reyes AE, Minniti AN, Inestrosa NC. Is there a role for copper in neurodegenerative diseases? Mol Aspects Med 2005;26:405–20.

26. Maecke HR, Hofmann M, Haberkorn U. (68)Ga-labeled peptides in tumor imaging. J Nucl Med 2005;46(Suppl 1):172S–8S.

27. Rau R. Have traditional DMARDs had their day? Effectiveness of parenteral gold compared to biologic agents. Clin Rheumatol 2005;24:189–202.

28. Nedorost S, Wagman A. Positive patch-test reactions to gold: patients' perception of relevance and the role of titanium dioxide in cosmetics. Dermatitis 2005;16(2):67–70.

29. van Roon EN, van de Laar MA, Janssen M, Kruijsen MW, Jansen TL, Brouwers JR. Parenteral gold preparations. Efficacy and safety of therapy after switching from aurothioglucose to aurothiomalate. J Rheumatol 2005;32:1026–30.

30. Umbreit J. Iron deficiency: a concise review. Am J Hematol 2005;78:225–31.

31. Chertow GM, Mason PD, Vaage-Nilsen O, Ahlmen J. Update on adverse drug events associated with parenteral iron. Nephrol Dial Transplant 2006;21:378–82.

32. Bailie GR, Clark CA, Lane CE, Lane PL. Hypersensitivity reactions and death associated with intravenous iron preparations. Nephrol Dial Transplant 2005;30:1443–9.

33. Saadeh CE, Srkalovic G. Acute hypersensitivity reaction to ferric gluconate in a premedicated patient. Ann Pharmacother 2005;39:2124–7.

34. Cuciti C, Mayer DC, Arnette R, Spielman FJ. Anaphylactoid reaction to intravenous sodium ferric gluconate complex during pregnancy. Int J Obstet Anesth 2005;14:362–4.

35. Lewis DF. Magnesium sulfate: the first-line tocolytic. Obstet Gynecol Clin North Am 2005;32:485–500.

36. Samol JM, Lambers DS. Magnesium sulfate tocolysis and pulmonary edema: the drug or the vehicle? Am J Obstet Gynecol 2005;192:1430–2.

37. Mehta R, Petrova A. Intrapartum magnesium sulfate exposure attenuates neutrophil function in preterm neonates. Biol Neonate 2006;89:99–103.

38. Hung JW, Tsai MY, Yang BY, Chen JF. Maternal osteoporosis after prolonged magnesium sulfate tocolysis therapy: a case report. Arch Phys Med Rehabil 2005;86:146–9.

39. Magee LA, Miremadi S, Li J, Cheng C, Ensom MH, Carleton B, Côté AM, von Dadelszen P. Therapy with both magnesium sulfate and nifedipine does not increase the risk of serious magnesium-related maternal side effects in women with preeclampsia. Am J Obstet Gynecol 2005;193:153–63.

40. Ohtake T, Negishi K, Okamoto K, Oka M, Maesato K, Moriya H, Kobayashi S. Manganese-induced Parkinsonism in a patient undergoing maintenance hemodialysis. Am J Kidney Dis 2005;46:749–53.

41. Brownawell AM, Berent S, Brent RL, Bruckner JV, Doull J, Gerschwin EM, Hood RD, Matanoski GM, Rubin R, Weiss B, Karol MH. The potential adverse health effects of dental amalgam. Toxicol Rev 2005;24:1–10.

42. Bigham M, Copes R. Thiomersal in vaccines: balancing the risk of adverse effects with the risk of vaccine-preventable disease. Drug Saf 2005;28:89–101.

43. Parker S, Todd J, Schwartz B, Pickering L. Thimerosal-containing vaccines and autistic spectrum disorder: a critical review of published original data. Pediatrics 2005;115:200.

44. Bigham M, Copes R. Thiomersal in vaccines: balancing the risk of adverse effects with the risk of vaccine-preventable disease. Drug Saf 2005;28:89–101.

45. Miller MA, Coon TP, Greethong J, Levy P. Medicinal mercury presents as appendicitis. J Emerg Med 2005;28:217.

46. Lee-Wong M, Resnick D, Chong K. A generalized reaction to thimerosal from an influenza vaccine. Ann Allergy Asthma Immunol 2005;94:90–4.

47. Kashani MN, Gorouhi F, Behnia F, Nazemi MJ, Dowlati Y, Firooz A. Allergic contact dermatitis in Iran. Contact Dermatitis 2005;52(3):154–8.

48. Lai DW, Saver JL, Araujo JA, Reidi M, Tobis J. Pericarditis associated with nickel hypersensitivity to the Amplatzer occluder device: a case report. Catheter Cardiovasc Interv 2005;66:424–6.

49. Raison-Peyron N, Guillard O, Khalil Z, Guilhou JJ, Guillot B. Nickel-elicited systemic contact dermatitis from a peripheral intravenous catheter. Contact Dermatitis 2005;53:222–5.

50. Abdulah R, Myazaki K, Nakazawa M, Koyama H. Chemical forms of selenium for cancer prevention. J Trace Elem Med Biol 2005;19:141–50.

51. Rayman MP. Selenium in cancer prevention: a review of the evidence and mechanism of action. Proc Nutr Soc 2005;64:527–42.

52. Gromer S, Eubel JK, Lee BL, Jacob J. Human selenoproteins at a glance. Cell Mol Life Sci 2005;62:2414–37.

53. Graham C. The role of silver in wound healing. Br J Nurs 2005;14:S22, S24, S26.

54. Lansdown AB. A guide to the properties and uses of silver dressings in wound care. Prof Nurse 2005;20:41–3.

55. Davenport K, Keeley FX. Evidence for the use of silver-alloy urethral catheters. J Hosp Infect 2005;60:298–303.

56. Chaby G, Viseaux V, Poulain JF, De Cagny B, Denoeux JP, Lok C. Topical silver sulfadiazine-induced acute renal failure. Ann Dermatol Venereol 2005;132:891–3.

57. Brandt D, Park B, Hoang M, Jacobe HT. Argyria secondary to ingestion of homemade silver solution. J Am Acad Dermatol 2005;53:S105–7.

58. Tchernitschek H, Borchers L, Geurtsen W. Non-alloyed titanium as bioinert metal—a review. Quintessence Int 2005;36:523–30.

59. Schuh A, Thomas P, Kachler W, Goske J, Wagner L, Holzwath U, Forst R. Allergic potential of titanium implants. Orthopäde 2005;34:327–8, 330–3.

60. Rowin J, Lewis SL. Copper deficiency myeloneuropathy and pancytopenia secondary to overuse of zinc supplementation. J Neurol Neurosurg Psychiatry 2005;76:750–1.

R.H.B. Meyboom

23   Metal antagonists

The chelating agents dimercaprol (British Anti-Lewisite, BAL), succimer (meso-DMSA), unithiol (DMPS), D-penicillamine, N-acetyl-D-penicillamine, calcium disodium ethylenediaminetetraacetate, calcium trisodium or zinc trisodium diethylenetriaminepentaacetate, deferoxamine, deferiprone (L1), triethylenetetraamine (trientine), N-acetylcysteine, and Prussian blue have been reviewed (1[R]).

Although the pathogenesis of Alzheimer's disease is largely unknown, since the concentrations of metals such as iron, aluminium, zinc, and copper are increased or dysregulated in the brain tissues of these patients, metal-mediated oxidative injury is likely to play a role and chelators may become a future treatment (2[R]). Recently, a novel approach to chelation therapy has been proposed, using nanoparticles (3[R]). Nanoparticles made of natural or artificial polymers, ranging in size from about 10 to 1000 nm, conjugated to chelators, can cross the blood-brain barrier, locally chelate metals, and be subsequently excreted from the brain together with the complexed metal.

IRON CHELATORS

Deferasirox   (SEDA-29, 236)

Deferasirox (ICL670), a hydroxyphenyltriazole derivative, is a tridentate selective iron chelator, two molecules of which form a stable complex with each iron atom. Animal studies have suggested that the kidney is a potential target for adverse effects, but there is as yet no evidence of progressive renal damage. It also produces

a dose dependent *increase in β_2 microglobulin*, typically transient, the clinical relevance of which is uncertain (4[r]). With limited experience, the adverse events that have so far been recorded include *headache, nausea*, and *diarrhea* (5[r]).

Deferiprone   (SED-15, 1054; SEDA-27, 233; SEDA-28, 256; SEDA-29, 237)

In her book *The drug trial*, Miriam Shuchman exposed the complex relationships between medical researchers, pharmaceutical companies, fellow scientists, doctors, and patients, and the dramatic conflicts that can occur when doubts arise about the efficacy or safety of a drug, the drug in question being deferiprone (6[R]). Hoffbrand has reviewed this major controversy, taking into account the perspective of the patients' therapeutic need for the drug (7[R]).

A major aim of iron chelation is to keep body iron stores sufficiently low to prevent accumulation of iron in the tissues, in particular in the heart and endocrine organs. A reasonable estimate is that iron concentrations should at any time be less than 7 mg/g dry tissue weight, but is not certain what the critical threshold is (4[r]). Deferiprone has a relatively short half-life (1.5 hours), necessitating thrice-daily dosing. At doses of 75 mg/kg/day deferiprone reduces serum ferritin concentrations when they are above 3000 µg/l; however, in patients with thalassemia and ferritin concentrations below 2500 µg/l, there is no significant change. Tissue concentrations are less affected, and in about half of the patients the iron concentrations in the liver and heart remain above the threshold for toxicity.

Observational studies In 44 children under 6 years of age with thalassemia major taking deferiprone 75 mg/kg/day and not receiving

Side Effects of Drugs, Annual 30
J.K. Aronson (Editor)
ISSN: 0378-6080
DOI: 10.1016/S0378-6080(08)00023-8

deferoxamine, deferiprone was withdrawn in 10 patients (13 episodes), usually about 10 months after the start of treatment, because of *thrombocytopenia* or *arthralgia*, and was permanently withdrawn in two (8[CR]). In 23 patients there was a red-brown discoloration of the urine from the first week of treatment. There were no other urinary complaints. Four patients had *arthralgia* of the knees and in one also of the ankles; there was no swelling; the time to onset ranged from 21 days to 1 year. Deferiprone was interrupted and restarted in all four; two patients relapsed. In one patient permanent dosage reduction was needed (only 28% of the original dose). As many as 20 patients had one or more episodes of *thrombocytopenia*, with platelet counts of $50-150 \times 10^9$/l; there were no episodes of bleeding. The onset of thrombocytopenia ranged from 3 months to 1 year. There were 26 episodes of thrombocytopenia below 100×10^9/l, requiring withdrawal of deferiprone, in two cases permanently. Two of the 44 patients had *neutropenia* with white cell counts of $0.5-1.5 \times 10^6$/l; there were no cases of *agranulocytosis*.

Since deferiprone 75 mg/kg/day is not always sufficient, a dosage of 100 mg/kg/day has been studied for over 2 years in 12 patients with thalassemia major aged 15–36 years (9[CR]). There were transient *rises in serum aspartate transaminase activity* in eight patients, three had *gastrointestinal discomfort*, and two had *arthralgia*. In 9 of the 12 patients, iron concentrations after 2 years were less than 15 mg/g dry weight (a concentration that has been seen in patients taking deferoxamine without signs of cardiac damage). There was a poor correlation between the serum ferritin concentrations and liver iron, as has been found in previous studies.

In 15 patients taking deferiprone for iron chelation in sickle cell anemia three withdrew from the study, one because of adverse effects (*nausea, vomiting,* and *fatigue*); possible adverse effects in the other 12 patients were not mentioned (10[cR]).

Deferoxamine   *(SED-15, 1058; SEDA-27, 233; SEDA-28, 256; SEDA-29, 237)*

Pregnancy   The hemodynamic changes that take place during pregnancy demand increased

cardiac performance. If the heart is compromised, as can happen in hemochromatosis, forward failure can occur.

• A 30-year-old Greek woman with β-thalassemia had serious heart failure during pregnancy (11[Cr]). Deferoxamine had been withdrawn when pregnancy was diagnosed, when the serum hemoglobin was above 10 mg/dl. However, in the 22nd week of gestation, dilated cardiomyopathy required intravenous deferoxamine 50 mg/kg/day on 5 days a week, and she was also given furosemide, potassium, and digoxin. Her cardiac function improved and at 31 weeks a healthy child (2080 g) was born, without malformations.

PENICILLAMINE AND RELATED DRUGS

Penicillamine   *(SED-15, 2729; SEDA-27, 235; SEDA-28, 257; SEDA-29, 238)*

The decreasing interest in penicillamine for the treatment of rheumatoid arthritis has been illustrated in recent reviews, in which little or no reference is made to penicillamine as a DMARD (12[R], 13[R]). Nor does it have a place in the management of pulmonary fibrosis (14[R]) or biliary cirrhosis (15[R]). On the other hand, in the treatment of Wilson's disease and various forms of acute and chronic metal poisoning, penicillamine is still being used.

Observational studies   Long-term follow-up data in 88 children with Wilson's disease, including 43 taking penicillamine, have been reported (16[cr]). The drug was withdrawn in seven cases because of adverse effects: *bone marrow suppression* in three, *hematuria* in two, a *rash* in one, and *hemolytic anemia* in one. *Hemolytic anemia* is a poorly documented adverse effect of penicillamine and it is unfortunate that in this case no details were given. In three more children with adverse effects the drug was continued; two had a *rash* and one *drowsiness*.

Hematologic   Of 29 Indian patients with severe Wilson's disease, all using penicillamine (full dose 750 mg/day) who were followed for 2 years to evaluate prognostic factors, 14 had progressive deterioration (group A) and 15 consistent improvement (group B) (17[CR]). In 13 patients (8 in group A and 5 in group B) penicillamine was withdrawn on 26 occasions. In two patients penicillamine was permanently withdrawn because of persistent hematological adverse effects (not specified). In the remainder the drug was temporarily withdrawn for a variety of reasons, notably *hematological events* and *paradoxical worsening of the symptoms of Wilson's disease*, but also financial constraints or poor understanding of the need for regular life-long use. When the full dose of penicillamine was given initially, there was paradoxical worsening in four patients (three in group A, one in group B). Two patients in group A died during the study, both of septicemia (organism not specified).

- A 35-year-old woman with Wilson's disease had to stop taking penicillamine (250 mg/day) after 3 weeks because of leukopenia and fever (18[A]).

Skin   *Pemphigus foliaceus* has again been attributed to penicillamine (19[CR]).

- A Japanese patient with systemic sclerosis developed pemphigus foliaceus while taking penicillamine (dose not specified) and prednisolone. A direct immunofluorescence test showed intercellular space deposits of IgG, and the ELISA index to anti-desmoglein 1 antibodies was raised to 115 (reference range <20). Withdrawal of penicillamine resulted in improvement of the skin lesions and a remarkably rapid fall in the titer of Dsg 1 antibodies, suggesting that the production of these antibodies required constant exposure to the drug.

The typical high-dose degenerative dermatosis associated with penicillamine, which is characterized by *elastosis perforans serpiginosa* and *pseudo-pseudoxanthoma elasticum*, has been described in three more patients (20[CR], 21[CR]). The long delay before proper management of the disorder illustrates a lack of awareness of the possible effects on the skin of the long-term treatment with penicillamine.

- A 25-year-old woman who had taken penicillamine (dose unspecified) for Wilson's disease for 14 years and developed pseudoxanthoma elasticum-like lesions (20[CR]). There was hyperkeratotic reddish brown papules in a semicircle of about 5 cm around a central area of atrophic skin in the in the neck and yellow "plucked chicken" lesions in the neck and axillae. A biopsy showed elastosis perforans serpiginosa, with focal acanthosis, parakeratosis, and transepidermal elimination

of elastotic material in the epidermis. The dermis contained thickened elastic fibers with small lateral projections with a toothbrush-like aspect, surrounded by a granulomatous infiltrate with giant cells, some engulfing elastic fibers. Ultrastructural histology showed altered elastic fibers with an electron-lucent core and branching protrusions, and collagen fibres with uneven calibres and sometimes fragmentation. Topical glucocorticoids and tretinoin were ineffective, and penicillamine was replaced by zinc, after which a few new smaller lesions developed for up to 3 months.

- A 25-year-old woman with Wilson's disease, who had taken penicillamine 1.2 g/day for 16 years, developed an asymptomatic plaque in the neck, with red keratotic papules suggestive of elastosis perforans serpiginosa (20[CR]). A biopsy showed increased amounts of enlarged and fragmented elastic fibers in the upper reticular dermis and a mild polymorphous infiltrate with lymphocytes, histiocytes, and neutrophils. Ultrastructural examination showed elastic fibers with abnormal electron-lucent cores and angular branches with lateral budding. Penicillamine was replaced by zinc, but no outcome information was given.

- A 10-year-old girl started taking penicillamine 1 g daily for Wilson's disease (21[CR]). After about 20 years she developed skin laxity in the axillae, groins, and abdomen, multiple yellowish 2–3 mm papules with a "plucked skin" appearance in her neck, and denuded nodules in the perianal area. A biopsy showed transepidermal elimination of thickened elastic fibers with prominent lateral protrusions and the typical "lumpy-bumpy" or "bramble bush" appearance. No follow-up information was given.

POLYSTYRENE SULFONATES
(SED-15, 2894; SEDA-27, 236; SEDA-28, 259; SEDA-29, 239)

Respiratory   *Pneumonitis* due to aspiration of sodium polystyrene sulfonate has been reported (22[A]).

- A 63-year-old woman with hyperkalemia (6.2 mmol/l) was given sodium polystyrene sulfonate (Kayexalate) but became unresponsive the morning after admission and died. Postmortem examination showed changes of pneumonitis attributed to aspiration of Kayexalate, particles of which were found in the alveoli.

This adverse effect has rarely been reported before (23[A], 24[A]). It is a definitive ("between-the-eyes") anecdotal adverse effect of type 1, in which there is tissue deposition of the drug or a metabolite (25[HR]), since when it is seen in the alveoli sodium polystyrene sulfonate has a characteristic microscopic appearance that is virtually diagnostic. However, the authors suggested that an innocent bystander effect was possible, since the pneumonitis could have been due to aspirated gastric acid.

Drug abuse   *Electrolyte abnormalities* have been reported in a patient who abused sodium polystyrene sulfonate (26[A]).

- A 65-year-old Chinese woman developed progressive peripheral edema, uncontrolled hypertension, muscle weakness, tetany, and weight gain of 5 kg over 3 weeks. She had a history of hypertension, treated with nifedipine 10 mg tds and atenolol 100 mg/day, and chronic renal insufficiency due to diabetic nephropathy. She had previously been given sodium polystyrene sulfonate (Kayexalate®) for hyperkalemia, but stopped taking it because it was unpalatable. She denied vomiting and diarrhea or recent use of laxatives, diuretics, or herbal medicines. She weighed 62.5 kg, her blood pressure was 180/110 mmHg, and she had a grade II/VI cardiac systolic murmur and grade III pitting edema of both legs. Her hemoglobin was 7.9 g/dl, she had hypokalemia (2.6 mmol/l), hypomagnesemia (0.49 mmol/l), hypocalcemia (ionized Ca^{++} 0.90 mmol/l), and mild hypernatremia (146 mmol/l). There was a mild respiratory and metabolic alkalosis. A chest X-ray showed moderate cardiomegaly with pulmonary congestion. Electrocardiography showed T wave flattening and left ventricular hypertrophy. Investigations suggested an extra-renal cause for the hypokalemia and she admitted to having taken sodium polystyrene sulfonate (Resonium-A®) 15 g qds for the past 3 weeks because she was trying to avoid another episode of hyperkalemia. Sodium polystyrene sulfonate was withdrawn, water and dietary sodium restriction were implemented, and she was given amlodipine 5 mg/day, ramipril

2.5 mg/day, and intravenous supplements of potassium (KCl 60 mmol/day), magnesium (MgSO$_4$ 16 mmol/day), and calcium (CaCl$_2$ 9 mmol/day). Her body weight and blood pressure fell.

The authors calculated that this patient had taken 1200 g of sodium polystyrene sulfonate, equivalent to 4800 mmol of sodium.

OTHER CHELATORS

DP-b99

DP-b99 is a newly developed lipophilic cell-permeable derivative of BAPTA (biaminoethane tetra-acetic acid), which selectively modulates the distribution of metal ions in a hydrophobic environment and has a high affinity for calcium, zinc, and copper ions. It is being tested as a neuroprotectant in ischemic stroke. After intravenous administration *phlebitis* of varying severity is common and more so in younger patients (27[cr]).

Ethylene diamine tetra-acetic acid (EDTA)   *(SED-15, 000; SEDA-27, 234)*

In a review of complementary therapies in the treatment of peripheral arterial disease, it was again emphasized that there is insufficient evidence to determine the effectiveness of intravenous chelation therapy with EDTA, while adverse reactions can occur (28[R]).

References

1. Blanusa M, Varnai VM, Piasek M, Kostial K. Chelators as antidotes of metal toxicity: therapeutic and experimental aspects. Curr Med Chem 2005;12(23):2771–94.

2. Gaeta A, Hider RC. The crucial role of metal ions in neurodegeneration: the basis for a promising therapeutic strategy. Br J Pharmacol 2005;146:1041–59.

3. Liu G, Garrett MR, Men P, Zhu X, Perry G, Smith MA. Nanoparticle and other metal chelation therapeutics in Alzheimer disease. Biochim Biophys Acta 2005;1741:246–52.

4. Porter JB. Monitoring and treatment of iron overload: state of the art and new approaches. Semin Hematol 2005;42(Suppl 1):S14–8.

5. Cappellini MD. Iron-chelating therapy with the new oral agent ICL670 (Exjade). Best Pract Res Clin Haematol 2005;18:289–98.

6. Shuchman M. The drug trial. Toronto: Random House Canada; 2005.

7. Hoffbrand AV. Research conduct and the case of Nancy Olivieri. Lancet 2005;366:1432–3.

8. Naithani R, Chandra J, Sharma S. Safety of oral iron chelator deferiprone in young thalassaemics. Eur J Haematol 2005;74:217–20.

9. Taher A, Sheikh-Taha M, Sharara A, Inati A, Koussa S, Ellis G, Dhillon AP, Hoffbrand AV. Safety and effectiveness of 100 mg/kg/day deferiprone in patients with thalassemia major: a two-year study. Acta Haematol 2005;114:146–9.

10. Voskaridou E, Douskou M, Terpos E, Stamoulakatou A, Meletis J, Ourailidis A, Papassotiriou I, Loukopoulos D. Deferiprone as an oral iron chelator in sickle cell disease. Ann Hematol 2005;84:434–40.

11. Tsironi M, Ladis V, Margellis Z, Deftereos S, Kattamis Ch, Aessopos A. Impairment of cardiac function in a successful full-term pregnancy in a homozygous beta-thalassemia major: does chelation have a positive role? Eur J Obstet Gynecol Reprod Biol 2005;120:117–8.

12. Sokka T, Hannonen P, Mottonen T. Conventional disease-modifying antirheumatic drugs in early arthritis. Rheum Dis Clin N Am 2005;31:729–44.

13. Choy EHS, Smith C, Dore CJ, Scott DL. A meta-analysis of the efficacy and toxicity of combining disease-modifying anti-rheumatic drugs in rheumatoid arthritis based on patient withdrawal. Rheumatology 2005;44:1414–21.

14. Bouros D, Antoniou KM. Current and future therapeutic approaches in idiopathic pulmonary fibrosis. Eur Respir J 2005;26:693–702.

15. Kaplan MM, Gershwin ME. Primary biliary cirrhosis. N Engl J Med 2005;353:126–73.

16. Dhawan A, Taylor RM, Cheeseman P, De Silva P, Katsiyiannakis L, Mieli-Vergani G. Wilson's disease in children: 37-year experience and revised King's score for liver transplantation. Liver Transplant 2005;11:441–8.

17. Prashanth LK, Taly AB, Sinha S, Ravishankar S, Arunodaya GR, Vasudev MK, Swamy HS. Prognostic factors in patients presenting with severe neurological forms of Wilson's disease. Q J Med 2005;98:557–63.

18. Chan KH, Cheung RTF, Au-Yeung KM, Mak W, Cheng TS, Ho SL. Wilson's disease with depression and parkinsonism. J Clin Neurosci 2005;12:303–5.

19. Nagao K, Tanikawa A, Yamamoto N, Amagai M. Decline of anti-desmoglein 1 IgG ELISA scores by withdrawal of D-penicillamine in drug-induced pemphigus foliaceus. Clin Exp Dermatol 2005;30:43–5.

20. Becuwe C, Dalle S, Ronger-Savle S, Skowron F, Balme B, Kanitakis J, Thomas L. Elastosis perforans serpiginosa associated with pseudo-pseudoxanthoma elasticum during treatment of Wilson's disease with penicillamine. Dermatology 2005;210:60–3.

21. Choi H-J, Lee D-K, Chang S-E, Lee M-W, Choi J-H, Moon K-C, Koh J-K. An iatrogenic dermatosis with ulceration. Clin Exp Dermatol 2005;30:463–4.

22. Idowu MO, Mudge M, Ghatak NR. Kayexalate (sodium polystyrene sulfonate) aspiration. Arch Pathol Lab Med 2005;129(1):125.

23. Haupt HM, Hutchins GM. Sodium polystyrene sulfonate pneumonitis. Arch Intern Med 1982;142:379–81.

24. Fenton JJ, Johnson FB, Przygodzk RM, Kalasinsky VF, Al-Dayel F, Travis WD. Sodium polystyrene sulfonate (kayexalate) aspiration: histologic appearance and infrared microspectrophotometric analysis of two cases. Arch Pathol Lab Med 1996;120(10):967–9.

25. Aronson JK, Hauben M. Anecdotes that provide definitive evidence. BMJ 2006;333(7581):1267–9.

26. Chen CC, Chen CA, Chau T, Lin SH. Hypokalaemia and hypomagnesaemia in an oedematous diabetic patient with advanced renal failure. Nephrol Dial Transplant 2005;20(10):2271–3.

27. Rosenberg G, Angel I, Kozak A. Clinical pharmacology of DP-b99 in healthy volunteers: first administration to humans. Br J Clin Pharmacol 2005;60:7–16.

28. Pittler MH, Ernst E. Complementary therapies for peripheral arterial disease: systematic review. Atherosclerosis 2005;181:1–7.

Pam Magee

24

Antiseptic drugs and disinfectants

BISBIGUANIDES

Chlorhexidine   (SED-15, 714; SEDA-27, 239; SEDA-28, 261; SEDA-29, 241)

Placebo-controlled studies   Hospital-acquired infections, notably those caused by methicillin-resistant *Staphylococcus aureus* (MRSA), are a major public health concern. Thus, new prevention strategies targeting MRSA have been developed. Various formulations of chlorhexidine have significant efficacy against catheter-related infections and as a standard skin disinfectant in surgical patients, although allergic reactions have been reported (SEDA-26, 258; SEDA-27, 239; SEDA-28, 261). As a hand-washing agent, chlorhexidine also reduces cross-transmitted nosocomial infection. Combined with nasal mupirocin, chlorhexidine body washing reduces the rate of MRSA ventilator-associated pneumonia.

In a multicenter, double-blind, randomized, placebo-controlled study, two decontamination regimens were assessed in the prevention of acquired infections in 515 high-risk intubated patients in intensive care (1^C):

- topical polymyxin + tobramycin ($n = 130$);
- nasal mupirocin ointment with chlorhexidine body washing ($n = 130$);
- the two regimens combined ($n = 129$);
- matching placebo (topical placebo and/or nasal placebo + liquid soap; $n = 126$).

There were fewer acquired infections with the combined regimens than with either regimen alone or placebo. There were no differences between either regimen alone and placebo. There were *allergic reactions* in six patients who received chlorhexidine and six patients who received the liquid soap. There was no intolerance to the nasal ointment. The polymyxin + tobramycin regimen was withdrawn in 37 patients, mostly because the serum tobramycin concentration exceeded 2 mg/l. Body washing was discontinued in nine patients receiving chlorhexidine and in eight patients receiving the liquid soap.

Mouth   Chlorhexidine is the most commonly used mouthwash for chemical plaque control. Its use is becoming widespread as an adjuvant treatment of mechanical control, particularly in individuals with compromised oral hygiene. However, several adverse effects that limit patients' acceptance of mouth rinsing have been identified—*brown staining of the teeth*, an *unpleasant taste*, and rarely *painful desquamation of the oral mucosa*. Alternative formulations of chlorhexidine and other chemical plaque controls have therefore been developed to minimize adverse effects.

The effects of three oral sprays containing chlorhexidine, benzydamine hydrochloride, and chlorhexidine plus benzydamine hydrochloride on plaque and gingivitis have been compared (2^c). Chlorhexidine and chlorhexidine + benzydamine hydrochloride sprays were equally effective and the benzydamine hydrochloride spray alone was less effective. The chlorhexidine/benzydamine hydrochloride spray caused a *burning sensation*.

Commercial formulations of chlorhexidine mouthwash include other active ingredients, in an attempt to improve their effectiveness and reduce adverse effects. Using a double-blind crossover design, three different commercial formulations of 0.12% chlorhexidine digluconate mouthwash were compared for their

Side Effects of Drugs, Annual 30
J.K. Aronson (Editor)
ISSN: 0378-6080
DOI: 10.1016/S0378-6080(08)00024-X

effects on dental plaque, supragingival calculus, and dental staining. Changes in gingival and dental staining indices were not affected differently by the three products, but *tongue staining* was more frequent with the product that contained cetylpyridinium chloride (3ᶜ).

Chlorphenesin

Chlorphenesin (3-(4-chlorphenoxy)-1,2-propane-diol) is an antimicrobial agent with antifungal, antibacterial, and anticandidal activity. There have been two cases of *contact allergy* attributed to chlorphenesin because of positive skin tests (4ᶜ). The authors estimated the incidence of such reactions, based on their overall experience, at 0.02% per year.

IODOPHORS *(SEDA-15, 1896; SEDA-27, 240; SEDA-28, 262; SEDA-29, 242)*

Polyvinylpyrrolidone

Endocrine   The use of iodinated skin disinfectants in the perinatal period and in mothers during pregnancy or at delivery can result in significant iodine overload in the neonate and transient *hypothyroidism* (SEDA-25, 277; SEDA-28, 263). Severe hypothyroidism requiring levothyroxine replacement therapy has been reported in a neonate after prolonged use of an iodinated skin disinfectant (5ᴬ).

- In a boy born at 25 weeks gestation, neonatal screening for hypothyroidism on day 4 after delivery was normal (thyroid-stimulating hormone, TSH, <20 mU/l). On day 10, septic thrombophlebitis of the scalp with abscess formation, probably secondary to an intravenous catheter, was treated with intravenous antibiotics and topical povidone iodine, polysporin, and saline compresses. The povidone iodine was discontinued after 20 days and thyroid function tests showed a marked increase in TSH (455 mU/l) and a reduction in free thyroxine concentration (0.51 ng/dl). Transient hypothyroidism secondary to iodine overload was diagnosed. There were no clinical signs of hypothyroidism. Ultrasonography of the thyroid gland showed enlargement of the two lobes and the isthmus, with increased vascularity. Levothyroxine 25 micrograms/day was started on day 39. Thyroid-stimulating hormone and free thyroxine concentrations returned to the reference range after 10 days of levothyroxine therapy and withdrawal of povidone iodine. The levothyroxine was withdrawn on day 65.

Thyroid hormones play a major role in postnatal brain development and linear growth. This case of severe transient hypothyroidism after the use of povidone iodine skin disinfectant suggests that neonatal iodine exposure should be minimized whenever possible and that TSH should be routinely measured soon after exposure to iodinated skin disinfectants. This is especially important in preterm neonates, in whom skin permeability is high, the thyroid gland is particularly sensitive to the antithyroid effects of iodine excess, and the clinical signs of hypothyroidism are difficult to recognize.

References

1. Camus C, Bellissant E, Sebille V, Perrotin D, Garo B, Legras A, Renault A, Le Corre P. Prevention of acquired infections in intubated patients with the combination of two decontamination regimens. Crit Care Med 2005;33:307–14.
2. Bozkurt FY, Ozturk M, Yetkin Z. The effects of three oral sprays on plaque and gingival inflammation. J Periodontol 2005;76:1654–60.
3. Bascones A, Morante S, Mateos L, Mata M, Poblet J. Influence of active ingredients on the ef-

fectiveness of non-alcoholic chlorhexidine mouthwashes: a randomized controlled trial. J Periodontol 2005;76:1469–75.
4. Brown VL, Orton DI. Two cases of facial dermatitis due to chlorphenesin in cosmetics. Contact Dermatitis 2005;52(1):48–9.
5. Khashu M, Chessex P, Chanoine J-P. Iodine overload and severe hypothyroidism in a premature neonate. J Pediatr Surg 2005;40:E1–4.

Tore Midtvedt

25   Penicillins, cephalosporins, other beta-lactam antibiotics, and tetracyclines

"Just as there are fundamental principles underlying mathematics, I am convinced that a code of universal rights and rules, most notably the right of life itself, exists independently of human ethics"

F. Schätzing, *The Swarm* (2004, ISBN 3462033748)

The increasing rate of antibiotic resistance in an increasing number of microbial species world wide has been addressed almost yearly in this chapter of SEDA as the most serious adverse effect of antimicrobial drugs. Over the years attitudes to this problem have altered. The World Health Organization, the European Union, and several other countries have started to collect data about levels of resistance in important groups of pathogens, and international study groups have been established for the rapid interchange and evaluation of these data. It is also recognized that with the increasing worldwide emergence of microbial antibiotic resistance, there is a pressing need for novel or alternative sources of antimicrobial agents (1[R]). Of the many agents that have been tested, the most promising seem to come from life itself, echoing Pasteur's dictum, "La vie empêche la vie". All types of animals—mammals, amphibians, birds, fish, insects—produce antimicrobial peptides to protect themselves, and the same holds true for many micro-organisms (2[R]). These peptides or "autobiotics" may have affected our fight against infections.

However, we should by now have recognized that the spread—vertical as well as horizontal—of genes that code for resistance is a major mechanism in nearly all microbial species. In order to avoid further breakdown in sensitivity—as we have seen with our "old" antimicrobial drugs—we have to use new agents far more responsibly than we have used the old ones. Philosophically, the key point has recently been stressed by Woose: "Modern society desperately needs to learn how to live in harmony with the biosphere" (3[R]).

BETA-LACTAM ANTIBIOTICS

(SED-15, 478; SEDA-27, 242; SEDA-28, 267; SEDA-29, 267)

Nervous system   The neurotoxic effects of beta-lactam antibiotics have been reviewed (4[R]).

Hematologic   *Neutropenia* due to beta-lactam antibiotics has been reviewed (5[R]). It usually occurs after high-dose therapy lasting more than 10 days, and the frequency rises with cumulative dose. It is often preceded by a fever or rash, usually lasts less than 10 days, and is uncommonly associated with infectious complications or death. Although any beta-lactam can cause neutropenia, there seems to be a high incidence associated with the prolonged use of cefepime or piperacillin + tazobactam.

Three patients with endocarditis and septic shock had presumed beta-lactam-induced bleeding (6[A]).

Cross-reactivity in penicillin and cephalosporin hypersensitivity reactions

Possible cross-reactivity between penicillins and cephalosporins was discussed in SEDA-

Side Effects of Drugs, Annual 30
J.K. Aronson (Editor)
ISSN: 0378-6080
DOI: 10.1016/S0378-6080(08)00025-1

28 (p. 261). There are now new data. In a meta-analysis, using Medline and EMBASE databases and the key words "cephalosporin", "penicillin", and "cross-sensitivity" for the years 1960–2005, 219 articles were found, of which nine served as sources for an evidence-based analysis (7^M). First-generation cephalosporins have cross-allergy with penicillins, but cross-allergy is negligible with second- and third-generation cephalosporins; this is also most probably true for fourth-generation cephalosporins (8^c). The value of emphasizing the role of chemical structure has been underlined in a case report.

- *A 39-year-old woman developed anaphylactic shock a few minutes after taking a tablet of cefuroxime axetil 500 mg (9^A). Skin tests confirmed that she was allergic to cefuroxime, and the reaction was defined as probable according to the Naranjo probability scale. A structure-activity relation study was performed using skin testing. She was sensitized to beta-lactam antibiotics with a methoxylimino group, but not to similar compounds that lack this chemical group (for example amoxicillin, penicillin G, and penicillin V). Intravenous amoxicillin was well tolerated.*

The authors suggested that an approach based on structure-activity relations could help physicians and pharmacists in advising patients with allergic reactions.

A similar approach to studying the tolerability of other beta-lactams has been used in patients with a history of aminopenicillin-induced rash (10^c). Skin testing was followed by oral challenge to identify beta-lactams that patients with confirmed delayed-type non-immunoglobulin E-mediated allergic hypersensitivity to aminopenicillins could tolerate. Of 71 patients, 69 tolerated cephalosporins without an aminobenzyl side-chain (such as cefpodoxime or cefixime) and 51 also tolerated phenoxymethylpenicillin. The authors concluded that skin tests and drug challenge tests can help in determining individual cross-reactivity. Beta-lactam-specific IgE has good specificity but poor sensitivity (11^C). More sensitive methods should therefore be developed.

In a survey of 83 patients who reported penicillin allergy and were given a cephalosporin, seven had an adverse reaction (12^C). Six of these reported a definite history of an immediate reaction to penicillin, including urticaria. Of 62 patients who reported that their penicillin reaction had been delayed, probable,

or unknown, only one had a reaction to a cephalosporin. The risk of a reaction was highest with second-generation cephalosporins and least with fourth-generation cephalosporins. The presence of an aminobenzyl ring in the cephalosporin molecule increased the risk.

There have been reports of presumed IgE-mediated hypersensitivity reactions of individual cephalosporins without cross-reactivity to other beta-lactam antibiotics.

- *A 51-year-old woman had anaphylactic shock 10 minutes after an intravenous dose of cefodizime 1 g, having tolerated intramuscular cefodizime 11 months before (13^A). Skin tests with major and minor penicillin determinants, amoxicillin, ampicillin, benzylpenicillin, cefamandole, cefotaxime, ceftriaxone, ceftazidime, and cefuroxime were all negative. Cefodizime produced wheal, maximum diameter 10 mm, surrounded by erythema after 20 minutes.*
- *A 3-year-old girl had an anaphylactic reaction 20 minutes taking a second oral dose of ceftibuten 135 mg, which she had tolerated 6 months before (14^A). Prick and intradermal skin tests with standard concentration of major and minor determinants, amoxicillin, ampicillin, penicillin G, penicillin V, cefaclor, cefotaxime, ceftriaxone, and cephalexin were all negative. There was a positive response to prick testing with ceftibuten.*

In both cases, although the authors did not detect specific IgE to cefodizime they attributed this to the fact that the tests were carried out some time after the reactions, and they suggested that the reactions were IgE-mediated. They also suggested that the lack of cross-reactivity with other beta-lactams emphasized the role of the IgE epitope present on R1 side-chain in inducing immediate hypersensitivity.

Tables 1 and 2 show penicillins and cephalosporins that are structurally similar and for which cross-reactivity is more likely. The author of an extensive review of the evidence reached the following conclusions (15^R):

- *If a patient has a reaction to a penicillin or cephalosporin that was not IgE-mediated and was not serious, it is safe to give repeated courses of that antibiotic and related antibiotics; only IgE-mediated reactions are likely to become more severe with time and to result in anaphylaxis.*
- *If the rash is non-urticarial and non-pruritic, it is almost certain that it is not IgE-mediated and the risk of recurrence of the same rash with repeated courses of the same antibiotic*

Table 1. *Structural similarities in the 7-position side-chains of some penicillins and cephalosporins (15^{MR})*

Similar structures			Dissimilar structures	
Related	Related	Related	Not related	
Penicillin G	Amoxicillin	Cefepime	Cefazolin	Cefamandole
Cefoxitin	Ampicillin	Cefetamet	Cefdinir	Cefixime
Cephaloridine	Cefaclor	Cefotaxime	Cefonicid	Cefmetazole
Cephalothin	Cefadroxil	Cefpirome	Cefoperazone	Cefotiam
	Cefatrizine	Cefpodoxime	Cefotetan	Ceftazidime
	Cefprozil	Cefteram	Cefsulodin	Ceftibuten
	Cephalexin	Ceftizoxime	Cefuroxime	Cephapirin
	Cephradine	Ceftriaxone		Moxalactam

Table 2. *Structural similarities in the 3-position side-chains of some cephalosporins (15^{MR})*

Similar structures							Dissimilar structures
Related	Related	Related	Related	Related	Related	Related	Unrelated
Cephradine	Cefmetazole	Cephapirin	Ceftazidime	Cefuroxime	Cefdinir	Ceftibuten	Cefatrizine
Cefadroxil	Cefoperazone	Cefotaxime	Cefsulodin	Cefoxitin	Cefixime	Ceftizoxime	Cefotiam
Cephalexin	Cefotetan	Cephalothin					Cefpodoxime
	Cefamandole						Cefprozil
							Ceftibuten
							Ceftriaxone
							Cefonicid
							Cefepime
							Cefotiam
							Cefazolin
							Cephaloridine
							Cefaclor

is not increased; in uncertain cases, elective penicillin skin testing is advisable.

- If the patient has a history that is consistent with a severe IgE-mediated reaction to a penicillin, cephalosporins with a similar 7-position side chain on the beta-lactam ring (Table 1) should be used with caution.
- If the allergic reaction followed administration of ampicillin or amoxicillin, cephalosporins with a similar side chain (Table 1) should be used with caution.
- Other cephalosporins with different side-chains are not more likely to produce allergic reactions in penicillin-allergic patients than among non-allergic patients.
- A cephalosporin can be given to a patient who has had a non-IgE-mediated adverse reaction to a penicillin, i.e. a type II, III, IV, or unclassified reaction, such as hemolytic anemia, serum sickness, contact dermatitis, or a morbilliform or maculopapular rash; in un-

certain cases, elective penicillin skin testing is advisable.

- When patients give a history of penicillin allergy, it is advisable to question this information, because very often the drug was not actually taken or a recognized non-immunological adverse effect (for example vomiting, diarrhea, or a non-specific rash) occurred.
- Penicillin skin testing can be useful to identify allergic patients, and testing is about 60% predictive of clinical hypersensitivity.
- Cephalosporins cause allergic or immune-mediated reactions among about 1–3% of patients, even if they are not allergic to penicillins.
- The incidence of allergic reactions to cephalosporins among penicillin-allergic patients, attributable to cross-reactive antibodies, varies with the side-chain similarity of the cephalosporin to the penicillin.

- *For first-generation cephalosporins, the risk is 0.4%; for cefuroxime, cefpodoxime, and cefdinir the risk is nearly zero.*
- *A patient who has an allergic reaction to a specific cephalosporin probably should not use that cephalosporin again; however, the risk of a drug reaction when a different cephalosporin is given appears to be very low or non-existent if the side-chains of the drugs are not similar.*
- *Penicillin skin testing is not predictive of cephalosporin allergy unless the side-chain of the penicillin is similar to the side-chain of the cephalosporin.*

In a retrospective review of 101 patients who underwent penicillin skin tests, 92 had a negative result and five had a positive result; in four the test result was indeterminate (16[c]). Of patients with negative skin tests 49% were given a penicillin-based drug and 48% a cephalosporin; there were no serious adverse reactions. There was a 96% reduction in the use of vancomycin and a 96% (23/24) reduction in the use of fluoroquinolones in patients with negative skin tests.

Skin tests with commercially available haptens to major and minor determinants (benzylpenicilloyl poly-l-lysine and a mixture of minor determinants), penicillin G, injectable amoxicillin, and ampicillin and cephalosporins, if they have been incriminated by the patient, have typically been used in the diagnosis of allergy to beta-lactam antibiotics. However, both benzylpenicilloyl poly-l-lysine and mixtures of minor determinants have been withdrawn commercially in most countries. The likely effect of this withdrawal on the diagnosis of beta-lactam allergy has been retrospectively analysed in 824 patients (mean age 37 years, 254 men and 570 women) (17[c]). There was a positive skin test response in 136 (16.5%), of whom six (4.4% of those with positive skin test responses) had positive skin test responses to benzylpenicilloyl poly-l-lysine only, nine (6.6%) to a mixture of minor determinants only, and five (3.7%) to both without a positive reaction to other beta-lactams. There were positive skin tests to other beta-lactams in 116 (85.3%), of whom about 30% of those with positive skin test responses also had positive responses to benzylpenicilloyl poly-l-lysine, a mixture of minor determinants, or both. Thus, had benzylpenicilloyl poly-l-lysine and a mixture of minor determinants not

been available, the diagnosis would not have been made in 20 patients, who could not otherwise have been identified. In another study it was estimated that a misdiagnosis would have occurred in 47% of 463 patients in the absence of benzylpenicilloyl poly-l-lysine and a mixture of minor determinants (18[c]). Although there were differences between the results of these two studies, both sets of authors concluded that major and minor determinants are necessary in the investigation of allergy to beta-lactams.

Drug contamination   The administration of piperacillin + tazobactam or co-amoxiclav can result in detectable amounts of *Aspergillus* galactomannan antigen in the plasma (SEDA-29, 248), since some beta-lactam antibiotics may contain galactomannan. In a study of 39 batches of four different beta-lactam antibiotics galactomannan was not detected in nine batches of piperacillin, whereas it was detected in all 10 batches of amoxicillin and co-amoxiclav and in six of 10 batches of piperacillin + tazobactam (19[cE]). Within each four groups of drugs, all the batches came from the same company. The real size of this problem is not known, but it is large enough for regulatory agencies to start taking action.

CARBAPENEMS   (SED-15, 638; SEDA-27, 246; SEDA-29, 246)

Drug–drug interactions   Interactions of carbapenems with *valproic acid* are so common that the Ministry of Health and Welfare in Japan has banned co-administration. There have been many reports of seizures in epileptic patients due to lowered plasma concentrations of valproic acid, including a child with a neurodegenerative disorder and epilepsy, in whom valproate serum concentrations fell rapidly on two occasions when meropenem was used (20[A]).

- A 21-year-old woman was given valproic acid 1000 mg/day as a continuous intravenous infusion for generalized tonic–clonic seizures (serum valproate concentration 53 µg/ml) (21[A]). After 13 days she was given intravenous meropenem 1 g tds, and 2 days later, when she was afebrile, had numerous myoclonic episodes involving her arms and face (valproate concentration 42 µg/ml). The dose of valproic acid was increased to 2880 mg/day. Two days later, she had a generalized tonic–clonic seizure and despite the increased dosage the valproate concentration was 7 μg/ml. The dose of valproic acid was increased to 3600 mg/day, but the serum concentration remained below 10 μg/ml. Meropenem was withdrawn and the serum valproate concentration rose to 52 μg/ml.

There are several possible mechanisms for this interaction (22[E], 23[E], 24[E]), such as reduced plasma protein binding and inhibition of the enterohepatic circulation of valproic acid and valproic acid glucuronide. The results of a retrospective study in 39 patients suggested that the most critical mechanism is inhibition by carbapenems of the hydrolysis of valproic acid glucuronide in the liver (25[C]). There was an interaction of meropenem with valproic acid in all patients, leading to a fall in valproic acid concentration by an average of 66% within 24 hours. The authors concluded that to avoid neurological deterioration, meropenem and valproate should not be co-administered. This may also be true for all carbapenems, although data on doripenem are still lacking.

Ertapenem

Ertapenem has been reviewed (26[R], 27[R]).

Nervous system   Carbapenems rarely cause *seizures*, which can be fatal (28[A]). The risk is increased by a previous stroke (29[A]).

- An 85-year-old man was given ertapenem 500 mg/day for a urinary tract infection and had three seizures on day 4. A CT scan of the brain showed peripheral and central brain atrophy and an old infarct. He was given a different antimicrobial drug and the seizures did not recur.
- A 71-year-old man was given ertapenem 500 mg/day for a urinary tract infection and had four seizures on day 5, each accompanied by loss of consciousness. A CT scan of the brain showed old right-sided temporal–parietal and occipital infarcts. He was given a different antimicrobial drug. He had further seizures the next day and was given antiepileptic drugs. He had no recurrence thereafter.

The presence of underlying pathology, such as an old stroke, increases the risk of seizures when carbapenems are given (30[R]). The message is clear: a previous stroke should be a contraindication to the use of ertapenem.

Imipenem

Observational studies   In a comparison of intravenous imipenem + cilastatin (500 mg 6-hourly) and intravenous piperacillin + tazobactam (4 g 6-hourly) + amikacin (20 mg/kg/day) in 290 patients the incidences of drug-related adverse events were 13 and 6% respectively, with no differences in moderate or severe adverse events nor in those that caused withdrawal of antibiotic therapy (31[c]).

Metabolism   Cilastatin prevents the metabolism of imipenem by renal tubular dipeptidase, which also hydrolyses the glutathione metabolite cysteinylglycine. In patients taking imipenem + cilastatin, *plasma concentrations of cysteinylglycine were significantly increased*, while cysteine concentrations fell and homocysteine concentrations were unchanged (32[c]). The clinical significance of this is not clear.

Hematologic   *Pure white cell aplasia* has been reported in a patient taking imipenem + cilastatin (33[A]).

CEPHALOSPORINS   *(SED-15, 688; SEDA-27, 245; SEDA-28, 268; SEDA-29, 246)*

Hematologic   Drug-induced immune *hemolytic anemia* has been reviewed (34[R]). Twelve cephalosporins have been implicated the most common being cefotetan and ceftriaxone.

Cefaclor

Immunologic   Typical *anaphylactic reactions* to beta-lactams usually involve the skin and the respiratory and cardiovascular systems, and commonly present with urticaria, angioedema, dyspnea, wheeze, dizziness, syncope, and hypotension. Gastrointestinal symptoms, including nausea, vomiting, diarrhea, and abdominal cramp, can occur, but mucosal lesions are rarely detected or indeed sought.

- A 27-year-old man visited a local clinic complaining of fatigue and arthralgia (35[A]). He was given paracetamol, cefaclor, and diclofenac, and 20 minutes later developed generalized itching, oral dysesthesia, and dyspnea, followed by hypotension and loss of consciousness. He was successfully treated with adrenaline and an intravenous glucocorticoid, but 15 hours after admission developed epigastric pain, nausea, and vomiting. Gastroduodenoscopy showed generalized ulcers with white exudates and petechiae from the bulb to the second part of the duodenum; histology of the duodenal ulcers showed eosinophilic infiltration. His symptoms resolved with a proton pump inhibitor. Total IgE was 160 IU/ml. Specific IgE antibodies were negative to 11 common allergens. Aspirin intolerance was excluded by a negative inhalation challenge with sodium tolmetin and oral challenges with paracetamol and diclofenac were also negative.

The authors concluded that cefaclor was the most probable cause of the anaphylaxis.

Cefepime

Nervous system   Cefepime is a fourth-generation cephalosporin with a broad antibacterial spectrum. It often causes neurotoxicity and neuropsychiatric adverse effects (SEDA-26, 264; SEDA-27, 245; SEDA-28, 269) and new reports continue to appear. Seven patients developed reversible cefepime-induced *encephalopathy* with a peculiar electroencephalographic pattern, characterized by semiperiodic diffuse triphasic waves (36[c]). Abnormal electroencephalography was also found in a US patient (37[A]). Most often, these types of adverse effects occur in patents with reduced renal function (37[A], 38[A]), but they can occur in patients with normal renal function (39[c]). In a 79-year-old patient with normal renal function subtle mental status changes during cefepime therapy were shown by electroencephalography to be due to non-convulsive status epilepticus (40[A]). In three other patients non-convulsive status epilepticus due to cefepime was associated with varying degrees of renal impairment (41[A]). Cefepime toxicity should be suspected whenever a patient taking the drug has a change in mental status or myoclonus.

Cefoperazone

Hematologic   *Agranulocytosis* has been attributed to cefoperazone in a patient with end-stage renal insufficiency (42[A]).

Cefprozil

Skin   A *rash* has been attributed to cefprozil in a patient with infectious mononucleosis (43[A]).

Ceftriaxone

Nervous system   *Pseudotumor cerebri* has been attributed to ceftriaxone (44[A]).

Hematologic   *Hemolytic anemia* associated with ceftriaxone-dependent antibodies has been described in a patient with hemoglobin SC disease (45[Ar]) and in one with sickle cell anemia (46[Ar]). In the former it was fatal.

Biliary tract   Of 50 children who were given ceftriaxone 13 developed abnormal biliary sonography suggestive of *biliary sludge* (so-called pseudolithiasis) (47[A]). Susceptibility was independent of age, weight, and sex. In another similar study, 19 of 33 children developed ultrasonographic biliary sludge within 10 days of treatment with intravenous ceftriaxone 100 mg/kg/day; all were asymptomatic (48[A]).

This effect of ceftriaxone, which usually occurs in children (SEDA-29, 246) and can occur at doses as low as 50 mg/kg/day (49[r]), is rarely symptomatic. However, it can occasionally result in cholelithiasis, as in the case of a 7-year-old boy (50[A]). This adverse effect has been reviewed in the context of a 53-year-old man who was given intravenous ceftriaxone 2 g every 12 hours and became jaundiced after 7 days (51[AR]). Ultrasonography showed biliary sludge and cholelithiasis without cholecystitis. Ceftriaxone was withdrawn, the jaundice subsided, and the liver function test results normalized within 14 days.

In neurosurgical patients the symptoms of biliary pseudolithiasis can mimic those of raised intracranial pressure (52[r]).

Urinary tract   *Nephrolithiasis* has been attributed to ceftriaxone in a child with acute pyelonephritis (53[AR]) and in another with septic arthritis (54[AR]). In the latter the stones were composed of 90% ceftriaxone; in other words this is a between-the-eyes adverse effect of type 1 (55[RH]).

Immunologic   A *hypersensitivity reaction* has been reported in a patient taking ceftriaxone (56[A]).

- A 50-year-old man developed fever, headache, nausea, vomiting, myalgia, arthralgia, and a pruritic skin rash 4 days after the start of a course of ceftriaxone 4 g/day for 21 days for meningitis. His temperature was 38.8 °C, heart rate 110/minute, and blood pressure 120/70 mmHg. He had extensive erythroderma, petechiae, and desquamation, edema on the face, and painful subconjunctival hyperemia and hemorrhages. His leukocyte count was 24×10^9/l with 8% eosinophils, the C-reactive protein 98 mg/l, and the erythrocyte sedimentation rate 30 mm/hour. All other investigations were normal or negative. After treatment with prednisone 48 mg/day for 3 days the syndrome resolved.

Cefuroxime

Cardiovascular   *Angina and myocardial infarction* can occur in the absence of angiographically stenosed coronary arteries, because of arterial vasospasm during a drug-induced allergic reaction. This rare condition is called the Kounis syndrome, and it has been reported in a 70-year-old woman after intravenous cefuroxime (57[C]). The authors suggested that individuals in whom there is increased mast cell degranulation may be more susceptible to this effect.

Lactation   The safety of cefuroxime during lactation has been studied prospectively in 38 women (58[C]). Women taking cefalexin ($n = 11$) were used as controls and were matched for indication, duration of treatment, and age. The frequencies of adverse effects in the infants were not significantly different (OR = 0.92; 95% CI = 0.94, 1.06). All adverse effects were minor and self-limiting and did not necessitate interruption of breast-feeding.

MONOBACTAMS   *(SED-15, 2378; SEDA-27, 247; SEDA-29, 247)*

Aztreonam

Skin   The term *erythroderma* or *generalized exfoliative dermatitis* is used to describe any inflammatory skin disease that involves the whole or most of the skin surface. There is usually a poor correlation between the clinical presentation and the histological findings, because the specific cutaneous changes of a dermatosis or a drug reaction are obscured by nonspecific changes caused by the erythroderma itself. Erythroderma is uncommon but can be life-threatening.

- A 73-year-old woman was given intravenous clindamycin 600 mg 6-hourly and 7 days later developed generalized erythema with intense pruritus, malaise, and chills (59[A]). The eruptions started on the trunk and spread rapidly over the entire surface of the skin, including the palms and soles. Clindamycin was withdrawn and she was given dexchlorpheniramine and methylprednisolone. She improved slowly, and her symptoms resolved in 12 days. She was given aztreonam and ceftriaxone, which were well tolerated. Two years later, she was given aztreonam 500 mg 8-hourly for a urinary tract infection and developed the same symptoms and signs. Serial skin prick tests and intradermal tests with aztreonam and clindamycin on different days produced delayed reactions (aztreonam at 6–8 hours and clindamycin at 12 hours).

On the basis of the skin tests and the history, the authors identified aztreonam and clindamycin as the cause of these skin reactions. As there are no structural analogies between aztreonam and clindamycin, coincidental sensitization seems more likely than cross-reactivity.

PENICILLINS   *(SED-15, 2756; SEDA-26, 262; SEDA-27, 244)*

Co-amoxiclav and clavulanic acid

Liver   Drug-induced *jaundice* is a serious adverse effect that can lead to acute liver failure and death. In most cases, antimicrobial drugs are the drugs that are most commonly involved. However, in a study from China, Chinese herbal medicines were most commonly involved, accounting for almost 25% of cases (60[M]), and in a US study paracetamol (acetaminophen) was top of the list (61[R]).

In a recent study in Southwest England over 66 months during 1998–2004, 800 patients presented to a jaundice referral system serving a community of 400 000 (62[R]). Of these, 28 cases were related to drugs (mean age 69 years, 17 men), most often antimicrobial drugs ($n = 21$). Co-amoxiclav ($n = 9$) and flu-cloxacillin ($n = 7$) were the main culprits, with incidence rates per 100 000 prescriptions of 9.91 and 3.60 respectively. Jaundice due to co-amoxiclav was more common in elderly men (age 65 years; M:F = 7:2). The authors suggested that an alternative to co-amoxiclav should be used if possible in men over the age of 60 years.

The hepatotoxic profile of co-amoxiclav has been further evaluated in a prospective study from Spain (63[R]). In data from all cases of he-patotoxicity reported to the Spanish Registry, co-amoxiclav was implicated in 69 patients (36 men, mean age 56 years), representing 14% of all reported cases. The predominant pattern of lesion was hepatocellular damage, and the mean time lapse between the start of therapy and the onset of jaundice was 16 days. Multiple logistic regression analysis iden-tified advanced age as being associated with the cholestatic/mixed type of injury. There was an unfavourable outcome in 7% of the patients. The lesson is the same as that from England: co-amoxiclav should be used with care in el-derly men.

Immunologic   Although there have been many reports of allergic reactions and cross-reactivity to penicillins, there have been few reports of *allergic reactions* to clavulanic acid, which contains a beta-lactam ring, but differs from penicillin G and penicillin V in its second ring, which is an oxazolidine instead of a thiazolidine ring (64[A]). Clavulanic acid shares this ring with cloxacillin.

- A 46-year-old woman with a history of allergy to co-amoxiclav was challenged with a single tablet; 30 minutes later she developed itching, wheals, and flares, which started on her groins and armpits but then spread over her entire body within a few minutes (65[A]). Radioallergosorbent tests for specific IgE to penicillin V, penicillin G, amox-icillin, and ampicillin were all negative. Skin prick tests and intradermal tests to amoxicillin, peni-cillin major determinant (penicilloyl polylysine), and penicillin minor determinant were also nega-tive. Oral challenge with progressively increasing doses of amoxicillin up to 500 mg gave no reac-tions. However, 10 minutes after she took a half a capsule of co-amoxiclav 500/125 mg she de-veloped itching, wheals, and flares. Her symptoms were relieved by adrenaline, a glucocorticoid, and an antihistamine. A histamine release test was neg-ative for amoxicillin, but positive for co-amoxiclav

and clavulanic acid alone. Skin prick tests were positive with the combination, but negative with cloxacillin, tazobactam, and sulbactam. Specific IgE determination 2 months later was positive with penicillin V, but negative with penicillin G, amox-icillin, and ampicillin. Skin prick tests to amox-icillin, penicillin major and minor determinants, and penicillin V were all negative. She refused oral challenge with clavulanic acid.

In this case, allergy to clavulanic acid was demonstrated by specific IgE antibody concen-trations, skin prick tests, a histamine release test, and oral challenge. The results of the skin prick tests with cloxacillin and the other beta-lactamase inhibitors almost certainly excluded the oxazolidine ring as the epitope responsi-ble for sensitization, and this is consistent with previous reports of clavulanic acid allergy, in most of which type I sensitization has been demonstrated by skin prick tests (66[c]), although delayed reactions have also been described (67[c]). The authors also suggested that sensiti-zation to penicillin V, which occurred in this case, might have been due to repeated exposure during the months of evaluation.

Lactation   The safety of co-amoxiclav dur-ing lactation has been studied prospectively in 67 women (58[C]). Women taking amoxicillin ($n = 40$) were used as controls and were matched for indication, duration of treatment, and age. There were adverse effects in 15 in-fants and the frequency increased with dosage. In the control group three infants had adverse effects (RR = 2.99; 95% CI = 0.92, 9.7). All the adverse effects were minor and self-limiting and did not necessitate interruption of breast-feeding.

Piperacillin

Skin   *Acute generalized exanthematous pus-tulosis* (AGEP) has been reported in a patient taking piperacillin + sodium tazobactam (68[A]).

Drug–drug interactions   An interaction of piperacillin+tazobactam with *methotrexate* has been described (69[A]).

- A 50-year-old woman with Burkitt's lymphoma was given one cycle of chemotherapy with IVAC (ifosfamide, etoposide, and high-dose cytarabine) and on day 10 developed febrile neutropenia and cavitating pneumonia due to *Pseudomonas aeruginosa*. She was given piperacillin + tazobactam (dose not stated) empirically. She then had a cycle of CPDOX-M (cyclophosphamide, doxorubicin, vincristine, and high-dose methotrexate), during which a drug interaction was suspected. Cytotoxic methotrexate concentrations were sustained for 8 days and did not fall below 0.05 µmol/l until piperacillin + tazobactam was withdrawn. During a second cycle of CPDOX-M, piperacillin + tazobactam was not administered and the serum methotrexate concentrations were lower. Her serum creatinine concentration was the same during the two cycles, and concurrent medications, aside from piperacillin + tazobactam, did not differ. Methotrexate total body clearance fell to 3% of normal in the presence of piperacillin + tazobactam.

This interaction has been reported only once before (70[c]). However, it has been forecast from experiments in monkeys and rabbits. In *Rhesus* and *Cynomolgus* monkeys, penicillin and methotrexate share a common secretory system in the kidney and penicillin blocks methotrexate secretion (71[E]). Piperacillin blocks the renal excretion of methotrexate and its main metabolite 7-hydroxymethotrexate in rabbits by an effect on the tubular transport mechanism for organic acids (72[E]).

In general, it would be wise to think of possible interactions when the combination of piperacillin+tazobactam is given with weak organic acids that are excreted renally.

TETRACYCLINES AND GLYCYLCYCLINES   (SED-15, 3330; SEDA-27, 247; SEDA-28, 270; SEDA-29, 248)

℞ *Tetracyclines, chemically-modified tetracyclines, and their non-antimicrobial properties*
(SEDA-23, 255; SEDA-25, 278; SEDA-26, 266)

Ever since the tetracyclines were introduced half a century ago, their non-antimicrobial effects have been well recognized and have been looked on as side effects. However, in the last 15 years, these biological actions of tetracyclines have been studied in greater detail and

in a wide variety of areas, such as inflammation, proteolysis, angiogenesis, apoptosis, ionophoresis, and bone metabolism. Clinical trials have also been performed in many different non-microbial fields, and there have been more than 300 reports. An excellent review was published in 2006 (73[R]). Here I shall briefly comment on some recent reports, including "old" tetracyclines as well as chemically modified tetracyclines (CMTs), i.e. tetracyclines with greatly reduced antimicrobial activity but increased inhibitory effects on matrix metalloproteases (MMPs), enzymes that are primarily responsible for deposition of extracellular matrix proteins.

Diabetic proteinuria   Because matrix metalloproteases contribute to the pathogenesis of diabetic proteinuria, 35 patients with overt diabetic nephropathy (proteinuria over 300 mg/day) were given doxycycline 100 mg/day for 2 months (74[C]). There was a statistically significant reduction in proteinuria, and it increased when doxycycline was withdrawn. Further studies are necessary to determine the long-term effects, the optimal dosage, and the optimal duration of treatment.

Periodontitis   In a rat model of pulp infection in the mandibular first molar, CMT-3, a potent inhibitor of matrix metalloproteases, affected pulp and periapical inflammation, increased the rate of spread of necrosis in the root channels, and increased the rate of periapical lesion formation (75[E]). This might be of substantial clinical value, since some inhibitors of matrix metalloproteases, especially doxycycline, are used in some countries to prevent periodontal inflammation.

Metastatic colorectal cancer   In a complicated model of metastatic colorectal cancer in mice, inhibition of matrix metalloproteases was associated with significantly fewer and smaller liver tumors (76[E]). The authors concluded that after resection of colorectal tumors, inhibition of matrix metalloproteases may be clinically beneficial in preventing recurrence.

Breakthrough endometrial bleeding   The endometrial environment in contraceptive users is characterized by increased production of matrix metalloproteases. In an in vitro model doxycycline only moderately and in a cell-specific *manner reduced expression of matrix metallo-proteases without inducing their activity (77[E]). The clinical relevance of these findings is unclear.*

Tendinopathy   *Increased activity of matrix metalloproteases and subsequent degradation of extracellular matrix are supposed to be implicated in the pathogenesis of tendinopathy. In an experimental study in tendons in rats' tails doxycycline inhibited pericellular matrix generation (78[E]). The authors hypothesized that this could be beneficial in the treatment of tendinopathy in humans. In another study, related to tendon repair in rats, doxycycline at clinically relevant serum concentrations impaired healing processes in experimentally induced Achilles tendon injuries (79[E]). It currently seems reasonable to conclude that matrix metalloprotease inhibitors should be used with great care in sports medicine, since it is uncertain that these results can be extrapolated from rats' tails to athletes' Achilles tendons.*

Metamfetamine adverse effects   *Metamfetamine can be associated with behavioral changes and neurotoxicity. In a recent study, minocycline ameliorated behavioral changes and neurotoxicity in mouse brain dopaminergic terminals after the administration of metamfetamine (80[E]). The authors suggested that minocycline may be useful in the treatment of several symptoms associated with metamfetamine abuse, although this may be merely a pipe dream.*

Conclusions   *The future for tetracyclines and chemically modified tetracyclines is very exciting. However, a common feature of all of these new approaches is that there are many uncertainties about long-term beneficial and adverse effects. However, one thing is certain— increased use will create increased microbial resistance. Even though chemically modified tetracyclines have minor, if any, antimicrobial properties, they might increase resistance to the old tetracyclines. Microbes most commonly get rid of tetracyclines, and most probably also chemically modified tetracyclines, by efflux mechanisms. If so, they might be just as good inducers of resistance as the old ones.*

The adverse effects profiles of oral doxycycline and minocycline have been systematically reviewed (81[M]). Between 1966 and 2003, a total of 130 and 333 adverse events were published in case reports of doxycycline and minocycline respectively. In 24 doxycycline studies ($n = 3833$) and 11 minocycline studies ($n = 788$), adverse events occurred in 0–61% and 12–83% respectively. Gastrointestinal adverse events were most common with doxycycline; central nervous system and gastrointestinal adverse events were most common with minocycline. The FDA MedWatch data contained 628 events for doxycycline and 1099 events for minocycline reported in the USA from January 1998 to August 2003, during which time 47 630 000 new prescriptions for doxycycline and 15 234 000 new prescriptions for minocycline were dispensed, yielding event rates of 13 per million for doxycycline and 72 per million for minocycline.

Doxycycline   *(SEDA-27, 247; SEDA-28, 270)*

Placebo-controlled studies   In a randomized, placebo-controlled study in 150 patients with chronic meibomian gland dysfunction, doxycycline 20 or 200 mg bd both increased tear production and reduced symptoms (82[C]). However, the high-dose group reported adverse effects more often than the low-dose group (18 versus 8, 39 versus 17%).

Teeth   Four patients with brucellosis developed *yellow-brown discoloration of permanent teeth* after taking doxycycline 200 mg/day for 30–45 days (83[A]). In all cases, the staining completely resolved and the teeth recovered their original color after abrasive dental cleaning. The authors suggested that staining of the permanent dentition associated with doxycycline may be much commoner than reported, especially if the drug is taken during the summer months, and that strict avoidance of sunlight exposure during high-dose, long-term doxycycline therapy may prevent this complication.

Gastrointestinal   Doxycycline can cause *esophageal ulcers*, which may respond to proton pump inhibitors and sucralfate (84[A]).

- In a 15-year-old girl esophageal ulceration was attributed to doxycycline 100 mg/day (85[A]).

• A 46-year-old woman with rosacea took doxycycline 50 mg/day and after 48 hours developed
retrosternal chest pain and dysphagia due to two
benign esophageal ulcers, which responded to
omeprazole and sucralfate (86^A).

This is a rare complication—of all cases of
esophageal ulcers attributed to drugs, doxycycline has been implicated in 1 in about 4000. It
can occur in children (87^A).

Of 1442 patients with chronic prostatitis due
to *Ureaplasma urealyticum* 63 were randomized to azithromycin 4.5 g over 3 weeks or
doxycycline 100 mg bd for 21 days; five patients who took doxycycline had *nausea* (88^C).

Nails   *Discoloration of the nails* is rarely attributed to doxycycline and has previously been
reported as being painful (89^A, 90^A).

• An 11-year-old-boy developed painless brown discoloration of the nails after taking doxycycline
100 mg/day for 15 days; the thumbs were particularly affected (91^A). The discoloration resolved
within 1 month after withdrawal.

Minocycline   *(SED-15, 2349; SEDA-26,*
265; SEDA-27, 247; SEDA-28, 271)

Nervous system   *Intracranial hypertension*
has been attributed to lithium and minocycline
in a child (92^A).

Respiratory   *Pleurocarditis and eosinophilic
pneumonia* have been associated with minocycline in a 37-year-old man (93^A).

Mouth   Minocycline can cause *discoloration
of the soft tissues of the mouth*, but this has often been attributed to staining of the underlying
bone.

• A 45-year-old Caucasian woman developed pigmentation of the gums, lips, and nail beds after
taking minocycline 100 mg bd for 6 months (94^A).
Biopsies from the gums and lips showed increased
melanin and melanocytes in the epithelium and
melanin and melanophages in the connective tissues. Nine months after withdrawal of minocycline
there was marked reduction in the pigmentation.

Skin   *Sweet's syndrome* is an acute febrile
neutrophilic dermatosis marked by non-pruritic,
painful, reddish nodules, most often on the
head and neck, the chest, and/or the arms,
accompanied by fever, arthralgias, and leukocytosis. Histopathology shows a diffuse dermal
neutrophilic infiltration. The pathogenesis is
not understood, but there is always prompt
resolution of the symptoms and lesions with
glucocorticoid therapy. Sweet's syndrome due
to minocycline was first reported in 1991 (95^A),
since when several reports have appeared (96^A,
97^A).

The authors of a systematic review concluded that granulocyte colony-stimulation factor (G-CSF), tretinoin (all-trans retinoic acid,
ATRA), and vaccines met two of three criteria
for an association with drug-induced Sweet's
syndrome (98^M). There were sufficient data for
an association with G-CSF and tretinoin and
plausible pharmacological mechanisms. Vaccines met the qualitative criteria and also had
a plausible pharmacological mechanism. For
minocycline, however, the authors concluded
that the evidence was of high quality, but the
quantity of evidence was small and a plausible
pharmacological mechanism was lacking.

Long-term minocycline often results in *pigmentation* of the skin, nails, bones (99^A), thyroid, mouth, and eyes; on the skin, the blue-
black pigmentation develops most often on the
shins, ankles, and arms. In one 15-year-old girl
bilateral discoloration on the legs was limited
to the subcutaneous adipose tissues and completely spared the dermis; unusually for this
form of hyperpigmentation, there was a negative stain for iron (100^A).

Immunologic   Over the years several reports
of minocycline-induce *lupus-like syndrome*
have been published. In 1999, Schrodt and
Callen were the first to describe cutaneous polyarteritis nodosa in a 15-year-old girl after 9
months of minocycline therapy for acne vulgaris (101^A).

• An 18-year-old girl used minocycline for acne for
1 year at age 15 (102^A). At age 18, she had a
flare-up and took minocycline 100 mg/day. About
4–6 weeks later she developed flu-like symptoms,
tender pink nodules on her legs, and a raised
antinuclear antibody (ANA) titer (1:240) with a
nuclear pattern. Her aspartate and alanine transaminase activities were slightly raised. Extractable

nuclear antigen, antinative DNA antibodies, anticardiolipin antibodies, and lupus anticoagulant were all negative, and complement C3 and C4 concentrations were normal. A punch biopsy of one of the nodules showed a medium-sized artery surrounded by a mixed infiltrate containing predominantly lymphocytes and histiocytes and occasional eosinophils, with disruption of the vessel and fibrin deposition. Minocycline was withdrawn and her symptoms gradually abated. About 2 months later her ANA titer was 1:80 and it became normal after another 2 months. After 8 months all of her symptoms had resolved.
- In a 17-year-old boy minocycline-associated lupus-like syndrome presented with a polyarthropathy, odynophagia, and a flu-like illness (103[A]).
- A 19-year-old woman, who was taking an oral contraceptive and minocycline 100 mg bd, abruptly developed a nodular rash, with multiple violaceous, tender, subcutaneous nodules, 0.5–2 cm in diameter, over her lower legs (104[A]). The overlying skin was slightly warm but non-tender. The lesions resolved after treatment with a glucocorticoid for 1 week but then recurred with bilateral ankle pain, stiffness, and swelling. Perinuclear antineutrophilic cytoplasmic antibodies (pANCA) were positive in a titer of 1:256. A skin biopsy showed necrotizing vasculitis of the small vessels of the dermis, panniculitis characterized by vascular wall neutrophil infiltration, hyalinizing necrosis, and intravascular thrombi, and granuloma formation characterized by epithelioid giant cells.

Minocycline-induced immunological syndromes, such as cutaneous polyarteritis nodosa and lupus-like syndrome, tend to occur in young women, usually after a prolonged period of minocycline therapy. Several cases of minocycline-induced lupus-like syndrome have also been described after restarting treatment. The results of laboratory tests are often similar in minocycline-induced polyarteritis nodosa and lupus-like syndrome, i.e. positive ANA titers, normal concentrations of complement, and absence of antibodies to native DNA.

Minocycline can cause perinuclear antineutrophil cytoplasmatic antibodies (pANCA), but the mechanisms are far from clear. It has been postulated that the drug or some of its metabolites may interact with the immune system, and that either drug or metabolites can act as haptens and induce an immune response against myeloperoxidases, enzymes that are involved in the metabolism of minocycline (105[R]). It may be more than a coincidence that other drugs that can cause a lupus-like syndrome, such as hydralazine and procainamide, are also substrates for myeloperoxidases (106[E], 107[E]).

Genes may also play a part in minocycline-related autoimmune phenomena. All of 13 patients with pANCA positive titers and minocycline-related lupus were either HLA-DR4 or HLA-DR2 positive (108[c]). Four had also cutaneous involvement. However, biopsies were not performed, and a diagnosis of polyarteritis nodosa could not be made.

It seems reasonable to assume that minocycline-induced cutaneous polyarteritis nodosa is more common than reported. In some cases the patients stopped taking minocycline themselves and in all cases rapid improvement of symptoms followed withdrawal of medication.

Tetracycline

Nervous system *Intracranial hypertension* is a well described adverse effect of tetracyclines.

- A 22-year-old girl who took tetracycline 500 mg 6-hourly for 3 days developed *intracranial hypertension with esotropia* (109[A]).
- A 24-year-old woman developed intracranial hypertension after taking oral tetracycline (110[A]). She had severely reduced visual acuity, papilledema, and concentric impaired visual fields. She was treated with acetazolamide and recurrent lumbar punctures and recovered, but without improvement in either acuity or visual fields.

Sensory systems *Ocular pigmentation* has not previously been attributed to oral tetracycline hydrochloride.

- A 48 year old healthy white man developed green crystals on the conjunctivae of both eyes after taking tetracycline 500 mg/day for several months for acne vulgaris (111[A]). Tetracycline was identified in a conjunctival biopsy.

This was a between-the-eyes adverse effect of type 1 (55[RH])

Teeth Tetracycline-induced *staining of the teeth* has been treated successfully with a porcelain laminate veneer (112[A]).

Tigecycline

The adverse effects of tigecycline have been reviewed; *nausea and vomiting* are the main adverse effects and can be managed with antiemetics (113[R], 114[R], 115[R]).

Comparative studies   In a double-blind study in 1116 adults with complicated skin infections, in which tigecycline was compared with vancomycin + aztreonam, the main adverse effects of tigecycline were *nausea* (35%), *vomiting* (20%), *diarrhea* (8.5%), and "*dyspepsia*" (3.7%); tigecycline also *prolonged the activated partial thromboplastin time and the prothrombin time* in about 3% and caused *increased transaminase activities* in 1–2% (116[C]). It is not clear whether two other report from the same group of similar study in 573 and 543 patients overlap with this (117[C], 118[C]), but the adverse effects of tigecycline were similar in the three studies.

Gastrointestinal   In a pooled analysis of two phase 3, double-blind comparisons of intravenous tigecycline and imipenem + cilastatin in 1642 adults with complicated intra-abdominal infections, *nausea* (24% tigecycline, 19% imi-penem + cilastatin), *vomiting* (19% tigecycline, 14% imipenem + cilastatin), and *diarrhea* (14% tigecycline, 13% imipenem + cilastatin) were the most common adverse events (119[M]).

In one of those studies, intravenous tigecycline (100 mg initially then 50 mg every 12 hours) and imipenem + cilastatin (500 + 500 mg 6-hourly or adjusted for renal dysfunction) for 5 to 14 days was compared in 825 patients (120[C]). Tigecycline was as efficacious as imipenem + cilastatin but caused more adverse effects, of which nausea (31 versus 5%), vomiting (26 versus 19%), and diarrhea (21 versus 19%) were the most common.

Food-drug interactions   In two pharmacokinetic studies of tigecycline food increased the maximum tolerated single dose from 100 to 200 mg (121[C]).

References

1. Levy SB, Marshall B. Antibacterial resistance worldwide: causes, challenges and responses. Nat Med 2004;10(12 Suppl):S122–9.
2. Diep DB, Skaugen M, Salehian Z, Holo H, Nes IF. Common mechanisms of target cell recognition and immunity for class II bacteriocins. Proc Nat Acad Sci 2007;104:2384–9.
3. Woose CP. A new biology for a new century. Mol Biol Rev 2004;68:173–86.
4. Chow KM, Hui AC, Szeto CC. Neurotoxicity induced by beta-lactam antibiotics: from bench to bedside. Eur J Clin Microbiol Infect Dis 2005;24(10):649–53.
5. Peralta G, Sanchez-Santiago MB. Neutropenia secundaria a betalactámicos. Una vieja compañera olvidada (Beta-lactam-induced neutropenia. An old forgotten companion). Enferm Infecc Microbiol Clin 2005;23(8):485–91.
6. Mellerup MT, Bruun NE, Nielsen JD. Increased bleeding tendency induced by beta-lactam antibiotics. Ugeskr Laeger 2005;167(25–31):2790–1.
7. Pichichero ME, Casey JR. Safe use of selected cephalosporins in penicillin-allergic patients: a meta-analysis. Otolaryngol Head Neck Surg 2007;136:340–7.
8. Moreno E, Davila I, Laffond E, Macias E, Isodoro M, Ruiz A, Lorente F. Selective im-mediate hypersensitivity to cefepime. J Investig Allergol Clin Immunol 2007;17:52–4.
9. Hasdenteufel F, Luyasu S, Renaudin JM, Trechot P, Kanny G. Anaphylactic chock associated with cefuroxime axetil: structure-activity relationships. Ann Pharmacother 2007;41:1069–72.
10. Trcka J, Seitz CS, Bröcker EB, Gross GE, Trautmann A. Aminopenicillin-induced exanthema allows treatment with certain cephalosporins or phenoxymethylpenicillin. J Antimicrob Chemother 2007;60:107–11.
11. Lucena Fontaine C, Mayorga C, Bouscuet PJ, Arnoux B, Torres MJ, Bianca M, Demoly P. Relevance of the determination of serum-specific IgE antibodies in the diagnosis of immediate beta-lactam allergy. Allergy 2007;62:47–52.
12. Fonacier L, Hirschberg R, Gerson S. Adverse drug reactions to a cephalosporins in hospitalized patients with a history of penicillin allergy. Allergy Asthma Proc 2005;26(2):135–41.
13. Romano A, Viola M, Gueant-Rodriguez RM, Valluzzi RL, Gueant JL. Selective immediate hypersensitivity to cefodizime. Allergy 2005;60(12):1545–6.
14. Atanasković-Marković M, Cirković Velicković T, Gavrović-Jankulović M, Ivanovski P, Nestorović B. A case of selective IgE-

mediated hypersensitivity to ceftibuten. Allergy 2005;60(11):1454.

15. Pichichero ME. A review of evidence supporting the American Academy of Pediatrics recommendation for prescribing cephalosporin antibiotics for penicillin-allergic patients. Pediatrics 2005;115(4):1048–57.

16. Nadarajah K, Green GR, Naglak M. Clinical outcomes of penicillin skin testing. Ann Allergy Asthma Immunol 2005;95(6):541–5.

17. Bousquet PJ, Co-Minh HB, Arnoux B, Daures JP, Demoly P. Importance of mixture of minor determinants and benzylpenicilloyl poly-L-lysine skin testing in the diagnosis of beta-lactam allergy. J Allergy Clin Immunol 2005;115(6):1314–6.

18. Matheu V, Pérez-Rodriguez E, Sánchez-Machin I, de la Torre F, García-Robaina JC. Major and minor determinants are high-performance skin tests in *β*-lactam allergy diagnosis. J Allergy Clin Immunol 2005;116(5):1167–8.

19. Aubry A, Porcher R, Bottero J, Touratier S, Leblanc T, Brethon B, Rousselit P, Raffoux E, Menotti J, Derouin F, Ribaud P, Sulahian A. Occurrence and kinetics of false-positive *Aspergillus* galactomannan test results following treatment with beta-lactam antibiotics in patients with hematological disorder. J Clin Microbial 2006;44:389–94.

20. Santucci M, Parmeggiani A, Riva R. Seizure worsening caused by decreased serum valproate during meropenem therapy. J Child Neurol 2005;20(5):456–7.

21. Coves-Orts FJ, Borrás-Blasco J, Navarro-Ruiz A, Murcia-López A, Palacios-Ortega F. Acute seizures due to a probable interaction between valproic acid and meropenem. Ann Pharmacother 2005;39(3):533–7.

22. Hobara N, Kameya H, Hokama N, Ohshiro S. Altered pharmacokinetics of sodium valproate by simultaneous administration of imipenem/cilastatin sodium. Jpn J Hosp Pharm 1998;24:464–72.

23. Kojima S, Nadai M, Kitaichi K, Wang L, Nabeshima T, Hasegawa T. Possible mechanism by which the carbapenem antibiotic panipenem decreases the concentration of valproic acid in plasma in rats. Antimicrob Agents Chemother 1998;42:3136–40.

24. Nakajima Y, Mizobuchi M, Nakamura M, Takagi H, Inagaki HI, Kominami G, Koike M, Yamaguchi T. Mechanism of the drug interaction between valproic acid and carbapenem antibiotics in monkeys and rats. Drug Metab Dispos 2004;32:1381–91.

25. Spriet L, Goyens J, Meersseman W, Wilmer A, Willems L, van Paesschen W. Interaction between valproate and meropenem: a retrospective study. Ann Pharmacol 2007;41:1130–6.

26. Keating GM, Perry CM. Ertapenem: a review of its use in the treatment of bacterial infections. Drugs 2005;65(15):2151–78.

27. Zhanel GG, Johanson C, Embil JM, Noreddin A, Gin A, Vercaigne L, Hoban DJ. Ertapenem: review of a new carbapenem. Expert Rev Anti Infect Ther 2005;3(1):23–39.

28. Seto AH, Song JC, Guest SS. Ertapenem-associated seizures in a peritoneal dialysis patient. Ann Pharmacother 2005;39(2):352–6.

29. Saidel-Odes L, Borer A, Riesenberg K, Smolyakov R, Schlaeffer F. History of cerebrovascular events: a relative contraindication to ertapenem treatment. Clin Infect Dis 2006;43:262–3.

30. Calandra G, Lydick E, Carrigan J, Weiss L, Guess H. Factors predisposing to seizures in seriously ill patients receiving antibiotics: experience with imipenem/cilastatin. Am J Med 1988;84:911–8.

31. Sanz MA, Bermúdez A, Rovira M, Besalduch J, Pascual MJ, Nocea G, Sanz-Rodríguez C, for the COSTINE Study Group. Imipenem/cilastatin versus piperacillin/tazobactam plus amikacin for empirical therapy in febrile neutropenic patients: results of the COSTINE study. Curr Med Res Opin 2005;21(5):645–55.

32. Badiou S, Bellet H, Lehmann S, Cristol JP, Jaber S. Elevated plasma cysteinylglycine levels caused by cilastatin-associated antibiotic treatment. Clin Chem Lab Med 2005;43(3):332–4.

33. Kalambokis G, Vassou A, Bourantas K, Tsianos EV. Imipenem–cilastatin induced pure white cell aplasia. Scand J Infect Dis 2005;37(8):619–20.

34. Arndt PA, Garratty G. The changing spectrum of drug-induced immune hemolytic anemia. Semin Hematol 2005;42(3):137–44.

35. Shirai T, Mori M, Uotani T, Chida K. Gastrointestinal disorders in anaphylaxis. Intern Med 2007;46(6):315–6.

36. Bragatti JA, Rossato R, Ziomkowski S, Kliemann FA. Encefalopatia induzida por cefepime: achados clinicos e eletroencefalograficos em sete pacientes (Cefepime-induced encephalopathy: clinical and electroencephalographic features in seven patients). Arq Neuropsiquiatr 2005;63(1):87–92.

37. Lam S, Gomolin IH. Ceepime neurotoxicity: case report, pharmacokinetic considerations, and literature review. Pharmacotherapy 2006;26:1169–74.

38. Lin CM, Chen YM, Po HL, Hseuh IH. Acute neurological deficit caused by cefipime: a case report and review of literature. Acta Neurol Taiwan 2006;15:279–82.

39. Capparelli FJ, Diaz MF, Hiavnika A, Wainsztein NA, Leigurda R, Del Castillo ME. Cefepime and cefixime-induced encephalopathy in a patient with normal renal function. Neurology 2005;65:1840.

40. Maganti R, Jolin D, Rishi D, Biswas A. Nonconvulsive status epilepticus due to cefepime in a patient with normal renal function. Epilepsy Behav 2006;8(1):312–4.

41. Fernandez-Torre JL, Martinez-Martinez M, Gonzalez-Rato J, Maestro I, Alonso I, Rodrigo E, Horcajada JP. Cephalosporin-induced nonconvulsive status epilepticus: clinical and

electroencephalographic features. Epilepsia 2005;46(9):1550–2.

42. Balkarova OV, Fomin VV, Kozlovskaia LV. Agranulocytosis due to cefoperazon treatment in a patient with terminal renal failure. Ter Arkh 2005;77(6):76–8.

43. Baciewicz AM, Chandra R. Cefprozil-induced rash in infectious mononucleosis. Ann Pharmacother 2005;39(5):974–5.

44. Goenaga Sánchez MA, Sánchez Haya E, Martínez Soroa I, Millet Sampedro M, Garde Orbáiz C. Pseudotumor cerebri probably due to ceftriaxone. An Med Interna 2005;22(3):147–8.

45. Bell MJ, Stockwell DC, Luban NL, Shirey RS, Shaak L, Ness PM, Wong EC. Ceftriaxone-induced hemolytic anemia and hepatitis in an adolescent with hemoglobin SC disease. Pediatr Crit Care Med 2005;6(3):363–6.

46. Corso M, Ravindranath TM. Albuterol-induced myocardial ischemia in sickle cell anemia after hemolysis from ceftriaxone administration. Pediatr Emerg Care 2005;21(2):99–101.

47. Ceran C, Oztoprak I, Cankorkmaz L, Gumuş C, Yildiz T, Koyluoglu G. Ceftriaxone-associated biliary pseudolithiasis in paediatric surgical patients. Int J Antimicrob Agents 2005;25(3):256–9.

48. Ozturk A, Kaya M, Zeyrek D, Ozturk E, Kat N, Ziylan SZ. Ultrasonographic findings in ceftriaxone: associated biliary sludge and pseudolithiasis in children. Acta Radiol 2005;46(1):112–6.

49. Avci Z, Karadag A, Odemis E, Catal F. Re: Pediatric ceftriaxone nephrolithiasis. J Urol 2005;174(3):1153.

50. Costa DL, Barbosa MD, Barbosa MT. Cholelithiasis associated with the use of ceftriaxone. Rev Soc Bras Med Trop 2005;38(6):521–3.

51. Bickford CL, Spencer AP. Biliary sludge and hyperbilirubinemia associated with ceftriaxone in an adult: case report and review of the literature. Pharmacotherapy 2005;25(10):1389–95.

52. Evliyaoglu C, Kizartici T, Bademci G, Unal B, Keskil S. Ceftriaxone-induced symptomatic pseudolithiasis mimicking ICP elevation. Zentralbl Neurochir 2005;66(2):92–4.

53. Tasic V, Sofijanova A, Avramoski V. Nephrolithiasis in a child with acute pyelonephritis. Ceftriaxone-induced nephrolithiasis and biliary pseudolithiasis. Pediatr Nephrol 2005;20(10):1510–1, 1512–3.

54. Gargollo PC, Barnewolt CE, Diamond DA. Pediatric ceftriaxone nephrolithiasis. J Urol 2005;173(2):577–8.

55. Aronson JK, Hauben M. Anecdotes that provide definitive evidence. BMJ 2006;333(7581):1267–9.

56. Akcam FZ, Aygun FO, Akkaya VB. DRESS like severe drug rash with eosinophilia, atypic lymphocytosis and fever secondary to ceftriaxone. J Infect 2006;53(2):e51–3.

57. Mazarakis A, Koutsojannis CM, Kounis NG, Alexopoulos D. Cefuroxime-induced coronary artery spasm manifesting as Kounis syndrome. Acta Cardiol 2005;60(3):341–5.

58. Benyamini L, Merlob P, Stahl B, Braunstein R, Bortnik O, Bulkowstein M, Zimmerman D, Berkovitch M. The safety of amoxicillin/clavulanic acid and cefuroxime during lactation. Ther Drug Monit 2005;27(4):499–502.

59. Gonzalo-Garilo MA, de Argila D. Erythroderma due to aztreonam and clindamycin. J Investig Allergol Clin Immunol 2006;16:210–1.

60. Li B, Wang Z, Fang JJ, Xu CV, Chen WX. Evaluation of prognostic markers in severe drug-induced liver disease. World J Gastroenterol 2007;13:628–32.

61. Lewis JH, Ahmed M, Shobassy A, Palese C. Curr Opin Gastroenterol 2006;22:223–33.

62. Hussaini SH, O'Brien CS, Despott EJ, Dalton HR. Antibiotic therapy; a major cause of drug-induced jaundice in southwest England. Eur J Gastroenterol Hepatol 2007;19:15–20.

63. Lucena MI, Andrade RJ, Fernandez MC, Pachkoria K, Pelaez G, Duran JA, Villar M, Rodrigo L, Romero-Gomez M, Planas R, Barriocanal A, Costa J, Guarner C, Blanco S, Navarro JM, Pons F, Castiella A, Avila S, Spanish Group for the Study of Drug-Induced Liver Disease (Grupo de Estudio para las Hepatopatias Asociadas a Medicamentos (GEHAM)). Determinants of the clinical expression of amoxicillin–clavulanate hepatotoxicity: a prospective series from Spain. Hepatology 2006;44(4):850–6.

64. Edwards RG, Dewdney JM, Dobrzanski RJ, Lee D. Immunogenicity and allergenicity studies on two beta-lactam structures, a clavam, clavulanic acid, and a carbapenem: structure-activity relationships. Int Arch Allergy Appl Immunol 1988;85:184–9.

65. Gonzales de Olano D, Losada PA, Caballer BdeL, Vazquez Gonzales AC, Diegues Pastor MC, Cuevas Agustin M. Selective sensitization to clavulanic acid and penicillin V. J Investig Allergol Clin Immunol 2007;17:119–21.

66. Raison-Peyron N, Messaad D, Bousquet J, Demoli P. Selective immediate hypersensitivity to clavulanic acid. Ann Pharmacother 2003;37:1146–7.

67. Kamphof WC, Rustemeyer T, Bruyzeel DP. Sensitization to clavulanic acid in Augmentin. Contact Dermatitis 2002;47:47.

68. Grieco T, Cantisani C, Innocenzi D, Bottoni U, Calvieri S. Acute generalized exanthematous pustulosis caused by piperacillin/tazobactam. J Am Acad Dermatol 2005;52(4):732–3.

69. Zarychanski R, Wlodarczyk K, Ariano R, Bow E. Pharmacokinetic interaction between methotrexate and piperacillin/tazobactam resulting in prolonged toxic concentrations of methotrexate. J Antimicrob Chemother 2006;58:228–30.

70. Yamamoto K, Sawada Y, Matsushita Y, Moriwaki K, Bessho F, Iga T. Delayed elimination of methotrexate associated with piperacillin administration. Ann Pharmacother 1997;31:1261–2.

71. Williams WM, Chen TS, Huang KC. Effect of penicillin on the renal tubular secretion of methotrexate in the monkey. Cancer Res 1984;44:1913–7.

72. Iven H, Brasch H. Influence of the antibiotics piperacillin, doxycycline and tobramycin on the pharmacokinetics of methotrexate in rabbits. Cancer Chemother Pharmacol 1986;17:218–22.

73. Sapardin AN, Fleischmajer R. Tetracyclines: nonantibiotic properties and their clinical implications. Am Acad Dermaol 2006;54:258–65.

74. Naini AE, Harandi AA, Moghtaderi J, Bastani B, Amiran A. Doxycycline: a pilot study to reduce diabetic proteinuria. Am J Nephrol 2007;27:269–73.

75. Tjäderhane L, Hotakainen T, Kinnunen S, Ahonen M, Salo T. The effect of chemical inhibition of matrix metalloproteases on the size of experimentally induced apical periodontitis. Int Endod J 2007;40:282–9.

76. Nicoud IB, Jones CM, Pierce JM, Earl TM, Matrisian LM, Chari RS, Gordon DL. Warm hepatic ischemia-reperfusion promotes growth of colorectal carcinoma micrometastases in mouse liver via matrix metalloprotease-9 induction. Cancer Res 2007;15:272–8.

77. Li R, Luo X, Archer DF, Chegini N. Doxycycline alters the expression of matrix metalloproteases in the endometrial cells exposed to ovarian steroid and proinflammatory cytokines. J Reprod Immunol 2007;73:118–29.

78. Arnoczky SP, Lavagnino M, Egerbacher M, Caballero O, Gardner K. Matrix metalloproteases inhibitors prevent a decrease in the mechanical properties of stress-deprived tendons: an in vitro experimental study. Am J Sport Med 2007;35:763–9.

79. Pasternak B, Fellenius M, Aspenberg P. Doxycycline impairs tendon repair in rats. Acta Orthop Belg 2006;72:756–60.

80. Zhang L, Kitaichi K, Fujimoto Y, Nakayama H, Shimizu E, Iyo M, Hashimoto K. Protective effects of minocycline on behavioural changes and neurotoxicity in mice after administration of methamphetamine. Prog Neuropsychopharmacol Biol Psychiatry 2006;30:1381–9.

81. Smith K, Leyden JJ. Safety of doxycycline and minocycline: a systematic review. Clin Ther 2005;27(9):1329–42.

82. Yoo SE, Lee DC, Chang MH. The effect of low-dose doxycycline therapy in chronic meibomian gland dysfunction. Korean J Ophthalmol 2005;19(4):258–63.

83. Ayaslioglu E, Erkek E, Oba AA, Cebecioğlu E. Doxycycline-induced staining of permanent adult dentition. Aust Dent J 2005;50(4):273–5.

84. Grgurević I, Marusić S, Banić M, Buljevac M, Crncevic-Urek M, Cabrijan Z, Kardumz D, Kujundzić M, Lesnjaković I, Tadić M, Loncar B. Doxycycline induced esophageal ulcers: report of two cases and review of the literature. Lijec Vjesn 2005;127(11–12):285–7.

85. Passalidou P, Giudicelli H, Moreigne M, Khalfi A. Doxycycline-induced esophageal ulceration. Arch Pediatr 2006;13(1):90–1.

86. Fernándeza MA. Úlcera esofágica y doxiciclina. Aten Primaria 2005;36:224.

87. Pociello Almiñana N, Vilar Escrigas P, Luaces Cubells C. Esofagitis por doxiciclina. A propósito de dos casos. An Pediatr (Barc) 2005;62(2):171–3.

88. Skerk V, Mareković I, Markovinović L, Begovac J, Skerk V, Barsić N, Majdak-Gluhinić V. Comparative randomized pilot study of azithromycin and doxycycline efficacy and tolerability in the treatment of prostate infection caused by *Ureaplasma urealyticum*. Chemotherapy 2006;52(1):9–11.

89. Coffin SE, Puck J. Painful discoloration of the fingernails in a 15-year-old boy. Pediatr Infect Dis J 1993;12:702–3. 706.

90. Yong CK, Prendiville J, Peacock DL, Wong LT, Davidson AG. An unusual presentation of doxycycline-induced photosensitivity. Pediatrics 2000;106:E13.

91. Akcam M, Artan R, Akcam FZ, Yilmaz A. Nail discoloration induced by doxycycline. Pediatr Infect Dis J 2005;24(9):845–6.

92. Jonnalagadda J, Saito E, Kafantaris V. Lithium, minocycline, and pseudotumor cerebri. J Am Acad Child Adolesc Psychiatry 2005;44(3):209.

93. Hidalgo Correas FJ, de Andrés Morera S, Ramallal Jiménez de Llano M, Garrote Martínez FJ, García Díaz B. Pleurocarditis y neumonía eosinofílica inducida por minociclina: a propósito de un caso. Farm Hosp 2005;29(2):145–7.

94. LaPorta VN, Nikitakis NG, Sindler AJ, Reynolds MA. Minocycline-associated intra-oral soft-tissue pigmentation: clinicopathologic correlations and review. J Clin Periodontol 2005;32(2):119–22.

95. Mensing H, Kowalzick L. Acute febrile neutrophilic dermatosis (Sweet's syndrome) caused by minocycline. Dermatologica 1991;182:43–6.

96. Thibaut MJ, Bilick RC, Srolovitz H. Minocycline-induced Sweet's syndrome. J Am Acad Dermatol 1992;27:801–4.

97. Khan Durani B, Jappe U. Drug-induced Sweet's syndrome in acne caused by different tetracyclines: case report and review of the literature. Br J Dermatol 2002;147:558–62.

98. Thompson DF, Montarella KE. Drug-induced Sweet's syndrome. Ann Pharmacother 2007;41:802–11.

99. Hepburn MJ, Dooley DP, Hayda RA. Minocycline-induced black bone disease. Orthopedics 2005;28(5):501–2.

100. Rahman Z, Lazova R, Antaya RJ. Minocycline hyperpigmentation isolated to the subcutaneous fat. J Cutan Pathol 2005;32(7):516–9.

101. Schrodt BJ, Callen JP. Polyarteritis nodosa attributable to minocycline treatment for acne vulgaris. Pediatrics 1999;103:146–9.

102. Tehrani R, Nash-Goelitz A, Adams E, Dahiya M, Eilers D. Minocycline-induced cutaneous polyarteritis nodosa. J Clin Rheumatol 2007;13(3):146–9.

103. Leydet H, Armingeat T, Pham T, Lafforgue P. Lupus induit par la minocycline. Rev Med Interne 2006;27(1):72–5.

104. Culver B, Itkin A, Pischel K. Case report and review of minocycline-induced cutaneous polyarteritis nodosa. Arthritis Rheum 2005;53(3):468–70.

105. Angulo JM, Sigal LH, Espinoza LR. Coexistent minocycline-induced systemic lupus erythematosus and autoimmune hepatitis. Semin Arthritis Rheum 1998;28:187–92.

106. Hughes GRV. Recent development in drug-associated systemic lupus erythematosus. Adverse Drug React Bull 1987;123:460–3.

107. Yamamoto K, Kawanishi S. Free radical production and site-specific DNA damage induced by hydralazine in the presence of metal ions of peroxidase/hydrogen peroxide. Biochem Pharmacol 1991;41:905–13.

108. Dunphy J, Oliver M, Rand AL, Lovell CR, McHugh NJ. Antineutrophil cytoplasmic antibodies and HLA class II alleles in minocycline-induced lupus-like syndrome. Br J Dermatol 2000;14:461–7.

109. Santos FX, Parolin A, Lindoso EM, Santos FH, Sousa LB. Hipertensão intracraniana com manifestações oculares associada ao uso de tetraciclina: relato de caso. Arq Bras Oftalmol 2005;68(5):701–3.

110. Altinbas A, Hoogstede HA, Bakker SL. Intracranial hypertension with severe and irreversible reduced acuity and impaired visual fields after oral tetracycline. Ned Tijdschr Geneeskd 2005;149(34):1908–12.

111. Morrison VL, Kikkawa DO, Herndier BG. Tetracycline induced green conjunctival pigment deposits. Br J Ophthalmol 2005;89(10):1372–3.

112. Chen JH, Shi CX, Wang M, Zhao SJ, Wang H. Clinical evaluation of 546 tetracycline-stained teeth treated with porcelain laminate veneers. J Dent 2005;33(1):3–8.

113. Garrison MW, Neumiller JJ, Setter SM. Tigecycline: an investigational glycylcycline antimicrobial with activity against resistant gram-positive organisms. Clin Ther 2005;27(1):12–22.

114. Rello J. Pharmacokinetics, pharmacodynamics, safety and tolerability of tigecycline. J Chemother 2005;17(Suppl 1):12–22.

115. Scheinfeld N. Tigecycline: a review of a new glycylcycline antibiotic. J Dermatolog Treat 2005;16(4):207–12.

116. Ellis-Grosse EJ, Babinchak T, Dartois N, Rose G, Loh E, Tigecycline 300 cSSSI Study Group. The efficacy and safety of tigecycline in the treatment of skin and skin-structure infections: results of 2 double-blind phase 3 comparison studies with vancomycin–aztreonam. Clin Infect Dis 2005;41(Suppl 5):S341–53.

117. Sacchidanand S, Penn RL, Embil JM, Campos ME, Curcio D, Ellis-Grosse E, Loh E, Rose G. Efficacy and safety of tigecycline monotherapy compared with vancomycin plus aztreonam in patients with complicated skin and skin structure infections: results from a phase 3, randomized, double-blind trial. Int J Infect Dis 2005;9(5):251–61.

118. Breedt J, Teras J, Gardovskis J, Maritz FJ, Vaasna T, Ross DP, Gioud-Paquet M, Dartois N, Ellis-Grosse EJ, Loh E, Tigecycline 305 cSSSI Study Group. Safety and efficacy of tigecycline in treatment of skin and skin structure infections: results of a double-blind phase 3 comparison study with vancomycin–aztreonam. Antimicrob Agents Chemother 2005;49(11):4658–66.

119. Babinchak T, Ellis-Grosse E, Dartois N, Rose GM, Loh E, Tigecycline 301 Study Group, Tigecycline 306 Study Group. The efficacy and safety of tigecycline for the treatment of complicated intra-abdominal infections: analysis of pooled clinical trial data. Clin Infect Dis 2005;41(Suppl 5):S354–67.

120. Oliva ME, Rekha A, Yellin A, Pasternak J, Campos M, Rose GM, Babinchak T, Ellis-Grosse EJ, Loh E, 301 Study Group. A multicenter trial of the efficacy and safety of tigecycline versus imipenem/cilastatin in patients with complicated intra-abdominal infections [Study ID Numbers: 3074A1-301-WW; ClinicalTrials.gov Identifier: NCT00081744]. BMC Infect Dis 2005;5:88.

121. Muralidharan G, Micalizzi M, Speth J, Raible D, Troy S. Pharmacokinetics of tigecycline after single and multiple doses in healthy subjects. Antimicrob Agents Chemother 2005;49(1):220–9.

Natascia Corti and Alexander Imhof

26 Miscellaneous antibacterial drugs

AMINOGLYCOSIDE ANTIBIOTICS *(SED-15, 118; SEDA-27, 251; SEDA-28, 274; SEDA-29, 253)*

Drug–drug interactions In a prospective study in 80 patients with cystic fibrosis and normal renal function, the combination of aminoglycosides with the polymyxin antibiotic *colistin* may have increased the risk of nephrotoxicity; in a multiple linear regression model there was a strong correlation between the use of aminoglycosides and reduced renal function, which was potentiated by colistin (1[C]).

Gentamicin *(SED-15, 1500; SEDA-29, 253)*

Sensory systems An intraocular injection of a high dose of gentamicin given by mistake led to severe *retinal damage*, which was at first misdiagnosed as central retinal artery occlusion; the damage was completely reversed by vitrectomy (2[A]).

Urinary tract Four women presented with a *Bartter-like syndrome*, with hypokalemia, metabolic alkalosis, hypomagnesemia, hypermagnesiuria, hypocalcemia, and hypercalciuria, after receiving gentamicin 1.2–2.6 g (3[c]). The syndrome lasted for 2–6 weeks after withdrawal of gentamicin.

  Acute tubular necrosis occurred in an adolescent with cystic fibrosis receiving intravenous gentamicin and ceftazidime (4[A]).

Neomycin

Sensory systems *Eighth nerve damage* from aminoglycosides can occur after topical administration.

- A 60-year-old man with a perforated tympanic membrane developed total hearing loss after the application of a cream containing neomycin, triamcinolone, gramicidin, and nystatin (5[A]).

Tobramycin *(SED-15, 3437; SEDA-29, 254)*

Sensory systems

Eyes A 59-year-old woman developed severe *erythema, edema, and exudation in the left eye and eyelid, with ocular pruritus*, after treatment with tobramycin 0.3% eye drops for several days after cataract removal (6[A]). Skin patch testing was positive and there was no response to the excipients. The symptoms subsided within 1 month after withdrawal of the eye drops.

Ears *Vestibular damage* without hearing loss has been reported with tobramycin.

- A 59-year old woman, a lung transplant recipient with sputum positive for *Pseudomonas aeruginosa*, taking tacrolimus and sirolimus, developed acute renal insufficiency and ataxia with bilateral vestibular system paresis but no hearing loss after using inhaled tobramycin 300 mg every 12 hours for 2 weeks (7[A]). After withdrawal, renal function improved but the vestibular symptoms never fully resolved.

Urinary tract In a double blind, randomized, controlled trial once-daily versus thrice-daily intravenous tobramycin was compared in 219

Side Effects of Drugs, Annual 30
J.K. Aronson (Editor)
ISSN: 0378-6080
DOI: 10.1016/S0378-6080(08)00026-3

patients with cystic fibrosis and pulmonary exacerbations (8[C]). In children once-daily treatment was significantly less nephrotoxic than
thrice daily administration ($n = 61$ versus 64).
However, the study was not powered to detect
differences in toxicity.

- Bone cement impregnated with tobramycin and cefazolin, which was placed into an infected total
knee arthroplasty, led to renal insufficiency in an
85-year-old man with pre-existing renal impairment (9[A]).

CHLORAMPHENICOL AND RELATED DRUGS   *(SED-15, 706; SEDA-29, 254)*

Chloramphenicol

Hematologic   *Paroxysmal nocturnal hemoglobinuria* occurred after 6 weeks of oral chloramphenicol therapy for treatment of a hip
prosthesis infection with *Bacillus fragilis* in a
78-year-old man (10[A]).

FLUOROQUINOLONES   *(SED-15, 1396; SEDA-27, 254; SEDA-28, 276; SEDA-29, 254)*

Metabolism   There was a higher rate of *hyperglycemia* with gatifloxacin or levofloxacin
compared with ceftriaxone in a retrospective
chart review of 17 000 patients (11[c]). Sulfonylurea therapy was identified as an independent
risk factor for hypoglycemia.

Teratogenicity   There was no increased risk
of overall malformations after prenatal exposure to fluoroquinolones in a database cohort
study of 217 women before or during pregnancy
(12[c]). However, there were more cases of bone
malformations in the children of women who
had been exposed before or during the first 30
days of pregnancy.

Ciprofloxacin   *(SED-15, 783; SEDA-29, 255)*

Nervous system   Ciprofloxacin might have
prolonged a *seizure* associated with electroconvulsive therapy in a patient with a urinary tract
infection (13[A]).

- A 43-year old woman developed a subacute confu-
sional state and involuntary movements after being
given ciprofloxacin, cephalexin, and co-amoxiclav
after an insect bite (14[A]). The antibiotics were
withdrawn. She later had two generalized tonic–
clonic seizures.

Sensory systems   Precipitation of topical ciprofloxacin on the corneal surface can delay
recovery from viral ocular surface infection
(15[A]).

- A 27-year-old man with an ophthalmic infection
with adenovirus type 3 had worse eye symptoms
within a week of treatment with 0.3% ciprofloxacin
ophthalmic solution. The ocular symptoms resolved after ciprofloxacin had been withdrawn and
white corneal precipitates had been scraped off.

Urinary tract   A 58-year-old woman developed *acute renal insufficiency* after taking ciprofloxacin 1 g without any other identifiable risk
factor (16[A]). Renal biopsy showed no evidence
of interstitial nephritis, but there were tubular
lesions and deposits of a brown-yellowish substance, which was identified as ciprofloxacin
salt. The outcome was favorable.

Skin   An 80-year-old woman taking ciprofloxacin developed *acute generalized exanthematous pustulosis* mimicking a bullous drug
eruption (17[A]).

Musculoskeletal   A 35-year-old man developed discomfort in his left medial thigh 3 days
after taking ciprofloxacin 500 mg bd for pneumonia; *rupture of the adductor longus tendon*
was confirmed by MRI (18[A]).

Drug–drug interactions   In eight patients
with non-Hodgkin's lymphoma ciprofloxacin
co-administration with *cyclophosphamide* resulted in a significantly lower exposure to
cyclophosphamide and in a lower ratio of
the AUCs of cyclophosphamide and its active
metabolite 4-hydroxycyclophosphamide (19[c]).
The authors postulated that ciprofloxacin inhibited CYP3A2, which is involved in the
conversion of cyclophosphamide to 4-hydroxy-
cyclophosphamide.

Gatifloxacin   *(SED-15, 1482;*
SEDA-29, 256)

Nervous system   Of five patients who devel-oped suspected drug-induced *aseptic meningi-tis*, one had been treated for *Salmonella* gas-troenteritis with ciprofloxacin (20[Ac]). Symp-toms of nervous system disease, including psychomotor excitement and deterioration of auto and allopsychical orientation, occurred after 4 days. She had a concomitant urticar-ial rash and considerable swelling of the face. Ciprofloxacin was immediately withdrawn and her symptoms improved.

Metabolism   In an observational study of spontaneous adverse events reports gatifloxacin was associated with much higher rates of *hy-poglycemia* and *hyperglycemia* (477 reports per 10^7 retail prescriptions) compared with ciprofloxacin (4 reports), levofloxacin (11 re-ports), and moxifloxacin (36 reports) (21[c]).

In four pivotal studies in 867 children, low concentrations of fasting and non-fasting glu-cose occurred more often in children taking gatifloxacin (5.8%) than in those taking co-amoxiclav (2.5%) (22[C]).

Gatifloxacin 600 mg intravenously has been associated with a serious episode of hypo-glycemia after cardiopulmonary bypass (23[A]).

Severe hyperglycemia occurred in a non-diabetic patient with progressive renal dys-function who took gatifloxacin 200 mg/day for 9 days (24[A]). Gatifloxacin was withdrawn and blood glucose concentrations returned to normal within several days after intensive treat-ment with insulin.

Susceptibility factors

Children   In a pharmacokinetic study in 111 children taking gatifloxacin oral suspension or tablets 5, 10, or 15 mg/kg, the most common adverse events were vomiting (17%), headache (3%), and rash (4%) (25[c]). Three had tran-siently increased liver function tests, up to seven times the upper limit of the reference range.

Drug–drug interactions   A 77-year old wom-an took gatifloxacin 400 mg/day for pneumonia together with *calcium carbonate* 500 mg and a multivitamin formulation and failed to im-prove (26[A]). The time of administration of

gatifloxacin was changed and her symptoms improved 2 days later. However, plasma con-centrations of gatifloxacin were not measured. Reduced absorption of quinolones by divalent and trivalent cations such as aluminium, mag-nesium, calcium, iron, and zinc occurs by the formation of insoluble chelates.

Levofloxacin   *(SED-15, 2047;*
SEDA-29, 257)

Nervous system   *Increased seizure activity* has been associated with the use of levofloxacin.

- A 75-year-old man with Alzheimer's disease, chronic renal insufficiency, and seizures was given levofloxacin 500 mg/day for 1 week for a urinary tract infection and developed increased seizure ac-tivity over 3 days; the seizure activity ceased after withdrawal of levofloxacin (27[A]).
- A 73-year old man with community-acquired pneumonia took oral levofloxacin after complet-ing treatment with intravenous ceftriaxone and 2 days later became disoriented and confused; the symptoms regressed completely after withdrawal of levofloxacin (28[A]).

Liver   Acute fulminant fatal *hepatic failure* has been reported in a patient taking lev-ofloxacin (29[A]).

- A 55-year-old woman with asymptomatic he-patitis B infection was given oral levofloxacin 500 mg/day for 10 days for an upper respiratory tract infection. On day 12 she developed mixed hepatocellular and cholestatic liver damage, with transaminases 20 tomes the upper limit of the refer-ence range. Despite supportive treatment she died 12 weeks later.

Skin   Cases of *toxic epidermal necrolysis* have been reported in patients taking levofloxacin.

- An 87-year-old woman developed a pruritic rash on her trunk and limbs 3 hours after taking a single dose of levofloxacin followed by a gener-alized seizure (30[A]). A skin biopsy confirmed the diagnosis of toxic epidermal necrolysis. She had developed a rash after taking ciprofloxacin several years before, which had probably sensitized her to levofloxacin.
- A 15-year-old boy developed fatal toxic epider-mal necrolysis, with a pruritic rash, fever, and joint pains, after taking levofloxacin 500 mg/day for 9 days (31[A]). The exfoliation progressed to involve 80% of the body surface and he died despite sup-portive treatment.

Musculoskeletal A 19-year-old man developed *rhabdomyolysis* with swelling and weakness of the arms and creatine kinase activity up to 16 546 U/l having taken ofloxacin and then levofloxacin for periorbital cellulitis; the symptoms improved after withdrawal of levofloxacin (32[A]).

Immunologic A 33-year old Japanese man developed a severe *anaphylactic reaction* 10 minutes after taking his first dose of levofloxacin with mefenamic acid and L-carbocysteine orally; patch tests only showed a reaction to levofloxacin (33[A]).

Drug–drug interactions Levofloxacin and ciprofloxacin reduced the renal clearance of procainamide and N-acetylprocainamide (acecainide) (34[c]).

Moxifloxacin *(SED-15, 2392; SEDA-29, 257)*

Nervous system Moxifloxacin has been reported to cause *coma* (35[A]).

- A 56 year old woman with Child–Pugh A grade alcoholic cirrhosis became comatose after taking oral moxifloxacin 400 mg/day for 8 days. After intravenous treatment with gammahydroxybutyrate (GHB) she became conscious and oriented.

Quinolones inhibit the binding of GABA to its receptor and gammahydroxybutyrate is structurally similar to GABA.

Immunologic Although moxifloxacin is chemically different from other fluoroquinolones, in six patients with hypersensitivity to different fluoroquinolones there was cross-reactivity between moxifloxacin, ciprofloxacin, levofloxacin, and ofloxacin, confirmed by skin tests (36[c]).

Drug–drug interactions In five cases an interaction of moxifloxacin with *warfarin* was suspected to be the cause of a raised international normalized ratio (INR), with clinically significant hemorrhage in one; in three cases the interaction was assessed as probable and in two as possible (37[c]).

Norfloxacin *(SED-15, 2583; SEDA-29, 258)*

Skin A 40-year-old man developed *toxic epidermal necrolysis* 10 days after the end of a 14-day course of norfloxacin 800 mg/day (38[A]). He had typical cutaneous and mucous lesions and recovered after treatment with oral prednisolone and fluids.

Drug–drug interactions The AUC of *mycophenolic acid* after a single dose was reduced by 10% when norfloxacin was given concomitantly (39[c]).

Ofloxacin *(SED-15, 2597; SEDA-29, 258)*

Skin A 40-year-old woman developed *Sweet's syndrome* after taking ofloxacin for 3 days for watery bloody diarrhea in the course of Crohn's disease (40[A]). She had a fever (38.6 °C), rash, abdominal tenderness, and painful joints. Her symptoms resolved spontaneously 3 days after withdrawal of ofloxacin.

Sparfloxacin *(SED-15, 3172; SEDA-29, 259)*

Nails *Blue-black discoloration of the nails* occurred in three patients taking sparfloxacin; the discoloration gradually moved distally and disappeared within 6 months (41[c]).

During treatment for tuberculosis with sparfloxacin, streptomycin, ethambutol, and pyrazinamide a 36-year-old man developed an exaggerated sunburn-like rash with painful onycholysis of the fingernails and toenails; after withdrawal of sparfloxacin and substitution of rifampicin, the symptoms improved (41[A]).

GLYCOPEPTIDES *(SEDA-27, 259; SEDA-28, 280; SEDA-29, 260)*

Dalbavancin *(SEDA-29, 260)*

Comparative studies Dalbavancin has been compared with vancomycin in an open, multicenter, phase 2 study in 67 patients with catheter-related septicemia (42[C]). Intravenous dalbavancin was given to 33 patients as a single dose of 1000 mg followed by a dose of 500 mg 1 week later. The most common medication related adverse events were *diarrhea* (7%), *constipation* (6%), *fever* (6%), and *oral candidiasis* (4%).

Teicoplanin   *(SED-15, 3305; SEDA-29, 260)*

Immunologic   A 76-year-old man receiving intramuscular teicoplanin 400 mg/day for septic arthritis due to *Staphylococcus aureus* developed a vasculitis with cutaneous and renal involvement (43[A]). On day 17, tender purpura appeared in his legs, and there was concomitant impairment of renal function. A skin biopsy showed the typical features of a *leukocytoclastic vasculitis*. Teicoplanin was withdrawn and he was given flucloxacillin and prednisolone. The purpura resolved and renal function recovered partly.

Vancomycin   *(SED-15, 3593; SEDA-29, 261)*

Immunologic   *Hypersensitivity reactions* to vancomycin have been described.

- A 56-year-old white woman developed a drug-induced hypersensitivity syndrome after receiving intravenous vancomycin 2 g/day for 20 days for methicillin-resistant *Staphylococcus aureus* (44[A]). She developed a fever and a maculopapular rash, which progressed to purpuric erythema multiforme without mucosal lesions, associated with pharyngitis, leukocytosis, and eosinophilia. There was organ involvement, with raised liver enzymes and creatinine. She was given methylprednisolone for 2 month until the laboratory findings and cutaneous lesions normalized.
- In a 45 year old Caucasian woman acute interstitial nephritis and hepatitis did not improve after withdrawal of vancomycin and empirical glucocorticoid administration, but the rash resolved and renal function recovered after a 5-day course of ciclosporin (45[A]).
- A 76-year-old man developed progressive itching, soreness, photophobia, and lacrimation in the left eye 3 days after completing a 2-week course of 5% vancomycin eye-drops after cataract surgery (46[A]). Vancomycin skin tests were positive and his

symptoms resolved after treatment with an antihistamine and systemic and topical glucocorticoids.

KETOLIDES   *(SED-15, 1976; SEDA-27, 260; SEDA-28, 281; SEDA-29, 262)*

Telithromycin

Observational studies   In an open multicenter study in 432 patients with community-acquired pneumonia given telithromycin 800 mg/day for 7 days, *diarrhea* was reported in 8.1% and nausea in 5.8% (47[c]). Six patients discontinued treatment because of *allergic reactions, abdominal pain, vomiting, vertigo*, or *increased alanine transaminase activity*, which were considered possibly related to telithromycin. Two patients had non-significant *prolongation of the QT interval*.

Placebo-controlled studies   In three randomized, double blind, multicenter studies in 609 patients who took telithromycin 800 mg/day for 5 days for exacerbations of chronic bronchitis, *diarrhea* and *nausea* occurred in 6.4 and 4.8% respectively (48[M]). One patient had QT_c *interval prolongation* from 488 to 531 ms, which returned to baseline after the end of therapy.

Skin   An 18-year-old woman with infectious mononucleosis developed a *pruritic rash* after treatment with co-amoxiclav (49[A]). Treatment was switched to telithromycin, and the rash started to resolve but worsened again, with the development of additional headache and joint pains. The antibiotic was withdrawn and the symptoms and the rash resolved with supportive therapy with antihistamines and methylprednisolone.

Drug–drug interactions   A possible interaction of *verapamil* with telithromycin has been reported (50[A]).

- A 76-year-old woman took telithromycin 800 mg/day for nasal congestion and malaise in additional to verapamil 180 mg/day among others. Two days later she developed profound hypotension and a junctional rhythm at 30/minute. A temporary pacemaker was necessary.

LINCOSAMIDES   *(SED-15, 2063;*
SEDA-27, 260; SEDA-28, 281; SEDA-29, 263)

Clindamycin

Skin   In a retrospective study of drug reactions in children with various ear, nose, and throat infections, seven of 62 reported cases of skin reactions were attributed to clindamycin (51[c]).

MACROLIDE ANTIBIOTICS
(SED-15, 2183; SEDA-27, 261; SEDA-28, 282;
SEDA-29, 263)

Azithromycin   *(SED-15, 389;*
SEDA-29, 264)

Cardiovascular   *Polymorphous ventricular tachycardia* has been attributed to azithromycin (52[A]).

- A 51-year-old woman took azithromycin 500 mg for an upper respiratory tract infection shortly after a dose of over-the-counter pseudoephedrine. Two hours later she had two syncopal events due to polymorphous ventricular tachycardia without QT interval prolongation. Azithromycin was withdrawn and the ventricular tachycardia abated after 10 hours. She was symptom-free 1 year later.

Liver   Liver damage has been attributed to azithromycin (53[A]).

- A 75-year-old woman took azithromycin 500 mg/day for 3 days and developed jaundice, fatigue, and diarrhea. She had a history of allergy to penicillin, morphine, and pethidine. Transaminases, bilirubin, and alkaline phosphatase were raised. Liver biopsy showed centrilobular necrosis consistent with a drug reaction. Two months later her liver function tests had returned to baseline.

Skin   In a randomized, multicenter, double-blind study *rash* was reported in 2.5% of patients after a single dose of azithromycin for acute otitis media (54[C]).

- A 5-year-old child developed Stevens–Johnson syndrome 3 days after starting a course of azithromycin and improved after treatment with a glucocorticoid for 28 days (55[A]).

Clarithromycin   *(SED-15, 799;*
SEDA-29, 265)

Sensory systems   An 81-year-old woman developed irreversible *sensorineural hearing loss* in the right ear 3 days after starting low-dose clarithromycin for an acute exacerbation of chronic obstructive pulmonary disease (56[A]).

Skin   Various eruptions have been attributed to clarithromycin.

- A 68-year-old woman developed a fixed drug eruption on the tongue after taking clarithromycin for 4 days for an acute upper respiratory infection (57[A]). The erythematous violaceous patch over the posterior dorsum of the tongue resolved 15 days after withdrawal of the drug.
- A 29-year-old woman with tonsillitis was given clarithromycin and developed a pruritic rash after 48 hours (58[A]). Despite switching to amoxicillin her condition worsened, with the appearance of bullous lesions on her abdomen, a fever of 40 °C, peeling of 70% of the body surface, and mucosal involvement. Stevens–Johnson syndrome was diagnosed. She recovered with residual scars on the skin and ophthalmic lesions.

Drug–drug interactions   Clarithromycin can inhibit the metabolism of other drugs.

- An 85-year old woman, who was taking carbamazepine, fluoxetine, a benzodiazepine, an ACE inhibitor, a statin, and a coumarin anticoagulant, developed confusion and asterixis, with raised liver enzymes and an increased international normalized ratio (INR) after taking clarithromycin for 10 days for a respiratory infection (59[A]).

This presentation was associated with *carbamazepine* and *coumarin* toxicity caused by an interaction with clarithromycin.

In a 77-year-old man a life-threatening pharmacokinetic interaction of clarithromycin with *nifedipine* was suspected as the cause of vasodilatory shock (60[A]).

Erythromycin   *(SED-15, 1237;*
SEDA-29, 265)

Liver   Liver damage due to erythromycin is well described.

- After two doses of erythromycin ethylsuccinate, following unsuccessful treatment with penicillin for a respiratory illness, a 10-year-old previously healthy girl developed liver damage (61[A]). Liver biopsy showed moderate panlobular parenchymatous degeneration with cholestasis due to numerous intracellular and intraductal bile plugs. She recovered completely 6–8 weeks after withdrawal of erythromycin.

Drug–drug interactions   Co-administration of modified-release erythromycin 999 mg in an adolescent taking methylphenidate and *bupropion* was associated with an acute myocardial infarction (62[A]). Co-administration of erythromycin may have inhibited CYP3A4-dependent metabolism of bupropion, leading to raised plasma bupropion concentrations and excessive vasospasm due to the sympathetic effect of methylphenidate and bupropion.

Co-administration of erythromycin tds increased exposure to *quetiapine* 200 mg bd significantly in Chinese patients by inhibition of the CYP3A4-dependent metabolism of quetiapine; the C_{max} rose by 68% and the AUC by 129% (63[C]). Intra individual variability was large and so a fixed modification of the dosage regimen could not be recommended.

Roxithromycin   *(SED-15, 3083;*
SEDA-29, 266)

Nails   A 22-year-old office worker developed *onycholysis* after taking roxithromycin 150 mg bd for 8 weeks for chronic sinusitis (64[A]).

NITROFURANTOIN   *(SED-15, 2542;*
SEDA-27, 264; SEDA-28, 284; SEDA-29, 266)

Respiratory
DoTS classification:
Reaction: Nitrofurantoin-induced lung disease
Dose relation: Hypersusceptibility reaction
Time course: Late
Susceptibility factors: Female sex

Nitrofurantoin causes *acute lung injury* more often than any other drug. Acute respiratory reactions include dyspnea, cough, interstitial pneumonitis, and pleural effusion; interstitial pneumonitis and fibrosis are common chronic reactions (SEDA-25, 310). In a retrospective analysis of 18 patients with chronic nitrofurantoin-induced lung disease (median age 72 years, range 47–90; 17 women) the median daily dosage of nitrofurantoin was 100 mg (range 50–200) (65[C]). The onset of symptoms occurred after a median duration of 23 months (range 10–144). Although the clinical and radiological presentation is non-specific, there are characteristic features on CT that are distinctly different from those seen in idiopathic pulmonary fibrosis. Most patients with chronic nitrofurantoin-induced lung disease will improve, either on withdrawal of nitrofurantoin alone or with the addition of a glucocorticoid. However, it is not uncommon for residual infiltrates to persist in the long term.

Hematologic   A 74-year-old white man developed *agranulocytosis* after a short course of nitrofurantoin 100 mg qds (66[A]). On day 5 the total white blood cell count and granulocyte count fell to 1.9×10^9/l and 0.5×10^9/l respectively. Nitrofurantoin was withdrawn and replaced with cefuroxime and 2 days later the total white blood cell count and granulocyte count had increased to 2.5×10^9/l and 1.1×10^9/l respectively.

Salivary glands   Nitrofurantoin can cause *parotitis* (67[A]).

Skin   *Stevens–Johnson syndrome* and *toxic epidermal necrolysis* are more common in the setting of a compromised immune system.

- Stevens–Johnson syndrome occurred in a 24-year-old HIV-positive pregnant woman who took nitrofurantoin for 2 days (68[A]).

Treatment with nitrofurantoin is rarely associated with a *lupus-like syndrome*.

- A 71-year-old woman developed a lupus-like syndrome associated with hepatitis after taking nitrofurantoin for 5 years; her symptoms rapidly improved with systemic glucocorticoid therapy (69[A]). The symptoms resolved after withdrawal of nitrofurantoin.

OXAZOLIDINONES   *(SED-15, 2645; SEDA-27, 264; SEDA-28, 284; SEDA-29, 266)*

Linezolid is the first of an entirely new class of antibiotics in decades, the oxazolidinones. It has a spectrum of activity against virtually all important Gram-positive pathogens. The unique mechanism of action of linezolid makes cross-resistance with other antimicrobial agents unlikely. Linezolid is marketed in intravenous and oral formulations and the latter has 100% systemic availability. Since its first approval and marketing in March 2000 in the USA, linezolid has gained approval for use in many other countries for the treatment of community-acquired and nosocomial pneumonia, complicated and uncomplicated skin and soft-tissue infections, and infections caused by methicillin-resistant *Staphylococcus aureus* and vancomycin-resistant enterococci, including cases with concurrent bacteremia (70[r]).

Observational studies   In a retrospective analysis in 42 patients receiving linezolid for osteomyelitis, the clinical cure rate was 55% in the 20 patients who received therapy for at least 6 weeks. Adverse events included *gastrointestinal disturbances* (15%), *thrombocytopenia* (10%), *anemia* (10%), *neutropenia* (5%), and *rash* (5%) (71[c]).

Nervous system   Long-term use of linezolid can be associated with *severe peripheral and optic neuropathy* (72[R]). In most cases, the optic neuropathy resolved after withdrawal of linezolid but the peripheral neuropathy did not. The duration of therapy rather than the indication for treatment seems to be the most important factor.

Linezolid-induced *peripheral neurotoxicity* has been reported (73[A], 74[A]).

- A 70-year-old man took linezolid for 10–12 days and complained of numbness in his toes. Nerve conduction studies showed sensory motor axonal damage. During the next 5 months he develop progressive perineal anesthesia without fecal incontinence or urinary tract disorder. Spinal cord MRI and nerve biopsy were normal. The hemoglobin was 8.5 g/dl. Linezolid was withdrawn after 24 weeks of therapy. The perineal anesthesia disappeared after 8 months, but the neuropathy persisted.
- A 45-year-old woman complained of bilateral, predominantly left-sided paresthesia of the toes after taking linezolid for 6 months. One week later,

linezolid was withdrawn because of a glove-and-stocking neuropathy without abnormal ankle reflexes. Nerve conduction studies were compatible with a sensory axonal neuropathy. Two weeks after withdrawal of linezolid, she reported subjective improvement of the sensory perception. After 3 months minor bilateral paresthesia persisted.
- A 38-year-old man presented with bilateral isolated lower limb dysesthesia after taking linezolid for 2 months. Linezolid was withdrawn and voriconazole was continued while the neurological signs improved. Spinal MRI and lumbar puncture were normal; a search for antineuronal antibodies in serum and CSF was negative. After 6 months the paresthesia persisted.
- A 42-year-old woman developed a severe irreversible sensory polyneuropathy after a 6-month course of linezolid.

Sensory systems   Two patients undergoing long-term treatment (both 11 months) with linezolid for pneumonia had *reduced visual acuity, dyschromatopsia*, and *cecocentral scotomata* characteristic of toxic optic neuropathy (75[A]). Visual function slowly recovered 3–4 months after withdrawal of linezolid.

- A 56-year-old man developed a toxic optic neuropathy after long-term treatment with linezolid 600 mg bd for 12 months then 600 mg/day for 44 months (76[A]). Linezolid was withdrawn and he noted subjective visual improvement within several weeks.
- A 27-year-old woman developed an optic and peripheral neuropathy after taking linezolid for 154 days for osteomyelitis (77[A]). A glucocorticoid exacerbated the visual loss. Withdrawal of linezolid resulted in marked improvement.

Metabolism   *Hyperlactatemia* and *metabolic acidosis* are adverse effects of linezolid that could be related to impaired mitochondrial function. Linezolid-induced lactic acidosis occurred in a 70-year-old man during the first 7 days of treatment with linezolid (78[A]). Mitochondria were studied from three patients, in whom weakness and hyperlactatemia developed during therapy with linezolid (79[c]). The results suggested that linezolid interferes with mitochondrial protein synthesis, probably because of similarities between bacterial and mitochondrial ribosomes.

Hematologic   Linezolid has been associated with dose-dependent and time-dependent reversible *myelosuppression* (including anemia, leukopenia, thrombocytopenia, and pancytopenia). The mechanism for the anemia is thought to be inhibition of mitochondrial respiration. The thrombocytopenia appears to result from immune-mediated platelet destruction. It is now recommended that complete blood counts be monitored weekly in patients who take linezolid, especially those who take it for more than 2 weeks. In children, thrombocytopenia is less common; however, the complete blood count should be monitored weekly while children are taking linezolid. Vitamin B_6 50 mg/day may prevent or modify the course of linezolid-associated cytopenias. Two patients developed dyserythropoietic anemia, strikingly similar to chloramphenicol-associated myelotoxicity, after taking linezolid for 25–28 days (80[A]).

In a retrospective case-control study of linezolid in 91 patients with end-stage renal disease, of whom 28 were receiving hemodialysis at the start of therapy, and patients with non-end-stage renal disease, the former had significantly more frequent severe thrombocytopenia (79 versus 43%) and anemia (71 versus 37%) (81[c]). Survival analysis for thrombocytopenia or death showed significant differences between the groups.

In a retrospective study patients taking linezolid with lower pre-treatment hematological values were at greater risk not only of anemia but also thrombocytopenia (82[c]).

Immunologic   Linezolid-related *leukocytoclastic vasculitis* occurred in a 68-year-old man after 7 days of treatment with linezolid 600 mg bd (83[A]).

Drug dosage regimens   Linezolid crosses the blood–retina barrier in non-inflamed eyes. The vitreous concentration in 12 adults after a single 600 mg oral dose rose exponentially with time and 33% of the late group achieved sufficient MIC_{90} concentrations for the common pathogens found in postoperative endophthalmitis (84[c]). The vitreous linezolid concentration correlated strongly with the interpolated serum concentration. Adequate concentrations might therefore be achieved with an altered dosage regimen to achieve higher serum steady-state concentrations.

Drug–drug interactions   Linezolid is a monoamine oxidase inhibitor, and particular attention has been paid to the question of whether *drugs that are metabolized by monoamine oxidase* interact with linezolid (85[M]).

Linezolid interacts with *selective serotonin reuptake inhibitors* (SSRIs) and other sympathomimetic drugs, resulting in the serotonin syndrome. There have been two cases of serotonin syndrome due to interaction of linezolid with venlafaxine (86[A]), one case in a patient taking linezolid, amitriptyline, and paroxetine (87[A]), and one in a patient taking linezolid, citalopram, and mirtazapine (88[A]). In a retrospective study 12 patients (mean age 53 years) were found with linezolid-associated serotonin syndrome (89[c]). All had taken linezolid concomitantly with an SSRI. The onset of syndrome was 9.5 days after the introduction of linezolid and was directly correlated with age. The symptoms resolved in 2.9 days. Citalopram was associated with delayed resolution. There was a trend towards a longer resolution time the longer the half-life of the interacting drug.

Encephalopathy in a 74-year-old woman was attributed to an interaction of linezolid with *hydroxyzine* (73[A]).

POLYMYXINS

Colistin   *(SED-15, 2891; SEDA-27, 265; SEDA-28, 285; SEDA-29, 268)*

Two different forms of colistin are available for clinical use. Colistin sulfate is administered orally for bowel decontamination and is used topically as a powder for the treatment of bacterial skin infections; colistimethate sodium (also called colistin methanesulfate, pentasodium colistimethanesulfate, colistin sulfamethate, and colistin sulfonyl methate) is given intravenously and intramuscularly. Both formulations have been used in aerosols. However, colistimethate sodium is associated with fewer adverse effects, such as *chest tightness, throat irritation,* and *cough,* than colistin sulfate (90[A]).

Respiratory   Treatment with aerosolized colistin can be complicated by *bronchoconstriction* and *chest tightness.* Colistin caused bronchospasm in 20 patients with cystic fibrosis chronically infected with *Pseudomonas aeruginosa* in a placebo-controlled clinical trial with a crossover design testing colistin 75 mg in

4 ml of saline solution and a placebo solution of the same osmolarity using a breath-enhanced nebulizer for administration (91[C]). However, treatment with inhaled beta$_2$-adrenoceptor agonists before the start of treatment can prevent bronchoconstriction (92[R]).

Nervous system   The most common adverse effects of colistin are nephrotoxicity and neurotoxicity. Neurological toxicity is associated with *dizziness, weakness, facial and peripheral paresthesia, vertigo, visual disturbances, confusion, ataxia*, and *neuromuscular blockade*, which can lead to respiratory failure or apnea. The incidence of colistin-associated neurotoxicity reported in earlier literature was about 7%, paresthesia constituting the main adverse event. Neurotoxic events related to colistin occur more often in patients with cystic fibrosis (29% of patients who receive colistin experience paresthesia, ataxia, or both). Neurological toxicity is dose-related and is usually reversible after early withdrawal.

Intraventricular administration of colistin, especially in high doses, can cause *convulsions* (92[R]).

Urinary tract   Nephrotoxicity has been reported in 20% of 317 courses of colistin therapy and is mainly due to *acute tubular necrosis*. The risk of nephrotoxicity increases in the setting of pre-existing renal dysfunction and with increasing doses. Serum concentrations and toxicity appear to be a function of glomerular filtration rate (93[A]). Renal toxicity is dose-related and is usually reversible after early withdrawal. However, there are a few published reports of irreversible nephrotoxicity after withdrawal of colistin (91[R]).

In a prospective, observational, cohort study in 21 patients who received intravenous colistin for at least 7 days (median daily dose 17.7 mg and median duration of treatment 15 days), three patients developed nephrotoxicity (94[C]). The cumulative dose of colistin correlated with the difference in serum creatinine concentrations between the start and end of treatment.

- A 57-year-old man developed acute renal insufficiency after receiving colistin 250 mg intravenously every 6 hours for 4 days (94[A]).
- A 35-year-old man who received colistin 6 MU intravenously divided into three daily doses had no adverse effects. However, during two subsequent courses 1 month and 4 months later he developed acute renal insufficiency (95[A]).

In both of these episodes, renal function returned to normal values within 3–5 days after colistin withdrawal and despite the continuation of all other drugs.

In an observational retrospective cohort study of 17 patients who received intravenous colistin for more than 4 weeks, 19 courses of prolonged treatment were identified (96[c]). The mean duration of administration was 43 days, and the mean cumulative dose was 190 million IU. The median creatinine concentration rose by 220 µmol/l during treatment compared with baseline but returned to near baseline at the end of treatment.

Skin   *Hypersensitivity reactions, rash, urticaria, generalized itching*, and *fever* can occur during therapy with colistin, the incidence of allergic reactions being 2% (92[R]).

- A 27-year-old woman developed an allergic contact dermatitis after having both ears pierced followed by prophylactic application of an ointment containing colistin sulfate and bacitracin (97[A]). The eruption responded to a glucocorticoid ointment. Patch tests showed positive reactions to colistin sulfate and bacitracin.

Susceptibility factors   Intravenous colistin methanesulfonate is converted in vivo to colistin, and these two compounds have substantially different pharmacokinetics, antibacterial activities, and adverse effects. Patients who are currently receiving colistin methanesulfonate are often in intensive care units, have multiple organ dysfunctions, and receive renal replacement therapy.

- A 53-year-old woman weighing 110 kg undergoing continuous venovenous hemodiafiltration was given intravenous colistin methanesulfonate 150 mg (equivalent to 2.46 mg/kg ideal body weight) every 24 hours, reduced to 150 mg/48 hours after 14 days (98[A]). Each dose was given as a 30-minute infusion. The maximum concentration of colistin in plasma occurred 30 minutes after completion of the infusion, consistent with relatively rapid conversion to colistin. The terminal plasma half-lives of colistin methanesulfonate and colistin were 6.83 and 7.52 hours respectively. The total clearance of colistin methanesulfonate was 49 ml/minute and its volume of distribution was 11 liters. From 0 to 8 hours after dosing, 20% of the dose was recovered in the dialysate as colistin methanesulfonate and 6.9% as colistin. The hemodiafiltration clearances of colistin methanesulfonate and colistin were similar (11 and 12 ml/minute).

Drug–drug interactions   For the interaction of colistin with *aminoglycoside antibiotics*, see above.

Mupirocin

In a systematic review only one study reported any adverse events, primarily *rhinorrhea* and *itching at the application site*, in 4.8% of mupirocin recipients and 4.8% of placebo recipients (99[M]). Although five patients withdrew because of adverse events, only one of these patients was receiving mupirocin.

STREPTOGRAMINS   *(SED-15, 3182; SEDA-27, 265; SEDA-28, 285; SEDA-29, 269)*

Pristinamycin

Pristinamycin is a mixture of water-insoluble pristinamycin IA and pristinamycin IIA, derived from *Streptomyces pristinaespiralis*. The former is a group B streptogramin (a peptidic macrolactone or depsipeptide), and the latter is a group A streptogramin (a polyunsaturated macrolactone). Group A and group B streptogramins are both bacteriostatic by reversible binding of the 50S subunit of 70S bacterial ribosomes. Together, however, they are synergistic and bactericidal.

In a retrospective chart review of 27 patients with osteoarticular infections, there were adverse effects of pristinamycin in eight cases; seven were *gastrointestinal disturbances* and there was one instance of an *allergic rash*, which required drug withdrawal (100[c]).

Skin   *Toxic epidermal necrolysis* has been reported in a patient receiving pristinamycin (101[A]).

- A 75-year-old man developed a rash 4 hours after the start of treatment with pristinamycin. Extensive epidermal detachment was noted 48 hours later, with a positive Nikolsky's sign, and it progressed to cover 40% of the body surface. Skin biopsy confirmed toxic epidermal necrolysis, with subepidermal blistering and numerous necrotic keratinocytes. Re-epithelialization occurred in 3 weeks. Two weeks later pristinamycin

was given again and 2 hours later he developed a high fever with a generalized rash and large blisters associated with erosions in the buccal and ophthalmic mucosa. The blisters progressively covered the entire body surface. A skin biopsy confirmed toxic epidermal necrolysis. He died of multiorgan failure.

Quinupristin/dalfopristin

Quinupristin/dalfopristin is a semisynthetic injectable combination of streptogramins. Each is bacteriostatic against staphylococci and streptococci. Adverse effects include *infusion-site reactions* (42%), *infusion-site pain* (40%), *edema* (17%), *arthralgias* (47%), *myalgias* (6%), *gastrointestinal effects* (3–5%), *rash* (2.5%), *headache* (1.6%), *pruritus* (1.5%), and *hyperbilirubinemia* (25%) (102[R], 103[R]).

Hematologic   Quinupristin/dalfopristin is rarely associated with hematological adverse events, but *reticulocytopenia* has recently been reported (104[A]).

- A 52-year-old woman developed a reticulocytopenia after receiving quinupristin/dalfopristin 750 mg intravenously every 8 hours for 4 weeks. Before therapy, the hemoglobin concentration was 13 g/dl and it fell to 6.8 g/dl, with an absolute reticulocyte count of 2.4×10^9/l (reference range 28.4–150). Quinupristin/dalfopristin was withdrawn and doxycycline 100 mg orally bd was started. Four days later, the absolute reticulocyte count was 146×10^9/l. She completed her course of doxycycline without further complications.

Virginiamycin   *(SEDA-26, 293; SEDA-27, 268; SEDA-28, 288; SEDA-29, 273)*

Virginiamycin is a growth-promoting streptogramin antibacterial used as a feed additive in animals.

Drug tolerance (antibacterial resistance)
The use of virginiamycin has been linked to selection of *Enterococcus faecium* organisms resistant to quinupristin/dalfopristin. Because virginiamycin has been used in animals, but streptogramins have been used infrequently in human medicine, an animal origin of resistance has been suggested, and spread of this resistance via the food chain to humans is probable (105[E]).

SULFONAMIDES, TRIMETHOPRIM, AND CO-TRIMOXAZOLE *(SED-15, 3216, 3510; SEDA-27, 266; SEDA-28, 285; SEDA-29, 270)*

Trimethoprim and co-trimoxazole

Nervous system   *Aseptic meningitis* is a rare adverse reaction to co-trimoxazole.

- A 46-year-old African–American man with AIDS was admitted on two different occasions within 3 weeks with signs and symptoms of meningitis after using co-trimoxazole (106[A]).

Endocrine   Co-trimoxazole 14–16 mg/kg orally every 12 hours for 3 weeks in dogs *reduced total and free T4 concentrations and increased the TSH concentration*, conditions that would be compatible with hypothyroidism (107[E]). However, hypothyroidism has not been attributed to co-trimoxazole in humans.

Hematologic   Atovaquone+azithromycin and co-trimoxazole have been compared in a randomized, double-blind, placebo-controlled trial for 2 years in 366 HIV-infected children aged 3 months to 19 years (108[C]). Grade 3 and grade 4 hematological adverse events during co-trimoxazole therapy were *neutropenia* (9.3%), *thrombocytopenia* (8.8%), and *anemia* (2.2%).

- A 40-year-old man developed neutropenia, severe thrombocytopenia, and a fever, with a diffuse erythematous maculopapular rash after taking co-trimoxazole twice daily (109[A]).

Neutropenia is the most frequent adverse effect of co-trimoxazole in sub-Saharan Africa. In a prospective cohort study the incidence of hematological disorders was estimated during the first 6 months of a zidovudine-containing highly-active antiretroviral therapy regimen in 498 sub-Saharan African adults taking co-trimoxazole (110[C]). There was an unexpectedly high incidence of grade 3–4 neutropenia shortly after the introduction of zidovudine. Almost all of the persistent cases disappeared after co-trimoxazole was withdrawn. This suggests an interaction between these two drugs in sub-Saharan Africans.

Liver   In a retrospective study of suspected hepatic adverse drug reactions with fatal outcomes received by the Swedish Adverse Drug Reactions Advisory Committee (SADRAC) from 1966 to 2002, six patients (median age 55 years, range 17–87; three men) taking co-trimoxazole died because of *liver failure* (four hepatocellular, one cholestatic, one mixed); the median duration of treatment was 10 (3–22) days (111[cS]).

Pancreas   Drug-related acute *pancreatitis* is uncommon.

- A 53-year-old woman repeatedly developed pancreatitis after co-trimoxazole; a causal relation was confirmed by relapse after rechallenge (112[A]).

Skin   In a randomized, single-blind study in 59 patients with active ocular toxoplasmosis randomly assigned to pyrimethamine + sulfadiazine or co-trimoxazole, adverse reactions were limited to one patient in each treatment group, in both cases a *rash* (113[C]).

Urticarial vasculitis is characterized by the association of urticarial papules lasting for more than 24 hours with histological cutaneous vasculitis.

- A 30-year-old woman developed urticarial, purpuric, and necrotic cutaneous lesions of the legs after taking oral co-trimoxazole for 2 weeks (114[A]).

In a randomized, double-blind, placebo-controlled comparison of atovaquone + azithromycin and co-trimoxazole for 2 years in 366 HIV-infected children aged 3 months to 19 years, 26% of those who took co-trimoxazole had moderate rashes and two had life-threatening rashes (108[C]).

- A 70-year-old Asian man developed toxic epidermal necrolysis within a few hours of the first dose of trimethoprim for a urinary tract infection (115[A]). His skin became sore and itchy and he developed large blisters involving the trunk, buttocks, thighs, and perineum (about 60% of the body surface area).

Drug–drug interactions   Trimethoprim is a selective inhibitor of CYP2C8 in vitro. *Rosiglitazone* is predominantly metabolized in the liver by CYP2C8. The effect of trimethoprim on rosiglitazone metabolism in vitro has been determined in pooled liver microsomes and in a randomized crossover study in eight healthy subjects, who took a single dose of rosiglitazone 8 mg before and after taking trimethoprim 200 mg bd for 5 days (116[Ec]). Trimethoprim significantly inhibited the metabolism of rosiglitazone in vitro and in vivo it increased the AUC of rosiglitazone by 31% and the half-life by 27%. There was also a reduction in the plasma concentration of rosiglitazone metabolites. Trimethoprim should therefore be used with caution in patients with type 2 diabetes who are also taking rosiglitazone.

In 15 renal transplant recipients a single dose of co-trimoxazole did not affect the pharmacokinetics of *sirolimus* (117[c]).

OTHER ANTIMICROBIAL DRUGS

Daptomycin   (SED-15, 1053; SEDA-27, 267; SEDA-28, 287; SEDA-29, 271)

Daptomycin is a cyclic lipopeptide antibiotic used in the treatment of serious Gram-positive infections, including those caused by methicillin-resistant *Staphylococcus aureus* and vancomycin-resistant enterococci. In clinical trials, the most common adverse effects included gastrointestinal disorders, for example *constipation* (6%), *nausea* (6%), and *diarrhea* (5%), *injection site reactions* (6%), *headache* (5%), and *rash* (4%) (85[M]).

Nervous system   Daptomycin has been associated with *neuropathy* in a few cases in phase 2 clinical studies (85[M]). The dose in these studies (3 mg/kg bd) was higher than in phase 3 studies. Pooled laboratory data showed no differences in hematological measurements, blood chemistry, or hepatobiliary function between daptomycin and comparative antibiotics.

⌐ *Muscle damage from daptomycin*

Muscle pain and increased creatine kinase activity have been a concern in patients taking

daptomycin. In phase 3 trials, rises in creatine kinase activity occurred in 15 of 534 (2.8%) daptomycin-treated patients compared with 10 of 558 (1.8%) comparator-treated patients (118[R]). In 13 cases the rises reversed within about 7–10 days after withdrawal.

• *A 52-year-old man developed a severe myopathy after taking daptomycin 500 mg/day (6.5 mg/kg/day) for osteomyelitis (119[A]). He had also taken simvastatin, which was withdrawn when he started to take daptomycin. The baseline creatine kinase activity was 102 U/l (reference range 25–220). Nine days into the course, he developed generalized muscle pain and weakness, progressing to the point where he could not get out of bed. The creatine kinase activity was 20 771 U/l, urinalysis was negative for blood, and serum creatinine was 80 μmol/l. Daptomycin was withdrawn and he was admitted to the intensive care unit for close monitoring and hydration. He gradually recovered his muscle strength over the next 48 hours, with resolution of pain, although the creatine kinase activity was still 2700 U/l on day 14. Two weeks later the creatine kinase activity had normalized and all his muscle symptoms had resolved.*

Another case of daptomycin-related raised serum creatine kinase activity was reported in a randomized comparison of daptomycin 4 mg/kg every 24 hours intravenously, vancomycin, or a semi-synthetic penicillin (120[C]). The patient had arm pain and weakness during the second week of treatment with daptomycin. Daptomycin was withdrawn and all the clinical and laboratory abnormalities rapidly resolved. This was one of two cases (0.4%) of rises in creatine kinase activity leading to withdrawal of daptomycin among all 534 patients treated in phase 3 studies of daptomycin.

Creatine kinase activity should be monitored weekly in patients receiving daptomycin. Daptomycin should be withdrawn in patients who develop an otherwise unexplained myopathy with raised creatine kinase activity (over 5 times the upper limit of the reference range) or an isolated marked increase (over 10 times). Patients with abnormal findings who do not meet these criteria should be monitored closely, especially if they are taking other agents that can cause muscle damage, such as statins (85[R]).

Susceptibility factors   Daptomycin has linear pharmacokinetics at doses of 0.5–6 mg/kg, but in 20% of adults given 8 mg/kg intravenously there is non-linear accumulation. Daptomycin is highly protein-bound and is distributed mainly in the extracellular fluid. In a study of daptomycin concentrations collected from serum and inflammatory blisters, the mean concentrations at 1 and 2 hours were 9.4 and 14.5 µg/ml respectively (118[R]).

The pharmacokinetics of daptomycin 4 mg/kg have been studied in moderately obese adults (BMI over 25 and under 40 kg/m^2), morbidly obese adults (BMI 40 kg/m^2 and over), and a non-obese control group matched for sex, age, and renal function (121[C]). The terminal plasma half-life, the fraction of the dose excreted unchanged in the urine, and renal clearance were not affected by obesity. The volume of distribution and total plasma clearance were higher in the obese subjects. The rates of change of volume and clearance with increasing BMI were greater when they were expressed in absolute terms than when they were normalized for total or ideal body weight. This suggests that increases in body mass associated with obesity are proportionally higher than the corresponding increases in volume and clearance. C_{max} and AUC were respectively 25 and 30% higher in the obese subjects.

Fosmidomycin   *(SED-15, 1450;*
SEDA-27, 268; SEDA-28, 287; SEDA-29, 272)

Fosmidomycin inhibits 1-deoxy-D-xylulose 5-phosphate reductoisomerase, a key enzyme in the non-mevalonate pathway of isoprenoid biosynthesis. It thus inhibits the synthesis of isoprenoids by *Plasmodium falciparum* and suppresses the growth of multidrug-resistant strains in vitro. Studies in Africa of fosmidomycin as monotherapy have shown excellent tolerance.

Susceptibility factors   In 50 children with *Plasmodium falciparum* malaria given consecutively shortened regimens of artesunate + fosmidomycin (1–2 and 30 mg/kg respectively every 12 hours) the most frequent adverse events before day 7 were gastrointestinal (7/12), mostly abdominal pain (n = 5), but not diarrhea or loose stools (122[c]). However, there were two cases of transient rises in alanine transaminase activity, in an 8-year-old girl (up to 96 U/l on day 2 from 24 U/l on admission) and in a 10-year-old boy (up to 157 from 26 U/l).

Ramoplanin   *(SEDA-28, 288;*
SEDA-29, 273)

Ramoplanin is the first in a new class of antimicrobials, a glycolipodepsipeptide produced by fermentation of *Actinoplanes* spp (123[CR]). It blocks bacterial cell wall biosynthesis by interfering with peptidoglycan production. It inhibits the N-acetylglucosaminyltransferase-catalysed conversion of lipid intermediate I to lipid intermediate II, a step that occurs before transglycosylation and transpeptidation. Ramoplanin is currently being investigated for the treatment of diarrhea associated with *Clostridium difficile*. Oral ramoplanin is not systemically absorbed and reaches high concentrations in the feces.

Gastrointestinal   In a placebo-controlled study the occurrence of adverse events was similar with ramoplanin and placebo (123[CR]). The adverse events considered possibly related to ramoplanin included *diarrhea* (n = 3), *abdominal pain* (n = 2), and *dyspepsia, flatulence*, and *nausea* (n = 1 each).

References

1. Al-Aloul M, Miller H, Alapati S, Stockton PA, Ledson MJ, Walshaw MJ. Renal impairment in cystic fibrosis patients due to repeated intravenous aminoglycoside use. Pediatr Pulmonol 2005;39(1):15–20.
2. Zhang J, Li M, Lin X. A case report of injecting gentamicin intraocularly by mistake being misdiagnosed as central retinal artery occlusion. Yan Ke Xue Bao 2005;21(2):88–91.
3. Chou CL, Chen YH, Chau T, Lin SH. Acquired Bartter-like syndrome associated with gentamicin administration. Am J Med Sci 2005;329(3):144–9.
4. Kennedy SE, Henry RL, Rosenberg AR. Antibiotic-related renal failure and cystic fibrosis. J Paediatr Child Health 2005;41(7):382–3.
5. Thomas SP, Buckland JR, Rhys-Williams SR. Potential ototoxicity from triamcinolone, neomycin, gramicidin and nystatin (Tri-Adcortyl) cream. J Laryngol Otol 2005;119(1):48–50.
6. Gonzalez-Mendiola MR, Balda AG, Delgado MC, Montano PP, De Olano DG, Sanchez-Cano M. Contact allergy from tobramycin eyedrops. Allergy 2005;60(4):527–8.
7. Ahya VN, Doyle AM, Mendez JD, Lipson DA, Christie JD, Blumberg EA, Pochettino A, Nelson L, Bloom RD, Kotloff RM. Renal and vestibular toxicity due to inhaled tobramycin in a lung transplant recipient. J Heart Lung Transplant 2005;24(7):932–5.
8. Smyth A, Tan KH, Hyman-Taylor P, Mulheran M, Lewis S, Stableforth D, Knox A. Once versus three-times daily regimens of tobramycin treatment for pulmonary exacerbations of cystic fibrosis—the TOPIC study: a randomised controlled trial. Lancet 2005;365(9459):573–8.
9. Curtis JM, Sternhagen V, Batts D. Acute renal failure after placement of tobramycin-impregnated bone cement in an infected total knee arthroplasty. Pharmacotherapy 2005;25(6):876–80.
10. Diskin C. Paroxysmal nocturnal hemoglobinuria after chloramphenicol therapy. Mayo Clin Proc 2005;80(10):1392, 1394.
11. Mohr JF, McKinnon PS, Peymann PJ, Kenton I, Septimus E, Okhuysen PC. A retrospective, comparative evaluation of dysglycemias in hospitalized patients receiving gatifloxacin, levofloxacin, ciprofloxacin, or ceftriaxone. Pharmacotherapy 2005;25(10):1303–9.
12. Wogelius P, Norgaard M, Gislum M, Pedersen L, Schonheyder HC, Sorensen HT. Further analysis of the risk of adverse birth outcome after maternal use of fluoroquinolones. Int J Antimicrob Agents 2005;26(4):323–6.
13. Kisa C, Yildirim SG, Aydemir C, Cebeci S, Goka E. Prolonged electroconvulsive therapy seizure in a patient taking ciprofloxacin. J ECT 2005;21(1):43–4.
14. Azar S, Ramjiani A, Van Gerpen JA. Ciprofloxacin-induced chorea. Mov Disord 2005;20(4):513–4.
15. Patwardhan A, Khan M. Topical ciprofloxacin can delay recovery from viral ocular surface infection. J R Soc Med 2005;98(6):274–5.
16. Montagnac R, Briat C, Schillinger F, Sartelet H, Birembaut P, Daudon M. Fluoroquinolone induced acute renal failure. General review about a case report with crystalluria due to ciprofloxacin. Nephrol Ther 2005;1(1):44–51.
17. Hausermann P, Scherer K, Weber M, Bircher AJ. Ciprofloxacin-induced acute generalized exanthematous pustulosis mimicking bullous drug eruption confirmed by a positive patch test. Dermatology 2005;211(3):277–80.
18. Mouzopoulos G, Stamatakos M, Vasiliadis G, Skandalakis P. Rupture of adductor longus tendon due to ciprofloxacin. Acta Orthop Belg 2005;71(6):743–5.
19. Afsharian P, Mollgard L, Hassan Z, Xie H, Kimby E, Hassan M. The effect of ciprofloxacin on cyclophosphamide pharmacokinetics in patients with non-Hodgkin lymphoma. Eur J Haematol 2005;75(3):206–11.
20. Kepa L, Oczko-Grzesik B, Stolarz W, Sobala-Szczygiel B. Drug-induced aseptic meningitis in suspected central nervous system infections. J Clin Neurosci 2005;12(5):562–4.
21. Frothingham R. Glucose homeostasis abnormalities associated with use of gatifloxacin. Clin Infect Dis 2005;41(9):1269–76.
22. Pichichero ME, Arguedas A, Dagan R, Sher L, Saez-Llorens X, Hamed K, Echols R. Safety and efficacy of gatifloxacin therapy for children with recurrent acute otitis media (AOM) and/or AOM treatment failure. Clin Infect Dis 2005;41(4):470–8.
23. Brogan SE, Cahalan MK. Gatifloxacin as a possible cause of serious postoperative hypoglycemia. Anesth Analg 2005;101(3):635–6.
24. Blommel AL, Lutes RA. Severe hyperglycemia during renally adjusted gatifloxacin therapy. Ann Pharmacother 2005;39(7–8):1349–52.
25. Capparelli EV, Reed MD, Bradley JS, Kearns GL, Jacobs RF, Damle BD, Blumer JL, Grasela DM. Pharmacokinetics of gatifloxacin in infants and children. Antimicrob Agents Chemother 2005;49(3):1106–12.
26. Mallet L, Huang A. Coadministration of gatifloxacin and multivitamin preparation containing minerals: potential treatment failure in an elderly patient. Ann Pharmacother 2005;39(1):150–2.
27. Bird SB, Orr PG, Mazzola JL, Brush DE, Boyer EW. Levofloxacin-related seizure activity in a patient with Alzheimer's disease: assessment of potential risk factors. J Clin Psychopharmacol 2005;25(3):287–8.
28. Hakko E, Mete B, Ozaras R, Tabak F, Ozturk R, Mert A. Levofloxacin-induced delirium. Clin Neurol Neurosurg 2005;107(2):158–9.
29. Coban S, Ceydilek B, Ekiz F, Erden E, Soykan I. Levofloxacin-induced acute fulminant hepatic failure in a patient with chronic

hepatitis B infection. Ann Pharmacother 2005;39(10):1737–40.

30. Christie MJ, Wong K, Ting RH, Tam PY, Sikaneta TG. Generalized seizure and toxic epidermal necrolysis following levofloxacin exposure. Ann Pharmacother 2005;39(5):953–5.

31. Islam AF, Rahman MD. Levofloxacin-induced fatal toxic epidermal necrolysis. Ann Pharmacother 2005;39(6):1136–7.

32. Hsiao SH, Chang CM, Tsao CJ, Lee YY, Hsu MY, Wu TJ. Acute rhabdomyolysis associated with ofloxacin/levofloxacin therapy. Ann Pharmacother 2005;39(1):146–9.

33. Takahama H, Tsutsumi Y, Kubota Y. Anaphylaxis due to levofloxacin. Int J Dermatol 2005;44(9):789–90.

34. Bauer LA, Black DJ, Lill JS, Garrison J, Raisys VA, Hooton TM. Levofloxacin and ciprofloxacin decrease procainamide and N-acetylprocainamide renal clearances. Antimicrob Agents Chemother 2005;49(4):1649–51.

35. Koehler G, Haimann A, Laferl H, Wenisch C. Rapid reversible coma with intravenous gamma-hydroxybutyrate in a moxifloxacin-treated patient. Clin Drug Investig 2005;25(8):551–4.

36. Gonzalez I, Lobera T, Blasco A, del Pozo MD. Immediate hypersensitivity to quinolones: moxifloxacin cross-reactivity. J Investig Allergol Clin Immunol 2005;15(2):146–9.

37. Elbe DH, Chang SW. Moxifloxacin-warfarin interaction: a series of five case reports. Ann Pharmacother 2005;39(2):361–4.

38. Sahin MT, Ozturkcan S, Inanir I, Filiz EE. Norfloxacin-induced toxic epidermal necrolysis. Ann Pharmacother 2005;39(4):768–70.

39. Naderer OJ, Dupuis RE, Heinzen EL, Wiwattanawongsa K, Johnson MW, Smith PC. The influence of norfloxacin and metronidazole on the disposition of mycophenolate mofetil. J Clin Pharmacol 2005;45(2):219–26.

40. Ozdemir D, Korkmaz U, Sahin I, Sencan I, Kavak A, Kucukbayrak A, Cakir S. Ofloxacin induced Sweet's syndrome in a patient with Crohn's disease. J Infect 2006;52(5):e155–7.

41. Mahajan VK, Sharma NL. Photo-onycholysis due to sparfloxacin. Australas J Dermatol 2005;46(2):104–5.

42. Raad I, Darouiche R, Vazquez J, Lentnek A, Hachem R, Hanna H, Goldstein B, Henkel T, Seltzer E. Efficacy and safety of weekly dalbavancin therapy for catheter-related bloodstream infection caused by Gram-positive pathogens. Clin Infect Dis 2005;40(3):374–80.

43. Logan SA, Brown M, Davidson RN. Teicoplanin-induced vasculitis with cutaneous and renal involvement. J Infect 2005;51(3):e185–6.

44. Yazganoglu KD, Ozkaya E, Ergin-Ozcan P, Cakar N. Vancomycin-induced drug hypersensitivity syndrome. J Eur Acad Dermatol Venereol 2005;19(5):648–50.

45. Zuliani E, Zwahlen H, Gilliet F, Marone C. Vancomycin-induced hypersensitivity reaction with acute renal failure: resolution following cyclosporine treatment. Clin Nephrol 2005;64(2):155–8.

46. Hwu JJ, Chen KH, Hsu WM, Lai JY, Li YS. Ocular hypersensitivitiy to topical vancomycin in a case of chronic endophthalmitis. Cornea 2005;24(6):754–6.

47. Fogarty CM, Patel TC, Dunbar LM, Leroy BP. Efficacy and safety of telithromycin 800 mg once daily for 7 days in community-acquired pneumonia: an open-label, multicenter study. BMC Infect Dis 2005;5(1):43.

48. Fogarty C, Zervos M, Tellier G, Aubier M, Rangaraju M, Nusrat R. Telithromycin for the treatment of acute exacerbations of chronic bronchitis. Int J Clin Pract 2005;59(3):296–305.

49. Wargo KA, McConnell V, Jennings M. Amoxicillin/telithromycin-induced rash in infectious mononucleosis. Ann Pharmacother 2005;39(9):1577.

50. Reed M, Wall GC, Shah NP, Heun JM, Hicklin GA. Verapamil toxicity resulting from a probable interaction with telithromycin. Ann Pharmacother 2005;39(2):357–60.

51. Rallis E, Balatsouras DG, Kouskoukis C, Verros C, Homsioglou E. Drug eruptions in children with ENT infections. Int J Pediatr Otorhinolaryngol 2006;70(1):53–7.

52. Kim MH, Berkowitz C, Trohman RG. Polymorphic ventricular tachycardia with a normal QT interval following azithromycin. Pacing Clin Electrophysiol 2005;28(11):1221–2.

53. Baciewicz AM, Al-Nimr A, Whelan P. Azithromycin-induced hepatotoxicity. Am J Med 2005;118(12):1438–9.

54. Arguedas A, Emparanza P, Schwartz RH, Soley C, Guevara S, de Caprariis PJ, Espinoza G. A randomized, multicenter, double blind, double dummy trial of single dose azithromycin versus high dose amoxicillin for treatment of uncomplicated acute otitis media. Pediatr Infect Dis J 2005;24(2):153–61.

55. Schmutz JL, Barbaud A, Trechot P. Azithromycin and Stevens–Johnson syndrome. Ann Dermatol Venereol 2005;132(8–9 Pt 1):728.

56. Coulston J, Balaratnam N. Irreversible sensorineural hearing loss due to clarithromycin. Postgrad Med J 2005;81(951):58–9.

57. Alonso JC, Melgosa AC, Gonzalo MJ, Garcia CM. Fixed drug eruption on the tongue due to clarithromycin. Contact Dermatitis 2005;53(2):121–2.

58. Khaldi N, Miras A, Gromb S. Toxic epidermal necrolysis and clarithromycin. Can J Clin Pharmacol 2005;12(3):e264–8.

59. Leclercq V, Lacaille S, Delpierre S, Karoubi E, Legrain S. Avoidable adverse event: carbamazepine encephalopathy when introducing clarithromycin. Rev Med Interne 2005;26(10):835–6.

60. Geronimo-Pardo M, Cuartero-del-Pozo AB, Jimenez-Vizuete JM, Cortinas-Saez M, Peyro-Garcia R. Clarithromycin–nifedipine interaction as possible cause of vasodilatory shock. Ann Pharmacother 2005;39(3):538–42.

61. Karthik SV, Casson D. Erythromycin-associated cholestatic hepatitis and liver dysfunction

in children: the British experience. J Clin Gastroenterol 2005;39(8):743–4.

62. George AK, Kunwar AR, Awasthi A. Acute myocardial infarction in a young male on methylphenidate, bupropion, and erythromycin. J Child Adolesc Psychopharmacol 2005;15(4):693–5.

63. Li KY, Li X, Cheng ZN, Zhang BK, Peng WX, Li HD. Effect of erythromycin on metabolism of quetiapine in Chinese suffering from schizophrenia. Eur J Clin Pharmacol 2005;60(11):791–5.

64. Sharma NL, Mahajan VK. Onycholysis: an unusual side effect of roxithromycin. Indian J Dermatol Venereol Leprol 2005;71(1):49–50.

65. Mendez JL, Nadrous HF, Hartman TE, Ryu JH. Chronic nitrofurantoin-induced lung disease. Mayo Clin Proc 2005;80(10):1298–302.

66. Roberts AD, Neelamegam M. Agranulocytosis associated with nitrofurantoin therapy. Ann Pharmacother 2005;39(1):198.

67. Gervilla-Cano J, Otal-Bareche J, Torres-Justribo M, Duran-Rabes J. Nitrofurantoin associated parotiditis. Med Clin (Barc) 2005;125(13):519.

68. Shilad A, Predanic M, Perni SC, Houlihan C, Principe D. Human immunodeficiency virus, pregnancy, and Stevens–Johnson syndrome. Obstet Gynecol 2005;105(5 Pt 2):1254–6.

69. Salle V, Lafon B, Smail A, Cevallos R, Chatelain D, Andrejak M, Ducroix JP. Nitrofurantoin-induced lupus-like syndrome associated with hepatitis. Rev Med Interne 2006;27(4):344–6.

70. Wilcox MH. Update on linezolid: the first oxazolidinone antibiotic. Expert Opin Pharmacother 2005;6(13):2315–26.

71. Aneziokoro CO, Cannon JP, Pachucki CT, Lentino JR. The effectiveness and safety of oral linezolid for the primary and secondary treatment of osteomyelitis. J Chemother 2005;17(6):643–50.

72. Rucker JC, Hamilton SR, Bardenstein D, Isada CM, Lee MS. Linezolid-associated toxic optic neuropathy. Neurology 2006;66(4):595–8.

73. Ferry T, Ponceau B, Simon M, Issartel B, Petiot P, Boibieux A, Biron F, Chidiac C, Peyramond D. Possibly linezolid-induced peripheral and central neurotoxicity: report of four cases. Infection 2005;33(3):151–4.

74. Zivkovic SA, Lacomis D. Severe sensory neuropathy associated with long-term linezolid use. Neurology 2005;64(5):926–7.

75. McKinley SH, Foroozan R. Optic neuropathy associated with linezolid treatment. J Neuroophthalmol 2005;25(1):18–21.

76. Kulkarni K, Del Priore LV. Linezolid induced toxic optic neuropathy. Br J Ophthalmol 2005;89(12):1664–5.

77. Saijo T, Hayashi K, Yamada H, Wakakura M. Linezolid-induced optic neuropathy. Am J Ophthalmol 2005;139(6):1114–6.

78. Kopterides P, Papadomichelakis E, Armaganidis A. Linezolid use associated with lactic acidosis. Scand J Infect Dis 2005;37(2):153–4.

79. Soriano A, Miro O, Mensa J. Mitochondrial toxicity associated with linezolid. N Engl J Med 2005;353(21):2305–6.

80. Dawson MA, Davis A, Elliott P, Cole-Sinclair M. Linezolid-induced dyserythropoiesis: chloramphenicol toxicity revisited. Intern Med J 2005;35(10):626–8.

81. Saijo Wu VC, Wang YT, Wang CY, Tsai IJ, Wu KD, Hwang JJ, Hsueh PR. High frequency of linezolid-associated thrombocytopenia and anemia among patients with end-stage renal disease. Clin Infect Dis 2006;42(1):66–72.

82. Grau S, Morales-Molina JA, Mateu-de Antonio J, Marin-Casino M, Alvarez-Lerma F. Linezolid: low pre-treatment platelet values could increase the risk of thrombocytopenia. J Antimicrob Chemother 2005;56(2):440–1.

83. Saez de la Fuente J, Escobar Rodriguez I, Perpina Zarco C, Bartolome Colussi M. Linezolid-related leukocytoclastic vasculitis. Med Clin (Barc) 2005;124(16):639.

84. Ciulla TA, Comer GM, Peloquin C, Wheeler J. Human vitreous distribution of linezolid after a single oral dose. Retina 2005;25(5):619–24.

85. Stein GE. Safety of newer parenteral antibiotics. Clin Infect Dis 2005;41(Suppl 5):S293–302.

86. Bergeron L, Boule M, Perreault S. Serotonin toxicity associated with concomitant use of linezolid. Ann Pharmacother 2005;39(5):956–61.

87. Morales-Molina JA, Mateu-de Antonio J, Grau Cerrato S, Marin Casino M. Likely serotoninergic syndrome from an interaction between amitryptiline, paroxetine, and linezolid. Farm Hosp 2005;29(4):292–3.

88. DeBellis RJ, Schaefer OP, Liquori M, Volturo GA. Linezolid-associated serotonin syndrome after concomitant treatment with citalopram and mirtazepine in a critically ill bone marrow transplant recipient. J Intensive Care Med 2005;20(6):351–3.

89. Morales-Molina JA, Mateu-de Antonio J, Marin-Casino M, Grau S. Linezolid-associated serotonin syndrome: what we can learn from cases reported so far. J Antimicrob Chemother 2005;56(6):1176–8.

90. Michalopoulos A, Kasiakou SK, Falagas ME. The significance of different formulations of aerosolized colistin. Crit Care 2005;9(4):417–8.

91. Alothman GA, Ho B, Alsaadi MM, Ho SL, O'Drowsky L, Louca E, Coates AL. Bronchial constriction and inhaled colistin in cystic fibrosis. Chest 2005;127(2):522–9.

92. Falagas ME, Kasiakou SK. Colistin: the revival of polymyxins for the management of multidrug-resistant gram-negative bacterial infections. Clin Infect Dis 2005;40(9):1333–41.

93. Daram SR, Gogia S, Bastani B. Colistin-associated acute renal failure: revisited. South Med J 2005;98(2):257–8.

94. Falagas ME, Fragoulis KN, Kasiakou SK, Sermaidis GJ, Michalopoulos A. Nephrotoxicity of intravenous colistin: a prospective evaluation. Int J Antimicrob Agents 2005;26(6):504–7.

95. Kallel H, Hamida CB, Ksibi H, Bahloul M, Hergafi L, Chaari A, Chelly H, Bouaziz M.

Suspected acute interstitial nephritis induced by colistin. J Nephrol 2005;18(3):323–6.

96. Falagas ME, Rizos M, Bliziotis IA, Rellos K, Kasiakou SK, Michalopoulos A. Toxicity after prolonged (more than four weeks) administration of intravenous colistin. BMC Infect Dis 2005;5(1):1.

97. Sowa J, Tsuruta D, Kobayashi H, Ishii M. Allergic contact dermatitis caused by colistin sulfate and bacitracin. Contact Dermatitis 2005;53(3):175–6.

98. Li J, Rayner CR, Nation RL, Deans R, Boots R, Widdecombe N, Douglas A, Lipman J. Pharmacokinetics of colistin methanesulfonate and colistin in a critically ill patient receiving continuous venovenous hemodiafiltration. Antimicrob Agents Chemother 2005;49(11):4814–5.

99. Kallen AJ, Wilson CT, Larson RJ. Perioperative intranasal mupirocin for the prevention of surgical-site infections: systematic review of the literature and meta-analysis. Infect Control Hosp Epidemiol 2005;26(12):916–22.

100. Ng J, Gosbell IB. Successful oral pristinamycin therapy for osteoarticular infections due to methicillin-resistant Staphylococcus aureus (MRSA) and other Staphylococcus spp. J Antimicrob Chemother 2005;55(6):1008–12.

101. Chanques G, Girard C, Pinzani V, Jaber S. Fatal pristinamycin-induced toxic epidermal necrolysis (Lyell's syndrome): difficulties in attributing causal association in the polymedicated intensive care unit patient. Acta Anaesthesiol Scand 2005;49(5):721–2.

102. Moellering RC, Linden PK, Reinhardt J, Blumberg EA, Bompart F, Talbot GH. The efficacy and safety of quinupristin–dalfopristin for the treatment of infections caused by vancomycin-resistant *Enterococcus faecium*. J Antimicrob Chemother 1999;44:251–61.

103. Nichols RL, Graham DR, Barriere SL, Rodgers A, Wilson SE, Zervos M, Dunn DL, Kreter B. Treatment of hospitalized patients with complicated gram-positive skin and skin structure infections: two randomized, multicentre studies of quinupristin/dalfopristin versus cefazolin, oxacillin or vancomycin. Synercid Skin and Skin Structure Infection Group. Antimicrob Chemother 1999;44:263–73.

104. Chan-Tack KM, Mehta S. Quinupristin–dalfopristin-induced reticulocytopenic anemia. South Med J 2005;98(12):1226–7.

105. Hershberger E, Oprea SF, Donabedian SM, Perri M, Bozigar P, Bartlett P, Zervos MJ. Epidemiology of antimicrobial resistance in enterococci of animal origin. J Antimicrob Chemother 2005;55(1):127–30.

106. Wambulwa C, Bwayo S, Laiyemo AO, Lombardo F. Trimethoprim–sulfamethoxazole-induced aseptic meningitis. J Natl Med Assoc 2005;97(12):1725–8.

107. Frank LA, Hnilica KA, May ER, Sargent SJ, Davis JA. Effects of sulfamethoxazole–trimethoprim on thyroid function in dogs. Am J Vet Res 2005;66(2):256–9.

108. Hughes WT, Dankner WM, Yogev R, Huang S, Paul ME, Flores MA, Kline MW, Wei LJ. Comparison of atovaquone and azithromycin with trimethoprim–sulfamethoxazole for the prevention of serious bacterial infections in children with HIV infection. Clin Infect Dis 2005;40(1):136–45.

109. Kocak Z, Hatipoglu CA, Ertem G, Kinikli S, Tufan A, Irmak H, Demiroz AP. Trimethoprim–sulfamethoxazole induced rash and fatal hematologic disorders. J Infect 2006;52(2):e49–52.

110. Moh R, Danel C, Sorho S, Sauvageot D, Anzian A, Minga A, Gomis OB, Konga C, Inwoley A, Gabillard D, Bissagnene E, Salamon R, Anglaret X. Haematological changes in adults receiving a zidovudine-containing HAART regimen in combination with cotrimoxazole in Cote d'Ivoire. Antivir Ther 2005;10(5):615–24.

111. Bjornsson E, Jerlstad P, Bergqvist A, Olsson R. Fulminant drug-induced hepatic failure leading to death or liver transplantation in Sweden. Scand J Gastroenterol 2005;40(9):1095–101.

112. Versleijen MW, Naber AH, Riksen NP, Wanten GJ, Debruyne FM. Recurrent pancreatitis after trimethoprim–sulfamethoxazole rechallenge. Neth J Med 2005;63(7):275–7.

113. Soheilian M, Sadoughi MM, Ghajarnia M, Dehghan MH, Yazdani S, Behboudi H, Anisian A, Peyman GA. Prospective randomized trial of trimethoprim/sulfamethoxazole versus pyrimethamine and sulfadiazine in the treatment of ocular toxoplasmosis. Ophthalmology 2005;112(11):1876–82.

114. Feiza BA, Samy F, Asma D, Rym B, Insaf M. Urticarial vasculitis. A case report after sulfamethoxazole–trimethoprim ingestion. Tunis Med 2005;83(11):714–6.

115. Mortimer NJ, Bermingham MR, Chapple SJ, Sladden MJ. Fatal adverse drug reaction to trimethoprim. Aust Fam Physician 2005;34(5):345–6.

116. Hruska MW, Amico JA, Langaee TY, Ferrell RE, Fitzgerald SM, Frye RF. The effect of trimethoprim on CYP2C8 mediated rosiglitazone metabolism in human liver microsomes and healthy subjects. Br J Clin Pharmacol 2005;59(1):70–9.

117. Bottiger Y, Brattstrom C, Backman L, Claesson K, Burke JT. Trimethoprim–sulphamethoxazole does not affect the pharmacokinetics of sirolimus in renal transplant recipients. Br J Clin Pharmacol 2005;60(5):566–9.

118. Oberholzer CM, Caserta MT. Antimicrobial update: daptomycin. Pediatr Infect Dis J 2005;24(10):919–20.

119. Echevarria K, Datta P, Cadena J, Lewis 2nd JS. Severe myopathy and possible hepatotoxicity related to daptomycin. J Antimicrob Chemother 2005;55(4):599–600.

120. Lipsky BA, Stoutenburgh U. Daptomycin for treating infected diabetic foot ulcers: evidence from a randomized, controlled trial comparing daptomycin with vancomycin or semi-synthetic

penicillins for complicated skin and skin-structure infections. J Antimicrob Chemother 2005;55(2):240–5.

121. Dvorchik BH, Damphousse D. The pharmacokinetics of daptomycin in moderately obese, morbidly obese, and matched nonobese subjects. J Clin Pharmacol 2005;45(1):48–56.

122. Borrmann S, Adegnika AA, Moussavou F, Oyakhirome S, Esser G, Matsiegui PB, Ramharter M, Lundgren I, Kombila M, Issifou S, Hutchinson D, Wiesner J, Jomaa H, Kremsner PG. Short-course regimens of artesunate–fosmidomycin in treatment of uncomplicated Plasmodium falciparum malaria. Antimicrob Agents Chemother 2005;49(9):3749–54.

123. Farver DK, Hedge DD, Lee SC. Ramoplanin: a lipoglycodepsipeptide antibiotic. Ann Pharmacother 2005;39(5):863–8.

Andreas H. Groll and Thomas J. Walsh

27 Antifungal drugs

ALLYLAMINES (SEDA-27, 284; SEDA-28, 294; SEDA-29, 280)

Terbinafine (SED-15, 3316; SEDA-29, 280)

Pulse-dose terbinafine has been compared with standard continuous-dose terbinafine for toenail onychomycosis in a double-blind, randomized, single-center, non-inferiority study in 306 volunteers randomized to terbinafine 250 mg/day for 3 months (continuous) or 500 mg/day for 1 week per month for 3 months (pulse) (1[C]). Continuous-dose terbinafine was more effective. The two regimens were equally well tolerated.

Sensory systems Terbinafine causes *taste loss* in 0.6–2.8% of patients. However, many so-called taste problems actually reflect olfactory problems, and the sole empirical study published on this topic, based on whole-mouth testing of a single subject, found no terbinafine-related deficit. Using well-validated taste and smell tests, chemosensory function in six patients complaining of taste disturbance after terbinafine were assessed and compared with six age-, race-, and sex-matched controls (2[C]). Taste function for sweet-, sour-, and bitter-tasting stimuli was significantly reduced in both the anterior and posterior lingual regions. For sodium chloride, the decrements were confined to the posterior region. Olfactory function was normal. These findings support anecdotal case reports of taste loss from terbinafine, demonstrate that all four major taste qualities are

affected, and suggest that olfactory dysfunction is not involved.

Skin Cutaneous adverse effects reportedly occur in 1–3% of patients taking terbinafine. The overwhelming majority of these reactions consist of mild to moderate *macular exanthems*. More serious skin disorders, such as *erythema multiforme, toxic epidermal necrolysis, Stevens–Johnson syndrome, erythema toxicum, cutaneous lupus erythematosus*, and *generalized pustular eruptions* are rare. *Acute generalized exanthematous pustulosis* (AGEP) is considered to be a clinical reaction pattern, 90% of cases of which are due to systemic drugs. It is a rare presentation of an adverse drug reaction most frequently triggered by antimicrobial drugs, including terbinafine. Further cases of acute generalized exanthematous pustulosis associated with oral terbinafine have been reported (3[A], 4[A]).

Susceptibility factors

Children Limited data suggest that the safety profile of terbinafine in children is not different from that observed in adults and that terbinafine is well tolerated in this population over short periods of time. Terbinafine has been approved for the treatment of tinea capitis in many countries worldwide, and provides good efficacy rates for *Trichophyton* tinea capitis using shorter regimens than griseofulvin.

The single dose and steady-state pharmacokinetics of terbinafine have been investigated in 22 otherwise healthy children aged 4–8 years with tinea capitis were comparable between children and adults for the administered dose; however, children had significantly lower values C_{max} and $AUC_{0\to24}$ when dose was corrected for weight (5[C]). Age accounted for about 50% of the variability in dose-normalized C_{max} and AUC. Adverse events consisted principally of headache ($n = 3$) and gastrointestinal complaints (altered eating habits, $n = 3$; loss of

Side Effects of Drugs, Annual 30
J.K. Aronson (Editor)
ISSN: 0378-6080
DOI: 10.1016/S0378-6080(08)00027-5

appetite, $n = 3$; stomach ache, $n = 4$; diarrhea, $n = 2$). There was a reduced neutrophil count in five children, thought to be related to terbinafine in two cases.

Drug–drug interactions   In a study of drugs that are co-prescribed with CYP2D6 inhibitors (bupropion, fluoxetine, paroxetine, and terbinafine) lists of patients taking both inhibitors and substrates of CYP2D6 were drawn from the prescription databases of three Norwegian primary pharmacies (6[M]). The highest frequencies of co-prescribed substrates were found for *paroxetine* (101 events per 267 patients, 38%), and *fluoxetine* (36 events per 110 patients, 33%). The drugs that were most often detected in combination with the inhibitors were *codeine* (116 events) and *metoprolol* (38 events). The frequency of co-prescribed substrates was comparatively low (3/96), codeine being co-prescribed with terbinafine in all three cases.

Drugs with long half-lives, such as terbinafine, have a potential for involvement in both long-lasting drug–drug interactions and interactions that can occur weeks after withdrawal.

- A 37-year-old white woman with normal CYP2D6 metabolic capacity taking amitriptyline, valproate, and olanzapine was given terbinafine and shortly after developed extreme dryness of the mouth, nausea, and dizziness, accompanied by a large increase in the serum concentrations of amitriptyline and nortriptyline (7[A]). Terbinafine was withdrawn and the dose of amitriptyline was reduced. Surprisingly, the serum concentrations of amitriptyline and nortriptyline did not return to baseline until about 6 months later.

Terbinafine is a highly potent competitive inhibitor of CYP2D6, an important intermediate enzyme in the metabolism of amitriptyline to nortriptyline. Nortriptyline is further metabolized to 10-hydroxy metabolites, mainly by CYP2D6. It is therefore likely that the concomitant use of terbinafine was the major cause of the increased serum concentrations of amitriptyline and nortriptyline. Based on the data of this case report, there is a risk of clinically significant drug–drug interactions for at least 3 months after withdrawal of terbinafine.

AMPHOTERICIN   *(SED-15, 192; SEDA-27, 276; SEDA-28, 295; SEDA-29, 280)*

Drug administration route

Home-based infusion therapy   The types and frequencies of adverse events associated with community-based amphotericin B infusion therapy have been analysed in 105 patients who received amphotericin B from a home-care provider (8[c]). A total of 113 courses of amphotericin B formulations were administered: liposomal amphotericin B, 41 courses (36%), amphotericin B deoxycholate, 31 courses (27%), amphotericin B lipid complex, 31 courses (27%), and amphotericin B colloidal dispersion, three courses (3%); an additional seven courses consisted of sequential therapy with two different formulations. Nephrotoxicity was associated with 46 (41%) courses, electrolyte abnormalities with 40 (35%) courses, venous access device complications with 12 (11%) courses, and infusion reactions with 13 (12%) courses. Nephrotoxicity occurred most often in those aged 60 years or older, solid organ transplant recipients, and those receiving concomitant ciclosporin. Only two (12%) of 17 courses in children under 13 years were associated with nephrotoxicity. Thirteen of all 113 courses resulted in patients requiring hospital admission owing to adverse events. Monitoring of electrolyte, serum creatinine, and blood urea nitrogen concentrations 2 or 3 times a week was adequate for identifying these events.

Amphotericin B Lipid Complex (ABLC)

Urinary tract   To investigate the renal safety of ABLC, the records of 3514 ABLC-treated patients with fungal infections registered in the CLEAR database were reviewed (9[C]). The median change in predicted creatinine clearance from baseline to the end of therapy was -3 (range -119 to 118) ml/minute; the serum creatinine concentration doubled in 13% of patients and new dialysis was needed for 3% of patients. Patients with underlying renal disease who had received prior antifungal therapy had a median creatinine clearance change of

0.5 (range −107 to 52) ml/minute. Despite an increased risk of renal impairment in recipients of allogeneic hemopoietic stem-cell transplants, only 17% had end-of-therapy doubling of serum creatinine concentrations, and the median change in creatinine clearance was −10 (range −107 to 108) ml/minute. In patients given ABLC concomitant treatment with potentially nephrotoxic agents and a baseline serum creatinine concentration of <176 μmol/l were predisposing factors for nephrotoxicity. These data support the notion that ABLC may be used safely to treat patients who are at increased risk of renal impairment.

Susceptibility factors

Children   The pharmacokinetics of ABLC have been investigated in 28 neonates (median weight 1.06, range 0.48–4.9 kg; median gestational age 27, range 24–41 weeks) with invasive candidiasis enrolled in a phase II multicenter trial (10[C]). They received intravenous ABLC 2.5 mg/kg/day ($n = 15$) or 5 mg/kg/day ($n = 13$) over 1 or 2 hours for a median of 21 (range 4–47) days. Population-based pharmacokinetic modelling of concentration data showed that the disposition of ABLC in neonates was similar to that observed in other age groups: weight was the only factor that influenced clearance. Based on these results and documented safety and efficacy, a daily dosage of 2.5–5.0 mg/kg for treatment of invasive *Candida* infections in neonates was recommended.

ABLC has also been assessed in 548 children and adolescents 0–20 years of age who were enrolled into the CLEAR registry. All had a cancer or had received a bone marrow, cord blood, or solid organ transplant and were receiving amphotericin B lipid complex for documented or suspected fungal infections (11[C]). Most were either intolerant of or refractory to conventional antifungal therapy, and almost one-half were neutropenic at the start of treatment. Of the 548 patients, 300 (55%) were transplant recipients and 393 (72%) had received one or more concomitant nephrotoxins. *Candida* and *Aspergillus* were the most commonly isolated species in patients with proven or probable infections. Response data were evaluable for 255 of the 285 patients with documented single or multiple pathogens. A complete response (cured) or partial response

(improved) was achieved in 55% of patients, and an additional 17% of patients had a stable outcome. There was no significant difference between the rates of new hemodialysis versus baseline hemodialysis. There were rises in serum creatinine of over 1.5 times baseline and over 2.5 times baseline values in 25 and 8.8% of all patients respectively.

Elderly people   ABLC has been evaluated retrospectively using the CLEAR database in 572 elderly patients (over 65 years of age) and 2930 controls (65 years or under) (12[C]). The patients were typically receiving ABLC for candidiasis, multiple fungal pathogen infections, and aspergillosis, or were being treated empirically. The median cumulative dose of ABLC in the two groups was similar. Despite higher median pretreatment serum creatinine concentrations among the elderly patients (150 versus 123 μmol/l), both groups had only a median change from baseline of 9 μmol/l by the end of therapy.

Monitoring therapy   The results of the Collaborative Exchange of Antifungal Research (CLEAR), an industry-supported registry of patients receiving ABLC for invasive fungal infections, have been published. The CLEAR database provides data on the efficacy and renal safety of ABLC in 3514 patients at over 160 institutions in the USA and Canada after regulatory approval (13[r]).

Within the CLEAR database, the efficacy and renal safety of ABLC were assessed in 398 patients with invasive aspergillosis (14[c]). The most common underlying conditions were hemopoietic stem-cell transplantation (25%), hematological malignancies (25%), and solid-organ transplants (27%). The most common reason for administration of ABLC was lack of response to prior antifungal therapy. Overall, 65% of patients had a favorable clinical response: 44% were cured or improved and 21% were stabilized. Clinical responses were similar in patients who received ABLC as either first-line or second-line therapy. Changes in serum creatinine concentrations were not clinically significant in most patients; however, dialysis was initiated in seven, of whom six had had prior antifungal therapy or had pre-existing renal disease.

Similarly, in over 900 patients with invasive candidiasis, clinical responses (cured or improved) were similar in patients infected with invasive *Candida albicans* and non-albicans *Candida* species (63 and 62% respectively) (15[C]). Compared with patients who received lower doses of ABLC, those who required higher doses of ABLC because of more severe infections did not develop significant renal impairment, as assessed by end-of-therapy changes in serum creatinine concentration from baseline (median 9, range −343 to 211 µmol/l), the incidence of serum creatinine doubling (16%), and the need for new dialysis (7%).

Intermediate-dose ABLC (3 mg/kg/day) as primary or salvage treatment of fungal infections has been assessed in 74 adults with hematological malignancies, of whom 45 received upfront therapy and 29 received salvage therapy for their infection (16[c]). Of 71 evaluable patients 48 responded, with complete responses in 40 (56%) and partial responses in eight (11%), and 15 (21%) died as a consequence of the fungal infection. In 40 patients with neutropenia-associated infection, rapid neutropenic recovery (at less than 10 days from study entry) was essential for a response (90 versus 32%). Treatment was well tolerated; 15% of the infusions were followed by infusion-related adverse events; there was nephrotoxicity in 7% of patients and 11% of withdrawals were due to toxicity.

Electrolytes were replaced when indicated by serum concentration measurements. The median duration of therapy was 14 days. The mean intravenous hydration and the mean diuresis were respectively 1530 and 1970 ml/m^2/day. Overall, 55 patients (71%) received a mean of 19 days of therapy without dose-limiting adverse events. Despite significant increases in mean serum creatinine concentrations and reductions in mean creatinine clearance, observed early in the whole population, in only six patients (7.8%) was therapy withdrawn because of renal insufficiency, which always recovered after withdrawal. In eight patients (10%) therapy was withdrawn because of infusion-related adverse effects. Seven patients died without evidence of DAMB-associated toxicity. This series confirms that adequate hydration (about 1500 ml/m^2/day) and careful electrolyte supplementation are simple measures that contain nephrotoxicity and permit DAMB therapy.

Drug formulations   The toxicity of amphotericin B deoxycholate has led to an increased preference for lipid formulations with more favorable safety profiles. However, many hospital formularies list both lipid and non-lipid formulations. A dispensing and administration error that caused amphotericin B deoxycholate to be given instead of liposomal amphotericin B resulted in death (19[A]).

Amphotericin B deoxycholate (DAMB)

Urinary tract   Hydration and sodium loading may reduce the *glomerular nephrotoxicity* that is associated with amphotericin B-deoxycholate (DAMB) (17[R]). A standardized protocol of hydration and electrolyte supplementation was studied prospectively in patients with hematological malignancies receiving empirical treatment, in order to evaluate its effect on DAMB-related renal toxicity (18[c]). In all, 77 consecutive patients received DAMB (1 mg/kg/day) in association with initial intravenous hydration of at least 1 l/m^2, containing at least 1 liter of 0.9% saline daily. Hydration was increased when serum creatinine concentrations increased by 20% from baseline.

Liposomal Amphotericin (L-AmB)

Observational studies   A dermatosis commonly known as *post kala-azar dermal leishmaniasis* can develop after treatment of human visceral leishmaniasis. In about 15% of cases the disfiguring lesions persist, sometimes for many years. The usefulness of LAMB 2.5 mg/kg/day for 20 days in the treatment of persistent post kala-azar dermal leishmaniasis has been evaluated in 12 Sudanese subjects, who were regularly screened for adverse effects; LAMB completely cleared the rash in 10 (83%) of the patients and caused no detectable adverse effects (20[c]).

Liver   In a retrospective matched case–control study, cases of *hepatotoxicity* among patients who underwent bone marrow transplantation

were investigated using multivariable logistic
regression modelling to evaluate the relation
between hepatotoxicity and exposure to antifungal medications (21^C). The unadjusted incidence of hepatotoxicity was 1.50 for liposomal
amphotericin B. In case–control analyses liposomal amphotericin B was associated with
a substantial increase in the risk of hepatotoxicity in these patients (OR = 3.33; 95%
CI = 1.61, 6.88); there was a smaller increase in risk for fluconazole (OR = 1.99; 95%
CI = 1.21, 3.26). Patients had greater rises in
serum transaminases associated with exposure
to larger cumulative doses of liposomal amphotericin B. In the follow-up analysis of patients
who developed hepatotoxicity and who continued to receive antifungal medication, one-third
of those who received liposomal amphotericin
B had marked increases in bilirubin concentrations, as opposed to 8% of patients treated with
fluconazole.

Susceptibility factors

Orthotopic liver transplantation   The prevalence of fungal infection after orthotopic liver
transplantation is 5–42%. The most commonly
isolated pathogens are *Candida* and *Aspergillus*
species. High-risk liver transplant recipients
are more susceptible to invasive fungal infections, with a prevalence of over 40% and
mortality rates of 78–100%; however, a strategy for fungal prophylaxis in this population
has not been defined. Among 100 consecutive
orthotopic liver transplantations followed for 28
months, 21 recipients (15 men, overall mean
age of 49, range 23–65 years) were considered
to be at high risk of fungal infections when
they had at least one of the following criteria:
acute liver failure, assisted ventilation for more
than 7 days, re-transplantation, re-laparotomy,
antibacterial therapy for more than 14 days,
transfusion requirements of over 20 units of
red blood cells, and/or biliary leakage (22^c).
This group received LAMB (1 mg/kg/day for
7–10 days). The one-year survival in the high-
risk group was 80%. The prevalence of invasive
fungal infections was 9.5%. No *Candida* infection was observed. Two patients developed
Aspergillus infection, in one case with a fatal
outcome. Adverse events related to the drug
were hypokalemia (*n* = 2), back pain (*n* = 3),
and renal dysfunction (*n* = 2). None of these

events required withdrawal of the prophylactic
regimen.

ANTIFUNGAL AZOLES   *(SED-15, 301; SEDA-27, 278; SEDA-28, 299; SEDA-29, 282)*

Drug–drug interactions with antifungal azoles   ✦

*Drug–drug interactions with antifungal azoles
are common and are usually based on one
of two mechanisms—inhibition of metabolism,
usually by CYP3A4, and inhibition of transport
by multidrug transporters.*

*To assess the frequency of potential drug
interactions with azole derivatives and the consequences of interactions between fluconazole
and other drugs in routine in-patient care, a
retrospective cohort study of patients with systemic fungal infections treated with an oral
or intravenous azole derivative was conducted
in a tertiary-care hospital (23^C). Of the 4185
admissions in which azoles (fluconazole, itraconazole, or ketoconazole) were given, 2941
(70%) admissions involved potential drug interactions, and in 2716 (92%) there were potential
interactions with fluconazole. The most frequent
interactions that were potentially moderate
or severe were co-administration of fluconazole with prednisone (25%), midazolam (18%),
warfarin (15%), methylprednisolone (14%), ciclosporin (11%), and nifedipine (10%). Charts
were reviewed for 199 admissions in which
patients were exposed to potential fluconazole drug interactions. While four adverse
events were attributed to fluconazole, none was
thought to have been due to a drug–drug interaction, although in one instance fluconazole
may have contributed. The authors concluded
that although fluconazole drug interactions
were very frequent they had few apparent clinical consequences.*

Anidulafungin   *In a placebo-controlled study
in 17 subjects anidulafungin (200 mg on day
1 then 100 mg/day on days 2–4) had no effect on the pharmacokinetics of voriconazole
(400 mg every 12 hours on day 1 then 200 mg
every 12 hours on days 2–4) (24^C). There were*

no dose-limiting or serious adverse events, and all adverse events were mild and consistent with the known safety profiles of the two drugs.

Antacids   The effects of an antacid suspension (aluminium hydroxide 220 mg + magnesium hydroxide 120 mg in 240 ml) on the oral absorption of itraconazole 200 mg from capsules has been investigated in a randomized, open, two-period, crossover study in 12 healthy Thai men (25^c). The t_{max} of itraconazole was prolonged and its C_{max} and AUC were markedly reduced by the antacid, implying that the antacid markedly reduced the speed and extent of itraconazole absorption.

Antihistamines   The effects of co-administration of ketoconazole 400–450 mg/day on the pharmacokinetics of ebastine 20 mg/day and loratadine 10 mg/day and on the QT_c interval have been evaluated in two placebo-controlled studies in healthy men (n = 55 and 62) (26^c). Neither ebastine nor loratadine alone altered the QT_c interval. Ketoconazole and placebo increased the mean QT_c by 6.96 ms in the ebastine study and by 7.52 ms in the loratadine study. Mean QT_c was statistically significantly increased during administration of both ebastine + ketoconazole administration (12.21 ms) and loratadine + ketoconazole (10.68 ms) but these changes were not statistically significantly different from the increases seen with placebo + ketoconazole (6.96 ms). Ketoconazole increased the mean AUC for ebastine 43-fold, and that of its metabolite carebastine 1.4-fold. It increased the mean AUC of loratadine 4.5-fold and that of its metabolite desloratadine 1.9-fold. No subjects withdrew because of electrocardiographic changes or drug-related adverse events. Thus, the larger effect of ketoconazole on the pharmacokinetics of ebastine was not accompanied by a correspondingly larger pharmacodynamic effect on cardiac repolarization.

Aripiprazole   Aripiprazole is mainly metabolized in vitro by CYP3A4 and CYP2D6. The effect of itraconazole 100 mg/day for 7 days on the pharmacokinetics of a single oral dose of aripiprazole 3 mg has been studied in 24 healthy adult men (27^E). Itraconazole increased the C_{max}, AUC, and terminal half-life of aripiprazole by 19, 48, and 19% respectively and of its main metabolite OPC-14857 by 19, 39, and 53%. Itraconazole reduced the oral clearance of aripiprazole in extensive metabolizers by 27%, with an even greater reduction (47%) in intermediate metabolizers. For C_{max}, there was no significant difference between extensive metabolizers and intermediate metabolizers, and the percent change by co-administration of itraconazole was less than 20% in both groups. For OPC-14857, the t_{max} in intermediate metabolizers was longer than that in extensive metabolizers, and the difference was amplified by itraconazole. The AUC was similarly affected by itraconazole in all genotypes. The urinary 6-beta-hydroxycortisol/cortisol concentration ratio was halved by itraconazole, consistent with inhibition of CYP3A4. However, the effect of CYP3A4 inhibition on the pharmacokinetics of aripiprazole was not thought to be clinically significant. On the other hand, there were definite differences in pharmacokinetics between CYP2D6 genotypes.

Atenolol   The effect of itraconazole 200 mg bd for 2 days on the pharmacokinetics of atenolol 50 mg has been investigated in 10 healthy volunteers in a randomized crossover study (28^c). Itraconazole increased the AUC of atenolol and the amount excreted in the urine by about 12%, suggesting a slight increase in systemic availability. However, it had no statistically significant effect on the pharmacodynamics of atenolol.

Ciclosporin   The outcomes in renal transplant patients have been monitored using simultaneous ciclosporin C0 and C2 concentration measurements (1998–9) and kin patients in whom only ciclosporin C2 concentrations were measured (29^c). The latter had higher ciclosporin C2 concentrations, AUCs, and drug doses during the immediate postsurgical period, and at 2 weeks and 4 and 6 months after transplantation. Six of the latter and none of the former had severe liver toxicity, characterized by jaundice and raised liver enzymes, with negative serological tests for CMV, HVC, and HVB. There was a correlation between aspartate transaminase activity and ciclosporin C2 concentrations and both normalized at 15–55 days after ciclosporin dosage reduction. High ciclosporin C2 concentrations, which have been recommended when the drug is used alone in renal transplantation, cannot be used in patients taking ketoconazole, because C2 does not reflect drug exposure and high C2 concentrations can cause liver toxicity.

Cyclophosphamide Cyclophosphamide is a prodrug that requires cytochrome P450-mediated activation to 4-hydroxycyclophosphamide. Agents that are frequently co-administered with cyclophosphamide in high-dose chemotherapy regimens were tested for inhibition of the activation of cyclophosphamide in human liver microsomes. The K_m and V_{max} of the conversion of cyclophosphamide to 4-hydroxycyclophosphamide were 93 $\mu mol/l$ and 4.3 $mg\cdot nmol/hour$ respectively; itraconazole was inhibitory at an IC_{50} of 5 $\mu mol/l$, which is higher than the usual plasma itraconazole concentration and was thus considered of no clinical relevance (30^E).

Dexloxiglumide Dexloxiglumide is a cholecystokinin CCK_1 receptor antagonist under investigation for functional gastrointestinal disorders; it is metabolized by CYP3A4 and CYP2C9. The effect of steady-state ketoconazole on the pharmacokinetics of dexloxiglumide and its primary metabolite O-demethyldexloxiglumide has been studied in healthy subjects in a randomized, two-period, crossover study (31^c). Ketoconazole increased dexloxiglumide C_{max} by 32% without affecting the C_{max} of changed O-demethyldexloxiglumide and increased the AUC of dexloxiglumide and O-demethyldexloxiglumide by 36%. There were no changes in the half-lives of dexloxiglumide or O-demethyldexloxiglumide.

Disopyramide The effect of fluconazole on the heart, and the interaction of fluconazole with disopyramide has been investigated in chick White Leghorns embryos (32^E). The drugs were injected into the air sac of each fertilized egg: fluconazole 0.4, 0.8, and 1.2 mg/egg alone, disopyramide 0.3 mg/egg alone, or fluconazole 0.4 mg/egg + disopyramide 0.3 mg/egg. Fluconazole 0.4 mg/egg had no effect on heart rate, but heart rate fell significantly after 0.8 and 1.2 mg/egg. The heart rate also fell significantly after fluconazole 0.4 mg/egg + disopyramide 0.3 mg/egg and there was a cardiac dysrhythmia. These experiments suggest that concurrent administration of fluconazole and Class I antidysrhythmic drugs may increase the

risk of cardiotoxicity by additive effects on QT prolongation.

Lipid lowering agents can cause rhabdomyolysis, which can be precipitated by concomitant use of fluconazole. Rhabdomyolysis has been reported in a patient taking atorvastatin and fluconazole (33^A).

Everolimus The effect of ketoconazole 200 mg bd for 8 days on the pharmacokinetics of a single dose of everolimus 2 mg has been investigated in a two-period, single-sequence, crossover study in 12 healthy subjects (34^C). Ketoconazole increased the C_{max} of everolimus 3.9-fold and the AUC 15-fold and prolonged the half-life from 30 to 56 hours. Everolimus did not alter ketoconazole predose concentrations. Given the magnitude of this drug interaction, ketoconazole should be avoided if possible in patients taking everolimus.

Fexofenadine The effects of itraconazole on the pharmacokinetics and pharmacodynamics of a single oral dose of fexofenadine 180 mg have been investigated in relation to the multidrug resistance gene MDR1 in seven healthy subjects with the 2677GG/3435CC (G/C) haplotype and seven with the 2677TT/3435TT (T/T) haplotype (35^c). One hour before the dose of fexofenadine, either 200 mg itraconazole or placebo was given in a double-blind, randomized, crossover manner with a 2-week washout period. Histamine-induced wheal and flare reactions were measured to assess the effects on the antihistamine response. In the placebo phase there was no difference between the two MDR1 haplotypes in the pharmacokinetics of either fexofenadine or itraconazole. However, after itraconazole pretreatment the differences in fexofenadine pharmacokinetics became statistically significant; the mean fexofenadine AUC in the T/T group was significantly higher than that in the G/C group and the oral clearance in the T/T group was lower than in the G/C group. Itraconazole pretreatment caused more than a 3-fold increase in the peak concentration of fexofenadine and the AUC to 6 hours compared with placebo. This resulted in significantly greater suppression of the histamine-induced wheal and flare reactions in the itraconazole pretreatment phase compared with placebo. Thus, the effect of these MDR1 haplotypes on fexofenadine disposition is magnified in the presence of itraconazole. Itraconazole pretreatment significantly altered the disposition of fexofenadine and thus its peripheral antihistamine effects.

Gefitinib   CYP3A4 is involved in the metabolism of gefitinib (Iressa, ZD1839). The in vitro metabolism of $[^{14}C]$-gefitinib 1–3 μmol/l has been investigated in human liver microsomes and a range of expressed human cytochrome P450 enzymes, with particular focus on the formation of O-desmethylgefitinib (M523595), the major metabolite in human plasma. Ketoconazole was used as a probe drug. While formation of M523595 was CYP2D6 mediated, the overall metabolism of gefitinib depended primarily on CYP3A4, and this was not obviously reduced in liver microsomes from CYP2D6 poor metabolizers (36^E).

When gefitinib 250 and 500 mg was administered in the presence of itraconazole, mean AUC increased significantly by 78 and 61% respectively (37^c). Although exposure to gefitinib is increased by co-administration with CYP3A4 inhibitors such as itraconazole, dosage reduction is not recommended due to the good tolerability profile of gefitinib.

Imatinib   A severe pustular eruption was associated with the concurrent use of voriconazole and imatinib in a patient with chronic myeloid leukemia (38^A). At the time of his skin eruption, the plasma concentrations of imatinib was raised. Imatinib is primarily metabolized by CYP3A4. Monitoring imatinib plasma concentrations may help in identifying patients at risk of severe toxicity.

Irinotecan   Ketoconazole inhibits the glucuronidation of the UGT2B7 substrates zidovudine and lorazepam, but its effect on UGT1A substrates is unclear. Co-administration of irinotecan and ketoconazole led to a significant increase in the formation of SN-38 (7-ethyl-10-hydroxycamptothecin), a UGT1A substrate (39^E). The contribution of ketoconazole to SN-38 formation by inhibition of SN-38 glucuronidation has been studied in pooled human liver microsomes and cDNA-expressed UGT1A isoforms (1A1, 1A7, and 1A9). Indinavir, which inhibits UGT1A1, was used as a positive control (39^E). Ketoconazole competitively inhibited SN-38 glucuronidation. Among the UGT1A isoforms screened, ketoconazole showed the highest inhibitory effect on UGT1A1 and UGT1A9, with K_i values of 3.3 μmol/l for UGT1A1 and 32 μmol/l for UGT1A9. This may be the basis for increased exposure to SN-38 when ketoconazole is co-administered with irinotecan.

Mefloquine   The effect of ketoconazole 400 mg/day for 10 days on the plasma concentrations of a single oral dose of mefloquine 500 mg has been studied in an open, randomized, twophase, crossover study in eight healthy Thai men (40^c). Ketoconazole increased mefloquine AUC, half-life, and C_{max} by 79, 39, and 64% respectively. The AUC and C_{max} of mefloquine's carboxylic acid metabolite were reduced by 28 and 31% respectively.

Nevirapine   Adverse events that occurred after initiation of nevirapine-based antiretroviral therapy have been investigated in HIV-infected Thai patients who did not receive fluconazole (group A, n = 225) or who received fluconazole 400 mg/week (group B, n = 392) or 200 mg/day (group C, n = 69) in a retrospective 6-month cohort study (41^C). The incidences of hepatitis were 2/225 (0.9%), 4/392 (1.0%), and 0/69 respectively; there were no significant differences in the frequencies of raised transaminases across the groups. Fluconazole treatment did not predict hepatitis, raised transaminases, or skin rashes. At 6 months after initiating nevirapine, 77–84% of patients were still taking it.

Paclitaxel   In guinea-pigs ketoconazole reduced the cumulative biliary excretion of paclitaxel and its metabolites up to 6 hours by 62% (42^E).

Ranolazine   The interactions of ranolazine, a new antianginal compound, with inhibitors and substrates of the CYP3A isoenzyme family have been studied in an open study and in four double-blind, randomized, multiple-dose studies in healthy adults. Ketoconazole increased ranolazine plasma concentrations and reduced the CYP3A4-mediated metabolic transformation of ranolazine, confirming that CYP3A4 is the primary metabolic pathway for ranolazine (43^c).

Risperidone   The effects of itraconazole 200 mg/day for 1 week on the plasma concentrations of risperidone 2–8 mg/day and its active metabolite 9-hydroxyrisperidone have been investigated in 19 patients with schizophrenia in relation to CYP2D6 genotype (44[c]). Dose-normalized plasma concentrations of risperidone and 9-hydroxyrisperidone were significantly increased by itraconazole and fell 1 week after withdrawal. However, the ratio of risperidone/9-hydroxyrisperidone, an index of CYP2D6 activity, was not altered. Itraconazole significantly increased the concentrations of risperidone by 69 and 75% in CYP2D6 extensive and poor metabolizers respectively; concentrations of risperidone plus 9-hydroxyrisperidone increased to a similar extent without a significant difference between CYP2D6 genotypes. There were no major pharmacodynamic effects. Thus, concentrations of both risperidone and 9-hydroxyrisperidone were significantly increased by the CYP3A inhibitor itraconazole, and this was independent of CYP2D6 activity, providing evidence that CYP3A is involved in the metabolism of risperidone and its metabolite.

Saint John's wort   The short-term and long-term effects of Saint John's wort (300 mg of LI 160 tds) on the pharmacokinetics of a single oral dose of voriconazole 400 mg have been investigated in a controlled, open study in 16 healthy men stratified for CYP2C19 genotype (45[c]). During the first 10 hours of the first day of administration of St John's wort, the AUC of voriconazole increased by 22% compared with control, but after 15 days the AUC was reduced by 59%, with a corresponding increase in oral voriconazole clearance. The baseline oral voriconazole clearance and the absolute increase in oral clearance were smaller in carriers of one or two deficient CYP2C19*2 alleles compared with wild-type individuals. Thus, co-administration of St John's wort leads to a short-term but clinically irrelevant increase followed by a prolonged extensive reduction in voriconazole exposure; CYP2C19 wild-type individuals may be at highest risk of potential voriconazole treatment failure.

Sildenafil   The effects of a single dose of sildenafil 3, 15, and 30 mg/kg and combined sildenafil + itraconazole 100 mg/kg on blood pressure, heart rate, and QT interval have been investigated in conscious beagle dogs (46[E]). There were no changes in blood pressure. Sildenafil 15 and 30 mg/kg increased heart rate from 0.5 to 6 hours after the dose and shortened the QT interval; these effects were significantly enhanced by itraconazole. This was attributed to inhibition of CYP3A4. Caution should therefore be taken when sildenafil is co-administered with itraconazole.

Sirolimus   An interaction between itraconazole and sirolimus has been reported in a primary renal allograft recipient (47[A]).

Tacrolimus   The interaction of itraconazole with tacrolimus in lung transplant recipients and the efficacy of itraconazole prophylaxis has been analysed in 40 patients who took prophylactic itraconazole 200 mg bd for the first 6 months after transplantation (48[c]). The mean dose of tacrolimus during itraconazole treatment was 3.26 mg/day compared with 5.74 mg/day (76% higher) after itraconazole was stopped. There were no differences in the rejection or fungal infection rates or in renal toxicity between the periods with and without itraconazole, although fewer positive fungal isolates were identified during itraconazole therapy.

Telithromycin   Itraconazole 200 mg/day increased the steady-state AUC of telithromycin 800 mg/day in a non-randomized, sequential, multiple-dose study in 34 healthy men (49[c]).

The effect of ketoconazole 400 mg/day for 5 days on the pharmacokinetics and pharmacodynamics (effect on the QT_c interval) of telithromycin 800 mg/day have been investigated using clarithromycin as a comparator in 32 subjects aged 60 years or over with renal impairment (50[C]). In those with creatinine clearances of 30–80 ml/minute ketoconazole increased telithromycin plasma concentrations to an extent similar to that for clarithromycin. There was no clinically significant prolongation of the QT_c interval.

Tretinoin   Tretinoin (all-trans-retinoic acid, ATRA) rarely causes hypercalcemia, but another case has been reported and attributed to inhibition of CYP3A4-mediated metabolism of tretinoin by voriconazole (51[A]).

Vincristine   *Another case of itraconazole-related vincristine neurotoxicity has been reported (52ᴬ).*

- *A 3-year-old boy with acute lymphoblastic leukemia received induction chemotherapy. On day 14, itraconazole 5 mg/kg was begun and 10 days later he developed paralytic ileus, neurogenic bladder, mild left ptosis, and absence of deep reflexes, with severe paralysis of the legs and mild weakness of the arms. Itraconazole withdrawal was followed by rapid improvement to normality within 6 weeks.*

Fluconazole   *(SED-15, 1377;*
SEDA-29, 286)

Liver   The *hepatotoxicity* of antifungal medications in bone marrow transplant recipients has been analysed in a retrospective matched-control study (21ᶜ). The unadjusted incidence of hepatotoxicity was 0.98 cases per 100 patient-days of exposure to fluconazole (OR = 1.99; 95% CI = 1.21, 3.26). In the follow-up analysis of patients who developed hepatotoxicity and who continued to take antifungal medications, 8% of those who took fluconazole developed marked increases in serum bilirubin concentration. Thus, fluconazole was associated with an increased risk of hepatotoxicity, independent of other treatments or patient characteristics. However, patients who develop hepatotoxicity appear to tolerate continued therapy with fluconazole.

Skin   *Erythema multiforme* associated with fluconazole has again been reported (53ᴬ).

Teratogenicity   Fluconazole is a teratogen in humans when used continuously at a dosage of 400–800 mg/day. Common features include *multiple synostosis* (including craniosynostosis and digital synostosis), *congenital heart defects, skeletal anomalies*, and recognizable *dysmorphic facial features* (SEDA-28, 306).

Another case of fluconazole *embryopathy* has been reported (54ᴬ).

- A 9-month-old boy was born to a 30-year-old woman following a 37-week pregnancy, which was complicated by maternal HIV infection and multiple drug exposures, including fluconazole

(400 mg/day) until the fifth month and then from 6 months to term, efavirenz, nevirapine, methadone, dapsone, pentamidine, and co-trimoxazole. At birth the infant had multiple congenital anomalies and at 9 months had craniosynostosis secondary to coronal and lambdoidal suture closures, a shallow orbital region, hypoplastic supraorbital ridges, hypertelorism, and mild ptosis. He had radioulnar synostosis and metacarpophalangeal–proximal interphalangeal symphalangism of D2-D5 bilaterally.

The potential of in utero exposure to fluconazole to initiate teratogenesis has been analysed in ICR (CD-1) mice (55ᴱ). Developmental phase specificity was determined by treating mice with single oral doses of 700 mg/kg on gestational days 8, 9, 10, 11, or 12. Control animals received vehicle on days 8–12. Day 10 was identified as the phase of maximal sensitivity for induction of cleft palate, the predominant teratogenic effect induced by fluconazole, when 50% of exposed fetuses were affected. After treatments on days 8, 9, 11, or 12, cleft palate occurred with lower frequencies: 12, 21, 29, and 2.7% respectively. There were anomalies of the middle ear apparatus in 15% of the fetuses that were exposed on day 8. A dysmorphic tympanic ring and absence of the incus were the more common ear anomalies recorded. Humeral length was reduced in 22% of fetuses that were exposed on day 10. The dose-response relation was investigated by treating animals with 0 (vehicle), 87.5, 175, or 350 mg/kg on day 10, coincident with the phase of peak teratogenic sensitivity. There was a clear dose-response relation and 175 mg/kg was the lowest dose at which cleft palate induction was observed, 7.6% of exposed fetuses being affected.

Susceptibility factors

Advanced HIV infection   In HIV-infected patients, fluconazole prophylaxis is associated with reductions in the rate of fungal infection. However, there are concerns about fluconazole prophylaxis and the risk of fluconazole-resistant infections. In a randomized, open comparison of oral fluconazole given continuously (200 mg 3 times weekly; the "continuous fluconazole arm"; n = 413) and fluconazole that was provided only for episodes of oropharyngeal candidiasis or esophageal candidiasis (the "episodic fluconazole arm"; $n = 416$) in HIV-infected persons with CD4+ T cell counts of under $150 \times 10^6/l$ and a history of orophayngeal candidiasis (56^C). The primary end point was the time to development of fluconazole-resistant orophayngeal or esophageal candidiasis, which was defined as a lack of response to fluconazole 200 mg/day for 14 or 21 days respectively. After 42 months, 17 subjects in the continuous fluconazole arm (4.1%) developed fluconazole-resistant orophayngeal or esophageal candidiasis, compared with 18 (4.3%) in the episodic fluconazole arm. There was no difference between treatments with regard to the time to development of a fluconazole-resistant infection within 24 months or before the end of the study. Continuous fluconazole therapy was associated with fewer cases of orophayngeal or esophageal candidiasis (0.29 versus 1.08 episodes per patient-year) and fewer invasive fungal infections. This study shows that fluconazole is not associated with a significant risk of fluconazole-resistant orophayngeal or esophageal candidiasis, compared with episodic fluconazole therapy in HIV-infected patients with access to active antiretroviral therapy.

Immunocompromised patients with esophageal candidiasis   Micafungin 150 mg/day and fluconazole 200 mg/day have been compared in a large randomized study in 523 patients with documented esophageal candidiasis aged 16 years and over (57^C). The median duration of therapy was 14 days. For the primary end point of endoscopic cure, the treatment difference was negligible (88% each), and the overall therapeutic response rate was 87%. The incidences of drug-related adverse events were 28% for micafungin and 21% for fluconazole. Therapy was withdrawn in six patients taking micafungin and two taking fluconazole; rash was the most common event that led to withdrawal.

High-risk very low birth weight infants   Daily versus twice-weekly fluconazole prophylaxis for up to 6 weeks have been investigated in a randomized, double-blind trial in 81 preterm infants who weighed under 1000 g at birth and with an endotracheal tube and/or central vascular catheter (58^C). There was *Candida* colonization in nine children and *Candida* sepsis in three, with no difference between treatments. All fungal isolates were sensitive to

fluconazole and no adverse effects were documented.

Itraconazole   *(SED-15, 1932; SEDA-29, 286)*

Nervous system   *Painful neuropathy* associated with itraconazole has been reported in a man with type 1 diabetes (59^A).

Liver   *Liver failure* requiring liver transplantation after itraconazole treatment for 3 weeks for toenail onychomycosis has been reported in a 25-year-old woman (60^A).

Immunologic   *Urticaria and angioedema* attributed to itraconazole have been reported (61^A).

Ketoconazole   *(SED-15, 1969; SEDA-26, 304)*

Because of erratic systemic availability, less target specificity, and the advent of alternative azoles, ketoconazole has few if any indications in current practice. However, it is a potent inhibitor of CYP 3A4, and has an important role as a probe for CYP3A4-mediated drug interactions, indicating the potential for interactions with other azoles.

Cardiovascular   Ketoconazole has not previously been thought to be prodysrhythmic without concomitant use of drugs that cause *prolongation of the QT interval*, but this has now been reported (62^A).

- A 63-year-old woman with coronary artery disease developed a markedly prolonged QT interval and torsade de pointes after taking ketoconazole for a fungal infection. Her QT interval returned to normal on withdrawal of ketoconazole. There were no mutations in her genes that encode cardiac IK_r channel proteins.

The authors concluded that because it blocks inward rectifier potassium channels (IK_r) channels, ketoconazole alone can prolong the QT interval and induce *torsade de pointes*. This calls for attention when ketoconazole is given to patients with risk factors for the long QT syndrome.

Susceptibility factors

Androgen-independent prostate cancer   The combination of high-dose ketoconazole+hydrocortisone is effective in androgen-independent prostate cancer. The median duration of response tends to be brief but a significant minority of patients have extended responses. Well characterized information about response and survival, especially in patients who have more durable responses has not been previously reported. The medical records of 78 patients with androgen-independent prostate cancer treated with high-dose ketoconazole + hydrocortisone between March 1991 and February 1999 were retrospectively reviewed and baseline clinical and laboratory factors predictive of a prolonged response and survival were identified (63[c]). The median baseline prostate specific antigen concentration before the start of therapy was 25 µg/l. The number of patients with none, 1–3, and more than three lesions on bone scan were 25, 35, and 18 respectively. The median and mean times to progression of prostate specific antigen were 6.7 and 15 months. Median and mean survival times were 38 and 42 months respectively. Response time and survival were highly correlated. A total of 34 (44%) men had a greater than 75% fall in prostate specific antigen. The median survival times in men with more versus less than a 75% reduction were 60 versus 24 months respectively. In a Cox proportional hazard regression, prolonged survival was predicted by percent fall in prostate specific antigen, extent of disease on bone scan, and baseline prostate specific antigen. Adverse effects were not reported.

Posaconazole   *(SED-15, 2905;*

SEDA-29, 286)

Posaconazole is a lipophilic antifungal triazole. In vitro it has potent broad-spectrum activity against opportunistic, endemic, and dermatophytic fungi, including organisms that are often refractory to existing agents, such as *C. glabrata, C. krusei, A. terreus, Fusarium* spp., and the *Zygomycetes* (17[R], 64[R]). Posaconazole is available as an oral suspension and achieves optimal exposure when taken in 2–4 divided doses with food or a nutritional

supplement. It has a large volume of distribution and a half-life of about 20 hours. Posaconazole is not metabolized by CYP450 isoenzymes but is primarily excreted unchanged in the feces. It inhibits CYP3A4, but has no effects on CYP1A2, CYP2C8, CYP2C9, CYP2D6, or CYP2E1; therefore, a limited spectrum of drug–drug interactions can be expected.

Posaconazole had good antifungal efficacy in phase II and III clinical trials in immunocompromised patients with oropharyngeal and esophageal candidiasis. It also showed promising efficacy as salvage therapy in a large phase II study. In the subset of 107 patients with invasive aspergillosis, 42% had a complete or partial response at end of treatment compared with 26% of a control cohort.

In two large randomized phase III studies in high-risk patients posaconazole had preventive efficacy, in particular against invasive *Aspergillus* infections, and a survival benefit in patients with acute myeloblastic leukemia/myelodysplastic syndrome undergoing remission induction chemotherapy.

Posaconazole has been well tolerated and is comparable to fluconazole. It has been approved in the EU for treatment of aspergillosis, fusariosis, chromoblastomycosis, and coccidioidomycosis refractory to or in patients intolerant of standard therapies; in addition, it has been approved for prophylaxis in high-risk patients with acute myeloblastic leukemia/myelodysplastic syndrome and allogeneic hemopoietic stem cell transplantation and graft-versus-host disease in both the EU and the USA. The recommended daily dosage for salvage treatment is 400 mg bd given with food; for patients who cannot take solid food, a dosage of 200 mg qds is recommended, preferably with a nutritional supplement. The dosage for prophylaxis is 200 mg tds.

Susceptibility factors

Impaired renal function   The pharmacokinetics and safety of a single oral dose of posaconazole 400 mg have been studied in healthy subjects and in those with mild, moderate, and severe chronic renal disease ($n = 6$ in each group) (65[c]). In those on hemodialysis a dose was given on a non-hemodialysis day, and another 6 hours before hemodialysis. Mild to moderate renal disease had no effect on the pharmacokinetics of posaconazole. Mean oral clearances before and during hemodialysis were comparable. Furthermore, the difference in the pre-dialysis and post-dialysis posaconazole concentrations was only about 3%, suggesting that posaconazole is not removed by hemodialysis. Protein binding was similar in all groups (about 98%) and was unaffected by hemodialysis. Posaconazole was generally well tolerated. These results show that dosage adjustments are not required in patients with disease.

Voriconazole   *(SED-15, 3688; SEDA-29, 287)*

Voriconazole is a synthetic antifungal triazole with activity against a wide spectrum of clinically important yeasts and moulds, including *Candida* spp., *Cryptococcus neoformans, Aspergillus* and other hyaline moulds, dematiaceous moulds, and dimorphic moulds. It undergoes complex hepatic metabolism and has the potential for drug–drug interactions mediated by CYP 3A4, CYP2C9, and CYP2C19.

Voriconazole had excellent clinical efficacy in phase II studies in patients with oropharyngeal and esophageal candidiasis, acute and chronic invasive aspergillosis, and infections with rare fungal pathogens. In phase III clinical trials, it was superior to conventional amphotericin B for first-line therapy of invasive aspergillosis, as effective as conventional amphotericin as first-line therapy for candidemia, and comparable to liposomal amphotericin as empirical antifungal therapy in patients with persistent neutropenia.

Voriconazole causes more *liver function test abnormalities* than fluconazole, and *photosensitization, hallucinations*, and *visual disturbances* can occur (17[R], 66[R]).

Comparative studies   In a multicenter, randomized, non-inferiority study, voriconazole (*n* = 283) was compared with a regimen of amphotericin followed by fluconazole (*n* = 139) for candidemia in non-neutropenic patients (67[C]). Voriconazole was not inferior to amphotericin + fluconazole in the primary efficacy analysis, with successful outcomes in 41% of patients in both treatment groups. Withdrawals due to all-cause adverse events were more frequent with voriconazole, although most were due to non-drug-related events and there were significantly fewer serious adverse events and cases of renal toxicity than with amphotericin + fluconazole.

Nervous system   *Painful peripheral neuropathy* associated with voriconazole has been reported (68[A]).

- A 43-year-old woman who had undergone liver transplantation received voriconazole for invasive deep sinus aspergillosis and developed intolerable pain in all limbs. Electromyography and nerve conduction studies suggested a demyelinating neuropathy. The symptoms and signs of neuropathy disappeared permanently soon after voriconazole withdrawal.

Skin   Severe retinoid-like *photosensitivity* (cheilitis and erythema, desquamation, and ulceration of light-exposed skin) has previously been reported. While the exact mechanisms of this phototoxicity are unknown, inhibition of retinoid metabolism or a direct phototoxic effect of voriconazole or one of its metabolites have been implicated (SEDA-29, 287). *Photoageing* caused by voriconazole has now been reported (69[A]).

- A 15-year-old girl developed cheilitis and erythema over the sun-exposed areas of her body after taking voriconazole for 5 weeks for a severe fungal infection. The lesions improved transiently before subsequent photodamage occurred to the backs of her forearms, the backs of her hands, and face. Voriconazole was withdrawn once the fungal infection had completely resolved and her blisters, erythema, and cheilitis resolved. However, she was left with solar elastosis, multiple lentigines, and ephelides on sun-exposed areas.

These cutaneous manifestations may represent a unique adverse event caused by voriconazole.

Pseudoporphyria is an uncommon blistering disorder. It has clinical and histological similarities to porphyria cutanea tarda but without changes in urine and serum porphyrin concentrations. Pseudoporphyria has many causes, including chronic renal insufficiency, ultraviolet radiation, and many medications. Pseudoporphyria has been attributed to voriconazole for the first time (70[A]).

Susceptibility factors

Children   In a retrospective case review of 21 children aged 5 to 16 years with cystic fibrosis and allergic bronchopulmonary aspergillosis, voriconazole, used as monotherapy or in combination with an immunomodulatory agent, resulted in significant improvement in pulmonary function and serology (71[c]). There were adverse effects in seven children: photosensitivity reactions ($n = 3$), nausea ($n = 2$), a rise in hepatic enzymes ($n = 1$) and hair loss ($n = 1$).

Renal disease   The pharmacokinetics of a single oral dose of voriconazole 200 mg have been studied in five patients with end-stage renal disease undergoing peritoneal dialysis (72[c]). The t_{max} occurred in plasma at 2.4 hours and in dialysate at 2.8 hours. The dialysate to plasma ratio was 0.66. Less than 1% of the dose was recovered in dialysate 24 hours after dosing. These results suggest that voriconazole penetrates peritoneal fluid well; there is minimal peritoneal clearance and therefore no dosage adjustment is needed for patients undergoing peritoneal dialysis.

Monitoring therapy   Steady-state trough plasma voriconazole concentrations were obtained in 25 recipients of allogeneic hemopoietic stem cell transplants, once ($n = 13$), twice ($n = 10$), or at least three times ($n = 2$), 5–18 (median 10) days after starting voriconazole or dosage modification (73[c]). The 41 voriconazole concentrations were 0.2–6.8 µg/ml; six were below 0.5 (possibly below the in vitro MIC_{90} for *Aspergillus* spp.). Voriconazole concentrations correlated with aspartate transaminase and alkaline phosphatase activities, but not with creatinine, bilirubin, or alanine transaminase. Since liver dysfunction is common after HSCT, it was not possible to determine whether the increases in aspartate transaminase and alkaline phosphatase activities were due to higher voriconazole concentrations. The authors concluded that trough voriconazole concentrations vary considerably between patients and they suggested monitoring concentrations in patients taking voriconazole for confirmed fungal infections and in those with increased aspartate transaminase or alkaline phosphatase activities.

ECHINOCANDINS   *(SED-15, 1197; SEDA-28, 309; SEDA-29, 288)*

The echinocandins act by non-competitive inhibition of the synthesis of 1,3-beta-D-glucan, which is a major constituent of the cell wall of many pathogenic fungi and plays a key role in cell division and cell growth. The current echinocandins (anidulafungin, Eraxis®, caspofungin, Cancidas®, and micafungin, Mycamine®) have potent and broad-spectrum antifungal activity against *Candida* and *Aspergillus* spp. without causing cross-resistance to existing agents. Their activity against other fungal pathogens in vitro is variable (17[R], 66[R]).

All three compounds have dose-independent pharmacokinetics with half-lives of 8–24 hours and are dosed once daily. They are highly protein bound (over 85–99%) and distribute into all major tissues, including the brain; concentrations in non-inflammatory CSF are low. The echinocandins are eliminated by chemical degradation and/or hepatic metabolism and are slowly excreted as inactive metabolites via the urine and feces; only small amounts are excreted into the urine unchanged. They lack significant potential for drug interactions mediated by CYP isozymes and are generally well tolerated.

The efficacy of the echinocandins against *Candida* spp has been documented in phase II and phase III studies in immunocompromised patients with superficial and invasive fungal infections (anidulafungin, caspofungin, and micafungin), as second-line therapy for invasive aspergillosis (caspofungin), as empirical antifungal therapy in granulocytopenic patients with persistent fever despite broad-spectrum empirical antibacterial therapy (caspofungin), and as prophylaxis in high-risk granulocytopenic patients following hemopoietic stem cell transplantation (micafungin) (66[R]). At the time of writing, anidulafungin is licensed in the USA for patients aged 18 years and over for primary therapy in non-neutropenic patients with invasive *Candida* infections and for esophageal candidiasis; caspofungin is licensed in the EU and the USA for patients aged 18 years and over for second-line therapy of definite or probable invasive aspergillosis, for primary therapy in patients with invasive *Candida* infections, and for empirical antifungal therapy in granulocytopenic patients with persistent fever. Micafungin is licensed only in the USA for prevention of *Candida* infections in patients undergoing hemopoietic stem cell transplantation and for treatment of esophageal candidiasis.

Anidulafungin   *(SEDA-29, 289)*

Drug–drug interactions

Ciclosporin   The effect of anidulafungin on ciclosporin metabolism has been studied in vitro, in pooled human hepatic microsomal protein fractions, and in vivo, in a multiple-dose, open study in 12 healthy volunteers (74[cE]). Anidulafungin 200 mg intravenously was followed by 100 mg/day intravenously on days 2–8. Ciclosporin 1.25 mg/kg bd was given orally on days 5–8. The in vitro addition of anidulafungin had no effect on ciclosporin metabolism by hepatic microsomes. In the clinical study, there were no dose-limiting or serious adverse events; there was a small increase in anidulafungin concentrations and drug exposure (22%) after 4 days of ciclosporin, but this was not considered to be clinically important.

Voriconazole   Co-administration of anidulafungin and voriconazole has been investigated in a placebo-controlled study in 17 healthy subjects (24[c]). Anidulafungin was administered intravenously (200 mg on day 1 then 100 mg/day on days 2–4) and voriconazole orally (400 mg every 12 hours on day 1 then 200 mg every 12 hours on days 2–4). There were no dose-limiting or serious adverse effects and all adverse events were mild and consistent with the known safety profiles of the two drugs. There was no pharmacokinetic interaction.

Caspofungin   *(SEDA-29, 289)*

Observational studies   The efficacy and safety of caspofungin as salvage therapy for invasive aspergillosis has been studied in patients enrolled in the Caspofungin Compassionate Use Study (75[C]). There was a favorable response in 20/45 patients, including nine and 11 with complete and partial responses respectively. One serious drug-related adverse event was reported in a patient with acute biphenotypic leukemia, who had an *anaphylactic*

reaction to caspofungin, characterized by stridor/dyspnea, facial swelling, and accentuation of a pre-existing skin rash about 10 minutes into the infusion; all the symptoms resolved within 15 minutes of withdrawal of caspofungin and the administration of diphenhydramine and hydrocortisone.

Caspofungin 50 mg/day for a median duration of 20 (range 8–64) days has been used as first-line therapy for proven or probable pulmonary fungal infection in 32 immunocompromised patients with hematological malignancies (median age 52 years) (76[c]). The overall response rate was 56% (18/32), with 12/18 complete responses and 6/18 partial responses. Granulocyte recovery and status of disease (remission/onset versus refractory/relapsed) were significantly associated with a favorable outcome. There were no clinical adverse events and only grades I and II transient *increases in serum alkaline phosphatase and/or transaminase activities* in 4/32 patients.

Susceptibility factors

Children   In 39 children aged 2–11 years and adolescents aged 12–17 years with neutropenia, caspofungin, 1 mg/kg/day or 50 or 70 mg/m^2/day, was generally well tolerated (77[C]). None developed a serious drug-related adverse event or were withdrawn because of toxicity.

In 13 infants in whom caspofungin was added to conventional antifungal drugs (amphotericin B and/or fluconazole or flucytosine) for refractory candidemia, 12 of whom were preterm, sterilization of blood cultures was achieved in 11 at a median time of 3 (range 1–21) days (78[c]). Adverse events included thrombophlebitis ($n = 1$), hypokalemia ($n = 2$), and raised liver enzymes ($n = 4$). Three infants had a second episode of candidemia and seven died.

Drug–drug interactions

Ciclosporin   In phase I studies of caspofungin + ciclosporin there were mild transient rises in alanine transaminase activity, although in two previous retrospective case series this combination did not result in a significant risk of clinically important hepatotoxicity (SEDA-29, 289). Of 31 patients given caspofungin after allogeneic stem cell transplantation as a second-line agent for treatment of invasive fungal infection ($n = 15$) or for fever of unknown origin ($n = 16$), 23 received caspofungin + ciclosporin without any major adverse effects; increases in aspartate transaminase activity were not clinically significant (79[c]).

Rifampicin   Caspofungin treatment failure has been reported in a patient with invasive candidiasis and concomitant rifampicin treatment (80[A]). Rifampicin is a non-specific inducer/activator of mixed-function oxygenases and may increase the metabolism of caspofungin, thereby leading to ineffective plasma concentrations.

Micafungin   (SEDA-29, 290)

Observational studies   In an open, non-comparative study, neonates, children, and adults with new or refractory candidemia were given micafungin for up to 42 days (81[c]). A total of 126 patients were evaluable and received at least five doses. There was a complete or partial response in 83% and serious adverse events related to micafungin were uncommon.

Comparative studies   In a large, randomized comparative study in 523 adults with esophageal candidiasis randomized to either intravenous micafungin 150 mg/day or fluconazole 200 mg/day for a median of 14 days, the incidences of drug-related adverse events were 28% for micafungin and 21% for fluconazole (57[c]). Six patients taking micafungin and two taking fluconazole withdrew, most commonly because of *rashes*.

In a sequential dose escalation study, 74 adults with cancer undergoing bone marrow or peripheral blood stem cell transplantation were given fluconazole 400 mg/day and either isotonic saline (control, $n = 12$) or micafungin 12.5–200 mg/day ($n = 62$) for up to 4 weeks (82[c]). The maximum tolerated dose of micafungin was not reached, based on the Southwest Oncology Group criteria for grade 3 toxicity; drug-related adverse events were rare. Common adverse events that were considered to be related to micafungin were *headache* (6.8%), *arthralgia* (6.8%),

hypophosphatemia (4.1%), *insomnia* (4.1%), *maculopapular rashes* (4.1%), and *other rashes* (4.1%). There was no clinical or kinetic evidence of an interaction of micafungin with fluconazole.

Susceptibility factors

Children   In a multicenter, phase I, open, sequential-group, dose-escalation study in 77 children with neutropenia micafungin was begun at a dosage of 0.5 mg/kg/day and increased to 1.0, 1.5, 2.0, 3.0, and 4.0 mg/kg/day (83[c]). The most common adverse events were *diarrhea* (20%), *epistaxis* (18%), *abdominal pain* (17%), and *headache* (17%). Nine patients had adverse events that were considered by the investigator to be possibly related to micafungin; of these, the most common were diarrhea, vomiting, and headache, each of which occurred in two patients. There was an inverse relation between age and micafungin clearance: in those aged 2–8 years, clearance was about 1.35 times that of patients 9 years of age and older.

Liver disease and renal disease   The pharmacokinetics and plasma protein binding of micafungin have been studied in patients with moderate hepatic dysfunction ($n = 8$), patients with creatinine clearances below 30 ml/minute ($n = 9$), and matched controls ($n = 8$ and 9 respectively) (84[c]). The AUC of intravenous micafungin was significantly lower in those with moderate hepatic dysfunction than in controls, but there was no difference in micafungin weight-adjusted clearance. The difference in AUC may have been due to differences in body weight. Renal dysfunction did not alter micafungin pharmacokinetics.

Drug–drug interactions   Micafungin had little or no effect on CYP3A4-related metabolism in human liver microsomes or MDR1 transport activity in MDR1-overexpressing LLC-GA5-COL150 cells (85[E]). Thus, micafungin is unlikely to cause drug–drug interactions by inhibition of CYP3A4 or MDR1. In similar in vitro studies, micafungin neither inhibited nor stimulated the metabolic activities mediated by CYP1A2, CYP2D6, CYP2E1, CYP2C9, or CYP2C19. The IC_{50} of micafungin against CYP3A4-mediated nifedipine oxidation was comparable with that of voriconazole and fluconazole, compatible with the finding that micafungin is a mild inhibitor of CYP3A4 (86^E, 87^E).

Ciclosporin   The effect of micafungin 100 mg/day on the pharmacokinetics of a single oral dose of ciclosporin 5 mg/kg have been stud-

ied in 27 subjects (88^c). Micafungin inhibited ciclosporin metabolism by only about 16%.

Tacrolimus   Intravenous micafungin 100 mg had no effect on the pharmacokinetics of oral tacrolimus 5 mg in 26 healthy volunteers (89^c).

References

1. Warshaw EM, Fett DD, Bloomfield HE, Grill JP, Nelson DB, Quintero V, Carver SM, Zielke GR, Lederle FA. Pulse versus continuous terbinafine for onychomycosis: a randomized, double-blind, controlled trial. J Am Acad Dermatol 2005;53(4):578–84.
2. Doty RL, Haxel BR. Objective assessment of terbinafine-induced taste loss. Laryngoscope 2005;115(11):2035–7.
3. Beltraminelli HS, Lerch M, Arnold A, Bircher AJ, Haeusermann P. Acute generalized exanthematous pustulosis induced by the antifungal terbinafine: case report and review of the literature. Br J Dermatol 2005;152(4):780–3.
4. Gréco M, Plantin P. Acute generalized exanthematous pustulosis (AGEP) induced by terbinafine with involuntary positive reintroduction. Eur J Dermatol 2005;15(2):116.
5. Abdel-Rahman SM, Herron J, Fallon-Friedlander S, Hauffe S, Horowitz A, Riviere GJ. Pharmacokinetics of terbinafine in young children treated for tinea capitis. Pediatr Infect Dis J 2005;24(10):886–91.
6. Molden E, Garcia BH, Braathen P, Eggen AE. Co-prescription of cytochrome P450 2D6/3A4 inhibitor-substrate pairs in clinical practice. A retrospective analysis of data from Norwegian primary pharmacies. Eur J Clin Pharmacol 2005;61(2):119–25.
7. Castberg I, Helle J, Aamo TO. Prolonged pharmacokinetic drug interaction between terbinafine and amitriptyline. Ther Drug Monit 2005;27(5):680–2.
8. Malani PN, Depestel DD, Riddell J, Bickley S, Klein LR, Kauffman CA. Experience with community-based amphotericin B infusion therapy. Pharmacotherapy 2005;25(5):690–7.
9. Alexander BD, Wingard JR. Study of renal safety in amphotericin B lipid complex-treated patients. Clin Infect Dis 2005;40(Suppl 6):S414–21.
10. Wurthwein G, Groll AH, Hempel G, Adler-Shohet FC, Lieberman JM, Walsh TJ. Population pharmacokinetics of amphotericin B lipid complex in neonates. Antimicrob Agents Chemother 2005;49(12):5092–8.
11. Wiley JM, Seibel NL, Walsh TJ. Efficacy and safety of amphotericin B lipid complex in 548 children and adolescents with invasive fungal infections. Pediatr Infect Dis J 2005;24(2):167–74.
12. Hooshmand-Rad R, Chu A, Gotz V, Morris J, Batty S, Freifeld A. Use of amphotericin B lipid complex in elderly patients. J Infect 2005;50(4):277–87.
13. Pappas PG. Amphotericin B lipid complex in the treatment of invasive fungal infections: results of the Collaborative Exchange of Antifungal Research (CLEAR), an industry-supported patient registry. Clin Infect Dis 2005;40(Suppl 6):S379–83.
14. Chandrasekar PH, Ito JI. Amphotericin B lipid complex in the management of invasive aspergillosis in immunocompromised patients. Clin Infect Dis 2005;40(Suppl 6):S392–400.
15. Ito JI, Hooshmand-Rad R. Treatment of Candida infections with amphotericin B lipid complex. Clin Infect Dis 2005;40(Suppl 6):S384–91.
16. Martino R, Cortes M, Subira M, Parody R, Moreno E, Sierra J. Efficacy and toxicity of intermediate-dose amphotericin B lipid complex as a primary or salvage treatment of fungal infections in patients with hematological malignancies. Leuk Lymphoma 2005;46(10):1429–35.
17. Groll AH, Glasmacher A, Just-Nuebling G, Maschmeyer G, Walsh TJ. Clinical pharmacology of antifungal compounds. Infect Dis Clin N Am 2003;17:159–91.
18. Girmenia C, Cimino G, Di Cristofano F, Micozzi A, Gentile G, Martino P. Effects of hydration with salt repletion on renal toxicity of conventional amphotericin B empirical therapy: a prospective study in patients with hematological malignancies. Support Care Cancer 2005;13(12):987–92.
19. Mohr JF, Hall AC, Ericsson CD, Ostrosky-Zeichner L. Fatal amphotericin B overdose due to administration of nonlipid formulation instead of lipid formulation. Pharmacotherapy 2005;25(3):426–8.
20. Musa AM, Khalil EA, Mahgoub FA, Hamad S, Elkadaru AM, El Hassan AM. Efficacy of liposomal amphotericin B (AmBisome) in the treatment of persistent post-kala-azar dermal leishmaniasis (PKDL). Ann Trop Med Parasitol 2005;99(6):563–9.

21. Fischer MA, Winkelmayer WC, Rubin RH, Avorn J. The hepatotoxicity of antifungal medications in bone marrow transplant recipients. Clin Infect Dis 2005;41(3):301–7.

22. Castroagudin JF, Ponton C, Bustamante M, Otero E, Martinez J, Tome S, Conde R, Segade FR, Delgado M, Brage A, Galban C, Varo E. Prospective interventional study to evaluate the efficacy and safety of liposomal amphotericin B as prophylaxis of fungal infections in high-risk liver transplant recipients. Transplant Proc 2005;37(9):3965–7.

23. Yu DT, Peterson JF, Seger DL, Gerth WC, Bates DW. Frequency of potential azole drug–drug interactions and consequences of potential fluconazole drug interactions. Pharmacoepidemiol Drug Saf 2005;14(11):755–67.

24. Dowell JA, Schranz J, Baruch A, Foster G. Safety and pharmacokinetics of coadministered voriconazole and anidulafungin. J Clin Pharmacol 2005;45(12):1373–82.

25. Lohitnavy M, Lohitnavy O, Thangkeattiyanon O, Srichai W. Reduced oral itraconazole bioavailability by antacid suspension. J Clin Pharm Ther 2005;30(3):201–6.

26. Chaikin P, Gillen MS, Malik M, Pentikis H, Rhodes GR, Roberts DJ. Co-administration of ketoconazole with H1-antagonists ebastine and loratadine in healthy subjects: pharmacokinetic and pharmacodynamic effects. Br J Clin Pharmacol 2005;59(3):346–54.

27. Kubo M, Koue T, Inaba A, Takeda H, Maune H, Fukuda T, Azuma J. Influence of itraconazole co-administration and CYP2D6 genotype on the pharmacokinetics of the new antipsychotic aripiprazole. Drug Metab Pharmacokinet 2005;20(1):55–64.

28. Lilja JJ, Backman JT, Neuvonen PJ. Effect of itraconazole on the pharmacokinetics of atenolol. Basic Clin Pharmacol Toxicol 2005;97(6):395–8.

29. Videla C, Vega J, Borja H. Hepatotoxicity associated with cyclosporine monitoring using C2 recommendations in adult renal recipients receiving ketoconazole. Transplant Proc 2005;37(3):1574–6.

30. de Jonge ME, Huitema AD, van Dam SM, Rodenhuis S, Beijnen JH. Effects of co-medicated drugs on cyclophosphamide bioactivation in human liver microsomes. Anticancer Drugs 2005;16(3):331–6.

31. Jakate AS, Roy P, Patel A, Abramowitz W, Persiani S, Wangsa J, Kapil R. Effect of azole antifungals ketoconazole and fluconazole on the pharmacokinetics of dexloxiglumide. Br J Clin Pharmacol 2005;60(5):498–507.

32. Yoshiyama Y, Kanke M. Toxic interactions between fluconazole and disopyramide in chick embryos. Biol Pharm Bull 2005;28(1):151–3.

33. Kahri J, Valkonen M, Bäcklund T, Vuoristo M, Kivistö KT. Rhabdomyolysis in a patient receiving atorvastatin and fluconazole. Eur J Clin Pharmacol 2005;60(12):905–7.

34. Kovarik JM, Beyer D, Bizot MN, Jiang Q, Shenouda M, Schmouder RL. Blood concentrations of everolimus are markedly increased by ketoconazole. J Clin Pharmacol 2005;45(5):514–8.

35. Shon JH, Yoon YR, Hong WS, Nguyen PM, Lee SS, Choi YG, Cha IJ, Shin JG. Effect of itraconazole on the pharmacokinetics and pharmacodynamics of fexofenadine in relation to the MDR1 genetic polymorphism. Clin Pharmacol Ther 2005;78(2):191–201.

36. McKillop D, McCormick AD, Millar A, Miles GS, Phillips PJ, Hutchison M. Cytochrome P450-dependent metabolism of gefitinib. Xenobiotica 2005;35(1):39–50.

37. Swaisland HC, Ranson M, Smith RP, Leadbetter J, Laight A, McKillop D, Wild MJ. Pharmacokinetic drug interactions of gefitinib with rifampicin, itraconazole and metoprolol. Clin Pharmacokinet 2005;44(10):1067–81.

38. Gambillara E, Laffitte E, Widmer N, Decosterd LA, Duchosal MA, Kovacsovics T, Panizzon RG. Severe pustular eruption associated with imatinib and voriconazole in a patient with chronic myeloid leukemia. Dermatology 2005;211(4):363–5.

39. Yong WP, Ramirez J, Innocenti F, Ratain MJ. Effects of ketoconazole on glucuronidation by UDP-glucuronosyltransferase enzymes. Clin Cancer Res 2005;11(18):6699–704.

40. Ridtitid W, Wongnawa M, Mahatthanatrakul W, Raungsri N, Sunbhanich M. Ketoconazole increases plasma concentrations of antimalarial mefloquine in healthy human volunteers. J Clin Pharm Ther 2005;30(3):285–90.

41. Manosuthi W, Chumpathat N, Chaovavanich A, Sungkanuparph S. Safety and tolerability of nevirapine-based antiretroviral therapy in HIV-infected patients receiving fluconazole for cryptococcal prophylaxis: a retrospective cohort study. BMC Infect Dis 2005;5:67.

42. Bun SS, Giacometti S, Fanciullino R, Ciccolini J, Bun H, Aubert C. Effect of several compounds on biliary excretion of paclitaxel and its metabolites in guinea-pigs. Anticancer Drugs 2005;16(6):675–82.

43. Jerling M, Huan BL, Leung K, Chu N, Abdallah H, Hussein Z. Studies to investigate the pharmacokinetic interactions between ranolazine and ketoconazole, diltiazem, or simvastatin during combined administration in healthy subjects. J Clin Pharmacol 2005;45(4):422–33.

44. Jung SM, Kim KA, Cho HK, Jung IG, Park PW, Byun WT, Park JY. Cytochrome P450 3A inhibitor itraconazole affects plasma concentrations of risperidone and 9-hydroxyrisperidone in schizophrenic patients. Clin Pharmacol Ther 2005;78(5):520–8.

45. Rengelshausen J, Banfield M, Riedel KD, Burhenne J, Weiss J, Thomsen T, Walter-Sack I, Haefeli WE, Mikus G. Opposite effects of short-term and long-term St John's wort intake on voriconazole pharmacokinetics. Clin Pharmacol Ther 2005;78(1):25–33.

46. Kim EJ, Seo JW, Hwang JY, Han SS. Effects of combined treatment with sildenafil and itraconazole on the cardiovascular system in

telemetered conscious dogs. Drug Chem Toxicol 2005;28(2):177–86.

47. Kuypers DR, Claes K, Evenepoel P, Maes B, Vandecasteele S, Vanrenterghem Y, Van Damme B, Desmet K. Drug interaction between itraconazole and sirolimus in a primary renal allograft recipient. Transplantation 2005;79(6):737.

48. Shitrit D, Ollech JE, Ollech A, Bakal I, Saute M, Sahar G, Kramer MR. Itraconazole prophylaxis in lung transplant recipients receiving tacrolimus (FK 506): efficacy and drug interaction. J Heart Lung Transplant 2005;24(12):2148–52.

49. Shi J, Montay G, Leroy B, Bhargava VO. Effects of itraconazole or grapefruit juice on the pharmacokinetics of telithromycin. Pharmacotherapy 2005;25(1):42–51.

50. Shi J, Chapel S, Montay G, Hardy P, Barrett JS, Sica D, Swan SK, Noveck R, Leroy B, Bhargava VO. Effect of ketoconazole on the pharmacokinetics and safety of telithromycin and clarithromycin in older subjects with renal impairment. Int J Clin Pharmacol Ther 2005;43(3):123–33.

51. Bennett MT, Sirrs S, Yeung JK, Smith CA. Hypercalcemia due to all trans retinoic acid in the treatment of acute promyelocytic leukemia potentiated by voriconazole. Leuk Lymphoma 2005;46(12):1829–31.

52. Bermudez M, Fuster JL, Llinares E, Galera A, Gonzalez C. Itraconazole-related increased vincristine neurotoxicity: case report and review of literature. J Pediatr Hematol Oncol 2005;27(7):389–92.

53. Dalle S, Skowron F, Ronger-Savle S, Balme B, Thomas L. Erythema multiforme induced by fluconazole. Dermatology 2005;211(2):169.

54. Lopez-Rangel E, van Allen MI. Prenatal exposure to fluconazole: an identifiable dysmorphic phenotype. Birth Defects Res A Clin Mol Teratol 2005;73(11):919–23.

55. Tiboni GM, Giampietro F. Murine teratology of fluconazole: evaluation of developmental phase specificity and dose dependence. Pediatr Res 2005;58(1):94–9.

56. Goldman M, Cloud GA, Wade KD, Reboli AC, Fichtenbaum CJ, Hafner R, Sobel JD, Powderly WG, Patterson TF, Wheat LJ, Stein DK, Dismukes WE, Filler SG, AIDS Clinical Trials Group Study Team 323, Mycoses Study Group Study Team 40. A randomized study of the use of fluconazole in continuous versus episodic therapy in patients with advanced HIV infection and a history of oropharyngeal candidiasis: AIDS Clinical Trials Group Study 323/Mycoses Study Group Study 40. Clin Infect Dis 2005;41(10):1473–80.

57. de Wet NT, Bester AJ, Viljoen JJ, Filho F, Suleiman JM, Ticona E, Llanos EA, Fisco C, Lau W, Buell D. A randomized, double blind, comparative trial of micafungin (FK463) vs. fluconazole for the treatment of oesophageal candidiasis. Aliment Pharmacol Ther 2005;21(7):899–907.

58. Kaufman D, Boyle R, Hazen KC, Patrie JT, Robinson M, Grossman LB. Twice weekly fluconazole prophylaxis for prevention of invasive Candida infection in high-risk infants of <1000 grams birth weight. J Pediatr 2005;147(2):172–9.

59. Singh R, Cundy T. Itraconazole-induced painful neuropathy in a man with type 1 diabetes. Diabetes Care 2005;28(1):225.

60. Srebrnik A, Levtov S, Ben-Ami R, Brenner S. Liver failure and transplantation after itraconazole treatment for toenail onychomycosis. J Eur Acad Dermatol Venereol 2005;19(2):205–7.

61. Schmutz JL, Barbaud A, Trechot P. Urticaria and angiodema due to itraconazole. Ann Dermatol Venereol 2005;132(4):403.

62. Mok NS, Lo YK, Tsui PT, Lam CW. Ketoconazole induced torsades de pointes without concomitant use of QT interval-prolonging drug. J Cardiovasc Electrophysiol 2005;16(12):1375–7.

63. Scholz M, Jennrich R, Strum S, Brosman S, Johnson H, Lam R. Long-term outcome for men with androgen independent prostate cancer treated with ketoconazole and hydrocortisone. J Urol 2005;173(6):1947–52.

64. Groll AH, Walsh TJ. Posaconazole: clinical pharmacology and potential for management of fungal infections. Expert Rev Anti Infect Ther 2005;3:467–87.

65. Courtney R, Sansone A, Smith W, Marbury T, Statkevich P, Martinho M, Laughlin M, Swan S. Posaconazole pharmacokinetics, safety, and tolerability in subjects with varying degrees of chronic renal disease. J Clin Pharmacol 2005;45(2):185–92.

66. Boucher HW, Groll AH, Chiou CC, Walsh TJ. Newer systemic antifungal agents: pharmacokinetics, safety and efficacy. Drugs 2004;64(18):1997–2020.

67. Kullberg BJ, Sobel JD, Ruhnke M, Pappas PG, Viscoli C, Rex JH, Cleary JD, Rubinstein E, Church LW, Brown JM, Schlamm HT, Oborska IT, Hilton F, Hodges MR. Voriconazole versus a regimen of amphotericin B followed by fluconazole for candidaemia in non-neutropenic patients: a randomised non-inferiority trial. Lancet 2005;366(9495):1435–42.

68. Tsiodras S, Zafiropoulou R, Kanta E, Demponeras C, Karandreas N, Manesis EK. Painful peripheral neuropathy associated with voriconazole use. Arch Neurol 2005;62(1):144–6.

69. Racette AJ, Roenigk Jr HH, Hansen R, Mendelson D, Park A. Photoaging and phototoxicity from long-term voriconazole treatment in a 15-year-old girl. J Am Acad Dermatol 2005;52(5 Suppl 1):S81–5.

70. Sharp MT, Horn TD. Pseudoporphyria induced by voriconazole. J Am Acad Dermatol 2005;53(2):341–5.

71. Hilliard T, Edwards S, Buchdahl R, Francis J, Rosenthal M, Balfour-Lynn I, Bush A, Davies J. Voriconazole therapy in children with cystic fibrosis. J Cyst Fibros 2005;4(4):215–20.

72. Peng LW, Lien YH. Pharmacokinetics of single, oral-dose voriconazole in peritoneal dialysis patients. Am J Kidney Dis 2005;45(1):162–6.

73. Trifilio S, Ortiz R, Pennick G, Verma A, Pi J, Stosor V, Zembower T, Mehta J. Voriconazole therapeutic drug monitoring in allogeneic hematopoietic stem cell transplant recipients. Bone Marrow Transplant 2005;35(5):509–13.

74. Dowell JA, Stogniew M, Krause D, Henkel T, Weston IE. Assessment of the safety and pharmacokinetics of anidulafungin when administered with cyclosporine. J Clin Pharmacol 2005;45(2):227–33.

75. Kartsonis NA, Saah AJ, Joy Lipka C, Taylor AF, Sable CA. Salvage therapy with caspofungin for invasive aspergillosis: results from the Caspofungin Compassionate Use Study. J Infect 2005;50(3):196–205.

76. Candoni A, Mestroni R, Damiani D, Tiribelli M, Michelutti A, Silvestri F, Castelli M, Viale P, Fanin R. Caspofungin as first line therapy of pulmonary invasive fungal infections in 32 immunocompromised patients with hematologic malignancies. Eur J Haematol 2005;75(3):227–33.

77. Walsh TJ, Adamson PC, Seibel NL, Flynn PM, Neely MN, Schwartz C, Shad A, Kaplan SL, Roden MM, Stone JA, Miller A, Bradshaw SK, Li SX, Sable CA, Kartsonis NA. Pharmacokinetics, safety, and tolerability of caspofungin in children and adolescents. Antimicrob Agents Chemother 2005;49(11):4536–45.

78. Natarajan G, Lulic-Botica M, Rongkavilit C, Pappas A, Bedard M. Experience with caspofungin in the treatment of persistent fungemia in neonates. J Perinatol 2005;25(12):770–7.

79. Trenschel R, Ditschkowski M, Elmaagacli AH, Koldehoff M, Ottinger H, Steckel N, Hlinka M, Peceny R, Rath PM, Dermoumi H, Beelen DW. Caspofungin as second-line therapy for fever of unknown origin or invasive fungal infection following allogeneic stem cell transplantation. Bone Marrow Transplant 2005;35(6):583–6.

80. Belmares J, Colaizzi L, Parada JP, Johnson S. Caspofungin treatment failure in a patient with invasive candidiasis and concomitant rifampicin treatment. Int J Antimicrob Agents 2005;26(3):264–5.

81. Ostrosky-Zeichner L, Kontoyiannis D, Raffalli J, Mullane KM, Vazquez J, Anaissie EJ, Lipton J, Jacobs P, van Rensburg JH, Rex JH, Lau W, Facklam D, Buell DN. International, open-label, noncomparative, clinical trial of micafungin alone and in combination for treatment of newly diagnosed and refractory candidemia. Eur J Clin Microbiol Infect Dis 2005;24(10):654–61.

82. Hiemenz J, Cagnoni P, Simpson D, Devine S, Chao N, Keirns J, Lau W, Facklam D, Buell D. Pharmacokinetic and maximum tolerated dose study of micafungin in combination with fluconazole versus fluconazole alone for prophylaxis of fungal infections in adult patients undergoing a bone marrow or peripheral stem cell transplant. Antimicrob Agents Chemother 2005;49(4):1331–6.

83. Seibel NL, Schwartz C, Arrieta A, Flynn P, Shad A, Albano E, Keirns J, Lau WM, Facklam DP, Buell DN, Walsh TJ. Safety, tolerability, and pharmacokinetics of Micafungin (FK463) in febrile neutropenic pediatric patients. Antimicrob Agents Chemother 2005;49(8):3317–24.

84. Hebert MF, Smith HE, Marbury TC, Swan SK, Smith WB, Townsend RW, Buell D, Keirns J, Bekersky I. Pharmacokinetics of micafungin in healthy volunteers, volunteers with moderate liver disease, and volunteers with renal dysfunction. J Clin Pharmacol 2005;45(10):1145–52.

85. Sakaeda T, Iwaki K, Kakumoto M, Nishikawa M, Niwa T, Jin JS, Nakamura T, Nishiguchi K, Okamura N, Okumura K. Effect of micafungin on cytochrome P450 3A4 and multidrug resistance protein 1 activities, and its comparison with azole antifungal drugs. J Pharm Pharmacol 2005;57(6):759–64.

86. Niwa T, Inoue-Yamamoto S, Shiraga T, Takagi A. Effect of antifungal drugs on cytochrome P450 (CYP) 1A2, CYP2D6, and CYP2E1 activities in human liver microsomes. Biol Pharm Bull 2005;28(9):1813–6.

87. Niwa T, Shiraga T, Takagi A. Effect of antifungal drugs on cytochrome P450 (CYP) 2C9, CYP2C19, and CYP3A4 activities in human liver microsomes. Biol Pharm Bull 2005;28(9):1805–8.

88. Hebert MF, Townsend RW, Austin S, Balan G, Blough DK, Buell D, Keirns J, Bekersky I. Concomitant cyclosporine and micafungin pharmacokinetics in healthy volunteers. J Clin Pharmacol 2005;45(8):954–60.

89. Hebert MF, Blough DK, Townsend RW, Allison M, Buell D, Keirns J, Bekersky I. Concomitant tacrolimus and micafungin pharmacokinetics in healthy volunteers. J Clin Pharmacol 2005;45(9):1018–24.

Oscar Ozmund Simooya

28 Antiprotozoal drugs

ANTIMALARIAL DRUGS

In several countries in which malaria is endemic, artemisinin-based combination therapies have now been adopted as first-line treatment for uncomplicated falciparum malaria, while quinine has been retained as the drug of choice for severe or complicated malaria. However, beyond these two regimens there is limited choice of available therapies, because of widespread malaria parasite drug resistance. This is a major challenge, particularly in resource-poor settings, where the need for safe and efficacious drugs must be counterbalanced by cost and availability. New compounds that meet these criteria are therefore needed and needed urgently. Current work is focused on the re-modelling of existing therapies, as typified by the quinolones and the peroxides; novel use of older drugs such as artemisinin derivatives; and the targeting of new parasite-specific targets (1[r]).

4-AMINOQUINOLINES (CHLOROQUINE AND CONGENERS) *(SEDA-27, 289; SEDA-28, 315; SEDA-29, 294)*

Chloroquine + proguanil
(SED-15, 722)

The use of chloroquine has diminished in recent years owing to widespread parasite drug resistance and it is now used mainly for prophylaxis in combination with proguanil.

Liver *Hepatotoxicity*, which is uncommon with either chloroquine or proguanil, has been reported after the use of a fixed-dose combination of chloroquine and proguanil (2[A]).

- A day before visiting the Indian subcontinent a 50-year-old French Caucasian woman began a course of a fixed-dose combination of proguanil (200 mg) + chloroquine (100 mg), one tablet daily for chemoprophylaxis. Four days later she developed vomiting, discolored stools, dark urine, and general fatigue. The chloroquine + proguanil was stopped immediately. A week later she developed severe nausea, headache, and conjunctival hemorrhages. There was no abdominal pain, fever, or rash. She had abnormal liver function tests, with aspartate transaminase activity of 335 U/l (reference range $\leqslant$35 U/l), alanine transaminase activity of 660 U/l ($\leqslant$41 U/l), and alkaline phosphatase activity of 744 U/l (60–279 U/l). Total bilirubin was 616 (34–222) μmol/l and direct bilirubin was 393 (17–68) μmol/l. There were bile salts and increased bile pigments in the urine. An abdominal scan was unremarkable and serology for hepatitis A, B, and C was negative. Liver biopsy was not performed. She had no known susceptibility factors for liver disease. She had previously taken chloroquine + proguanil in 1998, 2002, and 2003 and recalled experiencing severe abdominal discomfort on the last occasion. Her symptoms improved after withdrawal of chloroquine+proguanil and her liver function tests gradually returned to normal.

The temporal relation between drug therapy and the appearance of symptoms suggested an adverse reaction to chloroquine + proguanil. The abnormal liver function tests, negative tests for hepatitis, the absence of fever, and the resolution of symptoms after withdrawal all suggested a causal relation. The exact mechanism is not known but it could have been an allergic reaction after sensitization from previous exposures.

Hydroxychloroquine *(SED-15, 722; SEDA-29, 294)*

Hydroxychloroquine is being increasingly used to treat immune diseases, such as systemic lu-

Side Effects of Drugs, Annual 30
J.K. Aronson (Editor)
ISSN: 0378-6080
DOI: 10.1016/S0378-6080(08)00028-7

pus erythematosus, rheumatoid arthritis, and chronic graft-versus-host disease (GVHD). It commonly causes *gastrointestinal disturbances* and less commonly *retinal toxicity, itching, intravascular hemolysis, rashes*, and *bone marrow suppression*.

Musculoskeletal   Muscle and peripheral nerve toxicity is rare with hydroxychloroquine. Severe *vacuolar myopathy* has been reported (3^A).

- A 51-year-old man with a mantle cell carcinoma was initially treated with cyclophosphamide, doxorubicin, vincristine, and prednisolone and obtained remission for 2 years. His lymphoma recurred and he was given rituximab, with a poor response. He subsequently received a bone marrow graft from his son. Despite complete remission he developed graft-versus-host disease with scleroderma and fascial involvement. He was given various drugs for graft-versus-host disease, including mycophenolate mofetil, tacrolimus, prednisolone, 2'-deoxycoformycin, and hydroxychloroquine. His condition was moderately sensitive to prednisolone in doses of 60–120 mg/day. While taking prednisolone and tacrolimus he was given hydroxychloroquine 400 mg bd. He then developed progressive debilitating limb and respiratory muscle weakness. Glucocorticoids were suspected of causing this and were tapered, but without much effect, and he gradually became too weak to walk. The serum creatine kinase activity was normal and acetylcholine receptor antibodies were negative. Electromyography showed a severe, non-irritable myopathy and a sensory motor axonal polyneuropathy. Muscle biopsy showed a necrotizing, vacuolar myopathy, with many fibers containing autophagic and red-rimmed vacuoles, consistent with an amphiphilic drug-induced myopathy. Following withdrawal of hydroxychloroquine, his strength and function improved considerably. Later prednisolone and tacrolimus were reintroduced and he made a good recovery.

Monitoring therapy   Susceptibility factors for the development of toxic retinopathy with hydroxychloroquine include high daily doses, long duration of treatment, concomitant liver or kidney disease, and age over 60 years. Constant monitoring for retinal toxicity is therefore vital for the prevention of this potentially irreversible severe adverse effect. However, most methods for monitoring retinal toxicity, such as Amsler grid testing, color vision testing, and static perimetry, are subjective. Multifocal electronic retinography is a more objective test and offers multidimensional visualization of the retina. In a longitudinal study of 12 patients who had multifocal electronic retinography at baseline and at 12–24 months, serial recordings of retinal amplitudes and peak latencies showed that patients taking hydroxychloroquine had reduced retinal function while those who stopped taking it had improved retinal function (4^c). Multifocal electronic retinography therefore offers the possibility of detecting early changes in retinal function in patients taking hydroxychloroquine.

Mefloquine   *(SED-15, 2232; SEDA-29, 295)*

Comparative studies   Mefloquine alone has been compared with a combination of sulphalene + pyrimethamine (Metakelfin) plus quinine in 187 patients with uncomplicated malaria, randomized to either mefloquine 25 mg/kg ($n = 93$) or sulphalene + pyrimethamine plus quinine (sulphalene 1.25 mg/kg + pyrimethamine 25 mg/kg once on the first day, quinine 30 mg/kg/day in three doses; $n = 94$) (5^C). There was no significant difference between the cure rates in the two groups during the early follow-up period and there were no cases of recrudescence in the 135 subjects who completed the extended follow-up. Similarly, there was no difference in the parasite clearance time between the two groups, but patients who were given mefloquine had a shorter mean fever resolution time (36 versus 44 hours) and a shorter mean hospital stay (3.9 versus 4.6 days). Overall, the proportions of reported adverse effects was the same in the two groups, but patients treated with mefloquine had more central nervous system effects (29 versus 9.6%), including *sleep disturbances* (27 versus 9.6%).

Psychiatry   Severe *depression* has been attributed to mefloquine (6^A).

- A 48-year-old woman developed anxiety, tremor, depression, dry mouth, nausea, and marked weight loss. Physical examination, electrocardiography, chest X-ray, CT scan, and laboratory investigations were unremarkable. The Hamilton D score was 44 for 17 items. She had taken mefloquine 250 mg/week for 8 weeks for malaria prophylaxis, and after 2 weeks had started to feel unwell, with dysphoria, depression, and weakness. She was given fluoxetine 20 mg/day and alprazolam 1.5 mg/day. Her condition continued to deteriorate. The dose of fluoxetine was increased to 40 mg/day and flunitrazepam was added. She was later instead given milnacipran, a serotonin and noradrenaline reuptake inhibitor. Five months after the first course of mefloquine she had recovered sufficiently to return to work. However, she relapsed and she was eventually stabilized on venlafaxine 75 mg/day.

Mefloquine has been associated with a number of neuropsychiatric adverse effects, which are often mild and of short duration.

ENDOPEROXIDES   *(SED-15, 342; SEDA-27, 292; SEDA-28, 320; SEDA-29, 297)*

Artemisinin

Nervous system   Artemisinin, now widely used as an antimalarial drug, is also being explored for its potential in the treatment of cancer. In animals artemisinin can cause brainstem neurotoxicity. *Brainstem encephalopathy* has been attributed to artemisinin in a patient with cancer (7[A]).

- A 42-year-old woman with early breast carcinoma developed diplopia, dysarthria, and an ataxic gait. Her medications included tamoxifen 20 mg/day, fluoxetine 10 mg/day, and 2 weeks of herbal therapy for breast cancer. The herbs consisted of artemisinin tablets 200 mg bd and a daily combination containing *Paeonia alba, Atractylodes alba, Momordica, Cudrania, Cochichinensis, Sophora flavenisis*, and *Dioscorea*. She had conjugate downward gaze, prominent vertical nystagmus, dysarthric speech, bilateral incoordination of both legs and arms, and an unsteady wide-based gait. Laboratory investigations were unremarkable, but brain MRI scanning showed symmetrical punctate foci. There was no evidence of stroke, demyelinating disease, or metastasis. After withdrawal of artemisinin, her neurological symptoms rapidly resolved. A repeat MRI scan on day 7 showed improvement. Tamoxifen and fluoxetine were restarted without recurrent symptoms.

Tamoxifen infrequently causes reversible neurotoxicity, but at much higher doses ($\geqslant 160$ mg/m^2/day). There are no reports of similar adverse effects due to fluoxetine or the other herbal medications that the patient was taking. In animals, artemisinin derivatives cause degeneration and necrosis in the pons, medulla, and spinal cord, but not in cortical neurons or astrocytes. The MRI findings in this patient correlated closely with brainstem injury and mimicked that found in animal studies.

Artesunate

Controlled studies   Most artemisinin-based combination therapies in current use comprise an artemisinin derivative combined with a long-acting antimalarial drug. However, it has been argued that the prolonged presence of subtherapeutic doses of drugs in the body encourages the development of drug-resistant strains of parasite. It has therefore been proposed that, to avoid this, artemisinin derivatives be combined with compounds with short half-lives.

The combination of artesunate+clindamycin (2 mg/kg + 7 mg/kg 12 hourly for 3 days) has been compared with quinine + clindamycin (15 mg/kg + 7 mg/kg 12 hourly for 3 days) in 100 patients in a randomized comparison (8[C]). Asexual parasite clearance time was faster with artesunate + clindamycin (29 versus 46 hours), and patients who took artesunate+clindamycin also experienced a shorter time to fever clearance (21 versus 30 hours). Both regimens were well tolerated and no severe adverse events were recorded. However, one patient who took artesunate + clindamycin had diarrhea and two who took quinine + clindamycin developed diarrhea and tinnitus.

DRUGS USED IN THE TREATMENT OF *PNEUMOCYSTIS JIROVECI* INFECTIONS

Co-trimoxazole (trimethoprim + sulfamethoxazole)
(SED-15, 3510; SEDA-27, 296; SEDA-28, 322; SEDA-29, 297; see also Chapter 26)

Nervous system   *Tremors* and *chorea* have been attributed to co-trimoxazole in immuno-compromised adults and in a child with dihydrofolate reductase deficiency and have now been reported in an immunocompromised child with *Pneumocystis jiroveci* infection (9[A]).

- A girl aged 1.5 years, who was taking long-term azathioprine and methylprednisolone for an immunological lung disease, developed severe pneumonia. Azathioprine was withdrawn and ciprofloxacin, aciclovir, fluconazole, and co-trimoxazole (7.5 + 37.5 mg/kg/day) were added.

Pneumocystis jiroveci was grown from broncho-alveolar lavage fluid. The dose of co-trimoxazole was increased to 20 + 100 mg/kg/day. Five days later she developed involuntary movements consisting of diffuse, continuous, high-frequency, low-amplitude tremors associated with choreic movements. Laboratory investigations were within the reference ranges and electroencephalography showed no signs of epilepsy. A CT scan and lumbar puncture were also normal. On day 10 ciprofloxacin, aciclovir, fluconazole, and methylprednisolone were withdrawn but the symptoms persisted. On day 12, co-trimoxazole was withdrawn and all the abnormal movements disappeared within 3 days.

DRUGS USED IN THE TREATMENT OF OTHER PROTOZOAL INFECTIONS

Metronidazole   *(SED-15, 2323; SEDA-28, 323)*

Nervous system   *Neurotoxicity* has been attributed to metronidazole (10^A).

- A 20-year-old man with ulcerative colitis who had taken metronidazole 1500 mg/day for 2 years developed reduced visual acuity (2/10 bilaterally) and major impairment of red color discrimination, painful distal paresthesia, and dysarthria and impaired coordination in both hands. Pattern visual evoked potentials were absent but low amplitude flash visual evoked potentials were elicited with markedly prolonged latencies. An MRI scan of the brain and optic nerves showed increased signal intensities in the splenium, truncus, and genu of the corpus callosum but normal optic nerves. Metronidazole was withdrawn and he gradually improved. The painful paresthesia resolved within 3 months. Repeat brain scans after 2 and 8 months showed moderate resolution of the increased signal in the corpus callosum. After 14 months all the other symptoms and signs had normalized and pattern evoked visual latencies had normalized.

Multiple sclerosis is the most common disease associated with corpus callosum hyperintensities. However, in this case the reversibility of the symptoms and signs, the reversible non-contrasting MRI images, and the absence of new neurological complications pointed to a causal effect of metronidazole.

Pancreas   Metronidazole has been associated with *acute pancreatitis* in a few case reports. This association has been investigated in a large population-based case control study (11^C). Computer-based prescription records of 3083 cases of acute pancreatitis were compared with the records of 30 083 matched controls. The odds ratios for acute pancreatitis in those who had redeemed a prescription for metronidazole were 3.0 (95% CI = 1.4, 4.6), 1.8 (1.2, 2.9), and 1.1 (0.6, 1.8) within 30, 31–180, and 181–365 days before hospitalization or the index date respectively. Among those with a concomitant prescription for proton pump inhibitors and/or amoxicillin, macrolides, or tetracyclines the respective adjusted odds ratios were 8.3 (2.6, 26), 2.7 (1.4, 5.5), and 1.7 (0.6, 4.8).

Thus, metronidazole increases the risk of acute pancreatitis, with an intermediate time-course, and the risk is even higher when it is used in combination with other drugs used for the treatment of *Helicobacter pylori*.

Teratogenicity   Previous studies have found no association between metronidazole treatment and congenital abnormalities, but a new report has suggested a possible association of the use of vaginal metronidazole suppositories and *hydrocephalus* (12^C). The study was a population-based case-control comparison of 38 151 pregnant women who had newborn babies without congenital anomalies and 22 843 pregnant women who delivered babies or fetuses with congenital anomalies. Of the cases, 388 (1.7%) reported having used vaginal metronidazole compared with 570 (1.5%) in the control group (OR = 1.1; 95% CI = 1.0, 1.3). A further comparison of cases and controls showed an association between the use of vaginal metronidazole in the second and third months of gestation and hydrocephalus (OR = 11; 95% CI = 1.1, 105). However, this finding was based on only five cases and evaluation of medically recorded metronidazole treatment was non-confirmatory. This association has not previously been reported and requires further investigation.

Drug–drug interactions   The effect of 1 week of *Helicobacter pylori* eradication therapy with rabeprazole, clarithromycin, and metronidazole on CYP-dependent hepatic metabolism has been determined using the $[^{13}C]$aminophenazone (aminopyrine) breath test (13^c). The test was performed before treatment, immediately after treatment, and 1 month after treatment. There was no change in hepatic metabolic function during and after treatment.

Metronidazole has been reported to increase blood concentrations of *tacrolimus* (14^A).

- A 24-year-old man with a renal transplant, who had been stabilized on tacrolimus 4 mg bd (trough concentrations of 7–10 ng/ml) for 2 months and prednisolone 20 mg/day, developed severe diarrhea due to *Clostridium difficile*. He was given metronidazole 500 mg qds. Within 4–14 days his serum creatinine and tacrolimus trough concentrations rose to 292 µmol/l and 26.3 ng/ml. The dose of tacrolimus was reduced to 1 mg bd and after withdrawal of metronidazole the tacrolimus trough concentration fell to 9.4 ng/ml and the serum creatinine to 68 µmol/l.

℞ *Combination regimens in the eradication of Helicobacter pylori*

New antibiotic combinations and simpler regimens for eradicating Helicobacter pylori have been reported.

- *Twelve patients with duodenal ulcer who had previously been treated unsuccessfully with two regimens containing clarithromycin and metronidazole, were given a daily combination of rabeprazole 20 mg, levofloxacin 500 mg, and furazolidone 200 mg as a single dose for 10 days (15^c). Two patients discontinued treatment because of nausea and vomiting. After 90 days of treatment 10 patients were left in the study, in six of whom culture of gastric tissue fragments was obtained: 100 and 83% of the samples showed sensitivity to furazolidone and levofloxacin respectively. Eradication rates for Helicobacter pylori as determined per protocol and intention to treat were 100 and 83%.*
- *A 10-day regimen of esomeprazole 40 mg qds, tetracycline 500 mg qds, and metronidazole 500 mg qds has been studied in 20 patients with penicillin allergy, duodenal ulcer disease, and Helicobacter pylori infection (16^c). In 17 this was the first course of treatment and in three there had been*

prior treatment failure. Baseline and follow-up endoscopy was performed after 30 days or more of treatment for urease tests and biopsies for Helicobacter pylori. Eradication rates by intention to treat were 85% for first-time treatment and 100% for prior failure. Endoscopy was normal in 70% of all cases at follow-up and 85 and 100% of the patients had healed erosive gastritis and duodenal ulcers respectively. Three patients reported oral candidiasis which required drug withdrawal at days 6, 7, and 9. The symptoms resolved with fluconazole 100 mg/day and nystatin lozenges. In all three Helicobacter pylori was eradicated. One patient reported anorexia, nausea, and diarrhea. The combination of esomeprazole, tetracycline, and metronidazole is effective and well tolerated in patients with penicillin allergy.

- *Four different combinations for Helicobacter pylori eradication have been studied in patients with penicillin allergy (17^c). The regimens comprised:*
  - *first-line (n = 12)—metronidazole, omeprazole, and clarithromycin for 7 days;*
  - *second-line (n = 17)—metronidazole, ranitidine bismuth citrate, and tetracycline for 7 days;*
  - *third-line (n = 9)—rifabutin, clarithromycin, and omeprazole for 10 days;*
  - *fourth-line (n = 12)—levofloxacin, clarithromycin, and omeprazole for 10 days.*

  The outcome measure was a negative $[^{13}C]$urea breath test 8 weeks after completion of treatment. The eradication rates for the four groups were 58, 47, 11, and 100% for the four treatments. Compliance was generally good apart from the rifabutin-based regimen, which had adverse effects in 89% of the patients, including four cases of myelotoxicity.
- *Moxifloxacin-based regimens have been compared with comparable clarithromycin-based therapies in 320 patients with Helicobacter pylori (18^C). The regimens comprised:*
  - *moxifloxacin, amoxicillin, and esomeprazole;*
  - *moxifloxacin, tinidazole, and esomeprazole;*
  - *clarithromycin, amoxicillin, and esomeprazole;*
  - *clarithromycin, tinidazole, and esomeprazole.*

Each group had 80 patients. Eradication rates were 89, 92, 78, and 79%. Taste disturbance and bloating were less frequent in those who took moxifloxacin than in those who took the other treatments.

- *Failure of Helicobacter pylori eradication in childhood is common. The efficacy of amoxicillin, bismuth subcitrate, and omeprazole, with either nifuratel (n = 37) or furazolidone (n = 39) has been evaluated in 76 children aged 12–16 years who had failed one attempt at eradication using a metronidazole-containing triple regimen (19^c). Eradication rates were 33/37 with nifuratel and 34/39 with furazolidone. More patients who took furazolidone complained of severe anorexia than those who took nifuratel (eight versus one).*

MISCELLANEOUS DRUGS

Eflornithine   *(SED -15, 1207)*

Trypanosomiasis due to *Trypanosoma gambiense rhodesiense* is still a major public health problem in sub-Saharan Africa. Melarsoprol, an arsenical drug, has been used for many years for the treatment of trypanosomiasis despite its high frequency of adverse effects and resultant high case-fatality rate. Eflornithine (difluoromethylornithine) is an alternative.

Comparative studies   There has been a comparison of melarsoprol 2.2 mg/kg/day plus prednisolone 20 mg/day (*n* = 708) and eflornithine (400 mg/kg given as a slow intravenous infusion in four 3-hour doses daily for 14 days; *n* = 251) in patients with trypanosomiasis who presented with meningoencephalitis (20^C). *Acute reactive encephalopathy* occurred in 80 (11%) of those who took melarsoprol and in one (0.4%) who took eflornithine. Of those who took melarsoprol 25 (3.5%) died (23 because of acute reactive encephalopathy) while only two (0.8%) of those who took eflornithine died. *Fever, hypertension, macular rash, severe headache, peripheral neuropathy*, and *tremors* were more common in those who took melarsoprol, while *diarrhea* was more frequent in

those who took eflornithine. After 12 months of follow-up there was no significant difference between the rates of relapse.

Eflornithine is therefore effective and safer than melarsoprol for the treatment of trypanosomiasis. However, a simpler dosage regimen needs to be developed, as the staff needed to administer prolonged intravenous infusions may not be available in endemic regions.

Furazolidone   *(SED -15, 1454)*

Skin   *Non-pigmented fixed drug eruptions* have previously been attributed to furazolidone; they usually affect the palms, trunk, inguinal folds, and buttocks. Another case has been reported (21[A]).

- A 23-year-old man developed well circumscribed bright red macular patches on the palms and soles after taking furazolidone for an acute intestinal infection. There was no central blistering or telangiectasis. The lesions subsided within 7 days. On rechallenge with a quarter of the dose he developed acute edematous erythematous lesions at the same sites as before.

Melarsoprol   *(SED-15, 2243)*

Drug dosage regimens   Melarsoprol dosage regimens vary; usually 3 or 4 series of 3 or 4 injections of increasing doses are given, with rest periods of 7–10 days. Shorter regimens are desirable. In 2020 patients with human African trypanosomiasis who were treated with the shortened melarsoprol treatment schedule (2.2 mg/kg/day for 10 days) the cure rate 24 hours after treatment was 94%; 2 years later it was 86% (22[C]). However, 935 patients were lost to follow-up. The case fatality rate was 5.9%. Of the treated patients 8.7% had an encephalopathy that was fatal 46% of the time. The rates of severe bullous and maculopapular reactions were 0.8 and 6.8% respectively.

The 10-day melarsoprol regimen is effective and easier to administer than longer regimens. However, the high number of adverse events shows that the development of more effective and less toxic drugs remains a top priority.

References

1. Biagini GA, Oneill PM, Bray PG, Ward SA. Current drug development portfolio for antimalarial therapies. Curr Opin Pharmacol 2005;5(5):473–8.
2. Wielgo-Polanin R, Largace L, Gautron E, Diquet B, Lainé-Cessac P. Hepatotoxicity associated with the use of a fixed combination of chloroquine and proguanil. Int J Antimicrob Agents 2005;26(2):176–8.
3. Bolaños-Meade J, Zhou L, Hoke A, Corse A, Vogelsang G, Wagner KR. Hydroxychloroquine causes severe vacuolar myopathy in a patient with chronic graft-versus-host disease. Am J Hematol 2005;78:306–9.
4. Lai TYY, Chan W-M, Li H, Lai RYK, Lam DSC. Multifocal retinographic changes in patients receiving hydroxychloroquine therapy. Am J Ophthamol 2005;140(5):794–808.
5. Matteeli A, Saleri N, Bisoffi Z, Gregis G, Gaviera G, Visonà R, Tedoldi S, Scolari C, Marocco S, Gulletta M. Mefloquine versus quinine plus sulphalene–pyrimethamine (Metakelfin) for treatment of uncomplicated imported falciparum malaria acquired in Africa. Antimicrob Agents Chemother 2005;49(2):663–7.
6. Whitworth AB, Aichhorn W. First time diagnosis of depression. Induced by Mefloquine? J Clin Pyschopharmacol 2005;25(4):399–400.
7. Panossian LA, Garga NI, Pelletier D. Toxic brainstem encephalopathy after artemisinin treatment for breast cancer. Ann Neurol 2005;58(5):812–3.
8. Ramharter M, Oyakhirome S, Klouwenberg PK, Adégnika AA, Agnandji ST, Missinou MA, Matsiégui P-B, Mordmüller B, Borrmann S, Kun JF, Lell B, Krishna S, Graninger W, Issifou S, Kremsner P. Artesunate–clindamycin versus quinine–clindamycin in the treatment of *Plasmodium falciparum* malaria: a randomized controlled trial. Clin Infect Dis 2005;40:1777–84.
9. Bua J, Marchetti F, Barbi E, Sarti A, Ventura A. Tremors and chorea induced by trimethoprim–sulfamethoxazole in a child with *Pneumocystis* pneumonia. Pediatr Infect Dis J 2005;24(4):934–5.
10. De Bleecker JL, Leroy BP, Meire V. Reversible visual deficit and corpus callosum lesions due to metronidazole toxicity. Eur Neurol 2005;53(2):93–5.
11. Nørgaard M, Ratanajamit C, Jacobsen J, Skriver MV, Pedersen L, Sørensen HT. Metronidazole and risk of acute pancreatitis: a population-based case control study. Aliment Pharmacol Ther 2005;21:415–20.
12. Kazy J, Puhó E, Czeizel E. Teratogenic potential of metronidazole vaginal treatment during pregnancy. Eur J Obstet Gynaecol Reprod Biol 2005;123(2):174–8.
13. Giannini EG, Malfatti F, Botta F, Polegato S, Testa E, Fumagalli A, Mamone M, Savarino V, Testa R. Influence of 1-week *Helicobacter pylori* eradication therapy with rabeprazole, clarithromycin, and metronidazole on ^{13}C-aminopyrine breath test. Dig Dis Sci 2005;50(7):1207–13.
14. Page II RL, Klem PM, Rogers C. Potential elevation of tacrolimus trough concentrations with concomitant metronidazole therapy. Ann Pharmacother 2005;39(6):1109–13.
15. Coelho LGV, Moretzsohn LD, Vieira WLS, Gallo MA, Passos MCF, Cindr JM, Cerqueira MC, Vitiello L, Ribeiro ML, Mendonça S, Pedrazzoli-Júnior J, Castro LP. New once-daily, highly effective rescue triple therapy after multiple *Helicobacter pylori* treatment failures: a pilot study. Aliment Pharmacol Ther 2005;21(6):783–7.
16. Rodríguez-Torres M, Salgado-Mercado R, Ríos-Bedoya CF, Aponte-Rivera E, Marxuach-Cuétara AM, Rodríguez-Orengo JF, Fernández-Carbia A. High eradication rates of *Helicobacter pylori* infection with second-line combination of esomeprazole, tetracycline, and metronidazole in patients allergic to penicillin. Dig Dis Sci 2005;50(4):634–9.
17. Gisbert JP, Gisbert JL, Marcos S, Olivares D, Pajares JM. *Helicobacter pylori* first line treatment and rescue operations in patients allergic to penicillin. Aliment Pharmacol Ther 2005;22(10):1041–6.
18. Nista EC, Candelli M, Zocco MA, Cazzato IA, Cremonini F, Ojetti V, Santoro M, Finizio R, Pignataro G, Cammarota G, Gasbarrini G, Gasbarrini A. Moxifloxacin-based strategies for first line treatment of *Helicobacter pylori* infection. Aliment Pharmacol Ther 2005;21(10):1241–7.
19. Nijevitch AA, Shcherbakov PL, Sataev VU, Khasanov RSH, Al Khashash R, Tuygunov MM. *Helicobacter pylori* eradication in childhood after failure on initial treatment: advantage of quadruple therapy with nifuratel to furazolidine. Aliment Pharmacol Ther 2005;22(9):881–7.
20. Chappuis F, Udayraj N, Stietenroth K, Meussen A, Bovier PA. Eflornithine is safer than melarsoprol for the treatment of second stage *Trypanosoma brucei gambiense* human African trypanosomiasis. Clin Infect Dis 2005;1:748–51.
21. Tan C, Zhu WY. Furazolidine induced nonpigmenting fixed drug eruptions affecting the palms and soles. Allergy 2005;60(7):972–3.
22. Schmid C, Richer M, Miaka Mia Bilenge C, Josenando T, Chappuis F, Manthelot CR, Nangouma A, Doua F, Asumu P, Simarro PP, Burri C. Effectiveness of a 10 day melarsoprol schedule for the treatment of late stage human African trypanosomiasis: confirmation from a multinational study (IMPANEL II). J Infect Dis 2005;195:1922–31.

Brian J. Angus

29   Antiviral drugs

DRUGS ACTIVE AGAINST CYTOMEGALOVIRUS

Cidofovir   *(SED-15, 771; SEDA-27, 303; SEDA-28, 326)*

Skin   Topical cidofovir 1–3% has been successfully used for the treatment of oral warts in three HIV-positive patients with no adverse effects (1[A]). However, *ulceration and pain at the site of the lesion*, leaving the normal skin unharmed, were reported as the main adverse effect after topical application to high-grade vulval intraepithelial neoplasia in 12 women (2[A]).

Topical cidofovir 1% has also been used in the successful treatment of a refractory verruca in a child with acute lymphoblastic leukemia (3[A]).

- A 9-year-old girl who had had acute lymphoblastic leukemia since the age of 18 months, had maintenance chemotherapy (methotrexate 10–15 mg/day, mercaptopurine 50–90 mg/day, and intrathecal methotrexate with hydrocortisone) reintroduced for a fourth CNS relapse, and developed a verruca on the sole of her right foot. This was treated initially with curettage, but it recurred quickly and grew larger and more painful. Treatment with cryotherapy was ineffective. The verruca continued to enlarge and became more painful. It again failed to respond to gentle cryotherapy. Cidofovir 1% ointment was compounded from the parenteral formulation (Vistide®, Gilead, Foster City, CA, USA) in ointment (Merck and Co, Inc, Whitehouse Station, NJ, USA) and was applied once daily for 6 weeks, by which time the verruca had completely resolved. No adverse effects or local irritation were observed.

Urinary tract   Of 10 pediatric stem cell recipients with systemic adenovirus infections,

one-third had a *rise in serum creatinine* 50% above baseline despite pre- and post-dose intravenous hydration and pre-dose probenecid (4[A]). Renal tubular cell apoptosis is prevented by probenecid in vitro (5[E]).

DRUGS ACTIVE AGAINST HERPESVIRUSES   *(SEDA-27, 305; SEDA-28, 328, SEDA-29, 301)*

Aciclovir   *(SED-15, 29)*

Nervous system   It has been suggested that hemodialysis can be a useful diagnostic tool in the differential diagnosis between aciclovir-induced neurotoxicity and herpes encephalitis, as well as a fast and reliable treatment of drug-induced neurotoxicity (6[A]).

- A previously healthy 59-year-old woman developed right eye pain for 3 days and vesicle formation on her forehead. She received intravenous aciclovir 250 mg every 8 hours, but 48 hours later she became drowsy and lethargic, with incoherent speech and hallucinations. Her blood urea nitrogen concentration rose from 0.71 mmol/l on admission to 2.41 mmol/l, serum creatinine rose from 53.6 to 442 (reference range 51–115) μmol/l and the serum sodium concentration fell from 135 to 121 mmol/l. Electroencephalography showed mild diffuse cortical dysfunction, with more emphasis in the right hemisphere, and regional epileptiform activity in the bilateral frontal and right parietal regions. An MRI scan of her head was normal. Because of deteriorating renal function and the debilitating nature of the neurological symptoms, which were thought to be due to acyclovir toxicity, hemodialysis was initiated. The pre-hemodialysis trough plasma aciclovir concentration was 18 mg/l, compared with peak and trough concentrations of 5.5–13.8 mg/l and 0.2–1 mg/l respectively in adults who receive 5 mg/kg of acyclovir (7[S]). She underwent two 4-hour sessions of hemodialysis over 2 days. The post-hemodialysis plasma aciclovir concentration fell to 3 mg/l. Her conscious level improved and the blood urea nitrogen and serum creatinine

Side Effects of Drugs, Annual 30
J.K. Aronson (Editor)
ISSN: 0378-6080
DOI: 10.1016/S0378-6080(08)00029-9

concentrations fell to 6.1 mmol/l and 142 μmol/l respectively. She was well by the fifth day.

DRUGS ACTIVE AGAINST HEPATITIS VIRUSES
(SEDA-29, 301)

Adefovir   *(SED-15, 35)*

Observational studies   A total of 49 consecutive lamivudine-resistant hepatitis B e antigen-negative chronic hepatitis B patients were enrolled in a study of the effects of adefovir 10 mg/day plus lamivudine 100 mg/day (8[C]). After 52 weeks all had some hepatitis B virus DNA response and 57% had a complete virological response. There was a biochemical response in 76%. There were no serious adverse events.

Entecavir

Entecavir recently received FDA approval in the USA for use in treatment-naïve hepatitis B e antigen (HBeAg) positive patients and those with evidence of lamivudine resistance. Diminution of viral titers reached 7 $\log_{10}$ units (9[R]). There were no significant differences in adverse events compared with lamivudine. Most of the adverse events were mild or moderate and the incidences were comparable in the four treatment groups, 65–73% of patients describing at least one adverse event. One patient taking entecavir had asymptomatic *increases in alanine transaminase activity and bilirubin concentration*; the drug was withdrawn and the tests improved. Two patients withdrew from the study, one because of *lethargy and photosensitivity* after 5 months, which resolved 3 days after withdrawal, and the other because of acute HIV infection.

Lamivudine   *(SED-15, 1989)*

Comparative studies   Lamivudine is being increasingly used in chronic hepatitis B infec-

tion. However, resistance arises rapidly with monotherapy and lamivudine is not superior to interferon. Of 136 patients given pegylated interferon alpha-2b monotherapy 49 (36%) had lost HBeAg at the end of follow-up at week 78, compared with 46 (35%) of 130 who were given interferon in combination with lamivudine (10[C]). More of those in the combination group had cleared HBeAg at the end of treatment at week 52 (44 versus 29%) but they relapsed during follow-up. The patterns were similar when the response was assessed by suppression of serum hepatitis B virus (HBV) DNA or a change in alanine transaminase activity. Response rates (HBeAg loss) varied significantly by HBV genotype: genotype A 47%; genotype B 44%; genotype C 28%; genotype D 25%.

Lamivudine has been well tolerated in long term studies in hepatitis B positive patients; *malaise* and *fatigue* were the most common adverse effects (11[A]).

It has been suggested that lamivudine be used prophylactically in only those patients with breast cancer who have active HBV viral replication (12[A]).

Liver   Of 814 HBV eAg-positive patients two taking lamivudine monotherapy had *hepatic decompensation* after the end of treatment (13[A]). One received a liver transplant and made a full recovery; the other died.

Ribavirin   *(SED-15, 3036)*

The combined effects of ribavirin + interferon

The mechanism of the beneficial effect of adding ribavirin to interferon is not fully understood. Ribavirin monotherapy is not effective in hepatitis C. However, adding ribavirin to interferon increases the number of patients with a virological response although it also increases the number of adverse events. Both the benefits and harms of adding ribavirin to interferon for patients with chronic hepatitis C should be considered before therapy is started.

Systematic reviews   In a meta-analysis of 72 trials with a total of 9991 patients, ribavirin plus interferon significantly reduced morbidity plus mortality (OR = 0.46; 95% CI = 0.22, 0.96) and significantly improved sustained viral clearance in treatment-naive patients (RR = 0.72; 95% CI = 0.68, 0.76), relapsers (RR = 0.63; 95% CI = 0.54, 0.73), and non-responders (RR = 0.89; 95% CI = 0.84, 0.94) (14^M). This gave the following numbers needed to treat for beneficial effects (NNT_B): for reduction in mortality/morbidity 444 (302–5650); for clearing of HCV-RNA 4 (4–5); and for improving the histological response 8 (7–100).

This analysis also gave information about the increased toxicity of adding ribavirin, with the following numbers needed to harm (NNT_H): anemia 4 (4–5); leukopenia 4 (3–7); rash 11 (9–17); pruritus 13 (10–20); insomnia 14 (6–20); dosage reductions 14 (11–17); dermatitis 14 (8–50); dyspnea 17 (11–25); fatigue/weakness 17 (11–33); dry skin 20 (11–50); anorexia/ nausea 20 (13–50); dyspepsia 20 (13–50); pharyngitis 20 (13–100); cough 20 (14–33); and stopping treatment 50 (33–100).

Treatment with peginterferon alpha-2b + ribavirin can achieve a complete clinical response in about 75% of patients with hepatitis C-related vasculitis. A complete clinical response correlates with the eradication of the virus and requires a shorter treatment period than that previously reported for interferon alpha plus ribavirin (14 months) (15^M). The short course was well tolerated, although one patient withdrew because of neutopenia (16^C).

Observational studies

Chronic hepatitis D   Combination treatment of interferon alpha + ribavirin for chronic hepatitis D does not induce virological responses at a sufficient rate, despite its partial effectiveness in improving biochemical responses, and is not superior to interferon alpha monotherapy. Patients with chronic hepatitis D (n = 19) were treated with interferon alpha-2b (10 million U three times/week subcutaneously) and ribavirin (1000–1200 mg/day orally) for 24 months, with follow-up for at least 6 months (range 7–19) (17^C). All had compensated liver disease, raised transaminase activities, and hepatitis D virus RNA positivity at baseline. Genotypic analyses showed hepatitis D virus genotype I and hepatitis B virus genotype D. There were biochemical responses in eight patients (42%) at the end of treatment and in seven patients (37%) at the end of follow-up. Only eight patients at the end of treatment and four at the end of follow-up had sustained virological responses. There were flu-like symptoms, generally mild or moderate, in most of the patients. Two patients required a short-term dosage reduction from 10 to 5 MU because of leukopenia and thrombocytopenia and two patients had a drop in hemoglobin, which was managed with a reduction in the dosage of ribavirin.

Prevention of recurrence after liver transplantation   It has been postulated that there is a risk of increased severity of recurrent hepatitis C virus infection in living donor liver transplantation (LDLT) patients. Preventive therapy for this has been studied in 23 patients (18^C). All received interferon alpha-2b and ribavirin 1 month after transplantation and for 12 months after the first negative HCV RNA test. They were then observed without therapy for 6 months (Group 1). Therapy was continued for at least 12 months when the HCV-RNA test remained positive (Group 2). They were removed from the protocol if they could not continue therapy for 12 months because of adverse effects or could not start therapy because of early death. Eight patients were removed from the protocol (three died and two could not start because of their poor general condition). Nine patients were assigned to Group 1 and the other six to Group 2. The sustained virological response ratio was 39% (9/23). There was a significant difference between the groups in the histological activity score 1 year after therapy. No details were given of the adverse effects in the eight patients who were withdrawn.

Prediction of outcome   Hepatitis C virus (HCV) RNA kinetics have been studied on day 1 in 15 patients (nine and six of genotypes 1 and non-1 respectively) and at weeks 1, 4, and 12 in 53 patients (19 and 34 of genotypes 1 and non-1 respectively) during treatment with ribavirin + pegylated interferon α-2a (19^C). Patients with a sustained virological response

(SVR) had a significantly more pronounced mean log$_{10}$ decline from baseline in HCV RNA amounts at weeks 1 and 4 compared with patients who failed to achieve a sustained response, whereas there was no difference after day 1. For patients with a 2 log$_{10}$ reduction in HCV RNA amounts on day 7, the positive predictive value for a sustained virological response was 92%, whereas week 12 was the best time point for predicting a later non-response in patients who failed to achieve a 2 log$_{10}$ fall. In patients with genotype non-1 and a 2 log$_{10}$ fall in HCV RNA amounts the positive predictive value for a sustained virological response was 89% at week 1, and 79% at weeks 4 and 12. The corresponding negative predictive values for patients with genotype non-1 were 43, 40, and 100% respectively. Of the 60 patients, one withdrew from treatment after the second dose of pegylated interferon α-2a, four withdrew prematurely, one each at treatment weeks 8, 12, and 27 for unknown reasons, and one at week 16 for psychiatric reasons. One other patient withdrew at week 16 because of arthralgia. Dosage reduction was required in three patients because of thrombocytopenia or neutropenia, and in three others the dosage of ribavirin was reduced because of anemia.

Fulminant hepatitis C   *Pegylated interferon and ribavirin have been used successfully to treat fulminant hepatitis C infection; there were only mild self-limiting adverse effects, such as hemolytic anemia (20[A]).*

Nervous system   *Progressive multifocal leuko-encephalopathy in an HIV negative patient has been attributed to pegylated interferon alpha-2a + ribavirin (21[A]).*

Hematologic   *The anemia associated with peginterferon + ribavirin is thought to be a mixed form of ribavirin-induced hemolysis and interferon-induced myelosuppression. However in an 8-week study of 97 patients receiving peginterferon+ribavirin, while the mean hemoglobin fell significantly from 14.4 to 11.9 g/dl the serum erythropoietin responses were lower than seen in historical controls with iron deficiency (22[C]). The mean dosage of ribavirin was reduced from 986 to 913 mg/day. Only 74% maintained their dosage of ribavirin.*

Skin   *Dermatitis occurred in 36 patients who were given ribavirin + pegylated interferon (23[C]). Half of the patients had clinical symptoms within the first month of combination treatment, and the first signs typically appeared distant from the sites of peginterferon injection. All complained of generalized itch, and most had xerosis and erythemato-papulo-microvesicular lesions with a predilection for the extensor surfaces of the limbs and skin sites exposed to friction. Seven had skin biopsies with a superficial dermal perivascular inflammation with spongiosis and parakeratosis; erythrocyte extravasation, sparse keratinocyte necrosis, and extension of the inflammation to the interface were variable; the last of these occurred in the clinically more severe cases. Two patients developed specific skin signs that differed from the eczema-like pattern described above. One patient with generalized eczematous skin changes eventually developed malar hypertrichosis lanuginosa and bullous skin lesions with milia on the backs of both hands, leading to a diagnosis of porphyria cutanea tarda; one patient developed a bullous eruption with histological features of acantholytic dermatitis with a non-specific immunohistological profile.*

Five cases of Meyerson's syndrome (halo dermatitis), a benign eczematous rash around a pre-existing nevus, have been reported during treatment for hepatitis C (24[A], 25[A]). This syndrome has been reported with interferon alpha-2b but not ribavirin in other conditions and resolved on withdrawal of therapy.

There is a well established association between hepatitis C virus infection and porphyria cutanea tarda. However it is thought that ribavirin increases the risk by increasing iron overload via hemolysis. Two cases of porphyria cutanea tarda have been reported after treatment with ribavirin and interferon (26[A]).

There have been three reports of cutaneous sarcoidosis associated with pegylated interferon alpha plus ribavirin treatment (27[A]).

Drug–drug interactions   *The intracellular triphosphorylation and pharmacokinetics of lamivudine (3TC), stavudine (d4T), and zidovudine (ZDV) have been assessed in 56 patients co-infected with human immunodeficiency virus and hepatitis C virus receiving peginterferon alpha-2a (40KD) 180 micrograms/week plus* *either placebo or ribavirin 800 mg/day; there was no difference (28[C]).*

Management of adverse drug reactions   The *management with epoetin alpha and danazol of anemia during therapy with interferon and ribavirin has been reported (29[A]).*

- *A 50-year-old African–American man with chronic hepatitis C was initially given subcutaneous interferon alpha-2b (3 mU three times/week) and oral ribavirin 1200 mg/day. The pre-treatment hemoglobin was 14.3 g/dl. There was a good therapeutic response, but the hemoglobin fell firstly to 11.2 g/dl and then to 9.4 g/dl by week 42. This prompted a reduction in the dosage of ribavirin to 800 mg/day, and the hemoglobin rose to 11.8 g/dl. The antiviral therapy was withdrawn at week 48 and reintroduced 3 months later for a relapse. He was given subcutaneous peginterferon alpha-2a (180 micrograms/week) and oral ribavirin 1200 mg/day plus subcutaneous epoetin alpha 4000 U/week to prevent anemia and therefore the need to reduce the dose of ribavirin. Serum hemoglobin at the start of the second course of therapy was 14.7 g/dl and it remained stable throughout the first 12 weeks of therapy. However, at week 16, there was an abrupt fall in hemoglobin from 14.6 to 8.5 g/dl. The ribavirin was immediately withdrawn, the dosage of peginterferon was reduced, and the dosage of epoetin alpha was increased to 60 000 U/week. At week 18, the hemoglobin fell to 7.2 g/dl and the peginterferon was withdrawn. At week 20, the hemoglobin reached a nadir of 5.6 g/dl, requiring transfusion with 3 units of packed erythrocytes. The patient continued to require about 1 unit of blood every week despite continuing epoetin alpha, which was finally stopped at week 26. Erythropoietin antibodies became detectable by week 12 and peaked at week 24. Danazol 200 mg bd then 400 mg bd was started 8 weeks after the withdrawal of epoetin alpha. The hemoglobin then became stable at 9–10 g/dl for 24 weeks.*

DRUGS ACTIVE AGAINST HUMAN IMMUNODEFICIENCY VIRUS

Observational studies

Efficacy in middle-income countries   Chile began an expanded-access program to antiretroviral therapy in 2001 and a national cohort (the Chilean AIDS Cohort), was created to standard-ize treatment and evaluate the impact of the program; 4365 participants were enrolled by December 2004 (30[C]). At baseline, 48% had clinical AIDS, 26% were asymptomatic, 80% had a CD4 count under $200 \times 10^6/l$ and 58% were antiretroviral therapy-naive; the most frequent regimen was zidovudine + lamivudine + efavirenz. A 6-month follow-up study in 1057 patients showed a global mortality of 5% (0.5% if patients were asymptomatic at baseline and 8.3% if patients had baseline AIDS). There was a similar risk of death if the baseline CD4 count was $100–200 \times 10^6/l$ or under $200 \times 10^6/l$, but this increased to 4.8% (RR = 5.2) and 11% (RR = 12) if the CD4 count was $51–100 \times 10^6/l$ or under $51 \times 10^6/l$ respectively. Progression occurred in 2.9%. Severe toxicity was almost twice as common among women (13% of women and 6.5% of men). Therapy was withdrawn in 7.7% of patients because of adverse effects. Of patients taking zidovudine 6.9% stopped because of hematological toxicity, 6.8% of those taking stavudine stopped because of neuropathy, 9.3% of those taking nevirapine withdrew because of rash, and 4.6 and 12% of those taking indinavir or boosted indinavir respectively withdrew because of gastrointestinal toxicity. These results are similar to those in industrialized countries.

Drug dosage regimens

Structured treatment interruption   There has been increasing interest in structured treatment interruption in order to reduce the adverse effect of antiretroviral drugs. However, in 74 Thai patients with CD4 cell counts of under $350 \times 10^6/l$ and a plasma viral load of under 50 copies/ml who were randomized to either: (1) continuous therapy, (2) a CD4 cell count-guided theory, or (3) a week-on/week-off (WOWO) strategy, 31% of the patients in the WOWO group had virological failure (31[C]). Although the proportions of patients with a CD4 cell count below $350 \times 10^6/l$ were 100, 87, and 96% in treatment arms 1, 2, and 3 respectively and the percentages of weeks of antiretroviral use were 100, 41, and 70%, the adverse events were not significantly different among arms. The WOWO strategy is not recommended.

DRUGS ACTIVE AGAINST HUMAN IMMUNODEFICIENCY VIRUS: NUCLEOSIDE ANALOGUE REVERSE TRANSCRIPTASE INHIBITORS (NRTI)   *(SED-15, 2586; SEDA-27, 306; SEDA-28, 332; SEDA-29, 302)*

Abacavir   *(SED-15, 3; SEDA-27, 307; SEDA-29, 303)*

Immunologic   In the CNA30021 study abacavir 600 mg/day (*n* = 384) was compared with 300 mg bd (*n* = 386) in combination with lamivudine 300 mg and efavirenz 600 mg. The rates of adverse events, including abacavir *hypersensitivity reactions*, were similar in the two arms (9 versus 7%) (32^C).

Drug–drug interactions   The combination of abacavir + lamivudine + tenofovir in a triple-nucleoside regimen is no longer recommended (33^C). This is on the basis of a randomized, open, multicenter study of tenofovir disoproxil fumarate versus efavirenz, both administered once daily with the abacavir+lamivudine fixed-dose combination in 340 treatment-naïve subjects. The abacavir+lamivudine+tenofovir arm had an unacceptably high virological failure rate of 49% compared with 5% in the efavirenz arm at 12 weeks and the study was ended prematurely. Only 54% of the patients who failed had the typical K65R and M184V mutations on subsequent genotyping (34^C). The mechanism for this interaction is still unclear and there is no classical pharmacokinetic interaction. It has been hypothesized that the interaction occurs at the level of the intracellular nucleotide (33^C).

Didanosine   *(SED-15, 1113; SEDA-27, 307; SEDA-29, 303)*

Placebo-controlled studies   In a study of 168 patients with virological failure didanosine was compared with placebo in addition to optimized background treatment (35^C). The incidence of adverse events was similar in the two groups (38% with didanosine and 36% with placebo). Most of the adverse events were gastrointestinal (20%) or affected the nervous system (14%). Only five patients (4.5%) in the didanosine group and two (3.6%) in the placebo group complained of grade 1–2 *diarrhea*; no grade 3 diarrhea was reported. One patient in the didanosine group had a grade 2 *rise in serum lipase activity*, and one in the placebo group had a grade 3 rise.

Drug–drug interactions   *Tenofovir disoproxyl fumarate* significantly increases plasma didanosine concentrations by 40–50%. The efficacy of switching from 400 mg/day to 250 mg/day of didanosine (for patients weighing under 60 kg), has been confirmed by measuring intracellular concentrations, but there was no evidence of a kinetic interaction (36^C). The long intracellular half-lives of the drugs were also noted (7.5 days for tenofovir).

Racivir

Racivir is an unlicensed nucleoside reverse transcriptase inhibitor (racemic beta-2′,3′-dideoxy-5-fluoro-3′-thiacytidine), which is similar in structure to lamivudine. In six HIV positive subjects oral racivir in combination with stavudine and efavirenz was well tolerated at all doses tested (37^C). The maximum concentration (C$_{max}$) in serum at 200, 400, and 600 mg/day exceeded the 90% effective concentration for wild-type HIV-1. Viral loads fell in all dosage groups, with mean reductions from 1.13–1.42 log$_{10}$ units by day 4 and 2.02–2.43 log$_{10}$ units by day 14. HIV RNA amounts remained suppressed for more than 2 weeks in the absence of any additional therapy, with mean viral loads of 2.1–2.6 log$_{10}$ units below baseline to day 28. By day 35, HIV RNA amounts began to increase, but still remained >1 log$_{10}$ unit below baseline. The adverse events reported most often during the 14-day treatment period were *dizziness* (six, seven, nine, and five episodes in subjects taking racivir 200, 400, and 600 mg or lamivudine respectively) and *headache* (five, two, five, and one episode respectively) One subject taking racivir 600 mg reported "*heartburn*" possibly related to the drug. One subject taking racivir 600 mg withdrew on day 4 because of moderate *nausea and vomiting* associated with mild *dizziness*, possibly caused by racivir or efavirenz. Another subject taking racivir 200 mg developed significantly *raised creatinine kinase activity after exercise*. One subject, who had chronic hepatitis B and was taking racivir 400 mg, had *high aspartate and alanine transaminase activities* during the whole study, thought to be related to a flare of hepatitis B related to racivir.

Stavudine   *(SED-15, 3180)*

Fetotoxicity   Concerns continue about the toxicity of stavudine on the fetus. Five of ten infants born to ten pregnant women who took the drug during pregnancy developed grade 3 *neutropenia*, one developed *hypoglycemia*, and three developed *hyperkalemia* (38[r]).

DRUGS ACTIVE AGAINST HUMAN IMMUNODEFICIENCY VIRUS: NUCLEOTIDE ANALOGUE REVERSE TRANSCRIPTASE INHIBITORS

Tenofovir   *(SED-15, 3314; SEDA-29, 304)*

Urinary tract   *Acute irreversible renal insufficiency* has been reported with tenofovir (39[A]).

- A 39-year-old HIV-positive white man, developed acute renal insufficiency after taking lamivudine, zidovudine, and nevirapine for 2 weeks. His serum creatinine was 237 µmol/l. Renal ultrasound was normal and renal histology showed acute tubular necrosis with vacuolation of the proximal tubular cells and no evidence of focal or global glomerulosclerosis. All drugs were withdrawn but he required permanent dialysis.

Drug–drug interactions   See also didanosine.

In a population pharmacokinetic study of 192 HIV-infected patients a two compartment model fitted best (40[C]). This study also confirmed the increase in AUC over 24 hours for tenofovir induced by *lopinavir + ritonavir* and no observable effect of didanosine. Tenofovir plasma clearance was related to the body weight/serum creatinine ratio but not to serum creatinine or estimated GFR.

Tenofovir had no effect on the pharmacokinetics of saquinavir hard gel + ritonavir in 18 HIV-infected subjects (41[C]).

DRUGS ACTIVE AGAINST HUMAN IMMUNODEFICIENCY VIRUS: NON-NUCLEOSIDE REVERSE TRANSCRIPTASE INHIBITORS (NNRTI)   *(SED-15, 2553; SEDA-27, 308; SEDA-28, 334; SEDA-29, 305)*

Efavirenz   *(SED-15, 1204; SEDA-27, 309; SEDA-28, 334; SEDA-29, 305)*

Nervous system   Mild and clinically tolerable *neuropsychiatric disorders* can persist after a mean of 2 years after withdrawal of an efavirenz-based therapy (42[C]).

In a cross-sectional study, 60 patients taking an efavirenz-based approach were compared with 60 patients taking a protease inhibitor-containing regimen for at least 1 year. The mean times on treatment were 91 weeks and 120 weeks respectively. Mild *dizziness* (22%), *sadness* (37%), *mood changes* (27%), *irritability* (30%), *lightheadedness* (28%), *nervousness* (30%), *impaired concentration* (27%), *abnormal dreams* (48%), and *somnolence* (25%) were reported more often with efavirenz than the protease inhibitor. Of 60 patients 49 had plasma concentrations in the target range (1.0–4.0 mg/l). Efavirenz plasma concentrations were similar in subjects with and without neuropsychiatric disorders.

In a retrospective study in 134 patients taking efavirenz there were no significant differences in nervous system adverse effects or discontinuation rates between recreational substance (cocaine, ecstasy, cannabis) users and non-users (43[c]).

Metabolism   In a cross-sectional evaluation of 1018 HIV-infected patients treated with HAART during the previous 12 months in an Italian clinic, *isolated hypertriglyceridemia* was more common in 183 naive patients taking efavirenz compared with nevirapine, and both *hypertriglyceridemia and hypercholes-terolemia* appeared earlier (44^C). In the 295 antiretroviral-experienced patients, in whom an NNRTI was introduced for the first time, the frequency of raised triglyceride concentrations was higher and occurred earlier with efavirenz. In the 145 subjects taking salvage HAART, including an NNRTI plus a protease inhibitor-containing regimen, the rates of *hypertriglyceridemia, hypercholesterolemia*, and *hyperglycemia* were greater among patients taking efavirenz compared with nevirapine, and the time to peak metabolic alterations in hypercholesterolemia and hyperglycemia, but not hypertriglyceridemia, were more rapid in the whole efavirenz group. Comparing all of the 324 patients who took efavirenz with the 299 subjects who took nevirapine, the frequencies of raised triglyceride, cholesterol, and glucose concentrations were much higher in those taking efavirenz. There was some grade of *lipodystrophy* in 207 pretreated patients, but there was appreciable improvement after an NNRTI was introduced in patients taking efavirenz compared with those taking nevirapine.

Breasts   *Gynecomastia* was diagnosed in 13/324 (4%) patients who took efavirenz, compared with 2/299 (0.7%) subjects taking nevirapine (44^C).

Susceptibility factors

Genetic   Plasma efavirenz concentrations were increased in 40 of 100 subjects with the polymorphic homozygous genotype 516G>T at the gene encoding cytochrome CYP2B6 and 19% of subjects with the heterozygous genotype; 20% of those with the wild-type genotype had subtherapeutic concentrations of efavirenz (45^C). The CYP2B6-516 genotype, which is commoner in African–Americans, may help to identify subjects who will have plasma efavirenz concentrations that are outside the usual target range.

Drug–drug interactions   In patients who were taking the NNRTIs efavirenz and nevirapine, the apparent oral clearance (CL/F) of *lopinavir* increased by 39% (46^C). This is in line with an advised 33% dosage increment for lopinavir + ritonavir when combined with

NNRTIs. There was a 41% increase in indinavir clearance when it was co-administered with nevirapine or efavirenz (47^C).

The interactions of efavirenz, amprenavir, nelfinavir, indinavir, and ritonavir have been measured in 56 seronegative subjects (ACTG 5043) (48^C). African–American non-Hispanics had higher efavirenz AUCs than white non-Hispanics on day 14. The authors concluded that efavirenz reduced the AUC of amprenavir, but nelfinavir, indinavir, or ritonavir compensated for the induction of amprenavir metabolism by efavirenz. There were *rashes* in 11% of subjects but none was worse than grade 1. There was no relation between rash and amprenavir plasma concentration, but there were higher efavirenz concentrations in those with rashes. Efavirenz concentrations did not correlate with nervous system symptoms, possibly because those with more severe symptoms dropped out before the efavirenz AUCs were obtained on day 14.

Nevirapine   *(SED-15, 2498; SEDA-27, 310; SEDA-28, 334, SEDA-29, 305)*

Observational studies   In a Nigerian prospective, observational, cohort study, 50 antiretroviral drug-naive patients in stage 2 or stage 3 World Health Organization clinical classification were treated with generic brands of oral nevirapine (Nevimal, Cipla, Mumbai, India) 200 mg/day, lamivudine (Lamivir, Cipla) 150 mg bd, and stavudine (Stavir, Cipla) 40 mg bd (49^C). At week 48 the median CD4+ cell count increased by $186 \times 10^6/l$, the frequency of opportunistic infections fell by 82%, and the median body mass index increased by 4.8 kg/m^2. There were minor and transient adverse effects in 36%. The most comment adverse effect was a *rash* associated with nevirapine.

Liver   Boehringer Ingelheim have conducted an analysis of *hepatotoxicity* in all of their past controlled and uncontrolled studies (50^C). This analysis resulted in warnings that female sex and a higher CD4 cell count at the start of therapy increases the risk of hepatotoxicity, particularly during the first 6 weeks of treatment. They recommended against starting nevirapine in women with CD4 cell counts over $250 \times 10^6/l$ or in men with CD4 cell counts over $400 \times 10^6/l$.

Lactation   In 20 mother-infant pairs in a pharmacokinetic study in Botswana, maternal serum concentrations of nevirapine were high (median 9534 ng/ml) at a median of 4 hours after nevirapine ingestion, and the median breast-milk concentration of nevirapine was two-thirds of the serum concentration (51[C]). The median infant serum nevirapine concentration was 971 ng/ml, which is at least 40 times the 50% inhibitory concentration and similar to peak concentrations after a single 2-mg/kg dose of nevirapine. One infant had a *rash* 3 days after birth (and had also received oral nevirapine at birth), and four of the infants had either severe or life-threatening *neutropenia* or *anemia* at some time during breast-feeding.

DRUGS ACTIVE AGAINST HUMAN IMMUNODEFICIENCY VIRUS: PROTEASE INHIBITORS
(SED-15, 2965; SEDA-28, 335; SEDA-29, 306)

Amprenavir   *(SED-15, 211, SEDA-29, 306)*

In a study of the pharmacokinetics of oral amprenavir administered as soft gelatin capsules to 20 HIV-positive children, the most common adverse event was *nausea* (48[C]). The kinetics supported twice daily dosing with 20 mg/kg.

Atazanavir

Metabolism   In an analysis of a randomized comparison of atazanavir and nelfinavir in 467 patients cardiovascular risk modelling was used to estimate the impact of *dyslipidemia* (52[C]). Concentrations of total cholesterol and low-density lipoprotein cholesterol increased significantly more among patients who used nelfinavir (24 and 28%) than among those who used atazanavir (4 and 1%). Overall, the relative risk of coronary disease, adjusted for risk status,

age, and sex, was increased by 50% for nelfinavir versus atazanavir over the next 10 years in men or women, regardless of the presence or absence of other coronary risk factors.

Indinavir   *(SED-15, 1735; SEDA-27, 313; SEDA-28, 335; SEDA-29, 307)*

Drug–drug interactions   Co-administration of *efavirenz* or *nevirapine* increased the clearance of indinavir by 41%, irrespective of the presence or absence of ritonavir (47[C]). Women had a 48% higher apparent systemic availability of indinavir than men. Population pharmacokinetic modeling supported ritonavir boosting of indinavir.

In a meta-analysis of three studies (total $n = 26$) and in a randomized study of 16 patients indinavir concentrations were not reduced significantly by the herbal treatment *milk thistle* (53[M]).

Lopinavir + ritonavir   *(SED-15, 2159; SEDA-27, 314; SEDA-28, 336; SEDA-29, 307, 308)*

Endocrine   Six patients with pre-existing HIV-lipodystrophy developed symptomatic *Cushing's syndrome* when treated with inhaled fluticasone at varying doses for asthma while concurrently taking low-dose ritonavir-boosted protease inhibitor antiretroviral regimens for HIV infection (54[A]). Stimulation studies showed evidence of adrenal suppression in all patients. After withdrawal of inhaled fluticasone, four patients developed symptomatic hypoadrenalism, and three required oral glucocorticoid support for several months. Other complications included evidence of *osteoporosis* ($n = 3$), *crush fractures* ($n = 1$), and *exacerbation of pre-existing type 2 diabetes mellitus* ($n = 1$).

Drug–drug interactions   See also efavirenz and nevirapine

From 122 outpatients, 748 lopinavir and 748 ritonavir plasma concentrations were available for analysis (55[C]). The interaction between the drugs was described by a time-independent in-verse relation between exposure to ritonavir over a dosing interval and the apparent oral clearance (CL/F) of *lopinavir*. No patient char-acteristics, other than the use of NNRTIs had a significant effect on the pharmacokinetics of lopinavir combined with ritonavir.

From 186 patients in an Amsterdam clinic, 505 ritonavir plasma concentrations at a sin-gle time and 55 full pharmacokinetic profiles were available, resulting in a database of 1228 plasma ritonavir concentrations (56[C]). The con-comitant use of lopinavir resulted in a sig-nificant 2.7-fold increase in the clearance of ritonavir. No patient characteristics affected the pharmacokinetics of ritonavir.

In 45 HIV-positive patients taking lopina-vir+ritonavir plus efavirenz and 24 patients tak-ing lopinavir+ritonavir plus nucleoside/nucleo-tide reverse transcriptase inhibitors, lopinavir metabolism was induced by efavirenz by about 25% (57[C]).

Nelfinavir   *(SED-15, 2433; SEDA-27, 315; SEDA-28, 336; SEDA-29, 309)*

Metabolism   An insulin-modified frequent sampling intravenous glucose tolerance test was performed in HIV-infected children, of whom 33 were taking a protease inhibitor and 15 were not (58[C]). The former were also taking ritonavir ($n = 10$), nelfinavir ($n = 14$), indi-navir ($n = 2$), lopinavir + ritonavir ($n = 5$), ritonavir + nelfinavir ($n = 1$), and nelfinavir + saquinavir ($n = 1$). There were no differences between the two groups with respect to fast-ing serum insulin or C-peptide, homeostatic model assessment of insulin resistance, or a quantitative insulin sensitivity check index. In a multiple regression analysis, the insulin sensi-tivity index and disposition index of children taking a protease inhibitor were significantly lower than in children who were not. In those taking a protease inhibitor, insulin sensitivity correlated inversely with visceral adipose tissue area and visceral to subcutaneous adipose tissue ratio. There was *mildly impaired glucose toler-ance* in four of 21 subjects taking a protease inhibitor. These results suggest that protease inhibitor therapy reduces insulin sensitivity in HIV-infected children but also that it impairs

the beta-cell response to this reduction in in-sulin sensitivity and, in a subset of children, leads to the development of impaired glucose tolerance.

In a cross-sectional analysis of existing data-bases, 17 children with HIV infection were identified as having taken protease inhibitors, either ritonavir 20–30 mg/kg/day ($n = 9$) or nelfinavir 60–90 mg/kg/day ($n = 8$) for an av-erage of 711 days (59[C]). They were matched with 112 apparently healthy children admitted for minor surgical procedures. Plasma con-centrations of cholesterol, triglycerides, and insulin-like growth factor 1 (IGF-1) tended to be high in those who had taken a protease inhibitor. The plasma concentrations of omega-6 long-chain polyunsaturated fatty acids and in particular of the highly unsaturated 22:4 omega-6 and 22:5 omega-6, were significantly increased. Infected children also had increased delta-6 and delta-4 desaturase activities and de-creased delta-5 desaturase activity. The authors concluded that these children have a *metabolic* syndrome associated with significant changes in plasma fatty acid composition, similar to that observed in insulin resistance.

Drug–drug interactions   There was a clini-cally non-significant interaction between nel-finavir and *zidovudine* in a pharmacokinetic study in 46 patients (60[C]).

DRUGS ACTIVE AGAINST INFLUENZA VIRUSES: NEURAMINIDASE INHIBITORS

(SED-15, 2436; SEDA-27, 317; SEDA-28, 337; SEDA-29, 310)

Systematic review   Recent trials of the neu-raminidase inhibitors for influenza have been reviewed (61[R]). The percentage of patients with serious or minor adverse effects associ-ated with the administration of neuraminidase inhibitors was as follows for zanamivir: seri-ous or life-threatening reactions were *allergic or allergic-like reactions, dysrhythmias, bron-chospasm, dyspnea, facial edema, rash, seizure, syncope,* and *urticaria* (<1.5%). Minor ad-verse effects included *headache* (2%), *dizziness*

(2%), *nausea* (3%), *diarrhea* (adults, 3%; children, 2%), *vomiting* (adults, 1%; children, 2%), *sinusitis* (3%), *bronchitis* (2%), *cough* (2%), *other nasal signs and symptoms* (2%), and *infections* (ear, nose, and throat: adults, 2%; children, 5%).

For oseltamivir the serious or life-threatening events were *aggravation of diabetes, dysrhythmias, confusion, hepatitis, pseudomembranous colitis, pyrexia, rash, seizures, swelling of the face or tongue, toxic epidermal necrolysis*, and *unstable angina* (<1%) The minor effects were *insomnia* (adults, 1%), *vertigo* (1%), *nausea* (10%), and *vomiting* (9%). The adverse effects of oseltamivir prophylaxis were similar to those reported during treatment, but generally with lower incidences. More common with prophylactic use were *headache* (20%), *fatigue* (8%), *cough* (6%), and *diarrhea* (3%).

Oseltamivir

Observational studies   In a large Japanese prospective multicenter study during the influenza season of 2002–3 oseltamivir was given to 803 patients with influenza A and 684 patients with influenza B; amantadine was given to 676 patients with influenza A (62[C]). In each group, the duration of fever (body temperature over 37.5 °C) was significantly shorter in patients who were treated within 12 hours after the onset of symptoms than in those who were treated more than 12 hours after the onset. The type of influenza, the highest body temperature, and the time between the onset of symptoms and the start of treatment independently affected the duration of fever. Only minor adverse reactions were reported by 19 patients with influenza A given oseltamivir, eight patients given amantadine, and one patient with influenza B given oseltamivir.

In a model of cost effectiveness comparing annual influenza immunization against empirical amantadine and rapid testing followed by oseltamivir if the results are positive, antiviral therapy without immunization was associated with the lowest overall costs ($234 per person per year for amantadine, $237 for oseltamivir). The cost of annual immunization was $239

per person and was associated with 0.0409 quality-adjusted days saved, for a marginal cost-effectiveness ratio of $113 per quality-adjusted day gained or $41 000 per quality-adjusted life-year saved compared with antiviral therapy (63[H]). Adverse effects were included in the model at estimated baseline probabilities from published work. The adverse effects of influenza vaccine included minor effects, such as *local soreness at the injection site*, estimated at a probability of 0.64, and rarely *Guillain–Barré syndrome* (10^{-6}). The authors estimated that adverse effects other than Guillain–Barré syndrome lasted 2 days. Minor adverse effects due to drugs were also included with a probability of 0.09 for amantadine and 0.1 for oseltamivir.

Susceptibility factors

Liver disease   A single oral dose of oseltamivir 75 mg has been studied in 11 subjects with (all with cirrhosis, seven alcohol-induced) and paired controls. Mean BMI and estimated serum creatinine clearance were matched. In hepatic impairment the values of oseltamivir and oseltamivir carboxylate C_{max} were <6% and <19% lower and their AUCs 33% higher and <19% lower respectively. Thus, the metabolism of oseltamivir is not compromised in hepatic impairment and no dosage adjustment is required (64[C]).

DRUGS ACTIVE AGAINST RHINOVIRUSES

Pleconaril

In a placebo-controlled study of pleconaril in 827 patients with positive baseline nasal mucus cultures for rhinoviruses, those who were infected with viruses that are more highly susceptible to pleconaril (50% effective concentration <0.38 µg/ml) had a median 1.9–3.9 day reduction in symptom duration compared with placebo (65[C]). In contrast, subjects whose baseline virus isolate susceptibility was >0.38 µg/ml did not benefit from pleconaril. Adverse effects were not mentioned.

References

1. Husak R, Zouboulis CC, Sander-Bähr C, Hummel M, Orfanos CE. Refractory human papillomavirus-associated oral warts treated topically with 1–3% cidofovir solutions in human immunodeficiency virus type 1-infected patients. Br J Dermatol 2005;152(3):590–1.

2. Tristram A, Fiander A. Clinical responses to cidofovir applied topically to women with high grade vulval intraepithelial neoplasia. Gynecol Oncol 2005;99(3):652–5.

3. Tobin AM, Cotter M, Irvine AD, Kirby B. Successful treatment of a refractory verruca in a child with acute lymphoblastic leukaemia with topical cidofovir. Br J Dermatol 2005;152(2):386–8.

4. Muller WJ, Levin MJ, Shin YK, Robinson C, Quinones R, Malcolm J, Hild E, Gao D, Giller R. Clinical and in vitro evaluation of cidofovir for treatment of adenovirus infection in pediatric hematopoietic stem cell transplant recipients. Clin Infect Dis 2005;41(12):1812–6.

5. Ortiz A, Justo P, Sanz A, Melero R, Caramelo C, Guerrero MF, Strutz F, Muller G, Barat A, Egido J. Tubular cell apoptosis and cidofovir-induced acute renal failure. Antivir Ther 2005;10(1):185–90.

6. Hsu CC, Lai TI, Lien WC, Chen WJ, Fang CC. Emergent hemodialysis for acyclovir toxicity. Am J Emerg Med 2005;23(7):899–900.

7. Drugspedia. Acyclovir. http://drugspedia.net/prep/24898.html [last accessed 27 October 2007].

8. Vassiliadis T, Nikolaidis N, Giouleme O, Tziomalos K, Grammatikos N, Patsiaoura K, Zezos P, Gkisakis D, Theodoropoulos K, Katsinelos P, Orfanou-Koumerkeridou E, Eugenidis N. Adefovir dipivoxil added to ongoing lamivudine therapy in patients with lamivudine-resistant hepatitis B e antigen-negative chronic hepatitis B. Aliment Pharmacol Ther 2005;21(5):531–7.

9. Ocama P, Opio CK, Lee WM. Hepatitis B virus infection: current status. Am J Med 2005;118(12):1413.

10. Janssen HL, van Zonneveld M, Senturk H, Zeuzem S, Akarca US, Cakaloglu Y, Simon C, So TM, Gerken G, de Man RA, Niesters HG, Zondervan P, Hansen B, Schalm SW, HBV 99-01 Study Group, Rotterdam Foundation for Liver Research. Pegylated interferon alfa-2b alone or in combination with lamivudine for HBeAg-positive chronic hepatitis B: a randomised trial. Lancet 2005;365(9454):123–9.

11. Buti M, Jardi R, Rodriguez-Frias F, Valdes A, Schaper M, Esteban R, Guardia J. Changes in different regions of hepatitis B virus gene in hepatitis B 'e' antigen-negative patients with chronic hepatitis B: the effect of long-term lamivudine therapy. Aliment Pharmacol Ther 2005;21(11):1349–56.

12. Dai MS, Chao TY. Lamivudine therapy in HBsAg-carrying breast cancer patients undergoing chemotherapy: prophylactic or preemptive? Breast Cancer Res Treat 2005;92(1):95–6.

13. Lau GK, Piratvisuth T, Luo KX, Marcellin P, Thongsawat S, Cooksley G, Gane E, Fried MW, Chow WC, Paik SW, Chang WY, Berg T, Flisiak R, McCloud P, Pluck N, Peginterferon Alfa-2a HBeAg-Positive Chronic Hepatitis B Study Group. Peginterferon alfa-2a, lamivudine, and the combination for HBeAg-positive chronic hepatitis B. N Engl J Med 2005;352(26):2682–95.

14. Brok J, Gluud LL, Gluud C. Effects of adding ribavirin to interferon to treat chronic hepatitis C infection: a systematic review and meta-analysis of randomized trials. Arch Intern Med 2005;165(19):2206–12.

15. Cacoub P, Saadoun D, Sene D, Limal N, Piette JC. Treatment of hepatitis C virus-related systemic vasculitis. J Rheumatol 2005;32(11):2078–82.

16. Cacoub P, Saadoun D, Limal N, Sene D, Lidove O, Piette JC. PEGylated interferon alfa-2b and ribavirin treatment in patients with hepatitis C virus-related systemic vasculitis. Arthritis Rheum 2005;52(3):911–5.

17. Kaymakoglu S, Karaca C, Demir K, Poturoglu S, Danalioglu A, Badur S, Bozaci M, Besisik F, Cakaloglu Y, Okten A. Alpha interferon and ribavirin combination therapy of chronic hepatitis D. Antimicrob Agents Chemother 2005;49(3):1135–8.

18. Sugawara Y, Makuuchi M. Should living donor liver transplantation be offered to patients with hepatitis C virus cirrhosis? J Hepatol 2005;42(4):472–5.

19. Carlsson T, Reichard O, Norkrans G, Blackberg J, Sangfelt P, Wallmark E, Weiland O. Hepatitis C virus RNA kinetics during the initial 12 weeks treatment with pegylated interferon-alpha 2a and ribavirin according to virological response. J Viral Hepat 2005;12(5):473–80.

20. Yu ML, Hou NJ, Dai CY, Chang WY, Chuang WL. Successful treatment of fulminant hepatitis C by therapy with alpha interferon and ribavirin. Antimicrob Agents Chemother 2005;49(9):3986–7.

21. Lima MA, Auriel E, Wuthrich C, Borenstein NM, Koralnik IJ. Progressive multifocal leukoencephalopathy as a complication of hepatitis C virus treatment in an HIV-negative patient. Clin Infect Dis 2005;41(3):417–9.

22. Balan V, Schwartz D, Wu GY, Muir AJ, Ghalib R, Jackson J, Keeffe EB, Rossaro L, Burnett A, Goon BL, Bowers PJ, Leitz GJ, HCV Natural History Study Group. Erythropoietic response to anemia in chronic hepatitis C patients receiving combination pegylated interferon/ribavirin. Am J Gastroenterol 2005;100(2):299–307.

23. Lubbe J, Kerl K, Negro F, Saurat JH. Clinical and immunological features of hepatitis C treatment-

associated dermatitis in 36 prospective cases. Br J Dermatol 2005;153(5):1088–90.

24. Girard C, Bessis D, Blatire V, Guilhou JJ, Guillot B. Meyerson's phenomenon induced by interferon-alfa plus ribavirin in hepatitis C infection. Br J Dermatol 2005;152(1):182–3.

25. Conde-Taboada A, de la Torre C, Feal C, Mayo E, Gonzalez-Sixto B, Cruces MJ. Meyerson's naevi induced by interferon alfa plus ribavirin combination therapy in hepatitis C infection. Br J Dermatol 2005;153(5):1070–2.

26. Thevenot T, Bachmeyer C, Hammi R, Dumouchel P, Ducamp-Posak I, Cadranel JF. Occurrence of porphyria cutanea tarda during peginterferon/ribavirin therapy for chronic viral hepatitis C. J Hepatol 2005;42(4):607–8.

27. Hurst EA, Mauro T. Sarcoidosis associated with pegylated interferon alfa and ribavirin treatment for chronic hepatitis C: a case report and review of the literature. Arch Dermatol 2005;141(7):865–8.

28. Rodriguez-Torres M, Torriani FJ, Soriano V, Borucki MJ, Lissen E, Sulkowski M, Dieterich D, Wang K, Gries JM, Hoggard PG, Back D. Effect of ribavirin on intracellular and plasma pharmacokinetics of nucleoside reverse transcriptase inhibitors in patients with human immunodeficiency virus-hepatitis C virus coinfection: results of a randomized clinical study. Antimicrob Agents Chemother 2005;49(10):3997–4008.

29. Stravitz RT, Chung H, Sterling RK, Luketic VA, Sanyal AJ, Price AS, Purrington A, Shiffman ML. Antibody-mediated pure red cell aplasia due to epoetin alfa during antiviral therapy of chronic hepatitis C. Am J Gastroenterol 2005;100(6):1415–9.

30. Wolff MJ, Beltran CJ, Vasquez P, Ayala MX, Valenzuela M, Berrios G, Arredondo A. The Chilean AIDS cohort: a model for evaluating the impact of an expanded access program to antiretroviral therapy in a middle-income country—organization and preliminary results. J Acquir Immune Defic Syndr 2005;40(5):551–7.

31. Cardiello PG, Hassink E, Ananworanich J, Srasuebkul P, Samor T, Mahanontharit A, Ruxrungtham K, Hirschel B, Lange J, Phanuphak P, Cooper DA. A prospective, randomized trial of structured treatment interruption for patients with chronic HIV type 1 infection. Clin Infect Dis 2005;40(4):594–600.

32. Moyle GJ, DeJesus E, Cahn P, Castillo SA, Zhao H, Gordon DN, Craig C, Scott TR, Ziagen Once-Daily in Antiretroviral Combination Therapy (CNA30021) Study Team. Abacavir once or twice daily combined with once-daily lamivudine and efavirenz for the treatment of antiretroviral-naive HIV-infected adults: results of the Ziagen Once Daily in Antiretroviral Combination Study. J Acquir Immune Defic Syndr 2005;38(4):417–25.

33. Kuritzkes DR. Less than the sum of its parts: failure of a tenofovir–abacavir–lamivudine triple-nucleoside regimen. J Infect Dis 2005;192(11):1867–8.

34. Gallant JE, Rodriguez AE, Weinberg WG, Young B, Berger DS, Lim ML, Liao Q, Ross L, Johnson J, Shaefer MS, ESS30009 Study. Early virologic nonresponse to tenofovir, abacavir, and lamivudine in HIV-infected antiretroviral-naive subjects. J Infect Dis 2005;192(11):1921–30.

35. Molina JM, Marcelin AG, Pavie J, Heripret L, De Boever CM, Troccaz M, Leleu G, Calvez V, AI454-176 JAGUAR Study Team. Didanosine in HIV-1-infected patients experiencing failure of antiretroviral therapy: a randomized placebo-controlled trial. J Infect Dis 2005;191(6):840–7.

36. Pruvost A, Negredo E, Benech H, Theodoro F, Puig J, Grau E, Garcia E, Molto J, Grassi J, Clotet B. Measurement of intracellular didanosine and tenofovir phosphorylated metabolites and possible interaction of the two drugs in human immunodeficiency virus-infected patients. Antimicrob Agents Chemother 2005;49(5):1907–14.

37. Herzmann C, Arastèh K, Murphy RL, Schulbin H, Kreckel P, Drauz D, Schinazi RF, Beard A, Cartee L, Otto MJ. Safety, pharmacokinetics, and efficacy of $(+/-)$-beta-2′,3′-dideoxy-5-fluoro-3′-thiacytidine with efavirenz and stavudine in antiretroviral-naive human immunodeficiency virus-infected patients. Antimicrob Agents Chemother 2005;49(7):2828–33.

38. Blanche S. Safety of stavudine during pregnancy. J Infect Dis 2005;191(9):1567–8, 1568–9 [author reply].

39. Krummel T, Parvez-Braun L, Frantzen L, Lalanne H, Marcellin L, Hannedouche T, Moulin B. Tenofovir-induced acute renal failure in an HIV patient with normal renal function. Nephrol Dial Transplant 2005;20(2):473–4.

40. Jullien V, Treluyer JM, Rey E, Jaffray P, Krivine A, Moachon L, Lillo-Le Louet A, Lescoat A, Dupin N, Salmon D, Pons G, Urien S. Population pharmacokinetics of tenofovir in human immunodeficiency virus-infected patients taking highly active antiretroviral therapy. Antimicrob Agents Chemother 2005;49(8):3361–6.

41. Boffito M, Pozniak A, Kearney BP, Higgs C, Mathias A, Zhong L, Shah J. of pharmacokinetic drug interaction between tenofovir disoproxil fumarate and nelfinavir mesylate. Antimicrob Agents Chemother 2005;49(10):4386–9.

42. Fumaz CR, Munoz-Moreno JA, Molto J, Negredo E, Ferrer MJ, Sirera G, Perez-Alvarez N, Gomez Q, Burger D, Clotet B. Long-term neuropsychiatric disorders on efavirenz-based approaches: quality of life, psychologic issues, and adherence. J Acquir Immune Defic Syndr 2005;38(5):560–5.

43. Faggian F, Lattuada E, Lanzafame M, Antolini D, Concia E, Vento S. Recreational substance use and tolerance of efavirenz in HIV-1 infected patients. AIDS Care 2005;17(7):908–10.

44. Manfredi R, Calza L, Chiodo F. An extremely different dysmetabolic profile between the two available nonnucleoside reverse transcriptase inhibitors: efavirenz and nevirapine. J Acquir Immune Defic Syndr 2005;38(2):236–8.

45. Rodriguez-Novoa S, Barreiro P, Rendón A, Jiménez-Nacher I, González-Lahoz J, Soriano V. Influence of 516G>T polymorphisms at the gene encoding the CYP450-2B6 isoenzyme on efavirenz plasma concentrations in HIV-infected subjects. Clin Infect Dis 2005;40(9):1358–61.

46. Crommentuyn KM, Huitema AD, Brinkman K, van der Ende ME, de Wolf F, Beijnen JH, Athena study. Therapeutic drug monitoring of nevirapine reduces pharmacokinetic variability but does not affect toxicity or virologic success in the ATHENA study. J Acquir Immune Defic Syndr 2005;39(2):249–50.

47. Kappelhoff BS, Huitema AD, Sankatsing SU, Meenhorst PL, Van Gorp EC, Mulder JW, Prins JM, Beijnen JH. Population pharmacokinetics of indinavir alone and in combination with ritonavir in HIV-1-infected patients. Br J Clin Pharmacol 2005;60(3):276–86.

48. Morse GD, Rosenkranz S, Para MF, Segal Y, Difrancesco R, Adams E, Brizz B, Yarasheski KE, Reichman RC. Amprenavir and efavirenz pharmacokinetics before and after the addition of nelfinavir, indinavir, ritonavir, or saquinavir in seronegative individuals. Antimicrob Agents Chemother 2005;49(8):3373–81.

49. Idigbe EO, Adewole TA, Eisen G, Kanki P, Odunukwe NN, Onwujekwe DI, Audu RA, Araoyinbo ID, Onyewuche JI, Salu OB, Adedoyin JA, Musa AZ. Management of HIV-1 infection with a combination of nevirapine, stavudine, and lamivudine: a preliminary report on the Nigerian antiretroviral program. J Acquir Immune Defic Syndr 2005;40(1):65–9.

50. Leith J, Piliero P, Storfer S, Mayers D, Hinzmann R. Appropriate use of nevirapine for long-term therapy. J Infect Dis 2005;192(3):545–6; author reply 546.

51. Shapiro RL, Holland DT, Capparelli E, Lockman S, Thior I, Wester C, Stevens L, Peter T, Essex M, Connor JD, Mirochnick M. Antiretroviral concentrations in breast-feeding infants of women in Botswana receiving antiretroviral treatment. J Infect Dis 2005;192(5):720–7.

52. Grover SA, Coupal L, Gilmore N, Mukherjee J. Impact of dyslipidemia associated with Highly Active Antiretroviral Therapy (HAART) on cardiovascular risk and life expectancy. Am J Cardiol 2005;95(5):586–91.

53. Mills E, Wilson K, Clarke M, Foster B, Walker S, Rachlis B, DeGroot N, Montori VM, Gold W, Phillips E, Myers S, Gallicano K. Milk thistle and indinavir: a randomized controlled pharmacokinetics study and meta-analysis. Eur J Clin Pharmacol 2005;61(1):1–7.

54. Samaras K, Pett S, Gowers A, McMurchie M, Cooper DA. Iatrogenic Cushing's syndrome with osteoporosis and secondary adrenal failure in human immunodeficiency virus-infected patients receiving inhaled corticosteroids and ritonavir-boosted protease inhibitors: six cases. J Clin Endocrinol Metab 2005;90(7):4394–8.

55. Crommentuyn KM, Kappelhoff BS, Mulder JW, Mairuhu AT, van Gorp EC, Meenhorst PL, Huitema AD, Beijnen JH. Population pharmacokinetics of lopinavir in combination with ritonavir in HIV-1-infected patients. Br J Clin Pharmacol 2005;60(4):378–89.

56. Kappelhoff BS, Huitema AD, Crommentuyn KM, Mulder JW, Meenhorst PL, van Gorp EC, Mairuhu AT, Beijnen JH. Development and validation of a population pharmacokinetic model for ritonavir used as a booster or as an antiviral agent in HIV-1-infected patients. Br J Clin Pharmacol 2005;59(2):174–82.

57. Dailly E, Allavena C, Raffi F, Jolliet P. Pharmacokinetic evidence for the induction of lopinavir metabolism by efavirenz. Br J Clin Pharmacol 2005;60(1):32–4.

58. Bitnun A, Sochett E, Dick PT, To T, Jefferies C, Babyn P, Forbes J, Read S, King SM. Insulin sensitivity and beta-cell function in protease inhibitor-treated and -naive human immunodeficiency virus-infected children. J Clin Endocrinol Metab 2005;90(1):168–74.

59. Aldamiz-Echevarria L, Pocheville I, Sanjurjo P, Elorz J, Prieto JA, Rodriguez-Soriano J. Abnormalities in plasma fatty acid composition in human immunodeficiency virus-infected children treated with protease inhibitors. Acta Paediatr 2005;94(6):672–7.

60. Panhard X, Goujard C, Legrand M, Taburet AM, Diquet B, Mentre F, COPHAR 1-ANRS study group. Population pharmacokinetic analysis for nelfinavir and its metabolite M8 in virologically controlled HIV-infected patients on HAART. Br J Clin Pharmacol 2005;60(4):390–403.

61. Moscona A. Neuraminidase inhibitors for influenza. N Engl J Med 2005;353(13):1363–73.

62. Kawai N, Ikematsu H, Iwaki N, Satoh I, Kawashima T, Maeda T, Miyachi K, Hirotsu N, Shigematsu T, Kashiwagi S. Factors influencing the effectiveness of oseltamivir and amantadine for the treatment of influenza: a multicenter study from Japan of the 2002–2003 influenza season. Clin Infect Dis 2005;40(9):1309–16.

63. Rothberg MB, Rose DN. Vaccination versus treatment of influenza in working adults: a cost-effectiveness analysis. Am J Med 2005;118(1):68–77.

64. Snell P, Dave N, Wilson K, Rowell L, Weil A, Galitz L, Robson R. Lack of effect of moderate hepatic impairment on the pharmacokinetics of oral oseltamivir and its metabolite oseltamivir carboxylate. Br J Clin Pharmacol 2005;59(5):598–601.

65. Pevear DC, Hayden FG, Demenczuk TM, Barone LR, McKinlay MA, Collett MS. Relationship of pleconaril susceptibility and clinical outcomes in treatment of common colds caused by rhinoviruses. Antimicrob Agents Chemother 2005;49(11):4492–9.

V.V. Banu Rekha and Soumya Swaminathan

30 Drugs used in tuberculosis and leprosy

The authors of an observational study in 367 HIV-infected patients with 372 episodes of culture-confirmed tuberculosis analysed the factors that complicate antituberculosis therapy (1[C]). In 25% there was hepatic disease at the time of the diagnosis of tuberculosis or during antituberculosis therapy, and there were *rises in serum transaminases* to at least twice the upper limits of the reference ranges during the first month of antituberculosis therapy in 116 (31%) of the episodes. The most commonly reported adverse effects were *rash* (28%), *nausea* (26%), *leukopenia or neutropenia* (20%), *diarrhea* (19%), *vomiting* (19%), and *raised temperature* (17%). There was co-prescription of rifampicin with medications that interact with rifampicin during 270 episodes (72%).

Dapsone (SED-15, 1050; SEDA-26, 340; SEDA-28, 343; SEDA-29, 315)

Hematologic *Aplastic anemia* is a rare complication of dapsone, but a fatal case has been reported (2[A]).

- A 23-year-old Brazilian man was given dapsone, clofazimine, and rifampicin for lepromatous leprosy. After 10 months he had a severe episode of epistaxis associated with pancytopenia (hematocrit 8.3%, white cell count 1.3×10^9/l, 28% neutrophils, platelet count 5×10^9/l). Aplastic anemia was confirmed by a bone marrow biopsy. Despite numerous transfusions of platelets and packed red cell concentrates, he died from bleeding and nosocomial infection.

Late-onset aplastic anemia, as in this case, does not depend on the dose and duration of exposure to dapsone and is irreversible. Therefore, periodic hematological monitoring is recommended and patients should be educated about suggestive symptoms.

Pure red cell aplasia has been attributed to dapsone (3[A]).

- A 75-year-old man with type 2 diabetes taking glibenclamide developed granuloma annulare and was given dapsone 100 mg/day. A full blood count was normal, but 4 weeks later his hemoglobin was 3.6 g/dl, reticulocyte count 0.54%, MCV 109 fl, serum iron 27 µg/l, and serum ferritin 711 ng/l. Vitamin B_{12} and folic acid concentrations were normal. A bone marrow aspirate showed a normocellular marrow with profound erythroid hypoplasia. Pure red cell aplasia was diagnosed and linked to dapsone, which was withdrawn. After blood transfusion the hematological profile gradually returned to normal by day 8.

The frequency of *methemoglobinemia* and reduced cytochrome b5 reductase (Cb5r) activity have been studied in 15 children with acute lymphoblastic leukemia taking dapsone prophylaxis for *Pneumocystis jiroveci* and 10 taking co-trimoxazole (4[c]). At a mean of 6.6 weeks, three children taking dapsone developed symptomatic methemoglobinemia, defined as increased concentrations of methemoglobin in association with hypoxemia (oxygen saturation <95%). The other 12 were all asymptomatic. All the controls had normal methemoglobin concentrations. Cb5 reductase activities in two of the three symptomatic children were below 50% of normal, suggesting heterozygosity, which was confirmed by assessment of their parent's Cb5 reductase activities.

Heterozygosity for Cb5 reductase deficiency can predispose to methemoglobinemia, and such patients tend to be symptomatic at low methemoglobin concentrations. Heterozygotes

Side Effects of Drugs, Annual 30
J.K. Aronson (Editor)
ISSN: 0378-6080
DOI: 10.1016/S0378-6080(08)00030-5

should therefore be monitored closely for the possibility of methemoglobinemia.

Ethambutol   *(SED-15, 1282; SEDA-29, 316)*

℞ *Ethambutol-induced optic neuropathy*

> **DoTS classification:**
> *Reaction*: Optic neuropathy due to ethambutol
> *Dose-relation*: Collateral
> *Time-course*: Intermediate
> *Susceptibility factors*: Renal impairment, zinc deficiency

Optic neuropathy, which is primarily retrobulbar, is the most important adverse effect of ethambutol and takes two forms central and peripheral. The commoner is axial neuritis (central type), which involves the papillomacular bundle and results in reduced visual acuity, cecocentral scotoma, and blue-yellow color vision impairment. In periaxial neuritis (peripheral type) there is peripheral visual field loss, especially bitemporal defects, with sparing of visual acuity and red-green color vision impairment (5[A]). Rarely damage to the retina and macula has also been reported (6[A], 7[A]).

Presentation   *Ocular symptoms begin with bilateral progressive blurred vision or defects in color vision. However, some individuals are asymptomatic and abnormalities are detected only by tests of vision. A central scotoma is the most common visual field defect. Dyschromatopsia in the form of red-green color changes may be the earliest sign. Fundoscopy is usually normal.*

Mechanism   *The exact mechanism of ethambutol-induced ocular toxicity is not known, but there is an association with low serum zinc concentrations and reduced renal function (8[c], 9[A]).*

Dose relation   *Ocular toxicity due to ethambutol is dose related in the therapeutic range. At doses of over 50 mg/kg/day, over 40% of adults develop toxicity, compared with 0–3% at a dose of 15 mg/kg/day (10[M]).*

Time course   *The mean interval between the onset of therapy and the adverse effects is as short as 1.5 months or as long as 12 months after the start of therapy (10[M]).*

Ocular toxicity in elderly people   *Of 299 patients, mean age 63 years, taking ethambutol-containing multidrug therapy for Mycobacterium avium complex lung disease for a mean period of 16 months, 42% consulted an ophthalmologist and 10% stopped taking ethambutol at least temporarily (11[c]). Ethambutol-associated ocular toxicity was present only in patients who took daily treatment (6%), while none of the patients who took ethambutol intermittently reported this complication. Baseline ocular function was restored on withdrawal of ethambutol.*

Two elderly women taking ethambutol for atypical mycobacterial disease developed reduced visual acuity after 10 and 14 months (12[A]). At the start both developed severe bilateral visual loss with bitemporal hemianopia-like visual field disturbance, and ethambutol was withdrawn. However, there was no disc pallor or nerve fiber layer defect (NFLD) at any time during the follow-up period, and they both had good recovery of visual function at 18 and 19 months after the onset of optic neuropathy. The authors concluded that in patients with severe ethambutol optic neuropathy, as long as disc pallor and NFLD are not observed, good visual recovery can be expected even if severe visual loss persists for a long time.

Ocular toxicity in children   *There has been considerable reluctance to use ethambutol in young children, because of the potentially serious nature of ocular complications. Most international and national guidelines recommend that ethambutol should not be given to children younger than 5 or 7 years of age.*

In a recent review of several studies that carefully evaluated significant numbers of children taking ethambutol 15–30 mg/kg/day there was no evidence of ocular toxicity. Moreover, the cases reported in those with tuberculous meningitis could not be attributed to the drug, as the disease itself would often have been responsible. In only two of 3811 cases (0.05%) was ethambutol stopped because of fears of poorly documented ocular toxicity. These results endorse the safety of ethambutol in children of all ages.

Comparative ethambutol pharmacokinetics in adults and children   The reason for the low toxicity observed in children could be attributed to differences in drug pharmacokinetics between children and adults.

In adults, peak ethambutol concentrations after daily doses of 25 and 50 mg/kg were 5 and 10 μg/ml respectively (13^R). Serum concentrations were proportional to the dose. Less than 10% of the administered dose was present in the serum after 24 hours and there was no evidence of accumulation of the drug over more than 3 months.

There have been few studies of the pharmacokinetics of ethambutol in children. Serum concentrations in children taking doses of 15–35 mg/kg were lower than those in adults after similar doses (14^c). Furthermore, serum ethambutol concentrations were lower in younger than in older children. The serum concentrations reached in adults and children given similar doses of ethambutol were clearly different, suggesting that in order to achieve serum concentrations equivalent to those reached in adults given 15 mg/kg a child would require a dose of 25 mg/kg or more. However, factors such as the ratio of extracellular to intracellular and total body water, biotransformation, and elimination have also to be considered in interpreting the results. The authors speculated that delayed absorption of ethambutol could be the reason, and slow and incomplete absorption of ethambutol has been observed in children.

Recommended dosages   In the absence of overt ocular toxicity in children aged from under 1 to 18 years, who had taken ethambutol 15–30 mg/kg/day the following dosage regimens have been recommended (15^S):

- Daily treatment—20 mg/kg (range 15–25 mg/kg) for children of all ages. Increasing the dose beyond this range to compensate for deficiencies in serum concentrations might increase the risk of ethambutol ocular toxicity.
- Intermittent treatment—30 mg/kg (range 20–35 mg/kg) three times weekly or 45 mg/kg (range 40–50 mg/kg) twice weekly (as currently recommended for adults).

Just as in adults, care should be taken to establish that a child does not have renal disease, as this could lead to exposure to unacceptably high serum concentrations of ethambutol.

Isoniazid   *(SED-15, 1923; SEDA-28, 343; SEDA-29, 317)*

Liver   *Hepatotoxicity*, defined as aspartate transaminase activity more than five times the upper limit of the reference range, associated with the treatment of latent tuberculosis has been evaluated over 7 years in a retrospective study in adults (16^c). Of 3377 patients taking isoniazid, 19 had high aspartate transaminase activities (5.6 per 1000 patients). Only one of the 19 had prodromal symptoms associated with hepatotoxicity. After 1, 3, and 6 months of therapy the numbers of hepatotoxic events per 1000 patients were 2.75, 7.20, and 4.10 respectively. Age over 49 years and a baseline aspartate transaminase activity above the upper limit of normal were susceptibility factors. Moderate to severe hepatotoxicity often occurs without symptoms, which emphasizes the value of transaminase monitoring.

Rifampicin   *(SED-15, 3040; SEDA-27, 324; SEDA-28, 344; SEDA-29, 317)*

Comparative studies   The efficacy and safety of rifampicin + pyrazinamide versus isoniazid for the prevention of tuberculosis among people with or without HIV infection has been evaluated in a meta-analysis of three trials in HIV infected patients and three in HIV non-infected persons (17^M). The rates of tuberculosis and mortality were similar in the two groups, whether the subjects were HIV infected or not. However, both subgroup analyses showed a higher incidence of all severe adverse events in those who took rifampicin + pyrazinamide among non-HIV-infected persons (29 versus 7%) (see also *Liver* below).

Endocrine   Rifampicin-induced *hypothyroidism* has been reported in three euthyroid patients (18^A).

- A 62-year-old man with recurrent non-Hodgkin's lymphoma developed pulmonary tuberculosis, for which he received rifampicin. Within 2 weeks, his thyrotropin (TSH) concentration increased to 170 mU/l and the serum concentrations of thyroxine (T_4) and triiodothyronine (T_3) fell to 24 µg/l and 180 ng/l respectively. He was given thyroxine. After the course of rifampicin therapy had been completed, thyroxine was withdrawn and he remained euthyroid for 4 years.

- A 66-year-old woman with tuberculous peritonitis was given rifampicin and developed hypothyroidism (thyrotropin concentration 12.5 mU/l, T_4 48 µg/l, T_3 8.7 ng/l). She was given thyroxine for 3 months. Hypothyroidism developed again, and thyroxine was resumed for the duration of the course of rifampicin therapy and then withdrawn, after which she remained euthyroid for 42 months.
- A 56-year-old woman with liver abscesses and tuberculous lymphadenitis was given rifampicin and 2 weeks later developed a raised thyrotropin concentration of 21 mU/ml, for which she was given thyroxine. The hypothyroidism resolved on withdrawal of rifampicin. However on re-starting rifampicin she developed hypothyroidism within 4 weeks. She was again given thyroxine, which was withdrawn on completion of the course of rifampicin. She remained euthyroid for 12 months.

Hypothyroidism developed within 2 weeks of rifampicin therapy in these patients and resolved when it was withdrawn. Rifampicin increases thyroxine clearance, possibly by enhancing hepatic thyroxine metabolism and the biliary excretion of iodothyronine conjugates. In healthy volunteers rifampicin reduces circulating thyroid hormone concentrations without affecting thyrotropin, suggesting that rifampicin directly reduces thyroid hormone concentrations.

Hematologic   *Thrombocytopenia* has been reported in a patient taking rifampicin (19[A]).

- A 40-year-old man with multiple anesthetic plaques due to Hansen's multibacillary disease was given WHO multidrug therapy consisting of once-a-month supervised rifampicin 600 mg and clofazimine 300 mg along with unsupervised dapsone 100 mg/day and clofazimine 50 mg/day for 1 year. After 2 months he developed multiple ecchymoses and bleeding from the gums. His hemoglobin was 9.2 g/dl, total white cell count 10.5×10^9/l, platelet count 17×10^9/l; the bleeding and clotting times were normal. Dapsone was withdrawn and rifampicin and clofazimine were continued. However, within 24 hours he developed malaise and fatigue, with purpuric spots and ecchymoses all over the body. Although other hematological parameters were normal, the platelet count was 10×10^9/l. Rifampicin was withdrawn and he was given minocycline with clofazimine and dapsone. The platelet count improved in 3 weeks and the purpura and ecchymoses resolved within 1 week.

Rifampicin-induced thrombocytopenia is rare, but even a single monthly supervised dose can cause life-threatening thrombocytopenia.

Liver   Rifampicin + pyrazinamide for 2 months ($n = 153$) has been compared with a 6-month course of isoniazid ($n = 199$) for latent tuberculosis in HIV-negative contacts of patients with infectious pulmonary tuberculosis (20[C]). Treatment was withdrawn because of *hepatotoxicity* (transaminases over 5 times the upper limit of normal) in 10% of contacts who took rifampicin + pyrazinamide and in 2.5% of those who took isoniazid. This higher than expected rate of hepatotoxicity led to premature termination of the study. There were no cases of severe or fatal liver injury. Liver function tests normalized after withdrawal of treatment. The authors concluded that the use of rifampicin + pyrazinamide should only be considered when other regimens are unsuitable and that intensive monitoring of liver function is feasible.

Urinary tract   *Acute renal insufficiency* is a rare life-threatening complication of rifampicin. The Tuberculosis Research Centre in India has treated more than 8000 patients with pulmonary and extrapulmonary tuberculosis, including three who developed rifampicin-induced acute renal insufficiency (21[A]).

- A 25-year-old man with sputum-positive pulmonary tuberculosis was given a daily rifampicin-containing regimen and responded with negative sputum smears and cultures by the end of treatment. However, he relapsed after 5 months. Antituberculosis treatment was re-started with thrice-weekly isoniazid 600 mg, rifampicin 450 mg, ethambutol 1200 mg, and pyrazinamide 1500 mg. After 20 days, he complained of vomiting, anorexia, fever, and oliguria. His blood urea concentration was 62 mmol/l and serum creatinine 1529 µmol/l. Abdomen ultrasonography showed normal kidneys with increased cortical echoes. He was treated with three sessions of peritoneal dialysis, along with salt, protein, and fluid restriction. He refused renal biopsy. His renal function improved and after 4 weeks his blood urea was 15 mmol/l and serum creatinine 88 µmol/l. He was then successfully treated with isoniazid 300 mg/day, ethambutol 800 mg/day, and pyrazinamide 1500 mg/day.
- A 14-year-old boy with a brain tuberculoma was treated successfully with a rifampicin-containing daily regimen. He developed sputum-positive pulmonary tuberculosis 12 years later and was given thrice-weekly isoniazid 600 mg, rifampicin 450

mg, ethambutol 1200 mg and pyrazinamide 1500 mg. After 10 days he developed low back pain, anorexia, and vomiting. His blood urea concentration was 27 mmol/l and serum creatinine 356 µmol/l. Renal biopsy suggested immune complex deposition in the interstitium and blood vessels. Rifampicin was withdrawn, and isoniazid, ethambutol, and pyrazinamide were continued. Renal insufficiency was managed with peritoneal dialysis and salt, protein, and fluid restriction. His renal function returned to normal after 5 days (blood urea 9 mmol/l and serum creatinine 88 µmol/l).

- A 25-year-old man had taken irregular treatment with a rifampicin-containing regimen for 5 months about 1 year before being treated with thrice-weekly isoniazid 600 mg, rifampicin 450 mg, ethambutol 1200 mg, and pyrazinamide 1500 mg. After 10 days he complained of oliguria, facial puffiness, pedal edema, and vomiting. His blood urea concentration was 168 mg/dl and serum creatinine 1132 µmol/l. He refused renal biopsy. Rifampicin was withdrawn. With peritoneal dialysis and supportive measures, his renal function returned to normal in 1 month (blood urea 14 mmol/l and serum creatinine 88 µmol/l).

All three patients reported here had previously taken daily rifampicin-containing regimens. They developed acute renal insufficiency after re-treatment with an intermittent rifampicin regimen after 5 months to 11 years, which manifested within 10–20 days of starting re-treatment. Although rifampicin-dependent antibody titers in these patients were not measured, the sequence of events was highly suggestive of rifampicin-induced acute renal insufficiency. On withdrawal of rifampicin and dialysis and supportive care renal function returned to normal.

The mechanism postulated for immune-induced rifampicin nephrotoxicity is that antibodies accumulate during the antigen-free interval when there is a gap in treatment or during an intermittent dosage regimen. When rifampicin is re-administered there is an intense immune reaction. Immune complexes are deposited in the blood vessels or interstitium and cause glomerular endotheliosis, leading to tubular injury, thereby impairing renal function.

Drug–drug interactions   Induction of cytochromes P450, uridine diphosphate-glucuronosyltransferases, monoamine oxidases, and glutathione S-transferases by rifampicin can lead to drug interactions when it is co-administered with drugs that are metabolized by these pathways.

Atenolol   The effect of rifampicin on the pharmacokinetics of atenolol has been studied in healthy volunteers (22[c]). Rifampicin reduced the mean AUC of atenolol to 81% and increased renal clearance to 109%. Rifampicin pretreatment reduced the peak plasma concentration (C_{max}), AUC_{0-33h}, and the amount of atenolol excreted to 85, 81, and 86% of the respective placebo values. The average heart rate and diastolic blood pressure were slightly higher after rifampicin than after placebo. Thus, although the inducing effect of rifampicin may not have been at its maximum by day 6, it has only a minor effect on the pharmacokinetics of atenolol, evidenced by a slight reduction in its systemic availability.

Mycophenolate mofetil   In a heart–lung transplant recipient long-term rifampicin caused a more than two-fold reduction in dose-corrected mycophenolic acid exposure; subsequent withdrawal of rifampicin resulted in reversal of these changes after 2 weeks of washout (23[c]). The effect of rifampicin on the metabolism of mycophenolate mofetil may be explained by simultaneous induction of renal, hepatic, and gastrointestinal uridine diphosphate-glucuronosyl transferases and organic anion transporters, with subsequent inhibition of enterohepatic re-circulation.

Ritonavir/saquinavir   The efficacy and safety of concomitant use of rifampicin and regimens containing ritonavir/saquinavir (400/400 mg bd) have been studied in HIV-positive patients with tuberculosis (24[c]). Of 20 patients 15 withdrew mainly because of adverse reactions. Therapeutic concentrations of the drugs were achieved in the other five patients, with reduction of viral load

Tenofovir disoproxil fumarate   Rifampicin has major pharmacokinetic interactions with HIV protease inhibitors and non-nucleoside reverse transcriptase inhibitors (NNRTI), which complicates the management of those who are co-infected with HIV and tuberculosis. However, a pharmacokinetic study in 24 healthy subjects has shown no interaction of tenofovir 300 mg, an NNRTI, and rifampicin 600 mg (25[c]). The 95% confidence intervals for AUC and C_{min} were 0.84–0.92 and 0.80–0.91 respectively, while for C_{max} the confidence interval was 0.78–0.90, suggesting pharmacokinetic equivalence when tenofovir was given with or without rifampicin. One patient had a grade 3 rise in hepatic enzymes, which led to withdrawal of therapy.

References

1. Dworkin MS, Adams MR, Cohn DL, Davidson AJ, Buskin S, Horwitch C, Morse A, Sackoff J, Thompson M, Wotring L, McCombs SB, Jones JL. Factors that complicate the treatment of tuberculosis in HIV-infected patients. J Acquir Immune Defic Syndr 2005;39:464–70.
2. Goulart IM, Reis AC, De Rezende TM, Borges AS, Ferreira MS, Nishioka SA. Aplastic anaemia associated with multidrug therapy (dapsone, rifampicin and clofazimine) in a patient with lepromatous leprosy. Lepr Rev 2005;76:167–9.
3. Borrás-Blasco J, Conesa-García V, Navarro-Ruiz A, Devesa P, Matarredona J. Pure red cell aplasia associated with dapsone therapy. Ann Pharmacother 2005;39(6):1137–8.
4. Williams S, MacDonald P, Hoyer JD, Barr RD, Athale UH. Methemoglobinemia in children with acute lymphoblastic leukemia (ALL) receiving dapsone for Pneumocystis carinii pneumonia (PCP) prophylaxis: a correlation with cytochrome b5 reductase (Cb5R) enzyme levels. Pediatr Blood Cancer 2005;44:55–62.
5. Schild HS, Fox BC. Rapid-onset reversible ocular toxicity from ethambutol therapy. Am J Med 1991;90:404–6.
6. Kakisu Y, Adachi-Usami E, Mizota A. Pattern electroretinogram and visual evoked cortical potential in ethambutol optic neuropathy. Doc Ophthalmol 1987;67:327–34.
7. Lai TYY, Chan W-M, Lam DSC, Lim E. Multifocal electroretinogram demonstrated macular toxicity associated with ethambutol related optic neuropathy. Br J Ophthalmol 2005;89(6):774–5.
8. Jhamaria JP, Rajput VS, Luhadia SK, Bansal PP, Ved ML, Gandhi VC, Rajput VS. Ocular toxicity of ethambutol and its correlation with serum zinc levels. Lung India 1989;7(4):183–5.
9. Fang J-T, Chen Y-C, Chang M-Y. Ethambutol-induced optic neuritis in patients with end stage renal disease on hemodialysis: two case reports and literature review. Renal Fail 2004;2(26):89–93.
10. Donald PR, Maher D, Maritz JS, Qazi S. Ethambutol dosage for the treatment of children: literature review and recommendations. Int J Tuberc Lung Dis 2006;10:1318–30.
11. Griffith DE, Brown-Elliott BA, Shepherd S, McLarty J, Griffith L, Wallace Jr RJ. Ethambutol ocular toxicity in treatment regimens for Mycobacterium avium complex lung disease. Am J Respir Crit Care Med 2005;172:250–3.
12. Takada R, Takagi M, Oshima A, Miki A, Usui T, Hasegawa S, Abe H. Delayed visual recovery from severe ethambutol optic neuropathy in two patients with atypical mycobacterium infection. Neuro-Ophthalmology 2005;29:187–93.
13. Place VA, Thomas JP. Clinical pharmacology of ethambutol. Am Rev Respir Dis 1963;87:901–4.
14. Zhu M, Burman WJ, Starke JR, Stambaugh JJ, Steiner P, Bulpitt AE, Ashkin D, Auclair B, Berning SE, Jelliffe RW, Jaresko GS, Peloquin CA. Pharmacokinetics of ethambutol in children and adults with tuberculosis. Int J Tuberc Lung Dis 2004;8:1360–7.
15. World Health Organization. Ethambutol efficacy and toxicity. Literature review and recommendation for daily and intermittent dosage in children. Geneva, Switzerland: WHO; 2006.
16. Fountain FF, Tolley E, Chrisman CR, Self TH. Isoniazid hepatotoxicity associated with treatment of latent tuberculosis infection: a 7-year evaluation from a public health tuberculosis clinic. Chest 2005;128:116–23.
17. Gao XF, Wang L, Liu GJ, Wen J, Sun X, Xie Y, Li YP. Rifampicin plus pyrazinamide versus isoniazid for treating latent tuberculosis infection: a meta-analysis. Int J Tuberc Lung Dis 2006;10:1080–90.
18. Takasu N, Takara M, Komiya I. Rifampicin induced hypothyroidism in patients with Hashimoto's thyroiditis. N Engl J Med 2005;352(5):518–9.
19. Sudip D, Kumar RA, Arunasis M. Rifampicin induced thrombocytopenia. Ind J Dermatol 2006;51:222.
20. Tortajada C, Martínez-Lacasa J, Sánchez F, Jiménez-Fuentes A, De Souza ML, García JF, Martínez JA, Caylà JA. Is the combination of pyrazinamide plus rifampicin safe for treating latent tuberculosis infection in persons not infected by the human immunodeficiency virus? Int J Tuberc Lung Dis 2005;9:276–81.
21. Banu Rekha VV, Santha T, Jawahar MS. Rifampicin induced renal toxicity in the retreatment of patients with pulmonary TB—case report. JAPI 2005;53:811–3.
22. Lilja JJ, Juntti-Patinen L, Neuvonen PJ. Effect of rifampicin on the pharmacokinetics of atenolol. Basic Clin Pharmacol Toxicol 2006;98:555–8.
23. Kuypers DRJ, Verleden G, Naesens M, Vanrenterghem Y. Drug interaction between mycophenolate mofetil and rifampin:

possible induction of uridine diphosphate-glucuronosyltransferase. Clin Pharmacol Ther 2005;78:81–8.

24. Rolla VC, da Silva Vieira MA, Pereira Pinto D, Lourenco MC, de Jesus C da S, Goncalves Morgado M, Ferreira Filho M, Werneck-Barroso E. Safety, efficacy and pharmacokinetics of ritonavir 400 mg/saquinavir 400 mg twice daily plus ri-fampicin combined therapy in HIV patients with tuberculosis. Clin Drug Invest 2006;26:469–79.

25. Droste JAH, Verweij-Van Wissen CPWGM, Kearney BP, Buffels R, VanHorssen PJ, Hekster YA, Burger DM. Pharmacokinetic study of tenofovir disoproxil fumarate combined with ri-fampin in healthy volunteers. Antimicrob Agents Chemother 2005;49:680–4.

P.J.J van Genderen

31 Antihelminthic drugs

BENZIMIDAZOLES *(SED-15, 424; SEDA-27, 326; SEDA-29, 320)*

Albendazole, mebendazole, and thiabendazole

Comparative studies

Echinococcosis Human hydatid disease is caused by the metacestode of *Echinococcus granulosus*. There are few data on the treatment of pulmonary hydatid disease in children. Mebendazole and albendazole have been evaluated in 82 children with a total of 102 pulmonary hydatid cysts (1^c). Mebendazole was given as 50 mg/kg/day in three divided doses and albendazole was given as 10 mg/kg/day in two divided doses continuously or in cycles consisting of 4 weeks of treatment alternating with 2-week drug-free intervals. The duration of treatment was 1–36 months. While taking benzimidazoles eight patients had *raised liver enzymes*, three had *rash*, and one had *neutropenia*; all were reversible on withdrawal.

Sensory systems *Eye pain* has been attributed to albendazole in a patient with ocular cysticercosis (2^A).

- A 19-year-old Nepalese housewife with horizontal diplopia due to orbital cysticercosis was given albendazole 15 mg/kg/day for 8 days. After 3 days she developed nausea, vomiting, and distressing nocturnal left eye pain. She was reluctant to continue taking albendazole and her symptoms settled after a short course of oral analgesia. Later ocular examinations did not show any residual orbital cyst.

Hematologic *Pancytopenia* has again been attributed to albendazole (3^A).

- A 68-year-old man with a large cystic lung mass due to echinococcosis was given albendazole and 2 weeks later developed septic shock with severe pancytopenia. He died after 10 days with no marrow recovery. Autopsy was consistent with albendazole-induced pancytopenia.

The clearance of albendazole sulfoxide is impaired in liver disease, which was relevant in this case. The authors suggested that frequent serial monitoring of blood counts is warranted in patients with liver disease.

Liver In 76 children *Trichinella britovi* infection was benign and milder than in adults who had consumed the same amount of infected meat (4^c). The children were treated with mebendazole 25 mg/kg divided into three doses for 14 days. Those with severe symptoms were also treated with oral prednisolone 20 mg/day for 7 days. No child reported adverse effects attributable to mebendazole. *Liver enzymes rose* in a 14-year-old child after 10 days of treatment with mebendazole and returned to normal 7 days after withdrawal.

Teratogenicity The effects of mebendazole during pregnancy have been investigated in a case–control study in the mothers of babies born with congenital abnormalities and in matched control mothers of babies born without congenital abnormalities in the population-based data set of the Hungarian Case–Control Surveillance of Congenital Abnormalities between 1980 and 1996 (5^C). Of 38 151 women whose neonates had no defects, 14 had taken mebendazole during pregnancy; of 22 843 women whose neonates had congenital abnormalities, 14 had taken mebendazole for intestinal parasites during pregnancy (OR = 1.67; 95% CI = 0.7, 4.2). In six groups of different congenital abnormalities there was no higher

Side Effects of Drugs, Annual 30
J.K. Aronson (Editor)
ISSN: 0378-6080
DOI: 10.1016/S0378-6080(08)00031-7

prevalence of mebendazole use by the mothers. Mean gestational age was longer and mean birth weight higher in neonates born to mothers who had taken mebendazole. Thus, treatment with mebendazole during pregnancy was not significantly teratogenic or fetotoxic, although the numbers of treated cases and controls in this study were limited, which may have reduced the statistical power of this case–control study.

Diethylcarbamazine   *(SED-15, 1115; SEDA-27, 328; SEDA-28, 348; SEDA-29, 322)*

Drug dosage regimens   The dose of diethylcarbamazine is adjusted according to age, and the following regimen is used in the treatment of carriers of *Wuchereria bancrofti* microfilaria: 50 mg (1–2 years), 100 mg (3–4 years), 150 mg (5–8 years), 200 mg (9–11 years), 250 mg (12–14 years), and 300 mg for over 14 years. In the hope of improving adherence to therapy a simpler schedule has been studied: 100 mg (2–4 years), 200 mg (5–14 years), and 300 mg for over 14 years (6[c]). However, in asymptomatic carriers of microfilaria the incidence of adverse reactions in those aged 4–8 years was 50% with a dose of 150 mg and 67% with 200 mg. There were no life-threatening adverse reactions. *Fever, headache*, and *myalgia*, the most common adverse reactions, were mild and similar with both schedules.

Ivermectin   *(SED-15, 1946; SEDA-27, 329; SEDA-28, 349; SEDA-29, 323)*

Refusal to take ivermectin by Ugandan villagers with onchocerciasis has been associated with age and intercurrent medical conditions— younger patients and those with intercurrent conditions were more likely to take it (7[c]). The adverse effects of treatment were not implicated.

Observational studies   In a prospective open study in 20 Thai patients with cutaneous gnathostomiasis oral ivermectin 50, 100, 150, or 200 micrograms/kg was associated with the following adverse events: *malaise* (n = 7),

myalgia (6), *drowsiness* (6), *pruritus* (4), *nausea/vomiting* (4), *dizziness* (3), *diarrhea* (3), *a feeling of shortness of breath* (2), *palpitation* (2), *constipation* (1), *anorexia* (1), and *headache* (1) (8[c]). These adverse events were self-limiting and there were no serious adverse events. There were laboratory abnormalities in three patients. *Transient microscopic hematuria, pyuria*, and mildly *raised liver enzymes* were found in one patient each.

Sensory systems   Following the observation in a 3-year double-blind, randomized, controlled trial in Cameroon that transient visual problems can occur after treatment with ivermectin in onchocerciasis, ophthalmological examinations were carried out (9[c]). The visual complaints were significantly more frequent in those who had received high doses of ivermectin (for example 800 versus 150 microgram/kg annually).

Immunologic   Ivermectin eradicates the microfilariae of *Onchocerca volvulus*. The major drawback is that treatment is associated with *adverse host inflammatory responses*. The association of proinflammatory chemokines with the intensity of infection and clinical adverse reactions has been studied (10[c]) by measurement of chemokine serum concentrations in patients with *Onchocerca volvulus* following a single dose of ivermectin or placebo (ivermectin 100 micrograms/kg, n = 13; ivermectin 150 micrograms/kg, n = 8; ivermectin 200 micrograms/kg, n = 24; placebo, n = 37). Adverse reactions scores in patients increased significantly on the third day after ivermectin treatment, and were unchanged in those who took placebo. The adverse reactions scores were significantly related to the microfilarial density but not the dose of ivermectin or serum concentrations of proinflammatory chemokines.

Susceptibility factors

HIV infection   The adverse effects of a single dose of ivermectin 150 micrograms/kg for onchocerciasis have been compared in 1256 Ugandan patients with and without infection with human immunodeficiency virus (HIV-1) (11[c]). In those aged over 15 years, the frequency of adverse reactions was higher among those who were HIV-1 seropositive (53 versus 46%), but the difference was not statistically significant. However, the severity of the adverse reactions was significantly less in the HIV-1 positive patients.

Levamisole   *(SED-15, 2028; SEDA-27, 330; SEDA-28, 350; SEDA-29, 324)*

Observational studies

Colorectal cancer   Levamisole is used as an immunomodulating drug in colorectal cancer, usually in combination with 5-fluorouracil. The IGCS-COL multicenter randomized phase III study partly addressed the role of levamisole in the modulation of 5-fluorouracil as adjuvant systemic chemotherapy in patients with colorectal cancer (12[C]). There was no evidence of improvement of disease-free survival or overall survival advantage by adding levamisole; nor did the addition of levamisole produce any statistically significant effect on the adverse effects profile of 5-fluorouracil.

In another study in 598 patients with stage III colon cancer the addition of levamisole to adjuvant fluorouracil significantly worsened the prognosis (13[C]).

Nephrotic syndrome   It has been stressed that levamisole is generally well tolerated by children with steroid-dependent nephrotic syndrome (14[r], 15[R]). Adverse effects are uncommon but include *neutropenia, vasculitis, liver toxicity,* and *convulsions*; they are reversible after withdrawal of levamisole. In 40 children with idiopathic steroid-dependent minimal-change nephrotic syndrome levamisole 2.5 mg/kg on alternate days was compared with intravenous cyclophosphamide 500 mg/m^2/month for 6 months (16[c]). Prednisolone was gradually tapered. After withdrawal of treatment, five children in the levamisole and cyclophosphamide groups stayed in remission at 6 months, four versus two respectively at 1 year, three versus one at 2 years, and one in each group at 3 and 4 years of follow-up. Adverse effects were mild, and none of the patients withdrew because of adverse effects. In the 20 patients who took levamisole, *infections* occurred in 13 but only when glucocorticoids were used in conjunction. Nine patients had respiratory infections (acute bronchitis), two

had scalp infections, and one had a urinary tract infection. One developed *sialadenitis*. One had *personality changes* characterized by aggression and nervousness after the start of glucocorticoid therapy. None developed neutropenia but there was a *lower leukocyte count* during levamisole treatment.

Comparative studies

Brucellosis   Adding levamisole to conventional antibiotic therapy may improve anergy against *Brucella,* bacteria that can survive in phagocytic cells. This hypothesis has been investigated in patients with chronic brucellosis in Turkey (17[c]). A 6-week course of levamisole in addition to conventional antibiotic therapy in chronic brucellosis was not superior to conventional antibiotic treatment alone with respect to lymphocyte subgroup ratios and phagocytic function. Adverse effects were not reported.

Skin   *Fever and rash* have been attributed to levamisole (18[A]).

- A 33-year-old man with vitiligo was given oral betamethasone 5 mg/day and levamisole 150 mg/day on 2 consecutive days every week. After 3 months, topical fluocinolone acetonide cream (0.01%) was added. After 8 months, on one occasion, 12 hours after taking the oral drugs, he developed a fever (38.9 °C) with chills and rigor, followed by itching and redness of the skin over the palms, soles, and both legs. The rash resolved in 8 days. He restarted betamethasone and levamisole after 1 month and developed similar symptoms within 4–5 hours. Rechallenge with oral levamisole 150 mg caused a fever (38.9 °C) after 5 hours, followed by itching, redness and swelling of the lips, palms and soles.

Teratogenicity   In an analysis of a large population-based data set in the Hungarian Case–Control Surveillance of Congenital Abnormalities, 1980–96, there was no evidence of a higher rate of congenital abnormalities in children born to mothers who had taken oral levamisole during pregnancy (19[C]).

Praziquantel   *(SED-15, 2911; SEDA-27, 331; SEDA-28, 351; SEDA-29, 324)*

Pregnancy   In a prospective study eastern Sudan in 25 pregnant women with *Schistosoma* *mansoni* infection were given a single oral dose of praziquantel at 40 mg/kg, six in the first trimester, 12 in the second trimester, and seven in the third trimester (20[R]). There were no maternal deaths, stillbirths, or congenital abnormalities.

Drug–drug interactions   Serum concentrations of praziquantel fall when *glucocorticoids* are used simultaneously, which is usually the case in moderate to heavy infections; no mechanism has bee proposed for this effect (21[R]).

Suramin   *(SED-15, 3249; SEDA-27, 331; SEDA-28, 352; SEDA-29, 325)*

Because of serious toxicity suramin is rarely used nowadays as a macrofilaricidal drug for the treatment of onchocerciasis or for the treatment of African trypanosomiasis. However, its potential anti-tumor effects have renewed interest in suramin, in particular in the treatment of urological malignancies.

Observational studies

Bladder cancer   In a phase I open, non-randomized dose-escalation study intravesical suramin 10, 50, 100, and 150 mg/ml was studied in 12 patients with recurrent transitional cell bladder carcinoma (22[c]). Three patients had minor *rises in fasting blood glucose* and one had minor *lymphopenia* at the lowest dose. There were no serious adverse events and no patient complained of urinary symptoms related to treatment. There were no drug-related adverse events worse than grade 1. Systemic absorption of suramin was only found at the highest dose of 150 mg/ml.

Hormone-refractory prostate cancer   Combination chemotherapy with estramustine, docetaxel, and suramin has been studied in 42 patients with symptomatic progressive hormone-refractory prostate cancer (23[c]). Estramustine was given at an oral dosage of 10 mg/kg/day on days 1–21 every 28 days, docetaxel 70 mg/m^2 intravenously on day 2 every 28 days, and a total dose of 2150 mg of suramin was given in each cycle. Treatment was continued until disease progression or excessive toxicity. The median number of consecutive cycles was 8. The median time to progression was 57 weeks and median overall survival was 132 weeks. Most adverse events were moderate and were managed medically. Major adverse effects consisted of grade 3–4 *anemia* in 50%, *leukopenia* in 33%, and *thrombocytopenia* in 21%. The duration of leukopenia was generally less than 2 weeks and there were no deaths because of the sequelae of leukopenia. Severe neuropathy and gastrointestinal toxicity were uncommon, although there was moderate neuropathy in two patients. Six patients had a *rash*, a well-known adverse effect of suramin. Grade 3 or 4 non-hematological adverse effects included *edema* in three patients, *malaise* and/or *fatigue* in two, and *dyspnea* in three. Grade 1 or 2 adverse effects included *hyperglycemia, malaise/fatigue, peripheral edema, nausea*, and *anorexia*. Suramin dosage reduction was required in six patients because of adverse events (*rash, weakness*, and *thrombocytopenia*). There were no treatment-related deaths.

References

1. Dogru D, Kiper N, Ozcelik U, Yalcin E. Gocmen. Medical treatment of pulmonary hydatid disease: for which child? Parasitol Int 2005;54:135–8.

2. Wong YC, Goh KY, Choo CT, Seah LL, Rootman J. An unusual cause of acquired horizontal diplopia in a young adult. Br J Opthalmol 2005;89:390–1.

3. Opatrny L, Prichard R, Snell L, Maclean JD. Death related to albendazole-induced pancytopenia: case report and review. Am J Trop Med Hyg 2005;72(3):291–4.

4. Ozdemir D, Ozkan H, Akkoc N, Onen F, Gurler O, Sari I, Akar S, Birlik M, Kargi A, Ozer E, Pozio E. Acute trichinellosis in chil-

dren compared with adults. Pediatr Infect Dis J 2005;24:897–900.

5. Acs N, Banhidy F, Puho E, Czeizel AE. Population-based case-control study of mebendazole in pregnant women for birth outcomes. Congenital Anomalies 2005;45:85–8.

6. Pani SP, Das LK, Vanamail P. Tolerability and efficacy of a three-age class dosage schedule of diethylcarbamazine citrate (DEC) in the treatment of microfilaria carriers of *Wuchereria bancrofti* and its implications in mass drug administration (MDA) strategy for elimination of lymphatic filariasis (LF). J Commun Dis 2005;37(1):12–7.

7. Semiyaga NB, Lalobo O, Ndyomugyenyi R. Refusal to take ivermectin: the associated 'risk' factors in Hoima district, Uganda. Ann Trop Med Parasitol 2005;99(2):165–72.

8. Bussaratid V, Krudsood S, Silachamroon U, Looareesuwan S. Tolerability of ivermectin in gnathostomiasis. Southeast Asian J Trop Med Public Health 2005;36(3):644–9.

9. Fobi G, Gardon J, Kamgno J, Aimard-Favennec L, Lafleur C, Gardon-Wendel N, Duke BO, Boussinesq M. A randomized, double-blind, controlled trial of the effects of ivermectin at normal and high doses, given annually or three-monthly, against Onchocerca volvulus: ophthalmological results. Trans R Soc Trop Med Hyg 2005;99(4):279–89.

10. Fendt J, Hamm DM, Banla M, Schulz-Key H, Wolf H, Helling-Giese G, Heuschkel C, Soboslay PT. Chemokines in onchocerciasis patients after a single dose of ivermectin. Clin Exp Immunol 2005;142:318–26.

11. Kipp W, Bamhuhiiga J, Rubaale T, Kabagambe G. Adverse reactions to the ivermectin treatment of onchocerciasis patients: does infection with the human immunodeficiency virus play a role? Ann Trop Med Parasitol 2005;99(4):395–402.

12. De Placido S, Lopez M, Carlomagno C, Paoletti G, Palazzo S, Manzione L, Iannace C, Ianniello GP, De Vita F, Ficorella C, Farris A, Pistillucci G, Gemini M, Cortesi E, Adamo V, Gebbia N, Palmeri S, Gallo C, Perrone F, Persico G, Bianco AR. Modulation of 5-fluorouracil as adjuvant systemic chemotherapy in colorectal cancer: the IGCS-COL multicentre, randomised, phase III study. Br J Cancer 2005;93:896–904.

13. Schippinger W, Jagoditsch M, Sorre C, Gnant M, Steger G, Hausmaninger H, Mlineritsch B,

Schaberl-Moser R, Mischinger HJ, Hofbauer F, Holzberger P, Mittlbock M, Jakesz R, Austrian Breast and Colorectal Cancer Study Group. A prospective randomised trial to study the role of levamisole and interferon alfa in an adjuvant therapy with 5-FU for stage III colon cancer. Br J Cancer 2005;92(9):1655–62.

14. Davin JC, Merkus MP. Levamisole in steroid-sensitive nephrotic syndrome of childhood: the lost paradise? Pediatr Nephrol 2005;20:10–4.

15. Hodson EM, Craig JC, Willis NS. Evidence-based management of steroid-sensitive nephrotic syndrome. Pediatr Nephrol 2005;20:1523–30.

16. Donia AF, Ammar HM, El-Agroudy AE, Moustafa FE, Sobh MA. Long-term results of two unconventional agents in steroid-dependent nephrotic children. Pediatr Nephrol 2005;20:1420–5.

17. Dizer U, Hayat L, Beker CM, Gorenek L, Özgüven V, Pahsa A. The effect of the doxycycline–rifampicin and levamisole combination on lymphocyte subgroups and functions of phagocytic cells in patients with chronic brucellosis. Chemotherapy 2005;51:27–31.

18. Gupta R, Gupta S. Drug rash due to levamisole. Indian J Dermatol Venereol Leprol 2005;71(6):428–9.

19. Kazy Z, Pucho E, Czeizel E. Levamisol leheseges teratogenitasanak vizsgalata terhessegben. Orv Hetil 2005;146(49):2499–500.

20. Adam I, Elwasila E, Homeida M. Praziquantel for the treatment of schistosomiasis mansoni during pregnancy. Ann Trop Med Parasitol 2005;99(1):37–40.

21. Garcia HH, Del Bruto O. Neurocysticercosis: updated concepts about an old disease. Lancet Neurol 2005;4:653–61 [for the Cysticercosis Working Group in Peru].

22. Ord JJ, Streeter E, Jones A, Le Monnier K, Cranston D, Crew J, Joel SP, Rogers MA, Banks RE, Roberts ISD, Harris AL. Phase I trial of intravesical suramin in recurrent superficial transitional cell bladder carcinoma. Br J Cancer 2005;92:2140–7.

23. Safarinejad MR. Combination chemotherapy with docetaxel, estramustine and suramin for hormone refractory prostate cancer. Urol Oncol 2005;23:93–101.

S. Dittmann

32   Vaccines

Editor's note: Abbreviations

- *BCG: Bacillus Calmette Guérin*
- *DTaP: Diphtheria + tetanus toxoids + acellular pertussis*
- *HA: Hepatitis A*
- *HB: Hepatitis B*
- *HBV: Hepatitis B virus*
- *Hib: Hemophilus influenzae type b*
- *HPV: Human papilloma virus*
- *IPV: Inactivated polio vaccine*
- *MMR: measles + mumps + rubella*
- *MMRV: measles + mumps + rubella + varicella*
- *OPV: Oral polio vaccine*
- *Td: Diphtheria + tetanus toxoids (adult formulation)*
- *Tdap Diphtheria+tetanus toxoids+acellular pertussis (adult formulation)*

Combination vaccines/multiple immunizations   *(SEDA-29, 327)*

Combination vaccines versus concomitant administration of single vaccines   The safety and reactogenicity of a booster dose of hexavalent DTaP–HBV–IPV/Hib vaccine (GSK Biologicals; n = 4725) has been compared with the separate administration of DTaP–IPV/Hib and HBV vaccines (GSK Biologicals; n = 4474) in two open, randomized, multicenter studies (1[C]). In the first study (n = 1149), the incidences of symptoms were similar in the two groups; no serious adverse events were either reported within 4 days of immunization

or considered to be causally related to immunization. In the second study (n = 8050), in which fever was the only solicited symptom, the rectal temperature was 39.5 °C or over in 2.5 and 2.8% of the subjects respectively. Fever of 40.0 °C or more was rare (0.6%), and only two cases of febrile convulsions were recorded during the 4 days after immunization, both in the control group. Extensive swelling (defined as local injection-site swelling with a diameter over 50 mm, noticeable diffuse injection-site swelling, or a noticeably increased circumference of the injected limb) was reported after 2.3% of the booster vaccine doses, regardless of the vaccine used. Extensive swelling involving an adjacent joint was reported in 0.1% of subjects.

The authors concluded that the hexavalent combination DTaP–HBV–IPV/Hib vaccine and the DTaP–IPV/Hib and HBV vaccines administered separately have similar good reactogenicity and safety profiles when given as booster doses in the second year of life.

Pentavalent and heptavalent vaccines and apnea or bradycardia   The incidence and clinical significance of apnea or bradycardia after immunization with pentavalent (DTaP–Hib–IPV) and heptavalent (DTaP–Hib–IPV–HB) combination vaccines have been evaluated in respiratory stable preterm infants (2[C]). The medical records of 53 infants with a mean gestational age of 28 weeks, hospitalized in the neonatal intensive care unit of the University Children's Hospital in Basel from January 2000 to June 2003, were analysed. Clinical data were recorded for 72 hours before and after the first immunization. Of the 53 infants, seven had a transient recurrence or an increase in episodes of apnea or bradycardia after immunization. Five of these seven required interventions, ranging from tactile stimulation to bag-and-mask ventilation, but there were no serious consequences. The rate of fever over 38 °C after immunization was higher in affected

Side Effects of Drugs, Annual 30
J.K. Aronson (Editor)
ISSN: 0378-6080
DOI: 10.1016/S0378-6080(08)00032-9

infants than in those without recurrence of or increase in apnea or bradycardia. The authors recommended monitoring of all preterm infants after immunization in neonatal intensive care units.

Sudden infant death shortly after the administration of hexavalent vaccines   *This was discussed at length in SEDA-29 (p. 327). The conclusion was that the evidence does not support a causal association between sudden infant death syndrome (SIDS) and hexavalent vaccines. A case-control study on SIDS (GeSID) was carried out in Germany between 1998 and 2001 in 18 forensic pathology institutes covering half of Germany (3^C). Infants who were immunized after the introduction of the hexavalent vaccines in October 2000 were analysed separately. There were 129 deaths from SIDS during the period October 2000 to October 2001. Of these, 22 (17%) had received a hexavalent vaccine compared with 100 of 378 controls (27%). If immunization increased the risk of SIDS one would expect a higher immunization rate among the SIDS cases than among the controls. In this study the opposite was the case. More controls were immunized and the control infants started their immunization schedule earlier. Even when the data were restricted to the 14 days before death/interview, there was no increased risk of SIDS in temporal relation to immunization. This study has provided further evidence that immunization is not a risk factor for SIDS.*

Nervous system   The data from the Vaccine Adverse Event Reporting System included 54 reports of *Guillain–Barré syndrome* after immunization that occurred in the USA in 2004 (4^c). In 38 of the patients, Guillain–Barré syndrome occurred within 6 weeks, and the authors considered this suggestive of a causal association. The highest incidence within 6 weeks was observed in patients who received influenza vaccine ($n = 23$), followed by six cases after hepatitis vaccine (not distinguished into hepatitis A and hepatitis B). Two cases of Guillain–Barré syndrome were temporally related to Td vaccine (adult formulation). After other vaccines, including combination vaccines and concomitant administration of single vaccines, seven cases were reported. This study had many limitations, because it was based on

data from a passive surveillance system and no attempt was made to determine the incidence of Guillain–Barré syndrome in vaccinees compared with the healthy population.

Immunologic   There has been a systematic review of the risk of *allergic disease* after infant immunization (5^M). The authors searched MEDLINE from 1966 to March 2003 and bibliography lists from retrieved articles, and consulted experts in the field to identify all articles relating immunization (diphtheria, tetanus, and pertussis, measles, mumps, and rubella, and BCG vaccine) to allergy. The design and quality of the studies varied considerably. Many did not address possible confounders, such as the lifestyle factors, leaving them susceptible to bias. The studies that offered the strongest evidence, including the only randomized controlled trial published to date, suggested that infant immunization does not increase the risk of allergic disease. Furthermore, BCG does not seem to reduce the risk of allergies.

Drug formulations

Aluminium adsorbent   During trials in Gothenburg, Sweden, of aluminium-adsorbed diphtheria–tetanus/acellular pertussis vaccines from a single producer, persistent itching nodules at the immunization site were observed in an unexpectedly high frequency: in 645 children out of about 76 000 immunized (0.8%) after both subcutaneous and intramuscular injection.. The itching was intense and long-lasting. After a median of 4 years 75% still had symptoms. There was contact hypersensitivity to aluminium in 77% of the children with itching nodules and in 8% of their symptomless siblings who had received the same vaccines (6^C). The authors suspected that the high incidence of itching nodules was related to the injection technique used. Post-marketing surveillance data from other regions in Sweden, Denmark, and Norway have suggested that the incidence of itching nodules is low after correct intramuscular administration of aluminium-adsorbed vaccines manufactured by Statens Seruminstitut in Copenhagen, Denmark (7^r).

The effect of reducing the aluminium content of a combined reduced-antigen-content Tdap vaccine on immunogenicity and safety has been evaluated in 647 healthy adolescents aged 10–18 years (8^C). Of those enrolled, 224 (35%) received a Tdap formulation with aluminium 0.5 mg, 209 (32%) a formulation with aluminium 0.3 mg, and 214 (33%) a formulation with aluminium 0.133 mg. One month after administration of the booster dose, all the subjects were seroprotected against diphtheria and tetanus toxoids. All were seropositive for anti-filamentous hemagglutinin and anti-pertactin antibodies, but 4% of those who were initially seronegative in both reduced aluminium groups did not seroconvert for anti-pertussis toxin. Booster responses did not differ significantly between the groups for any antibody, but geometric mean concentrations of anti-pertussis toxin after booster immunization differed significantly between groups and fell when vaccine aluminium content was reduced. There were no clear differences between the study groups in local or general adverse effects. The most frequently reported symptoms after immunization were injection site pain (90–91%), fatigue (42–47%) and headache (41–45%). This study showed that the aluminium content has a specific influence on the immunogenicity of this Tdap vaccine.

Gelatine   Since approval of live varicella vaccine (Oka strain) in 1986 in Japan, the effectiveness and safety of the vaccine has been investigated. From 1994, infants have been given acellular pertussis vaccine combined with diphtheria and tetanus toxoid (DTaP) until 12 months of age, before the administration of live vaccines, such as measles, rubella, mumps, and varicella vaccines. Increasing numbers of anaphylactic/allergic reactions to those vaccines have since been reported. Almost all of these subjects had previously been given three or four doses of DTaP containing gelatine. Gelatine-associated allergic reactions were also reported with varicella vaccine, and gelatine-free live varicella vaccine was introduced in 1999. Removal of gelatine from the live vaccine resulted in a dramatic reduction in anaphylactic/allergic reactions to this vaccine. The reported rates of anaphylactic/allergic reactions to gelatine-containing and gelatine-free varicella vaccines and titers of IgE antibodies to gelatine in those who developed anaphylactic/allergic reactions have been compared (9^C). After the use of gelatin-containing varicella vaccine (1994–9,

1 410 000 distributed doses), 28 serious anaphylactic reactions and 139 non-serious allergic reactions were reported; in contrast, there were no serious and only five non-serious reactions after the use of gelatin-free vaccine (1999–2000, 1 300 000 distributed doses). All nine sera available from children with serious reactions tested positive for gelatin-specific IgE, whereas 55 of the 70 available from those with non-serious reactions were positive, with one false positive. There was no correlation between gelatin-specific IgE antibody titers and the severity of allergic reaction. Anti-varicella antibody titers after immunization were comparable.

Surveillance of adverse events following immunization

Standardized case definitions   The Brighton collaboration was launched in 2000 as a voluntary international organization to facilitate the development of case definitions for adverse events following immunization and guidelines for collection, analysis, and presentation of immunization safety data. We have previously reported (SEDA-28, 356) the first six standardized case definitions and guidelines: fever, generalized convulsive seizures, hypotonic–hyporesponsive episodes, intussusception, nodules at injection sites, and persistent crying. New working groups have now finalized and published the case definitions and guidelines for anaphylaxis (10^H), aseptic meningitis (11^H), encephalitis, myelitis, and acute disseminated encephalomyelitis (ADEM) (12^H), fatigue (13^H), local reactions (abscesses (14^H), cellulitis (15^H), induration (16^H), swelling (17^H)), rash (18^H), sudden infant death syndrome (SIDS) (19^H), idiopathic thrombocytopenia (20^H), and smallpox vaccine-associated adverse events following immunization (eczema (21^H), generalized vaccinia (22^H), vaccinia progressiva (23^H), inadvertent inoculation (24^H), and robust take (25^H)).

Compensation for vaccine injuries

Modified Vaccine Injury Compensation Program in the USA   The National Childhood

Vaccine Injury Act of 1986 established the National Vaccine Injury Compensation Programme as a federal no-fault compensation system for individuals who may have been injured by specific vaccines. This compensation program relies on a Vaccine Injury Table that lists the vaccines that are covered by the programme, as well as injuries, disabilities, illnesses, and conditions (including death) for which compensation may be awarded. To better reflect current scientific knowledge about vaccine injuries, the Vaccine Injury Table has been subsequently further modified. The last modification, which became effective on 1 February 2007, is shown in Table 1 (26[S]).

BACTERIAL VACCINES

Bacille Calmette–Guérin (BCG) vaccine   *(SED-15, 397; SEDA-27, 337; SEDA-28, 358)*

Susceptibility factors

BCG immunization in infants at risk of HIV infection   WHO has previously recommended that in countries with a high burden of tuberculosis, BCG vaccine should be given to all healthy infants as soon as possible after birth, unless the child presents with symptomatic HIV infection. However, recent evidence has shown that children who were HIV-infected when immunized with BCG at birth, and who later developed AIDS, were at increased risk of developing disseminated BCG disease. Further studies have contributed to updated WHO recommendations. In a prospective hospital-based surveillance study in the Western Cape Province, South Africa, the risk of disseminated BCG disease was found to be increased several hundred-fold in HIV-infected infants compared with the risk in HIV non-infected infants (27[C]). In a retrospective study in the Hospital de Niños "R. Gutiérrez" in Buenos Aires, Argentina, in 310 infants perinatally infected with HIV and immunized with BCG after birth, 28/310 (9 %) developed BCG disease, among them for cases of disseminated BCG (28[C]).

The updated WHO recommendations are as follows. Infants who are HIV-infected, with or without symptoms, and infants whose HIV infection status is unknown but who have signs suggestive of HIV infection and who are born to HIV-infected mothers should not be immunized (29[S]).

Meningococcal vaccine   *(SED-15, 2250; SEDA-27, 337; SEDA-28, 359; SEDA-29, 331)*

Nervous system   Menactra®, a quadrivalent conjugated meningococcal vaccine (serogroups A,C,W$_{135}$,Y), is licensed in the USA and recommended for routine immunization at age 11–12 years (SEDA-29, 331). To date, more than 12 million doses have been delivered. As of 30 April 2007, a total of 19 cases of *Guillain–Barré syndrome*, occurring within 6 weeks of immunization, had been reported to the US Vaccine Adverse Event Reporting System (VAERS) (30[S]). Analysis of the data could not exclude a slightly increased risk of Guillain–Barré syndrome after immunization, but this finding should be viewed with caution, given the limitations of the reporting system and the uncertainty of the background rate of Guillain–Barré syndrome and its potential for seasonal fluctuation. The manufacturer of the vaccine is planning further studies to evaluate the possible risk of Guillain–Barré syndrome after immunization with Menactra®.

Pneumococcal vaccine   *(SED-15, 2873; SEDA-28, 360; SEDA-29, 332)*

The Global Advisory Committee on Vaccine Safety (GACVS) has reviewed safety data from 62 studies, including randomized controlled trials and post-marketing studies (31[MS]). Since the 7-valent pneumococcal conjugate vaccine was licensed in 2000, and following its widespread use in the USA and more recently in Canada and some European countries, major safety concern have not been identified. The evidence on the safety of the vaccine is reassuring. However, as with the introduction of any new vaccine, further careful surveillance for possible rare and unexpected events is recommended.

Table 1. *Vaccine Injury Table (26^S)*

	Vaccine	Adverse event	Interval
I	Tetanus toxoid-containing vaccines (for example DTaP, Tdap, DTP-Hib, DT, Td, TT)	A. Anaphylaxis or anaphylactic shock B. Brachial neuritis C. Any acute complication or sequel (including death) of the above events	0–4 hours 2–28 days Not applicable
II	Pertussis antigen-containing vaccines (for example DTaP, Tdap, DTP, P, DTP-Hib)	A. Anaphylaxis or anaphylactic shock B. Encephalopathy or encephalitis C. Any acute complication or sequel (including death) of the above events	0–4 hours 0–72 hours Not applicable
III	Measles, mumps, and rubella virus-containing vaccines in any combination (for example MMR, MR, M, R)	A. Anaphylaxis or anaphylactic shock B. Encephalopathy or encephalitis C. Any acute complication or sequel (including death) of the above events	0–4 hours 5–15 days Not applicable
IV	Rubella virus-containing vaccines (for example MMR, MR, R)	A. Chronic arthritis B. Any acute complication or sequel (including death) of the above event	7–42 days Not applicable
V	Measles virus-containing vaccines (for example MMR, MR, M)	A. Thrombocytopenic purpura B. Vaccine-Strain Measles Viral Infection in an immunodeficient recipient C. Any acute complication or sequel (including death) of the above events	7–30 days 0–6 months Not applicable
VI	Polio live virus-containing vaccines (OPV)	A. Paralytic polio • in a non-immunodeficient recipient • in an immunodeficient recipient • in a vaccine associated community case B. Vaccine-strain polio viral infection • in a non-immunodeficient recipient • in an immunodeficient recipient • in a vaccine associated community case C. Any acute complication or sequel (including death) of the above events	 0–30 days 0–6 months Not applicable 0–30 days 0–6 months Not applicable Not applicable
VII	Polio inactivated virus-containing vaccines (for example IPV)	A. Anaphylaxis or anaphylactic shock B. Any acute complication or sequel (including death) of the above event	0–4 hours Not applicable
VIII	Hepatitis B antigen-containing vaccines	A. Anaphylaxis or anaphylactic shock B. Any acute complication or sequel (including death) of the above event	0–4 hours Not applicable
IX	*Hemophilus influenzae* (type b polysaccharide conjugate vaccines)	A. No condition specified for compensation	Not applicable
X	Varicella vaccine	A. No condition specified for compensation	Not applicable
XI	Rotavirus vaccine	A. No condition specified for compensation	Not applicable
XII	Vaccines containing live, oral, rhesus-based rotavirus	A. Intussusception B. Any acute complication or sequel (including death) of the above event	0–30 days Not applicable
XIII	Pneumococcal conjugate vaccines	A. No condition specified for compensation	Not applicable
XIV	Any new vaccine recommended by the Centers for Disease Control and Prevention for routine administration to children, after publication by the Secretary, HHS, of a notice of coverage	A. No condition specified for compensation	Not applicable

VIRAL VACCINES

Hepatitis B vaccine (including combination vaccines with HB component)   *(SED-15, 1600; SEDA-29, 332)*

Liver   Severe *jaundice* and *raised serum liver enzyme activities* have been reported after a dose of Twinrix® (combination HA/HB vaccine) (32[A]).

- A 26-year-old man had a raised concentration of immunoglobulin G and an antinuclear antibody titer of 1:320. Liver biopsy showed marked bridging liver fibrosis and chronic inflammation, compatible with autoimmune hepatitis. Treatment led to complete normalization of liver function tests. The patient had never had jaundice or abnormal liver function tests.

The authors suggested that the vaccine had induced an acute exacerbation of an unrecognized autoimmune hepatitis.

Human papilloma virus vaccine (HPV vaccine)   *(SED-15, 1699; SEDA-27, 338)*

The Global Advisory Committee on Vaccine Safety (GACVS) has reviewed the safety of human papilloma virus vaccines (both the tetravalent Gardasil® and the bivalent Cervarix®). Data from prelicensing randomized controlled trials and post-licensing surveillance reports from the two vaccine manufacturers and from the European Medicines Evaluation Agency (EMEA), the US Food and Drug Administration (FDA), and the US Centers for Disease Control and Prevention (CDC) were included (33[S]). The current evidence on the safety of HPV vaccines is reassuring. The reviewed data covered short-term local and systemic events, and long-term events up to 6 years after immunization, including events in pregnancy. *Injection-site reactions* and *muscle pain* were common. During adolescent vaccine campaigns, some mass sociogenic illnesses, such as post-immunization *dizziness* and *syncope*, have been reported. These events have been prevented by observing adolescents for 15 minutes

after immunization and encouraging good hydration. The Committee recommended good surveillance systems to identify possible rare adverse effects and specific adverse effects during pregnancy, as the target group includes women of reproductive age, although according to the Summary of Product Characteristics of the HPV vaccine Gardasil®, immunization of pregnant women is not recommended.

Influenza vaccine   *(SED-15, 1753; SEDA-26, 358; SEDA-28, 361; SEDA-29, 332)*

An update on Flumist®, a cold-adapted live attenuated influenza vaccine, was presented at the June 2007 meeting of the Global Advisory Committee on Vaccine Safety (GACVS) (34[S]). Studies in young children showed that it is effective against circulating H1N1 and H3N2 strains, including H3N2 strains that are antigenically dissimilar to the strain that is included in the annual vaccine. Efficacy has also been demonstrated against circulating B strains. However, there was a significantly increased incidence of medically significant episodes of wheezing within 42 days of immunization among children aged 6–23 months. The manufacturer has applied to extend the indication to children under 5 years of age, and this is under review by the FDA.

Musculoskeletal   *Macrophagic myofasciitis* has been observed in a patient who received annual injections of influenza vaccine for 4 years (35[A]).

- A 59-year-old woman developed slowly progressive pain in the right thigh over 2 years. She had previously complained of diffuse myalgia and polyarthralgia for 2 years. She had been immunized with influenza vaccines annually after the diffuse myalgia had developed. There was severe focal muscle tenderness in the right thigh without muscle weakness or wasting. Clinical chemistry and serology were all normal. Open biopsy of the right vastus lateralis muscle and fascia showed characteristics of macrophagic myofasciitis, with conspicuous infiltration of macrophages, stained with PAS and CD68, but not desmin and smooth muscle actin or CD1a and S100 protein. The macrophage infiltrates were multifocal, and lymphocytes were mostly CD8+ T cells. CD4+ T cells and CD45 cells were rare, and neither CD20+ B cells nor plasma cells were found. Prednisolone was given and the right thigh pain abated somewhat.

Japanese encephalitis vaccine

(SED-15, 1957, SEDA-26, 359; SEDA-28, 363; SEDA-29, 334)

The Global Advisory Committee on Vaccine Safety (GACVS) has considered a report from an Indian expert panel that assessed cases of serious adverse events after immunization campaigns (including about 9.3 million children aged 1–15 years) with the live attenuated SA-14-14-2 Japanese encephalitis vaccine (36[S]). A total of 65 serious adverse events were reported, 22 of which were fatal. Most of the serious adverse events were considered to be unrelated to the vaccine. Two clusters of *encephalitis-like syndromes* were detected; the cases in one cluster probably represented cases of natural Japanese encephalitis, and the cases in the second cluster were classified as acute encephalopathy syndrome of unknown cause. A thorough investigation into possible alternative causes was not conducted. The committee concluded that the type of clustering of encephalopathy/encephalitis cases made it unlikely that they had been related to the vaccine. The committee recommended that future immunization campaigns should be accompanied by better adverse event monitoring and investigations.

Measles–mumps–rubella (MMR) vaccine *(SED-15, 2207; SEDA-27, 338; SEDA-28, 363; SEDA-29, 335)*

Psychiatric

Autism   The hypothesis that MMR vaccine can cause autism has been discussed at length (SED-15, 2207; SEDA-25, 387; SEDA-26, 359; SEDA-27, 338, SEDA-28, 363). To date, the hypothesis has not been confirmed. However, the controversy, particularly in the USA, has not ended. A survey commissioned by "Generation Rescue" (a parent-founded, parent-funded, and parent-led organization of more than 350 families) was published in June 2007. Data were gathered by Survey USA, a national market-research company, which carried out a telephone survey of the parents of more than 17 000 children, aged 4–17 years, in five

counties in California (San Diego, Sonoma, Orange, Sacramento, and Marin) and four counties in Oregon (Multnomah, Marion, Jackson, and Lane) (37[c]). They asked parents whether their child had been immunized, and whether that child had one or more of the following diagnoses: attention deficit disorder (ADD), attention deficit hyperactivity disorder (ADHD), Asperger's syndrome, pervasive development disorder not otherwise specified, or autism. Among more than 9000 boys aged 4–17 years, they found that immunized boys were 155% more likely to have neurological disorders compared with their non-immunized peers. Immunized boys were 224% more likely to have ADHD, and 61% more likely to have autism. Older immunized boys in the 11–17 age bracket were 158% more likely to have a neurological disorder, 317% more likely to have ADHD, and 112% more likely to have autism. It is open for discussion whether these results, obtained by this method, can really make a substantial contribution to a scientific question.

Measles inclusion-body encephalitis (MIBE) due to measles vaccine virus   After natural measles infection, measles inclusion-body encephalitis (also referred to as subacute measles encephalitis, acute encephalitis of the delayed type, or immunosuppressive measles encephalitis) is a well-known complication associated with immunodeficiency. It typically develops within months of measles virus infection. Using RNA-templated sequencing, vaccine-strain measles virus has been implicated as the cause of death in three immunocompromised children with inclusion body encephalitis (SEDA-23, 350) and a further case has been reported (38[A]).

- A 21-month-old boy developed measles inclusion-body encephalitis 8.5 months after measles-mumps-rubella immunization. He had no history of immunodeficiency, measles exposure, or measles disease. He presented with status epilepticus, a fever of 39.5 °C, but no signs of meningism. A cranial CT scan showed swelling of the left temporal lobe with narrowing of the ipsilateral ventricle. He had primary immunodeficiency, characterized by a profoundly depressed CD8 cell count and dysgammaglobulinemia. A brain biopsy showed histopathological changes consistent with measles inclusion-body encephalitis, and measles antigens were detected by immunohistochemical staining. The presence of measles virus in the brain tissue was confirmed by reverse transcription polymerase chain reaction. The nucleotide sequence in the nucleoprotein and fusion gene regions was identical to that of the Moraten and Schwarz vaccine strains; the fusion gene differed from known genotype A wild-type measles viruses. Despite intensive medical interventions, neurological deterioration continued, and on hospital day 51, he died.

This is an excellent example of the fourth ("fingerprint") type of definitive anecdotal adverse drug reaction (39[H]).

Measles–mumps–rubella–varicella   vaccine
A recently developed quadrivalent measles–mumps–rubella–varicella vaccine (ProQuad®, referred to as MMRV), which includes a varicella component of increased potency, has been evaluated in a blind multicenter study in 480 healthy children aged 12–23 months, who were randomized to either MMRV + placebo or MMR + monovalent varicella vaccine (40[C]). Children who were randomized to MMRV + placebo received a second dose of MMRV 90 days later. *Measles-like rash* and *fever* during days 5–12 were more common after the first dose of combination MMRV (rash 5.9%; fever 28%) than after MMR + monovalent varicella vaccine (rash 1.9%; fever 19%). The incidences of other adverse events were similar between the groups. Response rates were over 90% to all vaccine components in both groups. Geometric mean titers to measles and mumps were significantly higher after one dose of MMRV than after MMR+varicella vaccine. The second dose of MMRV elicited slight to moderate increases in measles, mumps, and rubella antibody titers and a substantial increase in varicella antibody titer.

Mumps vaccine   *(SED-14, 1080; SEDA-27, 338)*

The Global Advisory Committee on Vaccine Safety (GACVS) has reviewed the data on the safety of mumps vaccine strains, particularly regarding the risk of vaccine-derived meningitis (41[S]). They noted that cases of *aseptic meningitis* and estimates of incidence rates have been reported after the use of Urabe, Leningrad–Zagreb, Hoshino, Torii, and Miyahara strains from various surveillance systems and epidemiological studies. The data up to now have shown low rates of aseptic meningitis and no cases of virologically proven meningitis after the use of the Jeryl–Lynn and RIT 4385 strains. Information about the Leningrad-3 strain is limited. No data were available to assess the safety of the S79 strain. There is still a lack of carefully designed studies to discriminate between potential strain variability and age-specific risk in different populations. GACVS welcomed the establishment of a repository of mumps vaccine strains at the National Institute for Biological Standards and Control, Potters Bar, UK, and has urged the acceleration of work to gain insight into the biological determinants of risk from different strains.

Poliomyelitis vaccine   *(SED-15, 2881; SEDA-28, 365)*

Nervous system

Imported vaccine-associated paralytic poliomyelitis   The USA has eliminated indigenous wild poliovirus transmission and, through a vaccine policy change from oral polio vaccine (OPV) to inactivated polio vaccine (IPV), vaccine-associated   paralytic   poliomyelitis (VAAP). The primary risk for polio disease for US residents is through travel abroad to countries were polio remains endemic or where polio outbreaks are occurring.

- A 22-year-old woman, who had never been immunized against poliomyelitis, was probably exposed during travel in Latin America through contact with an infant who had recently been immunized with OPV (42[A]). She developed paralytic poliomyelitis. Stool specimens were positive for Sabin-strain poliovirus type 2 and 3. Sixty days after the onset of weakness, she had residual weakness in both legs.

This is the first known occurrence of imported vaccine-associated paralytic poliomyelitis in an unimmunized US adult who travelled abroad.

Rotavirus vaccine   *(SED-15, 3082; SEDA-27, 338; SEDA-28, 365)*

Hematologic   The US Food and Drug Administration (FDA) has reported that five cases of *Kawasaki disease* (mucocutaneous lymph node syndrome of unknown etiology) have been identified in children under 1 year of age who received the Rotavirus (RotaTeq®) vaccine during clinical trials conducted before the vaccine was licensed (43S). Three cases of Kawasaki disease were detected after the vaccine was approved in February 2006 through the Vaccine Adverse Event Reporting System (VAERS). After learning about these reports, CDC identified an additional unconfirmed case through its Vaccine Safety Datalink (VSD) Project. The number of reports of Kawasaki disease does not exceed the number of cases expected based on the usual occurrence of Kawasaki disease in children. There is not a known cause-and-effect relation between receiving RotaTeq® or any other vaccine and the occurrence of Kawasaki disease. The Global Advisory Committee on Vaccine Safety (GACVS) has recommended that current and future studies should incorporate surveillance for Kawasaki disease after immunization (44S).

Gastrointestinal   The Global Advisory Committee on Vaccine Safety (GACVS) has reviewed data presented by the Centers for Disease Control and Prevention (CDC) and the FDA related to the risk of *intussusception*, which had been identified as associated with a previous rotavirus vaccine. With respect to Rotarix®, there was no evidence from any of the studies, which included over 30 000 vaccinees in trials and worldwide usage (about 5 million doses distributed), that there was an excess incidence of intussusception. The cases of intussusception that were reported did not show a pattern with regard to the time of onset after immunization consistent with a causal relation. The overall number of cases reported was much smaller than would have been expected based on applying rates for the normal incidence of intussusception to a population of the size immunized.

A study of RotaTeq® in over 30 000 individuals has been reported, and an observational cohort study of 44 000 immunized children is planned. Most of the data, especially from post-marketing studies and spontaneous reporting, relate to developed countries. There is no evidence that the rate of intussusception

is raised above background, and it is certainly much less than the rate previously observed with the vaccine that was withdrawn after an association with intussusception was described. The VAERS spontaneous reporting data also showed a lower than expected rate of intussusception. GACVS concluded that the data, particularly those from developed countries, are reassuring (45S). However, it was noted that the current data relate mainly to vaccines that are used in young children at the recommended age. It is important that intussusception should be monitored in developing countries as rotavirus vaccines are introduced, especially because infants are likely to present for their first dose of vaccine at slightly older ages on average than is the case in developed countries.

Smallpox vaccine   *(SED-15, 3150)*

Alternative smallpox vaccines have been developed because of concerns over biological weapons. Live, attenuated vaccinia virus vaccines derived from calf lymph were used to eradicate smallpox worldwide. However, well documented safety limitations prevent their widespread use in civilian in the absence of an outbreak. Of every million people immunized for smallpox, 14–52 had serious or life-threatening adverse reactions, and 1–2 per million primary vaccinees died. Furthermore, live attenuated vaccinia virus vaccine is contraindicated in up to 30% or more of the population, including infants, pregnant women, women who are breastfeeding, the immunocompromised, those with eczema or exfoliative skin disorders, people who live in the same house or are in intimate contact with people with the above conditions, and people with cardiovascular conditions.

A new smallpox vaccine derived from cell culture has been compared with a vaccine derived from calf lymph in 350 healthy adults (46C). All but one participant developed pock lesions. Vaccine-associated adverse reactions were similar between the groups. The cell-cultured vaccine was as immunogenic and safe as the calf-lymph-derived vaccine.

References

1. Saenger R, Maechler G, Potreck M, Zepp F, Knuf M, Habermehl P, Schuerman L. Booster vaccination with hexavalent DTPa–HBV–IPV/Hib vaccine in the second year of life is as safe as concomitant DTPa–IPV/Hib + HBV administered separately. Vaccine 2005;23:1135–43.

2. Schulzke S, Heininger U, Lücking-Famira M, Fahnenstich H. Apnea and bradycardia in preterm infants following immunization with penta- and heptavalent vaccines. Eur J Pediatr 2005;164:432–5.

3. Vennemann MM, Butterfass-Bahloul T, Jorch G, Brinkmann B, Findeisen M, Sauerland C, Bajanowski T, Mitchell EA, The GeSID Group. Sudden infant death syndrome: no increased risk after immunisation. Vaccine 2007;25(2):336–40.

4. Souayah N, Nasar A, Suri MF, Qureshi AI. Guillain–Barré syndrome following vaccination in the United States. Vaccine 2007;25:5253–5.

5. Koppen S, de Groot R, Neijens HJ, Nagelkerke N, van Eden W, Rümke HC. No epidemiological evidence for infant vaccinations to cause allergic disease. Vaccine 2004;25-6:3375–85.

6. Bergfors E, Trollfors B, Inerot A. Unexpectedly high incidence of persistent itching nodules and delayed hypersensitivity to aluminium in children after the use of adsorbed vaccines from a single manufacturer. Vaccine 2004;22:158.

7. Thierry-Carstensen B, Stellfeld M. Itching nodules and hypersensitivity to aluminium after the use of adsorbed vaccines from SSI. Vaccine 2004;22:1845.

8. Theeten H, Van Damme P, Hoppenbrouwers K, Vandermeulen C, Leback E, Sokal EM, Wolter J, Schuerman L. Effects of lowering the aluminium content of a DTPa vaccine on its immunogenicity and reactogenicity when given as a booster to adolescents. Vaccine 2005;23:1515–21.

9. Ozaki T, Nishimura N, Muto T, Sugata K, Kawabe S, Goto K, Koyama K, Fujita H, Takahashi Y, Akiyama M. Safety and immunogenicity of gelatine-free varicella vaccine in epidemiological and serological studies in Japan. Vaccine 2005;23:1205–8.

10. Rüggeberg JU, Gold MS, Bayas JM, Blum MD, Bonhoeffer J, Friedlander S, de Souza Brito G, Heininger U, Imoukhuede B, Khamesipour A, Erlewyn-Lajeunesse M, Martin S, Mäkelä M, Nell P, Pool V, Simpson N, The Brighton Collaboration Anaphylaxis Working Group. Anaphylaxis: case definition and guidelines for data collection, analysis, and presentation of immunization safety data. Vaccine 2007;25:5675–84.

11. Tapiainen T, Prevots R, Izurieta HS, Abramson J, Bilynsky R, Bonhoeffer J, Bonnet MC, Center K, Galama J, Gillard P, Griot M, Hartmann K, Heininger U, Hudson M, Koller A, Khetsuriani N, Khuri-Bulos N, Marcy SM, Matulionyte R, Schöndorf I, Sejvar J, Steele R, The Brighton Collaboration Aseptic Meningitis Working Group. Aseptic meningitis: case definition and guidelines for collection, analysis and presentation of immunization safety data. Vaccine 2007;25:5793–802.

12. Sejvar JJ, Kohl KS, Bilynsky R, Blumberg D, Cvetkovich T, Galama J, Gidudu J, Katikaneni L, Khuri-Bulos N, Oleske J, Tapiainen T, Wiznitzer M, The Brighton Collaboration Encephalitis Working Group. Encephalitis, myelitis, and acute disseminated encephalomyelitis (ADEM): case definitions and guidelines for collection, analysis, and presentation of immunization safety data. Vaccine 2007;25:5771–92.

13. Jones JF, Kohl KS, Ahmadipour N, Bleijenberg G, Buchwald D, Evengard B, Jason LA, Klimas NG, Lloyd A, McCleary K, Oleske JM, White PD, The Brighton Collaboration Fatigue Working Group. Fatigue: case definition and guidelines for collection, analysis, and presentation of immunization safety data. Vaccine 2007;25:5685–96.

14. Kohl KS, Ball L, Gidudu J, Hammer SJ, Halperin S, Heath P, Hennig R, Labadie J, Rothstein E, Schuind A, Varricchio F, Walop W, The Brighton Collaboration Local Reactions Working Group for Abscess at Injection Site. Abscess at injection site: case definition and guidelines for collection, analysis, and presentation of immunization safety data. Vaccine 2007;25:5821–38.

15. Halperin S, Kohl KS, Gidudu J, Ball L, Hammer SJ, Heath P, Hennig R, Labadie J, Rothstein E, Schuind A, Varricchio F, Walop W, The Brighton Collaboration Local Reaction Working Group for Cellulitis at Injection Site. Cellulitis at injection site: case definition and guidelines for collection, analysis, and presentation of immunization safety data. Vaccine 2007;25:5803–20.

16. Kohl KS, Walop W, Gidudu J, Ball L, Halperin S, Hammer SJ, Heath P, Hennig R, Rothstein E, Schuind A, Varricchio F, The Brighton Collaboration Local Reactions Working Group for Induration at or near Injection Site. Induration at or near injection site: case definition and guidelines for collection, analysis, and presentation of immunization safety data. Vaccine 2007;25:5839–57.

17. Kohl KS, Walop W, Gidudu J, Ball L, Halperin S, Hammer SJ, Heath P, Varricchio F, Rothstein E, Schuind A, Hennig R, The Brighton Collaboration Local Reaction Working Group for Swelling at or near Injection Site. Swelling at or near injection site: case definition and guidelines for collection, analysis and presentation of immunization safety data. Vaccine 2007;25:5858–74.

18. Beigel J, Kohl KS, Khuri-Bulos N, Bravo L, Nell P, Marcy SM, Warschaw K, Ong-Lim A, Poerschke G, Weston W, Lindstrom JA, Stoltman G, Maurer T, The Brighton Collaboration Rash Working Group. Rash including mucosal involvement: case definition and guidelines for

collection, analysis, and presentation of immunization safety data. Vaccine 2007;25:5697–706.
19. Jorch G, Tapiainen T, Bonhoeffer J, Fischer TK, Heininger U, Hoet B, Kohl KS, Lewis EM, Meyer C, Nelson T, Sandbu S, Schlaud M, Schwartz A, Varricchio F, Wise RP, The Brighton Collaboration Unexplained Sudden Death Working Group. Unexplained sudden death, including sudden infant death syndrome (SIDS), in the first and second years of life: case definition and guidelines for collection, analysis, and presentation of immunization safety data. Vaccine 2007;25:5707–16.
20. Wise RP, Bonhoeffer J, Beeler J, Donato H, Downie P, Matthews D, Pool V, Riise-Bergsaker M, Tapiainen T, Varricchio F, The Brighton Collaboration Thrombocytopenia Working Group. Thrombocytopenia: case definition and guidelines for collection, analysis, and presentation of immunization safety data. Vaccine 2007;25:5717–24.
21. Nell P, Kohl KS, Graham PL, Larussa PS, Marcy SM, Fulginiti VA, Martin B, Trolin I, Norton SA, Neff JM, The Brighton Collaboration Vaccinia Virus Vaccine Adverse Event Working Group for Eczema Vaccinatum. Eczema vaccinatum as an adverse event following exposure to vaccinia virus: case definition & guidelines of data collection, analysis, and presentation of immunization safety data. Vaccine 2007;25:5725–34.
22. Beigel J, Kohl KS, Brinley F, Graham PL, Khuri-Bulos N, Larussa PS, Nell P, Norton S, Stoltman G, Tebaa A, Warschaw K, The Brighton Collaboration Vaccinia Virus Vaccine Adverse Event Working Group for Generalized Vaccinia. Generalized vaccinia as an adverse event following exposure to vaccinia virus: case definition and guidelines for data collection, analysis, and presentation of immunization safety data. Vaccine 2007;25:5745–53.
23. Nell P, Kohl KS, Graham PL, Larussa PS, Marcy SM, Fulginiti VA, Martin B, McMahon A, Norton SA, Trolin I, The Brighton Collaboration Vaccinia Virus Vaccine Adverse Event Working Group for Progressive Vaccinia. Progressive vaccinia as an adverse event following exposure to vaccinia virus: case definition and guidelines of data collection, analysis, and presentation of immunization safety data. Vaccine 2007;25:5735–44.
24. Wenger P, Oleske JM, Kohl KS, Fisher MC, Brien JH, Graham PL, Larussa PS, Lipton S, Tierney B, The Brighton Collaboration Vaccinia Virus Adverse Event Working Group for Inadvertent Inoculation. Inadvertent inoculation as an adverse event following exposure to vaccinia virus: case definition and guidelines for data collection, analysis, and presentation of immunization safety data. Vaccine 2007;25:5754–62.
25. Graham PL, Larussa PS, Kohl KS, The Brighton Collaboration Vaccinia Virus Adverse Event Working Group for Robust Take. Robust take following exposure to vaccinia virus: case definition and guidelines of data collection, analysis, and

presentation of immunization safety data. Vaccine 2007;25:5763–70.
26. National childhood vaccine injury act. Vaccine injury table. http://www.hrsa.gov/vaccinecompensation/table.htm [last accessed 26 July 2007].
27. Hesseling AC, Marais BJ, Gie RP, Schaaf HS, Fine PEM, Godfrey-Faussett P, Beyers N. The risk of disseminated Bacille Calmette–Guérin (BCG) disease in HIV-infected children. Vaccine 2007;25:14–8.
28. Fallo A, Torrado L, Sanchez A, Cerqueiro C, Shadgrosky L, Lopez EL. Delayed complications of BCG vaccination in HIV-infected children. Presented at the International AIDS Society meeting 2005. http://www.who.int/vaccine_safety/topics/bcg/immunocompromised/index.html [last accessed 27 July 2007].
29. Global Advisory Committee on Vaccine Safety (GACVS). Revised BCG vaccination guidelines for infants at risk for HIV infection. Wkly Epidemiol Rec 2007;82:193–6.
30. Global Advisory Committee on Vaccine Safety. Meeting on 12–13 June 2007. Menactra and GBS. Wkly Epidemiol Rec 2007;82:256.
31. Global Advisory Committee on Vaccine Safety. Meeting on 29–30 November 2006. Safety of pneumococcal conjugate vaccines: update. Wkly Epidemiol Rec 2007;82:24.
32. Csepregi A, Treiber G, Röcken C, Malfertheiner P. Acute exacerbation of autoimmune hepatitis induced by Twinrix. World J Gastroenterol 2005;11:4114–6.
33. Global Advisory Committee on Vaccine Safety. Meeting on 12–13 June 2007. Safety of HPV vaccines. Wkly Epidemiol Rec 2007;82:255–6.
34. Global Advisory Committee on Vaccine Safety. Meeting on 12–13 June 2007. Influenza vaccines: update. Wkly Epidemiol Rec 2007;82:255–6.
35. Park JH, Na KS, Park YW, Paik SS, Yoo DH. Macrophagic myofasciitis unrelated to vaccination. Scand J Rheumatol 2005;34:65–7.
36. Global Advisory Committee on Vaccine Safety. Meeting on 29–30 November. Safety of Japanese encephalitis immunization in India. Wkly Epidemiol Rec 2007;82:23–4.
37. The California–Oregon Unvaccinated Children Survey. www.GenerationRescue.org [last accessed 26 July 2007].
38. Bitnun A, Shannon P, Durward A, Rota PA, Bellini WJ, Graham C, Wang E, Ford-Jones EL, Cox P, Becker L, Fearon M, Petric M, Tellier R. Measles inclusion-body encephalitis caused by the vaccine strain of measles virus. Clin Infect Dis 1999;29:855–61.
39. Aronson JK, Hauben M. Anecdotes that provide definitive evidence. BMJ 2006;332:1267–9.
40. Shinefield H, Black S, Digilio L, Reisinger K, Blatter M, Gress JO, Hoffman Brown ML, Eves KA, Klopfer SO, Schadel F, Kuter BJ. Evaluation of a quadrivalent measles, mumps, rubella and varicella vaccine in healthy children. Pediatr Infect Dis J 2005;24:665–9.
41. Global Advisory Committee on Vaccine Safety. Meeting on 29–30 November 2006. Safety of

mumps vaccine strains. Wkly Epidemiol Rec 2007;82:20–2.

42. Imported vaccine-associated paralytic poliomyelitis (VAAP)—United States, 2005. MMWR Morb Mortal Wkly Rep 2006;55:97–9.

43. US Food and Drug Administration. Information pertaining to labeling revision for Rotateq. June 15, 2007; http://www.fda.gov/cber/label/rotateqLBinfo.htm [accessed 16 August, 2007].

44. Kawasaki Disease and RotaTeq® Vaccine. http://www.cdc.gov/od/science/iso/concerns/kawasaki_disease_rotavirus.htm [last accessed 26 July 2007].

45. Global Advisory Committee on Vaccine Safety. Meeting on 12–13 June 2007. Safety of rotavirus vaccines. Wkly Epidemiol Rec 2007;82:256–7.

46. Greenberg RN, Kennedy JS, Clanton DJ, Plummer EA, Hague L, Cruz J, Ennis FA, Blackwelder WC, Hopkins RJ. Safety and immunogenicity of new cell-cultured smallpox vaccine compared with calf-lymph derived vaccine: a blind, single-centre, randomised controlled trial. Lancet 2005;365:398–409.

P.F.W. Strengers and E. van Twuyver

33 Blood, blood components, plasma, and plasma products

ALBUMIN (SED-15, 54; SEDA-28, 371; SEDA-29, 338)

The outcome of the SAFE study has not ended the debate about the clinical use of albumin (SEDA-29, 369). It is not safety that is being questioned but the clinical benefit, in particular the use of albumin in neonates or for indications other than fluid resuscitation (1[r], 2[r], 3[r]). The incidence of the adverse effects of albumin is low compared with artificial colloids (SEDA-29, 369). In particular, albumin does not impair coagulation (4[C]).

ANTICOAGULANT PROTEINS
(SED-15, 266; SEDA-28, 371; SEDA-29, 338)

Drotrecogin alfa (recombinant human activated protein C)

Hematologic The anticoagulant effects of drotrecogin alfa can cause *bleeding* and *thrombocytopenia* (5[Ac]).

- An 81-year-old woman with septic shock after laparotomy for ischemic bowel was given drotrecogin alfa (activated) 24 micrograms/kg/hour for 67.5 hours. Significant increases in activated partial thromboplastin time (aPTT) during infusion led to temporary discontinuation of the drug on two occasions. Coagulation parameters improved when the drug was withheld and worsened with each rechallenge.

Following this observation the medical records of 26 other patients who had received drotrecogin alfa were reviewed retrospectively. Nine had completed over 90% of the 96-hour course. Coagulopathy and bleeding resulted in early discontinuation in four and six patients respectively. There was an increase in aPTT from baseline to during infusion of drotrecogin alfa in 14 patients with complete data. There was a fall in median platelet count from baseline to during infusion in the six patients who bled during therapy, two of whom had platelet counts below $30 \times 10^9/l$ during administration. The authors recommended that patients receiving drotrecogin alfa should be closely monitored for altered coagulation and that temporary withdrawal should be considered when the INR is greater than 3.0, the platelet count less than $15 \times 10^9/l$, and the aPTT longer than 100 seconds.

Of seven patients with severe sepsis after hemopoietic stem cell transplantation who were given activated drotrecogin alfa, two had serious bleeding events (6[R]). The first had a non-fatal diffuse alveolar hemorrhage 2 days after administration and the second had a severe coagulopathy and had a fatal intracranial hemorrhage on the third day of drug infusion.

BLOOD TRANSFUSION (SED-15, 529; SEDA-28, 369; SEDA-29, 338)

Transfusion of blood components (red cell concentrates, platelet concentrates, or fresh frozen plasma) is associated with adverse reactions, some of them serious (SEDA-29, 338). *Non-hemolytic febrile transfusion reactions, acute hemolytic transfusion reactions, delayed hemolytic transfusion reactions, transfusion-related acute lung injury (TRALI), trans-*

Side Effects of Drugs, Annual 30
J.K. Aronson (Editor)
ISSN: 0378-6080
DOI: 10.1016/S0378-6080(08)00033-0

fusion associated graft-versus-host disease (TA-GVHD), transfusion-associated circulatory overload, severe acute anaphylactic transfusion reactions, anaphylactoid transfusion reactions, viral infections, bacterial contamination, and new allo-antibody formation are reported to organized national hemovigilance systems (7^R, 8^R, 9^R, 10^R). These national systems are in development and not all hospitals are participating, which makes comparison of reported data difficult.

In the Haemovigilance Report 2003 and 1993–2002 of the Japanese Red Cross Society, the frequency of reported adverse events was 1:1233 for platelets, 1:8074 for plasma, 1:7826 for red cells, and 1:2842 for whole blood for a total amount of 5 533 721 supplied units (platelets 706 346; plasma 1 461 312; red cells 3 357 538; whole blood 8525) (10^R). In another country, the risk of reactions rated as grade 2 (moderate to severe) or worse (life-threatening reactions or death after a transfusion reaction) was 0.12 per 1000 blood components (8^R). In two countries, the most common adverse event related to transfusion was *incorrect blood component transfusion (IBCT)*, termed "wrong blood" when a patient receives an incorrect group or a blood component intended for a different patient. Events of this type accounted for 55–81% of reported cases, with a risk of receiving a wrong red cell transfusion of about 1:31 959 units (7^R, 9^R). There were four transfusion related deaths; two were related to IBCT, of which one involved an ABO-incompatible red cell transfusion and one was caused by an inappropriate transfusion based on a result from the wrong patient. One patient died because of TRALI and one death was reported as an acute transfusion reaction (7^R).

A patient who had autologous blood predeposited received only allogeneic blood; no adverse events were reported (7^R). In this case blood was requested out of hours and no system was in place to alert the laboratory that autologous blood was available.

Respiratory   The number of reports of *transfusion-related acute lung injury (TRALI)* after transfusion of a blood component containing anti-granulocyte antibodies, anti-HLA antibodies, or biological active lipids of donor origin is increasing (SEDA-29, 339). Most cases are related to transfusion of plasma containing

blood components. One hemovigilance office reported that the 13 reported cases were related to platelets ($n = 4$), red cells ($n = 2$), fresh frozen plasma ($n = 6$), or whole blood ($n = 1$). In all 13 cases, the donors of the implicated component were female and all had leukocyte antibodies (7^R). In another report, 1.7% of the 5810 non-hemolytic transfusion reactions reported over 6 years were cases of TRALI. Of these, 11 were fatal (10^R). Retrospective computer-based screening showed that the incidence was 1:1000 to 1:2400 units of blood issued, supporting the view that TRALI is underdiagnosed and under-reported (11^c). Acute transient leukopenia has been proposed as a premonitory sign, based on a report of two patients with TRALI accompanied by a precipitous drop in leukocyte count (12^c). In critically ill patients with coagulopathy but without active bleeding, the benefit to harm balance of a liberal strategy of transfusion with fresh frozen plasma may not be favorable, and is particularly associated with acute lung injury (12^c).

Hematologic   *Purpura* after transfusion has been reported in two cases (7^R).

Immunologic   There have been reports of *hemolysis, anaphylaxis,* and *severe allergic reactions* to transfused red cells, fresh frozen plasma, or platelets. It was of particular concern that in 33% of the adverse reactions to fresh frozen plasma, including one death and two cases of serious morbidity, there did not appear to be a clear clinical indication for fresh frozen plasma (7^R).

High levels of long-term *microchimerism* were detected in patients transfused with leuko-reduced blood products after severe traumatic injury, which has implications for graft-versus-host disease and the safety of transfusion (13^c).

- A 67-year-old woman had life-threatening adverse effects and thrombocytopenia caused by anti-CD36 antibodies present in fresh frozen plasma (14^A).
- A 71-year-old immunocompetent man who underwent coronary artery bypass received 2 units of red cells and 22 days later was thought to have had transfusion-associated graft-versus-host disease (15^A). The diagnosis was confirmed by short tandem repeat analysis in combination with HLA typing, which seems to be a useful method for rapid diagnosis of this problem. He died 25 days after transfusion because of multiorgan failure and sepsis.

Infection risk   Further cases of *transmission of blood-borne pathogens* by transfusion have been reported, including one case of *hepatitis E* (7[R]), and one case of *HIV infection*, one case of *HGV infection*, and 12 cases of *hepatitis B infection* (10[R]).

Hepatitis viruses   The contribution of past transfusions to the risk of *hepatitis B* or *C* infection has been determined in 2120 endoscopy patients (16[C]). Although screening has almost completely eliminated hepatitis C, there was an unexpected association of infection with blood transfusion. The results suggested that other nosocomial risks for hepatitis C infection are involved, which should be actively investigated.

Parvovirus B19   In patients with hematological malignancies receiving 2123 blood cell preparations and blood products, 1% of the products tested positive for parvovirus B19, but there were no symptomatic infections probably because of the low viral load. Despite these results, testing for parvovirus B19 remains necessary because the disease caused by the infection can be severe (17[C]).

Variant Creutzfeldt–Jakob disease   A case of probable infection with variant Creutzfeldt–Jakob disease transmitted by blood transfusion has been identified (18[A]). The patient developed the infection 8 years after receiving a blood transfusion from a donor who developed variant Creutzfeldt–Jakob disease 20 months after donation. In animals leukodepletion does not reduce the infectivity of variant Creutzfeldt–Jakob disease but reduces the prion concentration in blood by 40% (19[E]). Universal leukodepletion also offers other benefits, such as reduction of transmission of cell-based viruses, including cytomegalovirus and human T cell lymphotropic virus, reduced rates of alloimmunization, reduced immunomodulation, and reduced rates of graft-versus-host disease (19[E]). A new filter has therefore been developed combining leukoreduction with removal of infectious prions from red blood cells (20[R]).

Yersinia enterocolitica   Fatal septic shock followed the transfusion of red cells contaminated with *Yersinia enterocolitica* (biotype 4 serovar O:3) for refractory anemia in a 71-year-old woman (21[A]).

Susceptibility factors   Current transfusion protocols in critically ill patients are associated with high rates of morbidity and mortality, transmission of infectious agents, and immunomodulation. Improvement of the clinical outcomes in critically ill patients after a restrictive transfusion strategy justifies revision of current transfusion protocols (22[R]).

Transfusion of platelet-pheresis concentrates significantly increased the serum concentration of the plasticizer di(2-ethylhexyl)phthalate (DEHP) in 12 adults with thrombocytopenia (23[c]). Reduction of the DEHP concentration is therefore desirable and can be accomplished by reducing the storage time, storage in an additive solution, or exchange of the storage medium before transfusion.

BLOOD SUBSTITUTES   *(SEDA-28, 370; SEDA-29, 340)*

Perfluorocarbons   *(SED-15, 3544; SEDA-29, 340)*

Nervous system   In 36 adults who underwent cardiac surgery the perfluorocarbon emulsion, AF0144 (Perflubron, Alliance Pharmaceutical Corp, San Diego, CA) 1.8 or 2.7 g/kg, was used in conjunction with acute normovolemic hemodilution (24[c]). Both doses of AF0144 increased cerebral blood flow but the numbers of *cerebral emboli* were greater in those who were given high-dose AF0144 compared with placebo during the time from aortic cannulation to aortic cross-clamp placement and from aortic cross-clamp placement to cross-clamp removal.

PLASMA PRODUCTS   *(SED-15, 2847; SEDA-29, 340)*

C1 inhibitor concentrate

Hereditary angioedema, caused by C1 inhibitor deficiency, causes recurrent angioedema of the skin, gastrointestinal tract, and other organs. Laryngeal edema can result in rapid asphyxiation, the most frequent cause of death in these patients. There are three possible emergency treatments: fresh frozen plasma, Solvent/Detergent-Plasma, and C1 inhibitor concentrate. The authors of a recent review have concluded that C1 inhibitor concentrate should be the preferred treatment for acute attacks (25[R]). *Allergic reactions* can occur but are extremely rare.

Fresh frozen plasma

Respiratory   *Pulmonary embolism* has been attributed to fresh frozen plasma that had been treated with methylthioninium chloride (methylene blue) in a 36-year-old obese man with homozygous factor V deficiency (26[A]). Solvent/Detergent FFP-related thrombosis seems to be associated with reduced activity of protein S and plasmin inhibitor. However, the concentrations of these factors in the fresh frozen plasma that was used in this case were not available.

PLASMA SUBSTITUTES
(SEDA-27, 353; SEDA-28, 371;

SEDA-29, 340)

Hematologic   Hemodilution with hydroxyethyl starch and dextrans can cause *coagulopathy*. Ex vivo addition of a fibrinogen concentrate improves the coagulopathy induced by hydroxyethyl starch and dextrans (27[E]), but in vivo studies are required to assess the clinical efficacy of doing this.

Dextrans   *(SED-15, 1082; SEDA-27, 353)*

Cardiovascular   Arterial hypotension following spinal anesthesia, possibly due to vasodilatation, relative hypovolemia, and reduced cardiac output, has been treated with a short-acting colloid, low-molecular weight (1 kDa) dextran, or Ringer's solution in a bolus injection in a randomized, non-blind, controlled study in 75 patients (28[c]). *Nausea* or *near-fainting* associated with marked *hypotension* or *bradycardia* was recorded predominantly in the dextran-treated group (20%).

Etherified starches   *(SED-15, 1237;*

SEDA-29, 340)

Adverse reactions related to etherified starches are *anaphylactic reactions, impaired coagulopathy, renal dysfunction*, and *pruritus* (4[R]). Hetastarch can cause reactions (*generalized pruritus, severe nausea*, and *hypotension*) due to allergy to latex (29[A]).

Polygelines   *(SED-15, 2888;*

SEDA-29, 341)

The Australian Adverse Drug Reactions Advisory Committee (ADRAC) has received 83 reports about succinylated gelatin (Gelofusine) since the product was first registered in 1998, 70 of which were of *hypotension* and/or *hypersensitivity reactions* (30[S]). In 27 of these reports, hypotension or anaphylactoid reactions were the only feature listed, while the remaining 43 mentioned signs and symptoms consistent with anaphylactoid reactions, including cardiac ($n = 10$), respiratory ($n = 18$) or cutaneous ($n = 35$) manifestations. In 60 reports, recovery was documented; one patient died after a cardiac arrest. ADRAC has received similar reports associated with other plasma expanders, albumin (Albumex), polygeline (Haemaccel), and dextran. In all cases, the number of reports of anaphylactoid reactions, as a proportion of the total reports, was similar to the proportion of reports of such reactions received for gelatin (Gelofusine). In view of the fact that saline and albumin have equivalent efficacy, ADRAC has commented that "the safety of colloids such as gelatin should be considered carefully in the initial choice of resuscitation fluid".

GLOBULINS

Antithymocyte globulin
(SEDA-29, 341)

Comparative studies   In renal transplant recipients who were treated with basiliximab (20 mg on days 0 and 4; $n = 235$) or pretransplant rabbit antithymocyte globulin ($n = 115$)

for a maximum of 2 weeks, the incidence of rejection was 15% with basiliximab and 8.5% with rabbit antithymocyte globulin (31^C). Wound complications occurred in 26 and 39% respectively, incisional hernias in 11 and 18%, wound infections in 11 and 17%, and lymphoceles in 11 and 16%.

Infection risk *Mucormycosis* is a rare but potentially lethal fungal infection after renal transplantation. To date, only five cases have been reported.

- A renal allograft recipient developed mucormycosis 18 months after transplantation following treatment for acute rejection with high dose glucocorticoids and antithymocyte globulin (32^A).

Tumorigenicity *Lymphoproliferative disorders* associated with Epstein–Barr virus infection after bone marrow transplantation can be fatal. Major risk factors are ex vivo T cell depletion or in vivo T cell depletion with either antithymocyte globulin or monoclonal anti-T cell antibodies. Of 23 transplant recipients who received equine ($n = 20$) or rabbit ($n = 3$) antithymocyte globulin as part of the preparatory regimen, all of those who received rabbit antithymocyte globulin developed a lymphoproliferative disorder associated with Epstein–Barr virus at 60–90 days after bone marrow transplantation; all three died of complications (33^c). There were no cases in those who received equine antithymocyte globulin. This suggests that patients who receive rabbit antithymocyte globulin as part of their preparatory regimens require close monitoring of the Epstein–Barr virus load and possible early intervention with antiviral therapy.

Immunoglobulins *(SED-15, 1719; SEDA-28, 372; SEDA-29, 343)*

Intravenous immunoglobulin is used in different doses in neurology, hematology, rheumatology, dermatology, ophthalmology, and other areas for a wide variety of disorders. Its mechanisms of action depend on the dose and the pathogenesis of the underlying disease (34^R). Intravenous immunoglobulin products (5 or 6%) are widely used for replacement therapy of immunoglobulin in patients with primary and secondary immune deficiencies and for immune modulation in patients with inflammatory and autoimmune diseases. Almost all formulations are produced by cold ethanol precipitation, but several methods are used to treat Cohn fraction II to obtain the different formulations. These products differ slightly, although they are therapeutically equivalent.

Additional antiviral steps are used in all formulations to prevent contamination of blood-borne agents, particularly with viruses. Viral transmission of hepatitis viruses and retroviruses has not been reported over the last years. Concern about transmission of variant Creutzfeldt–Jakob disease has not been justified by human-to-human transmission by intravenous immunoglobulin.

Because of the increased use of intravenous immunoglobulin, there has been an increased number of reports of serious adverse events, such as *aseptic meningitis, renal insufficiency (mostly transient), transient hyperviscosity syndrome, thromboembolic events including myocardial infarction* and *stroke, immune hemolysis, disseminated intravascular coagulation (DIC), acute respiratory distress syndrome (ARDS)*, and *transfusion-related acute lung injury (TRALI)* (35^R). The postulated mechanisms of action are speculative, and remain to be confirmed. These serious adverse events occur particularly in older patients, partly reflecting the increased use of intravenous immunoglobulin in higher dosages (2 g/kg) for anti-inflammatory or immunomodulatory indications, partly because a large proportion of patients with these diseases are significantly older that patients with immune deficiencies (usual doses of 400–600 mg/kg). In primary immune replacement therapy, adverse events such as *headache, backache, chills, fever, chest tightness*, and *shortness of breath*, are generally mild and transient and respond to anti-inflammatory/antipyretic drugs or adjustment of the infusion rate.

Observational studies   Experience with monthly, high-dose intravenous immunoglobulin in patients with different connective tissue diseases who failed to respond to standard therapies or for whom immunosuppressive drugs were contraindicated, the success rate was 70%, without serious adverse effects (36^A).

Placebo-controlled studies　In a multicenter, double-blind, placebo-controlled, dose-escalating study of the safety and efficacy of an experimental plasma-derived, donor-selected, polyclonal antistaphylococcal immunoglobulin with high titers of IgG directed against staphylococcal fibrinogen-binding proteins (INH-A21), 2% of the 505 infants had 13 drug-associated adverse events, of which seven involved changes in vital signs (*apnea, tachycardia, bradycardia, hypertension, and temperature changes*) (37[A]).

Cardiovascular　*Diffuse venous thromboembolism* was reported in a patient with streptococcal toxic syndrome after two courses of high-dose intravenous immunoglobulin (0.4 g/kg/day over 5 days and 8 days later 0.4 g/kg/day over 4 days) (38[A]). Several causes of immunoglobulin-mediated thrombosis have been postulated, including increased plasma and blood viscosity, platelet activation, cytokine-mediated vasospasm, and contamination with factor IX. The authors suggested that combined therapy, including other inhibitors of the inflammatory cascade such as analogues of activated protein C, should be administered to avoid relapse or complications such as thrombosis (38[A]).

Nervous system　*Stroke* has been attributed to intravenous immunoglobulin (39[A]).

- An 82-year-old woman with chronic inflammatory demyelinating polyneuropathy was treated over 10 years with 86 doses of intravenous immunoglobulin and had a stroke when she was given an 87th dose (increased from 40 to 50 g) over several hours.

Analysis of the factors that can contribute to the occurrence of stroke during or after the administration of intravenous immunoglobulin suggests that certain precautions need to be taken. Pre-existing thrombogenic susceptibility factors, such as age, atherosclerosis, and hypercoagulable and hyperviscosity conditions should be considered.

Hematologic　Severe *intravascular hemolysis*, possibly complicated by *disseminated intravascular coagulation*, is rare but was detected during post-marketing surveillance of WinRho®SDF, an intravenous human rhesus D immunoglobulin, in patients with idiopathic thrombocytopenic purpura (40[r]).

The incidence of *neutropenia* during 110 treatment courses in 104 children (average age 6.5 years) with idiopathic thrombocytopenic purpura has been studied retrospectively (41[c]). There were 64 courses of intravenous immunoglobulin (0.8–1 g/kg) and 46 treatment courses of anti-D immunoglobulin (50–75 micrograms/kg). Despite similar neutrophil counts at admission, 28% of those who were given intravenous immunoglobulin developed a neutrophil count below $1.5 \times 10^9/l$ compared with none of those who were given anti-D immunoglobulin. The disadvantages of treating idiopathic thrombocytopenic purpura with intravenous immunoglobulin are the occurrence of acute adverse effects: *flushing, headaches, chills, nausea, vomiting* in 1–15% of recipients, *aseptic meningitis* in 4–23%, and *renal insufficiency and failure* in 6% (mostly with sucrose-containing formulations) (42[R]).

Hyperviscosity with pseudohyponatremia has been attributed to high-dose intravenous immunoglobulin in a full-term child with hemolytic disease of the newborn (43[A]).

Liver　In 18 patients with Guillain–Barré syndrome standard high-dose intravenous immunoglobulin only has been compared with combined methylprednisolone plus high-dose intravenous immunoglobulin (44[A]). There were similar mild adverse effects in the two groups. There was *altered liver function*, the most common adverse effect, in two of those who were given intravenous immunoglobulin alone and in six in the combined treatment group. Headache occurred in two patients in both groups, suggesting that pre-infusion of a glucocorticoid does not prevent headache.

Drug formulations　In a controlled study with a new 10% formulation the risk of mild adverse reactions was higher than the 5% product (number of infusions: 9.6 versus 2.5%; number of patients with adverse reactions: 17 versus 8.6%) (45[A]).

Drug dosage regimens　In a double-blind randomized comparison of two different doses of intravenous immunoglobulin in myasthenia gravis (1 and 2 g/kg), there were many adverse events, such as *fever, chills, myalgia, headaches, nausea* or *vomiting, skin reactions, increased serum creatinine concentration*, and *increased serum transaminases*. However, most were minor and self-limiting and occurrence rates were similar between the two groups, except for headache, which was the most frequent adverse event and more common at the higher dose (46[C]).

Musculoskeletal   Of 217 children with Kawasaki disease retrospectively reviewed five developed a *polyarthropathy* after intravenous immunoglobulin at a mean of 10 days after the onset of fever and at a mean of 5.8 days after defervescence after the final dose of intravenous immunoglobulin (47[A]).

Interference with diagnostic tests   *Falsely high blood glucose readings* have been attributed to interference by WinRho®SDF, an intravenous human rhesus D immunoglobulin, or other maltose-containing intravenous immunoglobulin products when using systems that are not glucose-specific. The FDA released a safety alert about this issue for all maltose-containing intravenous immunoglobulins (48[S]). Another case of *false hyperglycemia* induced by a maltose-containing immunoglobulin solution was reported where the monitoring device using the principle of bioamperometry created a falsely high blood glucose reading by interference from maltose in the blood (49[R]).

COAGULATION PROTEINS
(SED-15, 845; SEDA-28, 375; SEDA-29, 345)

Factor VIIa

Recombinant factor VIIa was a useful adjunct in controlling active bleeding in children with Dengue hemorrhagic fever, when a platelet concentrate was not available (50[c]). No adverse events were considered to be related to the recombinant factor VIIa.

Cardiovascular   Serious complications of recombinant factor VIIa, such as *thromboembolic events*, occur but are rare (51[r]). The binding of recombinant factor VIIa to exposed tissue factor at the site of endothelial injury forms a complex that activates factor X, thereby producing thrombin. Atherosclerotic plaques express tissue factor, so that pharmacological doses of recombinant factor VIIa may cause acute thrombosis. If tissue factor is expressed on the surface of monocytes, as is the case in sepsis, widespread coagulation can occur and cause disseminated intravascular coagulation. Case series and dose-ranging studies have reported events of thrombosis, disseminated intravascular coagulation, and anaphylaxis at doses of recombinant factor VIIa of 5–120 micrograms/kg. In hemophiliac patients with inhibitors, for whom the product is indicated, it is estimated that one thrombotic event occurs for every 11 300 doses (52[R]). The frequency of thromboembolic events after the administration of recombinant factor VIIa 40 micrograms/kg to 108 patients with intracerebral hemorrhage was 7% compared with 2% with placebo ($n = 96$) (53[C]).

Susceptibility factors   The use of recombinant factor VIIa is associated with increased morbidity, with stroke and major thrombotic complications as risk factors (54[c]). Caution in cardiac surgery is recommended.

Factor VIII

Immunologic   The development of *antibodies* (so-called "inhibitors") to B-domain-deleted recombinant factor VIII concentrates has been studied in patients with severe hemophilia A (55[c]). Antibodies to fibrinogen, prothrombin, thrombin, factor V, factor XI, factor XII, the protein C system, and von Willebrand factor can cause bleeding or thrombosis (56[R]).

In a case-control study in 108 children with hemophilia A treated with recombinant factor VIII, prophylactic treatment had a protective effect on the development of inhibitors (57[C]).

One of 113 previously treated patients and 32 of 101 previously untreated patients developed inhibitors; of the latter, 16 had low titers and 16 had high titers. Immune tolerance induction therapy resulted in a disappearance of inhibitors in the majority, and at the end of the study inhibitors were still detectable in 7% of the 101 previously untreated patients.

In an open post-marketing surveillance study, 32 patients with hemophilia A received prophylaxis and 28 patients received on-demand treatment with recombinant factor VIII (ReFacto) over 6 months or 50 exposure days (58[C]). Surgical prophylaxis was evaluated in seven patients who required elective surgery. No new safety concerns appeared, although one previously treated patient developed a high-titer inhibitor, one minimally treated patient developed a low-titer inhibitor, and one previously untreated patient developed a transient low-titer inhibitor.

Factor IX

Hematologic   In a comparative study of two products containing double-inactivated factor IX, a high-purity factor IX concentrate and a prothrombin complex concentrate, in patients with hemophilia B, prothrombin complex concentrate caused increases in prothrombin fragment F1+2, and thrombin–antithrombin, illustrating the *coagulation activation properties* of the product. Although there were no thrombotic events, with repeated doses or in the presence of other thrombogenic susceptibility factors, such as liver disease, surgery, or prolonged immobilization, the potential thrombogenic activity of the concentrate should be considered (59[c]).

Immunologic   A neonate with severe hemophilia B with subgaleal and subdural hemorrhages was treated with a continuous infusion of recombinant factor IX 30–35 U/kg/hour; no thrombosis or inhibitor formation occurred (60[A]).

von Willebrand factor

Drug formulations   A new formulation of a von Willebrand factor concentrate containing only small amounts of factor VIII (Wilfactin®) was tested for its pharmacokinetic profile in patients with von Willebrand disease. The three virus inactivation/removal steps did not change the pharmacokinetic profile (61[c]).

ERYTHROPOIETIN AND DERIVATIVES   *(SED-15, 1243; SEDA-29, 346)*

Recombinant human erythropoietins (rHuEPO), epoetin alfa and epoetin beta (half-lives 8 hours)

and darbepoetin alfa (half-life 49 hours), are used to treat anemia in patients with chronic renal insufficiency and malignant diseases (SEDA-29, 346). Other uses include anemia in chronic heart failure, preoperative anemia, HIV treatment, and anemia after liver transplantation (62[A]).

The discovery that erythropoietin and its receptor play a significant role in tissues outside the hemopoietic system has fuelled interest in other indications, including cerebral ischemia, myocardial infarction, and chronic congestive heart failure (63[H]). In oncology, epoetin alfa and darbepoetin alfa are approved for patients with solid tumors and non-myeloid malignancies receiving chemotherapy, while the indication for epoetin beta is restricted to patients with solid tumors undergoing platinum-containing chemotherapy.

There is wide variation in dosage regimens in all patients. In patients with renal anemia, strategies with proven efficacy to reduce the rHuEPO requirement include iron supplementation, subcutaneous administration, correction of hyperparathyroidism, treatment of infections, and correction of aluminium intoxication (64[c]). In oncology, there is limited evidence that epoetins improve symptoms, fatigue, or the quality of life (62[R]).

The adverse effects are *thromboembolic complications, hypertension, and the production of anti-erythropoietin antibodies.* Systematic reviews of the effectiveness of erythropoietin in the treatment of patients with cancer showed that rHuEPO can reduce the need for red blood cell transfusion and increase hematological response rates, and that transfusion before epoetin alfa therapy increases the risks of future transfusions (65[M]).

Many questions remain to be investigated, including the effects on quality of life and symptoms, the effect of baseline hemoglobin concentrations on the use of rHuEPO, the role of iron replacement, the use of rHuEPO concentrations to guide therapy, the effect on anemia due to the underlying hematological malignancy, the delay in the treatment of mild anemia, tumor response, and survival (66[R], 67[R]).

Although there have been reports of experience with rHuEPO on preoperative autologous blood donation in young patients undergoing spinal surgery, caution in this off-label use in different transfusion policies is required (68[r]).

Cardiovascular Erythropoietin in patients with cancer was associated with a risk of *hypertension* (over 19% higher) and of *thromboembolic events* (over 58% more common) compared with controls, but the increases were not significant (66[R], 69[R]). Likewise, in patients with chronic renal anemia undergoing peritoneal dialysis, one of the most common adverse events was hypertension (70[C]).

Nervous system There may be an association between *headache* and epoetin beta (70[C]).

Hematologic Multiple doses of rHuEPO can produce adverse rheological effects, regardless of the increase in red cell mass; rHuEPO is procoagulant and predisposes to *thrombosis* (69[R]). Three trials of erythropoietin were stopped early because of a higher incidence of thrombotic events in the active treatment arm (71[S]).

Pure red cell aplasia has been reported after treatment with rHuEPO due to *anti-erythropoietin antibodies* (SEDA-29, 347) (72[A], 73[A]). There was no ethnic difference in the risk. Switching rHuEPO products was not beneficial, because of cross-reactivity (69[A]). However, epidemiological data, together with chemical and immunological data, support the hypothesis that leachates in the polysorbate 80 formulation from uncoated rubber syringe stoppers increase the risk of pure red cell aplasia associated with epoetin alfa (Eprex) (70[H]).

There have been no reports of pure red cell aplasia associated with the use of rHuEPO in patients with cancer, probably because of a reduction in immune competence, other therapies, and reduced time of exposure to the drug (69[R]).

Skin Fatal *erythema multiforme* and *drug rash with eosinophilia and systemic symptoms (DRESS)* has been reported after a single subcutaneous dose of epoetin alfa (74[A]).

Infection risk In patients with chronic renal anemia undergoing peritoneal dialysis, one of the most common adverse events was *peritonitis* (68[C]).

Tumorigenicity There is increasing evidence that rHuEPO supports and extends *tumor growth*, since tumor cells can use the erythropoietin system for growth and angiogenesis (67[R]).

SERINE PROTEASE INHIBITORS

Serine protease inhibitors are found in the plasma and some are manufactured by fractionation from plasma obtained from blood donors. In a substrate-based development programme, a specific and potent peptidomimetic inhibitor, BILN-2061, of the hepatitis C virus NS3 protease has been shown to lower serum HCV-RNA markedly in patients chronically infected with the HCV genotype 1, and less pronounced and more variable in patients with HCV genotypes 2 and 3. In a small prospective, multicenter, double-blind, placebo-controlled, proof-of-principle study in eight patients, adverse events that were possibly drug related included mild constitutional symptoms, such as a *drunken feeling, fatigue, somnolence*, and mild *gastrointestinal symptoms* (75[c]).

STEM CELLS *(SEDA-29, 347)*

Mesenchymal stem cells provide a source for models of differentiation, cell therapy, and regenerative medicine. There are increasing reports that they can be isolated from various adult mesenchymal tissues, such as synovium, periosteum, skeletal muscle, and adipose tissue, as well as bone marrow. Their properties can be affected by their preparation, which has not been properly controlled for in some studies (76[R]). Umbilical cord blood is an alternative source of hemopoietic stem cells.

Immunologic Graft-versus-host disease has been reported after stem cell transplantation (77[A]).

- An 11-year-old boy with severe chronic active Epstein–Barr virus infection underwent successful cord blood transplantation after consecutive failure of peripheral blood and bone marrow transplants from his HLA-mismatched mother. Cord blood cells from an unrelated donor were infused after conditioning with total body irradiation (12 Gy), melphalan (120 mg/m^2), and etoposide (600 mg/m^2). Complete remission without circulating EB virus DNA continued for 15 months after delayed hematological recovery, with renal bleeding, skin graft-versus-host-disease (grade II), dissemination of herpes zoster, and hepatospleno-megaly.

Increasing numbers of stem cell transplantations using non-myeloablative or reduced-intensity conditioning are being performed. Compared with conventional-intensity conditioning, reduced-intensity conditioning results in a higher incidence of *Epstein–Barr viremia* and *lymphoproliferative disease* after stem cell transplantation (78[c]). *Graft failure* is another serious complication (79[c]).

Immunologic   The expression of the minor histocompatibility antigen UGT2B17 has been implicated in graft-versus-host disease after HLA-identical hemopoietic stem cell transplantation. In 435 stem cell recipients there was no association with graft-versus-host disease, but UGT2B17 was an independent susceptibility factor for transplant-related mortality and lower survival after allogeneic HLA-identical hemopoietic stem cell in UGT2B17-deleted recipients (80[c]).

References

1. Pradel V. Conclusions are misleading. Crit Care Med 2005;33(4):914.
2. Seppelt I, Burrell A. Human albumin meta-analysis. Crit Care Med 2005;33(4):914–5.
3. Regtien JG, Stienstra Y, Ligtenberg JJ, van der Werf TS, Tulleken JE, Zijlstra JG. Morbidity in hospitalized patients receiving human albumin: a meta-analysis of randomized, controlled trials. Crit Care Med 2005;33(4):915.
4. Arellano R, Gan BS, Salpeter MJ, Yeo E, McCluskey S, Pinto R, Irish J, Ross DC, Doyle DJ, Parkin J, Brown D, Rotstein L, Witterick I, Matthews W, Yoo J, Neligan PC, Gullane P, Lampe H. A triple-blinded randomized trial comparing the hemostatic effects of large-dose 10% hydroxyethyl starch 264/0.45 versus 5% albumin during major reconstructive surgery. Anesth Analg 2005;100(6):1846–53.
5. Castelli EE, Culley CM, Fink MP. Challenge and rechallenge: drotrecogin alfa (activated)-induced prolongation of activated partial thromboplastin time in a patient with severe sepsis. Pharmacotherapy 2005;25(8):1147–50.
6. Pastores SM, Shaw A, Williams MD, Mongan E, Alicea M, Halpern NA. A safety evaluation of drotrecogin alfa (activated) in hematopoietic stem cell transplant patients with severe sepsis: lessons in clinical research. Bone Marrow Transplant 2005;36(8):721–4.
7. Serious Hazards of Transfusion Office, Manchester E. Serious Hazards of Transfusion (SHOT). Annual Report 2004. 2005.
8. TRIP Office, The Hague, The Netherlands. Transfusie Reacties in Patienten (TRIP). Rapport 2004. 2005.
9. National Haemovigilance Office, Dublin I. National Haemovigilance Office. Annual Report 2004. 2005.
10. Japanese Red Cross Blood Service Headquarters, Tokyo J. Haemovigilance Annual Report 2003 and 1993–2002. 2005.
11. Finlay HE, Cassorla L, Feiner J, Toy P. Designing and testing a computer-based screening system for transfusion-related acute lung injury. Am J Clin Pathol 2005;124(4):601–9.
12. Dara SI, Rana R, Afessa B, Moore SB, Gajic O. Fresh frozen plasma transfusion in critically ill medical patients with coagulopathy. Crit Care Med 2005;33(11):2667–71.
13. Lee TH, Paglieroni T, Utter GH, Chafets D, Gosselin RC, Reed W, Owings JT, Holland PV, Busch MP. High-level long-term white blood cell microchimerism after transfusion of leuko-reduced blood components to patients resuscitated after severe traumatic injury. Transfusion 2005;45(8):1280–90.
14. Morishita K, Wakamoto S, Miyazaki T, Sato S, Fujihara M, Kaneko S, Yasuda H, Yamamoto S, Azuma H, Kato T, Ikeda H. Life-threatening adverse reaction followed by thrombocytopenia after passive transfusion of fresh frozen plasma containing anti-CD36 (Naka) isoantibody. Transfusion 2005;45(5):803–6.
15. Sage D, Stanworth S, Turner D, Navarrete C. Diagnosis of transfusion-associated graft-vs.-host disease: the importance of short tandem repeat analysis. Transfusion Med 2005;15(6):481–5.
16. Tawk HM, Vickery K, Bisset L, Lo SK, Cossart YE. The significance of transfusion in the past as a risk for current hepatitis B and hepatitis C infection: a study in endoscopy patients. Transfusion 2005;45(5):807–13.
17. Plentz A, Hahn J, Knoll A, Holler E, Jilg W, Modrow S. Exposure of hematologic patients to parvovirus B19 as a contaminant of blood cell preparations and blood products. Transfusion 2005;45(11):1811–5.

18. Health Protection Agency U. New case of CJD associated with blood transfusion. www.hpa.org.uk, 2006.
19. Ludlam CA, Turner ML. Managing the risk of transmission of variant Creutzfeldt Jakob disease by blood products. Br J Haematol 2006;132(1):13–24.
20. Sowemimo-Coker S, Kascsak R, Kim A, Andrade F, Pesci S, Kascsak R, Meeker C, Carp R, Brown P. Removal of exogenous (spiked) and endogenous prion infectivity from red cells with a new prototype of leukoreduction filter. Transfusion 2005;45(12):1839–44.
21. Leclercq A, Martin L, Vergnes ML, Ounnoughene N, Laran JF, Giraud P, Carniel E. Fatal *Yersinia enterocolitica* biotype 4 serovar O:3 sepsis after red blood cell transfusion. Transfusion 2005;45(5):814–8.
22. Raghavan M, Marik PE. Anemia, allogenic blood transfusion, and immunomodulation in the critically ill. Chest 2005;127(1):295–307.
23. Buchta C, Bittner C, Heinzl H, Höcker P, Macher M, Mayerhofer M, Schmid R, Seger C, Dettke M. Transfusion-related exposure to the plasticizer di(2-ethylhexyl)phthalate in patients receiving plateletpheresis concentrates. Transfusion 2005;45(5):798–802.
24. Hill SE, Grocott HP, Leone BJ, White WD, Newman MF, Neurologic Outcome Research Group of the Duke Heart Center. Cerebral physiology of cardiac surgical patients treated with the perfluorocarbon emulsion, AF0144. Ann Thorac Surg 2005;80(4):1401–7.
25. Longhurst HJ. Emergency treatment of acute attacks in hereditary angioedema due to C1 inhibitor deficiency: what is the evidence? Int J Clin Pract 2005;59(5):594–9.
26. García-Noblejas A, Osorio S, Durán AI, Córdoba R, Nistal S, Aguado B, Loscertales J, Gómez N. Pulmonary embolism in a patient with severe congenital deficiency for factor V during treatment with fresh frozen plasma. Haemophilia 2005;11(3):276–9.
27. Fenger-Eriksen C, Anker-Moller E, Heslop J, Ingerslev J, Sorensen B. Thrombelastographic whole blood clot formation after ex vivo addition of plasma substitutes: improvements of the induced coagulopathy with fibrinogen concentrate. Br J Anaesth 2005;94(3):324–9.
28. Ewaldsson CA, Hahn RG. Bolus injection of Ringer's solution and dextran 1 kDa during induction of spinal anesthesia. Acta Anaesthesiol Scand 2005;49(2):152–9.
29. Ritchey RM, Helfand RF, Irefin SA, Argalious M, Tetzlaff JE. Hetastarch allergy and positive latex radioallergosorbent test in a patient suffering cardiovascular decompensation during multiple perioperative periods. Anesth Analg 2005;101(6):1709–12.
30. Anonymous. Colloids. Safety considerations important in choosing resuscitation fluids. WHO Newslett 2006;4:7.
31. Benavides C, Mahmoud KH, Knight R, Barcenas C, Kahan BD, Van Buren CT. Rabbit antithymocyte globulin: a postoperative risk factor

for sirolimus-treated renal transplant patients? Transplant Proc 2005;37(2):822–6.
32. Ahmad M. Graft mucormycosis in a renal allograft recipient. J Nephrol 2005;18(6):783–6.
33. Peres E, Savasan S, Klein J, Abidi M, Dansey R, Abella E. High fatality rate of Epstein–Barr virus-associated lymphoproliferative disorder occurring after bone marrow transplantation with rabbit antithymocyte globulin conditioning regimens. J Clin Microbiol 2005;43(7):3540–3.
34. Jolles S, Sewell WA, Misbah SA. Clinical uses of intravenous immunoglobulin. Clin Exp Immunol 2005;142(1):1–11.
35. Durandy A, Wahn V, Petteway S, Gelfand EW. Immunoglobulin replacement therapy in primary antibody deficiency diseases— maximizing success. Int Arch Allergy Immunol 2005;136(3):217–29.
36. Kamali S, Cefle A, Sayarlioglu M, Gul A, Inanc M, Ocal L, Aral O, Konice M. Experience with monthly, high-dose, intravenous immunoglobulin therapy in patients with different connective tissue diseases. Rheumatol Int 2005;25(3):211–4.
37. Bloom B, Schelonka R, Kueser T, Walker W, Jung E, Kaufman D, Kesler K, Roberson D, Patti J, Hetherington S, INH-A21 Phase II Study Team. Multicenter study to assess safety and efficacy of INH-A21, a donor-selected human staphylococcal immunoglobulin, for prevention of nosocomial infections in very low birth weight infants. Pediatr Infect Dis J 2005;24(10):858–66.
38. Geller JL, Hackner D. Diffuse venous thromboemboli associated with IVIg therapy in the treatment of streptococcal toxic shock syndrome: case report and review. Ann Hematol 2005;84(9):601–4.
39. Alexandrescu DT, Dutcher JP, Hughes JT, Kaplan J, Wiernik PH. Strokes after intravenous gamma globulin: thrombotic phenomenon in patients with risk factors or just coincidence? Am J Hematol 2005;78(3):216–20.
40. Gaines AR. Disseminated intravascular coagulation associated with acute hemoglobinemia or hemoglobinuria following Rh(0)(D) immune globulin intravenous administration for immune thrombocytopenic purpura. Blood 2005;106(5):1532–7.
41. Niebanck AE, Kwiatkowski JL, Raffini LJ. Neutropenia following IVIG therapy in pediatric patients with immune-mediated thrombocytopenia. J Pediatr Hematol Oncol 2005;27(3):145–7.
42. Shad AT, Gonzalez CE, Sandler SG. Treatment of immune thrombocytopenic purpura in children: current concepts. Paediatr Drugs 2005;7(5):325–36.
43. Tarcan A, Gokmen Z, Dikmenoglu N, Gurakan B. Pseudohyponatraemia and hyperviscosity due to IVIG therapy in a term newborn. Acta Paediatr 2005;94(4):509–10.
44. Odaka M, Tatsumoto M, Hoshiyama E, Hirata K, Yuki N. Side effects of combined therapy of methylprednisolone and intravenous immunoglobulin in Guillain–Barré syndrome. Eur Neurol 2005;53(4):194–6.

45. Matamoros N, de Gracia J, Hernandez F, Pons J, Alvarez A, Jimenez V. A prospective controlled crossover trial of a new presentation (10 vs. 5%) of a heat-treated intravenous immunoglobulin. Int Immunopharmacol 2005;5(3):619–26.

46. Gajdos P, Tranchant C, Clair B, Bolgert F, Eymard B, Stojkovic T, Attarian S, Chevret S, Myasthenia Gravis Clinical Study Group. Treatment of myasthenia gravis exacerbation with intravenous immunoglobulin: a randomized double-blind clinical trial. Arch Neurol 2005;62(11):1689–93.

47. Lee KY, Oh JH, Han JW, Lee JS, Lee BC. Arthritis in Kawasaki disease after responding to intravenous immunoglobulin treatment. Eur J Pediatr 2005;164(7):451–2.

48. US Food and Drug Administration. Important safety information on interference with blood glucose measurement following use of parenteral maltose/parenteral galactose/oral xylose-containing products. www.fda.gov, 2006.

49. Souza SP, Castro MC, Rodrigues RA, Passos RH, Ianhez LE. False hyperglycemia induced by polyvalent immunoglobulins. Transplantation 2005;80(4):542–3.

50. Chuansumrit A, Wangruangsatid S, Lektrakul Y, Chua MN, Zeta Capeding MR, Bech OM. Control of bleeding in children with dengue hemorrhagic fever using recombinant activated factor VII: a randomized, double-blind, placebo-controlled study. Blood Coagul Fibrinolysis 2005;16(8):549–55.

51. Roberts HR. Recombinant factor VIIa: how safe is the stuff? Can J Anaesth 2005;52(1):8–11.

52. MacLaren R, Weber LA, Brake H, Gardner MA, Tanzi M. A multicenter assessment of recombinant factor VIIa off-label usage: clinical experiences and associated outcomes. Transfusion 2005;45(9):1434–42.

53. Mayer SA, Brun NC, Begtrup K, Broderick J, Davis S, Diringer MN, Skolnick BE, Steiner T, Recombinant Activated Factor VII Intracerebral Hemorrhage Trial Investigators. Recombinant activated factor VII for acute intracerebral hemorrhage. N Engl J Med 2005;352(8):777–85.

54. Karkouti K, Beattie WS, Wijeysundera DN, Yau TM, McCluskey SA, Ghannam M, Sutton D, van Rensburg A, Karski J. Recombinant factor VIIa for intractable blood loss after cardiac surgery: a propensity score-matched case-control analysis. Transfusion 2005;45(1):26–34.

55. Tjernberg P, Vos HL, Castaman G, Bertina RM, Eikenboom JC. Dimerization and multimerization defects of von Willebrand factor due to mutated cysteine residues. J Thromb Haemost 2004;2(2):257–65.

56. Lollar P. Pathogenic antibodies to coagulation factors. Part II. Fibrinogen, prothrombin, thrombin, factor V, factor XI, factor XII, factor XIII, the protein C system and von Willebrand factor. J Thromb Haemost 2005;3(7):1385–91.

57. Santagostino E, Mancuso ME, Rocino A, Mancuso G, Mazzucconi MG, Tagliaferri A, Messina M, Mannucci PM. Environmental risk factors for inhibitor development in children

with haemophilia A: a case-control study. Br J Haematol 2005;130(3):422–7.

58. Smith MP, Giangrande P, Pollman H, Littlewood R, Kollmer C, Feingold J. A postmarketing surveillance study of the safety and efficacy of ReFacto (St Louis-derived active substance) in patients with haemophilia A. Haemophilia 2005;11(5):444–51.

59. Ruiz-Sáez A, Hong A, Arguello A, Echenagucia M, Boadas A, Fabbrizzi F, Minichilli F, Bosch NB. Pharmacokinetics, thrombogenicity and safety of a double viral inactivated factor IX concentrate compared with a prothrombin complex concentrate. Haemophilia 2005;11(6):583–8.

60. Guilcher GM, Scully MF, Harvey M, Hand JP. Treatment of intracranial and extracranial haemorrhages in a neonate with severe haemophilia B with recombinant factor IX infusion. Haemophilia 2005;11(4):411–4.

61. Goudemand J, Scharrer I, Berntorp E, Lee CA, Borel-Derlon A, Stieltjes N, Caron C, Scherrmann JM, Bridey F, Tellier Z, Federici AB, Mannucci PM. Pharmacokinetic studies on Wilfactin, a von Willebrand factor concentrate with a low factor VIII content treated with three virus-inactivation/removal methods. J Thromb Haemost 2005;3(10):2219–27.

62. Engert A. Recombinant human erythropoietin in oncology: current status and further developments. Ann Oncol 2005;16(10):1584–95.

63. Maiese K, Li F, Chong ZZ. New avenues of exploration for erythropoietin. JAMA 2005;293(1):90–5.

64. Kadiroglu AK, Yilmaz ME, Sit D, Kara IH, Isikoglu B. The evaluation of postdialysis L-carnitine administration and its effect on weekly requiring doses of rHuEPO in hemodialysis patients. Ren Fail 2005;27(4):367–72.

65. Couture F, Turner AR, Melosky B, Xiu L, Plante RK, Lau CY, Quirt I. Prior red blood cell transfusions in cancer patients increase the risk of subsequent transfusions with or without recombinant human erythropoietin management. Oncologist 2005;10(1):63–71.

66. Bohlius J, Langensiepen S, Schwarzer G, Seidenfeld J, Piper M, Bennett C, Engert A. Recombinant human erythropoietin and overall survival in cancer patients: results of a comprehensive meta-analysis. J Natl Cancer Inst 2005;97(7):489–98.

67. Djulbegovic B. Erythropoietin use in oncology: a summary of the evidence and practice guidelines comparing efforts of the Cochrane Review group and Blue Cross/Blue Shield to set up the ASCO/ASH guidelines. Best Pract Res Clin Haematol 2005;18(3):455–66.

68. Franchini M, Gandini G, Regis D, de Gironcoli M, Cantini M, Aprili G. Recombinant human erythropoietin facilitates autologous blood collections in children undergoing corrective spinal surgery. Transfusion 2004;44(7):1122–4.

69. Stasi R, Amadori S, Littlewood TJ, Terzoli E, Newland AC, Provan D. Management of cancer-related anemia with erythropoietic agents:

doubts, certainties, and concerns. Oncologist 2005;10(7):539–54.

70. Grzeszczak W, Sulowicz W, Rutkowski B, de Vecchi AF, Scanziani R, Durand PY, Bajo A, Vargemezis V, European Collaborative Group. The efficacy and safety of once-weekly and once-fortnightly subcutaneous epoetin beta in peritoneal dialysis patients with chronic renal anaemia. Nephrol Dial Transplant 2005;20(5):936–44.

71. Department of Health and Human Services FaDA, Center for Drug Evaluation and Research ODAC. Minutes of the Meeting of Tuesday, May 4, 2004. http://www.fda.gov?OHRMS/DOCKETS/ac/04/transcripts/4037T2.DOC, 24-6-2005.

72. Shinohara K, Mitani N, Miyazaki M, Sakuragi S, Matsuda K, Ogawara S, Saito T, Kaneoka H, Ooji T. Pure red-cell aplasia caused by the antibody to recombinant erythropoietin, epoetin-beta, in a Japanese patient with chronic renal failure. Am J Hematol 2005;78(1):15–20.

73. Praditpornsilpa K, Buranasot S, Bhokaisuwan N, Avihingsanon Y, Pisitkul T, Kansanabuch T, Eiam-Ong S, Chusil S, Intarakumtornchai T, Tungsanga K. Recovery from anti-recombinant-human-erythropoietin associated pure red cell aplasia in end-stage renal disease patients after renal transplantation. Nephrol Dial Transplant 2005;20(3):626–30.

74. Norgard N, Wall GC. Possible drug rash with eosinophilia and systemic symptoms syndrome after exposure to epoetin alfa. Am J Health Syst Pharm 2005;62(23):2524–6.

75. Reiser M, Hinrichsen H, Benhamou Y, Reesink HW, Wedemeyer H, Avendano C, Riba N, Yong CL, Nehmiz G, Steinmann GG. Antiviral efficacy of NS3-serine protease inhibitor BILN-2061 in patients with chronic genotype 2 and 3 hepatitis C. Hepatology 2005;41(4):832–5.

76. Sakaguchi Y, Sekiya I, Yagishita K, Muneta T. Comparison of human stem cells derived from various mesenchymal tissues: superiority of synovium as a cell source. Arthritis Rheum 2005;52(8):2521–9.

77. Ishimura M, Ohga S, Nomura A, Toubo T, Morihana E, Saito Y, Nishio H, Ide M, Takada H, Hara T. Successful umbilical cord blood transplantation for severe chronic active Epstein–Barr virus infection after the double failure of hematopoietic stem cell transplantation. Am J Hematol 2005;80(3):207–12.

78. Cohen J, Gandhi M, Naik P, Cubitt D, Rao K, Thaker U, Davies EG, Gaspar HB, Amrolia PJ, Veys P. Increased incidence of EBV-related disease following paediatric stem cell transplantation with reduced-intensity conditioning. Br J Haematol 2005;129(2):229–39.

79. Narimatsu H, Kami M, Miyakoshi S, Murashige N, Yuji K, Hamaki T, Masuoka K, Kusumi E, Kishi Y, Matsumura T, Wake A, Morinaga S, Kanda Y, Taniguchi S. Graft failure following reduced-intensity cord blood transplantation for adult patients. Br J Haematol 2006;132(1):36–41.

80. Terakura S, Murata M, Nishida T, Emi N, Akatsuka Y, Riddell SR, Morishima Y, Kodera Y, Naoe T. A UGT2B17-positive donor is a risk factor for higher transplant-related mortality and lower survival after bone marrow transplantation. Br J Haematol 2005;129(2):221–8.

M.C. Allwood and P.A. Ball

34 Vitamins, intravenous solutions, and drugs and formulations used in nutrition

VITAMINS *(SED-15, 3686)*

Drug–drug interactions

Multivitamins The systemic availability of *gatifloxacin* may be reduced by multivitamin formulations (1[A]).

- A 77-year-old white woman was given gatifloxacin for a hospital-acquired bacterial pneumonia. She was also taking calcium carbonate 500 mg bd and a multivitamin formulation containing minerals once a day. Three days later she was still febrile, coughing, and not responding clinically. It was noted that the tablet of gatifloxacin was being administered at the same time as the multivitamin tablet. The time of administration of gatifloxacin was changed to 6 hours after the multivitamin formulation, and 2 days later she improved clinically.

The systemic availability of gatifloxacin is reduced by concurrent administration of antacids that contain aluminium or magnesium, by dietary supplements that contain zinc, magnesium, and iron, and by multivitamin formulations that contain minerals and sucralfate. This case illustrates the need to recognize this potential interaction, which was probably due to the mineral content of the multivitamin formulation.

VITAMIN C (ASCORBIC ACID)
(SED-15, 351)

Drug–drug interactions A potentially life-threatening interaction between a complementary medicine, *amygdalin*, and vitamin C has been reported (2[A]). The case involved severe accidental cyanide poisoning after a single dose of amygdalin with therapeutic intent.

- A 68-year-old patient with cancer took a single dose of amygdalin 3 g and developed impaired consciousness, seizures, and severe lactic acidosis, and required intubation and ventilation. She was also taking vitamin C 4800 mg/day. She responded rapidly to hydroxocobalamin. The adverse drug reaction was rated probable on the Naranjo probability scale.

Amygdalin and laetrile (a synthetic form of amygdalin) are commonly used as alternative medicines in the treatment of cancer. Vitamin C increases the in vitro conversion of amygdalin to cyanide and reduces body stores of cysteine, which is used to detoxify cyanide. The authors concluded that an interaction with vitamin C was a plausible explanation for this life-threatening effect.

VITAMIN D ANALOGUES
(SED-15, 3669; SEDA-28, 388; SEDA-29, 354)

Mineral metabolism In a double-blind, placebo-controlled study in secondary hyperparathyroidism in children, intravenous calcitriol (1,25-dihydroxycolecalciferol) produced two consecutive $\geqslant 30\%$ *reductions in parathyroid hormone concentrations* in 11/21 patients compared with 5/26 in the placebo group (3[C]). There was a greater effect in 12 patients aged 2–12 years than in 35 patients aged 13–18 years, but this may have been an artefact, because the children in the lower age group received a larger dose per kg body weight. The major adverse effect was *hyperphosphatemia*, which limited the total dose.

Side Effects of Drugs, Annual 30
J.K. Aronson (Editor)
ISSN: 0378-6080
DOI: 10.1016/S0378-6080(08)00034-2

Vitamin E   (SED-15, 3677;

SEDA-29, 355)

Cardiovascular   A possible link between long-term use of vitamin E and an increased risk of *heart failure* has been identified from an extensive analysis of experimental and epidemiological data related to the possible prevention of cancer and cardiovascular events by vitamin E supplementation (4^C). In fact, clinical trials have generally failed to confirm benefits, possibly because of their relatively short duration. The objective of this study was to evaluate whether long-term supplementation with vitamin E reduces the risks of cancer, death from cancer, and major cardiovascular events. The study, HOPE-TOO (HOPE–The Ongoing Outcomes), was an extension of a randomized, double-blind, placebo-controlled international study (the Heart Outcomes Prevention Evaluation, HOPE, study) in patients aged at least 55 years with vascular disease or diabetes mellitus. Of the initial 267 centers that had enrolled 9541 patients in HOPE, 174 centers participated in HOPE-TOO. Of 7030 patients enrolled at these centers, 916 were already dead at the beginning of the extension study, 1382 refused to participate, 3994 continued to take part, and 738 agreed to passive follow-up (median duration 7.0 years). The intervention comprised a daily dose of natural source vitamin E 400 IU or matching placebo. The primary outcome measures were the incidences of cancer, cancer deaths, and major cardiovascular events (myocardial infarction, stroke, and cardiovascular deaths). Secondary outcomes included heart failure, unstable angina, and revascularization. Among all the HOPE patients, there were no significant differences in the primary analysis between vitamin E and placebo:

- for cancer incidence, 552 (11.6%) versus 586 (12.3%) respectively (RR = 0.94; 95% CI = 0.84, 1.06);
- for cancer deaths 156 (3.3%) versus 178 (3.7%) respectively (RR = 0.88; 95% CI = 0.71, 1.09);
- for major cardiovascular events 1022 (21.5%) versus 985 (20.6%) respectively (RR = 1.04; 95% CI = 0.96, 1.14).

However, one significant finding was that patients who took vitamin E had a higher risk of

heart failure (RR = 1.13; 95% CI = 1.01, 1.26) and hospitalization for heart failure (RR = 1.21; 95% CI = 1.00, 1.47). Similarly, among patients enrolled at the centers that participated in HOPE-TOO, there were no differences in cancer incidence, cancer deaths, or major cardiovascular events, but higher rates of heart failure and hospitalization for heart failure. The authors concluded that in patients with vascular disease or diabetes mellitus, long-term vitamin E supplementation does not prevent cancer or major cardiovascular events and may increase the risk of heart failure.

Pregnancy   Oxidative stress is related to an imbalance in the concentrations of harmful oxidants, such as free radicals. One condition in which oxidative stress may contribute is pre-eclampsia. It is therefore possible that the risk of pre-eclampsia is related to dietary intake of vitamins C and E, and this has been explored prospectively in 299 pregnant women who attended an antenatal clinic in Adelaide (5^C). The median intake of vitamin C was 188 mg/day and of vitamin E 6.74 mg/day. There was no relation between the intake of vitamin C and hypertensive disorders of pregnancy. However, there was an association between low vitamin E intake and an increased risk of hypertensive disorders (RR = 1.75; 95% CI = 1.11, 2.75). This effect was confirmed after adjusting for the confounding factors of maternal age and parity.

Drug–drug interactions   A potential interaction between vitamin E and *ciclosporin* has been reported in a retrospective study in heart transplant recipients (6^c). In a chart review of the first 29 heart transplant recipients who received antioxidant agents (vitamin C 500 mg bd and vitamin E 400 IU bd), 22 were taking ciclosporin and seven tacrolimus. The baseline ciclosporin trough concentration was 137 ng/ml and it fell significantly to 99 ng/ml (average fall 30%) after the start of antioxidant therapy. There were no significant changes in tacrolimus concentrations. More detailed pharmacokinetic analysis is required to clarify the exact mechanism of this interaction, but the authors recommended that more frequent ciclosporin concentration monitoring is warranted in patients taking vitamins C and E.

AMINO ACIDS

Arginine

Placebo-controlled studies   L-arginine is an amino acid that is commonly used to sustain and promote healthy heart function. According to Health Canada, patients who have previously had a heart attack should not use arginine supplements, because of recent evidence that there is an increased risk of death in these circumstances (7^S). In a randomized, double-blind, placebo-controlled study, 153 patients were randomly assigned after a first ST-segment elevation myocardial infarction to L-arginine or matching placebo for 6 months (8^C). The dosage of arginine was 1 g tds for 1 week, 2 g tds in week 2, and 3 g tds in subsequent weeks for 6 months. Six (8.6%) of those who took L-arginine died during the 6-month study period compared with none in the placebo group. Because of concerns about safety, the data and safety monitoring committee closed enrolment to the study. The authors proposed several possible mechanisms. The proposed beneficial mechanism of arginine is increased nitric oxide synthesis by vascular endothelium, since arginine is a substrate for the endothelial-specific isoform of nitric oxide synthase (eNOS). However, if there is deficiency of tetrahydrobiopterin, a co-factor for nitric oxide synthase, instead of generating nitric oxide eNOS becomes a source of reactive oxygen species, and this could be enhanced by arginine. Arginine supplementation also increases homocysteine production, which can result in worsening of endothelial function and atherosclerosis. Furthermore, if there is atherosclerosis, the inducible isoform of nitric oxide synthase (iNOS) is expressed, resulting in the production of peroxynitrite and consumption of nitric oxide, potentially worsening atherosclerosis. All arginine products are now required to carry a warning on their label about the risk of using them after myocardial infarction. Health Canada has advised that for patients who have not had a previous heart attack, taking arginine is unlikely to present a risk and may provide benefits by helping the body repair damaged vessels in the heart.

ENTERAL NUTRITION   *(SED-15, 1221; SEDA-27, 355; SEDA-28, 383)*

Comparative studies   In a meta-analysis of 30 randomized controlled trials, enteral nutrition was compared with early parenteral nutrition in hospital in-patients (9^M). Early nutrition was defined as the initiation of nutrition support within 96 hours of hospital admission, ICU admission, or surgery. Only studies in which hospital mortality, length of stay, and/or complications had been reported were included. The analysis excluded all non-English language studies and those associated with "immunonutrition", including arginine, nucleotides, omega-3 fatty acids, and glutamine; this poorly reflects recent practice in intensive care units, in which glutamine-containing parenteral nutrition solutions are being increasingly used. Of the 30 studies, 10 were in medical patients, 11 in surgical patients, and 9 in trauma patients. Parenteral nutrition was associated with a 7.9% increase in infective complications, a 3.5% increase in *catheter-related blood-stream infections*, a 4.9% increase in *non-infective complications*, and an *increase in the length of stay* by 1.2 days. There was no effect of nutrition type on mortality or on technical complications, but enteral nutrition was associated with an increased risk of *diarrhea*. The authors acknowledged that as nutritional support has become more interventional, the numbers of complications have increased, particularly in the more interventional forms of enteral nutrition. They also noted that enteral nutrition is generally associated with lower nutritional intake overall.

PARENTERAL NUTRITION
(SED-15, 2700; SEDA-27, 355; SEDA-28, 383; SEDA-29, 353)

Comparative studies   See above, under *Enteral nutrition.*

Management of adverse reactions   *Cholestasis and cholelithiasis* are common complications of parenteral nutrition. The frequency of cholestasis in neonates on long-term parenteral nutrition is still reported to be 7–13%, associated with increased mortality and septic complications. In a randomized, blind, controlled trial of parenteral nutrition in 38 neonates (25 premature, eight with necrotizing enterocolitis, and five after abdominal surgery), the hypothesis that cholecystokinin-octapeptide administered concurrently with parenteral nutrition would prevent gallstone formation was tested (10[c]). Parenteral nutrition was given for a mean of 33 days. Four patients developed gallstones, including three in the treatment group. Gallstone formation was not affected by cholecystokinin and was not related to the underlying diagnosis, birth weight, gestational age, or duration of parenteral nutrition. The four patients with gallstones and two others who were not in the study were then given a prolonged course of ursodeoxycholic acid (mean duration 11.6 months), with serial ultrasound examinations at 6-monthly intervals. In none was there any degree of gallstone dissolution. There were no reported adverse reactions to either cholecystokinin or ursodeoxycholic acid.

Fat emulsions

Fat emulsions were once considered to be primarily a high-density source of energy in parenteral nutrition, but attention is now being increasingly focussed on fat emulsions as a source of important biological precursors with wider effects. These may become particularly important in long-term therapy, such as parenteral nutrition at home. Clinoleic® (Baxter–Clintec, Maurepas, France) is prepared from a mixture of soy bean oil 20% and olive oil 80%. Compared with other fat emulsions on the market, it contains 60% monounsaturated fatty acids, around 20% less polyunsaturated fatty acids, and no medium-chain triglycerides. In a non-randomized observational study in 14 patients (median age 50, range 35–79, years; 8 men) receiving long-term parenteral nutrition at home the new emulsion produced significantly lower plasma α-linolenic acid concentrations, but did not affect overall essential fatty acid status (11[c]). There were no adverse effects. In particular, some adverse effects that are commonly reported with other lipid emulsions (shivering, nausea, tachycardia, pyrexia, and hypertension) were not reported, although this is difficult to interpret as it was not stated whether any of these patients had had these symptoms during previous administration of other emulsions. However, five patients had reported migraine without aura during previous infusions; of these, three claimed to feel consistently better with the new emulsion at 3 months.

References

1. Mallet L, Huang A. Coadministration of gatifloxacin and multivitamin preparation containing minerals: potential treatment failure in an elderly patient. Ann Pharmacother 2005;39:150–2.

2. Bromley J, Hughes BGM, Leong DCS, Buckley NA. Life-threatening interaction between complementary medicines: cyanide toxicity following ingestion of amygdalin and vitamin C. Ann Pharmacother 2005;39:1566–9.

3. Greenbaum LA, Grenda R, Qiu P, Restaino I, Wojtak A, Paredes A, Benador N, Melnick JZ, Williams LA, Salusky IB. Intravenous calcitriol for treatment of hyperparathyroidism in children on haemodialysis. Pediatr Nephrol 2005;20:622–30.

4. Lonn E. Effects of long-term vitamin E supplementation on cardiovascular events and cancer: a randomized controlled trial. JAMA 2005;293:1338–47.

5. Rumbold AR, Maats FHE, Crowther CA. Dietary intake of vitamin C and vitamin E and the development of hypertensive disorders of pregnancy. Eur J Obs Gynecol Reproduc Biol 2005;119:67–71.

6. Lake KD, Aaronson KD, Gorman LE, Pagani FD, Koelling TM. Effect of oral vitamin E and C therapy on calcineurin inhibitor levels in heart transplant recipients. J Heart Lung Transplant 2005;24:990–4.

7. Anonymous. L-arginine. Not for heart patients. WHO Newslett 2006;3:1.

8. Schulman SP, Becker LC, Kass DA, Champion HC, Terrin ML, Forman S, Ernst KV, Keleman MD, Townsend SN, Capriotti A, Hare JH, Gerstenblith G. L-arginine therapy in acute myocardial infraction. The Vascular Interaction with Age in Myocardial Infarction (VINTAGE MI) Randomized Clinical Trial. JAMA 2006;295:58–64.

9. Peter JV, Moran JL, Phillips-Hughes J. A meta-analysis of treatment outcomes of early enteral versus early parenteral nutrition in hospitalized patients. Crit Care Med 2005;33(1):213–20.

10. Tsai S, Strouse PJ, Drongowski RA, Islam S, Teitelbaum DH. Failure of cholecystokinin-octapeptide to prevent TPN-associated gallstone disease. J Pediatr Surg 2005;40:263–7.

11. Reimund JM, Rahmi G, Escalin G, Pinna G, Finck G, Muller CD, Duclos B, Baumann R. Efficacy and safety of an olive oil-based intravenous fat emulsion in adult patients on home parenteral nutrition. Aliment Pharmacol Ther. 2005;21(4):445–54.

Job Harenberg

35 Drugs affecting blood coagulation, fibrinolysis, and hemostasis

---

Editor's note: The clotting factors, such as factor VIII, and anticoagulant proteins, such as activated factor C, are included in Chapter 33.

Citrate   *(SED-15, 797)*

In recent years regional citrate has been used as an anticoagulant in hemodialysis and hemofiltration, particularly in patients with bleeding problems. Its clearance is not affected by renal insufficiency (1[c]).

Mineral balance   The main adverse effect of citrate is *hypocalcemia*, which can be prevented by intravenous administration of calcium (2[c], 3[c]). Regional citrate anticoagulation for single-needle hemodialysis has been evaluated in a retrospective study of its use in 41 single-needle hemodialysis procedures in 24 patients at risk of bleeding, using 4% trisodium citrate, $CaCl_2$ 1 mol/l, and calcium-free dialysate (4[c]). Safety was assessed by the percentage of procedures that were terminated prematurely or changed to another modality because of citrate-related complications and by the incidence of important hypocalcemia; efficacy was evaluated by visually assessing clot formation in the circuit. There was important hypocalcemia in 34% of the procedures and 5% were terminated prematurely. Anticoagulation was suboptimal in 17% of the procedures, but none of the systems clotted.

COUMARIN ANTICOAGULANTS
(SED-15, 983; SEDA-27, 358; SEDA-28, 391; SEDA-29, 358)

Gastrointestinal   Small bowel obstruction due to bleeding in a patient taking long-term warfarin has been reported (5[A]).

- A 53-year-old woman developed abdominal pain and vomiting while taking warfarin after aortic and mitral valve surgery. There was jejunal narrowing consistent with a stricture, probably as a result of submucosal bleeding. Warfarin was withdrawn and she was given heparin, with complete resolution of symptoms.

Hematologic   In the common database of the German spontaneous reporting system, 1164 reports of adverse drug reactions were registered that had been attributed to therapy with vitamin K antagonists during the period from 1990 to 2002 (phenprocoumon: 91%; warfarin: 8.3%; acenocoumarol: 0.9%) (6[S]). Among these reactions a *reduction in prothrombin time* was the most common (15%), followed by *gastrointestinal hemorrhage* (13%), *cerebral hemorrhage* (9.1%), *melena* (7.4%), and *increased hepatic enzymes* (7.3%). *Unspecified hemorrhage, intracranial hemorrhage*, and *hematomas* accounted for 6.0% each, *hepatitis* 5.7%, and *hematuria* 4.9%. There were 42 reports (3.0%) of *skin necrosis* and seven of *hepatic necrosis*. Altogether, there were 609 cases of drug-induced hemorrhage. On average 47 cases of hemorrhage were attributed to phenprocoumon or warfarin each year from 1990, with spikes in the numbers of cases in 1997 (107) and 2002 (110). During the entire period the amount of prescribing increased continuously. Total sales reached 132.2 million defined daily doses (DDDs) in 1997 and 190.0 million

Side Effects of Drugs, Annual 30
J.K. Aronson (Editor)
ISSN: 0378-6080
DOI: 10.1016/S0378-6080(08)00035-4

DDDs in 2001. It was therefore not surprising that the number of adverse reactions reports increased.

R. *Interactions of herbal medicines with warfarin*

In a meta-analysis of interactions of warfarin with other drugs, herbal medicines, Chinese herbal drugs, and foods 642 citations were retrieved, of which 181 eligible articles contained original reports on 120 drugs or foods (7[M]). Of all the reports, 72% described potentiation of the effect of warfarin, and the authors considered that 84% were of poor quality, 86% of which were single case reports. The 31 incidents of clinically significant bleeding were all single case reports. Relatively few anecdotal reports of adverse event–drug associations are followed up with formal studies (8[M]), and reports of interactions of warfarin with herbal medicines are no exception—most are based on anecdotal reports.

Drug interactions of warfarin with herbal preparations have been reviewed (9[R], 10[R]). In a systematic review, warfarin was the most common cardiovascular drug involved in interactions with herbal medicines (11[M]). Medicines that resulted in increased anticoagulation include *Allium sativum* (garlic), *Angelica sinensis* (dong quai), *Carica papaya* (papaya), curbicin (from *Cucurbita pepo* seed and *Serenoa repens* fruit), *Ginkgo biloba* (maidenhair), *Harpagophytum procumbens* (devil's claw), *Lycium barbarum* (Chinese wolfberry), *Mangifera indica* (mango) (12[A]), *Peumus boldus* (boldo) (13[A]), *Salvia miltiorrhiza* (danshen), *Trigonella foenum graecum* (fenugreek), and PC-SPES (a patented combination of eight herbs). Medicines that resulted in reduced anticoagulation include *Camellia sinensis* (green tea), milk prepared from *Hypericum perforatum* (St John's wort), and *Panax ginseng* (ginseng).

In a retrospective analysis of the pharmaceutical care plans of 631 patients, 170 (27%) were taking some form of complementary or alternative medicine and 99 were using a medicine that could interact with warfarin, the commonest being cod-liver oil and garlic (14[R]).

Allium sativum **(garlic)**   The interaction of garlic with warfarin has been reviewed (15[R]). Certain organosulfur components inhibit human platelet aggregation in vitro and in vivo; some garlic components have an anticoagulant effect and might thus enhance the effect of warfarin. However, there is only anecdotal evidence that this occurs. Two case reports have suggested that the combination of warfarin with garlic extract prolonged the clotting time and increased the international normalized ratio (INR). There have also been reports that garlic can cause postoperative bleeding and spontaneous spinal epidural hematoma. Garlic should be withdrawn 4–8 weeks before an operation or in those taking long-term warfarin.

Angelica sinesis **(dong quai)**   Although *Angelica sinesis* is a commonly used herbal medicine, there are no clinical data on drug interactions except for one report of a 46-year-old African–American woman with atrial fibrillation stabilized on warfarin who had a greater than two-fold increase in prothrombin time and INR after taking *Angelica sinesis* for 4 weeks (16[R]). *Angelica sinesis* extract and its active ingredient, ferulic acid, inhibit rat platelet aggregation in vivo. In rabbits oral administration *Angelica sinesis* root extract (2 g/kg bd) significantly reduced the prothrombin time when combined with warfarin (2 mg/kg), while the pharmacokinetics of warfarin were not altered (17[R]). However, in rats an aqueous extract of *Angelica sinesis* increased the activities of CYP2D6 and CYP3A (18[E]), and in in vitro studies components from *Angelica sinesis* root altered CYP3A4 and CYP1A activity, indicating a potential for drug interactions with CYP substrates. For example, a decoction or infusion of *Angelica sinesis* root inhibited CYP3A4-catalysed testosterone 6-beta-hydroxylation in human liver microsomes, whereas ferulic acid (0.5 µmol/l) from *Angelica sinesis* root significantly inhibited ethoxyresorufin O-methylase (CYP1A) activity. All of these findings suggest that precautionary advice should be given to patients who self-medicate with *Angelica sinesis* root preparations while taking long-term warfarin. Well-designed case-control studies are needed to evaluate these effects of *Angelica sinesis* root.

Camellia sinensis (green tea)   *Camellia sinensis has been anecdotally reported to reduce the effect of warfarin (19[A]).*

- *A 44-year-old white man taking warfarin had an INR of 3.8. He then drank green tea 0.5–1 gallon/day (4.5 l/day) for about 1 week and the INR fell to 1.37. He stopped drinking green tea and the INR rose to 2.55.*

Green tea is a source of vitamin K. Dry green leaves contain 1428 micrograms of vitamin K per 100 g of leaves compared with only 262 micrograms per 100 g of dry black tea leaves (20[r]). The amount of vitamin K ingested will obviously depend on the dilution and amount of tea leaves used to brew the tea and the quantity of tea consumed.

Cucurbita pepo   *Curbicin has been anecdotally reported to cause altered coagulation in the absence of anticoagulant therapy and to enhance the anticoagulant action of warfarin; however, the authors attributed this effect to the vitamin E that was also present in the curbicin tablets (21[A]).*

Ginkgo biloba   *There are anecdotal reports of possible interactions of ginkgo with warfarin (22[A]). However, formal, albeit small, studies in patients and healthy volunteers have not confirmed this. In an open, crossover, randomized study, 12 healthy men took a single dose of warfarin 25 mg either alone or after pretreatment with Ginkgo biloba for 7 days; ginkgo did not significantly affect clotting or the pharmacokinetics or pharmacodynamics of warfarin (23[c]). In a randomized, double-blind, placebo-controlled, crossover study, oral ginkgo extract 100 mg/day for 4 weeks did not alter the INR in 24 Danish out-patients (14 women and 10 men) taking stable, long-term warfarin, and the geometric mean dosage of warfarin did not change (24[C]).*

The mechanism for this interaction, if it occurs, is unknown, but both pharmacokinetic and pharmacodynamic mechanisms may be involved, given that ginkgo extracts can modulate various CYP isoenzymes and exert antiplatelet activity. Ginkgolides are also potent inhibitors of platelet-activating factor (25[A]). There are reports of postoperative bleeding and spontaneous hemorrhage attributed to consumption of gingko (26[A], 27[A]) and interactions have been described with antiplatelet drugs. For example, spontaneous hyphema occurred when ginkgo extract was combined with aspirin (acetylsalicylic acid) (28[A]) and fatal intracerebral bleeding was associated with the combined use of ginkgo extract and ibuprofen (29[A]). Ginkgo extract also enhanced the antiplatelet and antithrombotic effects of ticlopidine in rats, resulting in prolongation of the bleeding time by 150% (30[E]). However, in a double-blind, randomized, placebo-controlled study in 32 young healthy men oral ginkgo extract 120, 240, or 480 mg/day for 14 days did not alter platelet function or coagulation (31[A]). Bleeding attributed to ginkgo often occurs in elderly or postoperative patients who may have had impaired platelet function before the use of ginkgo.

Hypericum perforatum (St John's wort)   *An interaction of St John's wort with warfarin has been reported anecdotally, including 22 spontaneous reports of reduced warfarin effect after treatment with St John's wort submitted to regulatory authorities in Europe between 1998 and 2000 (32[R]). These interactions all resulted in unstable INR values, a reduction in INR being the most common effect. Although no thromboembolic episodes occurred, the reduction in anticoagulant activity was considered clinically significant. Anticoagulant activity was restored when St John's wort was withdrawn or the warfarin dose was increased.*

In a crossover study, healthy volunteers who took hypericum extract LI 160, 900 mg/day for 11 days before a single dose of phenprocoumon had a lower AUC of the unbound fraction than when they took placebo (33[c]).

In an open, three-way, crossover, randomized study in 12 healthy men who took a single dose of warfarin 25 mg alone or after pretreatment for 14 days with St John's wort, the apparent clearance of S-warfarin was 3.3 ml/minute before St John's wort was added and 3.7 ml/minute after (34[C]). The respective apparent clearances of R-warfarin were 1.8 and 2.4 ml/minute. The mean ratios of the apparent clearances were 1.29 (95% CI = 1.16, 1.46) for S-warfarin and 1.23 (1.11, 1.37) for R-warfarin. St John's wort did not affect the apparent volume of distribution or protein binding of either enantiomer of warfarin. The authors concluded that St John's wort induces the clearance of both enantiomers of warfarin. INR was slightly reduced as a result, but platelet aggregation was not altered.

These observations suggest that St John's wort increases the clearance of both warfarin and phenprocoumon, possibly because of induction of CYP isozymes, particularly CYP2C9 and CYP3A4.

Lycium barbarum (Chinese wolfberry)   *There has been a single anecdotal report of a possible interaction of Lycium barbarum with warfarin (35[AE]).*

- *A 61-year-old Chinese woman, previously stabilized on warfarin (INR 2–3), drank a concentrated Chinese herbal tea made from Lycium barbarum fruits (3–4 glasses/day) for 4 days; her INR rose to 4.1. Warfarin was withheld for 1 day and then restarted at a lower dose. She stopped drinking the tea, and 7 days later her INR was 2.4.*

In vitro studies showed that Lycium barbarum tea inhibited S-warfarin metabolism by CYP2C9; however, the inhibition was weak, with a dissociation constant of 3.4 g/l, suggesting that the observed interaction may have been caused by other mechanisms.

Panax ginseng   *Ginseng can reduce the effect of warfarin (36[R]), and there have been anecdotal reports of such an interaction (37[A], 38[A]). There have also been several formal studies of the pharmacokinetic and pharmacodynamic effects of ginseng on warfarin.*

The effects of American ginseng (Panax quinquefolium) have been studied in a double-blind, randomized, placebo-controlled trial in 20 young healthy subjects (39[C]). Warfarin was given for 3 days during weeks 1 and 4, and starting in week 2 the subjects were assigned to either ginseng or placebo. The peak INR fell significantly after 2 weeks of ginseng administration compared with placebo; the difference between ginseng and placebo was −0.19 (95% CI = −0.36, −0.07).

However, in an open, three-way, crossover, randomized study in 12 healthy men who took a single dose of warfarin 25 mg alone or after pretreatment for 7 days with ginseng, there was no change in the pharmacokinetics or pharmacodynamics of either S-warfarin or R-warfarin (35[C]).

In 20 healthy volunteers who took 100 mg of an extract of Panax ginseng standardized to

4% ginsenosides twice daily for 14 days there were no effects on CYP3A and this result was confirmed in in vitro studies (40[CE]).

The discrepancies between these studies could be explained by differing susceptibilities of different populations or by different effects of ginseng from different sources.

Both pharmacokinetic and pharmacodynamic components could play a role in an interaction of ginseng with warfarin. Ginseng extracts have an antiplatelet effect. Ginsenosides Rg3 and protopanaxadiol-type saponins were platelet-activating factor antagonists with IC_{50} values of 49–92 μmol/l (41[E]). Modulation of various CYP isoenzymes could also be a mechanism. In rats the pharmacokinetics and pharmacodynamics of warfarin after a single dose and at steady state were not altered by co-administered ginseng (42[E]). However, extensive in vitro and in vivo animal studies have shown that constituents of ginseng can modulate various CYP isoenzymes that metabolize warfarin. Ginsenoside Rd was weakly inhibitory against recombinant CYP3A4, CYP2D6, CYP2C19, and CYP2C9, whereas ginsenoside Re and ginsenoside Rf (200 μmol/l) increased the activity of CYP2C9 and CYP3A4 (43[E]). In rats, the standardized saponin of red ginseng was inhibitory on p-nitrophenol hydroxylase (CYP2E1) activity in a dose-related manner (44[E]).

Salvia miltiorrhiza (danshen)   *There have been anecdotal reports of enhanced anticoagulation and bleeding when patients taking long-term warfarin therapy consumed Salvia miltiorrhiza root (45[A], 46[A], 47[A]). As these patients were also taking other medications, the contribution of Salvia miltiorrhiza to the interaction was difficult to determine. However, the author of a systematic review concluded that danshen should be avoided in patients taking warfarin (48[M]).*

The direct anticoagulant activity of Salvia miltiorrhiza root itself may provide a partial explanation for the interactions. However, pharmacokinetic interactions may also play a role. Warfarin is mainly metabolized by CYP2C9 and to a smaller extent by CYP1A2 and CYP3A4. In mice oral, administration of an ethyl acetate extract of danshen caused a dose-related increase in liver microsomal 7-methoxyresorufin

O-demethylation activity, with a three-fold increase in warfarin 7-hydroxylation (49[E]). However, the aqueous extract had no effects. Immunoblot analysis of microsomal proteins showed that ethyl acetate extraction increased the proteins associated with CYP1A and CYP3A. At a dose corresponding to its content in the ethyl acetate extract, tanshinone IIA, the main diterpene quinone in Salvia miltiorrhiza, increased mouse liver microsomal 7-methoxyresorufin O-demethylation activity. These results suggest that there are inducing agents for mouse CYP1A, CYP2C, and CYP3A in ethyl acetate extracts but not in aqueous extracts of Salvia miltiorrhiza.

In rats treatment with Salvia miltiorrhiza root extract 5 g/kg bd for 3 days followed by a single oral dose of racemic warfarin increased the absorption rate constants, AUC, C_{max}, and half-life of warfarin but reduced the clearances and apparent volumes of distribution of both (R)-warfarin and (S)-warfarin (50[E]). A similar effect was observed during steady-state warfarin administration. The anticoagulant effect of warfarin was also potentiated. Salvia miltiorrhiza root extract itself had no effect on prothrombin time at this dose, suggesting that altered warfarin metabolism was a possible mechanism.

After a single oral dose of racemic warfarin 2 mg/kg in rats, an oral extract of Salvia miltiorrhiza 5 g/kg bd for 3 days significantly altered the pharmacokinetics of both R-warfarin and S-warfarin and increased the plasma concentrations of both enantiomers over a period of 24 hours and the prothrombin time over 2 days (51[E]). Steady-state concentrations of racemic warfarin during administration of 0.2 mg/kg/day for 5 days with extract of Salvia miltiorrhiza 5 g/kg bd for 3 days not only prolonged the prothrombin time but also increased the steady-state plasma concentrations of R-warfarin and S-warfarin. These results suggested that Salvia miltiorrhiza increases the absorption rate, exposure, and half-lives of both R-warfarin and S-warfarin, but reduces their clearances and apparent volumes of distribution.

In addition, Salvia miltiorrhiza root extract might change the plasma protein binding of warfarin. Both (R)-warfarin and (S)-warfarin bind to the so-called site I of albumin with high affinity. Salvia miltiorrhiza root extract was 50–70% bound by albumin and in vitro Salvia miltiorrhiza root extract displaced salicylate from protein binding, thereby increasing the unbound salicylate concentration (52[E]). However, kangen-karyu, a mixture of six herbs (peony root, Cnidium rhizome, safflower, Cyperus rhizome, Saussurea root, and root of Salvia miltiorrhiza), significantly increased the plasma warfarin concentration and prothrombin time in rats, but did not alter the serum protein binding of warfarin (53[E]). Further studies are required to explore the effects of Salvia miltiorrhiza root extract on the metabolism and plasma protein binding of drugs such as warfarin in humans.

Zingiber officinale (ginger)　Despite anecdotal reports of a possible interaction (54[A], 55[A]), several studies in rats and humans have shown no effect of ginger on warfarin pharmacokinetics or pharmacodynamics (15[R], 24[C], 56[E], 57[C]).

Herbal mixtures　When mixtures of herbs are used, as is common practice in the far East, it is not possible to be sure which component was responsible for a reported interaction.

PC-Spes　PC-Spes is a mixture of eight herbs: Chrysanthemum morifolium, Isatis indigotica, Glycyrrhiza glabra (licorice), Ganoderma lucidum, Panax pseudoginseng, Robdosia rubescens, Serenoa repens (saw palmetto), and Scutellaria baicalensis (skullcap). It has been reported to increase the INR in a 79-year-old man with prostate cancer taking warfarin, an effect that was attributed to inhibition of warfarin metabolism (58[A]). However, warfarin has also been found in formulations of PC-Spes (59[r]).

Quilinggao　Quilinggao, a popular Chinese mixture that contains a multitude of herbal ingredients (including Fritillaria cirrhosa and other Fritillaria species, Paeoniae rubra, Lonicera japonica, and Poncirus trifoliata, in many different brands), has been anecdotally reported to enhance the actions of warfarin (60[A]).

- A 61-year-old man taking stable warfarin therapy developed gum bleeding, epistaxis, and skin bruising 5 days after taking quilinggao. His international normalized ratio was above 6. His warfarin was withdrawn and the international normalized ratio normalized. Days later he tried taking quilinggao again, with a similar result.

The authors pointed out that several herbs in this mixture have anticoagulant activity.

Supercoumarins   *(SED-15, 984)*

Anticoagulant pesticides are used widely in agricultural and urban rodent control. The emergence of warfarin-resistant strains of rats led to the introduction of a group of anticoagulant rodenticides variously referred to as "supercoumarins", "superwarfarins", "single dose" rodenticides, or "long-acting" rodenticides (61[R]). This group includes the second generation 4-hydroxycoumarins brodifacoum, bromadiolone, difenacoum, and flocoumafen and the indanedione derivatives chlorophacinone and diphacinone. Most cases of anticoagulant rodenticide exposure involve young children, and so the amounts ingested are almost invariably small. In contrast, intentional ingestion of large quantities of long-acting anticoagulant rodenticides can cause anticoagulation for several weeks or months (62[A]). Occupational exposure has also been reported.

The greater potency and duration of action of long-acting anticoagulant rodenticides is attributed to: (i) their greater affinity for vitamin K epoxide reductase; (ii) their ability to disrupt the vitamin K epoxide cycle at more than one point; (iii) hepatic accumulation; and (iv) unusually long half-lives, due to high lipid solubility and enterohepatic recirculation. Substantial ingestion produces epistaxis, gingival bleeding, widespread bruising, hematomas, hematuria with flank pain, menorrhagia, gastrointestinal bleeding, rectal bleeding, and hemorrhage into any internal organ; anaemia can result. Spontaneous hemoperitoneum has been described. Severe blood loss can result in hypovolemic shock, coma, and death. The first clinical signs of bleeding can be delayed and patients can remain anticoagulated for several days (warfarin) or days, weeks, or months (long-acting anticoagulants) after ingesting large amounts.

There are now sufficient data in young children exposed to anticoagulant rodenticides to conclude that routine measurement of the international normalized ratio (INR) is unnecessary. In all other cases, the INR should be measured 36–48 hours after exposure. If the INR is normal at this time, even in the case of long-acting formulations, no further action is required. If active bleeding occurs, prothrombin complex concentrate (which contains factors II, VII, IX, and X) 50 units/kg, or recombinant activated factor VII 1.2–4.8 mg, or fresh frozen plasma 15 ml/kg (if no concentrate is available) and phytomenadione 10 mg intravenously (100 micrograms/kg for a child) should be given. If there is no active bleeding and the INR is under 4.0, no treatment is required; if the INR is 4.0 or higher phytomenadione 10 mg should be given intravenously.

HEPARINS   *(SED-15, 1590; SEDA-27, 358; SEDA-28, 391; SEDA-29, 361)*

Observational studies   A new entity of autoimmune sensorineural hearing loss has been proposed and treated with subcutaneous enoxaparin 2000 IU bd for 10 days in a placebo-controlled study in 30 patients (63[C]). All those who received enoxaparin had both subjective and objective improvement and there were no adverse effects.

Cardiovascular   *Cholesterol crystal embolism* is a rare complication of anticoagulant treatment of ulcerative atheroma of the great arteries and has been attributed to low-molecular-weight heparins in three cases (64[A]).

Electrolyte balance   Heparin-induced *hyperkalemia* is often forgotten until life-threatening dysrhythmias have occurred (65[A]).

Hematologic   A spinal–epidural hematoma occurred after combined spinal–epidural anesthesia in a woman who had been taking clopidogrel and had received perioperative dalteparin for thromboprophylaxis (66[A]). This occurred despite adherence to standard guidelines on the administration of low-molecular-weight heparin perioperatively and withdrawal of clopidogrel 7 days before the anesthetic.

Heparin-induced thrombocytopenia

DoTS classification:
Reaction: Heparin-induce thrombocytopenia, type II
Dose-relation: Hypersusceptibility
Time-course: Early persistent
Susceptibility factors: Renal disease for some forms of heparin, pretreatment with heparin

Heparin-induced thrombocytopenia (67[R]) has been recognized in adults for some time, but only recently in neonates and children (68[M]). There are two types. Type I is non-immunogenic, mild, and self-limiting. Type II is a severe immune reaction that leads to thrombocytopenia and often thromboembolic complications. The incidence of type II thrombocytopenia is 2–5% in adults and may be equally high in neonates and children. The mortality rate in adults is 7–30% and is unknown but potentially high in neonates. The cardinal sign is a fall in platelet count by 50% or a platelet count below 70–100 × 10^9/l. Treatment is immediate withdrawal of heparin and introduction of alternative anticoagulants, such as the direct thrombin inhibitors lepirudin and argatroban. The literature on heparin-induced thrombocytopenia has been reviewed in the context of a case in a neonate after heart surgery (69[AR]).

Dose relation   Heparin-induced thrombocytopenia can occur after minimal heparin exposure, including heparin flushes (70[A]).

Time-course   The fall in platelet count usually occurs 5–10 days after the first exposure to heparin.

Incidence   The most frequently suspected drug registered by the German spontaneous reporting system in cases of thrombocytopenia was unfractionated heparin (10[S]). Of 3291 adverse reactions reports 78% were associated with unfractionated heparin, 13% with enoxaparin, 11% with certoparin, 5.5% with dalteparin, 2.8% with heparin fractions, 2.5% with reviparin, and 1.2% with tinzaparin. Heparin-induced thrombocytopenia was the most common adverse effect (38%), followed by pulmonary embolism (11%), hematomas (6.8%), erythematous rashes (4.8%), and unspecified bleeding (4.5%). Injection site reactions were common (15%) and included skin necrosis and injection site necrosis in 1.8% of cases. Antibodies to heparin–platelet factor (PF)4 complex can be demonstrated in almost all patients with type II heparin-induced thrombocytopenia. There was a positive specific antibody result in 736 (59%) of 1245 cases.

The incidences of heparin-induced thrombocytopenia in surgical and medical patients receiving thromboprophylaxis with either unfractionated or low-molecular-weight heparin have been studied in a systematic review of all relevant randomized and non-randomized studies identified in MEDLINE (1984–2004), not limited by language, and from reference lists of key articles (71[M]). Heparin-induced thrombocytopenia was defined as a fall in platelet count to less than 50% or less than 100 × 10^9/l and a positive laboratory diagnostic assay, including enzyme-linked immunosorbent assay (ELISA), (14[C]) serotonin release assay, or adenosine triphosphate lumi-aggregometry. There were 15 eligible studies (7287 patients). The odds ratios were as follows:

- two randomized controlled trials (n = 1014): OR = 0.10 (95% CI = 0.01, 0.2);
- three prospective studies with non-randomized comparison groups (n = 1464): OR = 0.10 (95% CI = 0.03, 0.33);
- all 15 studies (including ten in which only thrombocytopenia was measured): OR = 0.47 (95% CI = 0.22, 1.02).

The absolute risks were 0.2% with low-molecular-weight heparin and 2.6% with unfractionated heparin.

In a retrospective study of 389 consecutive patients with subarachnoid hemorrhage, 59 (15%) met the clinical diagnostic criteria for heparin-induced thrombocytopenia type II (72[c]). The average platelet count nadir was 69 × 10^9/l. Women and patients with Fisher Grade 3 were at higher risk. There were systemic thrombotic complications in 37% compared with 7% of those without thrombocytopenia. There were more new hypodensities on CT scan in those with thrombocytopenia (66 versus 40%) and more deaths (29 versus 12%).

Case reports   Thrombocytopenia has been reported in a patient who received intraperitoneal heparin (73[A]).

- A 52-year-old man with end-stage renal disease and peritonitis associated with CAPD was given intraperitoneal heparin 1000 U/day for 7 days. His platelet count 13 days before this had been 260 × 10^9/l, but 14 days after the last dose of heparin he developed epistaxis and petechiae on his trunk and lower legs and the platelet count was 25 × 10^9/l. His platelet count spontaneously normalized over the next 7 days.

Heparin-induced thrombocytopenia was con-firmed by detection of antibodies against the heparin–PF4 complex using a serotonin release assay.

Thrombosis can occur when heparin causes a fall in the platelet count within the reference range if there are associated antibodies (74^A).

- *A 45-year-old man with pulmonary embolism was given heparin and developed massive thrombosis after insertion of a filter on day 3; the platelet count was 221 × 10^9/l. Heparin was replaced by argatroban on day 13 and the platelet count rose to 355 × 10^9/l on day 15. There were antibodies against complexes of heparin and platelet factor 4.*

Since 1992, miniaturized pulsatile air-driven ventricular assist devices, the so-called "Berlin Heart", have been used in children at many institutions (36 cases in North America in 19 different institutions). Heparin-induced thrombocytopenia can cause thrombosis in such devices (75^A).

- *A 13-month-old girl, weight 8.1 kg, who required support with a left ventricular assist device for cardiogenic shock of unclear cause, developed a persistent low-grade fever, heparin-induced thrombocytopenia, and impaired renal function. On post-implant day 10, the pump required replacement because of concerns about an inlet valve thrombus; the explanted device contained a nearly occlusive clot.*

Susceptibility factors

Children   There is less published experience with low-molecular-weight heparins in children than in adults, but the low frequency of significant bleeding appears to be similar. A child who received therapeutic doses of a low-molecular-weight heparin for a deep vein thrombosis spontaneously developed an intramural hemorrhage in the small bowel, leading to infarction, which required partial bowel resection (76^A).

Renal disease   Unlike unfractionated heparin, dalteparin is mainly cleared through the kidney and can therefore accumulate if renal function is impaired, increasing the risk of hemorrhage.

- *An 84-year-old woman with chronic renal insufficiency had angioplasty for a stenosis in a femorofibular bypass, developed a deep vein thrombosis, and was given dalteparin (77^A). After 4 days she developed a pronounced hematoma on her flank and her hemoglobin fell to 5.5 g/dl.*

Dalteparin was withdrawn and she was given protamine 2500 U and packed red blood cells. She had no further bleeding during treatment with unfractionated heparin and an oral anticoagulant

Dalteparin should be avoided in patients with severe renal impairment or used only with close monitoring of antifactor Xa activity. As an alternative, unfractionated heparin can be used, since renal impairment does not affect its short half-life.

Two patients with chronic kidney disease had retroperitoneal hematomas requiring blood transfusion after the administration of enoxaparin (78^A). Enoxaparin should be administered with great caution in patients with chronic kidney disease, especially if antiplatelet agents or other anticoagulants are administered concomitantly.

Complications   *Heparin-induced skin necrosis is an immune-complex phenomenon associated with heparin-induced thrombocytopenia (HIT); it can rarely occur in the presence of HIT IgG alone (serological HIT). It is thought to be caused by an antibody-mediated local prothrombotic condition associated with platelet activation and increased thrombin production. If skin necrosis occurs, treatment with an alternative thromboprophylactic agent should be considered.*

Skin necrosis has been reported in patients receiving tinzaparin (79^A), enoxaparin (80^A), and unfractionated heparin (81^A).

- *A 76-year-old man with polycythemia vera, hypertension, diabetes mellitus, hyperuricemia, atrial fibrillation, and chronic bronchitis, taking hydroxyurea, digoxin, allopurinol, and enalapril, was given prophylactic subcutaneous enoxaparin 60 mg bd (80^A). After 5 days he developed two symmetrical erythematous patches, 5 cm in diameter, on the abdominal wall at injection sites. The lesions enlarged over 24 hours and formed purplish-blue necrotic plaques 15 cm × 5 cm. The hemoglobin was 7.4 g/dl, the white blood cell count, 29 × 10^9/l, and the platelet count 1025 × 10^9/l; there was no significant change in the platelet count throughout the admission. The prothrombin time ratio was 1.17 and the thromboplastin time ratio 1.36. Protein C was normal but protein S was reduced to 56% (reference range 71–142%), with a low free protein S concentration (63%; reference range 72–139%) and normal total protein S (protein S deficiency type III). There were no IgG antiphospholipid antibodies, but IgM was raised. Heparin–platelet factor 4 (PF4) antibodies were also demonstrated. A skin biopsy showed* multiple fibrin thrombi in the dermal microvasculature with ischemic necrosis of the overlying epidermis. Enoxaparin was withdrawn, the lesions were treated locally, and there was complete healing after about 1 month.

- A 69-year-old woman with severe bronchopneumonia was given subcutaneous prophylactic unfractionated sodium heparin (5000 IU bd) (81[A]). By day 7 she had developed blistering skin lesions with central necrosis and surrounding erythema at the heparin injection sites. The platelet count was stable at $275 \times 10^9/l$ (range 196–338). There was a circulating IgG antibody against heparin–platelet factor 4 and anticardiolipin IgG antibodies. A skin biopsy showed extensive focal epidermal necrosis with marked neutrophil infiltration and extensive fibrin deposition within the small vessels of the dermis. All the lesions resolved within 5 day of withdrawal of heparin.

The association of heparin-induced skin necrosis with antibodies directed against heparin–PF4 is well-established, but the participation of other procoagulant factors has received little attention. The observation of heparin-induced skin necrosis should motivate a systematic search for the presence of anti-PF4 antibodies, but also for additional genetic or acquired procoagulant factors. Heparin-induced skin necrosis may be a marker of an increased risk of systemic arterial or venous thromboembolism.

Catastrophic antiphospholipid syndrome is a medical emergency characterized by thrombosis of multiple small vessels of the internal organs and the brain (82[A]). In one case hepatic, renal, and splenic artery thromboses, as well as cerebral venous thrombosis, were complicated by severe thrombocytopenia and hemolytic anemia. However, there were no antiplatelet-factor-4 antibodies, making heparin-induced thrombocytopenia unlikely.

Management   Lepirudin has been used in patients with heparin-induced thrombocytopenia in a prospective study in 205 patients with 120 historical controls (HAT-3) and in a combined analysis of all HAT study data (83[CM]). Patients with laboratory-confirmed thrombocytopenia were treated with lepirudin in three different aPTT-adjusted dose regimens and during cardiopulmonary bypass. Mean lepirudin maintenance doses were 0.07–0.11 mg/kg/hour. End points were new thromboembolic complications, limb amputations, and death and major bleeding. The combined end point occurred in 43 (21%) of those treated with lepirudin; 30 died, 10 underwent limb amputation, and 11 had new thromboembolic complications. There was major bleeding in 40 patients, seven during cardiopulmonary bypass. Combining all the prospective HAT trials (n = 403), after the start of lepirudin treatment, the combined end point occurred in 82 patients (20%), with 47 deaths, 22 limb amputations, 30 new thromboembolic complications, and 71 episodes of major bleeding. Compared with the historical controls, the combined end point after the start of treatment was significantly reduced (30 versus 52%), primarily because of a reduction in new episodes of thrombosis (12 versus 32%). Major bleeding was more frequent in the lepirudin-treated patients (29 versus 9.1%). Thus, the rate of new thromboembolic complications in patients with heparin-induced thrombocytopenia is low after lepirudin treatment. The rate of major bleeding of 18% might be reduced by reducing the starting dose to 0.1 mg/kg/hour.

Argatroban has been used in 13 patients who developed heparin-induced thrombocytopenia after exposure to heparin 10–13 000 U from an intravascular catheter or filter flush, with a mean exposure of 8 days (84[c]). They were compared with 10 historical controls who had received no direct thrombin inhibitors. The platelet count recovered to a mean of $207 \times 10^9/l$ (n = 12) after 5.5 days of argatroban therapy and to a mean of $127 \times 10^9/l$ (n = 8) 5 days after baseline in the control group. A composite end point of death, amputation, or new thrombosis within 37 days occurred in five argatroban-treated patients and four controls. Death was the most common untoward outcome (about 30% in each group). No argatroban-treated patient and two control patients had new episodes of thrombosis. Major bleeding was comparable.

Skin   Skin necrosis is a rare complication of subcutaneous low-molecular-weight heparin in association with thrombocytopenia (see special review above).

Fat necrosis   Subcutaneous fat necrosis has been attributed to heparin (85[A]).

- A 91-year-old woman with diabetes, hypertension, and unstable angina was given subcutaneous enoxaparin. After 5 days she developed extensive induration of the skin and subcutaneous fat of the upper part of the left breast and bruising of the overlying skin. There were a few patches of ecchymosis were over other parts of her body, but none at injection sites on the abdomen. Coagulation screen and platelet count were normal. Mammography showed asymmetrical nodular densities over the upper inner quadrant of the left breast and ultrasound of the area was consistent with fat necrosis.

Subcutaneous calcinosis   Accumulation of calcium in the skin is usually classified as a group of disorders referred to as calcinosis cutis. Calcinosis has been attributed to subcutaneous nadroparin (86[A]).

- A 92-year-old man developed multiple cutaneous plaques and nodules on the abdomen and right thigh after daily subcutaneous administration of nadroparin calcium for 5 months. The lesions were asymptomatic, firm, and roundish and measured up to 3 cm. Some were isolated and others were confluent, forming annular shapes. Most were ulcerated. Some developed an erythematous, yellow, annular border, with a darker ring inside. Histopathology showed marked hyperkeratosis, mild epidermal acanthosis, and central ulceration. Within the superficial and mid-dermis there were marked regressive-degenerative changes of the collagen fibers, leading to artefactual dermoepidermal and intradermal clefts, marked fragmentation of the elastic fibers, focal liponecrosis, and deposition of calcium salts.

Calcifying panniculitis is a rare form of calcinosis cutis that belongs to the spectrum of calciphylaxis that has almost invariably been described in patients with severe renal impairment. It has been reported in a patient with hyperparathyroidism and normal renal function who received subcutaneous nadroparin calcium and resolved after withdrawal (87[A]). The authors suggested that low-molecular-weight calcium-containing heparins should probably be used with caution in patients with hyperparathyroidism.

Immunologic   Eczematous lesions resulting from *type IV hypersensitivity reactions* are common cutaneous adverse effects of subcutaneous heparin. If anticoagulation is further required, intravenous heparin, heparinoids, or lepirudin can be used instead. However, these alternatives are not optimal in terms of practicability and safety profiles. As variation in the molecular weights of different heparin formulations has repeatedly been implicated in determining the frequency of sensitization, it has been suggested

that the pentasaccharide fondaparinux may provide a practicable and safe alternative, because of its low molecular weight (88[c]). Patients with cutaneous reactions after subcutaneous anticoagulant treatment ($n = 12$) underwent a series of in vivo skin allergy and challenge tests with unfractionated heparin, low-molecular-weight heparins (certoparin, dalteparin, enoxaparin, nadroparin, and tinzaparin), danaparoid, and fondaparinux. There was a high degree of cross-reactivity among heparins and heparinoids. In contrast, there was rarely cross-sensitization with fondaparinux. Molecular weight was a key determinant of sensitization to heparins and other oligosaccharides.

Lepirudin can be used safely for prophylaxis of recurrent venous thromboembolism throughout pregnancy in patients with hypersensitivity reactions to heparins (89[A]).

- A 26-year-old woman with recurrent venous thromboembolism, lupus pernio with antiphospholipid antibodies, and local intolerance to heparin, low-molecular-weight heparin, and danaparoid, was given phenprocoumon during pregnancy and was later switched to subcutaneous lepirudin 25 mg bid/day and acetylsalicylic acid 100 mg/day. At week 16 she developed lupus pernio, with painful lesions on the toes and fingers and later also on the cheeks and nose. Aspirin was withdrawn and she was given cortisone and morphine. Fetal examination was normal. At week 29, she was given intravenous lepirudin. At week 30 a healthy child was delivered by cesarean section. After delivery the lupus pernio resolved within 2 weeks and subcutaneous lepirudin was restarted, followed by phenprocoumon.

Infection risk   Following a cluster of cases of unexpected hospital-acquired *bacteremia* suspected to be related to intravenous heparin infusion, all cases of hospital-acquired primary bacteremia in low-risk patients were analysed over 4 years (90[c]). Of 1618 episodes of hospital-acquired bacteremia a peripheral intravenous line was the only risk factor in 96 (6%). These patients were divided into two groups: 60 patients with phlebitis and 36 without local signs of inflammation. The baseline features in the two groups were comparable, but there was a significant association between intravenous heparin use, the predominance of Gram-negative organisms (especially *Klebsiella*, *Serratia*, and *Enterobacter* species), and the absence of phlebitis. However, in spite of a clear statistical association, the mechanism whereby the heparin solution became contaminated with Gram-negative organisms was unknown. Following implementation of infection control methods in handling heparin, there were no more cases.

Pregnancy   There has been a systematic review of studies on the use of low-molecular-weight heparins for thromboprophylaxis and treatment of venous thromboembolism in pregnancy (91^M). Data on recurrence of venous thromboembolism and adverse effects were extracted and cumulative incidences calculated. Of 81 reports, 64 reporting 2777 pregnancies were included. In 15 studies (174 patients) the indication for low-molecular-weight heparin was treatment of acute venous thromboembolism, and in 61 studies (2603 pregnancies) it was thromboprophylaxis or an adverse pregnancy outcome. There were no maternal deaths. Venous thromboembolism and arterial thrombosis (associated with antiphospholipid syndrome) were reported in 0.86% of pregnancies (95% CI = 0.55, 1.28) and 0.50% of pregnancies (95% CI = 0.28, 0.84) respectively. There was significant *bleeding*, generally associated with primary obstetric causes, in 1.98% of pregnancies (95% CI = 1.50, 2.57), *allergic skin reactions* in 1.80% (95% CI = 1.34, 2.37), *heparin-induced thrombocytopenia* in 0%, *thrombocytopenia* (unrelated to heparin) in 0.11% (95% CI = 0.02, 0.32), and *osteoporotic fractures* in 0.04% (95% CI < 0.01, 0.20). Overall, live births were reported in 94.7% of pregnancies, including 85% in those who received low-molecular-weight heparin for recurrent pregnancy loss.

DIRECT THROMBIN
INHIBITORS   *(SED-15, 1142; SEDA-27, 359; SEDA-29, 362)*

Dabigatran

Dabigatran etexilate is a prodrug of dabigatran, a specific, competitive, reversible inhibitor of thrombin. Dabigatran etexilate is rapidly absorbed after oral administration and converted to dabigatran. Its half-life is about 8 hours after a single dose and 14–17 hours after multiple doses. It is cleared renally.

Hematologic   In a multicenter, parallel-group, double-blind study, 1973 patients undergoing total hip or knee replacement were randomized to oral dabigatran etexilate for 6–10 days starting 1–4 hours after surgery or to subcutaneous enoxaparin starting 12 hours before surgery (92^C). Major bleeding with dabigatran was dose-related; it was significantly lower with dabigatran 50 mg bd than with enoxaparin (0.3 versus 2.0%) but higher at higher doses, nearly reaching statistical significance at a dose of 300 mg/day (4.7%).

Lepirudin   *(SEDA-29, 362)*

Lepirudin, a recombinant hirudin, is a direct thrombin inhibitor approved world wide for the treatment of heparin-induced thrombocytopenia.

Immunologic   Lepirudin rarely causes *allergic reactions* after re-exposure (SEDA-29, 362). In a retrospective analysis of the medical records of 43 adults who had received at least two courses of lepirudin there were no cases of anaphylaxis or allergic reactions (93^c). On the first day of lepirudin therapy 10 patients had lower systolic blood pressures (by at least 20 mmHg) and four had systolic blood pressures of less than 100 mmHg. However, isolated asymptomatic falls in blood pressure after re-exposure to lepirudin most probably do not reflect anaphylactic reactions. Isolated and uncommon cases of anaphylaxis temporally related to lepirudin exposure should not preclude its use in patients with heparin-induced thrombocytopenia and past lepirudin exposure.

In two patients with a history of heparin-induced thrombocytopenia and anti-lepirudin antibodies who received argatroban and lepirudin intravenously, IgG reacting against lepirudin was not generated, in contrast to two patients on lepirudin, in whom *anti-lepirudin antibodies* developed (94^c).

Drug dosage regimens   Nine patients received lepirudin for thromboembolic disease according to the dosage recommendations approved by the European Agency for the Evaluation of Medicinal Products (EMEA): a 0.4

mg/kg bolus followed by 0.15 mg/kg/hour by intravenous infusion, adjusted to the activated partial thromboplastin time, aPTT, in order to maintain a patient:mean normal aPTT ratio of 1.5–2.5 (95^c). However, this dosage regimen turned out to be excessive. There were episodes of overdosage in eight cases, usually within the first 4 hours, after which the infusion was stopped for 2 hours and restarted at 50% of the previous dose. The dosage was then gradually reduced until equilibrium was achieved in the target range. The minimal maintenance infusion rate could be as low as 0.01 mg/kg/hour and the median rate was 0.04 mg/kg/hour. There were neither hemorrhagic nor thrombotic events. The authors suggested that a bolus dose of lepirudin should be omitted in patients who do not have massive, life-threatening thrombosis, especially in elderly patients, and that therapy should start with an initial infusion rate of 0.10 mg/kg/hour only.

Monitoring therapy   The robustness and sensitivity of the different methods of monitoring therapy with direct thrombin inhibitors have been assessed in an international collaborative study using a panel of plasma samples spiked with lepirudin and argatroban (96^E). Activated partial thromboplastin time and the TAS analyser with ecarin clotting time cards gave the most reproducible results.

The ecarin clotting time (ECT) specifically reflects inhibition of meizothrombin by direct thrombin inhibitors (97^E) and is prolonged by vitamin K antagonists. Concomitant use of vitamin K antagonists with direct thrombin inhibitors may affect the two published ecarin clotting time methods differently. In 12 samples of normal plasma and 12 samples of plasma from patients taking stable warfarin, to which lepirudin (100–3000 ng/ml), argatroban (300–3000 ng/ml), and melagatran (30–1000 ng/ml) were added, two different assay methods produced different results. Use of the ecarin clotting time ratio improved but did not abolish the differences between the methods.

Ximelagatran   *(SEDA-29, 363)*

Product withdrawal   Treatment with ximelagatran has been associated with mainly asymp-

tomatic rises in alanine transaminase activity during long-term use (>35 days), in a mean of 7.9% of patients in long-term clinical trials. Nearly all of the cases occurred within the first 6 months of therapy. Rare symptomatic cases have occurred. Owing to the unexplained relation between raised alanine transaminase, and in some cases a raised bilirubin, with a fatal outcome in three patients, as well as the occurrence of a cute coronary syndrome after termination of therapy, the US Food and Drug Administration did not license ximelagatran. Consequently, the manufacturers withdrew ximelagatran from the European market.

Comparative studies   Ximelagatran 36 mg bd has been compared with standard enoxaparin + warfarin for prevention of recurrent venous thromboembolism in a 6-month, double-blind, randomized, non-inferiority study, the Thrombin Inhibitor in Venous Thromboembolism (THRIVE) Treatment Study in 2489 patients with acute deep vein thrombosis, of whom about one-third had a concomitant pulmonary embolism (98^C). Major bleeding occurred in 1.3 and 2.2% of those who used ximelagatran and enoxaparin + warfarin respectively, and the deaths rates were 2.3 and 3.4%. Alanine transaminase activity rose to more than three times the upper limit of normal in 119 patients (9.6%) and 25 patients (2.0%) respectively. The increased enzyme activity was mainly asymptomatic. Retrospective analysis of locally reported adverse events showed a higher rate of serious coronary events with ximelagatran (10/1240 patients) compared with enoxaparin + warfarin (1/1249 patients).

Hematologic   In a meta-analysis of 12 randomized controlled trials of ximelagatran there was an absolute risk of major venous thromboembolism of 4.04 and 1.69% and of *major bleeding episodes* of 1.68 and 1.03% in prophylaxis and treatment trials respectively (99^M). In prophylaxis trials, there was significant excess mortality (OR = 2.5; 95% CI = 1.02, 6.13) and an excess of major bleeding episodes (OR = 1.41; 95% CI = 0.93, 2.14) in the whole ximelagatran group. There was an increase in the absolute risk of bleeding (from 1.04 to 3.03%) between postoperative

and preoperative administration of ximelagatran.

Hepatotoxicity of ximelagatran

DoTS classification:
Reaction: Liver damage due to
    ximelagatran
Dose-relation: Collateral
Time-course: Intermediate, with tolerance
Susceptibility factors: Other diseases
    (simultaneous acute illnesses)

In a double-blind, placebo-controlled study,
THRIVE III, patients with venous thromboembolism who had taken an anticoagulant for
6 months were randomized to extended secondary prevention with ximelagatran 24 mg bd
or placebo for 18 months without monitoring
(100^C). Death from any cause occurred in six
patients who took ximelagatran and seven who
took placebo; bleeding occurred in 134 and
111 patients respectively (HR = 1.19; 95%
CI = 0.93, 1.53). The cumulative risk of a
transient rise in the alanine transaminase activity to more than three times the upper limit
of the reference range was 6.4% with ximelagatran compared with 1.2% with placebo. The
main reason for withdrawal from the study was
a rise in serum alanine transaminase activity
(101^C).

In a double-blind, randomized study in 254
patients with non-valvular atrial fibrillation,
ximelagatran (n = 187) 20, 40, or 60 mg bd
was compared with warfarin (n = 67) (102^C).
Alanine transaminase increased in eight patients taking ximelagatran, but normalized with
continuous treatment or withdrawal.

Adjusted-dose warfarin and fixed-dose oral
ximelagatran 36 mg bd have been compared in
a double-blind, randomized, multicenter study
in 3922 patients with non-valvular atrial fibrillation and additional risk factors for stroke
(103^C). There was no difference between the
groups in the rates of major bleeding, but there
was more total bleeding (major and minor) with
warfarin (37 versus 47% per year; 95% CI for
the difference = 6, 14). Serum alanine transaminase activities rose to greater than three times
the upper limit of the reference range in 6%

of the patients who took ximelagatran, usually within 6 months, and typically improved
whether or not treatment continued; however,
there was one clear case of fatal liver disease
and one other suggestive case.

In a prospective analysis of 6948 patients
randomized to ximelagatran and 6230 patients randomized to a comparator (warfarin,
low-molecular-weight heparin followed by warfarin, or placebo), the alanine transaminase
activity rose to more than three times the upper
limit of the reference range in 7.9% of the patients who received ximelagatran and 1.2% in
the comparator group (104^C). The increase in
alanine transaminase occurred at 1–6 months
after the start of therapy, and there was recovery to less than twice the upper limit of the
reference range in 96% of patients, whether
they continued to take ximelagatran or not.
A raised alanine transaminase activity was
more common in those with simultaneous acute
illnesses (acute myocardial infarction or venous
thromboembolism). Combined rises in alanine
transaminase activity (to three times the upper
limit of normal) and total bilirubin concentration (to twice the upper limit of normal within
1 month of the rise in alanine transaminase),
regardless of cause, were infrequent, occurring
in 37 patients (0.5%) taking ximelagatran, of
whom one had a severe hepatic illness that appeared to be resolving when the patient died
from a gastrointestinal hemorrhage. No deaths
were directly related to hepatic failure caused
by ximelagatran.

DIRECT FACTOR Xa INHIBITORS

Rivaroxaban

Rivaroxaban,   5-chloro-N-({(5S)-2-oxo-3-[4-
(3-oxomorpholin-4-yl)phenyl]-1,3-oxazolidin-
5-yl}methyl)thiophene-2-carboxamide, an oral
direct inhibitor of factor Xa, has been investigated in a single-center, placebo-controlled,
single-blind, parallel-group, multiple-dose escalation study in healthy men aged 20–45 years,
body mass index 19–31 kg/m^2, who took rivaroxaban (n = 8 per dosage regimen) or
placebo (n = 4 per dosage regimen) on days
0 and 3–7 (105^C). Dosage regimens were 5 mg
once, twice, or three times a day, and 10, 20,

or 30 mg twice a day. There were no clinically relevant changes in bleeding time or other safety variables across all doses and regimens. There was no dose-related increase in the frequency or severity of adverse events. Maximum inhibition of factor Xa activity occurred after about 3 hours and inhibition was maintained for at least 12 hours at all doses. Prothrombin time, activated partial thromboplastin time, and HepTest were prolonged to a similar extent to inhibition of factor Xa activity. The half-life of rivaroxaban was 5.7–9.2 hours at steady state.

Hematologic   In a multicenter, parallel-group, double-blind, double-dummy study, 621 patients undergoing elective total knee replacement were randomly assigned to oral rivaroxaban (2.5, 5, 10, 20, and 30 mg bd), starting 6–8 hours after surgery, or subcutaneous enoxaparin (30 mg bd, starting 12–24 hours after surgery) (106[C]). Treatment was continued for 5–9 days. The frequency of *major postoperative bleeding* increased with increasing doses of rivaroxaban. Bleeding end points were lower for the 2.5–10 mg bd dosages compared with higher dosages.

Otamixaban

Placebo-controlled studies   The effects of otamixaban have been studied in 10 consecutive parallel groups of healthy men, of whom eight received escalating intravenous doses of otamixaban as 6-hour infusions (1.7–183 micrograms/kg/hour) and two received a bolus dose (30 or 120 micrograms/kg) with a 6-hour infusion (60 or 140 micrograms/kg/hour) (107[C]). Otamixaban was said to be "well tolerated". Plasma concentrations increased with increasing dose, were maximal at the end-of-infusion, and fell rapidly as the infusion was stopped. Anti-factor Xa activity coincided with otamixaban plasma concentrations and clotting time measurements followed the same pattern.

INDIRECT FACTOR Xa INHIBITORS   *(SEDA-27, 359; SEDA-28, 392; SEDA-29, 362)*

Fondaparinux   *(SED-15, 1437; SEDA-29, 362)*

Fondaparinux is a synthetic analogue of the unique pentasaccharide sequence that mediates the interaction of unfractionated heparin and low-molecular-weight heparin with antithrombin. Once the pentasaccharide–antithrombin complex binds factor Xa, the pentasaccharide dissociates from the antithrombin and can be reused. Thus, the indirect inhibitors are catalytic and result in antithrombin-mediated irreversible inhibition of free factor Xa. Fondaparinux binds antithrombin with high affinity, has nearly 100% availability after subcutaneous injection, and has a half-life of 17 hours, permitting once-daily administration. It is excreted unchanged in the urine, and dosages should be adjusted in patients with severe renal insufficiency.

Immunologic   In patients with *delayed-type hypersensitivity* to heparin, cross-reactions often occur. Ultra-low-molecular-weight heparins may be a therapeutic alternative in some cases, but not in all patients with delayed-type hypersensitivity skin reactions at subcutaneous heparin injection sites (108[A]).

- A 59-year-old woman developed localized pruritic skin lesions after receiving nadroparin for 3 days. Patch tests and prick and intracutaneous tests with heparin, low molecular weight heparins, fondaparinux, heparinoid, and xylanolpolyhydrogensulfates were positive to all except pentosanpolysulfate, a recombinant form of desirudin. Fondaparinux produced a progressive itchy erythematous infiltrated patch at the injection site. Hirudin was well tolerated.

THROMBOLYTIC AGENTS
(SED-15, 3402; SEDA-28, 392; SEDA-29, 361)

Streptokinase

Cardiovascular   The prognostic value of ventricular late potentials and the character of rhythm disturbances have been studied in 64 patients with acute coronary syndrome (109ᶜ). The overall rate of ventricular late potentials increased 8 hours after admission from 69 to 86%. In all cases of reperfusion dysrhythmias there was deterioration of signal-averaged electrocardiographic parameters and ventricular late potentials. However, in those who received thrombolysis the rate of ventricular late potentials was lower than in those who did not: 31 versus 48% on day 10 and in 11 versus 41% by the end of hospital treatment. Beta-blockers improved signal-averaged electrocardiography and cardiac rhythm variability in both groups.

Hemorrhage   Various *bleeding complications* have been reported after thrombolysis, including atraumatic compartment syndrome in the thigh (110ᴬ), bleeding into the neck (111ᴬ), and a duodenal hematoma (112ᴬ). Hemorrhagic stroke due to streptokinase is not uncommon and has again been reported (113ᴬ).

Immunologic   *Antistreptokinase antibody titers* have been determined in 47 consecutive streptokinase-naive patients with the acute coronary syndrome from Australian communities with endemic group A streptococcal infection, because of the implications for streptokinase thrombolysis (114ᶜ). Antistreptolysin O and anti-DNAse B titers were also determined. Indigenous patients were significantly more likely to have anti-streptokinase antibodies than the non-indigenous patients. Antistreptokinase antibody titers also correlated well with antistreptolysin O and anti-DNAse B titers. The authors concluded that streptokinase should not be used for thrombolysis in populations with endemic group A streptococcal infection.

In a double-blind, randomized study in 50 consecutive patients with acute myocardial infarction who were given streptokinase 1.5 or 2.5 million units and underwent angiography within 24 hours, the presence of antistreptokinase antibodies or the administration of an increased dose of streptokinase had no effect on improving the patency rate of the infarct-related artery (115ᶜ). A larger study is needed to confirm these observations.

The use of streptokinase as a preflush in non-heart-beating kidney donors did not cause the production of anti-streptokinase antibodies in 18 recipients of renal transplants (116ᶜ).

Angioedema is a rare acute and potentially fatal reaction to streptokinase, which should be diagnosed and treated quickly to guarantee the best prognosis (117ᴬ).

- A 65-year-old white man with a myocardial infarction was given streptokinase 1 500 000 U intravenously. After infusion of 1/6th of the dose, he developed progressive hoarseness and nasal obstruction, secondary to angioedema. The infusion was stopped immediately and he was given adrenaline and hydrocortisone. He rapidly developed respiratory difficulty and wheezing, requiring intubation He also had edema of the eyebrows, lips, and tongue and later developed hemolytic anemia, which was attributed to activation of complement as part of the anaphylactic reaction.

DRUGS THAT ALTER PLATELET FUNCTION   *(SEDA-25, 412; SEDA-27, 360; SEDA-28, 396; SEDA-29, 363)*

Anagrelide   *(SEDA-29, 364)*

Cardiovascular   *High-output heart failure* has been attributed to anagrelide in a patient with essential thrombocytosis; there was dramatic improvement after withdrawal of anagrelide (118ᴬ). Of 577 patients taking anagrelide, 14 developed CHF; 2 died suddenly (119ᶜ). In another study of 942 patients taking anagrelide for thrombocytosis, 15 died of cardiac causes (120ᶜ). The authors suggested that increased cardiac output was due to the positive inotropic activity through phosphodiesterase inhibition.

Urinary tract   *Renal tubular damage* has been attributed to anagrelide in a 60-year-old man with Crohn's disease and essential thrombocytosis (121ᴬ).

Dipyridamole   *(SED-15, 1140; SEDA-28, 397; SEDA-29, 365)*

Respiratory   A 69-year-old non-smoking woman with stable asthma developed sudden *bronchospasm* within minutes of receiving intravenous dipyridamole during a thallium stress test; it responded to intravenous aminophylline 150 mg (122ᴬ). The authors proposed that dipyridamole had increased circulating concentrations of adenosine, a bronchoconstrictor.

Glycoprotein IIb-IIIa inhibitors

(SED-15, 4; SEDA-27, 360; SEDA-28, 396; SEDA-29, 363)

Nervous system   The safety of abciximab in patients with prior stroke undergoing percutaneous coronary intervention has not previously been adequately studied. In a database review of 7244 consecutive interventions, 6190 had been performed with abciximab, including 515 in patients with a history of *stroke*, either recent ($n =$ 101) or remote (>2 years; $n = 414$) (123^C). The rate of stroke after intervention was significantly higher in those with a prior stroke (2.06 versus 0.35% for all stroke; 0.38 versus 0.03% for intracerebral hemorrhage). However, the incidence of intracerebral hemorrhage among the abciximab-treated patients was 0.065%, and a history of prior stroke did not increase the incidence.

Distal embolization is the main potential risk of carotid stenting, and techniques to minimize the risk are evolving. Between July 1998 and March 2002, 305 consecutive patients who underwent elective or urgent percutaneous carotid intervention at The Cleveland Clinic were followed. During this period, the practice of carotid stenting evolved from the routine use of glycoprotein IIb-IIIa inhibitors to the routine of an emboli-prevention device (124^C). In all, 199 patients received adjunctive glycoprotein IIb-IIIa inhibitors (91% abciximab), and 106 patients had an emboli-prevention device inserted (85% filter design, 15% occlusive balloon). At 30 days, the composite end point of neurological death, non-fatal stroke, and major bleeding, including intracranial hemorrhage, was significantly less among patients treated with emboli-prevention device than in those treated with glycoprotein IIb-IIIa inhibitors (0 versus 5.1%).

Hematologic   *Splenic rupture* with massive intra-abdominal hemorrhage, as a consequence of secondary bleeding into multiple pre-existing splenic infarctions, has been reported in a patient taking a glycoprotein IIb-IIIa antagonist (125^A).

Acute *thrombocytopenia*, which is sometimes severe and life-threatening, is a recognized adverse effect of the glycoprotein IIb-IIIa inhibitors.

DoTS classification:
Reaction: Abciximab and
    thrombocytopenia
Dose-relation: Hypersusceptibility
Time-course: First dose or early persistent
Susceptibility factors: Female sex;
    drug–drug interactions (heparin,
    acetylsalicylic acid, ticlopidine); renal
    disease

In contrast to other types of drug-induced thrombocytopenia, this complication can occur within a few hours of first exposure. Accumulating evidence has suggested that drug-dependent antibodies, which can be naturally occurring, are the cause of platelet destruction in such cases. The clinical aspects of thrombocytopenia that results from sensitivity to glycoprotein IIb-IIIa inhibitors and the evidence that the platelet destruction is antibody-mediated have been reviewed (126^R).

There have been 2780 international reports of adverse events in patients taking abciximab, including 1046 cases of thrombocytopenia (38%). Of 250 adverse events reports of patients treated with abciximab in Germany, there were 76 (30.4%) cases of thrombocytopenia and 93 (37%) of hemorrhage; 44 patients (18%) had both thrombocytopenia and hemorrhage (6^S). Abciximab is often used in combination with heparin, acetylsalicylic acid, or ticlopidine, and combination therapy leads to a greater risk of severe and lethal bleeding.

Thrombocytopenia that develops after percutaneous coronary intervention can cause hemorrhagic complications, requirement for blood product transfusions, and potentially thrombotic or ischemic complications. Thrombocytopenia in patients with acute myocardial infarction who undergo primary percutaneous coronary intervention has not previously been evaluated. In the CADILLAC study, 2082 patients who had an acute myocardial infarction within 12 hours without shock were prospectively randomized to receive balloon angioplasty with or without abciximab versus stenting with or without abciximab (127^C). Acquired thrombocytopenia, defined as a nadir platelet count below 100×10^9/l in patients who did not have baseline thrombocytopenia, developed in 50 of 1975 patients (2.5%). The independent predictors of acquired thrombocytopenia were a platelet count below 200×10^9/l on admission

(OR = 5.35; 95% CI = 2.91, 9.81), non-insulin-requiring diabetes mellitus (4.42; 2.19, 8.91), previous statin administration (OR = 3.19; 1.55, 6.57), and use of abciximab (2.06; 1.11, 3.83). Thrombocytopenia was *less* likely in those with a greater body mass index (0.90; 0.84, 0.97) and previous aspirin use (0.27; 0.11, 0.63). Patients who developed thrombocytopenia had significantly higher rates of major hemorrhagic complications than those who did not (10 versus 2.7%), greater requirements for blood transfusions (10 versus 3.9%), and longer hospital stays (median 4.8 versus 3.6 days), and they incurred higher costs (median $14 466 versus $11 629). All-cause mortality was markedly increased at 30 days in patients who developed thrombocytopenia (8.0 versus 1.6%) and at 1 year (10 versus 3.9%).

Bleeding complications were prospectively recorded in 344 consecutive patients who underwent percutaneous coronary intervention with adjunctive use of abciximab (128[C]). There was major bleeding in six patients (1.7%) one of whom had pulmonary hemorrhage and one intracranial hemorrhage. There was minor bleeding in 20 (5.8%). There was thrombocytopenia in 13 (3.9%), mild in four cases, severe in four, and profound in five. Female sex and the "bail-out" use of abciximab were susceptibility factors for bleeding complications.

Profound thrombocytopenia occurring 1 week after administration of abciximab is uncommon, self-limiting, and mostly uneventful (129[Ar]). However, a quick diagnosis is essential, since other forms of thrombocytopenia associated with concomitant antithrombotic therapies may be much more severe and require prompt treatment. Awareness of this reaction may avoid unnecessary and risky withdrawal of other antiplatelet drugs in the critical phase after coronary stenting.

Drug–drug interactions   In 30 patients with acute myocardial infarction undergoing percutaneous coronary intervention, abciximab significantly increased the concentration of the platelet activation marker P selectin, and reduced the dosage of *unfractionated heparin* that was required to prolong the aPTT by over 60 seconds (130[c]). When abciximab was withdrawn the heparin dosage requirement increased to a greater extent and reached the level found in the untreated patients, even when

platelet aggregation was still inhibited. The authors concluded that the increased platelet activation found at the end of abciximab treatment points to a procoagulant condition that should be carefully monitored and treated by altering the doses of anticoagulants and antiplatelet drugs.

THIENOPYRIDINES   *(SED-15, 821; SEDA-28, 397; SEDA-29, 365)*

From 1990 to 2002, 475 reports of adverse reactions due to clopidogrel and 691 due to ticlopidine were registered in the database of the German spontaneous reporting system (6[S]). The breakdowns are reported under separate headings below.

Clopidogrel

Hematologic

Bone marrow   Clopidogrel, an analogue of ticlopidine, was developed because it seemed to have fewer bone marrow adverse effects. In the German pharmacovigilance database thrombocytopenia was the most frequent adverse event attributed to clopidogrel (60 cases; 13%), followed by gastrointestinal hemorrhage (56 cases; 12%), anemia (38 cases; 8.0%), hematoma (29 cases; 6.1%), and melena (27 cases; 5.7%) (6[S]). White cell disorders were reported in only 8.9% of cases compared with 42% with ticlopidine: There were three reports of clopidogrel-associated thrombotic thrombocytopenic purpura (0.6%).

Hemorrhage   The use of antiplatelet agents in elderly patients with trauma significantly increases the risk of death when head injury involves intracranial hemorrhage. In a retrospective analysis, patients older than 50 years who had had a traumatic intracranial hemorrhage over the previous 4 years associated with the use of aspirin, clopidogrel, or a combination of the two were compared with a control group of patients who had had a hemorrhage but were not taking antiplatelet drugs (131[c]). There were no significant differences between the 90 patients and the 89 controls in terms of demographics, mechanism of injury, Injury Severity Score, Glasgow Coma Score, or hospital length of stay. The patients who were taking antiplatelet drugs had significantly more co-morbid conditions (71 versus 35%); 21 patients and eight controls died (23 versus 8.9%) and age over 76 years and a Glasgow Coma Score lower than 12 correlated significantly with increased mortality.

An epidural hematoma occurred after combined spinal–epidural anesthesia in an 80-year-old woman who was given clopidogrel and dalteparin (66[A]).

Liver   *Hepatotoxicity* has been attributed to clopidogrel (132[A]).

- A 74-year-old man with acute coronary syndrome was given clopidogrel 75 mg/day and pantoprazole 40 mg/day and 4 weeks later developed tea-coloured urine and jaundice. The serum bilirubin concentration was 91 µmol/l, alkaline phosphatase 172 IU/l, and alanine transaminase 212 IU/l; serum albumin concentration and coagulation tests were normal, but there was mild thrombocytopenia (135×10^9/l) and a low white cell count (3.8×10^9/l). Serological tests for acute viral causes of hepatitis were negative, as were autoantibody tests. Clopidogrel was withdrawn. After 5 days the liver biochemistry started to improve gradually and became normal after 4 weeks.

Immunologic   *Allergic rashes* are common in patients taking clopidogrel and can require withdrawal.

A severe *hypersensitivity syndrome* in a patient taking clopidogrel resolved on dechallenge and recurred on rechallenge (133[A]). The reaction included neutropenia, rash, fever, tachycardia, nausea, and vomiting. This presentation is very similar to the frequently reported hypersensitivity reactions to ticlopidine and very similar to a case involving clopidogrel reported previously.

In another case hypersensitivity to clopidogrel in a 62-year-old man was associated with fever, severe pruritus, raised liver enzymes, pancytopenia, and a rash, with erythematous macules and papules symmetrically distributed on the face, trunk, and limbs, but without mucosal lesions (134[A]).

Drug resistance   Resistance to aspirin and clopidogrel, which can have serious consequences, such as recurrent myocardial infarction, stroke, or death, has been reviewed (135[R]).

In its broadest sense, resistance refers to the continued occurrence of ischemic events despite adequate antiplatelet therapy and adherence to therapy. However, the lack of a standard definition of resistance and the lack of standard diagnostic methods has hampered identification and treatment. Attempts have been made to develop a more useful definition, with the goal of correlating laboratory tests with clinical outcomes, but there is no current definition that unites biochemical and clinical expressions of failed treatment. Rates of aspirin resistance are reported at 5–45%, depending on the study and the method of determining therapeutic failure. However, rather than characterizing patients as resistant or sensitive to a medication, resistance is probably better regarded as a continuous variable, similar to blood pressure. The mechanisms of resistance to antiplatelet drugs are incompletely defined, but there are specific clinical, cellular, and genetic factors that affect therapeutic failure, including failure to prescribe these medications despite appropriate indications and polymorphisms of platelet membrane glycoproteins. As new bedside tests are developed for the rapid and accurate measurement of the response to antiplatelet drugs, it may become easier to individualize antiplatelet drug therapy.

Management of adverse reactions   Type I allergic reactions to drugs may be amenable to desensitization. A protocol for clopidogrel desensitization over 8 hours has been described, using 15 doubling doses of oral clopidogrel to achieve a maintenance dose of 75 mg/day (Table 1) (136[A]).

- A 71-year-old man with a history of allergy to penicillin was given clopidogrel after intracoronary stenting. After 7 days he developed generalized pruritic erythematous macules, without dyspnea, hypotension, or mucosal or vesiculobullous lesions. Clopidogrel was withdrawn and he was given ticlopidine instead. However, 2 weeks later he developed severe neutropenia, fever, and sinusitis, and ticlopidine was withdrawn. IgE-mediated drug allergy to clopidogrel was diagnosed and he was deemed suitable for desensitization, which was successfully completed without adverse effects. He continued to take clopidogrel and had no recurrence.
- A 68-year-old woman with a history of allergy to penicillin was given clopidogrel after intracoronary stenting and after 3 days developed a pruritic maculopapular rash on her lower abdomen. Clopidogrel was withdrawn and the rash resolved with

Table 1. *Clopidogrel desensitization protocol (136[A])*

Desensitizing dose (mg)	Concentration (mg/ml)	Volume (ml)
0.005	0.5	0.01
0.010		0.02
0.020		0.04
0.040		0.08
0.080		0.16
0.160		0.32
0.300		0.60
0.600		1.20
1.200	5	0.24
2.5		0.5
5		1
10		2
20		4
40		8
75	75 mg tablet	1 tablet

Notes: Doses are given orally every 30 minutes if no adverse reaction occurs. The patient is monitored closely during the procedure, with equipment available to treat anaphylaxis. If any adverse reactions occur the protocol is adjusted. The patient is kept under observation for at least 1 hour after the last dose.

a short course of prednisone. Later, after repeat stenting, she was given ticlopidine and after 2 days developed a similar rash. The ticlopidine was withdrawn and the rash resolved with prednisone. She underwent out-patient oral desensitization to clopidogrel. After the 12th dose she felt flushing of her forearms without objective changes, and the procedure was successfully completed without further incident. She then took clopidogrel 75 mg/day with no recurrence.

• A 71-year-old woman with no drug allergies was given clopidogrel after abdominal aneurysm stenting and 3 weeks later developed an erythematous macular rash on her trunk, arms, and upper thighs. Clopidogrel was withdrawn and the rash resolved with a short course of prednisone. She was given ticlopidine and 1 week later developed a similar pruritic rash on her face and limbs with associated vomiting. Ticlopidine was withdrawn and the rash resolved spontaneously within 1 week. She underwent clopidogrel desensitization, but 3 weeks later she had mild generalized pruritus, easy bruising, and melena. Clopidogrel was withdrawn. She later underwent redesensitization to clopidogrel as an outpatient, but developed a pruritic erythematous rash on her lower abdomen 10 minutes after taking a dose of 5 mg. She was given oral cetirizine and after 30 minutes, when the pruritus and erythema had subsided, the desensitization protocol was restarted with a dose of 2.5 mg and was completed at the 40 mg dose (total cumulative dose

87 mg) with no further complications. She then took clopidogrel 75 mg/day without recurrence.

This case series suggests that patients who have had a type I allergic reaction to clopidogrel can be rapidly desensitized. Further studies in a larger number of patients are needed to confirm the safety and efficacy of this regimen.

Ticlopidine

Hematologic   In the German spontaneous reporting system there were 107 cases (16%) of *agranulocytosis*, 79 of *leukopenia* (111%) and 48 of *thrombocytopenia* (6.9%) (6[S]). Other important hematological adverse effects were *granulocytopenia* (43 cases; 6.2%), *anemia* (29 cases; 4.2%), *pancytopenia* (18 cases; 2.6%), *thrombotic thrombocytopenic purpura* (14 cases; 2.0%), and *bone marrow depression* (14 cases; 2.0%).

Liver   In the German spontaneous reporting system there were 283 cases (41%) of *liver and biliary system disorders* (6[S]). These included increases in hepatic enzymes (123 cases; 18%), hepatitis and cholestatic hepatitis (65 cases; 9.4%), and jaundice (23 cases; 3.3%).

Protamine   *(SED-15, 2964)*

Cardiovascular   *Coronary artery spasm* has been attributed to protamine (137[A]).

• A 65-year-old man suddenly developed severe systemic hypotension, with electrocardiographic ST segment elevation and widening of the QRS interval after receiving protamine to reverse heparin anticoagulation following cardiopulmonary bypass. He had a similar reaction after another small dose of protamine.

The authors suggested that this event was due to coronary artery spasm associated with an anaphylactic reaction induced by protamine, despite the absence of other evidence of anaphylaxis, such as cutaneous manifestations and bronchospasm.

References

1. Bauer E, Derfler K, Joukhadar C, Druml W. Citrate kinetics in patients receiving long-term hemodialysis therapy. Am J Kidney Dis 2005;46(5):903–7.
2. Ridel C, Mercadal L, Béné B, Hamani A, Deray G, Petitclerc T. Regional citrate anticoagulation during hemodialysis: a simplified procedure using Duocart biofiltration. Blood Purif 2005;23(6):473–80.
3. Bihorac A, Ross EA. Continuous venovenous hemofiltration with citrate-based replacement fluid: efficacy, safety, and impact on nutrition. Am J Kidney Dis 2005;46(5):908–18.
4. Baran-Furga H, Chmielewska K, Bogucka-Bonikowska A, Habrat B, Kortowski W, Bienkowski P. Citrate anticoagulation for single-needle hemodialysis: safety and efficacy. Ther Apheresis Dial 2005;9(3):1103–11.
5. Manu N, Martin L. Warfarin-induced small bowel obstruction. Clin Lab Haematol 2005;27(5):350–2.
6. Tiaden JD, Wenzel E, Berthold HK, Muller-Oerlinghausen B. Adverse reactions to anticoagulants and to antiplatelet drugs recorded by the German spontaneous reporting system. Semin Thromb Hemost 2005;31(4):371–80.
7. Holbrook AM, Pereira JA, Labiris R, McDonald H, Douketis JD, Crowther M, Wells PS. Systematic overview of warfarin and its drug and food interactions. Arch Intern Med 2005;165(10):1095–106.
8. Loke YK, Price D, Derry S, Aronson JK. Case reports of suspected adverse drug reactions – systematic literature survey of follow-up. BMJ 2006;332(7537):335–9.
9. Hu Z, Yang X, Ho PC, Chan SY, Heng PW, Chan E, Duan W, Koh HL, Zhou S. Herb-drug interactions: a literature review. Drugs 2005;65(9):1239–82.
10. Williamson EM. Interactions between herbal and conventional medicines. Expert Opin Drug Saf 2005;4(2):355–78.
11. Izzo AA, Di Carlo G, Borrelli F, Ernst E. Cardiovascular pharmacotherapy and herbal medicines: the risk of drug interaction. Int J Cardiol 2005;98(1):1–14.
12. Monterrey-Rodríguez J. Interaction between warfarin and mango fruit. Ann Pharmacother 2002;36(5):940–1.
13. Lambert JP, Cormier J. Potential interaction between warfarin and boldo–fenugreek. Pharmacotherapy 2001;21(4):509–12.
14. Ramsay NA, Kenny MW, Davies G, Patel JP. Complimentary and alternative medicine use among patients starting warfarin. Br J Haematol 2005;130(5):777–80.
15. Vaes LP, Chyka PA. Interactions of warfarin with garlic, ginger, ginkgo, or ginseng: nature of the evidence. Ann Pharmacother 2000;34(12):1478–82.
16. Page 2nd RL, Lawrence JD. Potentiation of warfarin by dong quai. Pharmacotherapy 1999;19(7):870–6.
17. Lo AC, Chan K, Yeung JH, Woo KS. Danggui (*Angelica sinensis*) affects the pharmacodynamics but not the pharmacokinetics of warfarin in rabbits. Eur J Drug Metab Pharmacokinet 1995;20(1):55–60.
18. Tang JC, Zhang JN, Wu YT, Li ZX. Effect of the water extract and ethanol extract from traditional Chinese medicines *Angelica sinensis (Oliv.) Diels, Ligusticum chuanxiong Hort. and Rheum palmatum L.* on rat liver cytochrome P450 activity. Phytother Res 2006;20(12):1046–51.
19. Taylor JR, Wilt VM. Probable antagonism of warfarin by green tea. Ann Pharmacother 1999;33(4):426–8.
20. Cheng TO. Green tea may inhibit warfarin. Int J Cardiol 2007;115(2):236.
21. Yue QY, Jansson K. Herbal drug curbicin and anticoagulant effect with and without warfarin: possibly related to the vitamin E component. J Am Geriatr Soc 2001;49(6):838.
22. Matthews MK. Association of *Ginkgo biloba* with intracerebral haemorrhage. Neurology 1998;5:1933.
23. Jiang X, Williams KM, Liauw WS, Ammit AJ, Roufogalis BD, Duke CC, Day RO, McLachlan AJ. Effect of ginkgo and ginger on the pharmacokinetics and pharmacodynamics of warfarin in healthy subjects. Br J Clin Pharmacol 2005;59:425–32.
24. Engelsen J, Nielsen JD, Hansen KF. Effekten af coenzym Q10 og *Ginkgo biloba* pa warfarindosis hos patienter i laengerevarende warfarinbehandling. Et randomiseret, dobbeltblindt, placebokontrolleret overkrydsningsforsog. Ugeskr Laeger 2003;165(18):1868–71.
25. Koch E. Inhibition of platelet activating factor (PAF)-induced aggregation of human thrombocytes by ginkgolides: considerations on possible bleeding complications after oral intake of *Ginkgo biloba* extracts. Phytomedicine 2005;12(1–2):10–6.
26. Destro MW, Speranzini MB, Cavalheiro Filho C, Destro T, Destro C. Bilateral haematoma after rhytidoplasty and blepharoplasty following chronic use of *Ginkgo biloba*. Br J Plast Surg 2005;58(1):100–1.
27. Bebbington A, Kulkarni R, Roberts P. *Ginkgo biloba*: persistent bleeding after total hip arthroplasty caused by herbal self-medication. J Arthroplasty 2005;20(1):125–6.
28. Rosenblatt M, Mindel J. Spontaneous hyphema associated with ingestion of *Ginkgo biloba* extract. N Engl J Med 1997;336(15):1108.
29. Meisel C, Johne A, Roots I. Fatal intracerebral mass bleeding associated with *Ginkgo biloba* and ibuprofen. Atherosclerosis 2003;167(2):367.

30. Kim YS, Pyo MK, Park KM, Park PH, Hahn BS, Wu SJ, Yun-Choi HS. Antiplatelet and antithrombotic effects of a combination of ticlopidine and *Ginkgo biloba* ext (EGb 761). Thromb Res 1998;91(1):33–8.
31. Bal Dit Sollier C, Caplain H, Drouet L. No alteration in platelet function or coagulation induced by EGb761 in a controlled study. Clin Lab Haematol 2003;25(4):251–3.
32. Henderson L, Yue QY, Bergquist C, Gerden B, Arlett P. St John's wort (*Hypericum perforatum*): drug interactions and clinical outcomes. Br J Clin Pharmacol 2002;54(4):349–56.
33. Maurer A, Johne A, Bauer S. Interaction of St. John's wort extract with phenprocoumon. Eur J Clin Pharmacol 1999;55:A22.
34. Jiang X, Williams KM, Liauw WS, Ammit AJ, Roufogalis BD, Duke CC, Day RO, McLachlan AJ. Effect of St John's wort and ginseng on the pharmacokinetics and pharmacodynamics of warfarin in healthy subjects. Br J Clin Pharmacol 2004;57(5):592–9. Erratum, 58 2004(1):102.
35. Lam AY, Elmer GW, Mohutsky MA. Possible interaction between warfarin and *Lycium barbarum* L. Ann Pharmacother 2001;35(10):1199–201.
36. Coon JT, Ernst E. *Panax ginseng*: a systematic review of adverse effects and drug interactions. Drug Saf 2002;25(5):323–44.
37. Janetzky K, Morreale AP. Probable interaction between warfarin and ginseng. Am J Health Syst Pharm 1997;54(6):692–3.
38. Rosado MF. Thrombosis of a prosthetic aortic valve disclosing a hazardous interaction between warfarin and a commercial ginseng product. Cardiology 2003;99(2):111.
39. Yuan CS, Wei G, Dey L, Karrison T, Nahlik L, Maleckar S, Kasza K, Ang-Lee M, Moss J. American ginseng reduces warfarin's effect in healthy patients: a randomized, controlled trial. Ann Intern Med 2004;141(1):23–7.
40. Anderson GD, Rosito G, Mohustsy MA, Elmer GW. Drug interaction potential of soy extract and *Panax ginseng*. J Clin Pharmacol 2003;43:643–8.
41. Jung KY, Kim DS, Oh SR, Lee IS, Lee JJ, Park JD, Kim SI, Lee HK. Platelet activating factor antagonist activity of ginsenosides. Biol Pharm Bull 1998;21(1):79–80.
42. Zhu M, Chan KW, Ng LS, Chang Q, Chang S, Li RC. Possible influences of ginseng on the pharmacokinetics and pharmacodynamics of warfarin in rats. J Pharm Pharmacol 1999;51(2):175–80.
43. Henderson GL, Harkey MR, Gershwin ME, Hackman RM, Stern JS, Stresser DM. Effects of ginseng components on c-DNA-expressed cytochrome P450 enzyme catalytic activity. Life Sci 1999;65(15):PL209–14.
44. Kim HJ, Chun YJ, Park JD, Kim SI, Roh JK, Jeong TC. Protection of rat liver microsomes against carbon tetrachloride-induced lipid peroxidation by red ginseng saponin

through cytochrome P450 inhibition. Planta Med 1997;63(5):415–8.
45. Izzat MB, Yim APC, El-Zufari MH. A taste of Chinese medicine! Ann Thorac Surg 1998;66:941–2.
46. Tam LS, Chan TYK, Leung WK, Critchley JAJH. Warfarin interactions with Chinese traditional medicines: danshen and methyl salicylate medicated oil. Aust NZ J Med 1995;25:258.
47. Yu CM, Chan JCN, Sanderson JE. Chinese herbs and warfarin potentiation by "danshen". J Int Med 1997;241:337–9.
48. Chan TY. Interaction between warfarin and danshen (*Salvia miltiorrhiza*). Ann Pharmacother 2001;35(4):501–4.
49. Kuo YH, Lin YL, Don MJ, Chen RM, Ueng YF. Induction of cytochrome P450-dependent monooxygenase by extracts of the medicinal herb *Salvia miltiorrhiza*. J Pharm Pharmacol 2006;58(4):521–7.
50. Lo AC, Chan K, Yeung JH, Woo KS. The effects of danshen (*Salvia miltiorrhiza*) on pharmacokinetics and pharmacodynamics of warfarin in rats. Eur J Drug Metab Pharmacokinet 1992;17(4):257–62.
51. Chan K, Lo AC, Yeung JH, Woo KS. The effects of danshen (*Salvia miltiorrhiza*) on warfarin pharmacodynamics and pharmacokinetics of warfarin enantiomers in rats. J Pharm Pharmacol 1995;47(5):402–6.
52. Gupta D, Jalali M, Wells A, Dasgupta A. Drug–herb interactions: unexpected suppression of free danshen concentrations by salicylate. J Clin Lab Anal 2002;16(6):290–4.
53. Makino T, Wakushima H, Okamoto T, Okukubo Y, Deguchi Y, Kano Y. Pharmacokinetic interactions between warfarin and kangen-karyu, a Chinese traditional herbal medicine, and their synergistic action. J Ethnopharmacol 2002;82(1):35–40.
54. Lesho EP, Saullo L, Udvari-Nagy S. A 76-year-old woman with erratic anticoagulation. Cleve Clin J Med 2004;71(8):651–6.
55. Anonymous. Medical mystery. A woman with too-thin blood. Why was the patient bleeding? What's her case mean to you? Heart Advis 2004;7(12):4–5.
56. Weidner MS, Sigwart K. The safety of a ginger extract in the rat. J Ethnopharmacol 2000;73(3):513–20.
57. Jiang X, Blair EY, McLachlan AJ. Investigation of the effects of herbal medicines on warfarin response in healthy subjects: a population pharmacokinetic–pharmacodynamic modeling approach. J Clin Pharmacol 2006;46(11):1370–8.
58. Davis NB, Nahlik L, Vogelzang NJ. Does PC-Spes interact with warfarin? J Urol 2002;167(4):1793.
59. Duncan GG. Re: Does PC-Spes interact with warfarin? J Urol 2003;169(1):294–5.
60. Wong ALN, Chan TYK. Interaction between warfarin and the herbal product quilinggao. Ann Pharmacother 2003;37:836–8.

61. Watt BE, Proudfoot AT, Bradberry SM, Vale JA. Anticoagulant rodenticides. Toxicol Rev 2005;24(4):259–69.

62. Rodrigo Casanova P, Rodríguez Fernández V, García Peña JM, Aguilera Celorrio L. Intento autolitico con superwarfarinas (Attempted suicide with superwarfarin). Rev Esp Anestesiol Reanim 2005;52(8):506–7.

63. Mora R, Jankowska B, Passali GC, Mora F, Passali FM, Crippa B, Quaranta N, Barbieri M. Sodium enoxaparin treatment of sensorineural hearing loss: an immune-mediated response? Int Tinnitus J 2005;11(1):38–42.

64. Calota F, Vilcea D, Intorcaciu M, Pairvanescu H, Enache D, Comanescu V, Vasile I, Scurtu S. Emboliile cu cristale de colesterol in cursul tratamentului cu heparine cu greutate molecular mic (Cholesterol crystal embolisation in the course of treatment with low-molecular-weight heparins). Chirurgia (Bucur) 2005;100(6):605–8.

65. Su HM, Voon WC, Chu CS, Lin TH, Lai WT, Sheu SH. Heparin-induced cardiac tamponade and life-threatening hyperkalema in a patient with chronic hemodialysis. Kaohsiung J Med Sci 2005;21(3):128–33.

66. Tam NL, Pac-Soo C, Pretorius PM. Epidural haematoma after a combined spinal–epidural anaesthetic in a patient treated with clopidogrel and dalteparin. Br J Anaesth 2006;96(2):262–5.

67. Arnold DM, Kelton JG. Heparin-induced thrombocytopenia: an iceberg rising. Mayo Clin Proc 2005;80(8):988–90.

68. McNulty I, Katz E, Kim KY, Shah PS, Ng E, Sinha AK. Heparin for prolonging peripheral intravenous catheter use in neonates. Cochrane Database Syst Rev 2005(4):CD002774.

69. Martchenke J, Boshkov L. Heparin-induced thrombocytopenia in neonates. Neonatal Netw 2005;24(5):33–7.

70. Frost J, Mureebe L, Russo P, Russo J, Tobias JD. Heparin-induced thrombocytopenia in the pediatric intensive care unit population. Pediatr Crit Care Med 2005;6(2):216–9.

71. Martel N, Lee J, Wells PS. Risk for heparin-induced thrombocytopenia with unfractionated and low-molecular-weight heparin thromboprophylaxis: a meta-analysis. Blood 2005;106(8):2710–5.

72. Hoh BL, Aghi M, Pryor JC, Ogilvy CS. Heparin-induced thrombocytopenia type II in subarachnoid hemorrhage patients: incidence and complications. Neurosurgery 2005;57(2):243–8.

73. Kaplan GG, Manns B, McLaughlin K. Heparin induced thrombocytopaenia secondary to intraperitoneal heparin exposure. Nephrol Dial Transplant 2005;20(11):2561–2.

74. Ishibashi H, Takashi O, Hosaka M, Sugimoto I, Takahashi M, Nihei T, Kawanishi J, Ishiguchi T. Heparin-induced thrombocytopenia complicated with massive thrombosis of the inferior vena cava after filter placement. Int Angiol 2005;24(4):387–90.

75. Eghtesady P, Nelson D, Schwartz SM, Wheeler D, Pearl JM, Cripe LH, Manning PB. Heparin-induced thrombocytopenia complicating support by the Berlin Heart. ASAIO J 2005;51(6):820–5.

76. Shaw PH, Ranganathan S, Gaines B. A spontaneous intramural hematoma of the bowel presenting as obstruction in a child receiving low-molecular-weight heparin. J Pediatr Hematol Oncol 2005;27(10):558–60.

77. Egger SS, Sawatzki MG, Drewe J, Krahenbuhl S. Life-threatening hemorrhage after dalteparin therapy in a patient with impaired renal function. Pharmacotherapy 2005;25(6):881–5.

78. Malik A, Capling R, Bastani B. Enoxaparin-associated retroperitoneal bleeding in two patients with renal insufficiency. Pharmacotherapy 2005;25(5):769–72.

79. Patel GK, Knight AG. Generalised cutaneous necrosis: a complication of low-molecular-weight heparin. Int Wound J 2005;2(3):267–70.

80. Toll A, Gallardo F, Abella ME, Fontcuberta J, Barranco C, Pujol RM. Low-molecular-weight heparin-induced skin necrosis: a potential association with pre-existent hypercoagulable states. Int J Dermatol 2005;44(11):964–6.

81. Patel R, Lim Z, Dawe S, Salisbury J, Arya R. Heparin-induced skin necrosis. Br J Haematol 2005;129(6):712.

82. Zeller L, Almog Y, Tomer A, Sukenik S, Abu-Shakra M. Catastrophic thromboses and severe thrombocytopenia during heparin therapy in a patient with anti-phospholipid syndrome. Clin Rheumatol 2006;25(3):426–9.

83. Lubenow N, Eichler P, Lietz T, Greinacher A, HIT Investigators Group. Lepirudin in patients with heparin-induced thrombocytopenia—results of the third prospective study (HAT-3) and a combined analysis of HAT-1, HAT-2, and HAT-3. J Thromb Haemost 2005;3(11):2428–36.

84. McNulty I, Katz E, Kim KY. Thrombocytopenia following heparin flush. Prog Cardiovasc Nurs 2005;20(4):143–7.

85. Das AK. Low-molecular-weight heparin-associated fat necrosis of the breast. Age Ageing 2005;34(2):193–4.

86. Giorgini S, Martinelli C, Massi D, Lumini A, Mannucci M, Giglioli L. Iatrogenic calcinosis cutis following nadroparin injection. Int J Dermatol 2005;44(10):855–7.

87. Campanelli A, Kaya G, Masouye I, Borradori L. Calcifying panniculitis following subcutaneous injections of nadroparin–calcium in a patient with osteomalacia. Br J Dermatol 2005;153(3):657–60.

88. Ludwig RJ, Schindewolf M, Alban S, Kaufmann R, Lindhoff-Last E, Boehncke WH. Molecular weight determines the frequency of delayed type hypersensitivity reactions to heparin and synthetic oligosaccharides. Thromb Haemost 2005;94(6):1265–9.

89. Harenberg J, Jorg I, Bayerl C, Fiehn C. Treatment of a woman with lupus pernio,

thrombosis and cutaneous intolerance to heparins using lepirudin during pregnancy. Lupus 2005;14(5):411–2.

90. Siegman-Igra Y, Jacobi E, Lang R, Schwartz D, Carmeli Y. Unexpected hospital-acquired bacteraemia in patients at low risk of bloodstream infection: the role of a heparin drip. J Hosp Infect 2005;60(2):122–8.

91. Greer IA, Nelson-Piercy C. Low-molecular-weight heparins for thromboprophylaxis and treatment of venous thromboembolism in pregnancy: a systematic review of safety and efficacy. Blood 2005;106(2):401–7.

92. Eriksson BI, Dahl OE, Buller HR, Hettiarachchi R, Rosencher N, Bravo ML, Ahnfelt L, Piovella F, Stangier J, Kalebo P, Reilly P, BISTRO II Study Group. A new oral direct thrombin inhibitor, dabigatran etexilate, compared with enoxaparin for prevention of thromboembolic events following total hip or knee replacement: the BISTRO II randomized trial. J Thromb Haemost 2005;3(1):103–11.

93. Cardenas GA, Deitcher SR. Risk of anaphylaxis after reexposure to intravenous lepirudin in patients with current or past heparin-induced thrombocytopenia. Mayo Clin Proc 2005;80(4):491–3.

94. Harenberg J, Jorg I, Fenyvesi T, Piazolo L. Treatment of patients with a history of heparin-induced thrombocytopenia and anti-lepirudin antibodies with argatroban. J Thromb Thrombolysis 2005;19(1):65–9.

95. Hacquard M, de Maistre E, Lecompte T. Lepirudin: is the approved dosing schedule too high? J Thromb Haemost 2005;3(11):2593–6.

96. Gray E, Harenberg J, ISTH Control of Anticoagulation SSC Working Group on Thrombin Inhibitors. Collaborative study on monitoring methods to determine direct thrombin inhibitors lepirudin and argatroban. J Thromb Haemost 2005;3(9):2096–7.

97. Fenyvesi T, Harenberg J, Weiss C, Jorg I. Comparison of two different ecarin clotting time methods. J Thromb Thrombolysis 2005;20(1):51–6.

98. Fiessinger JN, Huisman MV, Davidson BL, Bounameaux H, Francis CW, Eriksson H, Lundstrom T, Berkowitz SD, Nystrom P, Thorsen M, Ginsberg JS. THRIVE Treatment Study Investigators. Ximelagatran vs low-molecular-weight heparin and warfarin for the treatment of deep vein thrombosis: a randomized trial. JAMA 2005;293(6):681–9.

99. Iorio A, Guercini F, Ferrante F, Nenci GG. Safety and efficacy of ximelagatran: meta-analysis of the controlled randomized trials for the prophylaxis or treatment of venous thromboembolism. Curr Pharm Des 2005;11(30):3893–918.

100. Schulman S, Wahlander K, Lundstrom T, Clason SB, Eriksson H, THRIVE III Investigators. Secondary prevention of venous thromboembolism with the oral direct thrombin inhibitor ximelagatran. N Engl J Med 2003;349:1713–21.

101. Schulman S, Lundstrom T, Walander K, Billing Clason S, Eriksson H. Ximelagatran for the secondary prevention of venous thromboembolism: a complementary follow-up analysis of the THRIVE III study. Thromb Haemost 2005;94(4):820–4.

102. Petersen P, Grind M, Adler J, SPORTIF II Investigators. Ximelagatran versus warfarin for stroke prevention in patients with nonvalvular atrial fibrillation. SPORTIF II: a dose-guiding, tolerability, and safety study. J Am Coll Cardiol 2003;41:1445–51.

103. Albers GW, Diener HC, Frison L, Grind M, Nevinson M, Partridge S, Halperin JL, Horrow J, Olsson SB, Petersen P, Vahanian A, SPORTIF Executive Steering Committee for the SPORTIF V Investigators. Ximelagatran vs warfarin for stroke prevention in patients with nonvalvular atrial fibrillation: a randomized trial. JAMA 2005;293(6):690–8.

104. Lee WM, Larrey D, Olsson R, Lewis JH, Keisu M, Auclert L, Sheth S. Hepatic findings in long-term clinical trials of ximelagatran. Drug Saf 2005;28(4):351–70.

105. Kubitza D, Becka M, Wensing G, Voith B, Zuehlsdorf M. Safety, pharmacodynamics, and pharmacokinetics of BAY 59-7939—an oral, direct factor Xa inhibitor—after multiple dosing in healthy male subjects. Eur J Clin Pharmacol 2005;61(12):873–80.

106. Turpie AG, Fisher WD, Bauer KA, Kwong LM, Irwin MW, Kälebo P, Misselwitz F, Gent M, OdiXa-Knee Study Group. BAY 59-7939: an oral, direct factor Xa inhibitor for the prevention of venous thromboembolism in patients after total knee replacement. A phase II dose-ranging study. J Thromb Haemost 2005;3(11):2479–86.

107. Paccaly A, Ozoux ML, Chu V, Simcox K, Marks V, Freyburger G, Sibille M, Shukla U. Pharmacodynamic markers in the early clinical assessment of otamixaban, a direct factor Xa inhibitor. Thromb Haemost 2005;94(6):1156–63.

108. Maetzke J, Hinrichs R, Schneider L-A, Scharffetter-Kochanek K. Unexpected delayed-type hypersensitivity skin reactions to the ultra-low-molecular-weight heparin fondaparinux. Allergy 2005;60:413–5.

109. Tatarchenko IP, Pozdniakova NV, Petranin AIu, Morozova OI. Ventricular arrhythmias and cardiac late potentials inpatients with acute coronary syndrome after reperfusion therapy. Klin Med (Mosk) 2005;83(5):19–22 [in Russian].

110. Reuben A, Clouting E. Compartment syndrome after thrombolysis for acute myocardial infarction. Emerg Med J 2005;22(1):77.

111. Ahmed J, Philpott J, Lew-Gor S, Blunt D. Airway obstruction: a rare complication of thrombolytic therapy. J Laryngol Otol 2005;119(10):819–21.

112. Cahill RA, Siddique S, O'Connor J. Vomiting in the recently anticoagulated patient. Gut 2005;54(1):90, 102.

113. Nandhagopal R, Vengamma B, Krishnamoorthy SG, Rajasekhar D, Subramanyam G. Thalamic disequilibrium syndrome after thrombolytic

therapy for acute myocardial infarction. Neurology 2005;65(3):494.

114. Blackwell N, Hollins A, Gilmore G, Norton R. Antistreptokinase antibodies: implications for thrombolysis in a region with endemic streptococcal infection. J Clin Pathol 2005;58(9):1005–7.

115. Abuosa AM, Akhras F, Sorour K, El-Said G, El-Tobgy S, Kinsara AJ. Effect of pretreatment antistreptokinase antibody and streptococcal infection on the efficacy and dosage of streptokinase in acute myocardial infarction. Saudi Med J 2005;26(6):934–6.

116. Mi H, Gupta A, Gok MA, Asher J, Shenton BK, Stamp S, Carter V, Del Rio Martin J, Soomro NA, Jaques BC, Manas DM, Talbot D. Do recipients of kidneys from donors treated with streptokinase develop anti-streptokinase antibodies? Transplant Proc 2005;37(8):3272–3.

117. Oliveira DC, Coelho OR, Paraschin K, Ferraroni NR, Zolner Rde L. Angioedema related to the use of streptokinase. Arq Bras Cardiol 2005;85(2):131–4.

118. Engel PJ, Johnson H, Baughman RP, Richards AI. High-output heart failure associated with anagrelide therapy for essential thrombocytosis. Ann Intern Med 2005;143(4):311–3.

119. Anagrelide Study Group. Anagrelide, a therapy for thrombocythemic states: experience in 577 patients. Am J Med 1992;92:69–76.

120. Petitt RM, Silverstein MN, Petrone ME. Anagrelide for control of thrombocythemia in polycythemia and other myeloproliferative disorders. Semin Hematol 1997;34:51–4.

121. Rodwell GE, Troxell ML, Lafayette RA. Renal tubular injury associated with anagrelide use. Nephrol Dial Transplant 2005;20(5):988–90.

122. Cogen F, Zweiman B. Dipyridamole (Persantin)-induced asthma during thallium stress testing. J Allergy Clin Immunol 2005;115(1):203–4.

123. Deliargyris EN, Upadhya B, Applegate RJ, Kontos JL, Kutcher MA, Riesmeyer JS, Sane DC. Safety of abciximab administration during PCI of patients with previous stroke. J Thromb Thrombolysis 2005;19(3):147–53.

124. Chan AW, Yadav JS, Bhatt DL, Bajzer CT, Gum PA, Roffi M, Cho L, Agah R, Topol EJ. Comparison of the safety and efficacy of emboli prevention devices versus platelet glycoprotein IIb/IIIa inhibition during carotid stenting. Am J Cardiol 2005;95(6):791–5.

125. Friedrich EB, Kindermann M, Link A, Bohm M. Splenic rupture complicating periinterventional glycoprotein IIb/IIIa antagonist therapy for myocardial infarction in polycythemia vera. Z Kardiol 2005;94(3):200–4.

126. Aster RH. Immune thrombocytopenia caused by glycoprotein IIb/IIIa inhibitors. Chest 2005;127(2 Suppl):53S–9S.

127. Nikolsky E, Sadeghi HM, Effron MB, Mehran R, Lansky AJ, Na Y, Cox DA, Garcia E, Tcheng JE, Griffin JJ, Stuckey TD, Turco M, Carroll JD, Grines CL, Stone GW. Impact of in-hospital acquired thrombocytopenia in patients undergoing primary angioplasty for acute myocardial infarction. Am J Cardiol 15 2005;96(4):474–81.

128. Razakjr OA, Tan HC, Yip WL, Lim YT. Predictors of bleeding complications and thrombocytopenia with the use of abciximab during percutaneous coronary intervention. J Interv Cardiol 2005;18(1):33–7.

129. Trapolin G, Savonitto S, Merlini PA, Caimi MT, Klugmann S. Delayed profound thrombocytopenia after abciximab administration for coronary stenting in acute coronary syndrome. Case reports and review of the literature. Ital Heart J 2005;6(8):647–51.

130. Piorkowski M, Priess J, Weikert U, Jaster M, Schwimmbeck PL, Schultheiss HP, Rauch U. Abciximab therapy is associated with increased platelet activation and decreased heparin dosage in patients with acute myocardial infarction. Thromb Haemost 2005;94(2):422–6.

131. Ohm C, Mina A, Howells G, Bair H, Bendick P. Effects of antiplatelet agents on outcomes for elderly patients with traumatic intracranial hemorrhage. J Trauma 2005;58(3):518–22.

132. Chau TN, Yim KF, Mok NS, Chan WK, Leung VK, Leung MF, Lai ST. Clopidogrel-induced hepatotoxicity after percutaneous coronary stenting. Hong Kong Med J 2005;11(5):414–6.

133. Doogue MP, Begg EJ, Bridgman P. Clopidogrel hypersensitivity syndrome with rash, fever, and neutropenia. Mayo Clin Proc 2005;80(10):1368–70.

134. Comert A, Akgun S, Civelek A, Kavala M, Sarigul S, Yildirim T, Arsan S. Clopidogrel-induced hypersensitivity syndrome associated with febrile pancytopenia. Int J Dermatol 2005;44(10):882–4.

135. Wang TH, Bhatt DL, Topol EJ. Aspirin and clopidogrel resistance: an emerging clinical entity. Eur Heart J 2006;27(6):647–54.

136. Camara MG, Almeda FQ. Clopidogrel (Plavix) desensitization: a case series. Catheter Cardiovasc Interv 2005;65(4):525–7.

137. Lee S, Nikai T, Kanata K, Koshizaki M, Nomura T, Saito Y. A case of severe coronary artery spasm associated with anaphylactic reaction caused by protamine administration. Masui 2005;54(9):1043–6.

H.J. Fellows and H.R. Dalton

36 Gastrointestinal drugs

ANTACIDS *(SED-15, 243; SEDA-28, 401)*

Fetotoxicity Gastroesophageal reflux disease is a common problem in pregnancy. In an open multicenter study of a low-sodium formulation of Gaviscon (alginic acid, aluminium hydroxide, magnesium trisilicate, sodium bicarbonate) there were 10 adverse events out of 150 pregnancies, including three episodes of *fetal distress* (1[c]). Other studies of formulations that contain magnesium trisilicate have reported *fetal nephrolithiasis, hypotonia, respiratory distress, and cardiovascular impairment* if used in high doses and long term.

ANTIEMETICS AND DRUGS THAT AFFECT GASTROINTESTINAL MOTILITY
(SEDA-27, 362; SEDA-28, 401; SEDA-29, 371)

Domperidone *(SED-15, 1178)*

Nervous system Central adverse effects of domperidone, such as *oculogyric crisis*, are thought to be more common in infants because of the immature blood–brain barrier. However, in a systematic review of four trials of the use of domperidone in children with gastroesophageal reflux disease no adverse events were reported, implying that the risk is relatively low (2[M]).

Metoclopramide *(SED-15, 2317; SEDA-27, 362; SEDA-28, 401; SEDA-29, 371)*

Nervous system *Tardive dyskinesia* in an infant has been described for the first time after a 17-day course of metoclopramide for gastroesophageal reflux disease (3[A]). The dyskinesia lasted for 9 months after drug withdrawal.

5-HT$_3$ RECEPTOR ANTAGONISTS *(SED-15, 1365; SEDA-27, 363; SEDA-28, 402; SEDA-29, 372)*

Alosetron *(SEDA-29, 372)*

Gastrointestinal In 662 men with diarrhea-predominant irritable bowel syndrome treated with alosetron, *constipation* was the most frequent adverse event and it occurred most often at higher doses (4[c]). Constipation was mild to moderate in most cases and there were no reported complications; however, 4% withdrew from the study because of constipation. There were no cases of ischemic colitis.

Liver Symptomatic *liver damage* has been reported in a patient taking alosetron (5[A]).

- A 39-year-old white woman developed right upper quadrant pain, nausea, and malaise. Blood tests showed raised transaminases with a normal bilirubin. After withdrawal of therapy the enzymes returned to normal and there were no long-term complications.

HISTAMINE H$_2$ RECEPTOR ANTAGONISTS *(SED-15, 1629; SEDA-27, 363; SEDA-28, 403; SEDA-29, 373)*

Drug tolerance *Tachyphylaxis* occurs during prolonged intravenous use of histamine H$_2$ re-

Side Effects of Drugs, Annual 30
J.K. Aronson (Editor)
ISSN: 0378-6080
DOI: 10.1016/S0378-6080(08)00036-6

ceptor antagonists, mediated by an increase in the release of histamine (6^R).

PROTON PUMP INHIBITORS
(SED-15, 2973; SEDA-27, 364; SEDA-28, 403; SEDA-29, 373)

Comparative studies In a comparison of omeprazole and ranitidine in 390 patients with symptoms of heartburn, there were no serious adverse events thought to be related to either treatment (7^C). The most common adverse events were *headache* (7.5%), *respiratory infections* (8.2%), *diarrhea* (7.0%), and *abdominal pain* (6.6%), with similar frequencies in the two groups.

In a comparison of omeprazole and rabeprazole in 80 patients with gastric ulcers, adverse effects were similar in the two groups (5%) and included *abdominal pain, nausea, headache,* and, with omeprazole, *diarrhea* (8^c).

Lymphatic tissues *Adenomatoid hyperplasia* occurred in two patients treated with proton pump inhibitors for 5 years (9^A). In both cases the hyperplasia was transient and did not recur despite continuation of PPI therapy.

Immunologic In reports of *allergy* to proton pump inhibitors there seems to be some degree of cross-reactivity. Anaphylaxis in a patient taking lansoprazole was confirmed by skin prick testing; the patient cross-reacted to rabeprazole but no other PPIs (10^A). Only two other cases of allergy to lansoprazole have been reported, one with cross-reactivity to omeprazole. This is also the first report of sensitization to rabeprazole.

Susceptibility factors

Genetic Proton pump inhibitors are metabolized in the liver by CYP2C19 and there are rapid, intermediate, and slow metabolizers. When omeprazole was used to treat recurrent reflux esophagitis in 119 patients in whom CYP2C19 status had been identified there was no significant difference in serious adverse events across the different groups (11^c). Adverse events that required withdrawal were aggravation of allergic granulomatous angiitis, an

acute cardiac disorder, colorectal cancer, neurosensory deafness, pruritus, and rash. The last three resolved on withdrawal. Adverse events were reported in 70% of patients and included nasopharyngitis (14%), upper respiratory tract inflammation (9%), diarrhea (8%), headache (5%), arthralgia (4%), back pain (3%), insomnia (3%), and cystitis (3%).

Teratogenicity In a study of the effects of omeprazole, lansoprazole, and pantoprazole in 53 pregnant women there was no increased risk of congenital malformations (12^c). However, the rate of elective termination of pregnancy was significantly higher in those who had taken omeprazole and lansoprazole. The reason for this is unknown.

Management of adverse drug reactions
Omeprazole delays gastric emptying by up to 40%, potentially causing a worsening of dyspeptic symptoms and increasing proximal gastrointestinal bacterial overgrowth. In a randomised, double-blind, placebo-controlled study of the effect of co-administration of tegaserod, a 5-HT$_4$ receptor agonist, to aid gastric emptying in 40 patients, there were only a few minor adverse effects (diarrhea, anorexia, abdominal bloating, flu-like symptoms, joint pains, and vomiting) (13^c).

Esomeprazole   *(SED-15, 1252; SEDA-28, 403; SEDA-29, 373)*

Comparative studies Cysteamine is used to treat cystinosis, an autosomal dominant condition that causes renal insufficiency before the age of 10 if left untreated. However, it is ulcerogenic (and is used to stimulate duodenal ulcers in laboratory animals by causing hypergastrinemia). Symptoms are normally controlled with omeprazole. In 12 children esomeprazole was as effective as omeprazole in symptom control; the only adverse effects were *headache* and *oral sores* in one patient, not requiring withdrawal (14^c).

Omeprazole   *(SED-15, 2615;*
SEDA-28, 403)

In eradication of *Helicobacter pylori* in 23 patients, omeprazole 40 and 80 mg had a similar incidence of adverse effects (20%), including *diarrhea*, *taste disturbances*, and *dyspepsia* (15[C]).

Nutrition   *H. pylori* positive patients have significantly reduced daily vitamin C intake and significantly *low vitamin C plasma concentrations*. Treatment for 1 month with omeprazole 40 mg/day reduced the mean plasma vitamin C concentration by 12% in 29 patients, irrespective of whether they were *H. pylori* positive or negative (16[c]). The reason for this is not known.

Teratogenicity   Omeprazole is a class C drug according to the FDA classification of teratogenicity (animal studies show a risk but human studies are inadequate). The other PPIs are classified by the FDA as class B (animal studies show no risk and human studies are inadequate). There have been 12 reports to the FDA of birth defects after the mothers took omeprazole during pregnancy. These included anencephaly and hydrocephaly. However, a meta-analysis of omeprazole exposure during pregnancy showed no significant difference in the incidence of major malformations compared with the general population (1[M]).

Rabeprazole   *(SED-15, 3011; SEDA-28,*
404; SEDA-29, 374)

In a randomized open study in 176 patients with gastroesophageal reflux disease taking rabeprazole as required, adverse events were reported as *diarrhea* (6%), *bronchiectasis* (5%), *gastroenteritis* (5%), *cystitis* (4%), *abdominal pain* (3%), *nausea* (2%), *headaches* (2%), *vertigo* (2%), and *lower back pain* (2%) (17[c]).

Sucralfate   *(SED-15, 3209)*

Gastrointestinal   The only adverse effect of sucralfate when used to treat radiation proctitis in 51 patients was *diarrhea*, but the incidence was not reported (18[r]).

HELICOBACTER PYLORI
ERADICATION REGIMENS
(SED-15, 1586; SEDA-27, 366; SEDA-28, 405)

Observational studies   Adverse effects of triple therapy (clarithromycin 500 mg bd + amoxicillin 1 g bd + omeprazole 20 mg/day or esomeprazole 40 mg/day) for *Helicobacter pylori* eradication occurred in about 30% of 200 patients. Common adverse effects included *nausea and vomiting, constipation and diarrhea, metallic and bitter taste sensations, headache*, and mild *abdominal pain* (19[c]).

In 582 patients the most common adverse effects of the most popular eradication regimen (omeprazole + amoxicillin + clarithromycin) were mild only; they included *bitter taste, diarrhea, dizziness*, and *malaise* (20[c]).

Eradication therapy with rabeprazole + clarithromycin+metronidazole was well tolerated; only two of 10 patients in an observational study reported a *metallic taste* alone (21[c]).

Rabeprazole + amoxicillin + metronidazole was well tolerated when used for *H. pylori* eradication in 120 patients in a randomized controlled study (22[C]). Adverse effects occurred equally in those given rabeprazole 10 or 20 mg (30%). Common adverse effects included *diarrhea* (17%), *dizziness* (10%), and *nausea* (3%).

When a low-dose eradication regimen of omeprazole + amoxicillin (1.5 g/day) + clarithromycin (800 mg/day) was compared with a high-dose regimen of omeprazole+amoxicillin (2 g/day)+clarithromycin (1 g/day) in 225 patients, 1.8% of patients in the low-dose group withdrew because of adverse effects (*sleep disorder and vertigo*) and 0.9% of patients in the high-dose group withdrew because of *diarrhea* (23[C]). There were adverse events in 66% of the low-dose group and 61% of the high-dose group. These comprised *diarrhea, bitter taste*, and *reflux symptoms*. There were four severe adverse events, all in the low-dose group; these were *esophageal cancer, pyelonephritis, myelopathy*, and *erythrocytosis and bronchitis*, which were not thought to be due to the trial drugs.

Helicobacter pylori eradication therapy was evaluated in 458 patients using rabeprazole 20 mg/day + clarithromycin + amoxicillin for either 7 or 10 days (24[C]). There was no significant difference in adverse effects between the two groups. The most common adverse effects were a *metallic taste sensation* (19%), *oral mucositis* (19%), and *diarrhea* (7%). Symptoms were limited to the duration of treatment.

In 55 patients *Helicobacter pylori* eradication with lansoprazole + amoxicillin + clarithromycin (LAC) was compared with LAC and subsequently lying in the left lateral position and LAC plus cetraxate (25^c). Adverse events were more common in the group treated with LAC alone (70%). There were two serious adverse events, one case of *diarrhea* in the LAC plus cetraxate group and one case of *abdominal pain* in the LAC group. Common adverse events were *diarrhea, taste disturbances, nausea, constipation, eczema, headache, abdominal pain*, and *indigestion*.

In a randomized study of the treatment options for patients allergic to penicillin the regimens studied were: omeprazole + clarithromycin + metronidazole for 7 days (group 1, $n = 12$); ranitidine + bismuth + tetracycline + metronidazole for 7 days (group 2, $n = 17$); omeprazole + rifabutin + clarithromycin for 10 days (group 3, $n = 9$); and levofloxacin + clarithromycin + omeprazole for 10 days (group 4, $n = 2$) (26^c). Group 1 tolerated the treatment best—only 17% of patients had adverse events, these being *nausea* and *diarrhea*. In group 2 adverse events occurred in 53%, including *nausea, heartburn, diarrhea*, and *abdominal pain*. In group 3 there was a drop-out rate of 33%, primarily because of the adverse events experienced by 89%, including *arthralgia* (55%) and *myelosuppression* (44%). Group 4 had an adverse incident rate of 50%, including *anorexia* and *arthralgia*.

Rescue therapy for 12 patients who had two previous failed courses of *H. pylori* eradication therapy was studied using rabeprazole + levofloxacin + furazolidone; 17% of patients stopped taking the medication because of *nausea and vomiting*; 33% had *nausea and dizziness* but did not need to stop taking therapy (27^c).

Other combinations have been used, such as rifabutin + amoxicillin + omeprazole, but this regimen has significant adverse effects, including *leukopenia* and *thrombocytopenia* (27^c).

ANTIDIARRHEAL AGENTS
(SEDA-27, 367; SEDA-28, 406; SEDA-29, 374)

Placebo-controlled studies   L-histidine, an essential amino acid with antisecretory properties, has been evaluated in combination with a rice-based oral rehydration solution in a placebo-controlled study in a double-blind, randomized, placebo-controlled study in 126 men with cholera (28^C). *Transaminase activities rose* significantly in both groups and there was no significant difference between the two groups.

LAXATIVES AND ORAL BOWEL PREPARATIONS   *(SED-15, 2008; SEDA-27, 367; SEDA-28, 406; SEDA-29, 374)*

A carbon dioxide-releasing suppository containing sodium bicarbonate and potassium bitartrate in a polyethylene glycol base has been evaluated in 29 patients with chronic constipation (29^C). There was *anal irritation* in 14% of the patients, but there was no statistical difference from placebo. There was mild to moderate *pain* in 38% of those who took the active suppository compared with 14% of those who took placebo.

Ispaghula has been compared with a combination of polyethylene glycol + electrolytes in the treatment of chronic constipation (30^c). The main adverse effect of the former was a *dry mouth* (in 5% of patients) and of the latter *dizziness* (also in 5%). There were no serious adverse events.

The management of chronic constipation has been reviewed (31^R, 32^R). Psyllium can be associated with bloating if used in large quantities. Mechanical obstruction of the esophagus and colon has been reported and *anaphylactic reactions* occur occasionally. Lactulose has been associated with an increase in *abdominal discomfort* compared with placebo. Polyethylene glycol is used to treat chronic constipation, but causes *multiple electrolyte abnormalities, hypovolemia*, and *excessive stool frequency*; the precise incidence of these adverse effects is unclear. Stimulant laxatives, such as senna and bisacodyl, showed no significant difference in adverse events compared with other treatments for chronic constipation. Tegaserod, a 5-HT$_4$ receptor agonist used in chronic constipation, can also cause *diarrhea*; however, this tends to be mild and transient, and only 1% of patients discontinue treatment as a result.

Phosphates   *(SED-15, 2820;*
SEDA-29, 375)

Of 30 patients who underwent bowel preparation with sodium phosphate tablets (INKP-101) before colonoscopy, five had adverse events, including *abdominal tightness, headache, nausea and vomiting*, and *bradycardia* (33^c). The endoscopist rated bowel preparation as good in all cases, but it took up to 4 minutes per endoscopy to suction microcrystalline cellulose deposits from the tablets off the mucosa.

Adverse effects reported from the use of a low residue diet with LoSo bowel prep in 506 patients compared favorably with the more conventional clear liquid diet with a standard sodium phosphate regimen (34^C). There were adverse effects in 59%, commonly *cramping, bloating, vomiting, headaches, rectal burning, indigestion, flatulence*, and *fatigue*.

Electrolyte balance   Polyethylene glycol, polyethylene glycol plus bisacodyl, and sodium phosphate have been compared for bowel preparation in 231 patients (35^C). The most significant electrolyte changes occurred in those who received sodium phosphate, who had a significant *fall in serum potassium* (mean -1.06 mmol/l) and an *increase in serum phosphate* (mean 1.6 mmol/l) compared with patients who took the other bowel preparations. There was also an increase in serum sodium and a fall in serum calcium, although these were less marked and not statistically significant. There was no statistically significant difference in the number of patients with *cardiac dysrhythmias*, although only 50% of patients had cardiac monitoring. One patient who took polyethylene glycol alone had a cardiac arrest, preceded by a sinus bradycardia; there was spontaneous reversion to sinus rhythm; this event was not related to any electrolyte abnormality. There were minor adverse reactions in all three groups,

including *nausea and vomiting, insomnia, abdominal pain, bloating*, and *anal irritation*; there was no difference in incidence across the groups.

Urinary tract   The US FDA has issued an alert that *acute phosphate nephropathy* is a rare but serious adverse event associated with the use of oral sodium phosphates for bowel cleansing (36^S). Acute phosphate nephropathy has been documented in 21 patients who used an oral sodium phosphate tablet; older individuals, those with kidney disease or reduced intravascular volume, and those taking medicines that affect renal perfusion or function (diuretics, angiotensin converting enzyme inhibitors, angiotensin receptor antagonists, and possibly non-steroidal anti-inflammatory drugs) are at higher risk.

Susceptibility factors

Renal disease   Bowel preparation before colonoscopy can cause major fluid shifts and significant electrolyte disturbances, most commonly *hyperphosphatemia, hypocalcemia*, and *hyponatremia*. Deaths have also been reported. Pre-existing renal impairment is the most significant susceptibility factor for adverse events. Of 100 patients undergoing routine colonoscopy using sodium phosphate bowel preparation, 45 developed hyperphosphatemia (37^c). This effect correlated with increasing age, creatinine clearance, and the use of diuretics and angiotensin converting enzyme inhibitors/angiotensin II inhibitors. Patients with very high serum phosphate concentrations were more likely to have their colonoscopy in the afternoon; the reason for this is uncertain. There was hypokalemia in 26 patients and hypocalcemia in 16, all asymptomatic.

Two patients, one with end-stage renal disease and the other with moderate renal impairment developed hypocalcemia and hyperphosphatemia after treatment with phosphates (38^A).

- A 51-year-old woman took two 45-ml doses of Fleet Phospho-Soda and developed severe hypocalcemia and hyperphosphatemia, causing generalized weakness, perioral tingling, a positive Chvostek's sign, and a prolonged QT interval. The patient recovered after intravenous calcium and dialysis.

- A 57-year-old man took two 45-ml doses of oral sodium phosphate and developed significant hypocalcaemia and hyperphosphatemia. He remained asymptomatic and received oral supplementation.

The authors suggested that hypocalcemia had occurred secondary to hyperphosphatemia and recommended that care should be taken when choosing bowel preparation for patients with renal impairment.

Polyethylene glycol   *(SED-15, 1516; SEDA-29, 375)*

See Chapter 49.

AMINOSALICYLATES   *(SED-15, 138; SEDA-27, 367; SEDA-28, 408; SEDA-29, 377)*

Radiotherapy for prostatic carcinoma can cause proctitis, and it is thought that the chronic inflammation puts the patient at increased risk of rectal carcinoma, just as patients with ulcerative colitis are at risk of colorectal carcinoma. However, trials with mesalazine and olsalazine have failed to record any improvement in symptoms in patients with prostatic carcinoma and can on occasions exacerbate symptoms (39[r]).

Mesalazine (5-aminosalicyclic acid, mesalamine)   *(SEDA-28, 408; SEDA-29, 378)*

Placebo-controlled studies   In 16 patients with ulcerative colitis of recombinant peptides such as trefoil factor 3 enemas versus placebo and in combination with oral mesalazine there were no adverse events (40[c]).

In a randomized, double-blind study in 127 patients with mild to moderate ulcerative colitis, all of whom received oral mesalazine plus either mesalazine enemas or placebo enemas, 34% of those who were given mesalazine enemas had adverse events (41[C]). The most common of these were *diarrhea* (4%), *headache*

(4%), and *vomiting* (3%). 50% of patients in the placebo group had adverse effects, most commonly abdominal pain (4%). There were three serious adverse events (*bloody diarrhea* and *abdominal pain*), 4% in those given Pentasa and 2% in those given placebo. These were thought to be related to ulcerative colitis rather than adverse drug effects.

Urinary tract   The incidence of *nephrotoxicity* due to mesalazine has been estimated at one in 4000 treated patients in a retrospective case series compiled through a questionnaire system sent to renal physicians and gastroenterologists (42[R]). This is higher than previous estimates. Nephrotoxicity can occur at any time during therapy. Of patients who developed abnormal renal function after starting treatment 32% regained normal renal function on withdrawal, 53% had partial resolution, and 17% had persistent renal impairment. Of those with renal impairment secondary to mesalazine 10% progressed to end-stage renal insufficiency requiring renal replacement therapy. There was an increased chance of returning to normal renal function if the mesalazine had been started within the preceding year. Patients with mesalazine nephrotoxicity develop recurrent deterioration in renal function when rechallenged. The authors recommended regular monitoring of renal function, particularly within the first year of treatment.

In 153 patients the duration of treatment with mesalazine and increasing age were the most important significant predictors of creatinine clearance, the mean fall in which was estimated to be 0.3 ml/minute/year (43[c]). There were no cases of interstitial nephritis.

Skin   In a recent study of mesalazine, adverse effects occurred in only 1.5% of 156 patients; one patient had to stop the taking the drug because of a *rash* (44[C]).

Immunologic   Although mesalazine (5-aminosalicyclic acid) and aspirin (acetylsalicyclic acid) are structurally related, combined *hypersensitivity* is rare.

- A 28-year-old woman with Crohn's disease and combined aspirin and mesalazine hypersensitivity was successfully treated with a 3-day course of desensitization and was then able to tolerate a full dose of mesalazine (45[A]).

Drug formulations   Two mesalazine delivery systems, Asacol and Ipcol, have been compared (46[C]). Ipcol is an enteric-coated tablet that contains the same dose of mesalazine as Asacol and has a similar but slightly thinner enteric coating. Adverse effects were reported in 73% of 88 patients in each group and were mostly mild. However, two patients who took Asacol reported severe adverse events and a further two developed severe abdominal pain thought to be related to Asacol and necessitating withdrawal.

A formulation of mesalazine for once-daily dosing in ulcerative proctitis has been compared with twice-daily dosing of a conventional formulation in a randomized study in 99 patients (47[C]). Adverse events were reported in equal numbers of patients in the two groups, including abdominal pain, bloating, diarrhea, and rectal haemorrhage. Other symptoms included headache (17–18%) and bronchospasm.

Mesalazine pellets and tablets have been compared in a randomized trial in 233 patients with mild to moderate ulcerative colitis (48[C]). Adverse events were reported in 32% of patients taking the pellets and 36% of those taking the tablets. The drug had to be withdrawn in one patient taking the pellets and in four patients taking the tablets.

Rectal formulations of mesalazine are well tolerated, with only minor adverse events such as dizziness (3%) and rectal pain (1%) (49[M]).

Drug–drug interactions   Oral mesalazine potentiates the effect of oral *6-mercaptopurine*, although the mechanism is not known. In 17 patients taking mercaptopurine oral mesalazine increased the concentrations of 6-thioguanine nucleotides (50[c]). This interaction could cause increased myelosuppression, although this was not observed in this small case series.

Olsalazine

The use of olsalazine is limited by dose-related adverse effects, the most common being *diarrhoea*, which occurred in 10% of 156 patients (44[M]). It is believed to be secondary to the action of intact olsalazine on the small intestine, causing stimulation of secretion of bicarbonate, chloride, and water and inhibiting their absorption.

BILE ACIDS   *(SED-15, 515; SEDA-27, 369; SEDA-28, 409; SEDA-29, 378)*

Pregnancy   In a retrospective analysis of 12 years of experience of the use of ursodeoxycholic acid 15 mg/kg/day in women with intrahepatic cholestasis of pregnancy 32 patients were compared with 16 historical controls; there were no adverse effects in the mothers or their infants (51[c]).

PANCREATIC ENZYMES   *(SED-15, 2670; SEDA-26, 389)*

Immunologic   In a study of the role of pancreatic enzyme supplements in causing *IgE-mediated allergic reactions*, skin prick testing in 69 patients showed no significant difference between enzyme supplement recipients and controls (52[c]).

Orlistat   ℞

Orlistat is used in obese patients as an aid to weight reduction. The most frequent adverse effects that necessitate withdrawal include increased frequency and urgency of stools, fecal spotting, and incontinence. The latter occurs in about 25% of patients but usually responds well to loperamide (53[c]).

Systematic reviews   *In a systematic review of 23 placebo-controlled or comparative trials the incidence of gastrointestinal adverse events was consistently higher in those taking orlistat (54[C]). The adverse events associated with orlistat included loose and/or fatty stools, fecal urgency, uncontrolled oily discharge, increased defecation, fecal incontinence, flatus with discharge, nausea/vomiting, and abdominal pain. Orlistat was sometimes associated with lower serum concentrations of fat-soluble vitamins and/or a requirement for vitamin supplements. Most of the adverse effects were transient and mild to moderate in intensity, occurred early in treatment, and resolved spontaneously. There were no reports of changes in bone density or bone mineralization.*

In a systematic review of 28 randomized trials, 17 of which (10 041 patients) compared orlistat 120 mg tds with placebo or an inactive control along with a hypocaloric diet over 1 year, gastrointestinal adverse events were more common with orlistat than with placebo (RR = 1.46; 95% CI = 1.37, 1.55) (55^C).

Comparative studies   *Orlistat 360 mg/day (n = 71) and sibutramine 10 mg/day (n = 70) have been compared in a double-blind, randomized study in obese patients with diabetes mellitus, who had had diabetes for at least 6 months and who were taking diet alone or diet plus oral hypoglycemic drugs (56^C). Of the 133 patients who completed the study, 22 (34%) of those taking orlistat and nine (13%) of those taking sibutramine had adverse effects. All the adverse effects of orlistat were gastrointestinal, occurred early in treatment, were mild to moderate in intensity, were generally transient, and resolved spontaneously.*

In a similar double-blind, randomized, controlled comparison of orlistat and sibutramine by the same authors in 115 obese hypertensive patients, adverse effects occurred in 48% of the patients who took orlistat; all were gastrointestinal (57^C). The changes in vitamin concentrations were small and all mean vitamin and beta-carotene concentrations stayed within the reference ranges. No patients required vitamin supplements.

Nutrition   *There have been contradictory results in studies of the effects of orlistat on the absorption of various vitamins.*

In a double-blind, randomized, placebo-controlled study in 103 men and 70 women who took 30, 90, 180, or 360 mg or orlistat or for 8 weeks, plasma concentrations of vitamins D and E fell, although both remained within the reference ranges (58^C).

In an open, placebo-controlled, randomized, two-way, crossover study in 48 healthy volunteers aged 19–58 years orlistat reduced the absorption of beta-carotene by about one-third (59^C). The authors concluded that two-thirds of a supplementary dose of beta-carotene will be absorbed during orlistat treatment; and that this may be sufficient to achieve physiological concentrations of beta-carotene.

In an open, placebo-controlled, randomized, two-way, crossover study in 12 healthy volunteers (aged 20–44 years) orlistat significantly

reduced the absorption of vitamin E by about 43% according to the effect on C_{max} and 60% according to AUC (60^C). The absorption of vitamin A was not affected.

In 17 adolescents with body mass indexes above the 95th percentile for age, race, and sex who also had at least one obesity-related co-morbid condition orlistat 120 mg tds was given with a daily multivitamin supplement containing vitamin A 5000 IU, vitamin D 400 IU, vitamin E 300 IU, and vitamin K 25 micrograms (61^c). The absorption of vitamin A was not significantly altered, but absorption of alpha-tocopherol (vitamin E) was significantly reduced compared with baseline. Serum concentrations of vitamins A, E, and K did not change significantly. However, mean vitamin D concentrations were significantly reduced after 1 month of orlistat therapy, despite multivitamin supplementation. The authors concluded that it may be prudent to monitor vitamin D concentrations in patients who take orlistat, even when a multivitamin supplement is prescribed.

Liver   *Subacute liver failure has been reported in a patient taking orlistat (62^A).*

Drug–drug interactions

Ciclosporin   *Orlistat reduces the systemic availability of ciclosporin (63^A, 64^A, 65^A, 66^A, 67^M, 68^A), perhaps by interfering with its absorption in the small intestine (69^A), although the effect may be mediated indirectly by via reduced fat absorption rather than a direct drug–drug interaction (70^A). Co-administration of orlistat with ciclosporin is not recommended. However, if concomitant use is unavoidable, ciclosporin blood concentrations should be monitored more often, both after the addition of orlistat and on withdrawal.*

Levothyroxine   *It has been suggested that orlistat may inhibit the absorption of levothyroxine and thus cause hypothyroidism in patients taking replacement therapy (71^A).*

Metformin   *A possible interaction of orlistat with metformin has been reported.*

- *A 59-year-old obese woman with normal renal function, taking metformin 500 mg tds, took orlistat 120 mg tds for 3 months (72^A). She developed abdominal pain and diarrhea, for which she was* given cimetidine, and became weak and dizzy, with blurred vision, reduced consciousness, agitation, and confusion. Her pH was 6.5, bicarbonate 2 mmol/l, base deficit 38 mmol/l, and lactate 21 mmol/l. She required rehydration, bicarbonate, inotropic support and renal replacement therapy.

The authors suggested that chronic diarrhea induced by orlistat could have led to impaired renal function or that orlistat could have in-creased the absorption of metformin by reducing fat absorption.

Management of adverse drug reactions   In a double-blind, randomized placebo-controlled study in 10 obese patients, loperamide improved stool consistency and reduced continence problems during treatment with orlistat (73^c).

References

1. Richter J. Review article: the management of heartburn in pregnancy. Aliment Pharmacol Ther 2005;22:749–57.
2. Pritchard D, Baber N, Stephenson T. Should domperidone be used for the treatment of gastro-oesophageal reflux in children? Systematic review of randomised controlled trials in children aged 1 month to 11 years. Br J Clin Pharmacol 2005;59(6):725–9.
3. Mejia NL, Jankovic J. Metoclopramide-induced tardive dyskinesia in an infant. Mov Disord 2005;20(1):86–9.
4. Chang L, Ameen V, Dukes G, McSorley D, Carter E, Mayer E. A dose ranging, phased II study of the efficacy and safety of alosetron in men with diarrhoea predominant IBS. Am J Gastroenterol 2005;100(1):115–23.
5. Turgeon DK, Tayeh N, Fontana RJ. Acute hepatitis associated with alosetron (Lotronex). J Clin Gastroenterol 2005;39(7):641–2.
6. Brett S. Science review. The use of proton pump inhibitors for gastric acid suppression in critical illness. Crit Care 2005;9:45–50.
7. Armstrong D, Veldhuyzen van Zanten SJ, Barkun AN, Chiba N, Thomson AB, Smyth S, Sinclair P, Chakraborty B, White RJ, The CADET-HR Study Group. Heartburn-dominant, un-investigated dyspepsia: a comparison of 'PPI-start' and 'H2-RA-start' management strategies in primary care – the CADET-HR Study. Aliment Pharmacol Ther 2005;21:1189–202.
8. Ando T, Kato H, Sugimoto N, Nagao Y, Seto N, Hongo H, Kajikawa H, Isozaki Y, Shimozawa M, Naito Y, Yoshida N, Ishizaki T, Yoshikawa T. A comparative study on endoscopic ulcer healing of omeprazole versus rabeprazole with respect to CYP2C19 genotypic differences. Dig Dis Sci 2005;50(9):1625–31.
9. Rindi G, Fiocca R, Morocutti A, Jacobs A, Miller N, Thjodleifsson B, The European Rabeprazole Study Group. Effects of 5 years of treatment with rabeprazole or omeprazole on the gastric mucosa. J Gastroenterol Hepatol 2005;17(5):559–66.
10. Porcel S, Rodriguez A, Jimenez S, Alvarado M, Hernandez J. Allergy to lansoprazole: study of cross-reactivity among proton-pump inhibitors. Allergy 2005;60:1087–93.
11. Ohkusa T, Maekawa T, Arakawa T, Nakajima M, Fujimoto K, Hoshino E, Mitachi Y, Hamada S, Min T, Kawahara Y, Nagai T, Aoyama A, Yoshida N, Tadokoro K, Chida N, Konda Y, Seno H, Shimatani T, Inoue M, Sato N. Effect of CYP2C19 polymorphism on the safety and efficacy of omeprazole in Japanese patients with recurrent reflux oesophagitis. Aliment Pharmacol Ther 2005;21:1331–9.
12. Diav-Citrin O, Arnon J, Shechtman S, Schaefer C, Van Tonningegn M, Clementis M, De Santis M, Robert-Gnansia E, Valti E, Malm H, Ornoy A. The safety of proton pump inhibitors in pregnancy: a multicentre prospective controlled study. Aliment Pharmacol Ther 2005;21:269–75.
13. Tougas G, Earnest D, Chen Y, Vanderkoy C, Rojavin M. Omeprazole delays gastric emptying in healthy volunteers: an effect prevented by tegaserod. Aliment Pharmacol Ther 2005;22:59–65.
14. Dohil R, Fidler M, Barshop B, Newbury R, Sellers Z, Deutsch R, Schneider J. Esomeprazole therapy for gastric acid hyper secretion in children with cystinosis. Paediatr Nephrol 2005;20:1786–93.
15. Manes G, Pieramico O, Perri F, Vaira D, Giardullo N, Romano M, Nardone G, Balzano A. Twice daily standard dose of omeprazole achieves the necessary level of acid inhibition for *Helicobacter pylori* eradication. A randomised controlled trial using standard and double doses of omeprazole in triple therapy. Dig Dis Sci 2005;50(3):443–8.
16. Henry E, Carswell A, Wirz A, Fyffe V, McColl K. Proton pump inhibitors reduce the bioavailability of dietary vitamin C. Aliment Pharmacol Ther 2005;22:539–45.

17. Bour B, Staub J, Chousterman M, Labayles D, Nalet B, Nouel O, Pariente A, Tocque E, Bonnot-Marlier S. Long term treatment of gastro-oesophageal reflux disease patients with frequent symptomatic relapses using rabeprazole: on-demand treatment compared with continuous disease treatment. Aliment Pharmacol Ther 2005;21:805–12.

18. Hovdenak N, Sorbye H, Dahl O. Sucralfate does not ameliorate acute radiation proctitis: randomised study and meta-analysis. Clin Oncol 2005;17:485–91.

19. Sheu B, Kao A, Cheng H, Hunag S, Chen T, Lu C, Wu J. Esomeprazole 40 mg twice daily in triple therapy and the efficacy of *Helicobacter pylori* eradication related to CYP2C19 metabolism. Aliment Pharmacol Ther 2005;21:283–8.

20. Wong W, Xiao S, Hu P, Wang W, Gu Q, Huang J, Xia H, Wu S, Li C, Chen M, Lai K, Chan C, Lam S, Wong B. Standard treatment for *Helicobacter pylori* infection is suboptimal in non ulcer dyspepsia compared with duodenal ulcer in Chinese. Aliment Pharmacol Ther 2005;21(1):73–81.

21. Giannini E, Malfatti F, Botta F, Polegato S, Testa E, Fumagalli A, Mamone M, Savarino V, Testa R. Influence of 1 week *Helicobacter pylori* eradication therapy with rabeprazole, clarithromycin, and metronidazole on 13C-aminopyrine breath test. Dig Dis Sci 2005;50(7):1207–13.

22. Wong W, Huang J, Xia H, Fung F, Tong T, Cheung K, Ho V, Lai K, Chan C, Chan A, Hui C, Lam S, Wong B. Low dose rabeprazole, amoxicillin and metronidazole triple therapy for the treatment of *Helicobacter pylori* infection in Chinese patients. J Gastroenterol Hepatol 2005;20:935–40.

23. Kuwayama H, Luk G, Yoshida S, Nakamura T, Kubo M, Uemura N, Harasawa S, Kaise M, Sanuki E, Haruma K, Inoue M, Shimatani T, Meino H, Kawanishi M, Watanabe H, Nakashima M, Nakazawa S. Efficacy of a low dose omeprazole based triple therapy regimen for *Helicobacter pylori* eradication independent of cytochrome P450 genotype. Clin Drug Investig 2005;25(5):293–305.

24. Calvet X, Ducons J, Bujanda L, Bory F, Monserrat A, Gisbert J, Hp Study Group of the Asociación Española de Gastroenterología. Seven versus ten days of rabeprazole triple therapy for *Helicobacter pylori* eradication: a multicenter randomised trial. Am J Gastroenterol 2005;100(8):1696–701.

25. Kubota K, Shimizu N, Nozaki K, Takeshita Y, Ueda T, Imamura K, Hiki N, Yamaguchi H, Shimoyama S, MaFune K, Kaminishi M. Efficacy of triple therapy plus cetraxate for the *Helicobacter pylori* eradication in partial gastrectomy patients. Dig Dis Sci 2005;50(5):842–6.

26. Gisbert J, Gisbert J, Marcos S, Olivares D, Pajares J. *Helicobacter pylori* first line treatment and rescue options in patients allergic to penicillin. Aliment Pharmacol Ther 2005;22:1041–6.

27. Coelho L, Moretsohn L, Viera W, Gallo M, Passos M, Cindr J, Cerqueira M, Vitiello L, Ribeiro M, Mendonca S, Pedrazzoli-Junior J, Castro L. New once daily, highly effective rescue triple therapy after multiple *Helicobacter pylori* treatment failure: a pilot study. Aliment Pharmacol Ther 2005;21:783–7.

28. Rabbani G, Sack D, Ahmed S, Peterson J, Saha S, Marni F, Thomas P. Antidiarrhoeal effects of L-histidine-supplemented rice-based oral rehydration solution in the treatment of male adults with severe cholera in Bangladesh: a double-blind, randomised trial. J Infect Dis 2005;191:1507.

29. Lazzaroni M, Casini V, Bianchi Porro G. Role for carbon dioxide releasing suppositories in the treatment of chronic functional constipation. Clin Drug Invest 2005;25(8):499–505.

30. Wang H, Liang X, Yu Z, Zhou L, Lin S, Geraint M. A randomised, controlled comparison of low dose polyethylene glycol 3350 plus electrolytes with ispaghula hush in the treatment of adults with chronic functional constipation. Drugs R D 2005;6(4):221–5.

31. American College of Gastroenterology Chronic Constipation Task Force. An evidence based approach to the management of chronic constipation in North America. Am J Gastroenterol 2005;100(Suppl 1):S1–4.

32. Brandt L, Prather C, Quigley E, Schiller L, Schoenfeld P, Talley N. Systematic review on the management of chronic constipation in North America. Am J Gastroenterol 2005;100(Suppl 1):S5–22.

33. Khashab M, Rex D. Efficacy and tolerability of a new formulation of sodium phosphate tablets (INKP-101), and a new reduced sodium phosphate dose, in colon cleansing: a single centre open-label pilot trial. Aliment Pharmacol Ther 2005;21:465–8.

34. Delegge M, Kaplan R. Efficacy of bowel preparation with the use of a pre-packaged, low fibre diet with a low sodium, magnesium citrate cathartic vs a clear liquid diet with a standard sodium phosphate cathartic. Aliment Pharmacol Ther 2005;21:1491–5.

35. Huppertz-Hauss G, Bretthauer M, Sauer J, Paulsen J, Kjellevold O, Majak B, Hoff G. Polyethylene glycol versus sodium phosphate in bowel cleansing for colonoscopy: a randomised trial. Endoscopy 2005;37(6):537–41.

36. Anonymous. Bowel cleansing oral sodium phosphates. Risk of renal damage. WHO Newslett 2006;3:3.

37. Ainley E, Winwood P, Begley J. Measurement of serum electrolytes and phosphate after sodium phosphate colonoscopy bowel preparation: an evaluation. Dig Dis Sci 2005;50(7):1319–23.

38. Mishra R, Kaufman D, Mattern J, Dutta S. Severe hyperphosphataemia and hypocalcaemia caused by bowel preparation for colonoscopy using oral sodium phosphate in end stage renal disease. Endoscopy 2005;37:1259.

39. Jahraus C, Rubin D, Scherl E, Bettenhausen D. Inflammation's role in rectal cancer following prostate radiotherapy, and emerging evidence for

a protective role of balsalazide. Gastroenterology 2005;129(2):770–1.

40. Mahmood A, Melley L, Fitzgerald A, Ghosh S, Playford RJ. Trial of trefoil factor 3 enemas, in combination with oral 5-aminosalicyclic acid for the treatment of mild-to-moderate left sided ulcerative colitis. Aliment Pharmacol Ther 2005;21:1357–64.

41. Marteau P, Probert C, Lindgren S, Gassul M, Tan T, Dignass A, Befrits R, Midhagen G, Rademaker J, Foldager M. Combined oral and enema treatment with Pentasa is superior to oral therapy alone in patients with extensive mild/moderate active ulcerative colitis: a randomised, double blind, placebo controlled trial. Gut 2005;54:960–5.

42. Muller A, Stevens P, Mcintyre A, Ellison H, Logans R. Experience of 5-aminosalicylate nephrotoxicity in the United Kingdom. Aliment Pharmacol Ther 2005;21:1217–24.

43. de Jong DJ, Tielen J, Habraken CM, Wetzels JF, Naber AH. 5-Aminosalicylates and effects on renal function in patients with Crohn's disease. Inflamm Bowel Dis 2005;11(11):972–6.

44. Paoluzi O, Iacopini F, Pica R, Crispino P, Marcheggiano A, Consolazio A, Rivera M, Paoluzi P. Comparison of two different daily dosages (2.4 g vs. 1.2 g) of oral mesalazine in maintenance in ulcerative colitis patients: 1 year follow up study. Aliment Pharmacol Ther 2005;21:1111–9.

45. Paraskevopoulos I, Konstantinou G, Liatsos C. Desensitisation treatment of an aspirin and mesalamine sensitive patient with Crohn's disease. Inflamm Bowel Dis 2005;11(4):417–8.

46. Forbes A, Al-Damluji A, Ashworth S, Bramble M, Herbert K, Hos J, Kangs J, Przemioslo R, Shetty A. Multicentre randomised controlled clinical trial of Ipcol, a new enteric coated form of mesalazine, in comparison with Asacol in the treatment of ulcerative colitis. Aliment Pharmacol Ther 2005;21:1099–104.

47. Lamet M, Ptak T, Dallaire C, Shah U, Grace M, Spenard J, de Montigny D, Mesalamine Study Group. Efficacy and safety of mesalamine 1 g HS versus BID suppositories in mild to moderate ulcerative proctitis: a multicenter randomised study. Inflamm Bowel Dis 2005;11(7):625–30.

48. Marakhouski Y, Fixa B, Holoman J, Hulek P, Lukas M, Batovsky M, Rumyantsev V, Grigoryeva G, Stoltess M, Vieth M, Greinwald R, The International Salofalk Group. A double-blind dose escalating trial comparing novel mesalazine pellets with mesalazine tablets in active ulcerative colitis. Aliment Pharmacol Ther 2005;21:133–40.

49. Qureshi AI, Cohen RD. Mesalamine delivery systems: do they really make much difference? Adv Drug Deliv Rev 2005;57(2):281–302.

50. Gilissen L, Bierau J, Derijks L, Bos L, Hooymans P, van Gennip A, Stockbrugger R, Engels L. The pharmacokinetic effect of discontinuation of mesalazine on mercaptopurine metabolite levels in inflammatory bowel disease patients. Aliment Pharmacol Ther 2005;22:605–11.

51. Zapata R, Sandoval L, Palma J, Hernandez I, Ribalta J, Reyes H, Sedano M, Toha D, Silva JJ. Ursodeoxycholic acid in the treatment of intrahepatic cholestasis of pregnancy. A 12-year experience. Liver Int 2005;25(3):548–54.

52. Greise M, Dokupil K, Latzin P. Skin prick test reactivity to supplemental enzymes in cystic fibrosis and pancreatic insufficiency. J Paediatr Gastroenterol Nutr 2005;40:194–8.

53. Fox M, Stutz B, Menner D, Fried M, Schwizer W, Thumshirn M. The effects of loperamide on continence problems and anorectal function in obese subjects taking orlistat. Dig Dis Sci 2005;50(9):1576–83.

54. O'Meara S, Riemsma R, Shirran L, Mather L, ter Riet G. A systematic review of the clinical effectiveness of orlistat used for the management of obesity. Obes Rev 2004;5(1):51–68.

55. Hutton B, Fergusson D. Changes in body weight and serum lipid profile in obese patients treated with orlistat in addition to a hypocaloric diet: a systematic review of randomized clinical trials. Am J Clin Nutr 2004;80(6):1461–8.

56. Derosa G, Cicero AF, Murdolo G, Ciccarelli L, Fogari R. Comparison of metabolic effects of orlistat and sibutramine treatment in Type 2 diabetic obese patients. Diabetes Nutr Metab 2004;17(4):222–9.

57. Derosa G, Cicero AF, Murdolo G, Piccinni MN, Fogari E, Bertone G, Ciccarelli L, Fogari R. Efficacy and safety comparative evaluation of orlistat and sibutramine treatment in hypertensive obese patients. Diabetes Obes Metab 2005;7(1):47–55.

58. Tonstad S, Pometta D, Erkelens DW, Ose L, Moccetti T, Schouten JA, Golay A, Reitsma J, Del Bufalo A, Pasotti E, et al. The effect of the gastrointestinal lipase inhibitor, orlistat, on serum lipids and lipoproteins in patients with primary hyperlipidaemia. Eur J Clin Pharmacol 1994;46(5):405–10.

59. Zhi J, Melia AT, Koss-Twardy SG, Arora S, Patel IH. The effect of orlistat, an inhibitor of dietary fat absorption, on the pharmacokinetics of beta-carotene in healthy volunteers. J Clin Pharmacol 1996;36(2):152–9.

60. Melia AT, Koss-Twardy SG, Zhi J. The effect of orlistat, an inhibitor of dietary fat absorption, on the absorption of vitamins A and E in healthy volunteers. J Clin Pharmacol 1996;36(7):647–53.

61. McDuffie JR, Calis KA, Booth SL, Uwaifo GI, Yanovski JA. Effects of orlistat on fat-soluble vitamins in obese adolescents. Pharmacotherapy 2002;22(7):814–22.

62. Thurairajah PH, Syn WK, Neil DA, Stell D, Haydon G. Orlistat (Xenical)-induced subacute liver failure. Eur J Gastroenterol Hepatol 2005;17(12):1437–8.

63. Colman E, Fossler M. Reduction in blood cyclosporine concentrations by orlistat. N Engl J Med 2000;342(15):1141–2.

64. Le Beller C, Bezie Y, Chabatte C, Guillemain R, Amrein C, Billaud EM. Co-administration of orlist at and cyclosporine in a heart transplant recipient. Transplantation 2000;70(10):1541–2.

65. Schnetzler B, Kondo-Oestreicher M, Vala D, Khatchatourian G, Faidutti B. Orlistat decreases the plasma level of cyclosporine and may be responsible for the development of acute rejection episodes. Transplantation 2000;70(10):1540–1.
66. Errasti P, Garcia I, Lavilla J, Ballester B, Manrique J, Purroy A. Reduction in blood cyclosporine concentration by orlistat in two renal transplant patients. Transplant Proc 2002;34(1):137–9.
67. Asberg A. Interactions between cyclosporin and lipid-lowering drugs: implications for organ transplant recipients. Drugs 2003;63:367–78.
68. Evans S, Michael R, Wells H, Maclean D, Gordon I, Taylor J, Goldsmith D. Drug interaction in a renal transplant patient: cyclosporin–Neoral and orlistat. Am J Kidney Dis 2003;41:493–6.
69. Nägele H, Petersen B, Bonacker U, Rödiger W. Effect of orlistat on blood cyclosporin concentration in an obese heart transplant patient. Eur J Clin Pharmacol 1999;55:667–9.
70. Barbaro D, Orsini P, Pallini S, Piazza F, Pasquini C. Obesity in transplant patients: case report showing interference of orlistat with absorption of cyclosporine and review of literature. Endocr Pract 2002;8:124–6.
71. Madhava K, Hartley A. Hypothyroidism in thyroid carcinoma follow-up: orlistat may inhibit the absorption of thyroxine. Clin Oncol (R Coll Radiol) 2005;17(6):492.
72. Dawson D, Conlon C. Case study: metformin associated lactic acidosis; could orlistat be relevant? Diabetes Care 2003;26:2471–2.
73. Fox M, Stutz B, Menne D, Fried M, Schwizer W, Thumshirn M. The effects of loperamide on continence problems and anorectal function in obese subjects taking orlistat. Dig Dis Sci 2005;50(9):1576–83.

F. Braun and M. Behrend

37 Drugs that act on the immune system: cytokines and monoclonal antibodies

COLONY-STIMULATING FACTORS *(SEDA-26, 398; SEDA-27, 391; SEDA-28, 415; SEDA-29, 383)*

Granulocyte colony-stimulating factor (G-CSF) and granulocyte-macrophage colony-stimulating factor (GM-CSF) *(SED-15, 1542)*

Cardiovascular *Capillary leak syndrome* is caused by damage to endothelial cells, resulting in extravasation of plasma proteins and fluid from the capillaries into the extravascular space. This results in large amounts of extravascular lung water and pulmonary vascular permeability, necessitating mechanical ventilation. Capillary leak syndrome in which serial extravascular lung water measurements were performed has been reported in a patient receiving granulocyte colony-stimulating factor (1[Ar]).

- A 68-year-old woman with a stage IIIB diffuse large B cell lymphoma developed severe capillary leak syndrome during treatment with G-CSF after autologous hematological stem cell transplantation, having received chemotherapy before transplantation. She was given subcutaneous G-CSF 480 micrograms/day and treatment was withdrawn on day 11 when the absolute neutrophil count exceeded $500 \times 10^6/l$. She developed renal impairment from day 2, became somnolent, and developed leg edema. Her blood pressure was 98/45 mmHg, pulse 137/minute, central venous pressure 14 mmHg, respiratory rate 20/minute, and temperature 38.4 °C. A chest X-ray showed marked pulmonary congestion. She was given slow extended daily dialysis, noradrenaline, and dobutamine, but became more hypoxic and required mechanical ventilation. Her liver function deteriorated and she became icteric without hepatomegaly or ascites. Liver biopsy showed drug-induced hepatitis without veno-occlusive disease. Her extravascular lung water volume was increased. Continuous venovenous hemofiltration and hydrocortisone 100 mg tds were ineffective. Hypoxia, respiratory and metabolic acidosis, and hemodynamic instability worsened and she died.

Five other cases have been reported before. The white blood cell count at the onset was $0-90 \times 10^9/l$. The symptoms started on days 5–9 after the start of G-CSF treatment, and all the patients had fever. Mechanical ventilation was required in three and renal replacement therapy in four; two died.

Respiratory Exacerbation of prior pulmonary involvement can occur during recovery from neutropenia. G-CSF-related pulmonary toxicity has been documented in patients with cancers, and experimental models have suggested a therapeutic role for G-CSF. Of 20 patients who developed non-cardiac acute respiratory failure during G-CSF-induced recovery from neutropenia, all had *pulmonary infiltrates* during neutropenia followed by respiratory deterioration coinciding with recovery from neutropenia (2[c]). Half of the patients had received hemopoietic stem cell transplants. Mechanical ventilation was required in 16 patients, including 14 with acute respiratory distress syndrome (ARDS), five of whom died. Recommended therapy includes eliminating other causes, withdrawal of G-CSF, and early supportive management, including diagnostic confirmation and mechanical ventilation.

Side Effects of Drugs, Annual 30
J.K. Aronson (Editor)
ISSN: 0378-6080
DOI: 10.1016/S0378-6080(08)00037-8

INTERFERONS   *(SED-15, 1841;*

SEDA-26, 393; SEDA-27, 383; SEDA-28, 416;
SEDA-29, 384; see also Chapter 29)

Interferon alfa   *(SED-15, 1793;*
SEDA-29, 386)

Nervous system   *Multifocal leukoencephalopathy and sensory-motor polyneuropathy* have been reported after long-term interferon alfa therapy (3[A]).

- A 77-year-old man developed a progressive exercise-induced gait disturbance with right-sided predominance, non-systemic vertigo, muscle pain in both thighs after exercise, restless legs, stocking-type sensory disturbances bilaterally, and hypesthesia in the left arm. He had received intramuscular interferon alfa 2b 4.5–5 million units 3 times weekly for 18 years for hairy cell leukaemia. A brain MRI scan showed multiple non-enhancing T2-hyperintense lesions supratentorially, interpreted as vascular lesions. He was also taking pramipexole, levodopa, cabergoline, diltiazem, molsidomine, finasteride, and allopurinol. There was bilateral hypacusis, bilateral dysmetria, exaggerated biceps tendon reflexes on the right side, reduced biceps reflexes on the left, discrete proximal weakness in the left arm, proximal weakness in both legs, reduced ankle reflexes on the right, extensor plantar reflexes bilaterally, left-sided hemihypesthesia, stocking-type sensory disturbances bilaterally, and a tendency to fall during Romberg's test and Unterberger's treadmill test. Serum IgG antibodies against *Borrelia burgdorferi* were positive, but the cerebrospinal fluid was negative.

Interferon can cause multifocal leukoencephalopathy and sensorimotor polyneuropathy, in which case long-term interferon therapy should be reviewed.

Psychological   Neurocognitive performance has been studied in 70 patients receiving interferon alfa 2b (pegylated or conventional) and ribavirin, because impairment of concentration is common during antiviral therapy of chronic hepatitis C (4[c]). Repeated computer-based testing showed significantly increased reaction times. Accuracy measures, reflected by the number of false reactions, were affected only for the working-memory task. Cognitive performance returned to pre-treatment values after the end of therapy. Cognitive impairment was not significantly correlated with the degree of concomitant depression.

Psychiatric   Patients with a wide variety of medical illnesses have behavioral alterations, including *depression*, at rates 5–10 times higher than in the general population. Recent theories have proposed that inflammatory mediators, notably cytokines, are involved. Interferon alfa causes behavioral symptoms, including depression, fatigue, and cognitive dysfunction. The psychiatric effects of low-dose interferon alfa on brain activity have been assessed using functional MRI during a task of visuospatial attention in patients infected with hepatitis C virus (5[c]). Despite having symptoms of impaired concentration and fatigue, the 10 patients who received interferon alfa had similar task performance and activation of parietal and occipital brain regions to 11 control subjects infected with hepatitis C. However, in contrast to the controls, the patients who received interferon alfa had significant activation in the dorsal part of the anterior cingulate cortex, which correlated highly with the number of task-related errors; there was no such correlation in the controls. Consistent with the role of the anterior cingulate cortex in conflict monitoring, this activation of the anterior cingulate cortex suggests that interferon alfa might increase the processing of conflict or reduce the threshold for conflict detection, thereby signalling the need for mental effort to maintain performance.

Hematologic   Since 1994, there have been four case reports and one study of the development of *inhibitors directed against factor VIII* in patients receiving interferon alfa. However, all of the patients had additional risk factors for the development of factor VIII inhibitors—either a hematological malignancy or a history of hemophilia A. Thus, there has not been unequivocal evidence that interferon alfa alone is associated with the development of an autoantibodies to factor VIII.

- A 53-year-old black man with a 30-year history of asymptomatic hepatitis C infection developed cryoglobulinemic glomerulonephritis and was given peginterferon, ribavirin, and prednisone (6[A]). After 6 months he noted scleral bleeding, easy bruising, and large ecchymoses after minor trauma. There was no history of a bleeding disorder and he had never had blood transfusions. Other medications included hydrochlorothiazide, labetalol, furosemide, amlodipine, and pantoprazole, and he had no known drug allergies. The hematocrit was 28%, platelet count 200×10^9/l, creatinine 186 µmol/l, partial thromboplastin time 74 seconds, and prothrombin time 12 seconds. Factor VIII activity was <1% and an inhibitor was detected in a titer of 24 Bethesda units. Peginterferon and ribavirin were withdrawn and he was given prednisone 1 mg/kg/day. After 3 weeks, there is no change in the inhibitor titer. Prednisone was gradually tapered and withdrawn. He was given rituximab 375 mg/m^2/week for 1 month, with little effect. One month later, he received another 4-week course of rituximab and the inhibitor titers normalized.

Exposure to interferon in the setting of cryoglobulinemia may be a risk factor for the development of autoantibodies to factor VIII. The use of interferon, and particularly peginterferon, which has a longer half-life, may be hazardous in patients with this disorder. Repeated examination of such patients for the presence of factor VIII autoantibodies seems warranted.

Susceptibililty factors

Genetic   Genotype 4a hepatitis C virus is the most prevalent type in patients with Egyptian chronic active hepatitis, and confers poor sensitivity to standard interferon and interferon + ribavirin. Pegylated interferon alfa-2b ($n = 30$) and interferon alfa-2b ($n = 31$), both in combination with ribavirin 800–1200 mg/day, resulted in comparable safety and tolerability, but poor responses to antiviral therapy, which may be related to intrinsic resistance to the direct antiviral effect of interferon (7^c).

Management of adverse drug reactions   Antiviral pegylated interferon + ribavirin in patients with hepatitis C virus infection can result in thrombocytopenia, which has been successfully treated with rituximab (8^A).

- A 43-year-old Caucasian woman with hepatitis C infection (genotype 1b) received pegylated interferon + ribavirin for 11 months, during which toime her platelet count remained above 150 × 10^9/l. After 1 year the platelet count fell to 31 × 10^9/l and she developed bruising and petechiae. Interferon + ribavirin was withdrawn without improvement in the platelet count. After 1 month, the platelet count fell to 13 × 10^9/l. She was given intravenous immunoglobulin, with transient improvement, but the platelet count fell again and she had bruising and petechiae. She was given intravenous anti-Rhesus D 50 mg/kg and four infusions of rituximab 375 mg/m^2/week. After the second dose her platelet count rose to 249 × 10^9/l

and after the fourth dose it was 156 × 10^9/l. Pegylated interferon + ribavirin was restarted after the third infusion of rituximab.

Interferon beta   *(SED-15, 1831; SEDA-29, 393)*

Nervous system   There is an association between multiple sclerosis and *central nervous system tumors*.

- A 19-year-old woman with multiple sclerosis had a concomitant right intraventricular tumor, consistent with meningioma on an MRI scan (9^A). Two years after the start of treatment with interferon beta, a brain MRI scan showed enlargement of the intraventricular mass and a relative increase in the number of white matter lesions without significant clinical deterioration. She underwent almost total resection of the mass. A papillary meningioma was confirmed histologically.

This association could have been coincidental. However, meningiomas have been previously reported in two patients with multiple sclerosis, with progression during treatment with interferon-beta (10^A). Based on immunohistochemistry, the meningioma was speculated to have resulted from enhanced platelet-derived growth factor receptors and/or down-regulated transforming growth factor receptors on the tumor itself.

Endocrine   Conflicting data have been reported on the association between interferon beta therapy in multiple sclerosis and thyroid disease. In 106 patients (76 women) with multiple sclerosis who received interferon beta-1a or beta-1b for up to 84 (median 42) months, there was baseline thyroid autoimmunity in 8.5% and hypothyroidism in 2.8% (11^c). *Thyroid dysfunction* (80% hypothyroidism, 92% subclinical, 56% transient) developed in 24% (68% with autoimmunity) and autoimmunity in 23% (46% with dysfunction), without a significant difference between the two cytokines; 68% of the cases of dysfunction occurred within the first year. Thyroid dysfunction was generally subclinical and was transient in over half of cases. Autoimmunity was the only predictive factor for the development of dysfunction (relative risk = 8.9), but sustained disease was also significantly associated with male sex.

Immunologic   An international panel specialized in the treatment of multiple sclerosis has summarized the question of whether neutralizing *antibodies to interferon beta* develop in patients with multiple sclerosis (12[M]). They concluded that interferon beta can induce the development of antibodies that reduce or "neutralize" the biological activity of interferon beta. The extent of development of these antibodies differs amongst the available interferon beta products. Interferon beta-1b is associated with the highest incidence; of interferon beta-1a products, Avonex is associated with the lowest incidence. Neutralizing antibodies are clinically important, since the efficacy of interferon is reduced in patients with persistent and significant titers. Thus, optimal management of patients with multiple sclerosis should not only consider the relative efficacy and safety of interferon beta, but also their immunogenic potential. An international standardized assay for neutralizing antibodies is required and all patients with multiple sclerosis who receive interferon beta should be evaluated for their presence.

INTERLEUKINS   *(SED-15, 1842; SEDA-26, 397; SEDA-27, 390; SEDA-28, 424; SEDA-29, 394)*

Interleukin-2 (IL-2)   *(SEDA-29, 394)*

Interleukin-2 or interferon alfa are often used as first-line treatments in progressive metastatic renal cell carcinoma, which usually does not respond to chemotherapy and is only moderately sensitive to radiotherapy.

Drug dosage regimens   High-dose intravenous IL-2 can induce a 14% response rate with 5–8% durable complete remission, but toxicity frequently requires hospitalisation. Toxicity can be limited by subcutaneous administration but that is less effective. Therefore, efficacy of the combination of continuous subcutaneous low-dose IL-2 1 mIU/m^2+thalidomide 200 mg/day has been investigated in 22 patients with progressive metastatic renal cell cancers (13[c]). Adverse effects included fatigue ($n = 17$), sensory neuropathy ($n = 9$), dizziness ($n = 4$), deep vein thrombosis ($n = 4$) and constipation ($n = 3$). Fatigue was mainly mild. Sensory

neuropathy required a reduction in the dosage of thalidomide to 100 mg/day in three patients. Deep venous thrombosis was treated with anticoagulants in three of four cases. In one patient extensive caval thrombosis developed in the first week of treatment despite anticoagulant treatment for a deep vein thrombosis.

Denileukin diftitox

Denileukin diftitox is a genetically engineered fusion protein combining the enzymatically active domains of diphtheria toxin and the full-length sequence for interleukin-2 (IL-2). It targets lymphoma cells that express the high-affinity IL-2 receptor. In vitro, the retinoid X receptor retinoid bexarotene upregulated both the p55 and p75 subunits of the IL-2 receptor and enhanced five- to ten-fold the susceptibility of T cell leukemia cells to denileukin diftitox (14[cE]).

Hematologic   In a phase I trial, 14 adults with relapsed or refractory cutaneous T cell lymphomas received bexarotene 75, 150, 225, or 300 mg/day beginning 7 days before the first dose of denileukin diftitox 18 micrograms/kg/day for 3 days every 21 days (14[cE]). The overall response rate was 67% (four complete responses, four partial responses). There was modulation of IL-2 receptor expression at or above a bexarotene dose of 150 mg/day. Four patients had grade 2 or 3 *leukopenia* and two had grade 4 *lymphopenia*.

Interleukin-11 (IL-11)

Observational studies   In a phase I/II trial in 47 children (median age 11, range 0.7–26, years) with solid tumors or lymphomas following chemotherapy, recombinant human interleukin-11 (25–125 micrograms/kg/day) was given subcutaneously on days 6–33 (15[c]). The median numbers of days to an absolute platelet count of at least 50×10^9/l and platelet transfusions were 19, 21, 20, and 18 days and 3, 3, 4, and 2 days at dosages of 25, 50, 75 and 100 micrograms/kg/day respectively. The most common adverse events probably related to treatment included *tachycardia* (46%), *conjunctival injection* (46%), *edema* (30%), *pain* (23%), *rhinitis* (21%), *diarrhea* (21%), *cardiomegaly* (21%), *papilledema* (16%), and *periosteal bone changes* (11%). Increased plasma volume was thought to be the cause of the cardiomegaly.

Cardiovascular   Low-dose recombinant IL-11 therapy was associated with one case of *dysrhythmia* and one *transient ischemic attack* in 32 patients with bone marrow failure due to myelodysplastic syndromes, graft failure, chemotherapy, or aplastic anemia (16[c]).

Hematologic   Interleukin-11 was identified in 1990 (17[E]). It is a 19 kD protein consisting of 199 amino acids. The gene for IL-11 is located on chromosome 19q13.3-q13.4 and acts synergistically with IL-3, thrombopoietin, or stem cell factor to stimulate megakaryopoiesis (18[E], 19[E], 20[E], 21[R], 22[R]). Recombinant human interleukin-11 has been approved by the Food and Drug Administration for adults with solid tumors and lymphomas associated with severe chemotherapy-induced thrombocytopenia. However, *thrombocytopenia* is still the major dose-limiting adverse effect of myelosuppressive chemotherapy in children with solid tumors.

Interleukin-12 (IL-12)

Interleukin 12 is a cytokine with important regulatory functions, bridging innate and adaptive immunity. It has been proposed as an immune adjuvant for immunization therapy in infectious diseases and malignancies.

Immunologic   Dose-dependent systemic *activation of multiple inflammatory mediator systems* in humans has been studied after sucutaneous injection of recombinant human IL-12 (0.5 micrograms/kg/day) in 26 patients with renal cell cancers (23[c]). IL-12 induced degranulation of neutrophils, with significant rises in the plasma concentrations of elastase and lactoferrin at 24 hours. It also caused release of lipid mediators, as shown by a sharp increase in the plasma secretory phospholipase A2 activity. The dose of IL-12 should therefore not exceed 0.1 micrograms/kg/day, in order to avoid severe systemic inflammatory responses.

TUMOR NECROSIS FACTOR (TNF) ANTAGONISTS   *(SEDA-26, 399; SEDA-27, 393; SEDA-28, 425; SEDA-29, 395)*

Various treatments for psoriasis, including adalimumab, efalizumab, and infliximab, alefacept and etanercept, and pimecrolimus, have been reviewed in the light of clinical data, including the results of phase II and/or III studies (24[R]).

Adalimumab   *(SED-15, 2380; SEDA-28, 426; SEDA-29, 397)*

Adalimumab has been approved alone or in combination with methotrexate for the treatment of rheumatoid arthritis in the EU and USA; approval for the treatment of psoriasis, psoriatic arthritis, and ankylosing spondylitis is expected in the near future (25[M]). Adverse effects that have been reported in trials include *worsening or initiation of congestive heart failure*, *raised transaminases*, medically significant *cytopenias*, including pancytopenia, and a *lupus-like syndrome*. Other adverse effects include *asthma* (26[A]), *paresthesia* in the leg and foot drop (27[A]), and severe *oral epithelial dysplasia* (28[A]). Adalimumab *increases the risk of rare serious infections* two-fold, and it should not be used during periods of active infection. Its most notable infectious complication is reactivation of tuberculosis and screening is recommended. Deep fungal and other serious and atypical infections can also be promoted.

- A 61-year-old man with rheumatoid arthritis receiving adalimumab developed a sore throat (29[A]). Screening for tuberculosis using PPD was positive, and isoniazid was prescribed prophylactically for 6 months. After taking adalimumab for 8 months he developed tonsillar enlargement and nodular pulmonary lesions. Histopathological and microbial investigations established the diagnosis of tonsillar tuberculosis.

Tumorigenicity   Promotion of *lymphoma* is a rare adverse effect of adalimumab. There has been a report of follicular mucinosis associated with mycosis fungoides in a patient taking adalimumab (30[A]).

Alefacept

Tumorigenicity *Lymphoproliferative disorders* are more common in individuals taking immunosuppressive drugs, and mycosis fungoides has been reported in a 72-year-old patient with a psoriasiform dermatitis taking alefacept (31[A]). The authors suggested that alefacept should be used with caution in patients with known mycosis fungoides or an unclassified atypical lymphocytic infiltrate of the skin.

Etanercept   *(SED-15, 1279;*
SEDA-29, 397)

Favorable safety data have been observed in a phase III randomized controlled study (24-week studies) of etanercept in patients with chronic plaque psoriasis (32[C]).

Infection risk Etanercept has been used in two children with severe atopic dermatitis: it was minimally effective and was associated with complications. One patient developed a superinfection with methicillin-resistant *Staphylococcus aureus* (MRSA) and the other had viral-like symptoms followed by a generalized urticarial eruption (33[c]). This was a limited study, which the authors suggested should not rule out the use of biologicals for severe atopic dermatitis, but should encourage a larger controlled study.

Infliximab   *(SED-15, 1747;*
SEDA-29, 398)

Infliximab is a chimeric monoclonal antibody to tumor necrosis factor (TNF). It was initially approved by the Food and Drug and Administration in August 1998 for the treatment of moderately to severely active Crohn's disease in patients with an inadequate response to conventional therapies and those with enterocutaneous fistulae. The indications were expanded in June 2002 and April 2003 to include maintenance of clinical remission, treatment of enterocutaneous and rectovaginal fistulae, and maintaining fistula closure.

Infliximab is well tolerated in most patients, but can be associated with serious adverse effects. The major concerns are *infusion reactions, infections, autoimmune disorders*, and *malignancies*. Acute infusion reactions occur in 3.8–27% of patients and can cause flushing, palpitation, sweating, chest pain, hypotension/hypertension, or dyspnea (34[M]).

Observational studies In 23 patients with refractory autoimmune uveitis, who were given three infusions of inflixiamb at weeks 0, 2, and 6, 78% had clinical success, but only 50% continued infliximab therapy for at least 1 year (35[c]). There was an unexpectedly high rate of adverse events. Seven patients had serious adverse events, including three cases of serious *thrombosis*, two *vitreous hemorrhages*, one *malignancy*, one new-onset *congestive heart failure*, and two possible cases of drug-induced *lupus-like syndrome*.

Metabolism Body composition was assessed in patients with Crohn's disease before and after treatment with infliximab at 1 and 4 weeks (36[c]). There were significant *increases in body weight* at 4 weeks and serum leptin concentrations at 1 and 4 weeks. The increase in serum leptin occurred at 1 week, when there were no significant changes in weight and fat mass, and was associated with down-regulation of TNF alfa-regulated mediators, soluble TNF receptor type II, and soluble intercellular antiadhesion molecule-1. Moreover, infliximab significantly increased cholesterol concentrations at 1 week compared with the control patients, who received methylprednisolone.

Immunologic Profound *immunomodulation* induced by blockers of TNF alfa is associated with a relatively low incidence of immune-related complications, such as demyelinating disease and lupus-like syndrome. This contrasts sharply with the prominent induction of autoantibodies such as antinuclear antibodies (ANA) and anti-doublestranded DNA (anti-dsDNA) antibodies by TNF alfa blockers. This phenomenon has been recognized for several years, but the clinical and biological correlates of this antibody induction in autoimmune arthritis are not yet fully understood.

Antibody formation has been studied in patients with spondylarthropathy (n = 34) or rheumatoid arthritis ($n = 59$) who were treated with infliximab for 2 years and in 20 patients with spondylarthropathy who were treated with etanercept for 1 year (37^c). After 1 year, the infliximab-treated patients with spondylarthropathy or rheumatoid arthritis had new antinuclear antibodies in 41 and 62% respectively and anti-dsDNA antibodies in 49 and 71%. Only 10% of etanercept-treated patients with spondylarthropathy developed antibodies. Isotyping showed almost exclusively IgM or IgM/IgA anti-dsDNA antibodies, which disappeared on withdrawal of treatment. Neither infliximab nor etanercept induced other lupus-related antibodies, such as anti-ENA antibodies, antihistone antibodies, or antinucleosome antibodies, and there was no clinical evidence of lupus-like syndrome. Similarly, infliximab, but not etanercept, selectively increased IgM but not IgG anticardiolipin antibody titers. Thus, the prominent antinuclear antibody and anti-dsDNA autoantibody response is not a pure class effect of TNF alfa blockers, is largely restricted to short-term IgM responses, and is not associated with other serological or clinical signs of lupus. Similar findings with anticardiolipin antibodies suggest that modulation of humoral immunity may be a more general feature of infliximab treatment.

The overall incidence of *infusion reactions* to infliximab is about 5%. However, severe infusion reactions have been observed (38^A).

- A 53-year-old woman with a 13-year history of rheumatoid arthritis received infliximab 3 mg/kg for 9 months, with a 20% improvement. Infliximab was replaced by methotrexate 12 mg/week but was restarted about 2 years later. She developed a fever and skin rash 10 days after the first infusion, which responded to hydrocortisone 100 mg. Before the next infusion she was given an antihistmaine, olopatadine hydrochloride 10 mg/day. The infusion rate of infliximab was lowered to less than half of the usual rate during the next infusion, but 15 minutes after the infusion, she had a skin rash and pruritis, followed by dyspnea and a swollen throat. The infusion was immediately stopped and she was given 50% oxygen, and intravenous hydrocortisone 200 mg and methylprednisolone 125 mg. Her symptoms resolved completely within 2 hours.
- A 49-year-old woman with a 16-year history of rheumatoid arthritis received infliximab for 10 months and then methotrexate 10.5 mg/week; 2 years later she was switched to infliximab again. During the first infusion, her body temperature rose from 35.6 to 37.6 °C and then steadily fell to baseline after the end of treatment. There were

no adverse events during the second and third infusions, but 10 minutes after the start of the fourth infusion she started to sweat and looked pale. Her systolic blood pressure fell from 150 to 78 mmHg, but her heart rate was unchanged. There were no skin lesions or laryngeal swelling. The infusion was immediately stopped. She was given intravenous hydrocortisone 100 mg and recovered.

The mechanisms of these immunological reactions are unclear. Development of a human antichimeric antibody against infliximab has been speculated. Antichimeric antibody titers are often not measured when infliximab is given at intervals of 8 weeks or less, because the antibody is undetectable when infliximab is present in the serum. However, an antichimeric antibody was detected retrospectively in the serum of both patients immediately before infliximab was resumed.

Susceptibility factors

Genetic factors   Genetic studies have identified potential predictors of the response to infliximab. A −308 polymorphism in the promoter of the TNF alfa gene influences TNF alfa transcription. The association between the response to infliximab and the polymorphism in the TNF region at the lymphotoxin A locus is controversial. Allelic and genotype frequencies for the −308 TNF gene polymorphism have not been shown to be significantly different between responders and non-responders to infliximab, but non-responders tended to have a higher frequency of the rare TNF2 allele, which has been associated with increased production of TNF.

The NOD2 (or NOD2/CARD15) gene has recently been identified as a Crohn's disease susceptibility gene, and mutations in NOD2/CARD15 are associated with Crohn's disease. However, the hypothesis that mutations in NOD2/CARD15 indirectly alter TNF production and thereby influence differences in response to infliximab has not been substantiated.

The IgG Fc receptor gene, FCGR3A, encodes FcgRIIIa receptors expressed on macrophages and natural killer cells, and polymorphism in this gene is associated with varying affinity for IgG1 and potency in antibody-dependent cellular cytotoxicity, which has been

implicated as one mechanism of action of infliximab in Crohn's disease. Therefore, polymorphism in FCGR3A has been suggested to
predict the response to infliximab, which is an
IgG1 antibody. Individuals with the FCGR3A
genotype that is associated with a high affinity
for IgG1 were more likely to have a biological
and possibly a clinical response to infliximab
(34[M]).

Age   Older age was associated with reduced
response to infliximab in patients with Crohn's
disease in a European multicenter study, but
a clear correlation between age and response
could not be confirmed by other studies in the
USA and UK (34[M]). It is not clear why younger
patients have a better response to infliximab.

Drug dosage regimens   In carefully selected
patients, infliximab infusion administered at
home is safe and cost-effective. Infliximab infusion was performed at home in 10 children, who
received 59 infusions of 7.5–10 mg/kg/dose.
The calculated average savings per patient were
$1335/100 mg infliximab (39[c]). Home infu-
sions lasted 2–5 hours. Infusions could be
performed on any day of the week, and school
absenteeism was reduced. The average patient
satisfaction rating for home infusions was 9 on
a scale from 1 to 10 (10 = most satisfied).
Three patients had difficulty with intravenous
access and required multiple attempts, but all
were able to receive their infusions. One infusion was stopped because of arm pain above the
infusion site. This patient had his next infusion
in the hospital before returning to the home infusion program. There were no severe adverse
events (palpitation, blood pressure instability,
hyperemia, respiratory symptoms) during home
infusion.

Interactions with smoking   A negative affect
of smoking on the response to infliximab therapy has been reported in two studies from the
USA and UK (34[M]). Smokers with Crohn's disease had lower response rates to infliximab than
non-smokers (22 versus 73%) and were more
likely to relapse within 1 year of therapy. However, a large European study failed to confirm
this association.

MONOCLONAL ANTIBODIES
*(SED-15, 2380; SEDA-26, 402; SEDA-27, 378;
SEDA-28, 434; SEDA-29, 404)*

Abciximab

See Chapter 35.

Adalimumab

See *TNF antagonists* above.

Alemtuzumab (Campath-1H®)
(SED-15, 71; SEDA-29, 404)

Alemtuzumab, an anti-CD52 monoclonal antibody, is effective in B cell and T cell lymphoproliferative disorders.

Hematologic   In a phase II trial in 11 patients
alemtuzumab was given in a dose of 3 mg intravenously on day 1, followed by 10 mg on
day 3; if it was tolerated the dose was increased
to 30 mg on day 5 and was continued thrice
weekly for 12 weeks (40[c]). Five patients developed severe *neutropenia* and *thrombocytopenia*,
and three had prolonged *cytopenias*, including two with *severe marrow hypoplasia*. Three
had trilineage morphological *myelodysplasia*,
two with new clonal cytogenetic abnormalities. The exact mechanism of alemtuzumab-
associated hematological toxicity is unclear.
Cytomegalovirus infection can rarely cause cytopenias, but this by itself is not enough to
explain the severe cytopenias or myelodysplasia
in this series, as not all patients with these complications had cytomegalovirus reactivation or
disease. Four of five patients with grade IV cytopenias had PCR-confirmed cytomegalovirus
reactivation, either at the time of or within 2
weeks of clinical reactivation. In two cases the
pancytopenia occurred before ganciclovir had
been given. There was no apparent relation
between the dose of alemtuzumab and the development of cytomegalovirus reactivation. It
has bvenpostulated that activated CD4+ T cells
are required for normal hemopoiesis, which
may be one mechanism for the cytopenias that

are associated with alemtuzumab, especially in T cell lymphoproliferative disorders (41[E]). Regular monitoring for cytomegalovirus and, if cytopenias develop, for parvovirus and Epstein–Barr virus reactivation/infection and marrow examination (including cytogenetics) is recommended.

Alemtuzumab (30 mg subcutaneously thrice weekly for 12 weeks) has been reported to be active against HTL-1-induced chemoresistant adult T cell leukemia in a 63-year-old woman who had responded poorly to chlorambucil, cyclophosphamide, antiretroviral drugs, thalidomide, interferon alfa, and denileukin diftitox (42[A]). *Neutropenia* and asymptomatic *cytomegalovirus (CMV) reactivation* occurred during treatment and responded to filgrastim and valganciclovir respectively.

Infection risk   Infectious complications due to adenoviruses are of increasing concern after allogeneic stem cell transplantation. Recent reports in adults have implicated alemtuzumab as a risk factor for *adenovirus infection*. Of 111 children, 54 received antithymocyte globulin and 57 received alemtuzumab. In all, 35/111 patients (32%) were infected with an adenovirus, and 9/111 (8%) had adenovirus disease (43[c]). Adenovirus infection was more common in those who received alemtuzumab (23/57 versus 12/54), and disseminated adenovirus disease was more frequent in those who received alemtuzumab (8/57 versus 1/54). The presence of grade 3–4 graft-versus-host disease was a risk factor for adenovirus infection. These findings highlight the fact that adenovirus infection in children is a frequent complication after stem cell transplantation from donors and that alemtuzumab carries a higher risk of infection than antithymocyte globulin.

Anti-human CD40 Mab chimeric 5D12

Ligation of CD40 by CD154 is a critical step in the interaction between antigen presenting cells and T cells. In animals, antagonizing CD40L–CD40 reduced the severity of several autoimmune and inflammatory disorders, including experimental colitis (44[E]). The non-stimulatory antagonistic activity of Mab 5D12 (anti-human CD40) has been demonstrated in various in vitro studies using different CD40-bearing cell types and ch5D12 antagonist activity has been validated in vivo using various non-human primate disease models (45[E], 46[E], 47[E], 48[E]). Chimeric 5D12 (ch5D12) is a molecularly engineered human IgG4 antibody that contains the variable domains of the heavy and light chains of 5D12 (49[E]). It was constructed to reduce the potential for immunogenicity and to enhance the in vivo half-life of the 5D12 monoclonal antibody when used in humans.

Observational studies   In an open dose-escalation phase I/IIa study, ch5D12 was given to 18 patients with moderate to severe Crohn's disease in single intravenous doses of 0.3, 1, 3, and 10 mg/kg (50[c]). The most common adverse effects were *pyrexia, arthralgia, myalgia*, and *headache*. Arthralgia was common at baseline and during follow-up, and fell in frequency during follow-up. No subjects withdrew from the study because of adverse events. There was no clear dose relation for any single adverse event, with the possible exception of headache/migraine.

Gastrointestinal   There were serious adverse events in six patients who were given ch5D12 (three at a dose of 1 mg/kg, two at 3 mg/kg, and one at 10 mg/kg) (44[c]). Five events were considered possibly related to ch5D12. Five of six events were gastrointestinal, including two cases of *subileus* both in patients taking 1.0 mg/kg, two cases of Crohn's disease aggravated by 1.0 and 3.0 mg/kg, and one case of *abdominal pain aggravated* by 3.0 mg/kg. However, two events occurred at a time that suggested that a causal relation was very unlikely.

Basiliximab   (SED-15, 418; SEDA-29, 407)

Basiliximab, an anti-IL2 receptor antibody, is effective in combination with different maintenance regimens, reduces the incidence of acute transplant rejection, allows safe reduction of doses of glucocorticoids, and is associated with economic savings (51[M]). However, there is no evidence that it prolongs either patient or graft survival. Initial administration of basiliximab is associated with fewer adverse events than T cell depleting agents. However, life-threatening re-actions have been reported after re-exposure to basiliximab in recipients who lost graft function early after transplantation and therefore stopped taking all immunosuppressive agents.

Susceptibility factors

Age   In children induction therapy with basil-iximab may provide potential benefits by pre-venting early episodes of acute rejection and allowing delayed administration of calcineurin inhibitors or avoidance of glucocorticoids (52[M]). Whether this results in better long-term graft survival has still to be confirmed. How-ever, induction therapy has beneficial effects in high-risk recipients and allows avoidance of glucocorticoids and minimization of doses of calcineurin inhibitors. Anti-IL-2 receptor an-tibodies are increasingly preferred to rabbit antithymocyte globulin, because they are very well tolerated. However, anti-IL-2 receptor an-tibodies have not yet been proven to be more effective or to have less late toxicity than poly-clonal agents. Benefits in early outcomes and no increase in adverse events commend the use of IL-2 receptor antagonists as induction therapy after organ transplantation in children.

Infection risk   *Septic arthritis* typically oc-curs in young children, often from staphylo-coccal infection. However, with chronic im-munosuppression pathogens may be atypical. Although reported in adult transplant recipients, infection with *Myocbacterium hominis* has not previously been described in children.

• A 15-year-old African–American girl developed septic arthritis due to *Mycoplasma hominis* in her right hip 2 months after kidney transplantation (53[A]). The presentation was subtle and indolent, without fever or leukocytosis. Early immunosup-pression with basiliximab, prednisone, tacrolimus, mycophenolate mofetil, and thymoglobulin may have increased her susceptibility. She underwent joint incision and drainage, treatment for 8 weeks with doxycycline and levofloxacin guided by in vitro sensitivities, and reduced immunosuppres-sion. She was subsequently free of infection for 3 years with stable graft function on moderate im-munosuppression with prednisone, tacrolimus and mycophenolate mofetil.

Bevacizumab   *(SED-15, 2380; SEDA-29, 407)*

Bevacizumab is an anti-angiogenic agent that has been rationally designed to target vascular endothelial growth factor (VEGF), a key me-diator in angiogenesis. The principal adverse events seen in clinical trials are *hyperten-sion, proteinuria, arterial thrombosis, effects on wound healing, bleeding*, and *gastrointesti-nal perforation*. These events are for the most part mild to moderate intense and clinically manageable (hypertension, proteinuria, minor bleeding) or are uncommon (wound healing complications, gastrointestinal perforation, and arterial thrombosis). The adverse effects profile of bevacizumab makes it a suitable adjunct to standard chemotherapy, and it is now approved for use in the USA, the European Union, and other markets worldwide (54[M]). For the use of bevacizumab in the treatment of choroidal neo-vascularization see Chapter 47.

Hypertension has been associated with beva-cizumab (55[r]).

Skin   Bevacizumab significantly prolongs sur-vival when it is added to intravenous fluorou-racil-based chemotherapy in first-line metasta-tic colorectal cancer. Bevacizumab in combina-tion with chemotherapy that included fluoroura-cil+leucovorin 28–60 days after primary cancer surgery caused no increased risk of wound heal-ing complications compared with chemother-apy alone (56[c]). However, *wound healing com-plications* were more common in patients who had major surgery during bevacizumab therapy. Most of the patients who received bevacizumab had no complications.

Daclizumab   *(SED-15, 1047; SEDA-29, 408)*

Daclizumab is a humanized monoclonal anti-body against the interleukin-2 receptor. It is used to prevent acute rejection without increas-ing the risk of infection after kidney transplan-tation.

Observational studies   Daclizumab 2 mg/kg was given subcutaneously to 15 patients with sight-threatening, non-infectious intermediate uveitis, posterior uveitis, or panuveitis (57[c]). Subcutaneous daclizumab 1 mg/kg every 2 weeks was then continued for 6 months. The initial immunosuppression load was tapered over 8–12 weeks in a staggered fashion beginning with the first induction treatment. Ten of the patients reduced their concomitant immunosuppression load by at least 50% while maintaining their baseline visual acuity at 12 and 26 weeks. Subcutaneous daclizumab was well tolerated with no serious adverse events during the 6 months, although three patients had non-serious adverse events that were possibly related to daclizumab.

Infection risk   After heart transplantation, 434 recipients received ciclosporin, mycophenolate mofetil, and glucocorticoids as standard immunosuppression (58[C]). They were randomized to induction with five doses of daclizumab ($n = 216$) or placebo ($n = 218$). The primary end point, defined as moderate or severe cellular rejection, hemodynamically significant graft dysfunction, second transplantation, or death or loss to follow-up after 6 months, was reached by 48% of the placebo and 36% of the daclizumab group. The rate of rejection was lower with daclizumab (26%) than placebo (41%). However, more of those who were given daclizumab (six versus none) died of infections. Daclizumab is therefore not recommended after heart transplantation.

Efalizumab   *(SEDA-29, 409)*

Efalizumab is a humanized monoclonal antibody that binds to CD11a, the alpha subunit of lymphocyte function-associated antigen-1, and consequently inhibits T-cell activation (59[R]). Favorable safety data have been observed in a 24-week, phase III, randomized, controlled study of efalizumab in patients with chronic plaque psoriasis (60[C]).

Hematologic   Immune *thrombocytopenia* has been reported in association with the use of efalizumab for psoriasis (61[A]).

Skin   Although cutaneous adverse effects of efalizumab are common the pathogenic mechanisms have yet to be identified. Precise diagnosis is required, considering that cutaneous adverse events pose a challenge about whether treatment should be withdrawn (62[M]).

Dermatitis has been reported in a patient with psoriasis vulgaris taking efalizumab (63[A]).

Musculoskeletal   In randomized, double-blind, placebo-controlled trials, subcutaneous efalizumab 1 mg/kg once a week for 12 weeks significantly reduced disease activity in patients with chronic moderate-to-severe plaque psoriasis (60[M]). There were few serious adverse events or treatment withdrawals. The most common adverse events were *headache, chills, myalgia, pain*, and *fever*; these most often occurred within 2 days of administration, were most frequent after the first or second dose, and reduced in frequency over time.

Infection risk   In phase III clinical trials, patients with moderate-to-severe chronic plaque psoriasis received subcutaneous efalizumab 1 or 2 mg/kg/week or placebo (64[M]). The incidence and severity of infections during 12 weeks of therapy were comparable to those observed in patients who received placebo (29 versus 26%). Infections did not appear to increase in frequency with extended therapy of up to 27 months. Serious infections requiring hospitalization occurred in 1.1% of patients who received efalizumab.

In four placebo-controlled trials patients who received efalizumab for 13–60 weeks the most common adverse events were mild to moderate, self-limiting, flu-like symptoms that were most frequent after the first two doses of efalizumab (65[M]). By the third dose, the incidence was comparable to that with placebo. There were serious adverse events in 2.2 and 1.7% with efalizumab and placebo respectively. Non-serious adverse events that led to withdrawal were infrequent and similar to placebo (2.8 versus 1.8%).

Tumorigenicity   *Cervical cancer* occurred in a woman taking long-term efalizumab (66[A]).

^{99m}Tc fanolesomab

The FDA has issued a public health advisory note to inform patients and health-care providers that Palatin Technologies, the manufacturer of technetium-labelled (^{99m}Tc) fanolesomab (NeutroSpec) has voluntarily suspended marketing of this product, owing to serious safety concerns (67^S). Technetium fanolesomab is indicated for radiological imaging in patients with unclear signs and symptoms of appendicitis who are 5 years of age and older. The FDA received reports from Palatin Technologies of two deaths and 15 additional life-threatening adverse events within minutes of the administration of technetium fanolesomab. The symptoms included shortness of breath, low blood pressure, and cardiopulmonary arrest. The patients required resuscitation with intravenous fluids, blood pressure support, and oxygen. Most of them had pre-existing cardiac and/or pulmonary conditions that may have put them at higher risk. A review of all post-marketing reports showed an additional 46 patients who had adverse events that were similar but less severe. There is no evidence that patients who have already safely received the drug are at long-term risk.

Gemtuzumab ozogamicin   *(SED-15, 1488; SEDA-29, 409)*

Gemtuzumab ozogamicin is composed of a humanized anti-CD33 antibody conjugated with a cytotoxic antitumor antibiotic, calicheamicin. Binding of the anti-CD33 antibody portion of mylotarg to the CD33 antigen, a scialic acid-dependent adhesion protein found on the surface of more than 90% of leukemic myeloblasts but not on normal hemopoietic stem cells, results in the formation of a complex that is internalized. The chalicheamicin derivative is then released in the lysosomes of the myeloid cell, resulting in breaks in double-stranded DNA and cell death. Gemtuzumab ozogamicin (Mylotarg$^®$) was approved for monotherapy by the FDA in May 2000 for the treatment of patients over 60 years old with CD33+ acute myeloid leukemia in first relapse.

Observational studies   When combined with chemotherapy, gemtuzumab ozogamicin is currently used in lower doses, owing to the risk of *hepatotoxicity* and *veno-occlusive disease*. This could explain why there was no difference between combined therapy and gemtuzumab alone in term of complete remission or overall and relapse free survival rates. When gemtuzumab ozogamicin was given in a full dose of 9 mg/m^2 4 days after the start of intermediate-dose aracytin and mitoxantrone (MIDAM) in 17 patients with refractory ($n = 4$) or relapsed ($n = 13$) acute myeloid leukemmia, there was complete remission in 12 patients and partial remission in one (68^c). However, the median time to relapse and overall survival were short (3.3–6.8 and 5.4–5.9 months respectively). All the patients developed grade 4 *neutropenia* and *thrombocytopenia*. There was *hyperbilirubinemia* in 10 patients (two grade 1, four grade 2, two grade 3, and two grade 4). One patient died on day 29 with veno-occlusive disease, not having received low-dose prophylactic heparin. Of five patients who had received a previous autologous transplant, three developed hepatotoxicity (two grade 2 and one grade 3). All had *fever* during hospitalization except one. There were documented *infections* in nine patients, including infections with *Aspergillus* ($n = 2$) and *Fusobacterium* ($n = 1$). One patient died on day 12 with multiple organ failure.

Cardiovascular   Gemtuzumab ozogamicin was used as initial treatment in 12 patients with acute myeloid leukemia over the age of 65; the response rate was 27% (69^c). The adverse effects were acceptable, although five patients developed *cardiac toxicity*, three of whom had grade 3 and/or 4. One of these patients had underlying coronary artery disease and required coronary stent placement. Another developed hypoxia related to pulmonary edema several hours after completing the initial infusion and eventually died of respiratory and ventilatory complications. Another had a myocardial infarction after the second infusion, and one had chest pains half an hour after the initial infusion. It is therefore recommended that elderly patients be screened for cardiac diseases. Patients with coronary artery disease or cardiac dysfunction should not receive gemtuzumab ozogamicin.

Infliximab

See *Tumor necrosis factor (TNF) antagonists* above.

MLN02 (humanized monoclonal antibody to alpha$_4$ beta$_7$ integrin)

Selective blockade of interactions between leukocytes and vascular endothelium in the gut is a promising strategy for the treatment of inflammatory bowel diseases. MLN02 (0.5 and 2 mg/kg intravenously on days 1 and 29) was more effective than placebo in inducing clinical and endoscopic remission in patients with active ulcerative colitis in a multicenter, double-blind, placebo-controlled trial in 181 patients with active ulcerative colitis (70[C]). Eligible patients also received concomitant mesalazine or no other treatment. Clinical remission rates at week 6 were 33, 32, and 14% in those who received 0.5, 2 mg/kg, and placebo respectively. The corresponding proportions of patients who improved by at least 3 points on the ulcerative colitis clinical score were 66, 53, and 33%. There was endoscopic remission in 28, 12, and 8%. There were no substantial differences among the three groups in the prevalence of adverse events, but three patients who received MLN02 had noteworthy adverse events, as listed below.

Immunologic   *Antihuman antibodies* developed by week 8 in 44% of the patients who received MLN02 and 24% of patients were positive for antibody at a titer of greater than 1:125 (31[c]). One 50-year-old woman developed hives and mild angioedema during a second infusion of MLN02; she had MLN02 antibodies in a titer of 1:3125. However, out of 103 participants who received two infusions of MLN02, this patient was the only one in whom a clinically relevant infusion reaction developed.

Infection risk   Primary *cytomegalovirus infection* developed in a patient who was given MLN02 but improved without antiviral therapy (70[C]). Another patient developed lobar pneumonia 3 days after spinal surgery and was treated successfully.

Natalizumab

Natalizumab is a monoclonal antibody that targets alpha-4 integrin and inhibits leukocyte adhesion and migration into inflamed tissues.

Nervous system   Natalizumab was withdrawn from the market 3 months after its approval in February 2005 and was suspended from all clinical trials because of reports of a rare neurological disease, *progressive multifocal leukoencephalopathy*, associated with the JC virus, a human polyomavirus, in patients with multiple sclerosis being treated with natalizumab (71[A], 72[A], 73[A], 74[C]). The Food and Drug Administration asked that all clinical trials involving drugs that target a4b1/VLA-4 be suspended until the full results of the Tysabri™ safety data were completed (75[R]).

Omalizumab   *(SED-15, 2614)*

The safety of the anti-IgE monoclonal antibody omalizumab, given subcutaneously in a dose adjusted for body weight and serum IgE every 2 or 4 weeks, was given as an add-on treatment in 419 asthmatic patients in a randomized, placebo-controlled, double-blind study (76[C]). Suspected drug-related adverse effects were similar between the groups, with the exception of events classified as "general and administration site conditions", including *injection site reactions* (4.9% with omalizumab and 1.7% with placebo). The total incidence of injection site reactions (a known effect of omalizumab) was higher with omalizumab than with placebo (5.3 versus 1.3% respectively). There was one case of omalizumab-related severe pruritus, rash, and petechiae. There were no clinically important changes in laboratory tests or vital signs related to omalizumab. Overall, omalizumab was generally well tolerated, the most common drug-related adverse events being local injection site reactions.

Ranibizumab

See Chapter 47.

Rituximab   *(SED-15, 3069;*
SEDA-29, 410)

Rituximab is a monoclonal anti-CD20 antibody.

Tumorigenicity   *Merkel cell carcinoma* after therapy with rituximab and cladribine has been reported (77[A]).

- A 51-year-old woman with chronic lymphatic leukemia received 4 courses of cladribine and then another four courses in combination with rituximab. She developed a red lump on the right cheek 2 months after the last course. A Merkel cell carcinoma was diagnosed hsitologically and immunohistologically. It was treated by surgically resection followed by local adjuvant radiochemotherapy.

References

1. Deeren DH, Zachee P, Malbrain ML. Granulocyte colony-stimulating factor-induced capillary leak syndrome confirmed by extravascular lung water measurements. Ann Hematol 2005;84(2):89–94.
2. Karlin L, Darmon M, Thiery G, Ciroldi M, de Miranda S, Lefebvre A, Schlemmer B, Azoulay E. Respiratory status deterioration during G-CSF-induced neutropenia recovery. Bone Marrow Transplant 2005;36(3):245–50.
3. Finsterer J, Sommer O, Stiskal M. Multifocal leukoencephalopathy and polyneuropathy after 18 years on interferon alpha. Leuk Lymphoma 2005;46(2):277–80.
4. Kraus MR, Schafer A, Wissmann S, Reimer P, Scheurlen M. Neurocognitive changes in patients with hepatitis C receiving interferon alfa-2b and ribavirin. Clin Pharmacol Ther 2005;77(1):90–100.
5. Capuron L, Pagnoni G, Demetrashvili M, Woolwine BJ, Nemeroff CB, Berns GS, Miller AH. Anterior cingulate activation and error processing during interferon-alpha treatment. Biol Psychiatry 2005;58(3):190–6.
6. Herman C, Boggio L, Green D. Factor VIII inhibitor associated with peginterferon. Haemophilia 2005;11(4):408–10.
7. Derbala M, Amer A, Bener A, Lopez AC, Omar M, El Ghannam M. Pegylated interferon-alpha 2b-ribavirin combination in Egyptian patients with genotype 4 chronic hepatitis. J Viral Hepat 2005;12(4):380–5.
8. Weitz IC. Treatment of immune thrombocytopenia associated with interferon therapy of hepatitis C with the anti-CD20 monoclonal antibody, rituximab. Am J Hematol 2005;78(2):138–41.
9. Drevelegas A, Xinou E, Karacostas D, Parissis D, Karkavelas G, Milonas I. Meningioma growth and interferon beta-1b treated multiple sclerosis: coincidence or relationship? Neuroradiology 2005;47(7):516–9.
10. Batay F, Al-Mefty O. Growth dynamics of meningiomas in patients with multiple sclerosis treated with interferon: report of two cases. Acta Neurochir (Wien) 2002;144(4):365–8.
11. Caraccio N, Dardano A, Manfredonia F, Manca L, Pasquali L, Iudice A, Murri L, Ferrannini E, Monzani F. Long-term follow-up of 106 multiple sclerosis patients undergoing interferon-beta 1a or 1b therapy: predictive factors of thyroid disease development and duration. J Clin Endocrinol Metab 2005;90(7):4133–7.
12. Hartung HP, Munschauer III F, Schellekens H. Significance of neutralizing antibodies to interferon beta during treatment of multiple sclerosis: expert opinions based on the Proceedings of an International Consensus Conference. Eur J Neurol 2005;12(8):588–601.
13. Kerst JM, Bex A, Mallo H, Dewit L, Haanen JB, Boogerd W, Teertstra HJ, de Gast GC. Prolonged low dose IL-2 and thalidomide in progressive metastatic renal cell carcinoma with concurrent radiotherapy to bone and/or soft tissue metastasis: a phase II study. Cancer Immunol Immunother 2005;54(9):926–31.
14. Foss F, Demierre MF, DiVenuti G. A phase-1 trial of bexarotene and denileukin diftitox in patients with relapsed or refractory cutaneous T-cell lymphoma. Blood 2005;106(2):454–7.
15. Cairo MS, Davenport V, Bessmertny O, Goldman SC, Berg SL, Kreissman SG, Laver J, Shen V, Secola R, van de Ven C, Reaman GH. Phase I/II dose escalation study of recombinant human interleukin-11 following ifosfamide, carboplatin and etoposide in children, adolescents and young adults with solid tumours or lymphoma: a clinical, haematological and biological study. Br J Haematol 2005;128(1):49–58.
16. Tsimberidou AM, Giles FJ, Khouri I, Bueso-Ramos C, Pilat S, Thomas DA, Cortes J, Kurzrock R. Low-dose interleukin-11 in patients with bone marrow failure: update of the M D Anderson Cancer Center experience. Ann Oncol 2005;16(1):139–45.
17. Paul SR, Bennett F, Calvetti JA, Kelleher K, Wood CR, O'Hara Jr RM, Leary AC, Sibley B,

Clark SC, Williams DA, Yang Y-C. Molecular cloning of a cDNA encoding interleukin 11, a stromal cell-derived lymphopoietic and hematopoietic cytokine. Proc Natl Acad Sci USA 1990;87(19):7512–6.

18. Bruno E, Cooper RJ, Briddell RA, Hoffman R. Further examination of the effects of recombinant cytokines on the proliferation of human megakaryocyte progenitor cells. Blood 1991;77(11):2339–46.

19. McKinley D, Wu Q, Yang-Feng T, Yang YC. Genomic sequence and chromosomal location of human interleukin-11 gene (IL11). Genomics 1992;13(3):814–9.

20. Teramura M, Kobayashi S, Hoshino S, Oshimi K, Mizoguchi H. Interleukin-11 enhances human megakaryocytopoiesis in vitro. Blood 1992;79(2):327–31.

21. Du XX, Williams DA. Interleukin-11: a multifunctional growth factor derived from the hematopoietic microenvironment. Blood 1994;83(8):2023–30.

22. Du X, Williams DA. Interleukin-11: review of molecular, cell biology, and clinical use. Blood 1997;89(11):3897–908.

23. Portielje JE, Kruit WH, Eerenberg AJ, Schuler M, Sparreboom A, Lamers CH, Gratama JW, Stoter G, Huber C, Hack CE. Subcutaneous injection of interleukin 12 induces systemic inflammatory responses in humans: implications for the use of IL-12 as vaccine adjuvant. Cancer Immunol Immunother 2005;54(1):37–43.

24. Saini R, Tutrone WD, Weinberg JM. Advances in therapy for psoriasis: an overview of infliximab, etanercept, efalizumab, alefacept, adalimumab, tazarotene, and pimecrolimus. Curr Pharm Design 2005;11:273–80.

25. Scheinfeld N. Adalimumab: a review of side effects. Expert Opin Drug Saf 2005;4(4):637–41.

26. Bennett AN, Wong M, Zain A, Panayi G, Kirkham B. Adalimumab-induced asthma. Rheumatol (Oxf) 2005;44(9):1199–200.

27. Berthelot CN, George SJ, Hsu S. Distal lower extremity paresthesia and foot drop developing during adalimumab therapy. J Am Acad Dermatol 2005;53(5 Suppl 1):S260–2.

28. Leão JC, Duarte A, Gueiros LA, Carvalho AA, Barrett AW, Scully C, Porter S. Severe oral epithelial dysplasia in a patient receiving adalimumab therapy. J Oral Pathol Med 2005;34(7):447–8.

29. Efde MN, Houtman PM, Spoorenberg JP, Jansen TL. Tonsillar tuberculosis in a rheumatoid arthritis patient receiving anti-TNFalpha (adalimumab) treatment. Neth J Med 2005;63(3):112–4.

30. Dalle S, Balme B, Berger F, Hayette S, Thomas L. Mycosis fungoides-associated follicular mucinosis under adalimumab. Br J Dermatol 2005;153(1):207–8.

31. Schmidt A, Robbins J, Zic J. Transformed mycosis fungoides developing after treatment with alefacept. J Am Acad Dermatol 2005;2:355–6.

32. Papp KA, Tyring S, Lahfa M, Prinz J, Griffiths CEM, Nakanishi AM, Zitnik R, van de Kerkhof PCM. A global phase III randomized controlled trial of etanercept in psoriasis: safety, efficacy, and effect of dose reduction. Br J Dermatol 2005;152:1304–12.

33. Buka RL, Resh B, Roberts B, Cunningham B, Friedlander S. Etanercept is minimally effective in 2 children with atopic dermatitis. J Am Acad Dermatol 2005;53:358–9.

34. Su C, Lichtenstein GR. Are there predictors of Remicade treatment success or failure? Adv Drug Deliv Rev 2005;57(2):237–45.

35. Suhler EB, Smith JR, Wertheim MS, Lauer AK, Kurz DE, Pickard TD, Rosenbaum JT. A prospective trial of infliximab therapy for refractory uveitis: preliminary safety and efficacy outcomes. Arch Ophthalmol 2005;123(7):903–12.

36. Franchimont D, Roland S, Gustot T, Quertinmont E, Toubouti Y, Gervy MC, Deviere J, Van Gossum A. Impact of infliximab on serum leptin levels in patients with Crohn's disease. J Clin Endocrinol Metab 2005;90(6):3510–6.

37. De Rycke L, Baeten D, Kruithof E, Van den BF, Veys EM, De Keyser F. Infliximab, but not etanercept, induces IgM anti-double-stranded DNA autoantibodies as main antinuclear reactivity: biologic and clinical implications in autoimmune arthritis. Arthritis Rheum 2005;52(7):2192–201.

38. Sugiura F, Kojima T, Oba M, Tsuchiya H, Ishiguro N. Anaphylactic reaction to infliximab in two rheumatoid arthritis patients who had previously received infliximab and resumed. Mod Rheumatol 2005;15(3):201–3.

39. Condino AA, Fidanza S, Hoffenberg EJ. A home infliximab infusion program. J Pediatr Gastroenterol Nutr 2005;40(1):67–9.

40. Gibbs SD, Westerman DA, McCormack C, Seymour JF, Miles PH. Severe and prolonged myeloid haematopoietic toxicity with myelodysplastic features following alemtuzumab therapy in patients with peripheral T-cell lymphoproliferative disorders. Br J Haematol 2005;130(1):87–91.

41. Monteiro JP, Benjamin A, Costa ES, Barcinski MA, Bonomo A. Normal hematopoiesis is maintained by activated bone marrow CD4+ T cells. Blood 2005;105(4):1484–91.

42. Mone A, Puhalla S, Whitman S, Baiocchi RA, Cruz J, Vukosavljevic T, Banks A, Eisenbeis CF, Byrd JC, Caligiuri MA, Porcu P. Durable hematologic complete response and suppression of HTLV-1 viral load following alemtuzumab in zidovudine/IFN-{alpha}-refractory adult T-cell leukemia. Blood 2005;106(10):3380–2.

43. Myers GD, Krance RA, Weiss H, Kuehnle I, Demmler G, Heslop HE, Bollard CM. Adenovirus infection rates in pediatric recipients of alternate donor allogeneic bone marrow transplants receiving either antithymocyte globulin (ATG) or alemtuzumab (Campath). Bone Marrow Transplant 2005;36(11):1001–8.

44. van Kooten C, Banchereau J. CD40-CD40 ligand. J Leukocyte Biol 2000;67:2–17.

45. Laman JD, 't Hart BA, Brok HPM, et al. Protection of marmoset monkeys against EAE by treatment with a murine antibody blocking CD40 (mu5D12). Eur J Immunol 2002;32:2218–28.

46. Boon L, Brok HPM, Bauer J, et al. Prevention of experimental autoimmune encephalomyelitis in the common marmoset (*Callithrix jacchus*) using a chimeric antagonist Mab against human CD40 is associated with altered B-cell responses. J Immunol 2001;167:2942–9.

47. Haanstra KG, Ringers J, Sick EA, et al. Prevention of kidney allograft rejection using anti-CD40 and anti-CD86 in primates. Transplantation 2003;75:637–43.

48. Haegel-Kronenberger H, Haanstra K, Ziller-Remy C, et al. Inhibition of costimulation allows for repeated systemic administration of adenoviral vector in rhesus monkeys. Gene Ther 2004;11:241–52.

49. Boon L, Laman JD, Ortiz-Buijsse A, et al. Preclinical assessment of anti-CD40 Mab 5D12 in cynomolgus monkeys. Toxicology 2002;174:53–65.

50. Kasran A, Boon L, Wortel CH, Hogezand RA, Schreiber S, Goldin E, Boer M, Geboes K, Rutgeerts P, Ceuppens JL. Safety and tolerability of antagonist anti-human CD40 Mab ch5D12 in patients with moderate to severe Crohn's disease. Aliment Pharmacol Ther 2005;22(2):111–22.

51. Boggi U, Vistoli F, Signori S, Del Chiaro M, Amorese G, Barsotti M, Rizzo G, Marchetti P, Danesi R, Del Tacca M, Mosca F. Efficacy and safety of basiliximab in kidney transplantation. Expert Opin Drug Saf 2005;4(3):473–90.

52. Di Filippo S. Anti-IL-2 receptor antibody vs. polyclonal anti-lymphocyte antibody as induction therapy in pediatric transplantation. Pediatr Transplant 2005;9(3):373–80.

53. Mian AN, Farney AC, Mendley SR. Mycoplasma hominis septic arthritis in a pediatric renal transplant recipient: case report and review of the literature. Am J Transplant 2005;5(1):183–8.

54. Gordon MS, Cunningham D. Managing patients treated with bevacizumab combination therapy. Oncology 2005;69(Suppl 3):25–33.

55. Rosiak J, Sadowski L. Hypertension associated with bevacizumab. Clin J Oncol Nurs 2005;9(4):407–11.

56. Scappaticci FA, Fehrenbacher L, Cartwright T, Hainsworth JD, Heim W, Berlin J, Kabbinavar F, Novotny W, Sarkar S, Hurwitz H. Surgical wound healing complications in metastatic colorectal cancer patients treated with bevacizumab. J Surg Oncol 2005;91(3):173–80.

57. Nussenblatt RB, Peterson JS, Foster CS, Rao NA, See RF, Letko E, Buggage RR. Initial evaluation of subcutaneous daclizumab treatments for noninfectious uveitis: a multicenter noncomparative interventional case series. Ophthalmology 2005;112(5):764–70.

58. Hershberger RE, Starling RC, Eisen HJ, Bergh CH, Kormos RL, Love RB, Van Bakel A, Gordon RD, Popat R, Cockey L, Mamelok RD. Daclizumab to prevent rejection after cardiac transplantation. N Engl J Med 2005;352(26):2705–13.

59. Wellington K, Perry CM. Efalizumab. Am J Clin Dermatol 2005;6(2):113–8.

60. Menter A, Gordon K, Carey W, Hamilton T, Glazer S, Caro I, Li N, Gulliver W. Efficacy and safety observed during 24 weeks of efalizumab therapy in patients with moderate to severe plaque psoriasis. Arch Dermatol 2005;141:31–8.

61. Warkentin TE, Kwon P. Immune thrombocytopenia associated with efalizumab therapy for psoriasis. Ann Intern Med 2005;143(10):761–3.

62. Thielen AM, Kuenzli S, Saurat JH. Cutaneous adverse events of biological therapy for psoriasis: review of the literature. Dermatology 2005;211(3):209–17.

63. de Groot M, de Rie MA, Bos JD. Dermatitis during efalizumab treatment in a patient with psoriasis vulgaris. Br J Dermatol 2005;153(4):843–4.

64. Langley RG, Carey WP, Rafal ES, Tyring SK, Caro I, Wang X, Wetherill G, Gordon KB. Incidence of infection during efalizumab therapy for psoriasis: analysis of the clinical trial experience. Clin Ther 2005;27(9):1317–28.

65. Papp KA, Camisa C, Stone SP, Caro I, Wang X, Compton P, Walicke PA, Gottlieb AB. Safety of efalizumab in patients with moderate to severe chronic plaque psoriasis: review of clinical data. Part II. J Cutan Med Surg 2005;9(6):313–23.

66. Morse LG, Yarbrough L, Hogan DJ. Cervical cancer in a woman associated with long-term efalizumab therapy. J Am Acad Dermatol 2005;53(2):354–5.

67. Anonymous. Technetium (99mTc) fanolesomab. Suspended due to safety concerns. WHO Newslett 2006;1:9.

68. Chevallier P, Roland V, Mahe B, Juge-Morineau N, Dubruille V, Guillaume T, Vigouroux S, Moreau P, Milpied N, Garand R, Avet-Loiseau H, Harousseau JL. Administration of Mylotarg 4 days after beginning of a chemotherapy including intermediate-dose aracytin and mitoxantrone (MIDAM regimen) produces a high rate of complete hematologic remission in patients with CD33+ primary resistant or relapsed acute myeloid leukemia. Leuk Res 2005;29(9):1003–7.

69. Nabhan C, Rundhaugen LM, Riley MB, Rademaker A, Boehlke L, Jatoi M, Tallman MS. Phase II pilot trial of gemtuzumab ozogamicin (GO) as first line therapy in acute myeloid leukemia patients age 65 or older. Leuk Res 2005;29(1):53–7.

70. Feagan BG, Greenberg GR, Wild G, Fedorak RN, Paré P, McDonald JW, Dubé R, Cohen A, Steinhart AH, Landau S, Aguzzi RA, Fox IH, Vandervoort MK. Treatment of ulcerative colitis with a humanized antibody to the alpha4beta7 integrin. N Engl J Med 2005;352(24):2499–507.

71. Van Assche G, Van Ranst M, Sciot R, Dubois B, Vermeire S, Noman M, Verbeeck J, Geboes K, Robberecht W, Rutgeerts P. Progressive multifocal leukoencephalopathy after natalizumab therapy for Crohn's disease. N Engl J Med 2005;353(4):362–8.

72. Kleinschmidt-DeMasters BK, Tyler KL. Progressive multifocal leukoencephalopathy complicating treatment with natalizumab and interferon beta-1a for multiple sclerosis. N Engl J Med 2005;353(4):369–74.

73. Langer-Gould A, Atlas SW, Green AJ, Bollen AW, Pelletier D. Progressive multifocal leukoencephalopathy in a patient treated with natalizumab. N Engl J Med 2005;353(4):375–81.

74. Sandborn WJ, Colombel JF, Enns R, Feagan BG, Hanauer SB, Lawrance IC, Panaccione R, Sanders M, Schreiber S, Targan S, van Deventer S, Goldblum R, Despain D, Hogge GS, Rutgeerts P, International Efficacy of Natalizumab as Active Crohn's Therapy (ENACT-1) Trial Group, Evaluation of Natalizumab as Continuous Therapy (ENACT-2) Trial Group. Natalizumab induction and maintenance therapy for Crohn's disease. N Engl J Med 2005;353(18):1912–25.

75. Simmons DL. Anti-adhesion therapies. Curr Opin Pharmacol 2005;5(4):398–404.

76. Humbert M, Beasley R, Ayres J, Slavin R, Hebert J, Bousquet J, Beeh KM, Ramos S, Canonica GW, Hedgecock S, Fox H, Blogg M, Surrey K. Benefits of omalizumab as add-on therapy in patients with severe persistent asthma who are inadequately controlled despite best available therapy (GINA 2002 step 4 treatment): INNOVATE. Allergy 2005;60:309–16.

77. Robak E, Biernat W, Krykowski E, Jeziorski A, Robak T. Merkel cell carcinoma in a patient with B-cell chronic lymphocytic leukemia treated with cladribine and rituximab. Leuk Lymphoma 2005;46(6):909–14.

Felix Braun and Matthias Behrend

38 Drugs that act on the immune system: immunosuppressive and immunostimulatory drugs

Ciclosporin *(SED-15, 743; SEDA-27, 374; SEDA-28, 452; SEDA-29, 426)*

Cardiovascular Calcineurin inhibitors potentially contribute to the risk of cardiovascular events through the development of new-onset diabetes mellitus, hypertension, and hyperlipidemia. Trials have consistently shown a higher incidence of new-onset diabetes mellitus with tacrolimus, which has been borne out in large-scale registry analyses. However, the risk of hypertension is about 5% higher with ciclosporin than tacrolimus, as is the risk of hyperlipidemia ([1R]).

Nervous system *Neuropathies* and *myopathies* have been reported in patients taking ciclosporin, particularly in combination with statins, and can occur with ciclosporin alone.

- A 67-year-old woman taking ciclosporin developed rapidly progressive sensorimotor changes a few months after kidney transplantation ([2A]). The symptoms improved after ciclosporin withdrawal. Other causes were ruled out.

Electrolyte balance Drug-related *potassium-channel syndrome* is a rare disorder that can occur after the administration of drugs that open K_{ATP} channels, such as ciclosporin, nicorandil, or isoflurane. It can cause severe life-threatening complications, including hyperkalemia and cardiovascular disturbances. Administration of the K_{ATP} channel blocker glibenclamide can promptly reverse these abnormalities ([3A]).

Urinary tract Ciclosporin *nephrotoxicity* leads to impaired renal function and chronic allograft nephropathy, which is a major predictor of graft loss. P glycoprotein contributes substantially to ciclosporin nephrotoxicity. The TT genotype at the ABCB1 3435C→T polymorphism is associated with reduced expression of P glycoprotein in renal tissue and has been implicated as a susceptibility factor for ciclosporin nephrotoxicity. Ciclosporin nephrotoxicity in 18 of 97 patients completely recovered after switching to a calcineurin inhibitor-free regimen ([4C]). The P glycoprotein low expressor genotype 3435TT in the kidney donors, but not in the recipients, was over-represented in the cases of ciclosporin nephrotoxicity. Ciclosporin dosage, trough concentrations, and the concentration per dose ratio were not different between the groups. In a multivariate model that included several other non-genetic covariates, only the donor's ABCB1 3435TT genotype was strongly associated with ciclosporin nephrotoxicity.

Drug–drug interactions

Amisulpride The antipsychotic drug amisulpride is a substrate of P glycoprotein. Co-administration of ciclosporin in rats resulted in a larger and significantly longer antipsychotic effect, with higher amisulpride AUC in serum and brain; renal clearance was not affected ([5E]). Amisulpride is not metabolized by rat liver and so this interaction was probably caused by inhibition of P glycoprotein.

Ketamine Various neurological symptoms have been reported in liver transplant recipients taking ciclosporin. However, seizures in the perioperative period can be due to other factors.

Side Effects of Drugs, Annual 30
J.K. Aronson (Editor)
ISSN: 0378-6080
DOI: 10.1016/S0378-6080(08)00038-X

Many anesthetics have been reported to have both proconvulsant and anticonvulsant properties. Perioperative seizures occurred after liver transplantation in a child who was taking ciclosporin and who was given ketamine (6[A]).

- A 6-year-old boy weighing 12 kg underwent living related left lateral segment liver transplantation for cryptogenic cirrhosis with portal hypertension. Immunosuppression consisted of microemulsion ciclosporin 10 mg/kg/day, azathioprine, and prednisolone. One month after transplantation, the transaminase activities rose, without derangement of other liver function tests. He was cheerful and spontaneously breathing with a respiratory rate of 18/minute (oxygen saturation 98–100% on air), accepting oral feeding, moving around, and febrile. For liver biopsy he was given intravenous ketamine 7 mg/kg and intramuscular glycopyrrolate 0.01 mg/kg. He developed generalized tonic–clonic seizures, which were treated with intravenous midazolam 1 mg and thiopental 60 mg. A CT scan on the day after the event did not show any abnormality.

In this case ketamine was given 2 hours after the last dose of ciclosporin, close to its t_{max}. Caution is therefore recommended when ketamine is given to patients who are taking ciclosporin.

Vitamins Supplementation with vitamin C 500–1000 mg/day and vitamin E 300 mg/day reduced the trough concentrations of ciclosporin in a single-blind, crossover, randomized, placebo-controlled study in 10 renal transplant recipients (7[C]) and in a double-blind, placebo-controlled study in 56 renal transplant recipients (8[C]). Although this could have led to transplant rejection, in fact glomerular filtration rate improved significantly and serum creatinine concentrations fell slightly. Changes in vitamin C and vitamin E concentrations did not correlate with changes in ciclosporin trough concentrations or changes in serum creatinine concentrations. The mechanism of this effect is not known.

Management of adverse drug reactions
Switching from ciclosporin to tacrolimus is an alternative strategy in kidney transplant patients with chronic allograft dysfunction or ciclosporin intolerance, particularly since tacrolimus may be less nephrotoxic than ciclosporin and may prolong transplant function despite ciclosporin failure. Tacrolimus replaced ciclosporin-based immunosuppression in 133 transplant patients (114 kidney, 15 kidney–pancreas,

4 pancreas after kidney) who had progressive loss of renal function (71%) or ciclosporin intolerance (29%) not responding to ciclosporin dosage reduction (9[c]). Tacrolimus was begun in an oral dosage of 0.1 mg/kg bd and was adjusted to trough concentrations of 6–10 ng/ml. Tacrolimus was well tolerated but needed to be withdrawn in 23 cases—21 graft failures, one case of diabetes, and one case of clinical intolerance. Differential creatininemia fell significantly and tacrolimus improved symptoms of ciclosporin intolerance in all cases. Blood urea, creatinine clearance, blood total cholesterol, and triglycerides improved significantly, and the number of hypertensive patients was unchanged. During follow-up, four patients died, one had acute rejection, and 21 transplants failed. Graft failure was significantly more frequent in patients with advanced renal impairment before tacrolimus.

Cyclophosphamide *(SED-15, 1025; SEDA-27, 375; SEDA-28, 456; SEDA-29, 433)*

Pregnancy Cyclophosphamide is a pregnancy category D agent (see Table 1).

- A 37-year-old Caucasian woman with an infiltrating ductal breast carcinoma in situ was given doxorubicin and cyclophosphamide in the second and third trimesters and delivered a premature baby boy at 31 weeks (10[A]). The neonate had respiratory distress and failure. There were no physical anomalies, but the baby had neutropenia and anemia probably because of the chemotherapy. The infant grew and developed normally during his first year of life and remained in good health.

Everolimus (SDZ-RAD) *(SED-15, 1306; SEDA-28, 457; SEDA-29, 433)*

Everolimus is a mammalian target of rapamycin (mTOR) inhibitor used in immunosuppressive therapies for the prevention of acute and chronic rejection after solid organ transplantation.

Table 1. The FDA's classification of teratogenic drug
risk

Category	Description of risk
A	No fetal risk shown in controlled human studies
B	No human data available and animal studies show no fetal risk or Animal studies show a risk but human studies do not show fetal risk
C	No controlled studies on fetal risk available for humans or animals or Fetal risk shown in controlled animal studies but no human data available (the benefit of drug use must clearly justify the potential fetal risk in this category)
D	Studies show fetal risk in humans (use of the drug may be acceptable even with risks such as in life-threatening illness or when safer drugs are ineffective)
X	Risk to fetus clearly outweighs any benefits from the drug

Comparative studies   Everolimus 1.5 or 3
mg/day has been compared with mycophenolate mofetil 2 g/day in 523 de novo renal-
transplant recipients (11^C). Antibody-treated
acute rejection at 36 months was significantly
lower with everolimus 1.5 mg (9.8%) than
mycophenolate mofetil (18%). Withdrawal after adverse events was more frequent with
everolimus; *hemolytic–uremic syndrome, lymphoproliferative disease, proteinuria*, and *higher serum creatinine concentrations* occurred at
increased frequency compared with mycophenolate mofetil. The mean rise in creatinine over
the first 6 months was 3 μmol/l or more with
everolimus and 7 μmol/l with mycophenolate
mofetil. However, serum creatinine concentrations were lower throughout in those who
received mycophenolate mofetil. Death and
graft loss were more frequent with everolimus.

Management of adverse drug reactions
The mTOR-inhibitors (for example everolimus,
sirolimus) are associated with certain adverse
events such as lymphocele, arthralgia, edema,
and hyperlipidemia, the management of which
has been discussed (12^c). Withdrawal of everolimus is usually not necessary. Moderate lymphoceles can resolve spontaneously or after in-

stillation of povidone-iodine; severe lymphocele may require surgical intervention. Eyelid
and ankle edema respond to low-dose furosemide, preferably coupled with ciclosporin and
everolimus dosage reduction. Hyperlipidemia
responds to a statin. Everolimus dosage reduction, maintaining trough blood concentrations
at about 3 ng/ml, was effective in a case of bilateral multiple arthralgia.

Monitoring therapy   Monitoring everolimus
plasma concentrations may improve efficacy
and reduce adverse effects (13^M). There is
a good relation between the concentration of
everolimus and the pharmacological response.
The recommended target for trough concentration is 3–8 ng/ml; concentrations over 3 ng/ml
have been associated with a reduced incidence
of rejection and concentrations over 8 ng/ml
with increased toxicity. African–Americans
have higher apparent clearance rates. Hepatic
dysfunction reduces clearance and inhibitors or
inducers of CYP3A4 reduce or increase clearance.

Leflunomide   (SED-15, 2015; SEDA-28, 457; SEDA-29, 435)

Leflunomide is licensed in France for "active psoriatic rheumatism". Pharmacovigilance
studies have confirmed some severe adverse effects (hepatic, cutaneous, and hematological)
and have uncovered other previously unrecognized effects, such as *interstitial pneumonia,
hypertension, weight loss*, and *peripheral neuropathies*. In France, leflunomide costs nearly
10 times more than methotrexate and it has been
suggested that it should not be used to treat psoriatic arthropathy (14^r).

Respiratory   Imaging findings in 26 cases of
leflunomide-related acute lung injury were similar to those caused by other drugs, including diffuse or widespread patchy g*round-glass
opacities* and/or *consolidation*, often accompanied by *septal thickening and intralobular
reticular opacities* (15^c). Of 23 cases 13 had
pre-existing *interstitial pulmonary disease* on
chest X-ray or CT scan. The imaging findings were classified into four patterns: diffuse

alveolar damage, acute eosinophilic pneumonia, a hyper-reaction, and cryptogenic organizing pneumonia. Those with diffuse alveolar damage had a higher mortality rate, which did not reach conventional statistical significance.

Nervous system   Two patients taking leflunomide developed severe *sensorimotor axonal polyneuropathy* starting 5 months after the start of leflunomide therapy; the symptoms rapidly improved after withdrawing leflunomide (16^c). Of 12 patients with leflunomide-related neuropathy 10 were older than 60 years. The mean delay to the onset of neuropathy was 9 months. The neuropathy improved after withdrawal in seven patients.

Gastrointestinal   *Diarrhea* and *weight loss* are common adverse events in patients with rheumatoid arthritis taking leflunomide (17^A, 18^C). They occur mostly during the first 6 months of treatment, are generally mild, and rarely require treatment withdrawal. Two patients with rheumatoid arthritis developed severe diarrhea and important weight loss more than 12 months after starting to take leflunomide. The symptoms were caused by colitis, but one had ulcerative colitis and the other microscopic colitis. The symptoms improved after withdrawal of leflunomide, making a causal relation probable. However, the heterogeneous histopathological findings did not allow any definitive conclusions about mechanism.

Leflunomide-associated persistent diarrhea or weight loss can be more serious than has previously been reported. In such cases leflunomide should be withdrawn and colonic endoscopy is recommended. Given the long half-life of leflunomide a washout procedure with colestyramine should be considered whenever the problem is severe or persistent (17^c, 18^c).

Hair   In 51 patients with proliferative lupus nephritis major adverse events in those who were taking leflunomide were infections (mainly herpes zoster) and *alopecia* (18^c).

Teratogenicity   Leflunomide increases the risks of fetal death and teratogenic effects in animals. However, no major or minor malformations have been reported in humans, and leflunomide is classified in category X of fetal risk (Table 1) (19^M). A wash-out regimen

may reduce the risk of fetal harm. Conception scheduling or early pregnancy detection is required for better clinical counselling and the avoidance of unnecessary risk.

Mycophenolate mofetil   *(SED-15, 2402; SEDA-27, 376; SEDA-28, 458; SEDA-29, 445)*

Gastrointestinal   Adverse effects, mainly gastrointestinal, occur in up to 45% of patients who take mycophenolate mofetil. Dosage changes resulting from these adverse events may lead to subtherapeutic dosing and poor clinical outcomes. In a retrospective study, 772 renal transplant patients from 10 US transplant centers took mycophenolate mofetil and 50% ($n = 382$) had at least one gastrointestinal complication within the first 6 months after transplantation; 67% ($n = 255$) of these had multiple gastrointestinal complications (20^c). Of the patients with gastrointestinal complications, the dosage was adjusted or the drug was withdrawn in 39%, and they had a significantly higher incidence of acute rejections than patients without gastrointestinal complications (30 versus 19%). Mean treatment costs were higher in patients with gastrointestinal complications than in those without. The mean incremental cost for patients with gastrointestinal complications was US$3700 per patient during the 6 months after transplant, which was mainly attributable to costs of hospitalization.

In another series, 79% of 403 patients with 407 kidney transplants taking ciclosporin or tacrolimus, mycophenolate mofetil, and glucocorticoids had adverse events during the 100 days after transplant (21^c). In half of all cases serum alanine transaminase activity was raised, and in 21% it was over three times the upper limit of the reference range. Patients with delayed graft function showed increased incidences of gastrointestinal symptoms and thrombocytopenia. There were more cases of increased alanine transaminase activity and thrombocytopenia in patients taking ciclosporin and more gastrointestinal symptoms in patients taking tacrolimus. The dose of mycophenolate mofetil was reduced or the drug was withdrawn in 34% of all cases. In patients taking ciclosporin and a reduced dose of mycophenolate mofetil by day 21, the incidence of rejection during the next 21 days was 10 versus 0.6% in patients who took full-dose mycophenolate mofetil until day 21. Patients taking tacrolimus had no increased rejection frequency after the dose of mycophenolate mofetil was reduced.

Liver   *Hepatotoxicity* associated with mycophenolate mofetil has not previously been reported, and has been assessed after kidney transplantation in 79 patients taking 2 g/day (22[c]). There was a progressive increase in liver enzymes in 11 patients. The median age of those with hepatotoxicity was 29 (19–54) and 73% were men. None of the patients had hepatitis B or C, cytomegalovirus infection, or other possible causes of raised liver enzymes, and abdominal ultrasonography was normal. The liver enzyme activities normalized after withdrawal ($n = 6$) or a reduction in dosage ($n = 5$). The median time to the increase in liver enzymes was 28 (4–70) days and after a 50% reduction in dose or withdrawal, they returned to normal in 16 (4–210) days. There was a significant positive correlation between the duration of the abnormal activity and the recovery time.

Mycophenolate sodium

Gastrointestinal   Gastrointestinal adverse effects have been assessed in a prospective questionnaire study in de novo renal-transplant patients ($n = 130$) taking either mycophenolate mofetil ($n = 93$) or enteric-coated mycophenolate sodium ($n = 37$) (23[c]). During the first year after transplantation, there were gastrointestinal disorders in 31 patients taking mycophenolate mofetil (33%) and 12 taking enteric-coated mycophenolate sodium (34%). The incidences of *upper gastrointestinal disorders* (19 versus 14%) and *diarrhea* (19 versus 14%) were not significantly different.

Gastrointestinal symptoms have been analysed in 22 de novo kidney transplant recipients receiving basiliximab, enteric-coated mycophenolate sodium, ciclosporin microemulsion, and prednisolone with a mean follow-up of 7.9 months (24[c]). Gastrointestinal adverse effects at a mean daily dose of enteric-coated mycophenolate sodium of 1422 mg included *dyspepsia*

27%, *acid regurgitation* 18%, *epigastralgia* 9%, *nausea* 9%, *vomiting* 4.5%, and *poor appetite* 4.5%. In comparison, in historical studies mycophenolate mofetil 2 g/day caused dyspepsia in 3.1–40%, epigastralgia in 10%, nausea in 3.7–34%, and vomiting in 0.6%–11%.

Drug–drug interactions   *Rifampicin* induces the expression of a number of genes involved in multidrug resistance (P glycoprotein and multidrug resistance proteins 1 and 2), CYP3A4, uridine diphosphate-glucuronosyltransferases, monoamine oxidases, and glutathione S-transferases. In a heart-lung transplant recipient long-term rifampicin caused a more than two-fold reduction in dose-corrected exposure to mycophenolic acid; after withdrawal of rifampicin the effect reversed after 2 weeks (25[A]). The effect of rifampicin on the metabolism of mycophenolate can, at least in part, be explained by simultaneous induction of renal, hepatic, and gastrointestinal uridine diphosphate-glucuronosyltransferases and organic anion transporters, with subsequent functional inhibition of the enterohepatic recirculation of mycophenolic acid.

The pharmacokinetics of mycophenolic acid at 2 weeks, 1 month, 2 months, and 3 months after kidney transplantation have been studied in recipients who took additional *sirolimus* ($n = 13$) or *ciclosporin* ($n = 17$) (26[c]). Those who took sirolimus had significantly higher values of dose-normalized mycophenolic acid $AUC_{0–12}$ than those who took ciclosporin. Plasma concentration monitoring of mycophenolic acid is therefore advised in kidney recipients co-treated with sirolimus.

Pimecrolimus   (SED-15, 2833; SEDA-28, 460; SEDA-29, 449)

The benefits associated with pimecrolimus (Elidel) and tacrolimus (Protopic/Protopy) outweigh their risks, but the Committee for Medicinal Products for Human Use (CHMP) of the European Medicines Agency (EMEA) has advised that caution is required, in order to reduce the risks of skin cancer and lymphoma (27[S]). The CHMP began its safety review after reports of skin cancer and lymphoma in patients using pimecrolimus and tacrolimus, but was unable to establish a casual relation, and has asked for more long-term safety profile data. Meanwhile, the CHMP has advised that patients using the products should not stop using them or alter their treatment without first consulting their physician. Product information changes recommended by the CHMP aim to raise patient and prescriber awareness of the potential long-term risks associated with these drugs.

Placebo-controlled studies   The efficacy and the adverse effects of pimecrolimus in the treatment of moderate to severe atopic dermatitis have been investigated in a randomized controlled trial (28[C]). The short-term adverse events profile was favorable, with no apparent adverse effects in any major organ system. The study consisted of a pre-treatment phase, a 12-week, double-blind treatment phase (placebo or pimecrolimus tablets 10, 20, or 30 mg twice daily), and a 12-week post-treatment phase. The only adverse events that were related to the dose of pimecrolimus were *nausea* and a *hot feeling*.

Sirolimus (rapamycin)   *(SED-15, 3148; SEDA-27, 377; SEDA-28, 460; SEDA-29, 449)*

Respiratory   Sirolimus-associated *pneumonitis* has been described in renal transplant patients, but only in two cases after cardiac transplantation; one had a fatal outcome. In another heart recipient, sirolimus-associated interstitial pneumonitis resolved completely after sirolimus withdrawal and treatment with corticosteroids (29[A]).

Liver   *Hepatotoxicity* associated with sirolimus has been reported in a kidney graft recipient (30[A]).

- A 30-year-old man underwent kidney transplantation and immunosuppression with a glucocorticoid, ciclosporin, and sirolimus. Serum transaminase activities increased 16 months after transplantation. Liver biopsy showed non-specific changes consistent with drug-induced damage. Sirolimus was switched to mycophenolate mofetil, and the serum transaminase quickly normalized.

Skin   The cutaneous adverse effects of sirolimus are not well described and may have been underestimated. They include *acne*, *rash*, and a *leukocytoclastic vasculitis*. Sirolimus caused follicular acneiform eruptions in two renal allograft recipients (31[A]). It was severe and difficult to treat and resolved only after withdrawal of sirolimus. After liver transplantation, 23 of 60 recipients took sirolimus in dosages adjusted to target trough concentrations of 30 to <100 ng/l, combined with a calcineurin inhibitor and/or mycophenolate mofetil (32[c]). There were non-specific rashes in three patients, including one case of leukocytoclastic vasculitis, one of exfoliative forearm dermatitis requiring change of medication, and one of perivascular lymphocytic eosinophilic dermatitis that subsided after dosage reduction. There were mouth ulcers in three cases, associated with trough concentrations exceeding 100 ng/l. Acne improved in six patients after dosage reduction. Sirolimus was continued in 18 patients.

The skin, mucous membranes, nails, and hair were evaluated in 80 renal transplant recipients taking sirolimus (mean duration 18 months); 74 patients were also taking mycophenolate mofetil and a glucocorticoid (33[c]). There were cutaneous adverse events in 72 patients, and 20 had serious adverse events; six stopped taking sirolimus as a result. The most frequent effects were pilosebaceous apparatus involvement, including *acne-like eruptions* (46%), *scalp folliculitis* (26%), and *hidradenitis suppurativa* (12%); edematous complaints, including *chronic edema* (55%) and *angioedema* (15%); and mucous membrane disorders, including *aphthous ulceration* (60%), *epistaxis* (60%), *chronic gingivitis* (20%), and *chronic fissure of the lips* (11%). Nail disorders included *chronic onychopathy* (74%) and *periungual infections* (16%).

Urinary tract   Evidence that sirolimus can cause *nephrotoxicity* has been accumulating in the last few years, including observations of thrombotic microangiopathy (34[M]). Kidney recipients taking ciclosporin had higher creatinine concentrations when sirolimus was added compared with placebo or azathioprine (175 versus 137 µmol/l). There was delayed graft function in kidney recipients taking tacrolimus almost three times more often with than without sirolimus. Sirolimus may cause direct tubular or, to a lesser degree, glomerular toxicity and may also potentiate nephrotoxicity due to a calcineurin inhibitor.

Proteinuria associated with sirolimus has been reported after renal transplantation (35[A]). Three patients with type I diabetes developed proteinuria (1, 2, and 7 g/day) while taking sirolimus and low-dose tacrolimus after islet cell transplantation. The proteinuria resolved after sirolimus that was replaced by mycophenolate mofetil combined with an increased dosage of tacrolimus. Renal biopsy in one case showed only diabetic glomerulopathy. Five other islet cell recipients developed microalbuminuria while taking sirolimus; all resolved after switching to tacrolimus and mycophenolate mofetil.

Infection risk   Infection due to *Mycobacterium xenopi* is rare in renal transplant recipients but occurred in two renal transplant patients, one of whom had interstitial pneumopathy and one a pulmonary nodule (36[A]). Both had recently started to take sirolimus, which inhibits interleukin-12-induced proliferation of activated T lymphocytes, which is critical for the development of the cell-mediated immunity that protects against mycobacterial infection.

Susceptibility factors

Liver disease   Hepatic impairment can alter the clearance of sirolimus. In 18 adults with mild to moderate hepatic impairment who took a single oral dose of sirolimus 15 mg, the mean whole-blood sirolimus weight-normalized oral-dose clearance was significantly lower than in healthy controls (32 versus 36%) (37[c]).

Drug–drug interactions   The pharmacokinetics of sirolimus have been studied in 22 kidney transplant recipients taking either *ciclosporin* microemulsion or *tacrolimus* capsules twice a day (38[c]). Sirolimus (6 mg as a loading dose followed by 2 mg/day for at least 7 days) was given 6 hours after the morning dose of the calcineurin inhibitor. Ciclosporin produced higher sirolimus AUC, C_{max}, and C_{min} than tacrolimus.

Tacrolimus   *(SED-15, 3279; SEDA-27, 377; SEDA-28, 463; SEDA-29, 453)*

In a meta-analysis of randomized controlled trials of pimecrolimus and tacrolimus in the treatment of atopic dermatitis, the authors concluded that in the absence of studies that show long-term safety gains, any advantages over topical glucocorticoids is unclear (39[M]).

Ear, nose, throat   *Hearing impairment* in patients after organ transplantation has been reported in association with different immunosuppressants, and has a high incidence after liver transplantation. Of 521 patients with liver transplants, 25 had hearing aids, of whom only nine had either had hearing loss before transplantation or had risk factors such as ototoxic drugs (40[c]). Hearing loss occurred early (eight patients required an aid within 2 years after transplantation) and was bilateral in 14 patients. Nine patients had tinnitus and three had otalgia. Four reported a history of sudden deafness associated with high concentrations of calcineurin inhibitors. The proportion of patients taking tacrolimus was higher than those taking ciclosporin. The mechanism is not known.

Skin   Topical tacrolimus can cause *flushing*, caused by the small amount of alcohol that it contains. This reaction can be mistaken for allergy. Three patients using topical tacrolimus developed a flushing reaction after ingesting alcohol; withdrawal of topical tacrolimus resolved the alcohol-related skin reaction (41[A]).

Drug–drug interactions

Itraconazole   After lung transplantation in 40 patients, itraconazole 200 mg bd for 6 months reduced the mean dosage requirement of tacrolimus from 5.74 to 3.26 mg/day (42[c]). Monitoring of tacrolimus trough concentrations is therefore advised during co-administration of itraconazole.

Micafungin   Micafungin is a mild in vitro inhibitor of CYP3A, of which tacrolimus is a substrate. However, micafungin 100 mg intravenously had no effect on the pharmacokinetics of oral tacrolimus 5 mg in 26 patients (43[c]).

Temsirolimus (cell cycle inhibitor-779; CCI-779)   *(SED-15, 1306; SEDA-29, 460)*

Temsirolimus (CCI-779), an ester analogue of sirolimus, is an inhibitor of the mammalian target of rapamycin (mTOR).

Observational studies   Two intravenous doses of temsirolimus (75 or 250 mg weekly) have been compared in 109 heavily pretreated patients with locally advanced or metastatic breast cancer (44^c). Efficacy was similar with the two doses but toxicity was more common with the higher, especially grade 3 or 4 depression (10% of patients at the 250 mg dose, 0% at the 75 mg dose). The most common temsirolimus-related adverse events of all grades were *mucositis* (70%), *maculopapular rash* (51%), and *nausea* (43%). The most common clinically important grade 3 or 4 adverse events were *mucositis* (9%), *leukopenia* (7%), *hyperglycemia* (7%), *somnolence* (6%), *thrombocytopenia* (5%), and *depression* (5%).

Susceptibility factors   In 50 patients with advanced renal cancer given intravenous temsirolimus 25, 75, or 250 mg once a week, single versus multiple doses and body surface area were significant pharmacokinetic co-variates (45^c). For sirolimus, dose and hematocrit were significant co-variates. Age, sex, and race did not affect temsirolimus disposition. AUC correlated with adverse event severity for thrombocytopenia, pruritus, and hyperlipidemia. Exposure correlated with a specific subset of gene transcripts in peripheral blood monocytes after 16 weeks of therapy. Pharmacogenomic profiling of monocytes showed that altered ribonucleic acid transcript expression correlated with exposure, and these transcripts represent potential biomarkers of exposure to temsirolimus in peripheral blood.

THIOPURINES

Tumorigenicity   The risk of *lymphoma* may be increased by about fourfold in patients with inflammatory bowel disease taking thiopurines, as a result of the medications, the severity of the underlying disease, or a combination of the two (46^R).

Azathioprine   *(SED-15, 377; SEDA-27, 373; SEDA-28, 450; SEDA-29, 424)*

Psychiatric   Azathioprine has been newly associated with psychiatric adverse events (47^A).

- A 13-year-old boy with Wegener's granulomatosis developed incapacitating obsessive–compulsive symptoms and severe panic attacks 4 weeks after switching from cyclophosphamide to azathioprine. He had obsessions about dying, committing suicide, and harming others, obsessive negative thoughts about himself and others, compulsive behavior, severe panic attacks more than once a day, and sleep disturbances. He was given fluvoxamine 100 mg/day, but 18 months later the symptoms suddenly disappeared, 3 weeks after he switched from azathioprine to methotrexate. In the next 4 years, he had no relapse.

Psychiatric adverse effects have not previously been reported with azathioprine. Neither does the database of the WHO Uppsala Monitoring Centre mention obsessive–compulsive symptoms or panic attacks as a possible adverse effect of azathioprine. However, the time course in this case and the absence of symptoms before and after azathioprine therapy suggest a causal relation. It is possible that the combination of subtle cerebral dysfunction as a result of the vasculitis and the use of azathioprine may have caused the symptoms in this patient.

Liver   Thiopurines can cause liver damage, and the incidence varies in different studies. *Hepatotoxicity*, defined as alanine transaminase or alkaline phosphatase activities greater than twice the upper normal limit, was studied in 161 patients with inflammatory bowel disease over a median follow-up of 271 days (48^c). There was abnormal liver function in 21 patients (13%), hepatotoxicity in 16 (10%) after a median of 85 days, and thiopurines were withdrawn in five patients because of hepatotoxicity.

Nodular regenerative hyperplasia of the liver can occur with any of the purine analogues (azathioprine, 6-mercaptopurine, and 6-thioguanine). It has again been described in four patients with inflammatory bowel disease taking azathioprine (49^c). All had either abnormal liver function tests and/or a low platelet count. The biochemical and hematological abnormalities resolved after azathioprine withdrawal. Male sex was a major susceptibility factor. In another series, two patients taking azathioprine developed nodular regenerative hyperplasia; both were heterozygous for the TPMT*3A mutation (50[A]).

Susceptibility factors

Genetic　Deficiency of thiopurine S-methyltransferase (TPMT) predisposes to myelotoxicity, but its association with other adverse effects is less clear. Polymorphisms in the inosine triphosphatase (ITPA) gene may also be involved in thiopurine metabolism and tolerance. In a 6-month prospective study in 71 patients with Crohn's disease taking azathioprine, early drop-out within 2 weeks was associated with the ITPA polymorphism 94C→A and low TPMT activity (<10 nmol/ml of erythrocytes/hour) (51[c]). High-risk individuals, defined by the 94C→A polymorphism or low TPMT activity, were significantly more likely to drop out at any stage. Drop-outs attributed to azathioprine-related adverse effects ($n = 16$) were significantly associated with the 94C→A polymorphism. A time-to-event analysis over the 24-week study period showed a significant association between the time to drop-out and carriage of the ITPA 94C>A mutant allele. Therefore, patients with ITPA 94C→A mutations or low TPMT activity constitute a pharmacogenetic high-risk group for drop-out from azathioprine therapy and ITPA 94C→A appears to be a promising marker of predisposition to azathioprine intolerance.

6-Thioguanine

Thioguanine is used as an escape thiopurine for treating inflammatory bowel disease patients intolerant or refractory to azathioprine, 6-mercaptopurine, or methotrexate.

Liver　Out of 95 patients with inflammatory bowel disease who were intolerant of azathioprine or 6-mercaptopurine 20 stopped taking low-dose 6-thioguanine maintenance therapy (mean 25 mg) (52[c]). The reasons for withdrawal of 6-thioguanine were *gastrointestinal complaints* (31%), *malaise* (15%), and *hepatotoxicity* (15%). Of 75 patients who continued to take 6-thioguanine, seven had hepatotoxicity. Therefore, 6-thioguanine should be administered only in prospective trials.

Pregnancy　Data on the use of 6-thioguanine in pregnancy are rare and controversial. Two patients with Crohn's disease took low doses of 6-thioguanine throughout their pregnancies (53[A]). The two infants were healthy, without congenital abnormalities and or laboratory signs of myelosuppression or hepatocellular injury. The infants had significantly lower concentrations of 6-thioguanine nucleotides in their erythrocytes (ratio 1:12) than the mothers.

References

1. Jardine AG. Assessing the relative risk of cardiovascular disease among renal transplant patients receiving tacrolimus or cyclosporine. Transpl Int 2005;18(4):379–84.
2. Guennoc AM, Corcia P, Al Najjar A, Bergemer-Fouquet AM, Lebranchu Y, de Toffol B, Autret A. Neuromyopathie toxique induite par la ciclosporine. Rev Neurol (Paris) 2005;161(2):221–3.
3. Singer M, Coluzzi F, O'Brien A, Clapp LH. Reversal of life-threatening, drug-related potassium-channel syndrome by glibenclamide. Lancet 2005;365(9474):1873–5.
4. Hauser IA, Schaeffeler E, Gauer S, Scheuermann EH, Wegner B, Gossmann J, Acker-mann H. ABCB1 genotype of the donor but not of the recipient is a major risk factor for cyclosporine-related nephrotoxicity after renal transplantation. J Am Soc Nephrol 2005;16(5):1501–11.
5. Schmitt U, Abou El-Ela A, Guo LJ, Glavinas H, Krajcsi P, Baron JM, Tillmann C, Hiemke C, Langguth P, Härtter S. Cyclosporine A (CsA) affects the pharmacodynamics and pharmacokinetics of the atypical antipsychotic amisulpride probably via inhibition of P-glycoprotein (P-gp). J Neural Transm 2006;113(7):787–801.
6. Agarwal A, Raza M, Dhiraaj S, Saxena R, Singh PK, Pandey R. Is ketamine a safe anesthetic for percutaneous liver biopsy in a liver

transplant recipient immunosuppressed with cyclosporine? Anesth Analg 2005;100(1):85–6.

7. Blackhall MR, Fassett RG, Sharman JE, Geraghty DP, Coombes JS. Effects of antioxidant supplementation on blood cyclosporin A and glomerular filtration rate in renal transplant recipients. Nephrol Dial Transplant 2005;20(9):1970–5.

8. de Vries AP, Oterdoom LH, Gans RO, Bakker SJ. Supplementation with anti-oxidants vitamin C and E decreases cyclosporine A trough-levels in renal transplant recipients. Nephrol Dial Transplant 2006;21(1):231–2.

9. Cantarovich D, Renou M, Megnigbeto A, Giral-Classe M, Hourmant M, Dantal J, Blancho G, Karam G, Soulillou JP. Switching from cyclosporine to tacrolimus in patients with chronic transplant dysfunction or cyclosporine-induced adverse events. Transplantation 2005;79(1):72–8.

10. Kerr JR. Neonatal effects of breast cancer chemotherapy administered during pregnancy. Pharmacotherapy 2005;25(3):438–41.

11. Lorber MI, Mulgaonkar S, Butt KM, Elkhammas E, Mendez R, Rajagopalan PR, Kahan B, Sollinger H, Li Y, Cretin N, Tedesco H, B251 Study Group. Everolimus versus mycophenolate mofetil in the prevention of rejection in de novo renal transplant recipients: a 3-year randomized, multicenter, phase III study. Transplantation 2005;80(2):244–52.

12. Pascual J, Marcén R, Ortuño J. Clinical experience with everolimus (Certican): optimizing dose and tolerability. Transplantation 2005;79(9 Suppl):S80–4.

13. Mabasa VH, Ensom MH. The role of therapeutic monitoring of everolimus in solid organ transplantation. Ther Drug Monit 2005;27(5):666–76.

14. Anonymous. Leflunomide: new indication. In psoriatic rheumatism: too many risks, too little efficacy. Prescrire Int 2005;14(78):123–6.

15. Sakai F, Noma S, Kurihara Y, Yamada H, Azuma A, Kudoh S, Ichikawa Y. Leflunomide-related lung injury in patients with rheumatoid arthritis: imaging features. Mod Rheumatol 2005;15(3):173–9.

16. Gabelle A, Antoine JC, Hillaire-Buys D, Coudeyre E, Camu W. Neuropathie axonale sévère et léflunomide. Rev Neurol (Paris) 2005;161(11):1106–9.

17. Verschueren P, Vandooren AK, Westhovens R. Debilitating diarrhoea and weight loss due to colitis in two RA patients treated with leflunomide. Clin Rheumatol 2005;24(1):87–90.

18. Cui TG, Hou FF, Ni ZH, Chen XM, Zhang FS, Zhu TY, Zhao XZ, Bao CD, Zhao MH, Wang GB, Qian JQ, Cai GY, Li YN, Lu FM, Mei CL, Zou WZ, Wang H. Treatment of proliferative lupus nephritis with leflunomide and steroid: a prospective multi-center controlled clinical trial. Zhonghua Nei Ke Za Zhi 2005;44(9):672–6.

19. Casanova Sorní C, Romá Sánchez E, Pelufo Pellicer A, Poveda Andrés JL. Leflunomida: valoración del riesgo teratógeno en el primer trimestre de embarazo. Farm Hosp 2005;29(4):265–8.

20. Tierce JC, Porterfield-Baxa J, Petrilla AA, Kilburg A, Ferguson RM. Impact of mycophenolate mofetil (MMF)-related gastrointestinal complications and MMF dose alterations on transplant outcomes and healthcare costs in renal transplant recipients. Clin Transplant 2005;19(6):779–84.

21. Kahu J, Kyllonen L, Salmela K. Impact of mycophenolate mofetil intolerance on early results of kidney transplantation. Transplant Proc 2005;37(8):3276–9.

22. Balal M, Demir E, Paydas S, Sertdemir Y, Erken U. Uncommon side effect of MMF in renal transplant recipients. Ren Fail 2005;27(5):591–4.

23. Kamar N, Oufroukhi L, Faure P, Ribes D, Cointault O, Lavayssiere L, Nogier MB, Esposito L, Durand D, Rostaing L. Questionnaire-based evaluation of gastrointestinal disorders in de novo renal-transplant patients receiving either mycophenolate mofetil or enteric-coated mycophenolate sodium. Nephrol Dial Transplant 2005;20(10):2231–6.

24. Chang HR, Lin CC, Lian JD. Early experience with enteric-coated mycophenolate sodium in de novo kidney transplant recipients. Transplant Proc 2005;37(5):2066–8.

25. Kuypers DR, Verleden G, Naesens M, Vanrenterghem Y. Drug interaction between mycophenolate mofetil and rifampin: possible induction of uridine diphosphate-glucuronosyltransferase. Clin Pharmacol Ther 2005;78(1):81–8.

26. Büchler M, Lebranchu Y, Bénéton M, Le Meur Y, Heng AE, Westeel PF, le Guellec C, Libert F, Hary L, Marquet P, Paintaud G. Higher exposure to mycophenolic acid with sirolimus than with cyclosporine cotreatment. Clin Pharmacol Ther 2005;78(1):34–42.

27. Anonymous. Pimecrolimus and tacrolimus. Cautious use recommended. WHO Newslett 2006;3:4.

28. Wolff K, Fleming C, Hanifin J, Papp K, Reitamo S, Rustin M, Shear N, Silny W, Korman N, Marks I, Cherill R, Emady-Azar S, Paul C, Multicentre Investigator Group. Efficacy and tolerability of three different doses of oral pimecrolimus in the treatment of moderate to severe atopic dermatitis: a randomized clinical trial. Br J Dermatol 2005;152:1296–303.

29. Hamour IM, Mittal TK, Bell AD, Banner NR. Reversible sirolimus-associated pneumonitis after heart transplantation. J Heart Lung Transplant 2006;25(2):241–4.

30. Niemczyk M, Wyzgal J, Perkowska A, Porowski D, Paczek L. Sirolimus-associated hepatotoxicity in the kidney graft recipient. Transpl Int 2005;18(11):1302–3.

31. Kunzle N, Venetz JP, Pascual M, Panizzon RG, Laffitte E. Sirolimus-induced acneiform eruption. Dermatology 2005;211(4):366–9.

32. Schaffellner S, Jakoby E, Kniepeiss D, Stadlbauer V, Duller D, Iberer F, Tscheliessnigg KH. Center experience in liver transplantation (LTX): management of dermal side effects caused by

sirolimus. Int Immunopharmacol 2005;5(1):137–40.

33. Mahé E, Morelon E, Lechaton S, Sang KH, Mansouri R, Ducasse MF, Mamzer-Bruneel MF, de Prost Y, Kreis H, Bodemer C. Cutaneous adverse events in renal transplant recipients receiving sirolimus-based therapy. Transplantation 2005;79(4):476–82.

34. Marti HP, Frey FJ. Nephrotoxicity of rapamycin: an emerging problem in clinical medicine. Nephrol Dial Transplant 2005;20(1):13–5.

35. Senior PA, Paty BW, Cockfield SM, Ryan EA, Shapiro AM. Proteinuria developing after clinical islet transplantation resolves with sirolimus withdrawal and increased tacrolimus dosing. Am J Transplant 2005;5(9):2318–23.

36. Thaunat O, Morelon E, Stern M, Buffet P, Offredo C, Mamzer-Bruneel MF, Kreis H. *Mycobacterium xenopi* pulmonary infection in two renal transplant recipients under sirolimus therapy. Transpl Infect Dis 2004;6(4):179–82.

37. Zimmerman JJ, Lasseter KC, Lim HK, Harper D, Dilzer SC, Parker V, Matschke K. Pharmacokinetics of sirolimus (rapamycin) in subjects with mild to moderate hepatic impairment. J Clin Pharmacol 2005;45(12):1368–72.

38. Wu FL, Tsai MK, Chen RR, Sun SW, Huang JD, Hu RH, Chen KH, Lee PH. Effects of calcineurin inhibitors on sirolimus pharmacokinetics during staggered administration in renal transplant recipients. Pharmacotherapy 2005;25(5):646–53.

39. Ashcroft DM, Dimmock P, Garside R, Stein K, Williams HC. Efficacy and tolerability of topical pimecrolimus and tacrolimus in the treatment of atopic dermatitis: meta-analysis of randomised controlled trials. BMJ 2005;330:516–24.

40. Rifai K, Bahr MJ, Cantz T, Klempnauer J, Manns MP, Strassburg CP. Severe hearing loss after liver transplantation. Transplant Proc 2005;37(4):1918–9.

41. Knight AK, Boxer M, Chandler MJ. Alcohol-induced rash caused by topical tacrolimus. Ann Allergy Asthma Immunol 2005;95(3):291–2.

42. Shitrit D, Ollech JE, Ollech A, Bakal I, Saute M, Sahar G, Kramer MR. Itraconazole prophylaxis in lung transplant recipients receiving tacrolimus (FK 506): efficacy and drug interaction. J Heart Lung Transplant 2005;24(12):2148–52.

43. Hebert MF, Blough DK, Townsend RW, Allison M, Buell D, Keirns J, Bekersky I. Concomitant tacrolimus and micafungin pharmacokinetics in healthy volunteers. J Clin Pharmacol 2005;45(9):1018–24.

44. Chan S, Scheulen ME, Johnston S, Mross K, Cardoso F, Dittrich C, Eiermann W, Hess D, Morant R, Semiglazov V, Borner M, Salzberg M, Ostapenko V, Illiger H-J, Behringer D, Bardy-Bouxin N, Boni J, Kong S, Cincotta M, Moore L. Phase II study of temsirolimus (CCI-779), a novel inhibitor of mTOR, in heavily pretreated patients with locally advanced or metastatic breast cancer. J Clin Oncol 2005;23(23):5314–22.

45. Boni JP, Leister C, Bender G, Fitzpatrick V, Twine N, Stover J, Dorner A, Immermann F, Burczynski ME. Population pharmacokinetics of CCI-779: correlations to safety and pharmacogenomic responses in patients with advanced renal cancer. Clin Pharmacol Ther 2005;77(1):76–89.

46. McGovern DP, Jewell DP. Risks and benefits of azathioprine therapy. Gut 2005;54(8):1055–9.

47. van der HJ, Duyx J, de Langen JJ, van Royen A. Probable psychiatric side effects of azathioprine. Psychosom Med 2005;67(3):508.

48. Bastida G, Nos P, Aguas M, Beltrán B, Rubín A, Dasí F, Ponce J. Incidence, risk factors and clinical course of thiopurine-induced liver injury in patients with inflammatory bowel disease. Aliment Pharmacol Ther 2005;22(9):775–82.

49. Daniel F, Cadranel JF, Seksik P, Cazier A, Duong Van Huyen JP, Ziol M, Coutarel P, Loison P, Jian R, Marteau P. Azathioprine induced nodular regenerative hyperplasia in IBD patients. Gastroenterol Clin Biol 2005;29(5):600–3.

50. Breen DP, Marinaki AM, Arenas M, Hayes PC. Pharmacogenetic association with adverse drug reactions to azathioprine immunosuppressive therapy following liver transplantation. Liver Transpl 2005;11(7):826–33.

51. von Ahsen N, Armstrong VW, Behrens C, von Tirpitz C, Stallmach A, Herfarth H, Stein J, Bias P, Adler G, Shipkova M, Oellerich M, Kruis W, Reinshagen M, Schütz E. Association of inosine triphosphatase 94C>A and thiopurine S-methyltransferase deficiency with adverse events and study drop-outs under azathioprine therapy in a prospective Crohn disease study. Clin Chem 2005;51(12):2282–8.

52. de Boer NK, Derijks LJ, Gilissen LP, Hommes DW, Engels LG, de Boer SY, et al. On tolerability and safety of a maintenance treatment with 6-thioguanine in azathioprine or 6-mercaptopurine intolerant IBD patients. World J Gastroenterol 2005;11(35):5540–4.

53. de Boer NK, Van Elburg RM, Wilhelm AJ, Remmink AJ, Van Vugt JM, Mulder CJ, Van Bodegraven AA. 6-Thioguanine for Crohn's disease during pregnancy: thiopurine metabolite measurements in both mother and child. Scand J Gastroenterol 2005;40(11):1374–7.

J. Costa and M. Farré

39

Corticotrophins, corticosteroids, and prostaglandins

Editor's note: In this chapter adverse effects arising from the oral or intravenous administration of corticosteroids (glucocorticoids and mineralocorticoids) are covered in the section on systemic administration. Other routes of administration are dealt with in the sections after that; inhalation and nasal administration are dealt with in Chapter 16, topical administration to the skin in Chapter 14, and ocular administration in Chapter 47.

SYSTEMIC GLUCOCORTICOIDS

(SED-15, 906; SEDA-27, 414; SEDA-28, 471; SEDA-29, 480)

Placebo-controlled studies Patients taking glucocorticoids have an increased risk of infections, including those produced by opportunistic and rare pathogens. However, it has been suggested that glucocorticoid administration in severe community-acquired pneumonia could attenuate systemic inflammation and lead to earlier resolution of pneumonia and a reduction in sepsis-related complications. In a placebo-controlled study in 46 patients with severe community-acquired pneumonia who received protocol-guided antibiotic treatment hydrocortisone (intravenous 200 mg bolus followed by infusion at a rate of 10 mg/hour) for 7 days produced significant clinical improvement (1[c]). Adverse effects were not described.

Side Effects of Drugs, Annual 30
J.K. Aronson (Editor)
ISSN: 0378-6080
DOI: 10.1016/S0378-6080(08)00039-1

Cardiovascular *Obstructive cardiomyopathy* has been attributed to a glucocorticoid in a child with subglottal stenosis (2[A]).

- A 4-month-old boy (weight 4 kg) developed fever, nasal secretions, and stridor due to a subglottal granuloma. Dexamethasone 1 mg/kg/day was started and tapered over 1 week. The mass shrank to 25% of its original size but the symptoms recurred 2 weeks later. The granuloma was excised and dexamethasone 1 mg/kg/day was restarted. After 5 days he developed a tachycardia (140/minute) and a new systolic murmur. Echocardiography showed severe ventricular hypertrophy with dynamic left ventricular outflow tract obstruction. The dexamethasone was weaned over several days. Over the next 3 weeks several echocardiograms showed rapid resolution of the outflow tract obstruction and gradual improvement of the cardiac hypertrophy. After 8 months there was no further problem.

Nervous system Glucocorticoid-induced *spinal epidural lipomatosis* is not very common in children. Spinal magnetic resonance imaging was performed in 125 children with renal diseases (68 boys); they either had back pain or numbness, were obese, or had taken a cumulative dose of prednisone of more than 500 mg/kg; there was lipomatosis in five patients (3[c]).

Psychological and psychiatric Chronic glucocorticoid exposure is associated with reduced size of the hippocampus, resulting in *impaired declarative memory*. In 52 renal transplant recipients (mean age 45 years, 34 men and 18 women) taking prednisone (100 mg/day for 3 days followed by 10 mg/day for as long as needed; mean dose 11 mg/day) there was a major reduction in immediate recall but not delayed recall (4[c]). However, there was a significant correlation between mean prednisone dose and delayed recall.

In animals, phenytoin pretreatment blocks the effects of stress on memory and hippocampal histology. In a double blind, randomized, placebo-controlled trial 39 patients (mean age 44 years, 8 men) with allergies or pulmonary or rheumatological illnesses who were taking prednisone (mean dose 40 mg/day) were randomized to either phenytoin (300 mg/day) or placebo for 7 days (5^c). Those who took phenytoin had significantly smaller increases in a *mania* self-report scale. There was no effect on memory. Thus, phenytoin blocked the hypomanic effects of prednisone, but not the effects on declarative memory.

Endocrine   Iatrogenic *Cushing's syndrome* is a well-known adverse effect of glucocorticoids. It usually develops after prolonged exposure to excessive doses and its development after a single low dose is exceptional (6^A).

- A 45-year-old woman was given a single-dose of intramuscular triamcinolone acetonide 40 mg for acute laryngitis and 1 month later had to have a cushingoid appearance. Endocrinological tests confirmed hypothalamic–pituitary–adrenal (HPA) axis suppression. Eight months later, the cushingoid appearance had completely disappeared and HPA function had spontaneously recovered.

Musculoskeletal   Doses of prednisone of 7.5 mg/day can cause premature or exaggerated *osteoporosis*. However, it is unclear whether a dose of 5 mg/day has the same effect. In a double-blind, randomized, placebo-controlled, 8-week trial 50 healthy postmenopausal women (mean age 57 years) were randomly assigned to prednisone 5 mg/day or matching placebo for 6 weeks, followed by a 2-week recovery phase (7^c). Prednisone rapidly and significantly decreased serum concentrations of propeptide of type I N-terminal procollagen, propeptide of type I C-terminal procollagen, and osteocalcin, and free urinary deoxypyridinoline compared with placebo. These changes were largely reversed during the recovery period. In conclusion, low-dose prednisone significantly reduced indices of bone formation and bone resorption in postmenopausal women.

Osteoporosis is common in Crohn's disease, often because of glucocorticoids. Budesonide as controlled-release capsules is a locally acting glucocorticoid with low systemic availability. In a randomized study in 272 patients with Crohn's disease involving the ileum and/or ascending colon, budesonide and prednisolone were compared for 2 years in doses adapted to disease activity (8^c). There was active disease in 181, of whom 98 were glucocorticoid-naive; 90 had quiescent disease and were corticosteroid-dependent. Efficacy was similar in the two groups, but treatment-related adverse effects were less frequent with budesonide. The glucocorticoid-naive patients who took budesonide had smaller reductions in bone mineral density than those who took prednisolone (mean −1.04 versus −3.84%).

Pregnancy   The effects of a single antenatal dose of a glucocorticoid on prostanoids have been evaluated in 43 singleton pregnancies in women who were taking betamethasone or not (9^c). Betamethasone (dose not described) reduced maternal PGE_2 concentrations, with concomitant increases in the fetoplacental compartment. Umbilical cord thromboxane B_2 concentrations in the treated group were significantly lower than the non-treated group, resulting in a higher ratio of 6-keto$PGF_{1\alpha}$ to thromboxane B2. Considering the regulatory role of PGE_2 and PGI_2 in fetal lung development and neonatal transition homeostasis, these results suggest a mechanism, at least in part, for the beneficial effects of antenatal glucocorticoids on fetal lung maturation and neonatal cardiopulmonary homeostasis at birth.

In a retrospective study of the use of betamethasone every 12 hours versus 24 hours for anticipated preterm delivery in 909 pregnancies, three groups were identified: those who had not received antenatal glucocorticoids, those who had received betamethasone 12 hours apart, and those who received 24-hour dosing (10^c). There was significantly more maternal antibiotic use (90 versus 84%) and more neonatal surfactant use (40 versus 26%) in the 12-hour group compared with the 24-hour group. For all other outcomes there was no clinically significant difference.

Single versus multiple courses of antenatal glucocorticoids have been compared retrospectively in 704 pregnancies that resulted in preterm births at 24–32 weeks. There three groups: 294 neonates whose mothers had not received glucocorticoids, 257 who had received a single dose, and 153 who had received multiple doses. Multiple doses compared with a single dose was associated with increased positive maternal cultures (44 versus 31%), small for gestational age infants (35 versus 21%), and intraventricular haemorrhage (45 versus 34%) (11[c]).

Fetotoxicity   The long-term consequences of antenatal glucocorticoids have been evaluated in two studies. One evaluated the effects on psychological functioning and health-related quality-of-life in adulthood and the other assessed if the treatment could affect cardiovascular risk factors in adulthood.

In 192 adult offspring (mean age 31 years) of mothers who had taken part in a randomized controlled trial of antenatal betamethasone for the prevention of neonatal respiratory distress syndrome (87 exposed to betamethasone two doses 24 hours apart, and 105 exposed to placebo) there were no alterations in cognitive functioning, working memory and attention, psychiatric morbidity, handedness, or health-related quality-of-life in adulthood (12[c]).

In 534 individuals aged 30 years, whose mothers had participated in a double-blind, randomized, placebo-controlled trial of antenatal betamethasone (two intramuscular doses 24 hours apart) for the prevention of neonatal respiratory distress syndrome, there were no differences between those exposed to betamethasone and placebo in body size, blood lipids, blood pressure, plasma cortisol, prevalence of diabetes, or history of cardiovascular disease (13[c]). After the oral glucose tolerance test, those who had been exposed to betamethasone had higher plasma insulin concentrations at 30 minutes (61 versus 52 mIU/l) and lower glucose concentrations at 120 minutes (4.8 versus 5.1 mmol/l) than did those exposed to placebo. Antenatal exposure to betamethasone might result in insulin resistance in adult offspring, but has no effect on cardiovascular risk factors at 30 years of age.

Drug–drug interactions

Ritonavir   In healthy volunteers a low dose of ritonavir increases the plasma concentrations of fluticasone and reduces cortisol concentrations, probably due to increased systemic availability of fluticasone. Five cases of iatrogenic Cushing's syndrome with osteoporosis and secondary adrenal failure have been described in patients with HIV taking oral ritonavir and inhaled glucocorticoids (four fluticasone and one budesonide) (14[A]).

Diagnosis of adverse drug reactions   Osteoporosis and osteopenia are usually evaluated by measuring bone density using dual-energy X-ray absorptiometry (DXA). However, there is increased interest in measuring not only bone density but also some structural properties of the bone, such as elasticity and trabecular stiffness and connectivity, which are more closely related to bone strength. Quantitative ultrasound could theoretically provide information on bone structure, as has been suggested by a prospective study in patients with glucocorticoid-induced osteoporosis (15[c]), but further studies are needed to define the role of quantitative ultrasonography in the prediction of fracture and in the clinical management of glucocorticoid-induced osteoporosis.

PROSTAGLANDINS AND ANALOGUES   *(SED-15, 2955; SEDA-27, 414; SEDA-28, 471; SEDA-29, 480)*

Epoprostenol   *(SED-15, 1228)*

Drug–drug interactions   *Anticoagulants* and continuous intravenous infusion of epoprostenol are the standard treatments for primary pulmonary hypertension. However, their combined use increases the likelihood of hemorrhagic complications, as demonstrated in a retrospective study of 31 consecutive patients with primary pulmonary hypertension (mean age, 29 years, 10 men, 21 women), nine of whom had 11 bleeding episodes; nine episodes were cases of alveolar hemorrhage and two patients had severe respiratory distress (16[A]). The mean dose of epoprostenol at the time of the first bleeding episode was 89 ng/kg/minute. More of the patients who had a bleeding episode died (67 versus 41%).

Latanoprost   *(SED-15, 2002)*

Cardiovascular   *Coronary spasm* has been attributed to latanoprost (17[A]).

- A 58-year-old man with stable angina pectoris started to use latanoprost eye drops and over the next few days his angina worsened and occurred at rest. After 15 days, he had syncope during physical exercise. Angiography showed coronary spasm.

Sweat glands   Profuse *sweating* has been attributed to latanoprost (18[A]).

- A 55-year-old woman with primary chronic angle glaucoma was given latanoprost ophthalmic solution (0.005%, 1 drop/day). After 3 days, 1–2 hours after administration, she reported severe sweating involving the entire body and drenching all her clothes. The excessive sweating disappeared on withdrawal of latanoprost and did not occur when she was given bimatoprost. One month later, latanoprost was restarted and the severe sweating recurred on the first day of therapy. Latanoprost was withdrawn and bimatoprost was started again.

Misoprostol   *(SED-15, 2357)*

Observational studies   In a retrospective study in patients with pre-eclampsia undergoing cervical ripening the complications associated with vaginal misoprostol ($n = 95$) and dinoprostone ($n = 108$) vaginal inserts before induction of labor have been reported (19[c]). The incidence of *uterine hyperstimulation* requiring emergency cesarean section because of fetal heart rate abnormalities was significantly higher among patients who received misoprostol (18 versus 8.3%). The overall incidence of *abruptio placenta* was also significantly higher among those who received misoprostol (14 versus 1.9%).

Reproductive system   Several cases of *uterine rupture* due to misoprostol after second trimester have been reported. However, unexpectedly, administration of misoprostol for cervical ripening before surgical evacuation of a missed abortion reportedly produced *uterine rupture* in the first trimester (20[A]).

- A 30-year-old woman with amenorrhea for 8 weeks had vaginal bleeding probably secondary to a missed abortion. Transvaginal ultrasonography showed a single fetus of 6 weeks without cardiac activity. She was scheduled for dilatation and evacuation but 1 hour after a single oral dose of misoprostol 400 micrograms she developed severe abdominal pain, hypotension (70/40 mmHg), and abdominal distension and rebound tenderness. The hemoglobin concentration was 6.5 g/l. Emergency laparoscopy showed a 1.5 cm rupture of the left uterine horn.

She had had a previous cesarean section, but it is very unlikely that that contributed, because the uterine rupture occurred at a different site to the caesarean incision (low-flap transverse section).

Infection risk   There were four deaths in previously healthy women due to *endometritis* and *toxic shock syndrome* within 1 week after medically induced abortions with oral mifepristone 200 mg and vaginal misoprostol 800 micrograms; in two cases *Clostridium sordellii* was found (21[A]). Another similar case was reported in Canada in 2001. Endometritis and toxic shock syndrome associated with *C. sordellii* are rare. Of 10 cases identified by authors in the previous literature, eight occurred after the delivery of live-born infants, one after a medical abortion, and one was not associated with pregnancy. The cases produced an FDA alert with a "Dear Health Care Provider" letter from the manufacturer and publication of a "Dispatch" in the Morbidity and Mortality Weekly Report (22[S]).

Travoprost

Gastrointestinal   *Abdominal cramp* has been attributed to travoprost (23[A]).

- A 34-year-old woman with primary open-angle glaucoma began topical application of travoprost ophthalmic solution (0.004%, 1 drop/day) and 30 minutes later developed abdominal cramp that lasted for 2 hours. The same symptoms appeared on 3 days after drug administration. The pain disappeared after travoprost withdrawal.

In order to investigate this adverse effect, a series of single-blind trials were carried out with the informed consent of the patient (including rechallenge with travoprost and other prostaglandin analogues and dechallenges). Abdominal cramp did not develop after substitution of travoprost with latanoprost or isotonic saline, but recurred on rechallenge with travoprost.

References

1. Confalonieri M, Urbino R, Potena A, Piattella M, Parigi P, Puccio G, Della Porta R, Giorgio C, Blasi F, Umberger R, Meduri GU. Hydrocortisone infusion for severe community-acquired pneumonia: a preliminary randomized study. Am J Respir Crit Care Med 2005;171(3):242–8.
2. Balys R, Manoukian J, Zalai C. Left ventricular hypertrophy with outflow tract obstruction-a complication of dexamethasone treatment for subglottic stenosis. Int J Pediatr Otorhinolaryngol 2005;69(2):271–3.
3. Kano K, Kyo K, Ito S, Nishikura K, Ando T, Yamada Y, Arisaka O. Spinal epidural lipomatosis in children with renal diseases receiving steroid therapy. Pediatr Nephrol 2005;20(2):184–9.
4. Bermond B, Surachno S, Lok A, ten Berge IJ, Plasmans B, Kox C, Schuller E, Schellekens PT, Hamel R. Memory functions in prednisone-treated kidney transplant patients. Clin Transplant 2005;19(4):512–7.
5. Brown ES, Stuard G, Liggin JD, Hukovic N, Frol A, Dhanani N, Khan DA, Jeffress J, Larkin GL, McEwen BS, Rosenblatt R, Mageto Y, Hanczyc M, Cullum CM. Effect of phenytoin on mood and declarative memory during prescription corticosteroid therapy. Biol Psychiatry 2005;57(5):543–8.
6. Iglesias P, González J, Díez JJ. Acute and persistent iatrogenic Cushing's syndrome after a single dose of triamcinolone acetonide. J Endocrinol Invest 2005;28(11):1019–23.
7. Ton FN, Gunawardene SC, Lee H, Neer RM. Effects of low-dose prednisone on bone metabolism. J Bone Miner Res 2005;20(3):464–70.
8. Schoon EJ, Bollani S, Mills PR, Israeli E, Felsenberg D, Ljunghall S, Persson T, Haptén-White L, Graffner H, Bianchi Porro G, Vatn M, Stockbrügger RW, Matrix Study Group. Bone mineral density in relation to efficacy and side effects of budesonide and prednisolone in Crohn's disease. Clin Gastroenterol Hepatol 2005;3(2):113–21.
9. Cho S, Beharry KD, Valencia AM, Guajardo L, Nageotte MP, Modanlou HD. Maternal and feto-placental prostanoid responses to a single course of antenatal betamethasone. Prostaglandins Other Lipid Mediat 2005;78(1–4):139–59.
10. Haas DM, McCullough W, Olsen CH, Shiau DT, Richard J, Fry EA, McNamara MF. Neonatal outcomes with different betamethasone dosing regimens: a comparison. J Reprod Med 2005;50(12):915–22.
11. Ogunyemi D. A comparison of the effectiveness of single-dose vs multi-dose antenatal corticosteroids in pre-term neonates. Obstet Gynaecol 2005;25(8):756–60.
12. Dalziel SR, Lim VK, Lambert A, McCarthy D, Parag V, Rodgers A, Harding JE. Antenatal exposure to betamethasone: psychological functioning and health related quality of life 31 years after

inclusion in randomised controlled trial. BMJ 2005;331(7518):665.
13. Dalziel SR, Walker NK, Parag V, Mantell C, Rea HH, Rodgers A, Harding JE. Cardiovascular risk factors after antenatal exposure to betamethasone: 30-year follow-up of a randomised controlled trial. Lancet 2005;365(9474):1856–62.
14. Samaras K, Pett S, Gowers A, McMurchie M, Cooper DA. Iatrogenic Cushing's syndrome with osteoporosis and secondary adrenal failure in human immunodeficiency virus-infected patients receiving inhaled corticosteroids and ritonavir-boosted protease inhibitors: six cases. J Clin Endocrinol Metab 2005;90(7):4394–8.
15. Cepollaro C, Gonnelli S, Rottoli P, Montagnani A, Caffarelli C, Bruni D, Nikiforakis N, Fossi A, Rossi S, Nuti R. Bone ultrasonography in glucocorticoid-induced osteoporosis. Osteoporos Int 2005;16(8):743–8.
16. Ogawa A, Matsubara H, Fujio H, Miyaji K, Nakamura K, Morita H, Saito H, Kusano KF, Emori T, Date H, Ohe T. Risk of alveolar hemorrhage in patients with primary pulmonary hypertension—anticoagulation and epoprostenol therapy. Circ J 2005;69(2):216–20.
17. Marti V, Guindo J, Valles E, Domínguez de Rozas JM. Angina variante asociada con latanoprost. Med Clin (Barc) 2005;125(6):238–9.
18. Kumar H, Sony P, Gupta V. Profound sweating episodes and latanoprost. Clin Experiment Ophthalmol 2005;33(6):675.
19. Fontenot MT, Lewis DF, Barton CB, Jones EM, Moore JA, Evans AT. Abruptio placentae associated with misoprostol use in women with preeclampsia. J Reprod Med 2005;50(9):653–8.
20. Kim JO, Han JY, Choi JS, Ahn HK, Yang JH, Kang IS, Song MJ, Nava-Ocampo AA. Oral misoprostol and uterine rupture in the first trimester of pregnancy: a case report. Reprod Toxicol 2005;20(4):575–7.
21. Fischer M, Bhatnagar J, Guarner J, Reagan S, Hacker JK, Van Meter SH, Poukens V, Whiteman DB, Iton A, Cheung M, Dassey DE, Shieh WJ, Zaki SR. Fatal toxic shock syndrome associated with Clostridium sordellii after medical abortion. N Engl J Med 2005;353(22):2352–60.
22. Centers for Disease Control and Prevention. Clostridium sordellii toxic shock syndrome after medical abortion with mifepristone and intravaginal misoprostol—United States and Canada, 2001–2005. MMWR Morb Mortal Wkl Rep 2005;54:724.
23. Lee YC. Abdominal cramp as an adverse effect of travoprost. Am J Ophthalmol 2005;139(1):202–3.

M.N.G. Dukes

40   Sex hormones and related compounds, including hormonal contraceptives

Author's note: Sex hormones, particularly estrogens and progestogens, can be used separately or in combination, and for various purposes. It is often not possible to determine to which compound or combination a particular adverse reaction can be attributed; information on particular types of adverse effects may therefore need to be sought under a series of differing headings.

The year 2008 will mark the completion of half a century of use of hormonal contraceptives. It is true that in 1958 no national regulatory had yet approved the sale of these products, but in that year the first large-scale phase III trials with the pioneering product, which was to become known as Enovid, were under way, and when marketing licences began to be handed down from 1960 onwards many thousands of the women who were already involved in clinical trials became established users; experimentation merged silently into practice. It had of course already been known for two decades that progesterone could suppress ovulation in rabbits, and that finding was soon confirmed in other species. However, substantial progress towards the exploitation of this effect in humans had been delayed both by difficulties in developing a synthetic analogue to progesterone that could be taken orally and by forebodings (both toxicological and moralistic) about what effects the lifelong use of such a product might have.

Concerns ranging from possible carcinogenesis or teratogenesis to delay of the menopause or a universal collapse of moral standards were aired and could hardly be dismissed lightly, since there was no trustworthy means of predicting the long-term outcomes. Never before had vast populations of entirely healthy subjects been exposed for much of their adult lives to potent and almost continuous medication designed to interfere with physiological function. Because they were healthy there was no strictly medical benefit to outweigh whatever long-time harms might emerge. There had been virtually no opportunity to identify possible risk groups, susceptibility factors, or interactions.

After half a century of experience one is perhaps justified in breathing a sigh of relief on most counts. Yes, thromboembolism proved within the first 10 years to be a disagreeable and sometimes highly dangerous complication, but that risk was to a large extent contained by progressive reductions in dosage and by recognition of the susceptibility factors. Yes, there were contraindications and susceptibility factors that had not at first been recognized. However, many millions of women benefited very greatly from having taken, arm in arm with their innumerable sisters across the world, what was at first very much a step into the unknown.

GONADOTROPINS AND OVULATION-INDUCING DRUGS
(SED-15, 1536; SEDA-27, 420; SEDA-28, 480; SEDA-29, 493)

Reproductive system   Efforts continue to identify and reduce the risk of *ovarian hyperstimulation* in individual cases of in vitro

Side Effects of Drugs, Annual 30
J.K. Aronson (Editor)
ISSN: 0378-6080
DOI: 10.1016/S0378-6080(08)00040-8

fertilization, but it remains difficult to assess in advance the chance of this complication. In a study of the relevance of the serum concentration of human chorionic gonadotrophin in 849 IVF cycles there were no significant relations between hCG concentrations and the proportion of follicles yielding oocytes, the fertilization rate, blastulation rate, or the probabilities of embryo transfer, implantation, or clinical pregnancy (1[c]). This result again stresses the desirability of using moderate doses of hCG, which seems to reduce the risk of ovarian hyperstimulation while maintaining efficacy.

Urine-derived urofollitropin and recombinant FSH appear to be equally effective and well tolerated for induction of ovulation (2[R]). However, it is unclear whether human menopausal gonadotropins have a higher risk of overstimulation and ovarian hyperstimulation syndrome than urofollitropin in women with polycystic ovary syndrome.

Pregnancy   A US group, working prospectively, has sought to develop a prediction model to assess the risk of inducing high-order *multiple pregnancies* (triplets or more) by gonadotrophic stimulation of the ovaries in 849 consecutive infertile women who underwent a total of 1542 cycles of treatment with gonadotrophins without the use of in vitro fertilization (3[C]). Using a series of criteria considered to point to an increased risk of multiple pregnancy, treatment was cancelled in those cycles in which there appeared to be a substantially increased risk of multiple pregnancy. The use of this predictive routine was estimated to have reduced the number of overall treatment successes by some 8% (95% CI = 6.8, 9.2), but it very markedly reduced the number of high-order multiple pregnancies, by 285% (95% CI = 279, 291).

ESTROGENS   *(SED-15, 1253; SEDA-27, 422; SEDA-28, 481; SEDA-29, 494)*

Drug administration route   Transdermal estrogen for androgen-dependent prostatic cancer is increasingly preferred over the oral route because it avoids first-pass hepatic exposure. The effects of this form of treatment have been studied in an open phase II study in 24 men with

prostatic carcinoma who were progressing after primary hormonal therapy and who received transdermal estradiol 0.6 mg (administered as six 24-hour patches of 0.1 mg each) replaced every 7 days (4[c]). Three of the 24 had a confirmed reduction in prostate-specific antigen by more than half. Adverse effects were modest and there were no thromboembolic complications. The mean serum estradiol concentration rose from 17 (range 15–20) pg/ml to 461 (range 335–587) pg/ml. The total testosterone concentration remained stable in the anorchid range during treatment, but the free testosterone concentration fell as a result of increased sex hormone binding globulin. There were no changes in factor VIII activity, F 1.2, or resistance to activated protein C, but there was a modest *reduction in the concentration of protein S*.

Hormone replacement therapy (HRT)   *(SED-15, 1684, 1686, 1692; SEDA-27, 423; SEDA-28, 483; SEDA-29, 496)*

Assessment of the efficacy and safety of hormonal replacement therapy has always been bedevilled by the question of adherence to therapy, which is often poorly recorded. Particularly after the acute symptoms of the menopause have passed and been forgotten, some women lose their motivation to continue hormonal treatment. Added to this is the now incontrovertible evidence that HRT can in some cases be harmful, and presentation of the risks in the mass media has undoubtedly further reduced adherence. An Italian group examined this problem prospectively in 138 women who agreed to be enrolled in a longitudinal study intended to last for 24 months (5[c]). Only 72 were still taking the treatment after 1 year and only 56 at the end of the study, although only three reported that they had experienced no benefit. Type of work, surgical menopause, and previous use of oral contraceptives were significantly associated with better adherence. The occurrence of real or supposed adverse effects and a fear of breast cancer were the commonest reasons cited for early discontinuation.

Cardiovascular   A paradoxical finding in the Women's Health Initiative (WHI) study (SEDA-29, 496-7) was that while HRT resulted in an improvement in blood lipid concentrations there was no reduction in the incidence of coronary heart disease. A re-examination of the findings in 2005 generated the hypothesis that the key to the paradox could lie in effects on specific lipid subgroups rather than on lipids as a whole (6[cH]). This hypothesis was tested by an evaluation of differences in coronary calcification, lipids, and lipoprotein subclasses among menopausal HRT users and non-users in a longitudinal study. Lipoprotein subclasses and coronary artery calcification (the latter measured using electron beam computed tomography) were studied in HRT users (49%) and non-users in a total of 243 women from the Healthy Women Study, who were about 8 years postmenopausal. The distribution of calcification scores was not significantly different between users and non-users and neither were there differences between the groups as regards any LDL subclass. However, regardless of HRT use, women with detectable calcification of the coronary arteries had *higher concentrations of VLDL and small LDL particles, higher LDL particle concentration, and smaller mean LDL size* compared with women with no detectable calcification. The fact that HRT users had higher concentrations of VLDL particles (triglycerides) and did not have a better LDL subclass distribution could explain the fact that HRT was not associated with a difference in coronary calcification in this study or with a reduction in coronary heart disease risk in randomized clinical trials.

In 2001, as recalled in an earlier volume in this series (SEDA-26, 437), the randomized Heart and Estrogen/progestin Replacement Study (HERS) produced some evidence that in women with clinically manifest heart disease HRT might produce some early harm but confer some later benefit as regards coronary events. The picture is still incomplete, but it has been filled in to some extent by a prospective study of the effects of HRT on cardiovascular function over 1 year of treatment in 46 healthy postmenopausal women, mean age 55 years, who took either estrogen replacement therapy alone ($n = 23$) or progestogen+estrogen replacement therapy ($n = 23$) (7[c]). The doses used were 0.625 mg/day of conjugated equine estrogen with or without medroxyprogesterone acetate 2.5 mg/day. The controls were 25 health premenopausal women, mean age 35 years. Long-term estrogen-only replacement *increased the*

QT interval, QT dispersal, and the index of parasympathetic activity; there was also a small non-significant *increase in the incidence of dysrhythmias*. Long term use of progestogen + estrogen did not affect the QT interval, QT dispersion, or the frequencies of ventricular dysrhythmias or parasympathetic activity, but it did increase the incidence of *supraventricular tachycardias*. These findings support the idea that estrogen may directly modulate ventricular repolarization and that progestogens do not. Obviously, further work on a larger scale is required if the HERS study is to be followed up adequately.

Psychological   The mechanisms underlying the *mood changes* that are often associated with menstruation, the menopause, and hormonal therapy are not understood, but there is now some evidence that they have an association with the response to the neuroactive steroid pregnanolone and that progestogens and estrogens might alter this response. In a randomized, double-blind, crossover study 26 postmenopausal women with climacteric symptoms took oral estradiol 2 mg/day continuously for two cycles and either vaginal progesterone 800 mg or a placebo during the last 14 days of each cycle (8[c]). Before treatment and again at the end of each treatment cycle pregnanolone was administered intravenously, and its effects on saccadic eye velocity, saccade acceleration, saccade latency, and self-rated sedation were examined. During treatment with either estradiol alone or with added progesterone the effect of pregnanolone on saccadic eye movements and self-rated sedation was increased. Saccadic eye velocity, saccade acceleration, and sedation responses to pregnanolone were also increased in women who usually experienced cyclicity of mood during HRT treatment, but not in those with no history of mood cyclicity.

Hematologic   In 27 postmenopausal subjects who took estradiol for 8 weeks, either alone or in combination with the progestogen norethisterone, there was an *increase in plasma thromboxane beta₂ concentration*, possibly determined by platelet activation, which suggests an increased short-term risk of *thrombosis*; P-selectin expression was not affected (9[cr]).

It is not surprising to see further evidence emerging, this time from Japan, as to *why* the risk of venous thromboembolism during HRT is likely to be greater in hypertensive women than in others. In 38 hypertensive (but treated) women and 32 normotensive subjects, who took a course of conjugated equine estrogen 0.625 mg/day + medroxyprogesterone acetate 2.5 mg/day for 12 months, and 19 other hypertensive subjects and 15 normotensive women who took no hormone replacement at all, antithrombin concentrations in the hypertensive and normotensive women who took HRT fell significantly at 6 and 12 months, their D-dimer concentrations fell at 12 months, and their plasminogen concentrations fell at 6 and 12 months (10^c). There were no changes in hemostatic factors in either control group. This meticulous study must lead one to conclude that this form of HRT *activates blood coagulation and fibrinolysis* in both hypertensive and normotensive postmenopausal women. This may well be related to the risk of thromboembolic events.

Urinary tract   At various times evidence has appeared that HRT reduces the risk of urinary infections, while other reports have suggested that the risk is increased. The same seems to apply to *urinary incontinence*; it has often been stated that incontinence is reduced by HRT, but a brief report has shown that in some cases existing urinary incontinence becomes more frequent and severe (11^A).

Tumorigenicity

Breast cancer   Whatever the level of breast cancer risk presented by postmenopausal hormonal cancer therapy, there is little doubt that it varies with the precise regimen. It is true that this does not come clearly to the fore in all the relevant studies, but that may simply be because the question was not specifically examined. In a thoughtful study of data from the E3N-EPIC cohort investigation, the risk of breast cancer associated with HRT was assessed in 54 548 postmenopausal women (mean age at inclusion 53 years) who had not taken any HRT in the year before entering the investigation. There were 948 primary invasive breast cancers during follow-up over an average of 5.8 years, and a modestly increased overall breast cancer risk compared with non-users (RR = 1.2) (12^M). However, while the relative risk was only 1.1 (CI = 0.8, 1.6) for estrogens used alone it

was 1.3 (1.1, 1.5) when estrogens were used in combination with oral progestogens. The risk was significantly greater with HRT containing synthetic progestins than with HRT containing micronized progesterone, the relative risks being 1.4 (1.2, 1.7) and 0.9 (0.7, 1.2) respectively. When combined with synthetic progestins, both oral estrogen and transdermal/percutaneous estrogen were associated with a significantly increased risk; for transdermal/percutaneous estrogen, this was the case even when exposure was less than 2 years. These findings suggest that when estrogens used for HRT are combined with synthetic progestogens even short-term use may increase the risk of breast cancer. It also seems that micronized progesterone may be preferable to synthetic progestins for short-term HRT. Findings such as these need more follow-up if the safest form of HRT is to be clearly identified.

Meanwhile in Australia an attempt has been made to estimate the national incidence of breast cancer due to hormone replacement therapy and to come to grips with it. The investigators used the attributable fraction technique, with prevalence data derived from the 2001 Australian Health Survey and published rates of breast cancer relative risks from HRT. In Australia 12% of adult women are current HRT users, and 11 783 breast cancers were reported in 2001, of which 1066 (9%) were potentially attributable to HRT (13^{MR}). Restricting HRT to women under 65 years, withdrawing HRT after 10 years, or limiting combined estrogen and progesterone HRT to 5 years (but otherwise keeping prescription patterns to 2001 levels) were considered to be approaches that could reduce the annual national breast cancer case load by 280 (2.4%), 555 (4.7%), and 674 (5.7%) cases respectively.

Endometrial cancer   It has long been thought that HRT can reduce the risk of endometrial cancer (SEDA-29, 498), but that the effect is likely to vary with the drugs and doses used. It is conceivable that some forms of HRT might actually increase the risk of endometrial malignancy or that this could be a risk in certain subjects.

In a critical review of all the relevant evidence on combined estrogen + progestogen HRT about 15% of the endometrial biopsies taken from women on sequential HRT showed proliferative activity, including atypical endometrial hyperplasia in up to 1% of the cases (14[R]). Most biopsies taken from women taking continuous combined HRT show endometrial atrophy. About 2–3% of these women will have proliferative activity, usually without atypical hyperplasia. There was no increased risk of endometrial cancer in the extensive WHI and HERS studies, but various endogenous factors, such as obesity, diabetes mellitus, the distribution of estrogen receptors alpha and beta, and genetic polymorphisms for receptors and enzymes, might alter the endometrial effects of various types of HRT. These authors considered that there should be a liberal indication for endometrial biopsies when HRT is used. Since the incidence of atypical hyperplasia or carcinoma under unopposed estrogen therapy is 2–10%, this type of HRT should not be used in non-hysterectomized women. As far as the risk of endometrial cancer from any kind of HRT is concerned, the different molecular pathways of endometrial carcinogenesis (types 1 and 2 cancers) should be taken into account. These authors noted that tibolone leaves the endometrium unaffected.

Drug dosage regimens   The variety of hormonal replacement products is considerable, and many have closely similar records as regards both efficacy and safety. The principal merit of many of them is simply that they offer alternatives—a woman who does not react well to one may fare better with another, sometimes for no apparent reason. Some of the published comparisons serve little more than promotional purposes and the basic data produced merely underline the similarity of the various products.

One study illustrates the point and is typical of many—a comparison of three sequential regimens in what is described as a randomized double-blind study; however, the 1218 women involved during the first year and the 531 subjects who continued for a further year were spread over multiple centers in eight countries, which makes valid comparisons difficult (15[C]). The first regimen was 17-beta-estradiol 1 mg on days 1–14 and then either 17-beta-estradiol 1 mg + trimegestone 0.125 mg or 17-beta-estradiol 1 mg + trimegestone 0.25 mg on days 15–28. The second regimen was estradiol valerate 1 mg on days 1–16 and then estradiol valerate 1 mg + norethisterone 1 mg on

days 17–28. The authors thought that the bleeding profile was more favorable with 17-beta-estradiol 1 mg + trimegestone 0.25 mg than with the lower dose of trimegestone. However, both of the trimegestone regimens had a good protective effect on endometrial proliferation, and the higher dose had a lower incidence of proliferative endometrium with an overall favorable bleeding profile. The mean percentage of women who reported withdrawal bleeding during the week after withdrawal of progestogen was higher with 17-beta-estradiol 1 mg + trimegestone 0.25 mg, which had a more efficient progestogen effect on the endometrium and good predictability of bleeding. Although the authors expressed a preference for one product, the data showed that the mean numbers and average lengths of bleeding episodes were similar in the three groups.

Drug administration route

Intrauterine administration   The effects of the Fibroplant intrauterine device, which releases some 14 micrograms/day of levonorgestrel and is given alongside estrogen therapy, have been evaluated in an open study over 3 years in 150 perimenopausal and postmenopausal women, most of whom also took an estimated 1.5 mg of estradiol, released from a percutaneous administration form (16[c]). In all, 132 women (88%) were satisfied with the treatment and wanted to have a further intrauterine device inserted at the end of the study. Histological examination of endometrial biopsies from 101 women showed a predominantly inactive endometrium characterized by a pseudodecidual reaction of the endometrial stroma with endometrial atrophy, which is in keeping with the effects seen with progestogens. No specimens showed signs of proliferation. While one can accept this as evidence that the Fibroplant device is an acceptable means of administering levonorgestrel for hormone replacement therapy, one is bound to question the authors' further conclusion that it is less likely than other forms of administration to produce such systemic adverse effects as those involving the breast and cardiovascular system; it is hard to see how this could be so.

Transdermal administration   On current evidence it seems clear that in women with osteoporosis an increase in bone density can be obtained by giving estrogens transdermally in such low doses that there is little risk of endometrial hyperplasia (17[cr]).

HORMONAL CONTRACEPTIVES

(SED-15, 1642 et seq; SEDA-27, 426; SEDA-28, 487; SEDA-29, 499)

Oral contraceptives

Cardiovascular   Much of the evidence on the occurrence of *thromboembolic complications* with oral contraceptives or hormone replacement therapy has been gathered from European or American populations, and it can be helpful to identify data from other parts of the world, where factors such as body weight, climate, or diet could affect the incidence. When a Japanese group sought to obtain national data by mailing questionnaires to a large number of institutes monitoring these forms of treatment, 771 (71%) of 1083 institutes responded (18[M]). Follow-up questionnaires were sent to 39 institutions that reported having experienced in all 53 cases of thromboembolism during hormone therapy; 29 cases related to oral contraceptives and 13 to hormone replacement therapy, while 11 had taken other forms of hormone treatment. Of the 29 patients taking contraceptives, eight had developed arterial thromboembolism (including two with myocardial infarctions).

Nervous system   *Headache* was a prominent complaint during the use of the high-dose combined oral contraceptives that were originally introduced, and it often led users to become discouraged and to abandon the method. A systematic review of published data on the occurrence of headache with the more modest combination products now used has shown little indication that they have a clinically important effect on headache in most women (19[M]). Headache that occurs during early cycles of oral contraceptive use tends to improve or disappear with continued use. No clear evidence supports the common clinical practice of switching from one oral contraceptive to another in the hope of attaining a lower incidence of headache. However, manipulating the extent or duration of estrogen withdrawal during the cycle may provide benefit.

Urinary tract   There has always been some uncertainty as to whether the sporadic reports of *urinary tract infections* among users of hormonal contraceptives reflect an adverse effect or simply a different pattern of sexual behavior among major users of these products. Some have found an increased incidence of urinary infections, others have not. The effect of local estrogens has been explored in a pilot study in 30 young women taking oral contraceptives, mean age 23 years, with a long-standing history of recurrent urinary tract infections (20[c]). Vaginal estrogen therapy consisted of estriol 1 mg/day for 2 weeks and then twice a week for 2 weeks. The patients had a mean history of infection over 2.3 years, while the mean period of oral contraceptive use was 3.2 years. In the follow-up period of 11 months after treatment, 24 of the 30 reported no symptoms of cystitis and used no additional medications. There was normal bladder epithelium at control cystoscopy after estriol in all patients in whom trigonal metaplasia although vulnerable highly vascularized urothelium had been found at the initial investigation. These findings led the authors to conclude that in most young women taking oral contraceptives with a long-standing history of recurrent urinary infections a considerable infection-free period can be achieved after vaginal application of estrogen, perhaps because of improved bladder perfusion. However, they did not provide any new evidence as to whether urinary infections are a significant problem in young users of oral contraceptives.

Skin   Many types of skin reaction have been attributed to hormonal contraceptives, and it is not always clear which component of a product is responsible. However, a recent Japanese report has suggested that *erythema multiforme* may be induced by a product based on a progestogen alone (21[A]).

Male hormonal contraception

Endocrine   Attempts to develop a hormonal contraceptive for men have been in progress for at least 40 years, with only limited success. The most common problems have related to unreliability, slow onset of the effect, and *loss of libido*. It has been postulated that the

addition of dutasteride, a combined inhibitor of
5-alpha-reductase type I and type II, or a long-
acting gonadorelin receptor antagonist (acyline)
to combination testosterone + levonorgestrel
treatment may be advantageous in suppress-
ing spermatogenesis (22[cH]). In a phase I study,
22 men received intramuscular testosterone
enanthate 100 mg weekly for 8 weeks combined with one of the following: (1) oral levonorgestrel 125 micrograms/day; (2) oral levonorgestrel 125 micrograms/day + dutasteride
0.5 mg/day; (3) subcutaneous acyline 300
micrograms/kg every 2 weeks (as a comparator for any additional progestogenic effects);
or (4) oral levonorgestrel 125 micrograms/day
plus subcutaneous acyline 300 micrograms/kg
every 2 weeks. Serum gonadotropin concentrations were suppressed to a similar degree by
all four treatments, falling to nadirs of 1.2–
3.4% for FSH and 0.5–0.8% for LH. Serum
dihydrotestosterone concentrations were significantly reduced by dutasteride to a nadir
of 31% at week 7. There were no significant
differences in sperm concentrations across the
groups.

Sexual function   In the study mentioned above
under Endocrine, there was severe *oligospermia*
(0.1–3 million/ml) or *azoospermia* in none of
five and four of five men taking testosterone +
levonorgestrel; two of six and four of six of
those taking testosterone + levonorgestrel +
dutasteride; two of six and four of six of those
taking testosterone + acyline; and one of five
and three of five of those taking testosterone +
levonorgestrel + acyline. There was one non-
responder each with testosterone + levonorgestrel and testosterone + levonorgestrel +
acyline.

ANTIESTROGENS AND SELECTIVE ESTROGEN RECEPTOR MODULATORS
(SERMS)   *(SEDA-27, 429; SEDA-28, 490; SEDA-29, 502)*

Clomiphene   *(SED-15, 812)*

Teratogenicity   Various older reports suggested that when clomiphene is used to induce

ovulation, which may sometimes result in its
inadvertent use in unsuspected early pregnancy,
the fetus might be adversely affected or that
there might be a change in the sex ratio of the
offspring. In 1995 a US group produced evidence of a possible link between clomiphene
and *hypospadias* in male offspring (23[c]). This
possible link has been further examined in a
case-control study, based on records of 319
cases of hypospadias recorded in four counties of Denmark over 30 years and prescribing records over that time, and a comparable
control group (24[c]). There was no evidence
of a link between clomiphene and hypospadias.

Raloxifene   *(SED-15, 3019; SEDA-29, 503)*

Observational studies   Raloxifene was the
first selective estrogen receptor modulators
(SERMs) to be approved for use in the prevention and treatment of postmenopausal osteoporosis. An extensive literature review has
now provided a useful assessment of the benefit to harm balance of raloxifene (25[R]). The
findings were reassuring. One large fracture
prevention trial provided the best evidence
that raloxifene 60 mg/day for 3 years reduced the relative risk of vertebral fractures
by 30–50% in women with prevalent fractures
or osteoporosis. The extraskeletal effects of
raloxifene include a reduction in total cholesterol and low density lipoprotein cholesterol
concentrations. Raloxifene was not associated
with endometrial hyperplasia, and there was
a 72% reduction in the incidence of invasive
breast cancer. Adverse events associated with
raloxifene included an increase in the absolute
risk of venous thromboembolism and increased
risks of *hot flushes* (flashes) and *leg cramps*.
Compared with other therapies for osteoporosis, raloxifene has a smaller impact on bone
mineral density, a similar effect on the occurrence of vertebral fractures, and no effect
on the frequency of non-vertebral fractures. In
the present state of knowledge it seems clear
that raloxifene can be recommended for prevention of vertebral fractures in women with
osteopenia/osteoporosis who are not at high
risk of non-vertebral fractures and who do

not have a past history of venous thromboembolism.

Tamoxifen   (SED-15, 3296; SEDA-29, 503)

Tamoxifen versus aromatase inhibitors

While tamoxifen is still widely regarded as the standard adjuvant endocrine treatment for postmenopausal women with localized breast cancer, provided it is hormone receptor positive, there are problems with recurrence and adverse effects. Reservations have recently been expressed about the future place of tamoxifen, and the case has been made that it is time to move from tamoxifen to the oral aromatase inhibitors (26^r).

There has been a brief report of some of the results of the ATAC trial (part of the CORE study) in 9366 women, which was designed to continue for 5 years, part of which involved directly comparing tamoxifen with the aromatase inhibitor anastrozole (27^C). The conclusion was that anastrozole should be the preferred treatment in such cases. After a median follow-up of 68 months, anastrozole significantly prolonged disease-free survival (575 events with anastrozole versus 651 with tamoxifen; hazard ratio = 0.87; 95% CI = 0.78, 0.97), prolonged time to recurrence, and significantly reduced distant metastases (324 versus 375) and contralateral breast cancers. There were fewer withdrawals with anastrozole than with tamoxifen, apparently reflecting the fact that anastrozole was also associated with fewer adverse effects (especially gynecological problems and vascular events), although arthralgia and fractures were increased.

The roles of tamoxifen and the aromatase inhibitors as adjuvant therapy for early breast cancer in postmenopausal women have been reviewed, distinguishing three approaches: replacement of tamoxifen as adjuvant therapy for 5 years (early adjuvant therapy); sequencing of tamoxifen before or after an aromatase inhibitor during the first 5 years (early sequential adjuvant therapy); or the use of an aromatase inhibitor after 5 years of tamoxifen (extended adjuvant therapy) (28^R). Briefly, the conclusions were that at the time of the survey there was little to choose between the three methods in terms of the balance of benefit and harm. However, like others, the authors stressed that agents of this type are proving to be superior to tamoxifen in preventing recurrence of the disease.

There may well be a role for combined therapy with both tamoxifen and an aromatase inhibitor if an optimal benefit to harm balance is to be attained, as suggested by a study of a combination of tamoxifen and exemestane for 8 weeks in 33 postmenopausal women with breast cancer (29^c). There was a striking absence of endocrine adverse effects.

Others have suggested that patients be treated for a period with tamoxifen and then switched to anastrozole for follow up. A report on the ABCSG 8 trial and the ARNO 95 trial (both of which were prospective open studies) has provided information on this approach (30^C). Women with hormone-sensitive early breast cancer who had taken adjuvant oral tamoxifen 20 or 30 mg/day for 2 years were randomized to oral anastrozole 1 mg/day (n = 1618) or tamoxifen 20 or 30 mg/day (n = 1606) for the remainder of their adjuvant therapy. At a median follow-up of 28 months, there was a highly significant 40% reduction in the risk of an event with anastrozole compared with tamoxifen (67 versus 110 events; hazard ratio = 0.60; 95% CI = 0.44, 0.81). There were significantly more fractures but significantly fewer case of thrombosis in those who took anastrozole than in those who took tamoxifen. These data lend support to a switch from tamoxifen to anastrozole in patients who have taken adjuvant tamoxifen for 2 years.

Reproductive system   *The unwanted effects of tamoxifen on the endometrium (including induction of fibroids, polyps, and endometrial cancer) have long been of concern, and attempts are now being made to find ways of preventing or reversing these complications, or finding an alternative treatment that does not involve these risks. Again, promising experience with the aromatase inhibitors features prominently in current recommendations.*

In a prospective study in 77 consecutive women with postmenopausal breast cancer scheduled to start endocrine treatment for *breast cancer, using either tamoxifen or an aromatase inhibitor tamoxifen treatment significantly increased endometrial thickness and uterine volume after 3 months (31^c). In additional, tamoxifen induced endometrial cysts and polyps and increased the size of pre-existing fibroids. In contrast, aromatase inhibitors did not stimulate endometrial growth and were not associated with endometrial pathology. Furthermore, they reduced endometrial thickness and uterine volume in patients who had previously taken tamoxifen.*

This study has again confirmed that endometrial problems can be induced by tamoxifen early in the course of treatment; and that these problems do not arise with aromatase inhibitors, which may actually reduce the endometrial changes induced by tamoxifen. The idea that the new oral aromatase inhibitors might well replace tamoxifen in breast cancer was tentatively advanced in SEDA-26 (p. 445) and has now been supported by some of the material cited above, as well as by a panel consensus (32^R). Citing efficacy and safety data on anastrozole, exemestane, and letrozole, the authors concluded that third-generation aromatase inhibitors may be considered first-line therapy of hormone-receptor-positive advanced breast cancer in postmenopausal women and may also be used for preoperative therapy of breast cancer.

Comparative studies   One of the many controversies surrounding the use of tamoxifen in elderly women is whether after lumpectomy it should be accompanied by radiotherapy to potentiate the desired effect. It has been suggested that there is not a great deal of merit in adding radiotherapy to tamoxifen, since radiotherapy plus tamoxifen reduces local recurrence of breast cancer in elderly women compared with tamoxifen alone, but survival rates are not improved and benefits are offset by an increase in adverse effects (33^r).

Cardiovascular   While tamoxifen has often been held responsible for cases of *thrombosis* and *pulmonary embolism*, some such incidents may have been attributable to the primary condition being treated, and the risk must not be over-estimated (34^R).

The effect of tamoxifen 20 mg/day on the incidence of venous thromboembolism has been assessed in a placebo-controlled breast cancer prevention trial for 5 years in 5408 hysterectomized women (35^C). There were 28 incidents of thromboembolism on placebo and 44 on tamoxifen (hazard ratio = 1.63; 95% CI = 1.02, 2.63), 80% of which involved only superficial phlebitis, which accounted for all of the excess due to tamoxifen within 18 months from randomization. Compared with placebo, the risk of venous thromboembolism with tamoxifen was higher in women aged 55 years or older, those with a body mass index of 25 kg/m^2 or more, those with a raised blood pressure or a total cholesterol of 6.50 mmol/l (250 mg/dl) or greater, current smokers, and those with a family history of coronary heart disease, all familiar risk factors for venous complications. Of the 685 women with a coronary heart disease risk score of 5 or greater, one in the placebo arm and 13 in the tamoxifen arm developed venous thromboembolism. In a multivariate regression analysis, age in excess of 60 years, height of 165 cm or more, and a diastolic blood pressure of 90 mmHg or higher all had independent detrimental effects on the risk of venous thromboembolism during tamoxifen therapy, whereas transdermal estrogen therapy concomitant with tamoxifen was not associated with any excess risk (HR = 0.64; 95% CI = 0.23, 1.82). The authors concluded that the increased risk of venous thromboembolism during the use of tamoxifen was largely associated with the well-known risk factors for this condition, and that this information should be part of pre-treatment counselling.

Susceptibility factors

Genetic   Since tamoxifen is metabolized by CYP450 enzymes, including CYP3A5, and bearing in mind two genetic polymorphisms in CYP3A5 (CYP3A5*3 and CYP3A5*6), it has been suggested that the presence of such polymorphisms in some patients might have an effect on the incidence of adverse effects of tamoxifen. However, a recent study seems to have shown that this is not the case—the metabolism and adverse effects of tamoxifen were the same in subjects with these polymorphisms as in other women (36^c).

PROGESTOGENS   *(SED-15, 2930;*
SEDA-27, 433; SEDA-28, 493; SEDA-29, 505)

See *Implantable contraceptives* above.

PROGESTERONE ANTAGONISTS
(SEDA-27, 433; SEDA-28, 494;
SEDA-29, 506)

Observational studies   Various anti-progesto-genic routines for the termination of pregnancy continue to be compared. Of 354 women who were given mifepristone 200 mg in the clinic and then sent home with two tablets of miso-prostol 200 micrograms to take 48 hours later, 324 (91.5%) had a successful termination (37[c]). The most common adverse effects were *pain or cramps* (93%) and *nausea* (67%), followed by *weakness* (55%), *headache* (46%), and *dizzi-ness* (44%). Overall acceptability of the regi-men was high: 63% of women reported that it was "very satisfactory" and another 23% found it "satisfactory". There were no serious compli-cations and the simplified routine, with a much reduced duration of hospital care, was consid-ered acceptable.

Mifepristone   *(SED-15, 2344;*
SEDA-29, 506)

Gastrointestinal   The safety and effective-ness of a combination of mifepristone + miso-prostol in dealing with late uterine death have been studied using two different regimens, each in 20 women (38[c]). In one, misoprostol was ad-ministered both vaginally and orally and in the other it was given only vaginally. There was no difference in the efficacy of the two regi-mens, but oral misoprostol was associated with a higher incidence of gastrointestinal adverse effects.

Pregnancy   When dealing with pre-term rup-ture of the membranes it is important to know the relative safety records of oxytocin alone or oral mifepristone preceding intravenous oxy-tocin, since these are the main therapeutic al-ternatives. In 65 pregnant women with sponta-neous rupture of the membranes at or beyond the 36th week, who were randomly assigned to oxytocin alone or to oral mifepristone 200 mg followed by oxytocin infusion if there had been no induction within 18 hours, the average in-terval from start of induction to delivery was 1194 minutes for mifepristone + oxytocin and 771 minutes for oxytocin given alone (39[c]). Successful induction of labor with vaginal de-livery was achieved within 24 hours in 78% of those who were given mifepristone com-pared with 52% of those given oxytocin alone. However, there was more fetal distress with mifepristone+oxytocin (9 versus 2; RR = 4.36; 95%; CI = 1.02, 19) and a trend toward more cesarean births (7 versus 3; RR = 2.26; 95% CI = 0.64, 7.99). Eleven infants of women who had been given mifepristone (33%) but only three infants of women who had been given oxytocin alone (9.4%) had to be admitted to the neonatal intensive care unit because of a generally poor condition (RR = 3.56; 95% CI = 1.09, 12). The authors concluded that oral mifepristone 18 hours before oxytocin infusion did not improve the stimulation of labor in women with premature rupture of membranes near term and was associated with more adverse fetal outcomes than oxytocin alone.

ANABOLIC STEROIDS, ANDROGENS, AND RELATED COMPOUNDS   *(SED-15, 216;*
SEDA-27, 434; SEDA-28, 495; SEDA-29, 507)

Androgenic anabolic steroids

In earlier volumes in this series we have pointed to the serious doubt that now exists about whether so-called "androgen supplementation" in older men confers benefits that outweigh the potential harms. Much of the evidence adduced to support this treatment, such as an attempt to demonstrate its use as a supportive treatment in depression (40[c]), is also far from convinc-ing. Current evidence of the continuing misuse of anabolic steroids in professional sport is now more readily accessible in the popular me-dia than in medical journals. Whether recent press reports of *cardiomegaly* among profes-sional cyclists reflect an effect of training or the known cardiac effects of anabolic steroids is not clear.

Psychological   In a useful new review of the entire field there is particular reference to the contested evidence on the *behavioral effects* of these compounds (41[R]). The authors observed that certain of these complications, in particular *hypomania* and *increased aggressiveness*, have been confirmed in some, but not all, randomized controlled studies. Epidemiological attempts to determine whether anabolic steroids trigger violent behavior have failed, primarily because of high rates of non-participation. Studies of the use of anabolic steroids in different populations typically report a prevalence of repeated use of 1–5% among adolescents. The symptoms and signs of the use of anabolic steroids seem to be often overlooked by healthcare professionals, and the number of cases of complications is virtually unknown. The authors suggested that future epidemiological research in this area should focus on retrospective case-control studies and perhaps also on prospective cohort studies of populations selected for a high prevalence of anabolic steroid use, rather than large-scale population-based studies.

Oxandrolone

Susceptibility factors

Children   However much the medical use of anabolic steroids may have declined, when these products were introduced in the 1960s there were some seriously documented claims for efficacy in a very few conditions—in the treatment of aplastic anemia and to promote general recovery in victims of severe burns. In these circumstances the tissue-building properties of these compounds were said to promote recovery of tissue, countering the catabolic process that can follow injury or severe illness. This was thought to outweigh the undesired androgenic effects, which were especially marked in women and children. The use of oxandrolone has been restudied in a prospective comparative investigation in 61 children with 40% total body surface area burns (42[C]). They were randomized to receive oral oxandrolone 0.1 mg/kg bd ($n = 30$) or placebo ($n = 31$) for 12 months after the injury. Oxandrolone significantly improved lean body mass, bone mineral content,

and muscle strength. Serum IGF-1, T3 uptake, and free thyroxine index were significantly increased by oxandrolone. There were significant increases in height and weight during and after the end of treatment. A broader view of these problems from burns experts is needed for final assessment. The conclusion regarding effects on height must be regarded with some caution, since androgens can result in early closure of the epiphyses. However, the essential question must be whether recovery was accelerated or rendered more complete.

Testosterone

Placebo-controlled studies   A well-founded indication for the cautious use of androgens in women is to treat those who have much reduced sexual desire after a surgical menopause and are troubled by it. In a 24-week, randomized, double-blind, placebo-controlled, parallel-group, study, 447 women aged 24–70 years were randomized to receive placebo or transdermal testosterone patches in dosages of 150, 300, or 450 micrograms twice weekly, and 318 subjects completed the study (43[C]). There were marginally significant successes in restoring sexual desire and activity, but only in the two higher dose groups. There were no serious safety concerns, but adverse effects were not discussed in detail.

Tumorigenicity   It has been stressed in a recent and very extensive American review that the benefit to harm balance of androgen replacement has still not been adequately examined (44[R]). In an otherwise positive review of this form of treatment, it has been pointed out that androgens are growth factors for pre-existing *prostate cancer* (45[R]). Before therapy is begun, careful digital rectal examination and determination of the serum concentration of prostate-specific antigen (PSA) should be performed, in order to exclude evident or suspected prostate cancer. The first 3–6 months after starting testosterone therapy is the most critical time for monitoring effects on the prostate. It is therefore important to monitor PSA concentrations every 3 months for the first year of treatment; thereafter, regular monitoring during therapy is mandatory, primarily to ensure prostate safety but also with a view to cardiovascular and hematological safety.

In this connection it may also be noted that, following a joint meeting in 2004, the International Society of Andrology, the International Society for the Study of the Aging Male, and the European Association of Urology revised their earlier recommendations on the definition, diagnosis, and management of late onset hypogonadism (46[R]). While by no means rejecting androgen replacement therapy, the recommendations remain cautious and are explicitly intended to be regarded as provisional until larger-scale, long-term studies are available.

A particular reason for caution is the fact that in this age group there will be a fair proportion of subjects at risk of prostate cancer. It is possible that in these subjects testosterone might further increase the risk or actually precipitate the neoplasm. In a review of the medical records of six urology practices, men undergoing testosterone supplementation for sexual dysfunction or "rejuvenation" who were found to have prostate cancer after initiation of exogenous testosterone supplementation were identified (47[c]). Cases were analysed to determine the clinical and pathological parameters that characterized the presentation of prostate cancer. A total of 20 men were found to have prostate cancer after the start of testosterone therapy. Prostate cancer was detected within 2 years in 11 men (55%) and from 28 months to 8 years in the rest. The tumors were of moderate and high grade, being of Gleason sums 6, 7, and 8–10 in nine men (45%), six men (30%), and five men (25%) respectively. The median serum prostate specific antigen (PSA) concentration at diagnosis tended to be low, at 5.1 (range 1.1–329) ng/ml, and digital rectal examination was generally more sensitive than PSA in detecting the cancer. Patients seen by non-urologist physicians were monitored less often for prostate cancer during use of testosterone than those followed by urologists. The authors therefore concluded that prostate cancer may become clinically apparent within months to a few years after the start of testosterone treatment. In their view, physicians who prescribe testosterone supplements and patients who take them should be cognizant of this risk, and serum PSA testing and digital rectal examination should be performed frequently during treatment.

ANTIANDROGENS   *(SEDA-27, 435; SEDA-28, 497; SEDA-29, 510)*

Drug dosage regimens   The difficulty in weighing benefit against harm when selecting a regimen for patients with hormone-refractory prostate carcinoma is compounded by the fact that patients differ markedly in their needs and responses. This is underlined by the outcome of a panel study undertaken by the Society of Urologic Oncology (48[R]). However, its only firm recommendation, after considering all the medicinal alternatives, was that "management strategies should be targeted toward the individual patient".

Androgen suppression therapy is now increasingly being used intermittently in the hope of attaining an adequate effect on prostate cancer with a lower incidence of adverse effects. In a phase II study of this approach, 95 patients with recurrent or metastatic prostate cancer received cyclical 8-month periods of treatment with leuprolide acetate and nilutamide, with intermittent rest periods (49[C]). Recovery periods were progressively lengthened until the treatment failed to achieve normal prostate-specific antigen (PSA) concentrations. The 95 subjects received 245 cycles of treatment. The median duration of rest periods was 8 months and the median time to treatment failure was 47 months. There was testosterone recovery during rest periods in 117 cycles (61%). There was mild anemia in 33, 44, and 67% of cycles 1, 2, and 3 respectively. Sexual function recovered during the rest periods in 47% of cycles. There was no significant overall change in body mass index at the end of the treatment period. Osteoporosis was documented in at least one site, evaluated in 41 patients (37%). The results of this study suggest that intermittent use of androgen suppression has the potential to reduce adverse effects, allowing recovery of the hemoglobin concentration, permitting return of sexual function, and avoiding weight gain.

Bicalutamide

Endocrine   *Thyroid function* has been studied in 183 patients with prostate cancer who were being treated with continuous androgen deprivation therapy; 64 were being treated with a luteinizing hormone-releasing hormone (LHRH) agonist alone and 119 others with an LHRH agonist+bicalutamide 50 mg/day (50[c]). Treatment lasted an average of 43 months. Mean concentrations of T3 and free T4 were very similar to those in a control group of post-surgical patients without medicinal treatment or recurrence. However, the mean TSH concentration was 16 (4.4–120) mU/l in the controls and 18 (1.5–66) mU/l in the treated group, and the serum concentration of TSH was higher than 5 mU/l in six treated patients (2.1%). There was also a mild reduction in the free T4 serum concentration in treated patients. It therefore seems that androgen deprivation therapy with bicalutamide alters some thyroid function tests.

Breasts   In a series of studies from Italy an attempt was made to determine whether giving anastrozole 1 mg/day and/or tamoxifen 20 mg/day could prevent *gynecomastia* and *breast pain* due to bicalutamide 150 mg/day (51[C]). In a 48-week double-blind study tamoxifen reduced the symptoms but anastrozole did not. Longer-term work has to be performed.

Tumorigenicity   Adenocarcinoma of the breast due to flutamide has been reported (SEDA-29, 513). One can now add to this the case of a man taking bicalutamide who developed gynecomastia, which proceeded to *male breast cancer* (52[A]).

℞   *Finasteride*

Finasteride is a selective inhibitor of 5-alpha-reductase. It thereby reduces prostatic concentrations of dihydrotestosterone and so reduces prostatic size (53[R], 54[R], 55[R]). It is therefore used to treat benign prostatic hyperplasia (56[C], 57[R], 58[M], 59[M]) and in the prevention and treatment of prostate cancer (60[R]). It is poorly effective in patients with prostatic obstruction and small prostate glands (61[R]), but in patients with glands larger than 40 ml it produces significant symptomatic improvement.

The ability of finasteride to block the conversion of testosterone to dihydrotestosterone also makes it useful in both male-pattern baldness (62[R]) and hirsutism related to hyperandrogenism (for example, in polycystic ovary syndrome) in women (63[M]).

Many of the problems seen with finasteride have undoubtedly been due to its use in unnecessarily high doses. Particularly when it is used for cosmetic purposes there has been doubt as to how far dosages can be reduced while maintaining acceptable effects. Long-term information on its safety in women with hirsutism is sparse, and in principle it might adversely affect an unborn child (63[R]). The dose should certainly be kept as low as possible.

Observational studies

Prostate cancer   The effect of adding finasteride 5 mg/day to high-dose bicalutamide 150 mg/day has been studied in 41 men with advanced prostate cancer treated over a mean of 3.9 years (64[C]). The serum prostate-specific antigen (PSA) concentration was measured every 2 weeks until disease progression. At the first nadir of PSA, the median fall from baseline was 96.5%; a second nadir occurred in 30 of 41 patients, with a median fall of 98.5% from baseline. The median times to each nadir were 3.7 and 5.8 weeks respectively. The median time to treatment failure was 21 months. Adverse effects were minor, including gynecomastia. Sex drive was normal in 17 of 29 men at baseline and in 12 of 24 men at the second PSA nadir, but one-third of the men had spontaneous erections at both times. The authors concluded that finasteride provided additional intracellular androgen blockade when added to bicalutamide. The duration of control was comparable to that achieved with castration, with preserved sexual function in some patients.

Hirsutism   In women with hirsutism low doses of finasteride (2.5 mg/day) are generally well tolerated (65[R]). However, in a randomized study in 38 hirsute women finasteride 2.5 mg every 3 days was as effective as 2.5 mg/day and better tolerated (66[C]).

Comparative studies

Benign prostatic hyperplasia   The benefit of combining an alpha-adrenoceptor antagonist with a 5-alpha-reductase inhibitor has been assessed in men with benign prostatic hyperplasia (67[C]). Modified-release alfuzosin was more effective than finasteride, with no additional benefit in combining the drugs. The adverse effects

Table 1. *Adverse effects of finasteride with or without dibenyline in benign prostatic hyperplasia (68^C)*

Adverse effect	Fina-steride (%)	Dibeny-line (%)	Combi-nation (%)
Light-headedness	1.9	25	19
Nasal stuffiness	–	9.9	11
Impotence	9.3	17	17

of alpha-blockade were postural hypotension, hypotension, headache, dizziness, and malaise; the adverse effects of finasteride were ejaculatory disorders and impotence.

The therapeutic and adverse effects of dibenyline, finasteride, and a combination of the two in 190 patients with symptomatic benign prostatic hyperplasia have been evaluated (68^C). Adverse effects were more common with dibenyline than with finasteride alone or in combination with dibenyline. The drop-out rate was higher with dibenyline (16%) reported adverse effects are listed in Table 1.

In short-term studies the herbal preparation saw palmetto (Serenoa repens) and finasteride seem to give a similar degree of relief in benign prostatic hyperplasia (69^C). However, in a prospective 1-year comparative randomized trial in 64 men with category III prostatitis or chronic pelvic pain syndrome, in which finasteride 5 mg/day was compared with saw palmetto 325 mg/day, the mean NIH Chronic Prostatitis Symptom Index score fell from 24 to 18 with finasteride, but scarcely or not at all with saw palmetto (70^C). Adverse events included headache (n = 3) with saw palmetto and reduced libido (n = 2) with finasteride. Although one might envisage even more prolonged studies, these findings hardly suggest that saw palmetto is a serious replacement for finasteride, even though it is well tolerated.

Male-pattern baldness   In an open study in male-pattern baldness in 90 men, oral finasteride (1 mg/day for 12 months; n = 65) was compared with 5% topical minoxidil solution twice daily (n = 25); the cure rates were 80 and 52% respectively (71^c). The adverse effects were all mild and did not lead to withdrawal of treatment. Of the 65 men who took oral finasteride, six had loss of libido and one had an increase in body hair at other

sites. There was irritation of the scalp in one of those who used minoxidil. These adverse events disappeared as soon as the treatment was withdrawn. The laboratory data did not show any statistically or clinically significant changes from baseline values to the end point, except for the serum total testosterone concentration, which was increased, and free testosterone and serum prostate-specific antigen in the finasteride group, which were reduced from baseline.

Polycystic ovary syndrome   In 44 women with polycystic ovary syndrome treated with finasteride or flutamide for 6 months the adverse effects of flutamide were reduced libido, gastrointestinal disorders, and dry skin (72^C). Finasteride caused reduced libido, headache, and dry skin. Dry skin was reported in 68% of users of flutamide and in only 27% of users of finasteride.

Placebo-controlled studies

Benign prostatic hyperplasia   The effects of finasteride and placebo on quality of life have been evaluated for 12 months in a diverse population of 2342 men with benign prostatic hyperplasia (73^C). Symptom scores fell significantly at month 3 in those taking finasteride and continued to improve throughout the study. The incidence of drug-related sexual adverse experiences was significantly higher in the finasteride group, but led to withdrawal in only 1.5% of patients.

Prostate cancer   In 9060 men who had participated in the randomized, placebo-controlled Prostate Cancer Prevention Trial in the USA for 7 years, finasteride 5 mg/day either prevented or delayed the appearance of prostate cancer, with an overall reduction in cancer incidence of 25% (74^C). However, of the 757 tumors that occurred with finasteride, no less than 37% were classified as relatively malignant (Gleason grades 7, 8, 9, or 10), whereas in the placebo group of 1068 tumors only 22% received this grading. The absolute number of high-grade tumors was also rather higher in the finasteride group (n = 280) than in the placebo group (n = 237). Sexual adverse effects (reduced volume of ejaculate, erectile dysfunction, loss of libido, gynecomastia) were also significantly more common in the treated group than in those taking placebo, but in the finasteride group urinary problems, such as prostatic hyperplasia or problems with micturition, were markedly reduced. The authors suggested that "physicians can use these results to counsel men regarding the use of finasteride" but it is hard to see that it provides a simple choice.

Male-pattern baldness   *In an unusual study, finasteride 1 mg/day was used for 1 year to treat male-pattern baldness in nine subjects; each had an identical twin who received placebo (75^c). Finasteride significantly improved hair growth. There were no drug-related adverse events, either clinical or biochemical.*

Of 1553 men with male-pattern baldness who took finasteride 1 mg/day, all of whom had initially taken part in one of two 1-year placebo-controlled studies, 1215 continued into further controlled studies over another 4 years (76^C). There was durable improvement in scalp hair over 5 years and no new safety concerns were identified.

Hirsutism   *The effects of finasteride for 9 months on hirsutism and serum concentrations of basal gonadotropins, androgens, estrogen, and sex hormone-binding globulin have been studied in 18 women with idiopathic hirsutism (77^C). Nine took oral finasteride 7.5 mg/day and the other nine took placebo. Hirsutism improved significantly with finasteride after 6 and 9 months; placebo had no significant effect. Adverse effects were headache and modest depression during the first month. Libido did not change. Hirsute patients who took finasteride had a marked fall in dihydrotestosterone from the third month and a significant increase in serum testosterone concentrations from the sixth month of treatment.*

Cardiovascular   *The long-term effects and adverse effects of finasteride have been studied in a multicenter study of 3270 men (78^C). There was a background history of cardiovascular disease in 40% of the patients at baseline, and myocardial infarction was reported in 1.5% of those who took finasteride and 0.5% of those who took placebo, a significant difference.*

Sensory systems   *Cataract has been associated with finasteride therapy (79^A).*

- *A 43-year-old man developed impaired vision in both eyes over 3 months. Anterior subcapsular opacities were found in both eyes, necessitating cataract extraction. He had been taking finasteride 1 mg/day for 3 years to treat the early stage of male-pattern baldness.*

Endocrine   *In men finasteride had no affect on serum concentrations of luteinizing hormone, follicle-stimulating hormone, cortisol, or estradiol (80^C). In women finasteride had no effect on basal and gonadorelin-stimulated gonadotropin secretion, the pulsatility of luteinizing hormone secretion, or the concentrations of estradiol, prolactin, free testosterone, androstenedione, dehydroepiandrosterone sulfate, or sex hormone-binding globulin; there were significant reductions in plasma concentrations of cortisol, dihydrotestosterone, and 3-alpha-androstanediol glucuronide (81^C).*

Metabolism   *In men finasteride did not affect serum lipids, including total cholesterol, low density lipoproteins, high density lipoproteins, or triglycerides (80^C).*

Pancreas   *The incidence of acute pancreatitis as a suspected complication of finasteride treatment has been examined in a case-control study in a Danish regional population of 490 000 over 7 years (82^M). Of 302 men aged 60 and older with incident acute pancreatitis, three had been exposed to finasteride; of 2994 controls 37 had been exposed. After adjusting for alcohol-related diseases, gallstone disease, hyperlipidemia, hypercalcemia, and hyperparathyroidism, the authors found no evidence of an increased risk of acute pancreatitis in users of finasteride.*

Musculoskeletal   *Reversible severe myopathy during treatment with finasteride has been described in a 70-year-old man (83^A).*

Sexual function   *The main adverse effects associated with finasteride are loss of libido, erectile dysfunction, and reduced ejaculate volume. At an oral dose of 1 mg/day finasteride has no major adverse effects on measures of semen production or quality (84^R), although it can cause a slight reduction in the volume of ejaculate (62^R).*

In clinical trials 4.4% of patients taking finasteride and 2.2% of patients taking placebo experience sexual adverse effects. However, there is evidence that sexual adverse effects are less common in practice. In a multicenter questionnaire study of 186 Italian patients with androgenetic alopecia sexual adverse effects occurred in under 0.5% of subjects, as judged by the five-item International Index of Erectile Function; there was no adverse effect on erection after 4–6 months, making this an adverse effect of intermediate time course (85[c]).

There is a higher incidence of impaired sexual function in men who take finasteride compared with placebo (86[C], 87[C]) and there are reports of reduced libido (62[R], 88[r]). The incidence of erectile dysfunction has been estimated at 5% (89[R]), but it is difficult to estimate, since in many users of the drug other causes are present, including advanced age, heart disease, diabetes, hypertension, smoking, and hypercholesterolemia. Benign prostatic hyperplasia itself can also aggravate or even induce erectile dysfunction. A questionnaire study in New Jersey suggested that such pathological factors have a greater role in inducing erectile dysfunction than drugs such as finasteride and alpha-adrenoceptor antagonists, although the latter can clearly contribute (90[c]).

The long-term efficacy and safety of finasteride have been studied in 102 patients with benign prostatic hyperplasia (91[C]). Adverse experiences due to sexual dysfunction continued throughout the study, but the low continuous dropout rate may have reflected a natural process in this aged population, and not necessarily a drug-related effect.

The incidence and nature of adverse effects of finasteride on sexual function have been documented in The Proscar Long-term Efficacy and Safety Study (PLESS), a 4-year, randomized, double-blind, placebo-controlled trial in 3040 men, all of whom took finasteride 5 mg/day (92[C]). At screening, 46% of all the patients reported some history of sexual dysfunction. During the first year of the study, 15% of the finasteride-treated patients and 7% of the placebo-treated patients had sexual adverse events that were considered to be drug-related; during years 2–4 there was no between-group difference in the incidence of new sexual adverse events (7% in each group). Sexual adverse events resolved during continued therapy in 12% of those taking finasteride and 19% of those taking placebo.

In a long-term multicenter study of finasteride in 3270 men the numbers of serious adverse events and withdrawals because of adverse events were significantly higher with placebo (78[C]). Drug-related adverse effects in 1% or more of patients were reduced libido, ejaculation disorders, and impotence. A total of 273 patients, 165 (10%) taking finasteride and 108 (7%) taking placebo, reported a sexual adverse event during the treatment period, including change in libido, ejaculation disorders, impotence, or orgasmic dysfunction.

The effects of finasteride (n = 545), tamsulosin, or the proprietary herbal remedy Permison on sexual function have been studied in patients with lower urinary tract symptoms due to benign prostatic hyperplasia (93[c]). At 6 months tamsulosin and finasteride caused slight increases in sexual disorders and Permixon caused a slight improvement. Ejaculation disorders were the most frequently reported adverse effects after tamsulosin or finasteride.

Reproductive system   Of 65 women with idiopathic hirsutism who took either finasteride 5 mg/day or the long-acting gonadorelin agonist leuprorelin (3.75 mg monthly as an intramuscular depot), none had either menstrual abnormalities or other adverse effects (94[C]). However, adequate doses may not have been used, since the hirsutism score improved in only 36% of the patients who took leuprorelin and 14% of those who took finasteride. Serum concentrations of total testosterone, free testosterone, androstenedione, and dehydroepiandrosterone fell in patients treated with leuprorelin, but only serum total testosterone and free testosterone concentrations fell significantly with finasteride.

Breasts   Reversible painful gynecomastia has been reported as an adverse effect of finasteride in a dose as low as 1 mg/day (95[C]); it can be unilateral (96[Ar]) or bilateral (97[A]).

• A 23-year-old man who was taking finasteride 1 mg/day for 2 months for androgenetic alopecia developed painful enlargement of his right breast (98[A]). Treatment was withdrawn and resolution occurred after 2 months.

However, breast cancer can be misdiagnosed as benign gynecomastia (see below).

Tumorigenicity   *Striking evidence of the association of finasteride with male breast cancer comes from the Medical Therapy of Prostatic Symptoms (MTOPS) study, a National Institutes of Health (NIH)-sponsored comparison of finasteride, doxazosin, and the combination for the treatment of benign prostatic hyperplasia in about 3000 men. The rate of breast cancer among men who took finasteride either alone or with doxazosin was four in 1554, or nearly 200 times that of the general population; one man in the finasteride + doxazosin group and three in the finasteride-alone group developed male breast cancer (99^{cr}).*

- *A 53-year-old man developed unilateral gynecomastia following finasteride therapy for alopecia (100^A). On needle biopsy the mammary mass was diagnosed as adenocarcinoma on the basis of nuclear atypia and particularly because of cytoplasmic vacuolization, but excision biopsy showed only benign gynecomastia with no evidence of malignant change.*

Susceptibility factors

Age   *In 3040 men with benign prostatic hyperplasia the effects of finasteride 5 mg/day for 4 years were studied in those over and under 65 years (101^C). In both groups the drug was effective and there were no significant differences in cardiovascular adverse events between placebo and finasteride. There were significant differences between placebo and finasteride in the overall incidence of typical drug-related adverse events, but there were no specific differences associated with age. The principal events were impotence (8.8%), reduced libido (6.8%), reduced volume of ejaculate (3.5%), other disorders of ejaculation (1.5%), rash (0.6%), breast enlargement (0.5%), and breast tenderness (0.2%).*

Drug–drug interactions   *An interaction of finasteride with sibutramine has been described (102^A).*

- *A 30-year man who was being successfully treated for obesity with sibutramine started to take finasteride to treat alopecia. Soon afterwards he developed paranoid psychotic behavior. The reaction abated and disappeared when finasteride was withdrawn.*

The suggested mechanism of this interaction was that finasteride inhibited the hepatic metabolism of sibutramine, which then displaced finasteride from its plasma protein binding sites; inhibition of 5HT (serotonin) and noradrenaline reuptake by sibutramine then triggering the psychotic event.

Interference with diagnostic routines   *Finasteride reduces serum prostate-specific antigen concentrations (84^R, 89^R). In participants in the Prostate Cancer Prevention Trial who had an end of study biopsy (928 with cancer and 8620 with a negative biopsy) or an interim diagnosis of prostate cancer (n = 671) those who took finasteride had a median fall in PSA of 2% after year 1, while the controls had an increase of 3% (103^A). By the end of the study PSA had increased annually by 6% (placebo) and 7% (finasteride). In those with interim diagnoses PSA increased by 11% (placebo) and 15% (finasteride) each year before diagnosis. Cases with high grade disease (Gleason 7 and above) had greater increases in PSA than cases with low grade disease. The authors concluded that in men who have taken finasteride for more than 1 year the PSA concentration will need to be adjusted to determine whether it is in the reference range. In the Prostate Cancer Prevention Trial the adjustment factor required to preserve a median PSA concentration increased from 2 at 24 months to 2.5 at 7 years after the start of finasteride treatment.*

Flutamide   *(SED-15, 1427; SEDA-29, 513)*

Metabolism   A marked *rise in blood glucose concentration* must be a very rare effect of antiandrogen therapy, but a Japanese group has described two patients with prostate cancer with this complication (104^A).

- A 61-year-old man with a 7-year history of diabetes, well-controlled with diet and acarbose, developed prostate cancer and was given leuprorelin acetate and flutamide. After the second injection of leuprorelin his fasting glucose and hemoglobin A$_{1c}$ concentrations were markedly raised (23 mmol/l and 11% respectively).
- An 81-year-old man with no history of diabetes developed diabetes mellitus after using leuprorelin for prostate carcinoma for 6 months. His fasting glucose was 19 mmol/l and his HbA$_{1c}$ was 9.9%.

In both cases the blood glucose concentration was successfully corrected with a brief course of insulin and was thereafter maintained in the reference range using pioglitazone. This is encouraging, but the toxicity of pioglitazone must surely be borne in mind (see Chapter 42), especially in this type of elderly patient.

Liver Flutamide causes hepatotoxicity in some 0.36% of patients, and for this reason alone it should not be used in the absence of a serious indication. Whether bulimia nervosa in women justifies its use is open to doubt, since non-pharmacological methods of treatment are available. Furthermore, bulimia nervosa in women can be associated with raised serum testosterone concentrations. In a small double-blind study of the use of flutamide, citalopram, a combination of the two, or placebo in 31 women over 3 months, all the active treatments reduced the tendency to binge eating (105ᶜ). However, there was a moderate and reversible *increase in serum transaminase activities*, leading to withdrawal in two of the 19 subjects who were taking flutamide either alone or in combination.

MISCELLANEOUS COMPOUNDS

Tibolone *(SEDA-27, 437; SEDA-28, 499; SEDA-29, 514)*

Placebo-controlled studies Despite the still uncertain adverse effects profile of tibolone, it continues to be used in relieving the hot flushes caused by anti-estrogen therapy, and does so in doses that cause no additional problems. In a further double-blind, placebo-controlled study of oral tibolone 2.5 mg/day in 70 postmenopausal women taking tamoxifen after breast cancer surgery tibolone reduced the severity of hot flushes and perhaps also their incidence (106ᶜ).

References

1. Shapiro BS, Daneshmand ST, Garner FC, Aguirre M, Ross R, Morris S. Effects of the ovulatory serum concentration of human chorionic gonadotropin on the incidence of ovarian hyperstimulation syndrome and success rates for in vitro fertilization. Fert Steril 2005;84:93–8.
2. Van Wely M, Andersen CY, Bayram N, Van Der Veen F. Urofollitropin and ovulation induction. Treatm Endocrin 2005;4:155–65.
3. Tur R, Barri PN, Coroleu B, Buxaderas R, Parera N, Balasch J. Use of a prediction model for high-order multiple implantation after ovarian stimulation with gonadotropins. Fert Steril 2005;83:116–21.
4. Bland LB, Garzotto M, DeLoughery TG, Ryan CW, Schuff KG, Wersinger EM, Lemmon D, Beer TM. Phase II study of transdermal estradiol in androgen-independent prostate carcinoma. Cancer 2005;103:717–23.
5. Corrado F, D'Anna R, Caputo F, Cannata ML, Zoccali MG, Cancellieri F. Compliance with hormone replacement therapy in postmenopausal Sicilian women. Eur J Obstet Gynecol Reprod Biol 2005;118:225–8.
6. Mackey RH, Kuller LH, Sutton-Tyrrell K, Evans RW, Holubkov R, Matthews KA. Hormone therapy, lipoprotein subclasses, and coronary calcification: The Healthy Women Study. Arch Int Med 2005;165:510–5.
7. Gokce M, Karahan B, Yilmaz R, Orem C, Erdol C, Ozdemir S. Long term effects of hormone replacement therapy on heart rate variability, QT interval, QT dispersion and frequencies of arrhythmia. Int J Cardiol 2005;99:373–9.
8. Wihlback A-C, Nyberg S, Backstrom T, Bixo M, Sundstrom-Poromaa I. Estradiol and the addition of progesterone increase the sensitivity to a neurosteroid in postmenopausal women. Psychoneuroendocrinology 2005;30:38–50.
9. Oliveira RLS, Aldrighi JM, Gebara OE, Rocha TRF, D'Amico E, Rosano GMC, Ramires JAF. Postmenopausal hormone replacement therapy increases plasmatic thromboxane beta2. Int J Cardiol 2005;99:449–54.
10. Sumino H, Ichikawa S, Sawada Y, Sakamoto H, Kumakura H, Takayama Y, Sakamaki T, Kurabayashi M. Effects of hormone replacement therapy on blood coagulation and fibrinolysis in hypertensive and normotensive postmenopausal women. Thromb Res 2005;115:359–66.

11. Hendrix SL, Cochrane BB, Nygaard IE, Handa VL, Barnabei VM, Iglesia C, Aragaki A, Naughton MJ, Wallace RB, McNeeley SG, Waetjen LE. Estrogen therapy increased the incidence and severity of urinary incontinence symptoms in postmenopausal women. Evid Based Obstet Gynec 2005;7:149–50.

12. Fournier A, Berrino F, Riboli E, Avenel V, Clavel-Chapelon F. Breast cancer risk in relation to different types of hormone replacement therapy in the E3N-EPIC cohort. Int J Cancer 2005;114:448–54.

13. Coombs NJ, Taylor R, Wilcken N, Boyages J. HRT and breast cancer: impact on population risk and incidence. Eur J Cancer 2005;41:1775–8.

14. Horn L-C, Dietel M, Einenkel J. Hormone replacement therapy (HRT) and endometrial morphology under consideration of the different molecular pathways in endometrial carcinogenesis. Eur J Obstr Gynec Reprod Biol 2005;122:4–12.

15. Koninckx PR, Spielmann D. A comparative 2-year study of the effects of sequential regimens of 1 mg 17-beta-estradiol and trimegestone with a regimen containing estradiol valerate and norethisterone on the bleeding profile and endometrial safety in postmenopausal women. Gynecol Endocrinol 2005;21:82–9.

16. Wildemeersch D, Janssens D, Schacht E, Pylyser K, De Wever N. Intrauterine levonorgestrel delivered by a frameless system, combined with systemic estrogen: acceptability and endometrial safety after 3 years of use in peri- and postmenopausal women. Gynecol Endocrinol 2005;20:336–42.

17. Ettinger B, Ensrud KE, Wallace R, Johnson KC, Cummings SR, Yankov V, Vittinghoff E, Grady D, Ravn P. Ultralow-dose transdermal estradiol increased bone mineral density, with a low rate of endometrial hyperplasia. Evid Based Obstet Gynecol 2005;7:162–3.

18. Adachi T, Sakamoto S. Thromboembolism during hormone therapy in Japanese women. Sem Thromb Hemostas 2005;31:272–80.

19. Loder EW, Buse DC, Golub JR. Headache as a side effect of combination estrogen-progestin oral contraceptives: a systematic review. Am J Obstet Gynecol 2005;193:636–49.

20. Pinggera G-M, Feuchtner G, Frauscher F, Rehder P, Strasser H, Bartsch G, Herwig R. Effects of local estrogen therapy on recurrent urinary tract infections in young females under oral contraceptives. Eur Urol 2005;47:243–9.

21. Suzuki R, Matsumura Y, Kambe N, Fujii H, Tachibana T, Miyachi Y. Erythema multiforme due to progesterone in a low-dose oral contraceptive pill. Br J Dermatol 2005;152:370–1.

22. Matthiesson KL, Amory JK, Berger R, Ugoni A, McLachlan RI, Bremner WJ. Novel male hormonal contraceptive combinations: the hormonal and spermatogenic effects of testosterone and levonorgestrel combined with a 5alpha-reductase inhibitor or gonadotropin-releasing hormone antagonist. J Clin Endocrinol Metab 2005;90:91–7.

23. Wilcox AJ, Baird DD, Weinberg CR, Hornsby PP, Herbst AL. Fertility in men exposed prenatally to diethylstilbestrol. N Engl J Med 1995;332:1411–6.

24. Sorensen HT, Pedersen L, Skriver MV, Norgaard M, Norgard B, Hatch EE. Use of clomifene during early pregnancy and risk of hypospadias: population based case-control study. BMJ 2005;330:126–7.

25. Cranney A, Adachi JD. Benefit-risk assessment of raloxifene in postmenopausal osteoporosis. Drug Saf 2005;28:721–30.

26. Fricker J. Letrozole better than tamoxifen in postmenopausal women. Lancet Oncol 2005;6:247.

27. Bradbury J. Results of the ATAC (Arimidex, Tamoxifen, Alone or in Combination) trial after completion of 5 years' adjuvant treatment for breast cancer. Lancet 2005;365:60–2.

28. Mouridsen HT, Robert NJ. The role of aromatase inhibitors as adjuvant therapy for early breast cancer in postmenopausal women. Eur J Cancer 2005;41:1678–89.

29. Love RR, Hutson PR, Havighurst TC, Cleary JF. Endocrine effects of tamoxifen plus exemestane in postmenopausal women with breast cancer. Clin Cancer Res 2005;11:1500–3.

30. Jakesz R, Jonat W, Gnant M, Mittlboeck M, Greil R, Tausch C, Hilfrich J, Kwasny W, Menzel C, Samonigg H, Seifert M, Gademann G, Kaufmann M. Switching of postmenopausal women with endocrine-responsive early breast cancer to anastrozole after 2 years' adjuvant tamoxifen. Combined results of ABCSG trial 8 and the ARNO 95 trial. Lancet 2005;366:455–62.

31. Morales L, Timmerman D, Neven P, Konstantinovic ML, Carbonez A, Van Huffel S, Ameye L, Weltens C, Christiaens MR, Vergote I, Paridaens R. Third generation aromatase inhibitors may prevent endometrial growth and reverse tamoxifen-induced uterine changes in postmenopausal breast cancer patients. Ann Oncol 2005;16:70–4.

32. Joensuu H, Ejlertsen B, Lonning PE, Rutqvist L-E. Aromatase inhibitors in the treatment of early and advanced breast cancer. Acta Oncol 2005;44:23–31.

33. Anonymous. After lumpectomy, overall survival is similar with tamoxifen alone compared with tamoxifen plus radiotherapy in elderly women with early stage breast cancer. Evid Based Health Care 2005;9:79–80.

34. Goldhaber SZ. Tamoxifen: Preventing breast cancer and placing the risk of deep vein thrombosis in perspective. Circulation 2005;111:539–41.

35. Decensi A, Maisonneuve P, Rotmensz N, Bettega D, Costa A, Sacchini V, Salvioni A, Travaglini R, Oliviero P, D'Aiuto G, Gulisano M, Gucciardo G, Del Turco MR, Pizzichetta MA, Conforti S, Bonanni B, Boyle P, Veronesi U. Effect of tamoxifen on venous thromboembolic events in a breast cancer prevention trial. Circulation 2005;111:650–6.

36. Tucker AN, Tkaczuk KA, Lewis LM, Tomic D, Lim CK, Flaws JA. Management of late intrauterine death using a combination of mifepristone and misoprostol—experience of two regimens. Cancer Lett 2005;217:61–72.

37. Shannon CS, Winikoff B, Hausknecht R, Schaff E, Blumenthal PD, Oyer D, Sankey H, Wolff J, Goldberg R. Multicenter trial of a simplified mifepristone medical abortion regimen. Obstet Gynecol 2005;105:345–51.

38. Fairley TE, Mackenzie M, Owen P, Mackenzie F. Management of late intrauterine death using a combination of mifepristone and misoprostol—experience of two regimens. Eur J Obstet Gynecol 2005;118:28–31.

39. Wing DA, Guberman C, Fassett M. A randomized comparison of oral mifepristone to intravenous oxytocin for labor induction in women with prelabor rupture of membranes beyond 36 weeks' gestation. Am J Obst Gynecol 2005;192:445–51.

40. Orengo CA, Fullerton L, Kunik ME. Safety and efficacy of testosterone gel 1% augmentation in depressed men with partial response to antidepressant therapy. J Geriat Psychiatry Neurol 2005;18:20–4.

41. Thiblin I, Petersson A. Pharmacoepidemiology of anabolic androgenic steroids: a review. Fundam Clin Pharmacol 2005;19:27–44.

42. Przkora R, Jeschke MG, Barrow RE, Suman OE, Meyer WJ, Finnerty CC, Sanford AP, Lee J, Chinkes DL, Mlcak RP, Herndon DN, Pruitt Jr BA, Gamelli RL. Metabolic and hormonal changes of severely burned children receiving long-term oxandrolone treatment. Ann Surg 2005;242:384–91.

43. Braunstein GD, Sundwall DA, Katz M, Shifren JL, Buster JE, Simon JA, Bachman G, Aguirre OA, Lucas JD, Rodenberg C, Buch A, Watts NB. Safety and efficacy of a testosterone patch for the treatment of hypoactive sexual desire disorder in surgically menopausal women: a randomized, placebo-controlled trial. Arch Intern Med 2005;165:1582–9.

44. Hijazi RA, Cunningham GR. Andropause: is androgen replacement therapy indicated for the aging male? Ann Rev Med 2005;56:117–37.

45. Ebert T, Jockenhovel F, Morales A, Shabsigh R. The current status of therapy for symptomatic late-onset hypogonadism with transdermal testosterone gel. Eur Urol 2005;47:137–46.

46. Lunenfeld B, Saad F, Hoesl CE. ISA, ISSAM and EAU recommendations for the investigation, treatment and monitoring of late-onset hypogonadism in males: scientific background and rationale. Aging Male 2005;8:59–74.

47. Gaylis FD, Lin DW, Ignatoff JM, Amling CL, Tutrone RF, Cosgrove DJ. Prostate cancer in men using testosterone supplementation. J Urol 2005;174:534–8.

48. Chang SS, Benson MC, Campbell SC, Crook J, Dreicer R, Evans CP, Hall MC, Higano C, Kelly WK, Sartor O, Smith Jr JA. Society of Urologic Oncology position statement. Redefining the management of hormone-refractory prostate carcinoma. Cancer 2005;103:11–21.

49. Malone S, Perry G, Segal R, Dahrouge S, Crook J. Long-term side-effects of intermittent androgen suppression therapy in prostate cancer. Results of a phase II study. BJU Int 2005;96:514–20.

50. Morote J, Esquena S, Orsola A, Salvador C, Trilla E, Cecchini L, Raventos CX, Planas J, Catalan R, Reventos J. Effect of androgen deprivation therapy in the thyroid function test of patients with prostate cancer. Anti-Cancer Drugs 2005;16:863–6.

51. Boccardo F, Rubagotti A, Battaglia M, Di Tonno P, Selvaggi FP, Conti G, Comeri G, Bertaccini A, Martorana G, Galassi P, Zattoni F, Macchiarella A, Siragusa A, Muscas G, Durand F, Potenzoni D, Manganelli A, Ferraris V, Montefiore F, Trump DL. Evaluation of tamoxifen and anastrozole in the prevention of gynecomastia and breast pain induced by bicalutamide monotherapy of prostate cancer. Urol Oncol 2005;23:377.

52. Chianakwalam CI, McCahy P, Griffiths NJ. A case of male breast cancer in association with bicalutamide-induced gynaecomastia. Breast 2005;14:163–4.

53. Peters DH, Sorkin EM. Finasteride. A review of its potential in the treatment of benign prostatic hyperplasia. Drugs 1993;46(1):177–208.

54. Steiner JF. Finasteride: a 5 alpha-reductase inhibitor. Clin Pharm 1993;12(1):15–23.

55. Steiner JF. Clinical pharmacokinetics and pharmacodynamics of finasteride. Clin Pharmacokinet 1996;30(1):16–27.

56. Nickel JC, Fradet Y, Boake C, Pommerville PJ, Perreault J-P, Afridi SK, Elhilali MM, Barr RE, Beland GA, Bertrand PE, et al. Efficacy and safety of finasteride therapy for benign prostatic hyperplasia; results of a 2-year randomized controlled trial (the PROSPECT study). Can Med Assoc J 1996;155:1251–9.

57. Nickel JC. Long-term implications of medical therapy on benign prostatic hyperplasia end points. Urology 1998;51(Suppl A):50–7.

58. Edwards JE, Moore RA. Finasteride in the treatment of clinical benign prostatic hyperplasia: a systematic review of randomised trials. BMC Urol 2002;2:14.

59. Jimenez Cruz JF, Quecedo Gutierrez L, Del Llano Senaris J. Finasterida. Diez anos de uso clinico. Revision sistematica de la literatura. Actas Urol Esp 2003;27:202–15.

60. Reddy GK. Finasteride, a selective 5-alpha-reductase inhibitor, in the prevention and treatment of human prostate cancer. Clin Prostate Cancer 2004;2(4):206–8.

61. Ekman P. A risk-benefit assessment of treatment with finasteride in benign prostatic hyperplasia. Drug Saf 1998;18:161–70.

62. Libecco JF, Bergfeld WF. Finasteride in the treatment of alopecia. Expert Opin Pharmacother 2004;5(4):933–40.

63. Townsend KA, Marlowe KF. Relative safety and efficacy of finasteride for treatment of hirsutism. Ann Pharmacother 2004;38(6):1070–3.

64. Tay M-H, Kaufman DS, Regan MM, Leibowitz SB, George DJ, Febbo PG, Manola J, Smith MR, Kaplan ID, Kantoff PW, Oh WK. Finasteride and bicalutamide as primary hormonal therapy in patients with advanced adenocarcinoma of the prostate. Ann Oncol 2004;15:974–8.

65. Bayram F, Muderris I, Guven M, Ozcelik B, Kelestimur F. Low-dose (2.5 mg/day) finasteride treatment in hirsutism. Gynecol Endocrinol 2003;17:419–22.

66. Tartagni M, Schonauer MM, Cicinelli E, Petruzzelli F, De Pergola G, De Salvia MA, Loverro G. Intermittent low-dose finasteride is as effective as daily administration for the treatment of hirsute women. Fertil Steril 2004;82:752–5.

67. De Bruyne FMJ, Jardin A, Colloi D, Resel L, Witjes WPJ, Delauche-Cavallier MC, McCarthy C, Geffriaud-Ricouard C. Sustained release alfuzosin, finasteride and the combination of both in the treatment of benign prostatic hyperplasia. Eur Urol 1998;34:169–75.

68. Kuo HC. Comparative study for therapeutic effect of dibenyline, finasteride and combination drugs for symptomatic benign prostatic hyperplasia. Urol Int 1998;60:85–91.

69. Carraro JC, Raynaud JP, Koch G, Chisholm GD, Di Silverio F, Teillac P, Da Silva FC, Cauquil J, Chopin DK, Hamdy FC, Hanus M, Hauri D, Kalinteris A, Marencak J, Perier A, Perrin P. Comparison of phytotherapy (Permixon) with finasteride in the treatment of benign prostate hyperplasia: a randomized international study of 1098 patients. Prostate 1996;29(4):231–40.

70. Kaplan SA, Volpe MA, Te AE. A prospective 1-year trial using saw palmetto versus finasteride in the treatment of category III prostatitis/chronic pelvic pain syndrome. J Urol 2004;171:284–8.

71. Arca E, Acikgoz G, Tastan HB, Kose O, Kurumlu Z. An open, randomized, comparative study of oral finasteride and 5% topical minoxidil in male androgenetic alopecia. Dermatology 2004;209:117–25.

72. Falsetti L, De Fusco D, Eleftheriou G, Rosina B. Treatment of hirsutism by finasteride and flutamide in women with polycystic ovary syndrome. Gynaecol Endosc 1997;6:251–7.

73. Byrnes CA, Morton AS, Liss CL, Lippert MC, Gillenwater JY. Efficacy, tolerability, and effect on health-related quality of life of finasteride versus placebo in men with symptomatic benign prostatic hyperplasia: a community based study. CUSP Investigators. Community based study of Proscar. Clin Ther 1995;17:956–69.

74. Thompson IM, Goodman PJ, Tangen CM, Lucia MS, Miller GJ, Ford LG, Lieber MM, Cespedes RD, Atkins JN, Lippman SM, Carlin SM, Ryan A, Szczepanek CM, Crowley JJ, Coltman Jr CA. The influence of finasteride on the development of prostate cancer. New Engl J Med 2003;349:215–24.

75. Stough DB, Rao NA, Kaufman KD, Mitchell C. Finasteride improves male pattern hair loss in a randomized study in identical twins. Eur J Dermatol 2003;12:32–7.

76. Kaufman KD. Long-term (5-year) multinational experience with finasteride 1 mg in the treatment of men with androgenetic alopecia. Eur J Dermatol 2002;12:38–49.

77. Ciotta L, Cianci A, Calogero AE, Palumbo MA, Marletta E, Sciuto A, Palumbo G. Clinical and endocrine effects of finasteride, a 5α-reductase inhibitor in women with idiopathic hirsutism. Fertil Steril 1995;64:299–306.

78. Margerger MJ. Long-term effects of finasteride in patients with benign prostatic hyperplasia; a double-blind, placebo-controlled multicenter study. Urology 1998;51:677–86.

79. Chou S-Y, Kao S-C, Hsu W-M. Propecia-associated bilateral cataract. Clin Exp Ophthalmol 2004;32:106–8.

80. Gormley GJ, Stoner E, Rittmaster RS, Gregg H, Thompson DL, Lasseter KC, Vlasses PH, Stein EA. Effects of finasteride (MK-906), a 5 alpha-reductase inhibitor, on circulating androgens in male volunteers. J Clin Endocrinol Metab 1990;70(4):1136–41.

81. Fruzzetti F, de Lorenzo D, Parrini D, Ricci C. Effects of finasteride, a 5 alpha-reductase inhibitor, on circulating androgens and gonadotropin secretion in hirsute women. J Clin Endocrinol Metab 1994;79(3):831–5.

82. Floyd A, Pedersen L, Nielsen GL, Thorlacius-Ussing O, Sorensen HT. Risk of acute pancreatitis in users of finasteride: a population-based case-control study. J Clin Gastroenterol 2004;38:276–8.

83. Haan J, Hollander JMR, van Duinen SG, Saxena PR, Wintzen AR. Reversible severe myopathy during treatment with finasteride. Muscle Nerve 1997;20:502–4.

84. McClellan KJ, Markham A. Finasteride. A review of its use in male pattern hair loss. Drugs 1999;57:111–26.

85. Tosti A, Pazzaglia M, Soli M, Rossi A, Rebora A, Atzori L, Barbareschi M, Benci M, Voudouris S, Vena GA. Evaluation of sexual function with an International Index of Erectile Function in subjects taking finasteride for androgenetic alopecia. Arch Dermatol 2004;140:857–8.

86. Lam JS, Romas NA, Lowe FC. Long-term treatment with finasteride in men with symptomatic benign prostatic hyperplasia: 10-year follow-up. Urology 2003;61:354–8.

87. Lowe FC, McConnell JD, Hudson PB, Romas NA, Boake R, Lieber M, Elhilali M, Geller J, Imperto-McGinely J, Andriole GL, Bruskewitz RC, Walsh PC, Bartsch G, Nacey JN, Shah S, Pappas F, Ko A, Cook T, Stoner E, Waldstreicher J. Long-term 6-year experience with finasteride in patients with benign prostatic hyperplasia. Urology 2003;61:791–6.

88. Whiting DA, Olsen EA, Savin R, Halper L, Rodgers A, Wang L, Hustad C, Palmisano J. Efficacy and tolerability of finasteride 1 mg in men

aged 41 to 60 years with male pattern hair loss. Eur J Dermatol 2003;13:150–60.

89. Neal DE. Drugs in focus: finasteride. Presc J 1995;35:89–95.

90. Sadeghi-Nejad H, Sherman N, Lue J. Comparison of finasteride and alpha-blockers as independent risk factors for erectile dysfunction. Int J Clin Pract 2003;57:484–7.

91. Ekman P. Maximum efficacy of finasteride is obtained within 6 months and maintained over 6 years. Eur Urol 1998;33:312–7.

92. Wessells H, Roy J, Bannow J, Grayhack J, Matsumoto AM, Tenover L, Herlihy R, Fitch W, Labasky R, Auerbach S, Parra R, Rajfer J, Culbertson J, Lee M, Bach MA, Waldstreicher J. Incidence and severity of sexual adverse experiences in finasteride and placebo-treated men with benign prostatic hyperplasia. Urology 2003;61:579–84.

93. Zlotta AR, Teillac P, Raynaud JP, Schulman CC. Evaluation of male sexual function in patients with lower urinary tract symptoms (LUTS) associated with benign prostatic hyperplasia (BPH) treated with a phytotherapeutic agent (Permixon®), tamsulosin or finasteride. Eur Urol 2005;48:269–76.

94. Bayhan G, Bahceci M, Demirkol T, Ertem M, Yalinkaya A, Erden AC. A comparative study of a gonadotropin-releasing hormone agonist and finasteride on idiopathic hirsutism. Clin Exp Obstet Gynecol 2000;27:203–6.

95. Wade MS, Sinclair RD. Reversible painful gynaecomastia induced by low dose finasteride (1 mg/day). Australas J Dermatol 2000;41:55.

96. Ferrando J, Grimalt R, Alsina M, Bulla F, Manasievska E. Unilateral gynecomastia induced by treatment with 1 mg of oral finasteride. Arch Dermatol 2002;138:543–4.

97. Kim BJ, Kim YJ, Ro BI. Two cases of reversible bilateral painful gynecomastia induced by 1 mg oral finasteride (Propecia). Korean J Dermatol 2003;41:232–4.

98. Kim H, Kye K, Seo Y, Suhr K, Lee J, Park J. A case of unilateral idiopathic gynecomastia aggravated by low-dose finasteride. Korean J Dermatol 2004;42:643–5.

99. See SC, Ellis RJ. Male breast cancer during finasteride therapy. J Natl Cancer Inst 2004;96:338–9.

100. Zimmerman RL, Fogt F, Cronin D, Lynch R. Cytologic atypia in a 53-year-old man with finasteride-induced gynecomastia. Arch Pathol Lab Med 2000;124:625–7.

101. Kaplan SA, Holtgrewe HL, Bruskewitz R, Saltzman B, Mobley D, Narayan P, Lund RH, Weiner S, Wells G, Cook TJ, Meehan A, Waldstreicher J. Comparison of the efficacy and safety of finasteride in older versus younger men with benign prostatic hyperplasia. Urology 2001;57:1073–7.

102. Dogol Sucar D, Botelho Sougey E, Brandao Neto J. Psychotic episode induced by potential drug interaction of sibutramine and finasteride. Rev Bras Psiquiatr 2002;24:30–3.

103. Etzioni RD, Howlader N, Shaw PA, Ankerst DP, Penson DF, Goodman PJ, Thompson IM. Long-term effects of finasteride on prostate specific antigen levels: results from the prostate cancer prevention trial. J Urol 2005;174(3):877–81 [erratum, 2071].

104. Inaba M, Otani Y, Nishimura K, Takaha N, Okuyama A, Koga M, Azuma J, Kawase I, Kasayama S. Combination therapy with rofecoxib and finasteride in the treatment of men with lower urinary tract symptoms (LUTS) and benign prostatic hyperplasia. Metab Clin Exp 2005;54:55–9.

105. Sundblad C, Landen M, Eriksson T, Bergman L, Eriksson E. Effects of the androgen antagonist flutamide and the serotonin reuptake inhibitor citalopram in bulimia nervosa: a placebo-controlled pilot study. J Clin Psychopharmacol 2005;25:85–8.

106. Kroiss R, Fentiman IS, Helmond FA, Rymer J, Foidart JM, Bundred N, Mol-Arts M, Kubista E. The effect of tibolone in postmenopausal women receiving tamoxifen after surgery for breast cancer: a randomised, double-blind, placebo-controlled trial. BJOG 2005;112:228–33.

Kristien Boelaert

41 Thyroid hormones, iodine, and antithyroid drugs

THYROID HORMONES *(SED-15, 3409; SEDA-27, 442; SEDA-28, 505; SEDA-29, 520)*

Thyroid hormones (liothyronine, T3, and levothyroxine, T4) are prescribed for about 1% of the adult population in developed countries, and for 5–10% in those aged over 60 years (1[R], 2[c], 3[c]). Large studies have suggested that about 25% of those who take levothyroxine use doses sufficient to suppress serum TSH (3[c], 4[C]), and much attention has focused on the potential adverse effects of this degree of over-treatment.

Psychiatric There is a well recognized association between hypothyroidism and psychiatric illness, and previous case reports have suggested that *psychosis* and *mania* can be the result of starting thyroid hormone replacement at too high a dosage (5[c]). Two further cases of mania associated with levothyroxine have been reported (6[A], 7[A]), suggesting that caution should be exercised when prescribing levothyroxine, especially in elderly people.

Musculoskeletal Large meta-analyses (8[M], 9[M]) have shown that levothyroxine in TSH-suppressive doses is associated with a minor but statistically significant *reduction in bone mineral density*. However, the evidence that suppressive doses of levothyroxine represent a risk factor for clinically relevant end points, such as the incidence of fractures and mortality, is scanty (1[R]). Two small studies have shown that low doses of levothyroxine have no adverse effects on bone mass and do not lead to a higher prevalence of vertebral fractures, even if the serum TSH is fully suppressed (10[c], 11[c]).

Drug–drug interactions There has been a report that *orlistat*, used in the management of obesity, reduced the systemic availability of levothyroxine (12[A]).

In a small study, *imatinib*, a tyrosine kinase inhibitor used in the treatment of a number of neoplastic diseases, increased the doses of levothyroxine necessary for adequate replacement therapy (13[c]).

IODINE AND IODIDES *(SED-15, 1896; SEDA-28, 506)*

Gastrointestinal Lugol's iodine spray is being increasingly used during diagnostic endoscopy to detect early mucosal changes of esophageal carcinoma. Transient *acute gastric mucosal damage* induced by iodine spray has been reported (14[A]).

ANTITHYROID DRUGS *(SED-15, 3387; SEDA-27, 442; SEDA-28, 506; SEDA-29, 520)*

Hematologic
DoTS classification:
Reaction: Agranulocytosis due to thionamides
Dose-relation: Collateral
Time-course: Intermediate
Susceptibility factors: Not known

Drug-induced agranulocytosis is the most serious and indeed life-threatening disorder associated with thionamide therapy, with a reported mortality of 5–15%. In a previous study it was estimated that the incidences of neutropenia

Side Effects of Drugs, Annual 30
J.K. Aronson (Editor)
ISSN: 0378-6080
DOI: 10.1016/S0378-6080(08)00041-X

and agranulocytosis in England and Wales were 120 and 7 cases per million per year respectively (15[C]). Current users of drugs classed as "thyroid inhibitors" had the highest risks of neutropenia (adjusted OR = 35; 95% CI = 12, 100) and agranulocytosis (OR = 21; 95% CI = 3.3, ∞) compared with other classes of drug associated with this complication. In a further UK-based study between 1981 and 2003 there were 5.23 million prescriptions for thionamide drugs in England and Scotland, 94% of which were for carbimazole (16[C]). Neutrophil dyscrasias (agranulocytosis and neutropenia) accounted for 49% of all deaths ascribed to these drugs. They were more frequently fatal in those over 65 years, and from 1981 reports of neutrophil dyscrasias were significantly more frequent per prescription of propylthiouracil than carbimazole. These findings confirm that agranulocytosis is the most important complication of antithyroid drugs, remembering that neutropenia may in part reflect underlying hyperthyroidism rather than an adverse drug effect.

Administration of granulocyte colony-stimulating factor (G-CSF) is the standard treatment for antithyroid drug-induced agranulocytosis and is reported to shorten the recovery period (17[c]), although others have reported it to be ineffective in severe agranulocytosis (18[c]). In a further study the efficacy of G-CSF has been investigated in 109 patients with agranulocytosis caused by antithyroid drugs (19[c]). G-CSF significantly reduced the recovery period from 9.2 to 2.3 days. However, it was ineffective in symptomatic patients with granulocyte counts below $0.1 \times 10^9/l$.

Immunologic

Hypersensitivity syndrome   Allergic reactions manifesting as fever, urticaria or other rashes, and arthralgia occur in 1–5% of patients taking antithyroid drugs. There has been a report of methimazole-induced hypersensitivity syndrome associated with reactivation of human herpes virus 6 and cytomegalovirus (20[A]).

Vasculitis   Antithyroid drugs, especially propylthiouracil, can be associated with the development of antineutrophil cytoplasmic antibody (ANCA)-positive vasculitis, often manifesting as renal disease. Atypical presentations, with

pulmonary capillaritis (21[A]) and lupus-like syndrome (22[A]), have been described in individual cases. Furthermore, two cases of vasculitis have been associated with carbimazole, one presenting with eosinophilic granulomatous vasculitis localized to the stomach (23[A]) and another with p-ANCA positive vasculitis causing simultaneous acute renal insufficiency and massive pulmonary hemorrhage (24[A]).

The long-term effects of antithyroid drug treatment on the prevalence of ANCAs has been examined in 209 consecutive patients with hyperthyroidism who had been treated with antithyroid drugs, radioactive iodine, thyroidectomy, or a combination of these treatment options (25[c]). Overall 12 patients who were taking antithyroid drugs were positive for antineutrophil cytoplasmic antibodies to myeloperoxidase, proteinase-3, or human leukocyte elastase; four of these had ANCA-associated vasculitis. When 77 of the 209 patients who were retested after 3–6 years (and antithyroid drug treatment had been withdrawn), ANCA could still be detected in three of six who had previously tested positive; in addition one patient who had not taken antithyroid drugs had developed myeloperoxidase-associated ANCA. The presence of ANCA was highly associated with treatment with antithyroid drugs (OR = 12; 95% CI = 1.5, 93). This study highlights the fact that the presence of ANCA with or without vasculitis is associated with previous treatment with antithyroid drugs, possibly after years.

The mechanism of propylthiouracil-induced vasculitis has been investigated in two separate studies, suggesting that the avidity of myeloperoxidase-associated ANCA (26[c]) or the presence of anti-endothelial cell antibodies (AECA) (27[c]) may be associated with vasculitic disease activity.

Teratogenicity   Concerns about the safety of carbimazole in pregnancy have been raised, but the association between antithyroid drug administration in early pregnancy and congenital abnormalities remains unclear. Aplasia cutis congenita and choanal atresia have been reported in association with maternal carbimazole therapy, suggesting a causative link either with the drug or with underlying hyperthyroidism. Two further cases of choanal atresia in association with carbimazole treatment during the first trimester of pregnancy have been reported

$(28^A, 29^A)$; in one case there were marked facial dysmorphic features and failure of breast development, thought to be secondary to maternal use of carbimazole during pregnancy (28^A). These cases continue to highlight a possible link between carbimazole, or its active metabolite methimazole, and congenital abnormalities, and they reinforce the view that propylthiouracil is the drug of choice in early pregnancy. However, it should be noted that one of the major hazards of antithyroid drug use in pregnancy is over-treatment, and hence induction of fetal hypothyroidism and goiter. It is therefore important to monitor maternal thyroid status carefully and to use the lowest possible dose of antithyroid drug sufficient to maintain maternal euthyroidism.

Drug–drug interactions In a small randomized controlled study the combination of propylthiouracil 100 mg bd with *colestyramine* 4 g bd for 4 weeks led to a more rapid and complete fall in thyroid hormone concentrations in 30 patients with Graves' disease (30^c). The authors proposed that colestyramine reduced the total body pool of thyroid hormone by enhanced fecal loss, thus inducing a more rapid response to propylthiouracil.

References

1. Boelaert K, Franklyn JA. Thyroid hormone in health and disease. J Endocrinol 2005;187(1):1–15.
2. Kaufman SC, Gross TP, Kennedy DL. Thyroid hormone use: trends in the United States from 1960 through 1988. Thyroid 1991;1(4):285–91.
3. Parle JV, Franklyn JA, Cross KW, Jones SR, Sheppard MC. Thyroxine prescription in the community: serum thyroid stimulating hormone level assays as an indicator of undertreatment or overtreatment. Br J Gen Pract 1993;43(368):107–9.
4. Canaris GJ, Manowitz NR, Mayor G, Ridgway EC. The Colorado thyroid disease prevalence study. Arch Intern Med 2000;160(4):526–34.
5. Josephson AM, Mackenzie TB. Thyroid-induced mania in hypothyroid patients. Br J Psychiatry 1980;137:222–8.
6. El Kaissi S, Kotowicz MA, Berk M, Wall JR. Acute delirium in the setting of primary hypothyroidism: the role of thyroid hormone replacement therapy. Thyroid 2005;15(9):1099–101.
7. Goldstein BI, Levitt AJ. Thyroxine-associated hypomania. J Am Acad Child Adolesc Psychiatry 2005;44(3):211.
8. Faber J, Galloe AM. Changes in bone mass during prolonged subclinical hyperthyroidism due to L-thyroxine treatment: a meta-analysis. Eur J Endocrinol 1994;130(4):350–6.
9. Uzzan B, Campos J, Cucherat M, Nony P, Boissel JP, Perret GY. Effects on bone mass of long term treatment with thyroid hormones: a meta-analysis. J Clin Endocrinol Metab 1996;81(12):4278–89.
10. Appetecchia M. Effects on bone mineral density by treatment of benign nodular goiter with mildly suppressive doses of L-thyroxine in a cohort women study. Horm Res 2005;64(6):293–8.
11. Heijckmann AC, Huijberts MS, Geusens P, de Vries J, Menheere PP, Wolffenbuttel BH. Hip bone mineral density, bone turnover and risk of fracture in patients on long-term suppressive L-thyroxine therapy for differentiated thyroid carcinoma. Eur J Endocrinol 2005;153(1):23–9.
12. Madhava K, Hartley A. Hypothyroidism in thyroid carcinoma follow-up: orlistat may inhibit the absorption of thyroxine. Clin Oncol (R Coll Radiol) 2005;17(6):492.
13. de Groot JW, Zonnenberg BA, Plukker JT, Der Graaf WT, Links TP. Imatinib induces hypothyroidism in patients receiving levothyroxine. Clin Pharmacol Ther 2005;78(4):433–8.
14. Sreedharan A, Rembacken BJ, Rotimi O. Acute toxic gastric mucosal damage induced by Lugol's iodine spray during chromoendoscopy. Gut 2005;54(6):886–7.
15. van Staa TP, Boulton F, Cooper C, Hagenbeek A, Inskip H, Leufkens HG. Neutropenia and agranulocytosis in England and Wales: incidence and risk factors. Am J Hematol 2003;72(4):248–54.
16. Pearce SH. Spontaneous reporting of adverse reactions to carbimazole and propylthiouracil in the UK. Clin Endocrinol (Oxf) 2004;61(5):589–94.
17. Tajiri J, Noguchi S, Okamura S, Morita M, Tamura M, Murakami M, Niho Y. Granulocyte colony-stimulating factor treatment of antithyroid drug-induced granulocytopenia. Arch Intern Med 1993;153(4):509–14.
18. Tamai H, Mukuta T, Matsubayashi S, Fukata S, Komaki G, Kuma K, Kumagai LF, Nagataki S. Treatment of methimazole-induced agranulocytosis using recombinant human granulocyte

colony-stimulating factor (rhG-CSF). J Clin Endocrinol Metab 1993;77(5):1356–60.

19. Tajiri J, Noguchi S. Antithyroid drug-induced agranulocytosis: how has granulocyte colony-stimulating factor changed therapy? Thyroid 2005;15(3):292–7.

20. Ozaki N, Miura Y, Sakakibara A, Oiso Y. A case of hypersensitivity syndrome induced by methimazole for Graves' disease. Thyroid 2005;15(12):1333–6.

21. Pirot AL, Goldsmith D, Pascasio J, Beck SE. Pulmonary capillaritis with hemorrhage due to propylthiouracil therapy in a child. Pediatr Pulmonol 2005;39(1):88–92.

22. Ozkan HA, Ozkalemkas F, Ali R, Ozkocaman V, Ozcelik T. Propylthiouracil-induced lupus-like syndrome: successful management with oral corticosteroids. Thyroid 2005;15(10):1203–4.

23. Seve P, Stankovic K, Michalet V, Vial T, Scoazec JY, Broussolle C. Carbimazole induced eosinophilic granulomatous vasculitis localized to the stomach. J Intern Med 2005;258(2):191–5.

24. Calanas-Continente A, Espinosa M, Manzano-Garcia G, Santamaria R, Lopez-Rubio F, Aljama P. Necrotizing glomerulonephritis and pulmonary hemorrhage associated with carbimazole therapy. Thyroid 2005;15(3):286–8.

25. Slot MC, Links TP, Stegeman CA, Tervaert JW. Occurrence of antineutrophil cytoplasmic antibodies and associated vasculitis in patients with hyperthyroidism treated with antithyroid drugs: a long-term followup study. Arthritis Rheum 2005;53(1):108–13.

26. Gao Y, Ye H, Yu F, Guo XH, Zhao MH. Anti-myeloperoxidase IgG subclass distribution and avidity in sera from patients with propylthiouracil-induced antineutrophil cytoplasmic antibodies associated vasculitis. Clin Immunol 2005;117(1):87–93.

27. Yu F, Zhao MH, Zhang YK, Zhang Y, Wang HY. Anti-endothelial cell antibodies (AECA) in patients with propylthiouracil (PTU)-induced ANCA positive vasculitis are associated with disease activity. Clin Exp Immunol 2005;139(3):569–74.

28. Foulds N, Walpole I, Elmslie F, Mansour S. Carbimazole embryopathy: an emerging phenotype. Am J Med Genet A 2005;132(2):130–5.

29. Myers AK, Reardon W. Choanal atresia—a recurrent feature of foetal carbimazole syndrome. Clin Otolaryngol 2005;30(4):375–7.

30. Tsai WC, Pei D, Wang TF Wu DA, Li JC, Wei CL, Lee CH, Chen SP, Kuo SW. The effect of combination therapy with propylthiouracil and cholestyramine in the treatment of Graves' hyperthyroidism. Clin Endocrinol (Oxf) 2005;62(5):521–4.

R.C.L. Page

42   Insulin, other hypoglycemic drugs, and glucagon

INSULIN   *(SED-15, 1761; SEDA-27, 446; SEDA-28, 509; SEDA-29, 523)*

Cardiovascular   In 215 subjects with type 1 diabetes *atherosclerosis* was assessed using carotid intima media thickness (1[c]). There was a positive correlation with cumulative short-acting insulin exposure but no correlation with intermediate-acting insulin. There was no power to distinguish between analogues and regular insulin. A review of insulin therapy has suggested that hyperglycemia is important, based on the results of the DCCT study, in which the intensive control group had less progression of atherosclerosis than the conventional group. Most studies have shown a beneficial or neutral effect of exogenous insulin on cardiovascular disease and atherosclerosis, which is different to the epidemiological data on endogenous insulin, which show an increased cardiovascular risk with increasing insulin concentrations (2[R]).

Metabolism

Hypoglycemia   In a systematic review of short-acting analogues, 42 randomized controlled trials in 7933 patients with type 1, type 2, and gestational diabetes showed only minor differences in overall hypoglycemia (3[M]). The standardized mean differences of episodes per patient per month were −0.05 and −0.04 in adults with type 1 and type 2 diabetes respectively, comparing short-acting analogues with regular insulin. There were no differences between children and pregnant women with type 1 diabetes and women with gestational diabetes. The change in HbA$_{1c}$ was small. Hypoglycemia remains a clinical problem whether analogue or regular insulin is used.

Susceptibility factors

Age   The management of very young children with type 1 diabetes remains a challenge. The incidence of hypoglycemia has been assessed in 6309 children with type 1 diabetes living in Germany and Austria (4[C]). Despite modern care, young children aged 0–5 years had frequent episodes of severe hypoglycaemia (31/100 patient-years), significantly more than in children aged 5–7 and 7–9 years (20/100 and 22/100 patient-years respectively). The youngest children also had higher rates of severe hypoglycemia, regardless of treatment regimen. Of children under 5 years 71% were using three or more injections per day or a pump.

Drug administration route

Continuous subcutaneous insulin infusion (CSII)   The use of CSII for 6 or more months has been reported in 70 children aged 2–12 (mean 9.1) years (5[c]). A retrospective review of charts compared with the year before CSII showed a non-significant reduction in severe hypoglycemia associated with a slight fall in HbA$_{1c}$. There were two episodes of diabetic ketoacidosis, compared with none during the control period. There were no practical problems; the children did not play with the pumps.

In 100 children aged 1.6 to 18 years who had used a pump for 6 or more months data were obtained from the insulin pump memory: 10% missed meal-time boluses and 7% had programming and adjusting errors (6[c]). One child aged 16 years had an episode of severe hypoglycemia

Side Effects of Drugs, Annual 30
J.K. Aronson (Editor)
ISSN: 0378-6080
DOI: 10.1016/S0378-6080(08)00042-1

due to overdosing on meal boluses. There were no episodes of diabetic ketoacidosis.

Children under the age of 10 years often do well, as the pumps are under the control of their carers. The use of pumps in 10 preschool children aged 6 years and under appeared to be safe (7[c]). Hypoglycemia appeared to be reduced compared with twice-daily mixed insulin. The use of pumps in children appears to be safe with appropriate commitment from the patients and their carers.

Administration of insulin by inhalation

Exubera, an insulin powder with a particle size of < 7.5 μm combined with a dry powder carrier, is commercially available in the UK. Other inhaled formulations are in development, including AERx, which is a liquid, and ProMaxx, which uses proprietary technology to produce microspheres of 1–5 μm. Regardless of the system used for delivery systemic availability is low (under 20%), and so high dosages are required. There is also variation in absorption and the intraindividual coefficient of variation can be about 34%, although the absorption of subcutaneously administered insulin is also variable. Smoking can increase the absorption rate by as much as 50%; this is reversed on stopping smoking but will recur when smoking is restarted (8[R]).

In this and other reviews the lack of long-term data, which is particularly important for understanding the management of a chronic disease that requires many years of therapy for an individual, has been discussed. Data from 4-year open studies suggest that lung function does not deteriorate compared with subcutaneous insulin. However, patients with lung disease have usually been excluded from such studies (9[R], 10[R]).

In a single-dose comparison of healthy individuals with those with asthma the latter had reduced insulin absorption and greater intra-subject variation in insulin concentrations (10[R]). Antibodies to inhaled insulin continue to be a concern, although there has been no correlation with antibody titer and insulin dosage or the development of hypoglycemia. Presensitization may be important. Patients with type 2 diabetes who had not used insulin before starting to use inhaled insulin had a lower antibody response, despite the addition of subcutaneous insulin in 32% of participants by the end of the study (11[R]).

In 10 non-diabetic volunteers with upper respiratory tract infections there were no differences in insulin pharmacokinetics after a single dose of inhaled insulin (AERx) given during the infection compared with recovery (12[c]). The authors suggested that this shows that AERx can be continued safely in patients with upper respiratory tract infections. The dose used was small (equivalent to 6 units of short-acting insulin). Insulin dosage often increases substantially during illness and further experience in patients with diabetes would be required before establishing safety.

Management of adverse drug reactions

Secondary growth hormone insensitivity syndrome is thought to develop when chronic insulin deficiency and poor metabolic control occur in people with type 1 diabetes. High growth hormone concentrations are found in conjunction with low concentrations of IGF1.

Intensifying insulin therapy in people with poor metabolic control exacerbates retinopathy. In three cases progressive retinopathy followed intensified insulin therapy, and the authors suggested that subcutaneous octreotide may be of benefit in management (13[A]). The cases were managed concurrently with standard therapy, including laser photocoagulation. Octreotide reduced IGF1 concentrations and reduced insulin requirements. However its role in managing retinopathy was unclear. There was speculation that it may be helpful for macular edema.

Training for patients in diabetes management to allow for dietary flexibility improves glycemic control without increasing the risk of severe hypoglycemia. In an analysis of data from 96 hospitals in Germany a low concentration of HbA$_{1c}$ was associated with a high risk of hypoglycemia before treatment (14[C]). After treatment hypoglycemia did not correlate with HbA$_{1c}$; there were 0.11 episodes of severe hypoglycemia per patient per year in the highest quintile of HbA$_{1c}$ compared with 0.16 in the lowest. Before treatment the figures were 0.18 and 0.54 respectively.

ALPHA-GLUCOSIDASE INHIBITORS   *(SED-15, 85; SEDA-27, 452; SEDA-28, 514; SEDA-29, 526)*

Three alpha glucosidase inhibitors, acarbose, miglitol, and voglibose, have been reviewed (15[R]).

Comparative studies   In a comparison of voglibose and acarbose in 21 in-patients with type 2 diabetes who took part in a randomized crossover study of acarbose 150 mg/day and voglibose 0.9 mg/day, there was marked interindividual variation in response (16[c]). For both drugs efficacy was better in those with gastrointestinal adverse effects, such as *abdominal distention* and *flatulence*.

Acarbose

Observational studies   In a post-marketing surveillance study in 27 803 patients with diabetes mellitus (94% type 2), data were reported after 12 weeks. The doses of acarbose were low: 4.1% took less than 100 mg/day, 64% 100–250 mg/day, 32% 250–300 mg/day, and 0.1% more than 300 mg/day. Only 2.1% stopped therapy, mainly because of *gastrointestinal adverse events*. Tolerability appeared to be good and independent of age. Abnormal liver function was reported in 0.01%. The difference between these results and those of many controlled trials may in part be explained by the fact that higher doses have been used in most trials (17[C]).

Nutrition   In a 56-week study there was an association between the use of acarbose and *low vitamin B_6 concentrations*, which occurred in 33% of 240 patients taking acarbose compared with 23% of 119 patients taking placebo (18[c]). Calcium concentrations fell more often in those who took acarbose (28 versus 16%) but returned to normal by the end. These findings have not been reported elsewhere and do not appear to be clinically significant.

Liver   In a 78-week double-blind single center study 139 patients with type 2 diabetes were randomized to acarbose or placebo in addition to their usual therapy (19[c]). The mean dose of

acarbose at the end of the study was 680 mg. Two patients taking 600 mg or more developed *raised liver enzymes*, to more than three times the upper limit of normal.

In a 56-week study there was an association between the dose of acarbose in the range 50–300 mg tds and the development of abnormal liver function in 359 patients with type 1 (21%) and type 2 diabetes (18[c]). The patients took the maximum tolerated dose, and 30% took doses of 100 mg or less. Of the patents who were randomized to acarbose (*n* = 240), 8% developed abnormal liver function tests (alanine transaminase activity more than three times the upper limit of normal) compared with 1% of those who took placebo (*n* = 119). The dose of acarbose was 200–300 mg tds in those who developed abnormal liver function. Liver function recovered promptly on withdrawal.

AMYLIN ANALOGUES   *(SEDA-27, 453; SEDA-28, 514; SEDA-29, 526)*

Pramlintide

Placebo-controlled studies   In three studies in 477 patients with type 1 diabetes, pramlintide 30 or 60 micrograms three or four times a day (*n* = 281) was compared with placebo (*n* = 196) (20[M]). The patients continued to take insulin in a mean daily dose of 50 units/day (pramlintide) or 48 units/day (placebo). After 26 weeks 43% of those using pramlintide had problems with *nausea* and 16% had *anorexia* compared with 10 and 2% of those who used placebo (21[R]). A review of other studies showed that the rate of mild to moderate nausea was 9.5–59%, and that severe nausea was 0.7–8.5%. Most studies suggested that the nausea was transient (2–8 weeks) although most did not document the reduction in nausea.

Gastrointestinal   Pramlintide *slows gastric emptying* and it should not be used in those with gastroparesis. The manufacturer also recommends that analgesics should not be taken less than 1 hour before or 2 hours after pramlintide.

Drug–drug interactions   Pramlintide buffers to a pH of 4.0 and precipitates at a pH at above 5.5 and would not be expected to be compatible with *insulin*, which is buffered at pH 7.8. In an open study of 51 patients with type 1 diabetes, pramlintide was mixed in the same syringe as insulin (regular insulin and isophane insulin) (22[c]). The pharmacokinetics of insulin and pramlintide were not significantly altered. However, mixing pramlintide and insulin is not recommended.

BIGUANIDES   *(SED-15, 506; SEDA-27, 453; SEDA-28, 514; SEDA-29, 526)*

Metformin

Sensory systems   *Altered vision* has been attributed to metformin (23[A]).

- A 62-year-old man with diabetes was given metformin 750 mg bd and his blood glucose concentration fell from 22 to 15 mmol/l within 4 days. The dose of metformin was increased to 850 mg bd and the blood glucose concentration fell to 8.7 mmol/l over the next week. Within 2 days of starting therapy his vision became blurred. Slit lamp examination 2 weeks later showed cracked shaped lines on the lens. The cracks resolved spontaneously by 3 months.

Although the timing made metformin a possible candidate in this case, it is much more likely that the problem was caused by rapid changes in blood glucose concentration and the associated fluid shifts.

Liver   Reports of metformin-induced *hepatotoxicity* are rare.

- A 73-year-old Japanese woman, weight 33.5 kg, took nateglinide 270 mg/day and pioglitazone 15 mg/day for 6 months (24[A]). Her HbA$_{1c}$ concentration was 8.6% and fasting glucose 11.4 mmol/l. Metformin 250 mg bd was added and 3 weeks later she developed jaundice and fatigue. A few months before her liver function tests had been normal. Aspartate transaminase activity was 689 IU/l, alanine transaminase 772 IU/l, alkaline phosphatase 639 IU/l, and bilirubin 6.5 mg/dl. All oral therapy was withdrawn and insulin started. Her liver function improved over the next few weeks.

Pregnancy   Fetuses are exposed to therapeutic concentrations of metformin, which for part of the day may be higher than those found in the mother (25[c]). Although many women have become pregnant while taking metformin, until recently most have stopped taking it during pregnancy. A review of the safety of metformin therapy for the management of polycystic ovary syndrome has shown an increased frequency of malformations in children born to mothers who took metformin during pregnancy. This was a personal communication and no information was given about the malformations, the numbers, or how the data were collected. It was also not stated who gave the communication. Animal studies with excessive doses have shown anophthalmia, anencephaly, and delayed blastocyst development (26[E]).

Susceptibility factors

Renal disease   When to stop metformin in people with diabetes mellitus and abnormal renal function continues to be debated. It has been suggested that it should not be used in those with an eGFR (MDRD) of less than 60 ml/minute (27[R]). However, this would exclude many people who have been taking metformin for many years without apparent ill effect. Others have recommended using the Cockcroft–Gault equation (SEDA-29, 527), which is preferable.

Liver disease   The use of metformin in patients with non-alcoholic fatty liver disease has been reported in two trials (28[c], 29[c]). Patients had abnormal liver function tests, which improved during the studies. No-one withdrew because of worsening of liver function tests or lactic acidosis.

Drug formulations   Metformin XR uses a modified-release system to allow once-daily dosing. In 16 healthy volunteers aged 18–40 years, 1-week regimens of metformin XR 500, 1000, and 1500 mg/day, followed by either metformin XR 2000 mg/day or metformin IR 1000 mg bd during weeks 4 and 5, produced 137 adverse events (30[c]). These were mainly gastrointestinal, including abdominal pain, reduced appetite, diarrhea, nausea, and vomiting. There were similar adverse effects with metformin XR and IR. There was no relation between the dose of metformin XR and the number of events.

Drug overdose   *Lactic acidosis* associated with metformin continues to be reported and reviewed. Two children developed lactic acidosis when they took metformin for attempted suicide.

- A 40-kg 14-year-old girl was thought to have taken up to 63 g of metformin, 1050 mg of diclofenac, and 1400 mg of atenolol (31[A]). She had a Glasgow coma scale score of 5, a blood glucose concentration of 1.9 mmol/l, a pH of 7.1, a bicarbonate concentration of 10.6 mmol/l, and a base excess of −18.6 mmol/l. The peak lactate concentration was 38 mmol/l.
- A 15-year-old girl took 38 g of metformin (32[A]). Her pH was 7.29, bicarbonate 17 mmol/l, base excess −10 mmol/l, and blood glucose 9.2 mmol/l after receiving glucose from the rescue team. Her condition worsened—the bicarbonate fell to 15 mmol/l, the pH to 7.2, and the blood glucose to 2.7 mmol/l; the lactate rose to 8.7 mmol/l. The lactate concentration subsequently peaked at 21 mmol/l.

These two cases show that although metformin at recommended doses is not usually associated with hypoglycemia, severe hypoglycemia can occur at higher doses. Overdosage is also associated with lactic acidosis in people with normal renal function. Metformin interferes with the production and clearance of lactate by a variety of mechanisms, including a shift in intracellular redox potential from aerobic to anaerobic metabolism, increasing lactate production. In both of these cases lactate concentrations peaked several hours after ingestion of metformin. This needs to be considered when managing metformin overdose.

℞ *Dipeptidyl peptidase IV inhibitors*

Dipeptidyl peptidase IV (DPP IV) is an enzyme that is involved in the rapid metabolism of incretins, such as glucagon-like peptide. Inhibitors of DPP IV therefore extend the action of incretins. The incretins increase glucose-dependent insulin secretion from the pancreas, and so inhibition of DPP IV is a new therapeutic approach in the treatment of type 2 diabetes. Unlike the incretin mimetic analogues of glucagon-like peptide, which are given subcutaneously, inhibitors of DPP IV can be given orally.

Sitagliptin ([2R]-4-oxo-4-[3-(trifluoromethyl)-5,6-dihydro(1,2,4)triazolo(4,3-a)pyrazin-7(8H)-yl]-1-[2,4,5-trifluorophenyl]butan-2-amine) (33[c]) is the first inhibitor of DPP IV to have received a licence in the UK (in 2007).

There are other closely related DPP enzymes, such as DPP 8 and DPP 9. When these enzymes are inhibited in experimental animals multiorgan toxicity occurs. Sitagliptin appears to be highly selective for DPP IV and has 2600 times selectivity for DPP IV compared with DPP 8 and DPP 9. Compared with placebo, sitagliptin produces an approximately two-fold increase in postprandial active glucagon-like peptide 1 concentrations (34[R]).

Pharmacokinetics   *Sitagliptin is well absorbed and about 80% is excreted unchanged in the urine; the half-life is 8–14 hours (34[R]). Renal clearance averages 388 ml/minute and is largely uninfluenced by dose. The AUC is dose-dependent and is not affected by food. The pharmacokinetics are not affected by obesity (35[C]).*

Observational studies   *In 34 healthy men, mean age 33 years, weight 77 kg, single doses of sitagliptin 1.5–600 mg resulted in 79 adverse events, of which 19 were thought to be drug related; 14 occurred in those taking sitagliptin and five in those taking placebo (33[c]). Adverse events were reported to be mild to moderate and resolved without treatment. The study was designed to investigate the single-dose pharmacokinetics and pharmacodynamics of sitagliptin, and data on the nature of the adverse events were not given. However, it was reported that there were no cases of hypoglycemia, and blood counts and liver and renal function tests were reported as unaffected.*

Placebo-controlled studies   *In a placebo-controlled study in 521 patients with type 2 diabetes mellitus aged 27–76 years, sitagliptin 100 or 200 mg/day for 18 weeks significantly improved glycemic control (36[C]). Hypoglycemia and gastrointestinal adverse events were not significantly different between sitagliptin and placebo.*

Metabolism   *In a randomized, double-blind, placebo-controlled study in 741 patients sitagliptin 100 or 200 mg for 24 weeks caused no* changes in body weight, although those who took placebo lost 1.1 kg (37[C]). However, in other similar studies, body weight fell similarly with sitagliptin and placebo (36[C], 38[C]).

Drug–drug interactions   *In a placebo-controlled, multiple-dose, crossover study in 13 patients with type 2 diabetes, sitagliptin 50 mg bd and metformin 1000 mg bd did not alter the pharmacokinetics of each other (39[C]).*

INCRETIN MIMETICS
(SEDA-29, 528)

Exenatide

Metabolism   *Weight loss* has been reported with exenatide. It occurs regardless of initial weight and does not relate to the degree of nausea (see below), but exenatide reduces food intake (40[c]). In a 30-week study those who took 10 micrograms bd lost 2.8 kg and those who took 5 micrograms bd lost 1.6 kg compared with 0.3 kg in those who took placebo.

Mild or moderate *hypoglycemia* occurred with a similar frequency in patients with type 2 diabetes who took exenatide or placebo: 5.3% in those who took 10 micrograms bd, 4.5% in those who took 5 micrograms bd, and 5.3% in those who took placebo (41[C]). However, in a study in which exenatide was combined with metformin and a sulfonylurea in 733 subjects the incidence of hypoglycemia was greater in those who took exenatide (13% placebo, 19% 5 micrograms bd, and 28% 10 micrograms bd) (42[C]). The incidence of hypoglycemia was lowest in those who were taking the lowest dose of sulfonylurea. The effect of exenatide to stimulate insulin production is glucose dependent, and it is likely that the hypoglycemia observed in this study related to the non-glucose-dependent actions of sulfonylureas superimposed on the effect of exenatide. It is therefore appropriate in patients whose HbA$_{1c}$ concentration is close to target to reduce their dose of sulfonylurea when they start to take exenatide and to make further adjustments depending on response.

Gastrointestinal   *Nausea* due to exenatide has been reviewed.

> **DoTS classification:**
> *Reaction*: Nausea due to exenatide
> *Dose-relation*: Collateral
> *Time-course*: Intermediate
> *Susceptibility factors*: None known

The mechanism is not fully established, but possible mechanisms include delay in gastric emptying, activation of afferent nerves, and or central effects of GLP-1 receptor activation (43[R]). It is dose related in the therapeutic range of doses and is more likely to occur in the first eight weeks (44[R], 45[R]). Gradually increasing the dose of exenatide may be helpful (46[R]).

During continuous subcutaneous infusion of exenatide at different doses in 12 patients with type 2 diabetes nausea was the most common adverse effect (47[c]). The dose of exenatide appears to be important. In a placebo-controlled study in 156 patients (mean age 52 years, BMI 33–36 kg/m²) with type 2 diabetes who received exenatide for 28 days, nausea varied with dose 23% of those who took 2.5 micrograms bd, 26% of those who took 5 micrograms bd, 61% of those who took 7.5 micrograms bd, and 52% of those who took 10 micrograms bd (48[c]). The nausea was maximal during the first week (33%), falling to 6% by the end of the study.

In another placebo-controlled study, the incidence of nausea also fell with time (42[C]). Patients with type 2 diabetes (mean age 55 years; $n = 733$) taking metformin and a sulfonylurea took either exenatide 5 micrograms bd or placebo for 4 weeks. Those taking exenatide were then randomized to either 5 micrograms bd or 10 micrograms bd for 30 weeks. Nausea, the most frequent severe adverse event, occurred at similar rates in both groups—5% of those taking 5 micrograms bd and 3% of those taking 10 micrograms bd. The overall incidence of nausea was slightly higher at all times in those who took 10 micrograms bd, about 31% at the start of the study falling to about 10% compared with about 24% in those who took 5 micrograms bd, falling to 7%.

In 336 patients with type 2 diabetes who took metformin, 36% of those who were randomized to exenatide 5 micrograms bd and 45% of those who took 10 micrograms bd had nausea compared with 23% of those who took placebo

(41^C). The frequency of nausea fell during the study in all groups.

Immunologic *Antibodies* to exenatide have been found in several studies, with an incidence of 43% and 49% (41^C, 42^C). The development of antibodies did not appear to alter glycemic control or adverse events. The titers of antibodies were low (1/125). The long-term effects of these antibodies are unknown, but could include a reduced response to exenatide. There appears to be no cross-reaction between exenatide antibodies and native human GLP-1 (49^R).

Tumorigenicity GLP-1 increases beta-cell mass in animals. Thus, exenatide has the potential to cause *increased beta-cell mass* through augmented differentiation of precursor cells and inhibition of apoptosis (43^R). No malignant islet cell tumors were found in 130 mice and rats who received the equivalent human dose of 20 micrograms/day for 2 years (50^E). Long-term follow-up is required to ensure safety.

Drug administration route The concentration versus time profiles after subcutaneous injection of 10 micrograms of exenatide into the abdomen, arm, and thigh were similar in 28 people with type 2 diabetes, mean age 56 years (51^c). Long-term injection of insulin can cause local problems such as lipohypertrophy, and so rotation of injection sites is recommended. Similar problems have also been reported with growth hormone. It would therefore be wise to vary the injection site of exenatide, as systemic availability is comparable.

Drug–drug interactions

Digoxin In 21 healthy Asian men who took *digoxin* and exenatide there was no important change in digoxin exposure; C_{max} fell by 17% and t_{max} was prolonged by a median of 2.5 hours. No digoxin concentrations increased to more than 2.0 mg/l (52^c). The summary of product characteristics (SPC) for exenatide specifies that dosage adjustment is not required for paracetamol or digoxin.

Paracetamol In 40 healthy people aged 18–65 years the absorption of exenatide 10 micrograms was unaffected by *paracetamol* 1000 mg (53^c). However, the absorption of paracetamol

was reduced, depending on the timing of ingestion in relation to the injection of exenatide. When paracetamol was taken 1 hour before exenatide there was no change in plasma paracetamol concentrations. However, when it was taken at the same time as the injection or 1 or 2 hours after there was up to a 56% reduction in C_{max} and the t_{max} was prolonged from 0.6 hours to a maximum of 4.2 hours. Exenatide reduces the rate of gastric emptying.

Liraglutide

Gastrointestinal Of 210 patients with type 2 diabetes, 179 completed a randomized study of the effects of five different doses (0.045, 0.225, 0.45, 0.6, and 0.75 mg) or metformin 100 mg bd for 12 weeks after a 4-week metformin run-in phase. The numbers of people who reported *nausea and vomiting* were small (4%) and comparable to the incidence with metformin (6%) (54^c). Careful upwards titration allows higher doses (2 mg/day) to be tolerated (49^R).

Immunologic After the end of 12 weeks treatment no antibodies to liraglutide were detected (54^c).

SULFONYLUREAS *(SED-15, 3230; SEDA-27, 456; SEDA-28, 518; SEDA-29, 530)*

Management of adverse drug reactions Octreotide inhibits the secretion of various neuropeptides, including insulin. It thus helps reduce the hyperstimulation of endogenous insulin production by sulfonylureas. The use of octreotide to manage sulfonylurea-induced hypoglycemia has been reviewed (55^R). Intravenous or subcutaneous octreotide was used over a period of days as necessary in young children and adults. The authors suggested a management guideline based on the use of intravenous glucose supplemented with octreotide either to treat or prevent relapse of hypoglycemia.

Glibenclamide

Pregnancy In 70 patients with gestational diabetes randomized to insulin (*n* = 27), glibenclamide (*n* = 24), or acarbose (*n* = 19) satisfactory blood glucose concentrations were not achieved in five of the women allocated to glibenclamide compared with eight of those allocated to acarbose (56[C]). Babies who were large for gestational age were found in 3.7% (insulin), 25% (glibenclamide), and 10% (acarbose). Neonatal hypoglycemia occurred in eight of the babies whose mothers had taken glibenclamide compared with one each of those whose mothers had taken acarbose or insulin. There was therefore more macrosomia and hypoglycemia in the babies of women taking glibenclamide. However, glibenclamide is inexpensive and may be useful if other more appropriate therapies are unavailable during pregnancy.

Glimepiride

Liver *Hepatotoxicity* is a rare but recognized adverse effect of sulfonylureas (57[A]).

- A 65-year-old man developed jaundice 2 weeks after presenting with type 2 diabetes. He had been given glimepiride 2 mg/day. There was a stone in the common bile duct, which was treated with sphincterotomy. However, his liver function tests remained abnormal. Glimepiride was withdrawn, his liver function gradually normalized, and glimepiride was restarted. Liver function became abnormal once more and returned to normal within 1 month of withdrawal of glimepiride.

THAZOLIDINEDIONES (GLITAZONES) *(SED-15, 3380; SEDA-27, 457; SEDA-28, 519; SEDA-29, 531)*

The use and safety of thiazolidinediones have been reviewed. Liver damage is rare, while weight gain and fluid retention are common. The mechanisms for fluid retention are suggested to be a change in intestinal ion transport resulting in an increased plasma volume, vasodilatation causing reflex sympathetic activity activation, and increased vascular permeability (58[R]).

Pioglitazone

Metabolism In a randomized placebo-controlled study in 48 people with type 2 diabetes, aged 35–75 years, who took pioglitazone 45 mg/day or placebo for 24 weeks, those taking pioglitazone gained 3.88 kg at 6 months, compared with a reduction of 0.79 kg in those who took placebo (59[c]). Scans showed that this was mainly due to a generalized *increase in subcutaneous fat*. Visceral adipose tissue did not change significantly. Subjective ratings of hunger did not change and neither was there a change in metabolic rate. However, more sensitive measures are probably required, as the calorie change to cause this sort of weight gain is small (175 kcal/day).

Drug–drug interactions Pioglitazone is metabolized in vitro by several cytochrome P450 isozymes, CYP2C8, CYP2C9, and CYP3A4 (60[R]). The metabolites have about 40–60% of the hypoglycemic activity of pioglitazone and longer half-lives.

Gemfibrozil inhibits CYP2C8 and CYP2C9 in vitro, but in vivo it inhibits CYP2C8 but not CYP2C9. *Itraconazole* inhibits CYP3A4. In 12 volunteers aged 20–27 years weight 55–85 kg, who took gemfibrozil 600 mg, itraconazole 100 mg, both, or placebo at 0800 h and 2000 h for 4 days and a single dose of 15 mg of pioglitazone on day 3, gemfibrozil increased the mean AUC of unchanged pioglitazone about three-fold and the half-life from 8 to 23 hours (61[c]). There was no change in those taking itraconazole. In those taking the combination the mean AUC of pioglitazone increased four-fold and the half-life from 8 to 40 hours. Gemfibrozil inhibited the oxidative metabolism of pioglitazone, whereas itraconazole appeared to have no effect. This suggests that in vivo CYP2C8 may be more important than CYP3A4 in the metabolism of pioglitazone. Gemfibrozil should be used cautiously when it is combined with pioglitazone.

Rosiglitazone

Neuromuscular A *myopathy* has been reported in a man taking rosiglitazone, fenofibrate, and metformin (62[A]).

- A 75-year-old man with type 2 diabetes and no history of muscle injury or viral illness presented with a creatine kinase of 6897 (reference range 0–171) U/l, MB fraction 1%, myoglobin 902 (0–110) ng/ml, and creatinine 116 (30–70) μmol/l. He had had diabetes for 11 years and his creatine kinase had been 250–350 U/l during the previous 4 years. Simvastatin had been changed 15 weeks before to fenofibrate 200 mg/day for raised triglycerides, and rosiglitazone 2 mg bd had been added 3 weeks before. He was also taking metformin 1 g bd, phenprocoumon, valsartan, and inhaled sympathomimetics. The metformin was withdrawn because of the increased creatinine. Fenofibrate and rosiglitazone were withdrawn because of a suspected drug interaction.

It is possible that the combination of rosiglitazone with fenofibrate was responsible for the severe myopathy, although the possibility of a single drug cannot be excluded. Raised creatine kinase activity has been reported with troglitazone, and there has been a report of rhabdomyolysis in a patient with type 2 diabetes taking pioglitazone when fenofibrate was added.

Sensory systems   *Macular edema* has been associated with rosiglitazone (63[A]).

- A 55-year-old man with diabetes, taking regular insulin, glargine, rosiglitazone, atorvastatin, amlodipine, quinapril, hydrochlorohiazide, and sertraline, had proliferative retinopathy, neuropathy, and nephropathy. His vision was 20/30 OD and 20/25 OS. The dose of rosiglitazone was increased from 2 to 8 mg bd and 1 month later his vision was 20/80 OD and 20/70 OS. At the same time he developed peripheral edema. The dose of rosiglitazone was reduced to 2 mg bd and his vision improved to 20/25 OU and the macular edema resolved over the next 3 weeks.

There have been several other reports of this rare adverse effect of rosiglitazone, which has been added to the SPC. Caution should be taken and appropriate follow-up should take place when rosiglitazone is added to the therapy of someone at risk of macular edema.

- A 53-year-old Hispanic woman developed bilateral, painless, slowly progressive proptosis over 12 months (64[A]). She had taken rosiglitazone 8 mg for 18 months. She had also noticed weight gain of 9 kg and an increase in abdominal girth of 4 inches. The dose of rosiglitazone was gradually reduced, with no change in appearance. A CT scan of the orbits showed normal extraocular muscles. Thyroid function was normal.

The authors postulated that there had been an increase in orbital fat in parallel to the increase in abdominal fat. Rosiglitazone can reactivate thyroid inflammatory orbitopathy and treatment of orbital fibroblasts in culture with PPARγ agonists can stimulate thyrotropin hormone receptor expression and subsequently promote adipogenesis (65[E]).

Mineral balance   In 20 people with type 2 diabetes and hypertension taking glibenclamide 15 mg/day rosiglitazone 4 mg/day was added; *serum calcium and magnesium concentration rose* slightly at 26 weeks (66[c]). The significance of this is unknown.

Liver   *Cholestatic hepatitis* has been attributed to rosiglitazone (67[A]).

- A 52-year-old man with a history of heavy alcohol use took rosiglitazone for at least 30 days before developing jaundice. Liver histology showed cholestatic hepatitis with enlarged xanthomatous Kupffer cells and no evidence of cirrhosis.

The incidence of drug-induced liver injury with rosiglitazone has been calculated at 0.02% for alanine transaminase activity 10 times the upper end of the reference range and 0.001% for jaundice (68[R]). The above case report is unusual because, although liver damage is rare, hepatic necrosis occurs more commonly than cholestatic hepatitis.

Fertility   In a study of women with polycystic ovary syndrome, 23 of 25 women with oligomenorrhea, four of five with secondary amenorrhea, and two of three with polymenorrhea achieved regular menstrual cycles after taking rosiglitazone 4 mg/day for 24 weeks. It may be worth informing women that their *fertility may increase* (69[c]).

Drug–drug interactions   Rosiglitazone is not metabolized by CYP3A4 and interactions with drugs such as *ciclosporin* and *tacrolimus* are therefore not expected. Several studies have confirmed this.

Rosiglitazone 4 mg/day, increased to 8 mg/day after 1 week, was given to 10 patients with glucose intolerance who had received a renal transplant; ciclosporin and tacrolimus whole blood concentrations were unchanged (70[c]).

In 40 patients with post-transplant diabetes using rosiglitazone 4 mg/day, with increased doses as necessary, there were no significant interactions with tacrolimus or ciclosporin; the patients were followed for 3–12 months (mean 26 weeks) (71[c]).

In 22 patients with recent renal transplants using rosiglitazone 4 and 8 mg/day there were no significant changes in blood ciclosporin and tacrolimus concentrations (72[c]).

Rosiglitazone is mainly metabolized by the CYP2C8, and CYP2C9 has a minor role. *Trimethoprim* is a competitive inhibitor of CYP2C8 and it increases rosiglitazone concentrations, with increased risks of peripheral edema and pulmonary edema. Genotype may influence the ability of trimethoprim to inhibit CYP2C8 (73[cE]).

References

1. Muis MJ, Bots ML, Bilo HJG, Hoogma RPLM, Hoekstra JBL, Grobbee DE, Stolk RP. High cumulative insulin exposure: a risk factor of atherosclerosis in type 1 diabetes? Atherosclerosis 2005;181:185–92.
2. Gerstein HC, Rosenstock J. Insulin therapy in people who have dysglycemia and type 2 diabetes mellitus: can it offer both cardiovascular protection and beta-cell preservation? Endocrinol Metab Clin N Am 2005;34:137–54.
3. Plank J, Siebenhofer A, Berghold A, Jeitler K, Horvath K, Mrak P, Pieber TR. Systematic review and meta-analysis of short-acting insulin analogues in patients with diabetes mellitus. Arch Intern Med 2005;165:1337–44.
4. Wagner VM, Grabert M, Holl RW. Severe hypoglycemia, metabolic control and diabetes management in children with type 1 diabetes in the decade after the diabetes control and complications trial – a large scale multicentre study. Eur J Pediatr 2005;164:73–9.
5. Mack-Fogg JE, Orlowski CC, Jospe N. Continuous subcutaneous insulin infusion in toddlers and children with type 1 diabetes is safe and effective. Pediatr Diabetes 2005;6:17–21.
6. Pankowska E, Skorka A, Szypowska A, Lipka M. Memory of insulin pumps and their record as a source of information about insulin therapy in children and adolescents with type 1 diabetes. Diabetes Technol Ther 2005;7:308–14.
7. Jeha GS, Karaviti LP, Anderson B, O'Brian Smith E, Donaldson S, McGirk TS, Haymond MW. Insulin pump therapy in preschool children with type 1 diabetes mellitus improves glycemic control and decreases glucose excursions and the risk of hypoglycemia. Diabetes Technol Ther 2005;7:876–84.
8. Mandal TK. Inhaled insulin for diabetes mellitus. Am J Health-Syst Pharm 2005;62:1359–64.
9. Odegard PS, Capoccia KL. Inhaled insulin: Exubera. Ann Pharmacother 2005;39:843–53.
10. Harsch IA. Inhaled insulins: their potential in the treatment of diabetes mellitus. Treat Endocrinol 2005;4:131–8.
11. Fineberg SE, Kawabata T, Finco-Kent D, Liu C, Krasner A. Antibody response to inhaled insulin in patients with type 1 or type 2 diabetes. An analysis of initial phase II and III inhaled insulin (Exubera) trials and a two year extension trial. J Clin Endocrinol Metab 2005;90:3287–94.
12. McElduff A, Mather LE, Kam PC, Clauson P. Influence of acute respiratory tract infection on the absorption of inhaled insulin using the AERx insulin diabetes management system. Br J Clin Pharmacol 2005;59:546–51.
13. Frystyk J, Chantelau E. Progression of diabetic retinopathy during improved metabolic control may be treated with reduced insulin dosage and/or somatostatin analogue administration – a case report. Growth Horm IGF Res 2005;15:130–5.
14. Sämann A, Mühlhauser I, Bender R, Kloos Ch, Müller UA. Glycaemic control and severe hypoglycaemia following training in flexible, intensive insulin therapy to enable dietary freedom in people with type 1 diabetes: a prospective implementation study. Diabetologia 2005;48:1965–70.
15. Delorme S, Chiasson J-L. Acarbose in the prevention of cardiovascular disease in subjects with impaired glucose tolerance and type 2 diabetes mellitus. Curr Opinion Pharmacol 2005;5:184–9.
16. Fujisawa T, Ikegami H, Inoue K, Kawabata Y, Ogihara T. Effect of two α-glucosidase inhibitors, voglibose and acarbose, on postprandial hyperglycemia correlates with subjective abdominal symptoms. Metabolism 2005;54:387–90.
17. Spengler M, Schmitz H, Landen H. Evaluation of the efficacy and tolerability of acarbose in patients with diabetes mellitus. A post marketing surveillance study. Clin Drug Invest 2005;25:651–9.
18. Neuser D, Benson A, Brückner A, Goldberg RB, Hoogwerf BJ, Petzinna D. Safety and tolerability of acarbose in the treatment of type 1 and type 2 diabetes mellitus. Clin Drug Invest 2005;25:579–87.

19. Segal P, Eliahou HE, Petzinna D, Neuser D, Brückner A, Spengler M. Long-term efficacy and tolerability of acarbose treatment in patients with type 2 diabetes mellitus. Clin Drug Invest 2005;25:589–95.

20. Ryan GJ, Jobe LJ, Martin R. Pramlintide in the treatment of type 1 and type 2 diabetes mellitus. Clin Ther 2005;27:1500–12.

21. Ratner R, Whitehouse F, Fineman MS, Strobel S, Shen L, Maggs DG, Kolterman OG, Weyer C. Adjunctive therapy with pramlintide lowers HbA$_{1c}$ without concomitant weight gain and increased risk of severe hypoglycemia in patients with type 1 diabetes approaching glycemic targets. Exp Clin Endocrinol Diabetes 2005;113:199–204.

22. Weyer C, Fineman MS, Strobel S, Shen L, Data J, Kolterman OG, Sylvestri MF. Properties of pramlintide and insulin upon mixing. Am J Health-Syst Pharm 2005;62:816–22.

23. Tangelder GJM, Dubbleman M, Ringens PJ. Sudden reversible osmotic lens damage ("sugar cracks") after initiation of metformin. N Engl J Med 2005;353:2621–2.

24. Kutoh E. Possible metformin-induced hepatotoxicity. Am J Geriatr Pharmacother 2005;3:270–3.

25. Vanky E, Zahlsen K, Spigset O, Carlsen SM. Placental passage of metformin in women with polycystic ovary syndrome. Fertil Steril 2005;83:1575–8.

26. Brock B, Smidt K, Ovesen P, Schmitz O, Rungby J. Is metformin therapy for polycystic ovary syndrome safe during pregnancy? Basic Clin Pharmacol Toxicol 2005;96:410–2.

27. Fall PJ, Szerlip HM. Lactic acidosis: from sour milk to septic shock. J Intens Care Med 2005;20:255–71.

28. Bugianesi E, Gentilcore E, Manini R, Natale S, Vanni E, Villanova N, David E, Rizzetto M, Marchesini G. A randomised controlled trial of metformin versus vitamin E or prescriptive diet in non-alcoholic fatty liver disease. Am J Gastroenterol 2005;100:1082–90.

29. Schwimmer JB, Middleton MS, Deutsch R, Lavine JE. A phase 2 clinical trial of metformin as a treatment for non-diabetic paediatric non-alcoholic steatohepatitis. Aliment Pharmacol Ther 2005;21:871–9.

30. Timmins P, Donahue S, Meeker J, Marathe P. Steady-state pharmacokinetics of a novel extended-release metformin formulation. Clin Pharmacokinet 2005;44:721–9.

31. Harvey B, Hickman C, Hinson G, Ralph T, Mayer A. Severe lactic acidosis complicating metformin overdose successfully treated with high-volume venovenous hemofiltration and aggressive alkalization. Pediatr Crit Care Med 2005;6:598–601.

32. Lacher M, Hermanns-Clausen M, Haeffner K, Brandis M, Pohl M. Severe metformin intoxication with lactic acidosis in an adolescent. Eur J Pediatr 2005;164:362–5.

33. Herman GA, Stevens C, Van Dyck K, Bergman A, Yi B, De Smet M, Snyder K, Hilliard D, Tanen M, Tanaka W, Wang AQ, Zeng W, Musson D, Winchell G, Davies MJ, Ramael S, Gottesdiener KM, Wagner JA. Pharmacokinetics and pharmacodynamics of sitagliptin, an inhibitor of dipeptidyl peptidase IV, in healthy subjects: results from two randomized, double-blind, placebo-controlled studies with single oral doses. Clin Pharmacol Ther 2005;78(6):675–88.

34. Miller S, St Onge EL. Sitagliptin: a dipeptidyl peptidase IV inhibitor for the treatment of type 2 diabetes. Ann Pharmacother 2006;40(7–8):1336–43.

35. Herman GA, Bergman A, Liu F, Stevens C, Wang AQ, Zeng W, Chen L, Snyder K, Hilliard D, Tanen M, Tanaka W, Meehan AG, Lasseter K, Dilzer S, Blum R, Wagner JA. Pharmacokinetics and pharmacodynamic effects of the oral DPP-4 inhibitor sitagliptin in middle-aged obese subjects. J Clin Pharmacol 2006;46(8):876–86.

36. Raz I, Hanefeld M, Xu L, Caria C, Williams-Herman D, Khatami H, Sitagliptin Study 023 Group. Efficacy and safety of the dipeptidyl peptidase-4 inhibitor sitagliptin as monotherapy in patients with type 2 diabetes mellitus. Diabetologia 2006;49(11):2564–71.

37. Aschner P, Kipnes MS, Lunceford JK, Sanchez M, Mickel C, Williams-Herman DE, Sitagliptin Study 021 Group. Effect of the dipeptidyl peptidase-4 inhibitor sitagliptin as monotherapy on glycemic control in patients with type 2 diabetes. Diabetes Care 2006;29(12):2632–7.

38. Charbonnel B, Karasik A, Liu J, Wu M, Meininger G, Sitagliptin Study 020 Group. Efficacy and safety of the dipeptidyl peptidase-4 inhibitor sitagliptin added to ongoing metformin therapy in patients with type 2 diabetes inadequately controlled with metformin alone. Diabetes Care 2006;29(12):2638–43.

39. Herman GA, Bergman A, Yi B, Kipnes M, The Sitagliptin Study 012 Group. Tolerability and pharmacokinetics of metformin and the dipeptidyl peptidase-4 inhibitor sitagliptin when co-administered in patients with type 2 diabetes. Curr Med Res Opin 2006;22(10):1939–47.

40. Edwards CMB, Stanley SA, Davis R, Brynes AE, Frost GS, Seal LJ, Ghatei MA, Bloom SR. Exendin-4 reduces fasting and postprandial glucose and decreases energy intake in healthy volunteers. Am J Physiol Endocrinol Metab 2001;281:E155–61.

41. DeFronzo RA, Ratner RE, Han J, Kim DD, Fineman MS, Baron AD. Effects of exenatide (exendin-4) on glycemic control and weight over 30 weeks in metformin-treated patients with type 2 diabetes. Diabetes Care 2005;28:1092–100.

42. Kendall DM, Riddle MC, Rosenstock J, Zhuang D, Kim DD, Fineman MS, Baron AD. Effects of exenatide (exendin-4) on glycemic control over 30 weeks in patients with type 2 diabetes treated with metformin and a sulfonylurea. Diabetes Care 2005;28:1083–91.

43. Ahren B. Exenatide: a novel treatment of type 2 diabetes. Therapy 2005;2:207–22.

44. Barnett AH. Exenatide. Drugs Today 2005;41:563–78.

45. Keating GM. Exenatide. Drugs 2005;65:1681–92.

46. Sinclair EM, Drucker DJ. Glucagon-like peptide 1 receptor agonists and dipeptidyl peptidase IV inhibitors: new therapeutic agents for the treatment of type 2 diabetes. Curr Opin Endocrinol Diabetes 2005;12:146–51.

47. Taylor K, Kim D, Nielsen LL, Aisporna M, Baron AD, Fineman MS. Day-long subcutaneous infusion of exenatide lowers glycemia in patients with type 2 diabetes. Horm Metabol Res 2005;37:627–32.

48. Poon T, Nelson P, Shen L, Mihm M, Taylor K, Fineman M, Kim D. Exenatide improves glycemic control and reduces body weight in subjects with type 2 diabetes: a dose-ranging study. Diabetes Technol Ther 2005;7:467–72.

49. Nauck MA, Meier JJ. Glucagon-like peptide 1 and its derivatives in the treatment of diabetes. Regulatory Peptides 2005;128:135–48.

50. Hiles R, Carpenter T, Serota D, Schafer K, Ross P, Nelson D, Rebelatto M. Exenatide does not cause pancreatic islet cell proliferative lesions in rats and mice following 2-year exposure. Diabetes 2004;53(Suppl 2):A380.

51. Calara F, Taylor K, Han J, Zabala E, Carr EM, Wintle M, Fineman M. A randomized, open-label, crossover study examining the effect of injection site on bioavailability of exenatide (synthetic exendin-4). Clin Ther 2005;27:210–5.

52. Kothare PA, Soon DKW, Linnebjerg H, Park S, Chan C, Yeo A, Lim M, Mace KF, Wise SD. Effect of exenatide on the steady-state pharmacokinetics on digoxin. J Clin Pharmacol 2005;45:1032–7.

53. Blase E, Taylor K, Gao H, Wintle M, Fineman M. Pharmacokinetics of an oral drug (acetaminophen) administered at various times in relation to subcutaneous injection of exenatide (exendin-4) in healthy subjects. J Clin Pharmacol 2005;45:570–7.

54. Feinglos MN, Saad MF, Pi-Sunyert FX, An B, Santiago O. Effects of liraglutide (NN2211) a long acting GLP-1 analogue, on glycemic control and bodyweight in subjects with type 2 diabetes. Diabetic Med 2005;22:1016–23 [on behalf of Lirglutide Dose-response Study Group].

55. Lheureux PER, Zahir S, Penaloza A, Gris M. Bench-to-bench review: antidotal treatment of sulfonylurea-induced hypoglycemia with octreotide. Crit Care 2005;9:543–9.

56. Bertini AM, Silva JC, Taborda W, Becker F, Bebber FRL, Viesi JMZ, Aquim G, Ribeiro TE. Perinatal outcomes and the use of oral hypoglycaemic agents. J Perinat Med 2005;33:519–23.

57. Chounta A, Zouridakis S, Ellinas C, Tsiodras S, Zoumpouli C, Kopanaks S, Giamoarellou H. Cholestatic liver injury after glimepiride therapy. J Hepatol 2005;42:944–6.

58. Huang A, Raskin P. Thiazolidinediones and insulin. Treat Endocrinol 2005;4:205–20.

59. Smith SR, de Jonge L, Volaufova J, Li Y, Xie H, Bray GA. Effect of pioglitazone on body composition and energy expenditure: a randomized controlled trial. Metab Clin Exp 2005;54:24–32.

60. Kirchheiner J, Roots I, Goldammer M, Rosenkranz B, Brockmöller J. Effect of genetic polymorphisms in cytochrome P450 (CYP) 2C9 and CYP2C8 on the pharmacokinetics of oral antidiabetic drugs: clinical relevance. Clin Pharmacokinet 2005;44(12):1209–25.

61. Jaakkola T, Backman JT, Neuvonen M, Neuvonen P. Effects of gemfibrozil, itraconazole and their combination on the pharmacokinetics of pioglitazone. Clin Pharmacol Ther 2005;77:404–14.

62. Ledl M, Hohenecker J, Francesconi C, Roots I, Bauer MF, Roden M. Acute myopathy in a type 2 diabetic patient on combination therapy with metformin, fenofibrate and rosiglitazone. Diabetologia 2005;48:1996–8.

63. Colucciello M. Vision loss due to macular edema induced by rosiglitazone treatment of diabetes mellitus. Arch Ophthalmol 2005;123:1273–5.

64. Levin F, Kazim M, Smith TJ, Marcovici E. Rosiglitazone-induced proptosis. Arch Ophthalmol 2005;123:119–21.

65. Valyasevi RW, Harteneck DA, Dutton CM, Bahn RS. Stimulation of adipogenesis, peroxisome proliferator-activated receptor-gamma (PPARγ) and thyrotropin receptor by PPARγ agonists in human orbital preadipocyte fibroblasts. J Clin Endocrinol Metab 2002;87:2352–8.

66. Sarafidis PA, Lasaridis AN, Nilsson PM, Hitoglou-Makedou AD, Pagkalos EM, Yovos JG, Pliakos CI, Tourkantonis AA. The effect of rosiglitazone on urine albumin excretion in patients with type 2 diabetes mellitus and hypertension. Am J Hypertens 2005;18:227–34.

67. Menees SB, Anderson MA, Chensue SW, Moseley RH. Hepatic injury in a patient taking rosiglitazone. J Clin Gastroenterol 2005;39:638–40.

68. Slavin DE, Schlichting CL, Freston JW. Rating the severity of the medical consequences of drug-induced liver injury. Regulatory Toxicol Pharmacol 2005;43:134–40.

69. Yilmaz M, Karakoc A, Törüner FB, Cakir N, Tiras B, Ayvaz G, Arslan M. The effects of rosiglitazone and metformin on menstrual cyclicity and hirsutism in polycystic ovary syndrome. Gynecol Endocrinol 2005;21:154–60.

70. Viytovich MH, Simonsen C, Jenssen T, Hjelmesaeth J, Asberg A, Hartsmann A. Short-term treatment with rosiglitazone improves glucose tolerance, insulin sensitivity and endothelial function in renal transplant recipients. Nephrol Dial Transplant 2005;20:413–8.

71. Villanueva G, Baldwin D. Rosiglitazone therapy of posttransplant diabetes mellitus. Transplantation 2005;80:1402–5.

72. Pietruck F, Kribben A, Van TN, Patschan D, Herget-Rosenthal S, Janssen O, Mann K, Philipp T, Witzke O. Rosiglitazone is as safe and effective treatment option of new-onset diabetes

mellitus after renal transplantation. Transplant Int 2005;18:483–6.

73. Hruska MW, Amico JA, Langaee TY, Ferrell RE, Fitzgerald SM, Frye RF. The effect of trimethoprim on CYP2C8 mediated rosiglitazone metabolism in human liver microsomes and healthy subjects. Br J Clin Pharmacol 2005;59:70–9.

R.C.L. Page

43   Miscellaneous hormones

Calcitonin   *(SED-15, 595; SEDA-27, 465;*
SEDA-29, 539)

Mineral balance   Calcitonin can cause *ab-*
normalities of calcium balance.

- A 46-year-old woman with low back pain and osteoporosis took salmon calcitonin subcutaneously
100 U/day and calcium carbonate orally 1.5 g/day
for 7 days before developing nausea and facial
flushing (1[A]). Calcitonin was continued for a further 8 days and then stopped. The next day she
developed intermittent generalized convulsions.
She was subsequently found to have breast cancer with skeletal metastases and hypercalcemia
(3.9 mmol/l) without a reduced parathyroid hormone concentration (115 pg/ml). She was given
fluids and the hypercalcemia promptly resolved.

The authors suggested that this was the first
report of exogenous calcitonin causing hypercalcemia. There were several unknowns in this
case, including the calcium concentration before treatment and the concentration of PTHrp,
which would have helped to determine the
cause of the hypercalcemia. Calcitonin is usually associated with a reduction in calcium
concentration rather than a rise. The authors
postulated that calcitonin could alter PTHrp
concentrations, with different effects depending
on cell type. They also provided evidence of hypercalcemia caused by calcitonin in non-human
models (2[E]).

- A 72-year-old woman received calcitonin 100 IU
twice a week intramuscularly, calcitriol 0.25 micrograms bd, and daily calcium supplements for
3 years, before presenting with a raised calcium
concentration (2.7 mmol/l) and linear calcification
in the knee joints. The parathormone concentration
was raised (151 pg/ml; reference range 7–53) and
a parathyroid adenoma was demonstrated on ultrasound (3[A]).

Side Effects of Drugs, Annual 30
J.K. Aronson (Editor)
ISSN: 0378-6080
DOI: 10.1016/S0378-6080(08)00043-3

Primary hyperparathyroidism was the likely explanation in this patient, rather than a direct
effect of calcitonin.

Gonadotropins (gonadorelin and
analogues)   *(SED-15, 1536; SEDA-27,*
465; SEDA-28, 528; SEDA-29, 539)

Placebo-controlled studies   In a randomized,
placebo-controlled study in women who received leuprolide acetate depot 11.25 mg intramuscularly with tibolone 2.5 mg/day ($n = 36$),
leuprolide acetate depot 11.25 mg with placebo
($n = 37$), or a placebo injection with placebo
tablets ($n = 39$), irritable bowel syndrome related to the menstrual cycle improved in those
who received leuprolide (4[C]). There were *hot*
flushes in those who took leuprolide compared
with placebo; no data were given about the frequency of hot flushes, but there were no withdrawals because of this symptom. *Amenorrhea*
also occurred. Both flushing and amenorrhea
are expected adverse effects of leuprolide.

Endocrine   Gonadotropin-releasing hormone
analogues initially stimulate the pituitary gland,
resulting in *increased concentrations of luteiniz-*
ing hormone and testosterone in men. Subsequently, the pituitary receptors down-regulate
and testosterone concentrations fall. On withdrawal of the agonist the effects have been
thought to be reversible. However, they can
be sustained for substantial periods in men receiving prolonged courses for prostate cancer
(5[R]). Patients receiving intermittent androgen
therapy for prostate cancer were treated with leuprolide acetate 7.5 mg monthly and nilutamide
orally for 8 months. Full testosterone recovery
during the off treatment period was documented
in 61% of cycles. In cycles during which recovery occurred, the median time to recovery was
23 (4–61) weeks (6[c]).

In Japanese children with precocious puberty treated with leuprolide the time between the last injection and the median onset of menarche was 15 (range 3.6–63) months (7^C). The *age at menarche was higher* than that of the healthy population (13 versus 12 years).

For in vitro fertilization the use of triptorelin 0.1 mg/day, with early withdrawal, caused *suppressed endogenous luteinizing hormone* for 10–14 days after withdrawal (8^C).

Metabolism   Two men developed *hyperglycemia* after using leuprolide acetate.

- A 61-year-old Japanese man with prostate cancer had had well controlled diabetes for 6 years (HbA_{1c} less than 6.4%). He received leuprolide acetate subcutaneously 3.75 mg/month and oral flutamide 250 mg/day. Three weeks after the second injection his fasting glucose was 18 mmol/l and HbA_{1c} 8.0%.
- An 81-year-old Japanese man not known to have diabetes developed prostate cancer. His HbA_{1c} concentration was 5.1%. He received three injections of leuprolide acetate 3.75 mg/month subcutaneously then 11.25 mg every 3 months. After 7 months he complained of thirst and his blood glucose had increased to 19 mmol/l and HbA_{1c} to 9.9%.

There is increasing evidence of a link between low testosterone concentrations and type 2 diabetes mellitus (9^A).

Hematologic   A *coagulopathy* has been attributed to leuprolide (10^A).

- A 65-year-old man, with metastatic carcinoma of the prostate was treated with flutamide 250 mg/day orally followed after 6 days by 7.5 mg leuprolide intramuscularly. Two days later he developed bleeding and hematomas. His hemoglobin fell from 12.4 to 7.8 g/dl and he had a disseminated intravascular coagulopathy.

The timing in this case suggested that testosterone release may have occurred despite androgen blockade by flutamide. As a result, tumor cell growth and coagulopathy may have occurred. In some patients with prostate cancer taking fluoxymesterone (an androgenic hormone) there was activation of clotting (11^c).

Skin   *Granulomatous reactions* at leuprorelin injection sites have been previously reported. Three further cases in Japanese men have led to speculation that they occur more often in Japan because of the use of subcutaneous injection rather than intramuscular injection, which is used in Western countries (12^{cr}). The exact mechanism of this reaction is unknown, and whether it is due to the co-polymer or leuprorelin itself is debated. Local reactions can cause reduced efficacy (13^A).

Pregnancy   Of 34 women who conceived while receiving triptorelin acetate for infertility, five developed gestational diabetes (17%) compared with a background rate of 5% (14^c). The increased incidence could not be explained by obesity, as only one of these five women had a BMI over 35 kg/m^2; nor could it be explained by polycystic ovary syndrome. Larger studies are required to confirm this finding.

Teratogenicity   There was one case of polydactyly with no major defects (3.4%) in the children of 35 women who had conceived while using triptorelin (14^c). This was probably coincidental.

Drug dosage regimens   Intermittent courses of gonadotropin analogues for prostate cancer may reduce the frequency of adverse effects. In 95 patients who received 245 cycles of leuprolide acetate and nilutamide for 8 months, testosterone concentrations recovered during the rest periods (61% of cycles) and sexual function improved (47%) (6^c).

Somatropin (human growth hormone, hGH)   *(SED-15, 3163; SEDA-27, 466; SEDA-28, 528; SEDA-29, 540)*

Cardiovascular   Of 23 adolescent patients with growth hormone deficiency in childhood who were reassessed when they had reached adult bone age and completed puberty, eight were no longer thought to be growth hormone deficient and therapy was withdrawn (15^c). The other 15 had a 6-month break from growth hormone therapy and then restarted. Compared with a control group at the time of withdrawal, the eight patients without growth hormone deficiency had *increased thickness of the intima media*, which fell to normal values by 12 months. These results support the recommendation that children with idiopathic growth hormone deficiency should be retested after completion of growth to assess the need for continued administration of growth hormone.

Musculoskeletal   Of 35 children with achondroplasia randomized to either low-dose growth hormone (0.1 IU/kg/day) or high-dose growth hormone (0.2 IU/kg/day), two in the low-dose group developed *worsening of bow legs*, requiring surgery; one in the high-dose group developed incomplete paraplegia, requiring thoracic laminectomy, and another had surgery for a narrow foramen magnum (16[c]). There was no control group, and although it was thought that all the events had been related to the achondroplasia rather than the growth hormone, it is not known whether problems had been exacerbated.

- A girl with floating harbor syndrome (short stature, delayed bone age, typical facies, and delayed speech development) received growth hormone from the age of 3.5 years for 14 months (17[A]). At 6 years she developed an abnormal gait due to a tethered cord.

A tethered cord is a developmental abnormality that does not usually manifest until midchildhood. Floating harbor syndrome is associated with severe short stature, and tethered cord is not usually a manifestation. It is possible that altered growth velocity associated with growth hormone may have been implicated.

Death   Sudden unexplained death in Prader–Willi syndrome has been reported with and without growth hormone treatment. The reports in association with growth hormone have been in boys. Two deaths in girls have now been reported (18[A]).

- A 4-year-old girl with Prader–Willi syndrome had an adenoidectomy for severe snoring, and growth hormone was started at a dose of 0.24 mg/kg/week. Suddenly, 7 weeks later, she died at home of cardiorespiratory failure.
- A 9-year-old girl with trisomy 21 and Prader–Willi syndrome started growth hormone treatment 0.14 mg/kg/week. She had previously received growth hormone 0.28 mg/kg/week for 12 months at the age of 7 years, but therapy had been stopped at the family's request. Six months later she developed a respiratory infection and died.

In a review of sudden death in patients with Prader–Willi syndrome, those who received growth hormone were compared with those who had not (19[R]). Death between the ages of 3 and 15 years seemed to be more common in those who had received growth hormone than in those who had not. The dose of growth hormone, obesity, and respiratory problems may have been contributing factors. Six of seven patients who had received growth hormone died within 4 months of starting treatment.

Tumorigenicity   The safety of growth hormone treatment for idiopathic short stature has been discussed in two reports of studies involving pharmaceutical companies. The doses and durations of therapy varied. Comparison of adverse event rates with those in the background population did not show an increased risk of new malignancies. However, this was a post-marketing surveillance study and it is uncertain that it had sufficient power to detect a small increase in risk (20[R]). In a similar report, adverse events in patients with idiopathic short stature were compared with those in patients with growth hormone deficiency and Turner's syndrome (21[R]). While malignancy was not attributed to the use of growth hormone, long-term safety data are essential to establish whether there is a small increased risk of life-threatening events.

Japanese patients with growth hormone deficiency who had taken part in a placebo-controlled study ($n = 64$) were entered into an open 48-week study of growth hormone; one had a recurrence of *craniopharyngioma* and required withdrawal from the study (22[C]). Whether growth hormone was contributory is not known.

Drug formulations   The proprietary product hGH-Biosphere is a dry powder containing microspheres of growth hormone, which is reconstituted and injected subcutaneously. In eight patients with growth hormone deficiency who took part in a phase I/II study, there were two peaks of growth hormone concentration: the first was 0.83 μg/l at 7.7 hours and the second was 1.2 μg/l after 7.2 days (23[c]). The concentrations fell to baseline from days 10 to 28. There were no serious adverse events. One patient had fatigue, headache, and cramps, which resolved over 28 hours, one had myalgia, and two had erythema. The long-term suitability of long-acting growth hormone replacement is not known.

Growth hormone receptor antagonists *(SEDA-28, 529)*

Metabolism   Fasting glucose concentrations fell and HbA$_{1c}$ concentrations improved in people with acromegaly who used pegvisomant (24^c). This occurred in those with and without diabetes, although there was a larger change in the former. However, this was an uncontrolled study and some change may have occurred because of closer monitoring. Pegvisomant does not alter insulin concentrations directly but does so through its action in blocking the effects of growth hormone. Monitoring blood glucose concentrations in those with diabetes receiving pegvisomant is advisable, in order to ensure appropriate treatment when necessary.

Liver   In a non-randomized, open, 32-week study in 53 people with acromegaly, 48 of whom had previously received pegvisomant, all of whom had used octreotide LAR for at least 3 months, pegvisomant 10 mg/day subcutaneously was given 4 weeks after the last dose of octreotide and the dose was adjusted depending on IGF1 concentrations; 51 completed 12 weeks of the study and 49 completed 32 weeks (24^c). Three patients developed *abnormal liver function tests* but continued the study. In one the alanine transaminase activity rose to more than 7 times the upper limit of the reference at week 20, and in another it rose to more than 4.5 times at week 24; a third had fluctuating activity, but never more than 3.5 times the upper limit of the reference range. The dose of pegvisomant was not reduced and liver function returned to normal with continued therapy.

Tumorigenicity   In one patient who switched to pegvisomant, a large aggressive pituitary tumor continued to grow (24^c). A second patient, who had been treated initially with surgery and then with a dopamine receptor agonist and octreotide LAR for 4 years, switched to pegvisomant for 21 months and subsequently octreotide LAR for 18 months and had stable disease with a tumor volume of 1.33 cm^3. When pegvisomant was given again at week 32 the tumor increased in size to 2.24 cm^3. When pegvisomant was continued for a further 12 months there was no further growth. Regular long-term follow-up by scanning when using pegvisomant is advisable.

Somatostatin (growth hormone release-inhibiting hormone) and analogues *(SED-15, 3160; SEDA-27, 467; SEDA-28, 530; SEDA-29, 541)*

Endocrine   Of 7 infants with congenital chylothorax whose cases were reviewed, one had been treated with continuous intravenous somatostatin (60 micrograms/kg/day) at 33 days (25^{Ac}). Therapy was withdrawn after 10 days as the symptoms had improved. Thyroid function had been normal at 13 days but was found to be abnormal at 57 days, during routine screening for *congenital hypothyroidism* (T$_4$ 26 µg/l, TSH 116 mU/l). The infant had recurrent sepsis and received further somatostatin. Levothyroxine was given and thyroid function was monitored over several months. At 11 months thyroid function was normal, levothyroxine having been withdrawn at 8 months. The other six infants with chylothorax did not receive somatostatin and did not develop hypothyroidism. It was therefore thought that the somatostatin could have been responsible, although the mechanism was unclear. Somatostatin inhibits TSH secretion and is useful for treating TSH-secreting adenomas.

Octreotide

Hematologic   *Thrombosis of a splenic artery pseudoaneurysm* has been reported in a patient receiving octreotide (26^A).

• A 55-year-old woman with a history of chronic pancreatitis developed epigastric pain and melena and was found to have a splenic artery pseudoaneurysm expanding a pseudocyst. She was given an intravenous bolus of octreotide followed by an infusion of 50 micrograms/hour. A CT scan subsequently suggested thrombosis of the pseudoaneurysm, with segmental splenic infarction. Nine months later the pseudoaneurysm had recanalized.

The octreotide may have contributed by causing vasoconstriction. A case of thrombosis in a splenic artery pseudoaneurysm in a patient receiving somatostatin has previously been reported (27^c).

Gastrointestinal   Of 24 patients with hepatocellular carcinoma receiving octreotide LAR, 11 had mild *diarrhea* (28[c]). The effect of octreotide on bowel transit appears to be variable. In some patients, such as those with carcinoid syndrome, it is useful for the management of diarrhea.

In 10 non-acromegalic controls, 11 patients with acromegaly not receiving octreotide, and 11 receiving long-term octreotide subcutaneously, large bowel transit time was increased in acromegaly and prolonged further in those receiving octreotide (29[c]). The total fecal count of anerobic bacteria was higher and bile acid activity was increased in those who received octreotide. The use of octreotide in acromegaly increases the risk of gallstones.

Skin   There have been three cases of *lipoatrophy* in women taking subcutaneous octreotide for acromegaly (30[A]). One had used octreotide 600 micrograms/day for 6 years, another had used octreotide 300 micrograms/day for 30 months, and the third developed problems 4 years after using octreotide 800 micrograms/day. The patients were given intramuscular octreotide instead; in one the lipoatrophy regressed. The mechanism is not known. Long-term subcutaneous octreotide has been used less often since the development of long-acting somatostatin analogues, but when it is used follow-up for lipoatrophy is appropriate. No data were given as to whether the lipoatrophy affected the absorption of octreotide.

Urinary tract   Of 12 patients with ascites due to cirrhosis of the liver, who received subcutaneous octreotide 300 micrograms bd for 11 days, 11 had increased renal plasma flow and 10 had a reduced GFR (31[c]). Creatinine concentrations did not change. The effects of octreotide on the kidneys have been variably reported in previous studies. In patients with cirrhosis the effects are likely to be affected by the activated renin–angiotensin–aldosterone system.

Oxytocin and analogues   *(SED-15, 2657; SEDA-27,468; SEDA-28 531)*

Pregnancy   High-dose and low-dose oxytocin have been compared in augmentation or induction of labor (32[R]). There was large variation in the doses given in the studies reviewed, particularly among the high doses used. In some studies low-dose oxytocin resulted in higher rates of cesarean section but fewer fetal heart rate abnormalities. In one study women given high-dose oxytocin had a higher rate of cesarean sections as a result of fetal distress. Studies were often underpowered.

VASOPRESSIN AND ANALOGUES   *(SED-15, 3609; SEDA-27, 469; SEDA-28, 531; SEDA-29, 542)*

A review of the use of vasopressin and terlipressin for the management of septic shock has shown that the available data are limited and that randomized controlled trials are needed (33[R]). The possible adverse effects of vasopressin on organ function require further clarification. Vasopressin 0.23 U/minute in patients with hepatorenal syndrome did not appear to be associated with the adverse effects that occur at the lower doses that are used to treat other critically ill patients (34[c]). A maximum dose of 0.04 U/minute is recommended for the management of septic shock (33[R]).

Electrolyte balance   *Hyponatremia* has been attributed to vasopressin in children undergoing cardiac surgery (35[A]).

- A 36-week-old 2.3 kg girl undergoing cardiac surgery received vasopressin 0.0003 units/kg/minute, titrated up to a maximum dose of 0.0012 units/kg/minute. After 82 hours vasopressin was discontinued because of hyponatremia (sodium 117 mmol/l).
- A 3.6 kg boy born at term underwent cardiac surgery and received similar doses of vasopressin, which was discontinued after 60 hours because of a sodium concentration of 119 mmol/l.

The falls in sodium were gradual and resolved on withdrawal of vasopressin. The authors recommended that when vasopressin is used for more than 24 hours sodium concentrations should be monitored.

Desmopressin (N-deamino-8-D-arginine vasopressin, DDAVP)   *(SED-15, 1076; SEDA-29, 543)*

Electrolyte balance Electrolyte abnormalities are well described with desmopressin. However, further reports on the use of desmopressin in nocturnal enuresis have suggested that significant *hyponatremia* is rare, provided that guidelines are adhered to (36[c]) (37[c]).

- A 3.5-year-old girl with mild hemophilia A received desmopressin 0.3 micrograms/kg intravenously 30 minutes before adenotonsillectomy. She drank 600 ml of fluid within the first 10 hours and then received 300 ml of intravenous 5% dextrose in 0.45% saline. She developed hyponatremia, headache, nausea, and seizures.

This case is a reminder that even one dose can result in problems if fluid intake is inappropriate (38[A]).

The pharmacokinetics of one dose of desmopressin 400 micrograms have been investigated in 15 men and nine women with nocturia aged over 65 years (39[c]). They then entered a placebo-controlled crossover evaluation period. Peak concentrations occurred at 1–2 hours after administration and gradually fell over 6–7 hours. The women had significantly higher concentrations than the men, even after adjustment for body weight. Four women were withdrawn from the crossover period because of *hyponatremia*. Hyponatremia has been reported to be more common in elderly patients using desmopressin. Particular caution should be taken when treating older women.

Terlipressin   *(SEDA-29, 544)*

Cardiovascular In 32 patients undergoing carotid endarterectomy treated with renin–angiotensin inhibitors *hypotension* developed under general anesthesia (40[c]). They were randomized to received terlipressin 1 mg ($n = 16$) or noradrenaline infusion. Compared with baseline those who received terlipressin had reduced gastric mucosal perfusion for at least 4 hours. There was also reduced oxygen delivery and oxygen consumption index at 30 minutes and 4 hours in those who received terlipressin.

References

1. Chung SY, Chen TH, Lai SL, Huang CH, Chen WH. Hypercalcaemia and status epilepticus relates to salmon calcitonin administration in breast cancer. Breast 2005;14(5):399–402.
2. Fouchereau-Peron M, Arlot-Bonnemains Y, Moukhtar MS, Milhaud G. Calcitonin induces hypercalcemia in grey mullet and immature freshwater and sea-water adapted rainbow trout. Comp Biochem Physiol A 1987;87:1051–3.
3. Ozcajar L, Akinci A. Linear joint calcifications while treating osteoporosis: in flagrante delicto. Rheumatol Int 2005;25:154–5.
4. Palomba S, Orio F, Manguso F, Russo T, Falbo A, Lombardi G, Doldo P, Zullo F. Leuprolide acetate treatment with and without coadministration of tibolone in premenopausal women with menstrual cycle-related irritable bowel syndrome. Fertil Steril 2005;83:1012–20.
5. Heyns CF. Triptorelin in the treatment of prostate cancer. Clinical efficacy and tolerability. Am J Cancer 2005;4:169–83.
6. Malone S, Perry G, Segal R, Dahrouge S, Crook J. Long-term side-effects of intermittent androgen suppression therapy in prostate cancer: results of a phase II study. BJU Int 2005;96:514–20.
7. Tanaka T, Niimi H, Matsuo N, Fujieda K, Tachibana K, Ohyama K, Satoh M, Kugu K. Results of long-term follow-up after treatment of central precocious puberty with leuprorelin acetate: evaluation of effectiveness of treatment and recovery of gonadal function. The TAP-144-SR Japanese study group on central precocious puberty. J Clin Endocrinol Metab 2005;90:1371–6.
8. Simons AHM, Roelolofs HJM, Schmoutziguer APE, Roozenburg BJ, van't Hof-van den Brink EP, Schoonderwoerd SA. Early cessation of triptorelin in in vitro fertilization: a double-blind, randomized study. Fertil Steril 2005;83:889–96.
9. Inaba M, Otani Y, Nishimura K, Takaha N, Okuyama A, Koga M, Azuma J, Kawase I,

Kasayama S. Marked hyperglycemia after androgen-deprivation therapy for prostate cancer and usefulness of pioglitazone for its treatment. Metabolism 2005;54(1):55–9.

10. Bern MM. Coagulopathy, following medical therapy, for carcinoma of the prostate. Haematology 2005;10(1):65–8.

11. Al-Mondhiry H, Manni A, Owen J, Gordon R. Hemostatic effects of hormonal stimulation in patients with metastatic prostate cancer. Am J Hematol 1988;28:141–5.

12. Yasukawa K, Sawamura D, Sugawara H, Kato N. Leuprorelin acetate granulomas: case reports and review of the literature. Br J Dermatol 2005;152:1045–7.

13. Tonini G, Marioni S, Forleo V, Rustico M. Local reactions to luteinizing hormone releasing hormone analog therapy. J Pediatr 1995;126:159–60.

14. Mayer A, Lunenfeld E, Wiznitzer A, Har-vardi I, Bentov Y, Levitas E. Increased prevalence of gestational diabetes mellitus in in vitro fertilization pregnancies inadvertently conceived during treatment with long-acting triptorelin acetate. Fertil Steril 2005;84:789–92.

15. Calao A, Di Somma C, Rota F, Di Maio S, Salerno M, Klain A, Spiezia S, Lombardi G. Common carotid intima–media thickness in growth hormone (GH) deficient adolescents: a prospective study after GH withdrawal and restarting GH replacement. J Clin Endocrinol Metab 2005;90:2659–65.

16. Hertel NT, Eklöf O, Ivarsson S, Aronson S, Westphal O, Sipilä I, Kaitila I, Bland J, Veimo D, Müller J, Mohnike K, Neumeyer L, Ritzen M, Hagenäs L. Growth hormone treatment in 35 prepubertal children with achondroplasia: a five-year dose-response trial. Acta Paediatr 2005;94:1402–10.

17. Wiltshire E, Wickremesekera A, Dixon J. Floating-Harbor syndrome complicated by tethered cord: a new association and potential contribution from growth hormone therapy. Am J Med Genet A 2005;136(1):81–3.

18. Riedl S, Blümel P, Zwiauer K, Frisch H. Death in two female Prader–Willi syndrome patients during the early phase of growth hormone treatment. Acta Paediatr 2005;94:974–7.

19. Nagai T, Obata K, Tonoki H, Temma S, Murakamai N, Katada Y, Yoshino A, Sakazume S, Takahashi E, Sakuta R, Niikawa N. Cause of sudden, unexpected death of Prader–Willi syndrome patients with or without growth hormone treatment. Am J Med Genet A 2005;136(1):45–8.

20. Kemp SF, Kuntze J, Attie KM, Maneatis T, Butler MS, Frane J, Lippe B. Efficacy and safety results of long-term growth hormone treatment of idiopathic short stature. J Clin Endocrinol Metab 2005;90:5247–53.

21. Quigley CA, Gill AM, Crowe BJ, Robling K, Chipman JJ, Rose SR, Ross JL, Cassorla FG, Wolka AM, Wit JM, Rekers-Mombarg LTM, Cutler GB. Safety of growth hormone treatment in pediatric patients with idiopathic short stature. J Clin Endocrinol Metab 2005;90:5188–96.

22. Chihara K, Koledova E, Shimatsu A, Kato Y, Kohno H, Tanaka T, Teramoto A, Bates PC, Attanasio AF. An individualized GH dose regimen for long-term GH treatment in Japanese patients with adult GH deficiency. Eur J Endocrinol 2005;153:57–65.

23. Jostel A, Mukherjee A, Alenfall J, Smethurst L, Shalet S. A new sustained-release preparation of human growth hormone and its pharmacokinetic, pharmacodynamic and safety profile. Clin Endocrinol 2005;62:623–7.

24. Barkan AL, Burman P, Clemmons DR, Drake WM, Gagel RF, Harris PE, Trainer PJ, van der Lely AJ, Vance ML. Glucose homeostasis and safety in patients with acromegaly converted from long-acting octreotide to pegvisomant. J Clin Endocrinol Metab 2005;90:5684–91.

25. Maayan-Metzger A, Sack J, Mazkereth R, Vardi A, Kuint J. Somatostatin treatment of congenital chylothorax may induce transient hypothyroidism in newborns. Acta Paediatr 2005;94:785–9.

26. Tang LJ, Zipser S, Kang YS. Temporary spontaneous thrombosis of a splenic artery pseudoaneurysm in chronic pancreatitis during intravenous octreotide administration. J Vasc Interv Radiol 2005;16(6):863–6.

27. De Rone T, VanBeers B, de Canniere L, Trigaux JP, Melange M. Thrombosis of splenic artery pseudoaneurysm complicating pancreatitis. Gut 1993;34:1271–3.

28. Slijkuis WA, Stadheim L, Hassoun ZM, Nzeako UC, Kremers WK, Talwalkar JA, Gores GJ. Octreotide therapy for advanced hepatocellular carcinoma. J Clin Gastroenterol 2005;39:333–8.

29. Thomas LA, Veysey MJ, Murphy GM, Russell-Jones D, French GL, Wass JAH, Dowling RH. Octreotide induced prolongation of colonic transit increases fecal anaerobic bacteria, bile acid metabolizing enzymes, and serum deoxycholic acid in patients with acromegaly. Gut 2005;54:630–5.

30. Atmaca A, Erbas T. Lipoatrophy induced by subcutaneous administration of octreotide in the treatment of acromegaly. Exp Clin Endocrinol Diabetes 2005;113:340–3.

31. Kalambokis G, Economou M, Fotopoulos A, Bokharhii JA, Pappas C, Katsaraki A, Tsianos EV. The effects of chronic treatment with octreotide versus octreotide plus midodrine on systemic hemodynamics and renal hemodynamics and function in nonazotemic cirrhotic patients with ascites. Am J Gastroenterol 2005;100:879–85.

32. Patka JH, Lodolce AE, Johnston AK. High-versus low-dose oxytocin for augmentation or induction of labor. Ann Pharmacother 2005;39:95–101.

33. Delmas A, Leone M, Rousseau S, Albanèse J, Martin C. Clinical review: vasopressin and terlipressin in septic shock patients. Crit Care 2005;9:212–22.

34. Kiser TH, Fish DN, Obritsch MD, Jung R, Mac-
Laren R, Parikh CR. Vasopressin, not octreotide,
may be beneficial in the treatment of hepatorenal syndrome: a retrospective study. Nephrol Dial
Transplant 2005;20:1813–20.

35. Scheurer MA, Bradley SM, Atz AM. Vasopressin
to attenuate pulmonary hypertension and improve systemic blood pressure after correction of
obstructed total anomalous pulmonary venous return. J Thorac Cardiovasc Surg 2005;129:464–6.

36. Del Gado R, Del Gaizo D, Cennamo M, Au-
riemma R, Del Gado G, Verni M. Desmopressin
is a safe drug for the treatment of enuresis. Scand
J Urol Nephrol 2005;39:308–12.

37. Triantafyllidis A, Charalambous S, Papat-
soris AG, Papathanasiou A, Kalaitzis C,
Rombis V, Touloupidis S. Management of
nocturnal enuresis in Greek children. Pediatr
Nephrol 2005;20:1343–5.

38. Molnár Z, Farkas V, Nemes L, Reusz GS, Sza-
bó AJ. Hyponatraemic seizures resulting from inadequate post-operative intake following a single
dose of desmopressin. Nephrol Dial Transplant
2005;20:2265–7.

39. Hvistendahl GM, Riis A, Nørgaard JP,
Djurhuus JC. The pharmacokinetics of 400 µg
of oral desmopressin in elderly patients with
nocturia, and the correlation between the absorption of desmopressin and clinical effect. BJU Int
2005;95:804–9.

40. Morelli A, Tritapepe L, Rocco M, Conti G,
Orecchioni A, De Gaetano A, Picchini U,
Pelaia P, Reale C, Pietropaoli P. Terlipressin
versus norepinephrine to counteract anesthesia-
induced hypotension in patients treated with
renin–angiotensin system inhibitors: effects on
systemic and regional hemodynamics. Anesthesiology 2005;102:12–9.

44 Drugs that affect lipid metabolism

Ezetimibe *(SED-15, 1308; SEDA-27, 473; SEDA-28, 534; SEDA-29, 546)*

Ezetimibe selectively and potently blocks intestinal absorption of dietary and biliary cholesterol. In studies so far it has had an adverse events profile similar to that of placebo (SEDA-28, 534). Co-administration with statins has also been well tolerated (SEDA-29, 546).

Liver   In several studies of co-administration of ezetimibe with a statin there have been small numbers of patients with *raised serum transaminase activities* at or above three times the upper limit of the reference range.

- A 50-year-old woman with previous autoimmune thyroid disease taking atorvastatin developed acute hepatitis when she also was given ezetimibe (1[A]). Further investigations, including liver biopsy, showed a probable drug-induced autoimmune hepatitis.

Ezetimibe was considered to be the most likely causal agent, although atorvastatin could not be ruled out.

Fibrates *(SED-15, 1358; SEDA-27, 473; SEDA-28, 534; SEDA-29, 546)*

Liver   Fibrates are associated with raised liver enzyme activities and occasional reports of acute hepatitis and hepatic fibrosis. *Cirrhosis* has been reported for the first time with fenofibrate (2[A]).

Side Effects of Drugs, Annual 30
J.K. Aronson (Editor)
ISSN: 0378-6080
DOI: 10.1016/S0378-6080(08)00044-5

- A 62-year-old Indian man developed abnormal liver function tests after taking fenofibrate for 11 months. Liver biopsy confirmed the presence of cirrhosis; there was no steatosis or cholestasis.

Possible mechanisms of fenofibrate-induced liver injury include activation of peroxisome proliferation-activator receptors, a hypersensitivity reaction, and immune-mediated injury from cross-reactivity of the drug with autoantigens. The authors referred to six reported cases of hepatic fibrosis attributed to fenofibrate. Raised transaminase activities occur commonly with fenofibrate but are generally transient, reverse on withdrawal, and do not result in long-term injury. Fenofibrate should be withdrawn if higher than normal enzyme activities persist, and a liver biopsy should be considered if liver enzymes do not normalize after withdrawal.

Fish oils *(SED-15, 1364; SEDA-28, 535)*

Cardiovascular   Some of the beneficial effects of fish oils after acute myocardial infarction have been attributed to an antidysrhythmic effect on the heart (3[C]). However, the results of a randomized trial in 200 patients with implantable cardioverter defibrillators are at variance with this: the rate of cardioversion was higher in those taking fish oils 1.8 g/day than in a control group who took olive oil (4[C]). The lack of benefit and the suggestion that fish oil supplementation may increase the risk *of ventricular tachycardia* or *ventricular fibrillation* in some patients with implantable cardioverter defibrillators can reasonably be interpreted as evidence that the routine use of fish oil supplementation in patients with implantable cardioverter defibrillators and recurrent ventricular dysrhythmias should be avoided.

HMG-CoA reductase inhibitors

(SED-15, 1632; SEDA-27, 473; SEDA-28, 535; SEDA-29, 547)

The adverse effects of statins, especially as reported during 2005 and 2006, have been reviewed in the light of the ever increasing dosages that are being used to lower LDL cholesterol to a minimum (5[R]). In another review high doses of atorvastatin and simvastatin were specially emphasized (6[R]).

Observational studies   In a multicenter, open, phase III study in 104 Korean patients there were eight adverse drug reactions in six patients taking pitavastatin and 19 adverse drug reactions in 12 patients taking simvastatin (7[C]). However, there were no reports of serious reactions in either group.

Psychiatric   Some studies have shown increased risks of *violent death* and *depression* in subjects with reduced serum cholesterol concentrations. Serum and membrane cholesterol concentrations, the microviscosity of erythrocyte membranes, and platelet serotonin uptake have been determined in 17 patients with hypercholesterolemia (8[c]). There was a significant increase in serotonin transporter activity only during the first month of simvastatin therapy. This suggests that within this period some patients could be vulnerable to depression, violence, or suicide. This is an important paper, in that it explains why mood disorders are not regularly seen in clinical trials with statins, as has been summarized in a recent review (6[R]).

Hematologic   *Leukopenia* with oral ulceration has been attributed to atorvastatin in a patient with insulin allergy who had received a pancreatic transplant; the symptoms resolved on withdrawal (9[C]).

Liver   The results of randomized trials do not suggest that statins in standard doses are hepatotoxic. In none of the large randomized studies in which standard doses were assessed (atorvastatin 10 mg/day, fluvastatin 40–80 mg/day, pravastatin 40 mg/day, simvastatin 20–40 mg/day) was there any clear excess risk of hepatitis or any other serious liver-related adverse events. Long-term large randomized trials have confirmed an excess of

persistent rises in transaminases with atorvastatin 80 mg/day compared with lower doses or placebo, and similarly some excess with simvastatin 80 mg/day, but hepatitis and liver failure were not reported (5[R]).

Musculoskeletal

> **DoTS classification:**
> *Reaction*: Myopathy and rhabdomyolysis due to statins
> *Dose-relation*: Collateral
> *Time-course*: Intermediate
> *Susceptibility factors*: Drug interactions (for example, with fibrates)

All statins can cause *myopathy* and *rhabdomyolysis*, but not all statins are alike. For example, the evidence to date, based on almost 2 decades of experience, points to an extremely low risk of myopathy and rhabdomyolysis with lovastatin, and lovastatin 20 mg tablets are being considered for non-prescription availability in several countries (10[R]). Furthermore, muscle adverse effects do not necessarily occur after a change from one statin to another (11[A]).

• A 59-year-old woman taking pravastatin 20 mg/day tolerated immunosuppression with ciclosporin, prednisone, and mycophenolate mofetil for 4 years after heart transplantation. After switching from pravastatin to simvastatin she developed severe muscle weakness and laboratory evidence of muscle breakdown. The biochemical markers of rhabdomyolysis did not normalize until after repeat hemodialysis. Clinical improvement did not occur until after 5 months.

For all types of statin the risk is higher with higher doses in the therapeutic range. The risk is not clearly related to LDL-lowering efficacy; for example, cerivastatin was not particularly effective but was much more likely than other statins to cause rhabdomyolysis. Despite the fact that they can cause a myopathy, there is no clear evidence from randomized trials that statins cause myalgia, and reports of muscle cramp do not seem to be increased (5[R]). However, these assertions, which are based on results from randomized clinical trials, are difficult to reconcile with observations made in the Primo study (12[C]). This was an observational study in an unselected population in France taking high doses of various statins. Muscle symptoms were reported by 832 of 7924 patients (11%), with a median time of onset of 1 month after the start of statin therapy. Muscle pain prevented even moderate exertion during everyday activities in 315 patients (38%), while 31 (4%) were confined to bed or unable to work. Among individual statins fluvastatin was associated with the lowest rate of muscular symptoms (5.1%). Creatine kinase activity was not measured.

Drug dosage regimens   In a comparison of atorvastatin 80 and 10 mg/day in 10 001 patients adverse events related to treatment occurred in 406 of those who took 80 mg/day ($n = 4955$) compared with 289 of those who took 10 mg/day ($n = 5006$) (8.1 versus 5.8%) (13[C]). The respective rates of withdrawal because of treatment-related adverse events were 7.2 and 5.3%. Treatment-related myalgia was reported by 241 patients taking 80 mg/day and by 234 patients taking 10 mg/day (4.8 and 4.7% respectively). There were persistent rises in the activities of alanine transaminase, aspartate transaminase, or both in 60 patients taking 80 mg/day compared with nine taking 10 mg/day. There were five cases of rhabdomyolysis, two in those taking 80 mg/day and three in those taking 10 mg/day. At the start of the study 131 patients were excluded because of abnormal liver function tests, but in all the study showed that high-dose atorvastatin is relatively safe. This finding has been supported by the results of another study, in which the proportion of patients who developed rises in liver enzymes with atorvastatin 80 mg/day was low and comparable to the results of other similar studies (14[C]).

Drug interactions with statins

Pharmacokinetic interactions with statins can occur by inhibition or induction of CYP isozymes. Pharmacodynamic interactions can occur through additive effects on muscle. There have been more reports of both types of interactions.

Clarithromycin   *Macrolide antibiotics are potent inhibitors of CYP3A4 and amiodarone less potent. Severe myopathy has been attributed to the combination of simvastatin with clarithromycin and amiodarone (15[A]).*

- *A 56-year-old man taking simvastatin was given clarithromycin and amiodarone for pneumonia and a supraventricular tachycardia. He found it difficult to move and complained of general weakness and muscle pain. The blood creatine kinase activity was over 20 000 IU/l. Simvastatin was withdrawn on day 19 and during days 22–31 he steadily improved.*

Clopidogrel   *Clopidogrel is a prodrug that is converted to its active form by CYP3A4. The active drug irreversibly blocks one specific platelet adenosine 5'-diphosphate (ADP) receptor (P2Y12). As certain lipophilic statins (atorvastatin, lovastatin, simvastatin) are substrates of CYP3A4, drug interactions are possible. However, previous studies with atorvastatin have given variable results (SEDA-28, 536; SEDA-29, 548). In a recent study the inhibitory potency of clopidogrel on ADP-induced platelet activation was not attenuated when it was co-administered with atorvastatin (20 mg/day) for 5 weeks in 51 patients with acute coronary syndromes (16[A]). Atorvastatin had no effect on either clopidogrel-induced inhibition of platelet aggregation initiated by ADP 5 or 10 µmol/l or clopidogrel-induced reduction of the membrane expression of P-selectin and CD40L induced by ADP. The same authors found a similar result in a previous study with a lower dosage of atorvastatin (10 mg/day) (SEDA-29, 548).*

Colchicine   *Interactions of statins with colchicine have been reported.*

- *A 70-year-old man with hyperlipidemia and gout had been taking fluvastatin 80 mg/day for 2 years (17[A]). After taking colchicine 1.5 mg/day for acute gouty arthritis for 3 days he developed stomach ache and nausea followed by severe pains and weakness in his arms and legs. After 10 days he developed rhabdomyolysis and non-oliguric myoglobinuric acute renal insufficiency.*
- *A 65-year-old woman who had been taking pravastatin 20 mg/day for 6 years developed acute gout (18[A]). Her blood urea nitrogen and serum creatinine concentrations were 48 and 1.3 mg/dl respectively. She was given colchicine 1.5 mg/day but 20 days later developed symmetrical proximal muscle weakness in the legs. Examination, laboratory findings, and electromyelography suggested myopathy. The weakness improved 7 days after withdrawal of colchicine and pravastatin and the enzyme activities returned to normal. Colchicine 1 mg/day was restarted 5 days later and the myopathy did not recur.*

Colchicine is cleared by a different CYP450 isozyme than fluvastatin and pravastatin are, but another possible mechanism is synergistic myotoxicity, since colchicine causes myopathy by disrupting tubular function with subsequent vacuolization. Patients taking colchicine should be informed about possible muscular and gastrointestinal adverse effects and advised to stop.

Fluconazole   *Azoles are potent inhibitors of drug metabolism, and fluconazole has previously been reported to interact with simvastatin. A similar interaction with atorvastatin has now been reported (19ᴬ).*

- *A 76-year-old man taking antimicrobial drug treatment including fluconazole switched from pravastatin to atorvastatin 40 mg/day. After 1 week he began to feel tired and became oliguric, and on day 2 the serum myoglobin concentration was 16 120 µg/l. After 8 days in intensive care he died in multiorgan failure.*

Gemfibrozil   *In a randomized crossover study gemfibrozil increased the AUC of atorvastatin and its metabolites (20ᶜ). Low doses of atorvastatin should be used if gemfibrozil is co-administered.*

Rifampicin   *In a randomized crossover study rifampicin reduced the total AUC of atorvastatin and increased the Cₘₐₓ of 2-hydroxyatorvastatin acid by 68% (20ᶜ). It is advisable to increase the dosage of atorvastatin and preferable to administer it in the evening to guarantee adequate concentrations during the period of rapid cholesterol synthesis that occurs at night when rifampicin or other potent inducers of CYP3A4 are co-administered.*

References

1. Heyningen CV. Drug-induced acute autoimmune hepatitis during combination therapy with atorvastatin and ezetimibe. Ann Clin Biochem 2005;42:402–4.
2. Ahmed F, Petrovic L, Rosen E, Gonzalez R, Jacobson IM. Fenofibrate-induced cirrhosis. Dig Dis Sci 2005;50(2):312–3.
3. Marchioli R, Barzi F, Bomba E, Chieffo C, Di Gregorio D, Di Mascio R, Franzosi MG, Geraci E, Levantesi G, Maggioni AP, Mantini L, Marfisi RM, Mastrogiuseppe G, Mininni N, Nicolosi GL, Santini M, Schweiger C, Tavazzi L, Tognoni G, Tucci C, Valagussa F. Early protection against sudden death by *n* − 3 polyunsaturated fatty acids after myocardial infarction: time-course analysis of the results of the Gruppo Italiano per lo Studio della Sopravvivenza nell'Infarto Miocardico (GISSI)-Prevenzione. Circulation 2002;105(23):1897–903 [on behalf of the GISSI-Prevenzione Investigators].
4. Raitt MH, Connor WE, Morris C, Kron J, Halperin B, Chugh SS, McClelland J, Cook J, MacMurdy K, Swenson R, Connor SL, Gerhard G, Kraemer DF, Oseran D, Marchant C, Calhoun D, Shnider R, McAnulty J. Fish oil supplementation and risk of ventricular tachycardia and ventricular fibrillation in patients with implantable defibrillators: a randomized controlled trial. JAMA 2005;293(23):2884–91.
5. Armitage J. The safety of statins in clinical practice. Lancet 2007;370(9601):1781–90.
6. Waters DD. Safety of high-dose atorvastatin therapy. Am J Cardiol 2005;96(5A Suppl):69F–75F.
7. Park S, Kang HJ, Rim SJ, Ha JW, Oh BH, Chung N, Cho SY. A randomized, open-label study to evaluate the efficacy and safety of pitavastatin compared with simvastatin in Korean patients with hypercholesterolemia. Clin Ther 2005;27(7):1074–82.
8. Vevera J, Fisar Z, Kvasnicka T, Zdenek H, Starkova L, Ceska R, Papezova H. Cholesterol-lowering therapy evokes time-limited changes in serotonergic transmission. Psychiatry Res 2005;133(2–3):197–203.
9. Malaise J, Leonet J, Goffin E, Lefebvre C, Tennstedt D, Vandeleene B, Buysschaert M, Squifflet J. Pancreas transplantation for treatment of generalised allergy to human insulin in type I diabetes. Transplant Proc 2005;37:2839.
10. Wortmann RL, Tipping RW, Levine JG, Melin JM. Frequency of myopathy in patients receiving lovastatin. Am J Cardiol 2005;95(8):983–5.
11. Sochman J, Podzimkova M. Not all statins are alike: induced rhabdomyolysis on changing from one statin to another one. Int J Cardiol 2005;99(1):145–6.
12. Bruckert E, Hayem G, Dejager S, Yau C, Begaud B. Mild to moderate muscular symptoms with high-dosage statin therapy in hyperlipidemic patients—the PRIMO Study. Cardiovasc Drugs Ther 2005;19(6):403–14.

13. LaRosa JC, Grundy SM, Waters DD, Shear C, Barter P, Fruchart JC, Gotto AM, Greten H, Kastelein JJP, Shepherd J, Wenger NK. Intensive lipid lowering with atorvastatin in patients with stable coronary disease. N Engl J Med 2005;352(14):1425–35 [for the Treating to Target (TNT) Investigators].

14. Pedersen TR, Faergeman O, Kastelein JJP, Olsson AG, Tikkanen MJ, Holme I, Larsen ML, Bendiksen FS, Lindahl C, Szarek M, Tsai J. High-dose atorvastatin vs usual-dose simvastatin for secondary prevention after myocardial infarction. The IDEAL Study: a randomized controlled trial. JAMA 2005;294(19):2437–45 [for the Incremental Decrease in End Points Through Aggressive Lipid Lowering (IDEAL) Study Group].

15. Chouhan UM, Chakrabarti S, Millward LJ. Simvastatin interaction with clarithromycin and amiodarone causing myositis. Ann Pharmacother 2005;39(10):1760–1.

16. Mitsios JV, Papathanasiou AI, Elisaf M, Goudevenos JA, Tselepis AD. The inhibitory potency of clopidogrel on ADP-induced platelet activation is not attenuated when it is co-administered with atorvastatin (20 mg/day) for 5 weeks in patients with acute coronary syndromes. Platelets 2005;16(5):287–92.

17. Atasoyu EM, Evrenkaya TR, Solmazgul E. Possible colchicine rhabdomyolysis in a fluvastatin-treated patient. Ann Pharmacother 2005;39(7–8):1368–9.

18. Alayli G, Cengiz K, Canturk F, Durmus D, Akyol Y, Menekse EB. Acute myopathy in a patient with concomitant use of pravastatin and colchicine. Ann Pharmacother 2005;39(7):1358–61.

19. Kahri J, Valkonen M, Bäcklund T, Vuoristo M, Kivistö KT. Rhabdomyolysis in a patient receiving atorvastatin and fluconazole. Eur J Clin Pharmacol 2005;60(12):905–7.

20. Backman JT, Luurila H, Neuvonen M, Neuvonen PJ. Rifampin markedly decreases and gemfibrozil increases the plasma concentrations of atorvastatin and its metabolites. Clin Pharmacol Ther 2005;78(2):154–67.

Hans-Peter Lipp and Jörg Thomas Hartmann

45 Cytostatic and cytotoxic drugs

Editor's note: The wide range of cytostatic and cytotoxic drugs, the multitude of their adverse effects, and the fact that they are generally used in combinations of several agents all make it impossible to provide as detailed a review of the adverse effects of all the drugs in this field as the Annual gives in others. This year this chapter is devoted to a special review of the tyrosine kinase inhibitors.

Previous special reviews in this chapter have been as follows:

- Anthracyclines (SEDA-25, 533)
- Antimetabolites (SEDA-29, 551): Purine antagonists, pyrimidine antagonists, antifolate drugs, phsophatidylcholine antagonists, adenosine deaminase inhibitors
- Fluorouracil (SEDA-23, 476)
- Inhibitors of topoisomerase I and topoisomerase II (SEDA-27, 477)
- Paclitaxel (SEDA-21, 463)
- Platinum compounds (SEDA-26, 490)
- Vinca alkaloids (SEDA-28, 538)

℞ Tyrosine kinase inhibitors

Tyrosine kinase inhibitors are effective in the targeted treatment of various malignancies. Imatinib was the first to be introduced into clinical oncology, and it was followed by drugs such as gefitinib, erlotinib, sorafenib, sunitinib, and dasatinib. Although they share the same mechanism of action, namely competitive ATP inhibition at the catalytic binding site of tyrosine kinase, they differ from each other in the

spectrum of targeted kinases, their pharmacokinetics, and their adverse effects (1^r).

Skin and hair With variations from drug to drug, tyrosine kinase inhibitors cause skin toxicity, including folliculitis, in more than 50% of patients (2^R). Among the tyrosine kinase inhibitors that are so far commercially available, the agents that target EGFR, erlotinib and gefitinib, have the broadest spectrum of adverse effects on the skin and hair, including folliculitis, paronychia, facial hair growth, facial erythema, and varying forms of frontal alopecia. In contrast, folliculitis is not common during administration of sorafenib and sunitinib, which target VEGFR, PDGFR, FLT3, and others, whereas both agents have been associated with subungual splinter hemorrhages. Periorbital edema is a common adverse effect of imatinib (2^R).

Imatinib mesylate

Imatinib (STI571), an inhibitor of bcr-abl tyrosine kinase, has become the first-line agent in the treatment of the chronic phase of chronic myeloid leukaemia and of locally advanced and metastatic gastrointestinal stromal tumors (GISTs) that express the CD117 antigen. The recommended dosage is 400 mg/day for patients with chronic myeloid leukaemia and for GIST and 600 mg/day in the accelerated phase or blast crisis of chronic myeloid leukaemia. The dose should be taken once a day with a meal and a large glass of water.

Pharmacokinetics The mean absolute systemic availability of imatinib is about 98% (3^c). CYP3A4 plays a pivotal role in imatinib metabolism; N-demethylated imatinib is the main metabolite and is active (4^c). The plasma AUC for this metabolite is about 15% of the AUC of imatinib. Drug elimination is

Side Effects of Drugs, Annual 30
J.K. Aronson (Editor)
ISSN: 0378-6080
DOI: 10.1016/S0378-6080(08)00045-7

primarily mediated via the feces (5^R, 6^R). The half-lives of imatinib and N-demethylimatinib are 18–27 hours and 40–74 hours respectively. The peak concentrations average 3340 and 781 ng/ml, and trough concentrations 1540 and 508 ng/ml respectively (7^A). These values were not changed significantly in patients with end-stage renal disease or on hemodialysis. Dosage adjustment is not therefore necessary in patients with renal impairment (8^A). Imatinib can also be used in patients with even severely impaired hepatic function (9^c).

- A 58-year-old patient with decompensated alcoholic liver cirrhosis developed a well-differentiated hepatocellular carcinoma (10^A). Because of in vitro sensitivity of the cells to antibodies against c-kit and cytokeratin 7, imatinib was given in a dosage of 100 mg bd based on increased transaminases and cholestasis. A year later the tumor mass had disappeared as assessed by histology, perhaps because of tumor necrosis.

Imatinib is generally well tolerated. Besides mild to moderate hematological toxicity, its adverse effects include fluid retention, edema, nausea, and some skin disorders (11^A, 12^c). There have also been case reports of hepatitis.

Cardiovascular   It has been suggested that imatinib may have caused severe heart failure and left ventricular dysfunction in 10 patients with pre-existing conditions such as hypertension, diabetes mellitus, and coronary heart disease (13^R). Experimental studies have shown that imatinib induces apoptosis in isolated cardiac myocytes (13^R). Several trials and a database of six registration trials have therefore been reviewed.

- The Italian Cooperative Study Group—four consecutive studies of imatinib therapy in 833 patients with Philadelphia chromosome-positive chronic myeloid leukemia, observed for a median of 19–64 months (14^r). The overall cardiac mortality rate was 0.3%.
- The MD Anderson experience—clinical trials of imatinib from July 1998 to July 2006, with median follow-up of 5 years (15^r). In all the imatinib protocols, standard research monitoring procedures were conducted before treatment and at regular intervals. Electrocardiography, echocardiography, and chest radiography were conducted routinely before treatment and as clinically

indicated during follow-up. The eligibility criteria excluded patients with cardiac problems (NYHA classes III and IV). After reviewing all reported adverse events, particularly those that could be considered as having a cardiac origin, 22 patients (1.8%) were identified as having symptoms that could be attributed to congestive heart failure, of whom 12 had previously received interferon and three had received anthracyclines. They included nine patients reported elsewhere (13^R). Their median age was 70 (range 49–83) years. The median time from the start of imatinib therapy to a cardiac adverse event was 162 (range 2–2045) days. Eighteen patients had previous medical conditions that predisposed them to cardiac disease: congestive heart failure (n = 6), diabetes mellitus (n = 6), hypertension (n = 10), coronary artery disease (n = 8), dysrhythmias (n = 3), and cardiomyopathy (n = 1). Of the 22 patients, 15 underwent echocardiography or multiple gated acquisition (MUGA) scanning at the time of the event: nine of these 15 patients had low ejection fractions, and six of these nine had significant conditions that predisposed them to cardiac disease (three had coronary artery disease, two congestive heart failure, and one a cardiomyopathy). Of the 22 patients with symptoms of congestive heart failure, 11 continued to take imatinib with dosage adjustments and management of congestive heart failure without further complications. However, with the host of confounding factors involved in these patients, the occurrence of congestive heart failure related to the use of imatinib was reasonably unambiguous in only seven of the 1276 patients reviewed (0.5%).

- Novartis clinical database—six registration trials comprising 2327 patients who took imatinib as monotherapy. These trials represented 5595 patient-years of exposure to imatinib (average exposure 2.4 years). Twelve cases of congestive heart failure (0.5%) were considered to be incident cases (with no previous history of congestive heart failure or left ventricular dysfunction) with a possible or probable relation to imatinib. If these cases are related to the 5595 patients-years of imatinib exposure the incidence of congestive heart failure is 0.2% per year across all trials.

- In the largest international, randomized phase III study reported to date, 1106 patients with newly diagnosed chronic myeloid leukemia were randomized to either initial therapy with imatinib or the previous standard treatment of interferon plus cytosine arabinoside (16[r]). Both regimens were examined for cardiac safety according to an analysis of adverse events as described above. The incident cases of cardiac failure and left ventricular dysfunction, possibly or probably related to exposure to the study medication, was 0.04% per year (1 case in 2309 patient-years) for patients taking imatinib versus 0.75% per year (four cases in 536 patient-years of exposure) in patients taking interferon + cytosine arabinoside.

Imatinib therapy as a cause of congestive heart failure seems to be rare. When it occurs, the symptoms most commonly occur in elderly patients with pre-existing cardiac conditions and may often reflect predisposing cardiac compromise compounded by some element of fluid retention. Patients with a previous cardiac history should be monitored closely and treated aggressively with diuretics if they develop fluid retention.

Sensory systems   Imatinib often causes facial edema. In some patients, intense eyelid edema can result in ophthalmologic symptoms, including ptosis, blepharoconjunctivitis, visual obstruction, or even retinal edema. Inhibition of PDGFR leads to dysregulation of the tension between endothelial cells and the extracellular matrix. Severe periorbital edema may need surgical debulking of excess skin, fat, and edema of the lower eyelids, and can produce immediate improvement in visual function. In one case there was no recurrence 6 months after surgery (17[A]).

Mineral metabolism

Hypophosphatemia   In a retrospective analysis imatinib caused hypophosphatemia more often than expected. Hypophosphatemia was more pronounced in younger patients, who had taken higher doses imatinib. The underlying mechanism may include reduced activity of PDGFR. Impairment of bone turnover and osteomalacia may therefore be expected during imatinib therapy. Whether phosphate and vitamin D concentrations should be measured routinely during imatinib therapy, with the aim of prescribing phosphate if necessary, is a matter of current debate (18[c]).

Hematologic   Patients can develop myelosuppression during imatinib therapy, perhaps because of inhibition of c-kit, a cytokine that is involved in early hemopoiesis, inhibition of which can result in more than expected suppression of normal progenitors. It has not yet been elucidated why patients with hypereosinophilic syndrome or atypical chronic myelomonocytic leukemia experience imatinib-related neutropenia very rarely compared with patients with advanced chronic myeloid leukemia. However, there is some evidence that the more severe the myelosuppression with imatinib, the larger the response, suggesting that this adverse effect is a prognostic factor. It has therefore been proposed that imatinib-related myelosuppression may be a therapeutic effect on Philadelphia chromosome-positive clones rather than inhibition of normal hemopoiesis. Whereas empirical interruption of treatment or dosage modification may affect the outcome in chronic myeloid leukemia, some authors have suggested the use of G-CSF (for example filgrastim 300 micrograms subcutaneously 2 or 3 times a week) in patients who have myelosuppression at doses of imatinib of 300 mg/day (19[R]).

Liver   There have been a few case reports of hepatotoxicity in patients taking imatinib, so far exclusively in women. It has been proposed that high drug concentrations of imatinib may predispose to an increased risk of liver damage; however, it is not clear whether immunological idiosyncrasy (i.e. a hypersusceptibility reaction) or a metabolic disorder is the underlying reason.

- A 40-year-old woman with chronic myeloid leukemia in the chronic phase took imatinib mesylate because of resistance to interferon (20[A]). She achieved a complete clinical remission after 3 months but the molecular response was incomplete. Six months later she developed hepatitis without any evidence of active viral infection. Serum concentrations of imatinib were markedly raised (8107 ng/ml), although she had stopped taking it 6 days before. At that stage there was a complete molecular response. Several weeks later her hepatic function had recovered and she had a normal blood count with a normal differential count. Rechallenge with imatinib was not performed.

Skin   There is some evidence that the severity of skin reactions due to imatinib is dose-related in the therapeutic range of doses. Mild forms are common at doses of 200–600 mg/day, whereas severe eruptions have been described in patients taking higher doses (600–1000 mg/day) (21^c). Re-exposure to higher doses resulted in relapse of skin eruptions, which highlights the need for adequate dosage reduction in affected patients. In case series, imatinib mesylate has been reported to cause reversible hypopigmentation of the skin, which may be dose-related in the therapeutic range (22^c, 23^c). This benign adverse effect occurred within the first month of treatment. The underlying mechanism may involve a regulatory disorder in melanocyte development and survival, which depends on KIT and SCF (2^R).

- A 60-year-old white woman with a GIST took imatinib 400 mg/day for 2 months with lansoprazole 15 mg/day (24^c). She developed bilateral palpebral edema with hyperemic conjunctivae and labial edema. After withdrawal and reintroduction of both drugs, she developed generalized skin reactions, even at a low dose of imatinib and a concomitant glucocorticoid plus lansoprazole. When imatinib and lansoprazole were withdrawn, the skin toxicity did not progress.

The authors suggested that the skin effect may have result from (1) the well-known drug-related adverse effects of imatinib and lansoprazole on the skin and (2) inhibition of lansoprazole clearance by imatinib.

Drug–drug interactions   Imatinib is an inhibitor of some cytochrome P450 isozymes, such as CYP3A4, CYP2C9, and CYP2D6, and may affect the pharmacokinetics of substrates such as ciclosporin, warfarin, and some tricyclic antidepressants (25^E).

Management of adverse drug reactions   Supportive management of common imatinib-related adverse effects has been described (26^r). Severe nausea may require antiemetics (for example a 5HT$_3$ receptor antagonist or prochlorperazine). Diarrhea can be controlled by loperamide. Rashes may need topical or systemic steroids. Muscle cramps may need electrolyte substitution with magnesium and calcium. Bone aches may be alleviated with coxibs.

Dasatinib

Dasatinib (BMS-354825), a thiazole carboximide derivative, is structurally related to imatinib. It targets src kinase and imatinib-resistant bcr-abl kinase and has impressive activity in patients with chronic myeloid leukemia or Philadelphia chromosome-positive acute lymphoblastic leukemia (27^E, 28^C).

Although dasatinib has been approved for these indications in a dosage of 70 mg bd, the search for the optimal dose regimen continues (29^c). Preliminary data suggest that 100 mg/day may offer a more favorable benefit to harm balance in patients with chronic myeloid leukemia that is resistant to imatinib or in whom imatinib causes unacceptable adverse effects. Compared with conventional twice daily dosing, intermittent tyrosine kinase inhibition produces clinical remissions with improved safety, with the lowest incidence of pleural effusion (all grades), neutropenia (grades 3–4), and thrombocytopenia (grades 3–4). In addition, the use of dasatinib 100 mg/day makes dosage reductions less necessary than dosage schedules based on 50 mg bd (30^c), 140 mg/day, or 70 mg bd. However, the accelerated phase or blast crisis makes doses of up to 100 mg bd necessary.

The main adverse effects of dasatinib include grade 3/4 hematological toxicity (for example neutropenia and thrombocytopenia), liver abnormalities, diarrhea, headache, peripheral edema, and hypocalcemia. In addition, pleural effusion is of clinical concern and may need treatment with diuretics and thoracentesis or pleurodesis.

Pharmacokinetics   Dasatinib is well absorbed from the gastrointestinal tract (28^C). However, its solubility is pH dependent, and the AUC of dasatinib can be reduced significantly when antacids or famotidine are used concomitantly (by 55 and 61% respectively). Dasatinib undergoes extensive metabolism by CYP3A4 and has an active metabolite. Further enzymes involved in the metabolism of dasatinib include FMO-3 and UGT isozymes. Exposure to the active metabolite, which is equipotent with the parent compound, represents about 5% of the AUC of dasatinib. Dasatinib and its metabolites are primarily excreted via the feces. The half-life of the parent compound is 3–5 hours.

Skin   *The difference in targets between imatinib and dasatinib may explain the observed risk of panniculitis with the latter.*

- *A 55-year old woman with chronic myeloid leukemia did not have a major cytogenetic response to imatinib mesylate, even in a dose of 800 mg/day, because of the activation-loop mutation H396R (31[A]). When she was given dasatinib (70 mg bd) for 4 weeks she developed a fever (38.1 °C) and painful subcutaneous nodules with overlying erythema on her thighs. After withdrawal of dasatinib the rash resolved within 1 week. However, her symptoms recurred when dasatinib was restarted, with manifestations on the arms, legs, and vulva. Biopsy of the skin lesions showed a lobular panniculitis, with massive infiltration by polymorphonuclear leukocytes. Withdrawal and reintroduction together with prednisone (50 mg/day) successfully controlled the panniculitis.*

Nilotinib

Nilotinib (AMN 107) is a second-generation tyrosine kinase inhibitors with structural similarity to imatinib. It does not affect src kinase at therapeutic doses. Nilotinib is 20–50 times more potent than imatinib, which may encourage its use in patients who are refractory to imatinib (27[E]). Nilotinib is generally well tolerated, as has been shown in recent phase II studies (32[C], 33[c]). The most frequent grade 3/4 laboratory abnormalities in 316 patients included thrombocytopenia (29%), neutropenia (28%), and asymptomatic increases in lipase activity (15%). Pleural and pericardial effusions and pulmonary edema were rare (under 1%). Growth factors or platelet transfusions were required very rarely.

Gefitinib

Gefitinib is an anilinoquinazoline derivative, the first agent to have been introduced as a potent inhibitor of EGFR tyrosine kinase for the treatment of advanced non-small-cell lung cancer refractory or resistant to cytotoxic chemotherapy. Case series have shown significant radiographic regression and improvement of symptoms. A history of never smoking cigarettes and bronchoalveolar histology are significant predictors of a radiographic response to

gefitinib. In addition, there are higher response rates in Japanese versus non-Japanese subjects, in those of performance status 0 to 1, in women, and in those with adenocarcinoma histology and prior immunotherapy or hormonal therapy. If several of these characteristics are present simultaneously, higher response rates and a longer median survival time with gefitinib, or the structurally related erlotinib, can be expected (34[R]).

The recommended dose of gefitinib is 250 mg/day, and 500 mg/day causes increased toxicity without additional efficacy.

Pharmacokinetics   *The mean absolute systemic availability after oral administration averages 60% (35[c]). Gefitinib probably crosses the blood-brain barrier, which is favorable in patients with metastatic disease (36[A]). Its half-life is about 48 hours, and steady-state concentrations are achieved within 10 days. Hepatic metabolism via CYP3A4 and biliary excretion are the major routes of elimination, and renal excretion is of minor importance.*

Respiratory   *The most serious adverse effect of gefitinib is lung toxicity, including rapidly progressive dyspnea with a risk of severe hypoxemia and bilateral ground-glass attenuation on chest CT.*

Of 110 patients with non-small-cell lung cancer who took gefitinib over 3 months, 12 developed significant lung toxicity and five died from progressive complications, including chronic pulmonary fibrosis. The mechanism may involve impairment of healing of epithelium, since EGF is needed to regenerate damaged alveolar epithelial cells. Thus, any underlying lung damage (for example preexisting pulmonary fibrosis) may predispose to lung toxicity (37[c], 38[c]).

- *A 70-year-old woman with a long history of smoking developed a non-small-cell lung cancer, stage IV (39[A]). She was given radiotherapy and chemotherapy consisting of cisplatin and gemcitabine. However, she developed hemolytic–uremic syndrome, with raised LDH activity, hypoalbuminemia, reticulocytosis, and a high blood urea nitrogen concentration. When the disease progressed she was given gefitinib 250 mg/day, which resulted in improvement in tumor-related bone pain after several days. However, she developed a characteristic drug-related acneoid reaction and after 2 months developed progressive dyspnea and a dry cough, which gradually worsened. She had interstitial infiltrates in both lungs. Despite high-dose glucocorticoids, her condition worsened and she needed mechanical ventilation. She then developed hemodynamic instability and died.*

Gastrointestinal   During treatment with efitinib 250 mg/day about 40% of patients develop diarrhea grade 2, which can be successfully controlled in most cases by symptomatic treatment with loperamide. Patients are advised to take loperamide 4 mg immediately, followed by 2 mg after every loose bowel movement (up to a maximum of 10 mg/day). If the is response inadequate, withdrawal of gefitinib may be warranted (40^R).

Skin   Gefitinib-associated skin reactions correlate with an increased likelihood of radiographic tumor response and symptomatic improvement, similar to the structurally related erlotinib and the monoclonal antibody cetuximab. However, durable radiographic regression and improvement of symptoms have also been observed in patients with only mild forms of rash and diarrhea.

The combination of clindamycin 1% and benzoylperoxide 5% gel has been used with some success for the treatment of inflammatory pustular lesions. If gel formulations are not well tolerated, oral minocycline 100 mg bd can be used instead. The roles of topical retinoids, topical or systemic corticosteroids, or topical pimecrolimus creams have not been clearly elucidated. In patients with very dry skin, Eucerin cream, Cetaphil cream, Aquaphor healing ointment, or Big Balm can be helpful in treating fissures on the palms and soles (40^R).

EGFR ligands (for example TGFα, EGF, HB-EGF) are cytokines that are excreted by keratinocytes during wound healing. It is therefore possible that wound healing may be impaired during the administration of EGFR tyrosine kinase inhibitors. However, in contrast to some preclinical results, no interference with would healing was seen with gefitinib in a series of patients who underwent laparotomy with concomitant lysis of adhesions and skin incisions (41^A).

- *A 72-year-old man with a history of metastatic non-small-cell lung cancer required internal fixation for bone metastasis 2 months after he started to take gefitinib. A 4 cm skin incision on the left forearm was made for the procedure. He continued to take gefitinib until the day before surgery and*

resumed 24 hours after surgery. His skin wound healing was unremarkable.

Hair   EGFR tyrosine kinase inhibitors can cause a folliculitis, with a median time to onset of 7–10 days. Follicular papules and pustules rarely reach grade 3/4 severity, including the facial area, the forehead, and the upper chest and back. In contrast to juvenile acne, bacterial cultures of the initial primary lesions are usually negative (42^c). The mechanism has not been clearly elucidated but it may involve disordered regulation of keratinocyte biology and homeostasis of hair follicles related to EGFR inhibition. A further mechanism may be increased expression of p27Kip1 in basal and follicular keratinocytes and modified chemokine expression, resulting in greater skin inflammation. Withdrawal usually leads to rapid improvement and in some cases spontaneous reduction of symptoms has been observed in spite of continued treatment (2^R).

Inhibitors of EGFR tyrosine kinase can change scalp hair, slow hair growth, and cause frontal alopecia. In contrast, facial hair and eyelashes can grow progressively, particularly in women. It has been speculated that modification of the interaction between the EGFR-dependent and androgen-dependent signalling pathways may be the underlying mechanism (2^R).

Nails   Inhibitors of EGFR tyrosine kinase can cause paronychial inflammation with symptoms such as erythema, painful lateral fingernails or toenails and pyogenic granuloma-like lesions. These can resolve spontaneously and commonly disappear after treatment is withdrawn. Topical glucocorticoids, local antiseptics, avoiding cutting nails too short, and avoiding the use of shoes that are too tight have been advised to minimize paronychial inflammation (40^R).

Management of adverse drug reactions   Increased thromboxane B2 and sP-selectin has been observed in patients taking gefitinib. In one study there were fewer adverse effects in 12 patients who took low-dose aspirin with gefitinib than in 28 who took gefitinib alone (43^c). The addition of reduced the frequencies of rash and diarrhea while therapeutic efficacy was not affected. The authors suggested that some gefitinib-related adverse effects may be due to platelet activation.

Erlotinib

Erlotinib is the second inhibitor EGFR tyrosine kinase to have been approved for the treatment of locally advanced non-small-cell lung cancer after failure of at least one prior cytotoxic drug regimen (44[C]). It has also been approved for the first-line treatment of metastatic pancreatic cancer in combination with gemcitabine (45[C]).

Erlotinib should be taken in a dosage of 150 mg/day on an empty stomach at least 1 hour before or 2 hours after a meal.

The most common adverse effects of erlotinib include grade 3/4 rashes and diarrhea, which occur in 9 and 6% of patients respectively, and which warrant drug withdrawal in 1% of patients. Sun protection is generally recommended, because inhibition of EGFR in the skin potentiates the harmful effects of ultraviolet radiation. In patients with lower constitutive concentrations of melanin in the skin, for example Fitzpatrick skin phototypes I and II, higher sensitivity to ultraviolet radiation and a higher probability of more severely graded rash are expected (46[c]). Withdrawal of erlotinib has been recommended when signs of new or progressive unexplained pulmonary symptoms are observed, such as dyspnea, cough, and fever, in order to reduce the risk of interstitial lung disease.

Pharmacokinetics The absolute systemic availability of erlotinib averages 59% and is significantly increased by a meal. Antacids, proton pump inhibitors, and histamine H_2 receptor antagonists impair the absorption of erlotinib, because its solubility is reduced at pH values exceeding 5.0. More than 90% of a dose is metabolized in the liver, primarily by CYP3A4 and CYP1A2. OSI-420, the major metabolite, has antineoplastic activity. Excretion is mainly via the feces. The half-life averages 36 hours, and steady-state concentrations are reached within 7–8 days.

Skin In 42 patients with either unresectable or metastatic biliary cancer, erlotinib 150 mg/day orally produced mild (grade 1/2) rashes in all those who responded; three had grade 2/3 rashes, which required dosage reductions (47[c]).

Drug–drug interactions In a small study in patients with gliomas, the median plasma AUC of erlotinib was significantly reduced by enzyme-inducing antiepileptic drugs, although the dose of erlotinib had been doubled beforehand from 450 to 900 mg/day (48[c]). In contrast, the AUC of the active metabolite OSI-420 increased about threefold, which may have compensated for the reduction in exposure to the parent compound. Drug concentrations in the cerebrospinal fluid were 1–3% of the peak plasma concentrations.

Erlotinib is a potent inhibitor of CYP1A1 and UGT1A1 and a moderate inhibitor of CYP3A4 and CYP2C8. However, the relevance of these in vitro data to clinical practice has not been elucidated.

Lapatinib

Lapatinib, a 4-anilinoquinazoline derivative, is the first dual tyrosine kinase inhibitor. In contrast to erlotinib and gefitinib, it inhibits both the ErbB1/HER1 (EGFR) tyrosine kinase and the ErbB2/HER 2 tyrosine kinase simultaneously. It is used in patients with advanced metastatic breast cancer who are refractory to anthracyclines or taxanes together with trastuzumab (49[R]). It is given orally in a dose of (1.25 g/day on days 1–14 every 21 days) together with capecitabine (1.0 g/m^2 bd on days 1–14 every 21 days).

Lapatinib is generally well tolerated. Grade 3 diarrhea is dose-limiting, whereas adverse effects such as acneiform rash, nausea, and fatigue are moderate (grades 1–2).

Pharmacokinetics Lapatinib peak concentrations are reached after 3–4 hours (50[r]). Absorption is increased about three-fold when it is given with a meal, and administration on an empty stomach has been recommended, in contrast to the co-administered capecitabine, which should be taken with food. The half-life of lapatinib increases significantly from about 11 hours to 24 hours during repeated administration, probably because of inhibition of CYP3A4. Lapatinib crosses the blood–brain barrier, which may help in the treatment of brain metastases, which are of concern in about one-third of women with ErbB2 over-expression. Elimination is primarily by hepatic *metabolism and biliary excretion; renal excretion is minor. Recovery of lapatinib in the feces accounts for about 27% (3–67%) of an oral dose.*

Cardiovascular   *The incidence of cardiac toxicity with lapatinib appears to be low; in one study only 37 of 2812 women (1.3%) had a fall in left ventricular ejection fraction (LVEF) of at least 20% from baseline (50^r). The onset of reduced LVEF occurred within 9 weeks of treatment in 68% of cases and was rarely symptomatic and generally reversible and non-progressive. The duration of reduction in LVEF averaged 42 days.*

Drug–drug interactions   *Lapatinib is a substrate of CYP3A4, and successive increases in dose may be necessary up to 4.5 g/day in patients who take inducing agents, such as carbamazepine 200 mg bd, which reduced the AUC of lapatinib by about 72% (51^S).*

Lapatinib may inhibit the metabolism of other CYP3A4 substrates, including SN38, resulting in a significant increase in AUC and C_{max} (52^c).

Sunitinib

Sunitinib (SU 11248) is a multi-targeted tyrosine kinase inhibitor which is highly active in patients with advanced renal cell carcinoma and gastrointestinal stromal tumors (GIST) (53^R). The recommended dose is 50 mg/day, in a schedule of 4 weeks on treatment followed by 2 weeks off (54^R, 55^C, 56^C, 57^C). An alternative is continuous dosing with 37.5 mg/day.

The most commonly reported grade 3 adverse effects related to sunitinib include fatigue, stomatitis, hypertension, dermatitis, depigmentation of the hair and skin (probably due to the yellow color of the drug itself), subungual splinter hemorrhages, bleeding events (for example epistaxis), and gastrointestinal discomfort (for example nausea and diarrhea). Grade 3/4 laboratory abnormalities include neutropenia, thrombocytopenia, anaemia, and raised plasma lipase activity. Dosage modifications (for example from 50 to 37.5 or 25 mg/day) were primarily based on severe forms of fatigue or increased amylase and lipase activities (53^R).

Pharmacokinetics   *Oral sunitinib is well absorbed from the gastrointestinal tract. Drug exposure is slightly increased after food, but administration is generally feasible with or without food (58^c).*

Sunitinib is mainly metabolized by CYP3A4, producing a major metabolite with comparable antineoplastic activity and comprising 23–37% of total exposure. The active metabolite and other CYP3A4-mediated biotransformation products are mostly excreted via the feces; the renal route accounts for less than 20% of the dose. The half-lives of sunitinib and its major metabolite are 40–60 hours and 80–110 hours respectively. Accumulation of the parent compound and its active metabolite occurred during repeated daily administration up to 3- to 4-fold and 7- to 10-fold respectively. Steady-state concentrations are commonly achieved after 10–14 days (24^c, 54^R, 58^c).

The AUC of sunitinib and total drug exposure correlated significantly with the probability of a partial response in cytokine-refractory patients with renal cell carcinoma and with the time to progression and overall survival, according to pharmacokinetic and efficacy data from three studies. These data suggest that there is an association between increased exposure to the active drug in the plasma and the probability of clinical benefit.

Drug–drug interactions   *Sunitinib and its major metabolite do not appear to cause clinically important drug–drug interactions. However, the concomitant use of potent inducers of CYP3A4 (for example rifampicin) or inhibitors of CYP3A4 (e.g. ketoconazole) may warrant an increase in dosage to a maximum of 87.5 mg/day or a dosage reduction to a minimum of 37.5 mg/day. The concomitant use of St. John's wort is generally not recommended because of unpredictable drug concentrations (53^R).*

Endocrine   *Sunitinib has been related to an increasing frequency of hypothyroidism. Screening for signs of hypothyroidism is recommended, with frequent measurements of TSH concentrations every 2–3 months in order to start levothyroxine in time.*

In a prospective, observational cohort study in a tertiary-care hospital, there were abnormal serum TSH concentrations in 26 of 42 patients who took sunitinib for renal cell carcinoma or GIST. Persistent primary hypothyroidism, isolated TSH suppression, and transient mild rises in TSH were found in 36, 10, and 17% of patients respectively. There appears to be a correlation between the duration of use of sunitinib and suppressed TSH concentrations as well as a risk of hypothyroidism. Whether sunitinib induces destructive thyroiditis through follicular cell apoptosis has not been fully elucidated (59[c], 60[A], 61[c]).

Sorafenib

Sorafenib (BAY 43-9006) is a multi-targeted inhibitor of tyrosine kinase that inhibits c-RAF and b-RAF kinases as well as VEGFR-2, VEGFR-3, FLT-3, c-kit, and the PDGFR tyrosine kinase in vitro (53[R]). Sorafenib is effective in pretreated renal cell carcinoma and advanced Child A hepatocellular carcinoma.

The incidence of treatment-related grade 3/4 adverse events in phase I studies with sorafenib (n = 179) included hand–foot skin reactions (8%), hypertension (4%), diarrhea (2%), reduced hemoglobin concentration (3%), and fatigue (5%). There is some evidence that grade 2–3 hand–foot syndrome and/or diarrhea correlates with the increase of time to progression compared with patients without such signs of toxicity (62[c]).

Pharmacokinetics The recommended oral dose, 400 mg bd, should not be taken with a fat-rich meal, because of reduced absorption by about 38–49% compared to intake on an empty stomach. Sorafenib is metabolized to some extent by CYP3A4, resulting in a pyridine-N-oxide derivative with similar antineoplastic activity to the parent compound. Elimination is primarily via the feces, about 51% of the dose being excreted as unchanged drug (53[R], 63[R]).

Cardiovascular Grade 3 hypertension is very common in patients taking sorafenib. The median time of onset in patients taking the anti-VEGF antibody bevacizumab was 131 (range 7–316) days. Twelve of 20 patients who took with sorafenib had a rise in systolic blood pressure of at least 20 mmHg compared with baseline, with a median change of 21 mmHg after 3

weeks (42[c]). There as a significant inverse relation between increased systolic blood pressure and a reduction in catecholamines, suggesting a secondary response to the increase in blood pressure.

Tyrosine kinase inhibitors of the VEGF and PDGF receptor pathways may target the VHL hypoxia-inducible gene pathway, which results in inhibition of hypoxia-inducible factor (HIF)-induced gene products. The latter mediate physiological responses of the myocardium to ischemia, including myocardial remodelling, peri-infarct vascularization, and vascular permeability.

Tyrosine kinase inhibitor-induced inhibition of HIF may be associated with more severe myocardial damage than previously expected. Of 73 patients with advanced renal cell carcinoma and normal creatine kinase MB fraction and cardiac troponin T at baseline, 23% had a significant increase in creatine kinase and troponin T after 2–32 weeks, with symptoms in seven (64[c]). One patient had an acute coronary artery occlusion and myocardial infarction. Electrocardiographic changes and biochemical markers are important indicators, and both should be measured regularly irrespective of whether sunitinib or sorafenib is used.

Endocrine Patients with metastatic renal cell carcinoma commonly develop mild biochemical thyroid function test abnormalities while taking sorafenib. However, compared with sunitinib, which is associated with a high incidence of thyroid dysfunction, making routine monitoring necessary, patients taking sorafenib need thyroid function monitoring only if clinically indicated (65[c]).

Drug–drug interactions Theoretically, important drug interactions can be expected during the co-administration of potent CYP3A4 inducing agents (for example rifamycins, St. John's wort, phenytoin, carbamazepine) and CYP3A4 inhibitors (for example triazole antifungal drugs). However, the co-administration of ketoconazole 400 mg/day with sorafenib 50 mg/day did not result in changes in sorafenib pharmacokinetics, perhaps because sorafenib is a low-clearance drug (66[c]). It is also possible that reduced N-oxide formation may be compensated by a small increase in UGT1A9-mediated glucuronidation. Therefore, no dose adjustment appears to be warranted during co-administration of sorafenib with ketoconazole and probably structurally related triazole antifungal drugs.

In vitro, sorafenib inhibits some CYP isozymes, such as CYP2C9, CYP2B6, CYPC8, and some UGT isozymes, such as UGT1A1 and UGT1A9 (63^R). Co-administration of sorafenib with CPT-11, paclitaxel, or propofol is therefore not recommended until further data are available.

Pazopanib

Pazopanib is a potent, selective, broad-spectrum, multi-targeted inhibitor of receptor tyrosine kinases, including VEGFR-1, VEGFR-2, VEGFR-3, PDGFR-α/β, and c-kit. It is still under clinical investigation. Total disease control in patients with advanced renal cell carcinoma was 82%. The most common adverse events included rises in transaminases, diarrhea, fatigue, nausea, hair depigmentation, and hypertension. According to a recent interim analysis, adverse effects led to drug withdrawal in 5% of patients. Preliminary data suggest additional activity of the drug in ovarian cancer, with a comparable spectrum of adverse effects (67^c, 68^c).

OTHER DRUGS

Doxorubicin   *(SED-15, 245; SEDA-25, 533)*

Cardiovascular   Repeated cycles of doxorubicin 75 mg/m^2 intravenously followed by bevacizumab 15 mg/kg intravenously every 3 weeks have been studied in 17 patients with metastatic soft-tissue sarcomas (69^c). Dexrazoxane was also given when the total dose of doxorubicin was over 300 mg/m^2. In all, 85 cycles of doxorubicin + bevacizumab were administered; the median number of cycles was four. Six patients developed cardiac toxicity of grade 2 or worse: four had grade 2 (cumulative doxorubicin dose 75, 150, 300, 300 mg/m^2), one had grade 3 (total doxorubicin dose 591 mg/m^2), and one had grade 4 (total doxorubicin dose 420 mg/m^2). One patient with extensive lung disease died of recurrent bilateral pneumothorax, possibly related to treatment. The 12% response rate for these patients was no greater than that observed for single-agent doxorubicin.

References

1. Maitland ML, Ratain MJ. Terminal ballistics of kinase inhibitors: there are no magic bullets. Ann Intern Med 2006;145:702–3.
2. Robert C, Soria JC, Spatz A, Le Cesne A, Malka D, Pautier P, Wechsler J, Lhomme C, Escudier B, Boige V, Armand JP, Le Chevalier T. Cutaneous side-effects of kinase inhibitors and blocking antibodies. Lancet Oncol 2005;6:491–500.
3. Beumer JH, Natale JJ, Lagattuta TF, Raptis A, Egorin MJ. Disposition of imatinib and its metabolite CGP74588 in patients with chronic myelogenous leukemia and short-bowel syndrome. Pharmacotherapy 2006;26:903–7.
4. Dutreix C, Peng B, Mehring G, Hayes M, Capdeville R, Pokorny R, Seiberling M. Pharmacokinetic interaction between ketoconazole and

imatinib mesylate (Glivec) in healthy subjects. Cancer Chemother Pharmacol 2004;54:290–4.
5. Fausel CA. Novel treatment strategies for chronic myeloid leukaemia. Am J Health-Syst Pharm 2006;63:S15–20.
6. Garcia-Manero G, Faderl S, O'Brien S, Cortes J, Talpaz M, Kantarjian HM. Chronic myelogenous leukemia: a review and update of therapeutic strategies. Cancer 2003;98:437–57.
7. Schleyer E, Ottmann O-G, Illmer T, Pursche S, Leopold T, Bonin M, Freiberg-Richter J, Jenkel A, Platzbecker U, Bornhäuser M, Ehninger G, le Coutre P. Pharmakokinetik von Imatinib (STI571) und seinem Hauptmetaboliten N-Desmethyl-Imatinib. Tumordiagn Ther 2004;25:192–6.
8. Pappas P, Karavasilis V, Briasoulis E, Pavlidis N, Marselos M. Pharmacokinetics of imatinib me-

sylate in end stage renal disease. A case study. Cancer Chemother Pharmacol 2005;56:358–60.

9. Bauer S, Hagen V, Pielken HJ, Bojko P, Seeber S, Schütte J. Imatinib mesylate therapy in patients with gastrointestinal stromal tumors and impaired liver function. Anticancer Drugs 2002;13:847–9.

10. Ramadori G, Füzesi L, Grabbe E, Pieler T, Armbrust T. Successful treatment on hepatocellular carcinoma with the tyrosine kinase inhibitor imatinib in a patient with liver cirrhosis. Anticancer Drugs 2004;15:405–9.

11. De Arriba JJ, Nerín C, García E, Gómez-Aldaraví L, Vila B. Severe hemolytic anemia and skin reaction in a patient treated with imatinib. Ann Oncol 2003;14:962.

12. van Oosterom AT, Judson I, Verweij J, Stroobants S, Donato di Paola E, Dimitrijevic S, Martens M, Webb A, Sciot R, Van Glabbeke M, Silberman S, Nielsen OS, European Organisation for Research and Treatment of Cancer Soft Tissue and Bone Sarcoma Group. Safety and efficacy of imatinib (STI571) in metastatic gastrointestinal stroma tumours: a phase I study. Lancet 2001;358:1421–3.

13. Kerkelä R, Grazette L, Yacobi R, Iliescu C, Patten R, Beahm C, Walters B, Shevtsov S, Pesant S, Clubb FJ, Rosenzweig A, Salomon RN, Van Etten RA, Alroy J, Durand JB, Force T. Cardiotoxicity of the cancer therapeutic agent imatinib mesylate. Nat Med 2006;12:908–16.

14. Rosti G, Martinelli G, Baccarani M. In reply to "Cardiotoxicity of the cancer therapeutic agent imatinib mesylate". Nat Med 2007;13:15–6.

15. Atallah E, Kantarjian H, Cortes J. In reply to "Cardiotoxicity of the cancer therapeutic agent imatinib mesylate". Nat Med 2007;13:14–6.

16. Hatfield A, Owen S, Pilot PR. In reply to "Cardiotoxicity of the cancer therapeutic agent imatinib mesylate". Nat Med 2007;13:13–6.

17. Esmaeli B, Prieto VG, Butler CE, Kim SK, Ahmadi MA, Kantarjian HM, Talpaz M. Severe periorbital edema secondary to STI571 (Gleevec). Cancer 2002;95:881–7.

18. Berman E, Nicolaides M, Maki RG, Fleisher M, Chanel S, Scheu K, Wilson BA, Heller G, Sauter NP. Altered bone and mineral metabolism in patients receiving imatinib mesylate. N Engl J Med 2006;354:2006–13.

19. Sneed TB, Kantarjian HM, Talpaz M, O'Brien S, Rios MB, Bekele BN, Zhou X, Resta D, Wierda W, Faderl S, Giles F, Cortes JE. The significance of myelosuppression during therapy with imatinib mesylate in patients with chronic myelogenous leukemia in chronic phase. Cancer 2004;100:116–21.

20. Kikuchi S, Muroi K, Takahashi S, Kawano-Yamamoto C, Takatoku M, Miyazato A, Nagai T, Mori M, Komatsu N, Ozawa K. Severe hepatitis and complete molecular response caused by imatinib mesylate: possible association of its serum concentration with clinical outcomes. Leukemia Lymphoma 2004;45:2349–51.

21. Brouard M, Saurat JH. Cutaneous reactions to STI571. N Engl J Med 2001;345:618–9.

22. Tsao AS, Kantarjian H, Cortes J, et al. Imatinib mesylate causes hypopigmentation in the skin. Cancer 2003;98:2483–7.

23. Ugurel S, Hildenbrand R, Dippel E, Hochhaus A, Schadendorf D. Dose-dependent severe cutaneous reactions to imatinib. Br J Cancer 2003;88:1157–9.

24. Sessa C, Viganò L, Grasselli G, Trigo J, Marimon I, Lladò A, Locatelli A, Ielmini N, Marsoni S, Gianni L. Phase I clinical and pharmacological evaluation of the multi-tyrosine kinase inhibitor SU006668 by chronic oral dosing. Eur J Cancer 2006;42:171–8.

25. Kajita T, Higashi Y, Imamura M, Maida C, Fujii Y, Yamamoto I, Miyamoto E. Effect of imatinib mesilate on the disposition kinetics of ciclosporin in rats. J Pharm Pharmacol 2006;58:997–1000.

26. Elliott M, Mesa RA, Tefferi A. Adverse events after imatinib mesylate therapy. N Engl J Med 2002;9:712–3.

27. O'Hare T, Walters DK, Stoffregen EP, Jia T, Manley PW, Mestan J, Cowan-Jacob SW, Lee FY, Heinrich MC, Deininger MW, Druker BJ. In vitro activity of Ber-Abl inhibitors AMN107 and BMS-354825 against clinically relevant imatinib resistant Abl kinase domain mutants. Cancer Res 2005;65:4500–5.

28. Talpaz M, Shah NP, Kantarjian H, Donato N, Nicoll J, Paquette R, Cortes J, O'Brien S, Nicaise C, Bleickardt E, Blackwood-Chirchir MA, Iyer V, Chen TT, Huang F, Decillis AP, Sawyers CL. Dasatinib in imatinib-resistant Philadelphia chromosome-positive leukemias. N Engl J Med 2006;354:2531–41.

29. Soverini S, Martinelli G, Colarossi S, Gnani A, Rondoni M, Castagnetti F, Paolini S, Rosti G, Baccarani M. Second-line treatment with dasatinib in patients resistant to imatinib can select novel inhibitor-specific BCR-ABL mutants in Ph+ ALL. Lancet Oncol 2007;8:273–4.

30. Shah NP, Kim DW, Kantarjian HM, Rousselot P, Dorlhiac-Llacer PE, Milone JH, Bleickardt E, Francis S, Hochhaus A. Dasatinib 50 mg or 70 mg bid compared to 100 mg or 140 mg qd in patients with CML in chronic phase (CP) who are resistant or intolerant to imatinib: one-year result of CA180034. ASCO Annual Meeting Proceedings. J Clin Oncol 2007;25(June 20 Suppl):7004.

31. Assouline S, Laneuville P, Gambacorti-Passerini C. Panniculitis during dasatinib therapy for imatinib-resistant chronic myelogenous leukemia. N Engl J Med 2006;354:2623–4.

32. Kantarjian H, Giles F, Wunderle L, Bhalla K, O'Brien S, Wassmann B, Tanaka C, Manley P, Rae P, Mietlowski W, Bochinski K, Hochhaus A, Griffin JD, Hoelzer D, Albitar M, Dugan M, Cortes J, Alland L, Ottmann OG. Nilotinib in imatinib-resistant CML and Philadelphia chromosome-positive ALL. N Engl J Med 2006;354:2542–51.

33. Rosti G, le Coutre P, Bhalla K, Giles F, Ossenkoppele G, Hochhaus A, Gattermann N, Haque A, Weitzman A, Baccarani M, Kantarjian H. A phase II study of nilotinib administered

to imatinib resistant and intolerant patients with chronic myelogenous leukemia (CML) in chronic phase (CP). ASCO Annual Meeting Proceedings. J Clin Oncol 2007;25(June 20 Suppl):7007.

34. Cersosimo RJ. Gefitinib: a new antineoplastic for advanced non-small-cell lung cancer. Am J Health-Syst Pharm 2004;61:889–98.

35. Baselga J, Rischin D, Ranson M, Calvert H, Raymond E, Kieback DG, Kaye SB, Gianni L, Harris A, Bjork T, Averbuch SD, Feyereislova A, Swaisland H, Rojo F, Albanell J. Phase I safety, pharmacokinetic, and pharmacodynamic trial of ZD 1839, a selective oral epidermal growth factor receptor tyrosine kinase inhibitor, in patients with five selected solid tumor types. J Clin Oncol 2002;20:4292–302.

36. Villano JL, Mauer AM, Vokes EE. A case study documenting the anticancer activity of ZD1839 (Iressa) in the brain. Ann Oncol 2003;14:656–8.

37. Inomata S, Takahashi H, Nagata M, Yamada G, Shiratori M, Tanaka H, Satoh M, Saitoh T, Sato T, Abe S. Acute lung injury as an adverse event of gefitinib. Anticancer Drugs 2004;15:461–7.

38. Inoue A, Saijo Y, Maemondo M, Gomi K, Tokue Y, Kimura Y, Ebina M, Kikuchi T, Moriya T, Nukiwa T. Severe acute interstitial pneumonia and gefitinib. Lancet 2003;361:137–9.

39. Rabinowits G, Herchenhorn D, Rabinowits M, Weatge D, Torres W. Fatal pulmonary toxicity in a patient treated with gefitinib for non-small cell lung cancer after previous hemolytic–uremic syndrome due to gemcitabine. Anticancer Drugs 2003;14:665–8.

40. Shah NT, Kris MG, Pao W, Tyson LB, Pizzo BM, Heinemann MH, Ben-Porat L, Sachs DL, Heelan RT, Miller VA. Practical management of patients with non-small-cell lung cancer treated with gefitinib. J Clin Oncol 2005;23:165–74.

41. Govindan R, Behnken D, Read W, McLeod H. Wound healing is not impaired by the epidermal growth factor receptor-tyrosine kinase inhibitor gefitinib. Ann Oncol 2003;14:1330–1.

42. Veronese ML, Mosenkis A, Flaherty KT, Gallagher M, Stevenson JP, Townsend RR, O'Dwyer PJ. Mechanisms of hypertension associated with BAY 43-9006. J Clin Oncol 2006;24:1363–9.

43. Kanazawa S, Yamaguchi K, Kinoshita Y, Muramatsu M, Komiyama Y, Nomura S. Aspirin reduces adverse effects of gefitinib. Anticancer Drugs 2006;17:423–7.

44. Shepherd FA, Rodrigues Pereira J, Ciuleanu T, Tan EH, Hirsh V, Thongprasert S, Campos D, Maoleekoonpiroj S, Smylie M, Martins R, van Kooten M, Dediu M, Findlay B, Tu D, Johnston D, Bezjak A, Clark G, Santabárbara P, Seymour L, National Cancer Institute of Canada Clinical Trials Group. Erlotinib in previously treated non-small-cell lung cancer. N Engl J Med 2005;353:123–32.

45. Moore MJ, Goldstein D, Hamm J, Figer A, Hecht JR, Gallinger S, Au HJ, Murawa P, Walde D, Wolff RA, Campos D, Lim R, Ding K, Clark G, Voskoglou-Nomikos T, Ptasynski M, Parulekar W, National Cancer Institute of Canada Clinical Trials Group. Erlotinib plus gemcitabine compared of gemcitabine alone in patients with advanced pancreatic cancer. A phase III trial of the National Cancer Institute of Canada Clinical Trials Group (NCIC-CTG). J Clin Oncol 2007;25:1960–6.

46. Lai SE, Minnelly L, O'Keeffe P, Rademaker A, Patel J, Bennett CL, Lacouture ME. Influence of skin color in the development of erlotinib-induced rash: a report from the SERIES Clinic. ASCO Annual Meeting Proceedings. J Clin Oncol 2007;25(June 20 Suppl):9127.

47. Philip PA, Mahoney MR, Allmer C, Thomas J, Pitot HC, Kim G, Donehower RC, Fitch T, Picus J, Erlichman C. Phase II study of erlotinib in patients with advanced biliary cancer. J Clin Oncol 2006;24:3069–74.

48. Buie LW, Lindley C, Shih T, Ewend M, Smith JK, Skelton M, Kwock L, Morris D, Tucker C, Collichio F. Plasma pharmacokinetics and cerebrospinal fluid concentrations of erlotinib in high-grade gliomas: a novel, phase I, dose escalation study. ASCO Annual Meeting Proceedings. J Clin Oncol 2007;25(June 20 Suppl):2054.

49. Nelson MH, Dolder CR. Lapatinib: a novel dual tyrosine kinase inhibitor with activity in solid tumors. Ann Pharmacother 2006;40:261–9.

50. Terkola R. Lapatinib ditosylate (Tykerb). Eur J Oncol Pharm 2007;1:13–7.

51. GlaxoSmithKline. Tykerb. http://us.gsk.com/products/assets/us_tykerb.pdf.

52. Midgley R, Flaherty KT, Haller DG, Versola MJ, Smith DA, Koch KM, Pandite L, Kerr DJ, O'Dwyer PJ, Middleton MR. Phase I study of lapatinib, a dual kinase inhibitor, in combination with irinotecan 5-fluorouracil and leucovorin. ASCO Annual Meeting Proceedings. J Clin Oncol 2005;23(June 1 Suppl):3086.

53. Larkin J, Eisen T. Kinase inhibitors in the treatment of renal cell carcinoma. Crit Rev Oncol Hematol 2006;60:216–26.

54. Motzer RJ, Hoosen S, Bello CL, Christensen JG. Sunitinib maleate for the treatment of solid tumours: a review of current clinical data. Expert Opin Investig Drugs 2006;15:553–61.

55. Motzer RJ, Hutson TE, Tomczak P, Michaelson MD, Bukowski RM, Rixe O, Oudard S, Negrier S, Szczylik C, Kim ST, Chen I, Bycott PW, Baum CM, Figlin RA. Sunitinib versus interferon alfa in metastatic renal-cell carcinoma. N Engl J Med 2007;356:115–24.

56. Motzer RJ, Michaelson MD, Redman BG, Hudes GR, Wilding G, Figlin RA, Ginsberg MS, Kim ST, Baum CM, DePrimo SE, Li JZ, Bello CL, Theuer CP, George DJ, Rini BI. Activity of SU11248, a multitargeted inhibitor of vascular endothelial growth factor receptor and platelet-derived growth factor receptor, in patients with metastatic renal cell carcinoma. J Clin Oncol 2006;24:16–24.

57. Motzer RJ, Rini BI, Bukowski RM, Curti BD, George DJ, Hudes GR, Redman BG, Margolin KA, Merchan JR, Wilding G, Ginsberg MS,

Bacik J, Kim ST, Baum CM, Michaelson MD. Sunitinib in patients with metastatic renal cell carcinoma. JAMA 2006;295:2516–24.

58. Bello CL, Sherman L, Zhou J, Verkh L, Smeraglia J, Mount J, Klamerus KJ. Effect of food on the pharmacokinetics of sunitinib malate (SU11248), a multi-targeted receptor tyrosine kinase inhibitor: results from a phase I study in healthy subjects. Anticancer Drugs 2006;17:353–8.

59. Desai J, Yassa L, Marqusee E, George S, Frates MC, Chen MH, Morgan JA, Dychter SS, Larsen PR, Demetri GD, Alexander EK. Hypothyroidism after sunitinib treatment for patients with gastrointestinal stromal tumors. Ann Intern Med 2006;145:660–4.

60. de Groot JW, Links TP, van der Graaf WT. Tyrosine kinase inhibitors causing hypothyroidism in a patient on levothyroxine. Ann Oncol 2006;17:1719–20.

61. Rini BI, Tamaskar I, Shaheen P, Salas R, Garcia J, Wood L, Reddy S, Dreicer R, Bukowski RM. Hypothyroidism in patients with metastatic renal cell carcinoma treated with sunitinib. J Natl Cancer Inst 2007;99:81–3.

62. Strumberg D, Awada A, Hirte H, Clark JW, Seeber S, Piccart P, Hofstra E, Voliotis D, Christensen O, Brueckner A, Schwartz B. Pooled safety analysis of BAY 43-9006 (sorafenib) monotherapy in patients with advanced solid tumours: is rash associated with treatment outcome? Eur J Cancer 2006;42:548–56.

63. Hahn O, Stadler W. Sorafenib. Curr Opin Oncol 2006;18:615–21.

64. Schmidinger M, Vogl UM, Schukro C, Bojic A, Bojic M, Schmidinger H, Zielinski CC. Cardiac involvement in patients with sorafenib or sunitinib treatment for metastatic renal cell carcinoma. ASCO Annual Meeting Proceedings. J Clin Oncol 2007;25(June 20 Suppl):5110.

65. Tamaskar IR, Unnithan J, Garcia JA, Dreicer R, Wood L, Iochimescu A, Bukowski R, Rini B. Thyroid function test (TFT) abnormalities in patients (pts) with metastatic renal cell carcinoma (RCC) treated with sorafenib. ASCO Annual Meeting Proceedings. J Clin Oncol 2007;25(June 20 Suppl):5048.

66. Lathia C, Lettieri J, Cihon F, Gallentine M, Radtke M, Sundaresan P. Lack of effect of ketoconazole-mediated CYP3A inhibition on sorafenib clinical pharmacokinetics. Cancer Chemother Pharmacol 2006;57:685–92.

67. Friedlander M, Hancock KC, Benigno B, Rischin D, Messing M, Stringer CA, Tay EH, Kathman S, Matthys G, Lager JJ. Pazopanib (GW786034) is active in women with advanced epithelial ovarian fallopian tube and peritoneal cancers: initial results of a phase II study. ASCO Annual Meeting Proceedings. J Clin Oncol 2007;25(June 20 Suppl):5561.

68. Hutson TE, Davis ID, Machiels JP, de Souza PL, Hong BF, Rottey S, Baker KL, Crofts T, Pandite L, Figlin R. Pazopanib (GW786034) is active in metastatic renal cell carcinoma (RCC): interim results of a phase II randomized discontinuation trial (RDT). ASCO Annual Meeting Proceedings. J Clin Oncol 2007;25(June 20 Suppl):5031.

69. D'Adamo DR, Anderson SE, Albritton K, Yamada J, Riedel E, Scheu K, Schwartz GK, Chen H, Maki RG. Phase II study of doxorubicin and bevacizumab for patients with metastatic soft-tissue sarcomas. J Clin Oncol 2005;23(28):7135–42.

Sameh K. Morcos

46 Radiological contrast agents

TYPES OF CONTRAST AGENTS

Iodinated water soluble contrast media are of four types:

(a) high-osmolar ionic monomers (e.g. diatrizoate, iothalamate, metrizoate);

(b) low-osmolar ionic dimers (e.g. ioxaglate);

(c) low-osmolar non-ionic monomers (e.g. iopitridole, iohexol, iomeprole, iopamidole, iopromide, ioversol);

(d) iso-osmolar non-ionic dimers (e.g. iodixonal, iotrolan).

They are mainly used intravascularly, but can also be injected into body cavities, particularly the low-osmolar contrast agents. They are also suitable for oral or rectal administration. The high-osmolar water-soluble contrast agent diatrizoate (Gastrografin) is suitable only for oral or rectal administration.

There are also contrast agents that enhance the diagnostic information provided by ultrasound scanning and magnetic resonance imaging. The latter are mainly gadolinium-based, but new non-gadolinium paramagnetic contrast agents have recently become available. Ultrasound contrast agents are microbubbles that provide acoustic enhancement.

Adverse reactions to contrast media are generally few, and serious reactions are uncommon. Ultrasound contrast agents are particularly safe.

Water-soluble intravascular iodinated contrast agents *(SED-15, 1848; SEDA-27, 496; SEDA-28, 552; SEDA-29, 573)*

Adverse reactions to intravascular iodinated contrast agents can be minor, intermediate, or severe and life-threatening. All types of reactions to low-osmolar contrast media are at least five times less common than reactions to high-osmolar contrast media. These reactions have been extensively covered in previous issues of SEDA. Fortunately, very serious or fatal reactions to low-osmolar contrast media are rare.

The incidence of adverse reactions to low-osmolar non-ionic and ionic contrast media when used together or separately during percutaneous coronary intervention has been investigated retrospectively in 532 patients (mean age ~60 years) undergoing percutaneous coronary intervention ([1^C]). Patients were divided into two groups: those who underwent diagnostic angiography and "follow-on" percutaneous coronary intervention; and those who underwent "planned" percutaneous coronary intervention. The groups were subdivided on the basis of the use of the ionic agent ioxaglate (mean dose ~192 ml) or the non-ionic agent iopromide (mean dose ~210 ml). Allergy-like reactions occurred in nine of 150 patients (6.0%) who received the combination of ioxaglate and iopromide versus one of 93 (1.1%) who only received iopromide. There was no difference with respect to major adverse cardiac events (six with ioxaglate and iopromide versus four with iopromide alone). In the planned group, seven of 165 patients (4.2%) who received ioxaglate had an allergy-like reaction as opposed to none of 124 patients who received iopromide. All the reactions were mild. The incidence of a major adverse cardiac event was similar in the two groups (one with ioxaglate versus two with iopromide). The incidence of allergy-like reactions was similar with ioxaglate

Side Effects of Drugs, Annual 30
J.K. Aronson (Editor)
ISSN: 0378-6080
DOI: 10.1016/S0378-6080(08)00046-9

alone or in combination with iopromide. The authors concluded that while combining ionic and non-ionic contrast agents in the same procedure was not associated with any more adverse reactions than using an ionic contrast agent alone, the ionic contrast agent ioxaglate was associated with the majority of allergy-like reactions. They suggested that the lowest risk of an adverse event in coronary intervention is associated with the non-ionic agent iopromide used alone.

Nervous system   Intravenous iodinated contrast media can be associated with the minor adverse effects of *heat sensation* and *local pain*. In a prospective study of the incidence of these reactions with iodinated contrast media in a high concentration (370 mg I/ml, 342 patients, mean age 60 years) or a medium concentration (300 mg I/ml, 387 patients, mean age 62 years), the mean score for heat sensation was 4.46 with the high concentration and 3.44 with the medium concentration (2[c]). There was no significant difference in the incidence of adverse reactions (five of 342 patients with the high concentration, and two of 387 with the medium concentration) between the two groups. The authors concluded that high and medium concentrations of iodinated contrast medium can be used for CT studies with comparable safety, even though the heat sensation produced by a high concentration is greater than that produced by a medium concentration.

- An 18-month-old boy had a focal seizure and cerebral contrast retention 12 hours after cardiac catheterization (3[A]). An unenhanced cranial CT scan 1 hour after the seizure showed general cerebral edema and unilateral focal cerebral contrast retention, with sparing of the area supplied by the middle cerebral artery. The contrast medium disappeared over 48 hours, the cerebral edema resolved over several days, and he recovered fully 4 days after the seizure.

The authors concluded that contrast toxicity should be considered in any case of a new-onset neurological deficit arising after angiography or enhanced CT.

Gastrointestinal   Iodinated water-soluble contrast media can be used for imaging the gastrointestinal tract without important adverse effects (SEDA-26, 512). The safety of using different concentrations of the high-osmolar ionic

contrast agent diatrizoate (Gastrografin) in MR imaging of the small bowel has been investigated in 24 healthy volunteers (median age 24 years) (4[c]). They were randomized into four groups, and received 350 ml of diatrizoate in concentrations of 50, 25, 10, or 0%. The most frequent adverse reactions were *diarrhea*, *nausea*, and *lack of palatability*. There was a graded relation between increasing osmolality and the adverse effects score.

Pancreas   CT scanning enhanced with intravenous iodinated contrast medium which is widely used to diagnose *acute pancreatitis*, can lengthen the duration of pancreatitis and increase the incidence of local or systemic complications. However, the authors of a review of the literature concluded that there are no well-substantiated data to incriminate contrast media in worsening the course of acute pancreatitis (5[M]).

Skin   Fatal *toxic epidermal necrolysis* with involvement of the gastrointestinal tract after cardiac angiography has been reported (6[A]).

- A 62-year-old white man with chest pain underwent cardiac angiography which showed three-vessel coronary artery disease. He had a history of type 2 diabetes mellitus, hyperlipidemia, peripheral vascular disease, chronic renal insufficiency, and significant alcohol abuse in the distant past. He was allergic to penicillin. Two days after the procedure, he developed an extensive rash with blistering, which resolved spontaneously. He developed abdominal distension 2 months later and a CT scan showed only mild hepatomegaly. After the CT examination he developed a rash and became feverish; the rash resolved over several days. Before subsequent catheterization he was pretreated with prednisone 60 mg, diphenhydramine 25 mg, and ranitidine 150 mg. He was also given intravenous fluids and N-acetylcysteine (4 doses of 600 mg) because of pre-existing renal insufficiency (baseline creatinine 130 µmol/l). About 6 hours after catheterization, he developed a rash and became feverish but his vital signs remained normal. Within 2 days his skin began to slough near the folds in his neck and upper back in spite of treatment with diphenhydramine and sulfadiazine cream. The lesions progressed to involve 70% of the body surface area. His renal function also deteriorated and the serum creatinine rose to 210 µmol/l. Skin biopsies showed toxic epidermal necrolysis. A few days later he developed gastrointestinal bleeding, and endoscopy showed extensive sloughing of the esophageal and gastric mucosa. His general condition continued to deteriorate and he became oliguric and died.

Delayed allergy-like skin reactions can occur within a few days of contrast injection and tend to be commoner with non-ionic dimers than other types of contrast media (SEDA-22, 499). However, severe cases of toxic epidermal necrolysis complicating contrast medium injection are rare. It is now widely accepted that these reactions are T-cell mediated and represent type IV hypersensitivity reactions. Unfortunately, the case report did not include details of the type or the dose of the contrast medium used and whether the same contrast agent or different ones were used in the CT and angiographic examinations. Skin tests are useful in identifying the culprit agent, which should be avoided in future examinations and replaced by a different contrast agent that does not induce a reaction on skin testing. Glucocorticoid prophylaxis, even in a high dose, according to some reports, cannot prevent the occurrence of toxic epidermal necrolysis.

Contrast medium-induced nephrotoxicity

DoTS classification:
Reaction: Contrast medium-induced
    nephrotoxicity
Dose-relation: Collateral
Time-course: Intermediate
Susceptibility factors: Endogenous factors
    (pre-existing renal insufficiency,
    particularly if it is secondary to diabetes
    mellitus congestive heart failure,
    dehydration); drugs (nephrotoxic drugs,
    such as non-steroidal anti-inflammatory
    drugs; metformin; mannitol and
    diuretics, particularly loop diuretics);
    multiple repeat exposures to contrast
    media within a short period of time (72
    hours)

Contrast medium-induced nephrotoxicity has been extensively covered in previous issues of SEDA, and only reports with important new information have been included here.

Differences between agents   *One contentious issue is whether there is an important difference in the renal effects of iso-osmolar and* *low-osmolar contrast agents. In 129 patients with diabetes and pre-existing renal impairment undergoing angiography (the NEPHRIC study) there was a 3% incidence of nephrotoxicity with iodixanol (an iso-osmolar non-ionic dimer) and 26% with the low-osmolar non-ionic monomer iohexol (SEDA-27, 501). Several new comparative studies have been carried out since the NEPHRIC study, with mixed outcomes.*

Apart from two new reports concordant with the outcome of the NEPHRIC study, other studies have not confirmed a lower incidence of nephrotoxicity with iodixanol compared with low-osmolar contrast media. In one study there was a higher incidence of nephrotoxicity after the administration of ioxaglate (25%) compared with iodixanol (8.2%) in patients with renal impairment undergoing coronary angiography (7[C]). In a meta-analysis of 2727 patients from 16 double-blind, randomized, controlled studies (intra-arterial iodixanol or low-osmolar contrast media) the incidence of nephrotoxicity was 1.4% with iodixanol and 3.5% with low-osmolar contrast media (8[M]). Analysis of a subgroup of patients with diabetes mellitus and chronic kidney disease showed that the incidence of nephrotoxicity was 3.5% with iodixanol and 16% with low-osmolar contrast media. The authors concluded that renal impairment appears to be significantly less with iodixanol than low-osmolar contrast media in patients undergoing angiography. However, there were certain limitations to this study, including the dose of contrast agent, which was significantly higher in the low-osmolar contrast group (59 g I/examination) compared with iodixanol (55 g I/examination) and no data on the state of hydration in each group were available.

In a retrospective analysis of 52 526 patients who underwent coronary angiography and intervention the incidence of renal impairment within 12 months was significantly higher with iodixanol (1.8%) than ioxaglate (1%) (9[M]).

In 285 patients undergoing cardiac angiography iopamidol and iodixanol-320 produced the same incidence of nephrotoxicity: 19% with iopamidol and 12% with iodixanol (10[c]).

In a retrospective study of 225 patients with moderate to severe kidney disease, there were no differences in the rates of nephrotoxicity between iodixanol and the low-osmolar non-ionic monomer iobitridol (11[c]).

In a prospective randomized study of 414 patients with renal impairment (eGFR 45 ml/minute) undergoing cardiac angiography there was no significant difference in the incidence of nephrotoxicity between iopamidol and iodixanol (12^C). The incidence of nephrotoxicity, defined as a fall in eGFR by at least 25% from baseline, was 5.8% with iopamidol-370 and 10% with iodixanol.

In a randomized, multicenter trial (IMPACT) of 155 patients with renal impairment (GFR less than 60 ml/minute) undergoing CT examinations there was no difference in the rates of nephrotoxicity between equal of doses iodine (40 g) as either iopamidol-370 or iodixanol-320 intravenously at 4 ml/second: 2.6% after iodixanol and 0% after iopamidol (13^C).

In a prospective, randomized, double-blind comparison of iodixanol and iopromide (a nonionic monomer) in 64 patients with moderate to severe renal insufficiency undergoing excretory urography, one non-diabetic patient developed nephrotoxicity after iodixanol; there were no cases among those who were given iopromide (14^c).

In a study of the same design, iodixanol was compared with the non-ionic monomer iobitridol in 50 patients with severe chronic kidney disease undergoing cranial or body CT (15^c). The two groups received similar volumes of contrast (113 ml of iobitridol, 113 ml of iodixanol) and had similar baseline renal function. The incidence of nephrotoxicity was 17% in both groups.

The rate of nephrotoxicity in 100 consecutive patients with renal impairment undergoing multidetector row-computed tomography (MDCT) angiography with intravenous iodixanol 100 ml was 9%; all recovered renal function (16^c).

The cost-effectiveness of iodixanol was investigated in 125 patients at high risk of nephrotoxicity (17^c). The analyses were based on a randomized, prospective, multinational comparison of the nephrotoxic effects of iodixanol with those of a low-osmolar non-ionic contrast medium, iohexol. There were seven contrast media-related serious adverse reactions, of which six cases of acute renal failure developed after iohexol. Two patients who were given iodixanol had one non-serious reaction each. The mean hospitalization costs per patient were €489, €573, and €393 lower after iodixanol than after iohexol using Swedish, German,

and French unit prices respectively. The mean per-patient costs of treating adverse drug reactions were €371, €399, and €445 lower after iodixanol than after iohexol, using the respective unit prices. The authors concluded that the iodixanol appears to be cost-effective when compared with iohexol in patients at risk of nephrotoxicity.

Prevention   *CO_2 gas has been proposed for use instead of iodinated contrast media in angiographic examinations in patients at risk of nephrotoxicity (18^C). The effect of intra-arterial CO_2 with added ioxaglate (a low-osmolar ionic dimer) or ioxaglate alone on renal function in patients with suspected renal artery stenosis has been studied in a prospective randomized study in 123 patients who underwent renovascular intervention (n = 83) and/or renal angiography (n = 40). Patients with a serum creatinine concentration under 200 μmol/l (n = 82) were randomized prospectively to receive CO_2 with small added amounts of ioxaglate (200 mg I/ml, n = 37) or only ioxaglate (n = 45). Patients with serum creatinine concentrations over than 200 μmol/l (n = 41) were not randomized and initially received CO_2. Serum creatinine concentrations were measured 1 day before and 1 day, 2 days, and 2–3 weeks after the procedure. The amount of injected CO_2 did not relate to an increase in serum creatinine concentration. However, the amount of injected iodine correlated significantly with an increase in serum creatinine concentration and a reduction in estimated creatinine clearance after 2 days. Among the randomized patients, one in the CO_2 group and three in the ioxaglate group had a more than 25% increase in serum creatinine concentration within the first 2 days after the intervention. The authors concluded that the risk of nephrotoxicity is lower after injection of CO_2 with small amounts of added ioxaglate compared with a larger dose of ioxaglate alone. The larger the dose of administered iodinated contrast medium, the greater the risk of renal impairment.*

There is accumulating evidence that reactive oxygen species have a role in renal damage. Prophylactic administration of antioxidant drugs could prevent this. The correlation between the antioxidant capacity of the serum and the risk of nephrotoxicity has been examined in a prospective study of 193 patients with normal renal function who underwent cardiac catheterization. Eleven patients developed mild renal insufficiency. There was no significant difference in the baseline concentrations of antioxidant species between the patients who developed renal impairment and those who had no change in renal function. The authors concluded that baseline concentrations of antioxidant material do not predict the possible development of nephrotoxicity (19ᶜ).

Isotonic bicarbonate starting 1 hour before given at a rate of 3 ml/kg/hour and continued for 6 hours after exposure to contrast at a rate of 1 ml/kg/hour reduced the incidence of nephrotoxicity in 119 patients compared with isotonic saline hydration (SEDA-29, 577). The mechanism by which bicarbonate is protective is not fully understood, but it has been suggested that increasing the pH of the renal medulla and urine reduces the production of free radicals and protects the kidney from the oxidant injury that can be associated with contrast medium-induced nephrotoxicity.

A recent report has suggested that combining bicarbonate infusion with N-acetylcysteine, in a dose of 1200 mg bd for 48 hours starting 24 hours before administration of contrast medium (iodixanol ~170 ml) in 219 patients with pre-existing renal impairment offers better protection against nephrotoxicity than 0.9% saline (20ᶜ). The incidence of nephrotoxicity after angiography was 9.9% in the patients who received isotonic saline and acetylcysteine (n = 111) and 1.9% in those who received sodium bicarbonate and acetylcysteine (n = 108).

Immunologic   The mechanisms responsible for the *allergy-like adverse effects* of contrast media are uncertain. A possible role for cysteinyl-leukotrienes (cys-LT) in adverse reactions induced by non-ionic contrast media has been investigated in 39 patients who received iopromide (a non-ionic monomer) or iotrolan (a non-ionic dimer) for routine CT examination and whose leukocytes were analysed for the production of cysteinyl-leukotrienes (21ᶜ). Three patients who received iopromide and five who received iotrolan had adverse reactions. The reactors had increased concentrations of cysteinyl-leukotrienes in samples obtained before contrast injection (6764 pg/ml). In vitro iopromide and iotrolan induced significant production of cysteinyl-leukotrienes

compared with IL-3 stimulation. In vivo both media caused a significant rise in the concentrations of cysteinyl-leukotrienes 6 hours after contrast administration. This study has provided some evidence that cysteinyl-leukotrienes play a significant role in contrast reactions and suggests that leukotriene receptor antagonists could be used to treat or prevent these reactions.

The role of T cells in mediating contrast reactions has been investigated in 12 patients, 11 of whom had had delayed adverse reactions at 1–48 hours after contrast injection (22ᶜ). The reactions including generalized maculopapular eruptions, drug hypersensitivity syndrome with rash and eosinophilia, fever, and late-onset urticaria, and in one patient an acute reaction (facial edema and respiratory distress) shortly after contrast administration. Skin tests (skin prick, intradermal, and patch tests) were performed with various iodinated contrast media (high-osmolar ionic contrast agents, sodium meglumine amidotrizoate and meglumine ioxitalamate; a low-osmolar ionic dimer, ioxaglate; low-osmolar non ionic monomers, iopamidol, iobitridol, iopentol, iohexol, ioversol, and iopromide; and an iso-osmolar non-ionic dimer, iodixanol) and were read after 15 minutes, 24 hours, and 48 hours. Skin biopsies of positive test sites in 11 patients were evaluated immunohistologically. An immune reaction was inferred from a positive skin prick test (n = 2), a positive patch test (n = 10), or a positive intradermal test (n = 9) at 24 and 48 hours. Skin biopsies showed a T-cell infiltrate in the dermis with predominantly CD4+ T cells in 8 patients, CD8+ T cells in one patient, and equal numbers in another. Cross-sensitivities to several iodinated contrast media were observed in nine patients. Other drug allergies were noted in six. The authors concluded that delayed reactions to contrast media are most likely to be T-cell mediated immune reactions to these drugs.

Fetotoxicity   Transplacental passage of water-soluble contrast media can occur after intravascular administration. Iopromide, a non-ionic monomer, has been detected in the bowel and urine of a preterm infant, born 10 days after intravenous administration to his mother (23ᴬ).

- An obese 26-year-old primipara had threatened preterm labour at 27 weeks and 2 days later, because of acute dyspnea and low oxygen saturation, pulmonary CT angiography was performed with intravenous iopromide 370 mg I/ml (200 ml) to exclude pulmonary embolism, which was not detected. Ten days after angiography, the membranes ruptured spontaneously and 1 hour later a preterm boy was born vaginally. The baby had only mild respiratory distress and no goiter. A plain abdominal X-ray showed intraluminal gastrointestinal opacifications consistent with the presence of radiographic contrast material. The iopromide concentration was 0.13 ng/ml in a urine sample. The iopromide concentration in the CSF was 0.1 ng/ml. The urinary iodine concentration on day 8 of life was 880 µg/l (reference range <200 µg/l). Iodine containing solutions had not been used in the delivery room or during neonatal care. Serum free thyroxine concentrations were 11 and 12 ng/l on days 7 and 31 of life respectively (reference range 9–17 ng/l). The corresponding concentrations of TSH were 2.7 and 6.2 mU/l (95% age-specific confidence intervals 0.45–4.12 mU/l). Apart from persistent apnea, the further hospital course was uneventful. On follow-up at the corrected age of 4 months, the child showed normal neurodevelopment and thyroid function was normal.

The authors of the report concluded that contrast media can cross the placenta and accumulate in various fetal tissues in significant amounts, causing possible neonatal toxicity.

MRI CONTRAST MEDIA

Gadolinium salts   *(SED-15, 1469; SEDA-27, 504; SEDA-28, 561; SEDA-29, 578)*

℞ *Gadolinium-based contrast agents and nephrogenic systemic fibrosis*

Seven extracellular gadolinium-based contrast agents are currently available for use in ionic and non-ionic forms (Table 1). They are all chelates containing gadolinium ion (Gd^{+++}). The configuration of the molecules is either linear or cyclic.

The incidence of adverse events with these agents is low and serious reactions are rare. Their general safety has been discussed in detail in previous issues of SEDA. However, since January 2006 several reports have appeared suggesting that there may be a causal relation between their use and the condition of nephrogenic systemic fibrosis, which was originally known as nephrogenic fibrosing dermopathy.

This condition is characterized by scleroderma-like skin changes that mainly affect the limbs and trunk. The lesions can be itchy and painful. Induration of the skin can progress to flexion contractures of joints. The fibrotic changes can also affect other organs, such as skeletal muscle, heart, liver, and lungs. The disease can be aggressive in some patients, leading to serious physical disability or even death. No effective treatment is available. The gold standard for diagnosing nephrogenic systemic fibrosis is deep skin biopsy, which shows irregularly thickened bundles of collagen and increased deposition of mucin in the dermis. Between these bundles are deposited numerous spindle-shaped fibroblastic cells and large dendritic cells. The total number of cases of nephrogenic systemic fibrosis associated with gadolinium is currently about 120 patients of all ages, including children. Nephrogenic systemic fibrosis has been reported only in patients with acute or chronic severe renal insufficiency (glomerular filtration rate below 30 ml/minute), including patients on dialysis, patients with renal dysfunction due to the hepatorenal syndrome, or in the perioperative liver transplantation period. There have been no reports in patients with normal kidney function or with mild to moderate renal insufficiency. The dose of the agent varied from 0.1 to 0.50 mmol/kg. The onset of the disease varies from a few days to a few months after exposure (24[A], 25[A], 26[A], 27[A], 28[A], 29[A], 30[A], 31[A], 32[A]). The overwhelming majority (~90%) followed the administration of the non-ionic linear chelate gadodiamide (Omniscan); the other cases were observed with the non-ionic linear chelate gadoversetamide (OptiMark) and the ionic linear chelate gadopentate dimeglumine (Magnevist).

The strong association between nephrogenic systemic fibrosis and gadodiamide suggests that the stability of the chelate complex could be an important factor in triggering the development of nephrogenic systemic fibrosis. Extracellular gadolinium-based agents are eliminated from the body through the kidneys and half-life in patients with normal renal function is 1.5 hours. In patients with advanced renal impairment the half-life can be prolonged to 30 hours or more. Patients on hemodialysis would require three consecutive dialysis sessions over 6 days to remove 97% of the administered dose. Continuous ambulatory peritoneal dialysis for 20 days

Table 1. *Physicochemical characteristics of clinically available extracellular gadolinium-based contrast agents (33[H])*

Extracellular gadolinium-based contrast agent	Type	Thermodynamic stability constant	Conditional stability	Amount of excess chelate (mg/ml)	Kinetic stability (dissociation half-life at pH 1.0)
Gadoversetamide, Gd-DTPA-BMEA (OptiMark, Tyco, USA)	Non-ionic linear	17	15	28	Not available
Gadodiamide, Gd-DTPA-BMA (Omniscan, GE, USA)	Non-ionic linear	17	15	12	35 seconds
Gadobutrol, Gd-BT-DO3A (Gadovist, Schering, Berlin)	Non-ionic cyclic	22	Not available	Not available	24 hours
Gadoteridol, Gd-HP-DO3A (Prohance, Bracco, Italy)	Non-ionic cyclic	24	17	0.23	3 hours
Gadopentetate, Gd-DTPA (Magnevist, Schering, Berlin)	Ionic linear	22	18	0.4	10 minutes
Gadobenate, Gd-BOPTA (MultiHance, Bracco, Italy)	Ionic linear	23	18	None	Not available
Gadoterate, Gd-DOTA (Dotarem, Guerbet, France)	Ionic cyclic	26	18	None	>1 month

eliminates 69% of the injected dose. Transmetallation is likely to occur when the gadolinium–chelate complex remains in the body for a long period, as is the case in patients with end-stage renal disease, including those on dialysis. Transmetallation leads to release of free gadolinium through replacement of the Gd^{+++} within the chelate molecule by cations such as zinc or copper. Free gadolinium is highly toxic, and in animals it causes splenic degeneration, central lobular necrosis of the liver, and a variety of hematological abnormalities. It is therefore crucially important that Gd^{+++} should be strongly attached to a chelate to avoid toxicity.

The binding between the ligand and Gd^{+++} is weaker in the linear chelates (Magnevist, Omniscan, MultiHance, Optimark) than in the macrocyclic chelates (Dotarem, Gadovist, Prohance), and weaker in the non-ionic linear chelates (Omniscan and Optimark) than in the ionic linear chelates (Magnevist and Multi-Hance) (Table 1). The following measurements are used to assess the stability of the chelate molecules: thermodynamic stability constant, conditional stability, and kinetic stability (dissociation half-life under very acidic conditions, pH 1.0). The higher these measurements the higher is the stability of the molecule. In addition, the presence of excess chelate in the formulation is an indirect marker of low stability (Table 1). These markers indicate that the least stable formulations are the non-ionic linear chelates, which have the lowest thermodynamic and constant stability values and the highest amount of excess chelate compared with the other types of chelate. The most stable chelates are the macrocyclic ones, particularly the ionic macrocyclic chelate Dotarem, which has the highest stability values and no excess chelate.

The most likely hypothesis of the pathogenesis of nephrogenic systemic fibrosis so far is that free Gd^{+++} released from an unstable chelate deposits in the dermis and other organs, attracting circulating fibrocytes to these sites to initiate the process of fibrosis (33^H). Gadolinium has been found in the skin biopsies of patients with nephrogenic systemic fibrosis (34^A).

In response to the steady increase in the number of cases of nephrogenic systemic fibrosis after the administration of gadolinium-based agents the UK Commission on Human Medicines (CHM) together with the European Pharmacovigilance Working Party (PhVWP) of the Committee on Medicinal Products for Human Use (CHMP) recommended in a letter to health professionals on 7 February 2007 "Do not use Omniscan (gadodiamide) in patients with severe renal impairment (i.e. GFR below 30 ml/min/1.73 m^2) or in patients who have had, or who are awaiting, liver transplantation. Prescribers are also warned that gadodiamide should be used in neonates and infants up to 1 year of age only after careful consideration. Careful consideration should be given to the use of other gadolinium-based MRI contrast agents in patients with severe renal impairment (i.e. GFR below 30 ml/minute/ 1.73 m^2)" (35^S). The Food and Drug Administration (FDA) in the USA first notified healthcare professionals and the public about the gadolinium-related risks of nephrogenic systemic fibrosis in June 2006. Information on the risks was updated in December 2006. On 23 May 2007 the FDA asked manufacturers of all gadolinium-based contrast agents to add a new boxed warning to the product label, highlighting the risk of nephrogenic systemic fibrosis after exposure to a gadolinium-based contrast agents in patients with acute or chronic severe renal insufficiency (glomerular filtration rate below 30 ml/minute/1.73 m^2) and patients with acute renal insufficiency of any severity due to the hepatorenal syndrome or in the perioperative liver transplantation period. In these patients, avoid the use of a gadolinium-based contrast agent unless the diagnostic information is essential and not available with non-contrast enhanced magnetic resonance imaging. Nephrogenic systemic fibrosis can cause fatal or debilitating systemic fibrosis. Patients should be screened for kidney problems (history and or laboratory tests) before being given

one of these imaging agents. The recommended dose should not be exceeded and enough time should elapse to ensure that a dose has been eliminated from the body before the agent is used again (36^S).

Ultrasound contrast agents

Ultrasound contrast agents approved for clinical use are well tolerated, and serious adverse reactions are rare. Adverse events are usually minor (for example headache, nausea, altered taste, sensation of heat) and resolve spontaneously. These symptoms may not be related to the ultrasound contrast materials, as they have also been observed in placebo groups. Generalized *allergy-like reactions* are rare. To reduce the risks, the ultrasound scanning time and the acoustic output should be kept to the lowest level consistent with obtaining diagnostic information (37^R).

Cardiovascular   In a post-marketing analysis of more than 157 838 studies of the ultrasound contrast agent Sonovue® there were three (0.002%) fatal and 19 (0.012%) severe, non-fatal adverse reactions; of the latter, nine were cardiac events (four *bradycardia*, two *tachycardia*, three *myocardial ischemia*); 11 of these 19 patients received Sonovue for echocardiography (38^c). These results led to the addition of several contraindications to the use of Sonovue. Although a strong relation was established between the non-fatal cases and administration of Sonovue, a causal relation with the fatal cases is debatable. Therefore, the risk associated with the use of Sonovue should be judged carefully, taking into consideration the prevalence of adverse effects of other contrast media and diagnostic procedures used, particularly in cardiology.

Dobutamine stress echocardiography is widely used after myocardial infarction. It is safe, and severe adverse reactions are uncommon. However, *cardiac rupture* has been reported (39^A).

• A 57-year-old man with a history of hypertension had an inferior myocardial infarction and was referred for dobutamine stress echocardiography. An unnamed intravenous ultrasound contrast agent was used to improve endocardial visualization.

Resting echocardiographic images showed akinesia of the inferior and posterior basal segments without a pericardial effusion. At the peak dobutamine dose (40 µg/kg/minute), he had chest pain and ST segment elevation in the inferior leads. Simultaneously, extravasation of the contrast material into the pericardial cavity was detected by echocardiography. A few seconds later, electromechanical dissociation with cardiopulmonary arrest occurred. All attempts at cardiopulmonary resuscitation failed and he died.

This seems to have been the first report of acute cardiac rupture during dobutamine stress testing, diagnosed by the use of intravenous contrast echocardiography.

The ultrasound contrast agent ECHOVIST-200 has been used for hysterosonography with diagnostic success in 195 cases (40^c). The most common adverse effect during the procedure was abdominal pain, which was well tolerated by the patients. There were no other important adverse effects.

References

1. Juergens CP, Khaing AM, McIntyre GJ, Leung DYC, Lo STH, Fernandes C, Hopkins AP. Adverse reactions of low osmolar non-ionic and ionic contrast media when used together or separately during percutaneous coronary intervention. Heart Lung Circ 2005;14:172–7.
2. Masui T, Katayama M, Kobayashi S, Sakahara H. Intravenous injection of high and medium concentrations of computed tomography contrast media and related heat sensation, local pain, and adverse reactions. J Comput Assist Tomogr 2005;29:704–8.
3. Frye RE, Newburger JW, Nugent A, Sahin M. Focal seizure and cerebral contrast retention after cardiac catheterization. Pediatr Neurol 2005;32:213–6.
4. Borthne AS, Abdelnoor M, Hellund JC, Geitung JT, Jonn T, Storaas T, Gjesdal K, Klow N-E. MR imaging of the small bowel with increasing concentrations of an oral osmotic agent. Eur Radiol 2005;15:666–71.
5. Plock JA, Schmidt J, Anderson SE, Sarr MG, Roggo A. Contrast-enhanced computed tomography in acute pancreatitis: does contrast medium worsen its course due to impaired microcirculation? Langenbecks Arch Surg 2005;390:156–63.
6. Garza A, Waldman AJ, Mamel J. A case of toxic epidermal necrolysis with involvement of the GI tract after systemic contrast agent application at cardiac catheterization. Gastrointest Endosc 2005;62:638–42.
7. Jo SH, Youn TJ, Koo BK, Park JS, Kang HJ, Cho YS, Chung WY, Joo GW, Chae IH, Choi DJ, Oh BH, Lee MM, Park YB, Kim HS. Renal toxicity evaluation and comparison between Visipaque (iodixanol) and Hexabric (ioxaglate) in patients with renal insufficiency undergoing coronary angiography. The RECOVER study: a randomized controlled trial. J Am Coll Cardiol 2006;48:924–30.
8. McCullough PA, Bertrand ME, Brinker JA, Stacul F. A meta-analysis of the renal safety of isosmolar iodixanol compared with low osmolar contrast media. J Am Coll Cardiol 2006;48:692–9.
9. Liss P, Presson PB, Hansell P, Lagerqvist B. Renal failure in 57 925 patients undergoing coronary procedures using iso-osmolar or low-osmolar contrast media. Kidney Int 2006;70:1811–7.
10. Jingwei N, Ruiyan Z, Jiansheng Z, Xian Z, Weifeng S. Safety of isosmolar nonionic dimer during percutaneous coronary intervention. J Intervent Radiol 2006;15:327–9.
11. Briguori C, Colombo A, Airoldi F, Morici N, Sangiorgi GM, Violante A, Focaccio A, Montorfano M, Carlino M, Condorelli G, Ricciardelli B. Nephrotoxicity of low-osmolality versus iso-osmolality contrast agents: impact of N-acetylcysteine. Kidney Int 2006;68:2250–5.
12. Solomon RJ, Natarajan MK, Doucet S, Sharma SK, Staniloae CS, Katholi RE, Gelormini JL, Labinaz M, Moreyra AE, Investigators of the CARE Study. Cardiac Angiography in Renally Impaired Patients (CARE) study: a randomized double-blind trial of contrast-induced nephropathy in patients with chronic kidney disease. Circulation 2007;115(25):3189–96.

13. Barrett BJ, Katzberg RW, Thomsen HS, Chen N, Sahani D, Soulez G, Heiken JP, Lepanto L, Ni ZH, Nelson R. Contrast-induced nephropathy in patients with chronic kidney disease undergoing computed tomography: a double-blind comparison of iodixanol and iopamidol. Invest Radiol 2006;41(11):815–21.

14. Carraro M, Malalan F, Antonione R, Stacul F, Cova M, Petz S, Assante M, Grynne B, Haider T, Palma LD, Faccini L. Effects of a dimeric vs a monomeric nonionic contrast medium on renal function in patients with mild to moderate renal insufficiency: a double-blind, randomized clinical trial. Eur Radiol 1998;8:144–7.

15. Kolehmainen H, Soiva M. Comparison of Xenetix 300 and Visipaque 320 in patients with renal failure. Eur Radiol 2003;13:B32–3.

16. Becker CR, Reiser MF. Use of iso-osmolar nonionic dimeric contrast media in multidetector row computed tomography angiography for patients with renal impairment. Invest Radiol 2005;40:672–5.

17. Aspelin P, Aubry P, Fransson S-G, Strasser R, Willenbrock R, Lundkvist J. Cost-effectiveness of iodixanol in patients at high risk of contrast-induced nephropathy. Am Heart J 2005;149:298–303.

18. Liss P, Eklof H, Hellberg O, Hagg A, Bostrom-Ardin A, Lofberg A-M, Olsson U, Orndahl P, Nilsson H, Hansell P, Eriksson L-G, Bergqvist D, Nyman R. Renal effects of CO2 and iodinated contrast media in patients undergoing renovascular intervention: a prospective, randomized study. J Vasc Interv Radiol 2005;16:57–65.

19. Elias M, Swae'ed S, Shneor A, Turgman Y, Saliba W, Goldstein LH, Rosenfeld T. Serum antioxidant capacity and the risk of contrast medium nephropathy. Nephron Clin Pract 2005;99:3–7.

20. Briguori C, Airoldi F, Dandrea D, Bonizzoni E, Morici N, Focaccio A, Michev I, Montorfano M, Carlino M, Cosgrave J, Ricciardelli B, Colombo A. Renal Insufficiency Following Contrast Media Administration Trial (REMEDIAL): a randomized comparison of 3 preventive strategies. Circulation 2007;115:1211–7.

21. Bohm I, Speck U, Schild H. A possible role for cysteinyl-leukotrienes in non-ionic contrast media induced adverse reactions. Eur J Radiol 2005;55:431–6.

22. Kanny G, Pichler W, Morisset M, Franck P, Marie B, Kohler C, Renaudin J-M, Beaudouin E, Laudy JS, Moneret-Vautrin DA. T cell-mediated reactions to iodinated contrast media: evaluation by skin and lymphocyte activation tests. J Allergy Clin Immunol 2005;115:179–85.

23. Vanhaesebrouck P, Verstraete AG, De Praeter C, Smets K, Zecic A, Craen M. Transplacental passage of a nonionic contrast agent. Eur J Pediatr 2005;164:408–10.

24. Grobner T. Gadolinium—a specific trigger for the development of nephrogenic fibrosing dermopathy and nephrogenic systemic fibrosis? Nephrol Dial Transplant 2006;21:1104–8 [erratum, 1745].

25. Marckmann P, Skov L, Rossen K, Dupont A, Damholt MB, Heaf JG, Thomsen HS. Nephrogenic systemic fibrosis: suspected causative role of gadodiamide used for contrast-enhanced magnetic resonance imaging. J Am Soc Nephrol 2006;17:2359–62.

26. Maloo M, Abt P, Kashyap R, Younan D, Zand M, Orloff M, Jain A, Pentland A, Scott G, Bozorgzadeh A. Nephrogenic systemic fibrosis among liver transplant recipients: a single institution experience and topic update. Am J Transplant 2006;6:2212–7.

27. Broome DR, Girguis MS, Baron PW, Cottrell AC, Kjellin I, Kirk GA. Gadodiamide-associated nephrogenic systemic fibrosis: why radiologists should be concerned. AJR Am J Roentgenol 2007;188:586–92.

28. Khurana A, Runge VM, Narayanan M, Greene Jr JF, Nickel AE. Nephrogenic systemic fibrosis: a review of 6 cases temporally related to gadodiamide injection (Omniscan). Invest Radiol 2007;42:139–45.

29. Deo A, Fogel M, Cowper SE. Nephrogenic systemic fibrosis: a population study examining the relationship of disease development to gadolinium exposure. Clin J Am Soc Nephrol 2007;2:264–7.

30. Sadowski EA, Bennett LK, Chan MR, Wentland AL, Garrett AL, Garrett RW, Djamali A. Nephrogenic systemic fibrosis: risk factors and incidence estimation. Radiology 2007;243:148–57.

31. Marckmann P, Skov L, Rossen K, Heaf JG, Thomsen HS. Case-control study of gadodiamide-related nephrogenic systemic fibrosis. Nephrol Dial Transplant May 2007;4 [epub ahead of print].

32. Thomsen HS. Nephrogenic systemic fibrosis: a serious late adverse reaction to gadodiamide. Eur Radiol 2006;16:2619–21.

33. Morcos SK. Nephrogenic systemic fibrosis following the administration of extracellular gadolinium based contrast agents: is the stability of the contrast agent molecule an important factor in the pathogenesis of this condition? Br J Radiol 2007;80:73–6.

34. Boyd AS, Zic JA, Abraham JL. Gadolinium deposition in nephrogenic fibrosing dermopathy. J Am Acad Dermatol 2007;56:27–30.

35. Gadolinium-containing MRI contrast agents and nephrogenic systemic fibrosis (NSF). Available at: http://www.mhra.gov.uk/home/idcplg?IdcService=SS_GET_PAGE&useSecondary=true&ssDocName=CON2030229&ssTargetNodeId=221.

36. US Food and Drug Administration. Public health advisory: update on magnetic resonance imaging (MRI) contrast agents containing gadolinium and nephrogenic fibrosing dermopathy. Updated 22 December 2006 and 23 May 2007. Available at: http://www.fda.gov/cder/drug/InfoSheets/HCP/gcca_200705HCP.pdf.

37. Jakobsen JA, Oyen R, Thomsen HS, Morcos SK, Members of Contrast Media Safety Committee of European Society of Urogenital Radiology

(ESUR). Safety of ultrasound contrast agents. Eur Radiol 2005;15:941–5.

38. Dijkmans PA, Visser CA, Kamp O. Adverse reactions to ultrasound contrast agents: is the risk worth the benefit? Eur J Echocardiogr 2005;6:363–6.

39. Datino T, Garcia-Fernandez MA, Martinez-Selles M, Quiles J, Avanzas P. Cardiac rup-ture during contrast-enhanced dobutamine stress echocardiography. Int J Cardiol 2005;98:349–50.

40. Tamasi F, Weidner A, Domokos N, Bedros RJ, Bagdany S. ECHOVIST-200 enhanced hystero-sonography: a new technique in the assessment of infertility. Eur J Obstet Gynecol Reprod Biol 2005;121:186–90.

B.C.P. Polak

47   Drugs used in ocular treatment

DRUGS USED IN THE MANAGEMENT OF AGE-RELATED MACULAR DEGENERATION

Angiostatic drugs are currently used intravitreally in the treatment of age-related macular degeneration and other exudative and proliferative diseases. The risk of serious adverse events after intravitreal injection is low, but careful attention to injection technique and appropriate peroperative and postoperative monitoring are essential. The general risks of intravitreal injection of drugs were discussed in SEDA-29 (p. 581).

Bevacizumab   *(SED-15, 2380; SEDA-29, 407)*

Bevacizumab (Avastin®), a recombinant humanized monoclonal antibody against all isoforms of vascular endothelial growth factor (VEGF), was originally developed to treat metastatic carcinoma of the colon and the rectum. It is effective after intravitreal injection in patients with age-related macular degeneration and has been used off-label for neovascular and exudative ocular diseases in thousands of intravitreal injections world wide.

Observational studies   In an internet-based survey of the adverse effects of bevacizumab, a web address was distributed to the international community of vitreoretinal surgeons via e-mail; 70 centers from 12 countries participated and reported on 5228 patients (7113 injections) (1ᶜ). Adverse events included *corneal abrasions, lens injury, endophthalmitis, retinal detachment, inflammation or uveitis, cataract progression, acute loss of vision, central retinal artery occlusion, subretinal hemorrhages, retinal pigment epithelial tears, increased blood pressure, transient ischemic attacks, strokes*, and *death*. None of these adverse events exceeded a frequency of 0.21%. There did not seem to be an association between intravitreal bevacizumab and an increased risk of thromboembolic events, myocardial infarction, stroke, or hypertension, which can be associated with systemic administration of bevacizumab.

There were no cases of severe loss of vision or other adverse effects in a retrospective study of 48 patients, of whom 72% had previously been treated with either pegaptanib or photodynamic therapy, who received one or more intravitreal injections of bevacizumab for exudative age-related macular degeneration (2ᶜ). The average number of injections over the mean follow-up period of 34 weeks was 3.5, and mean visual acuity increased by 6.5 letters at 4 weeks and 5.3 letters at 24 weeks after the first injection.

Intravitreal bevacizumab improved visual acuity in 10 eyes with idiopathic choroidal neovascularization in which posterior subtenon triamcinolone injections over more than 3 months were not efficacious (3ᶜ). In one patient *conjunctival swelling* developed after the injection, but it resolved and did not occur after another injection.

In a prospective case series 102 eyes of 102 patients with neovascular age-related macular degeneration received monthly intravitreal bevacizumab (1.25 mg) until there was resolution of macular edema, subretinal fluid, and/or pigment epithelial detachment (4ᶜ). Most patients attained stability or improvement of their visual acuity. The injections were well tolerated in all and there were no cases of uveitis, glaucoma, or endophthalmitis, or systemic cardiovascular events.

Side Effects of Drugs, Annual 30
J.K. Aronson (Editor)
ISSN: 0378-6080
DOI: 10.1016/S0378-6080(08)00047-0

These observations suggest that there are no major serious problems with bevacizumab in the short term.

Ranibizumab

Ranibizumab (Lucentis®) is a specific, affinity-mature, recombinant, humanized, antivascular endothelial growth factor-A (anti-VEGF-A) antibody fragment, which binds all isoforms of VEGF-A, rendering them inactive; it is effective in the treatment of age-related macular degeneration after intravitreal injection (5R).

Observational studies   Two patients with serous pigment epithelial detachment and occult choroidal neovascularization associated with age-related macular degeneration developed *retinal pigment epithelial tears* within 4 weeks after intravitreal injection of ranibizumab (6c). In another observational study two patients had retinal pigment epithelial tears on follow-up visits at 1 month, confirmed by optical coherence tomography and by fluorescein or indocyanine green angiography (7c). The tears developed within 4 weeks after intravitreal injection of ranibizumab, a time course that suggested a causal role.

Placebo-controlled studies   In a 2-year, phase I/II, multicenter, randomized, single-masked, controlled study, patients with predominantly classical choroidal neovascularization secondary to age-related macular degeneration received either monthly intravitreal ranibizumab 0.5 mg (*n* = 106) or sham injections (*n* = 56); photodynamic therapy was performed 7 days before the injection (8c). At 12 months, 91% of the treated patients and 68% of the control patients had lost fewer than 15 letters of visual acuity. In those who had received ranibizumab there was a relatively high incidence of *endophthalmitis* (1.9%), which rose to 4.8% when all patients with presumed endophthalmitis were included; furthermore, 11% of those who received ranibizumab had *intraocular inflammation*. The numbers of *strokes* were similar in the two groups: 3.6% (photodynamic therapy) and 3.8% (ranibizumab).

In a multicenter, 2-year, double-masked, sham-controlled study 716 patients with age-related macular degeneration, with either minimally classical or occult choroidal neovascularization, were randomized to receive monthly intravitreal injections of ranibizumab 0.3 or 0.5 mg for 2 years or sham injections (9C). At 1 year, 95% of those who received ranibizumab 0.3 mg and 95% of those who received ranibizumab 0.5 mg had lost fewer than 15 letters, compared with 62% of those who received sham injections. Visual acuity improved by 15 letters or more in 25% of the 0.3 mg group and 34% of the 0.5 mg group, compared with 5% of the sham group. In those who received ranibizumab presumed *endophthalmitis* was identified in five patients and serious *uveitis* in six.

In a 2-year, multicenter, double-masked study 423 patients with predominantly classical neovascular age-related macular degeneration were assigned in a ratio of 1:1:1 to receive monthly intravitreal injections of ranibizumab 0.3 mg or 0.5 mg plus sham verteporfin therapy, or monthly sham injections plus active verteporfin therapy (10C). In all, 94% of those treated with ranibizumab 0.3 mg and 96% of those treated with ranibizumab 0.5 mg lost fewer than 15 letters, compared with 64% of those who were treated with verteporfin. Visual acuity improved by 15 letters or more in 36% of those who received 0.3 mg and 40% of those who received 0.5 mg, compared with 5.6% of those who received verteporfin. Presumed *endophthalmitis* occurred in two of those given ranibizumab 0.5 mg and serious *uveitis* in one.

Verteporfin and photodynamic therapy   ℞

Photodynamic therapy is a procedure that exploits the physical properties of chemical compounds that are activated by [laser] light and cause tissue oxidation and destruction (11R). It has antiangiogenic effects on subfoveal choroidal neovascular membranes, such as occur in age-related macular degeneration. Verteporfin (Visudyne®) is a photosensitizing protoporphyrin derivative, which has a high affinity for choroidal neovascular membranes and has been used intravenously in the treatment of subfoveal neovascularization secondary to age-related macular degeneration (12^R), pathological myopia (13^C), angioid streaks (14^c), and toxoplasmic retinochoroiditis (15^c). It has also been used to treat pterygium (16^c).

Photodynamic therapy with verteporfin over 1 and 2 years reduces the decline in visual acuity in patients with subfoveal neovascularization secondary to age-related macular degeneration. In choroidal neovascularization secondary to pathological myopia, verteporfin was also significantly better than placebo in reducing visual acuity after 1 year, but not after 2 years: however, choroidal lesions were significantly smaller in verteporfin recipients after 2 years.

Verteporfin has been generally well tolerated by most patients in randomized trials. Common adverse events were injection-site reactions, pain in the back, chest, and elsewhere, nausea, photosensitivity reactions, weakness, and hypercholesterolemia, each affectin 1–10% of patients (17^R).

Placebo-controlled studies　The adverse effects of verteporfin have been studied in a systematic review of three similar multicenter, 24-month, double-masked, randomized, placebo-controlled trials in 948 patients (18^M). The percentages of patients who had at least one ocular or non-ocular adverse event were similar with verteporfin and placebo (92 and 89% respectively). The only clinically relevant ocular adverse events that had a higher incidence with verteporfin were visual disturbances (22 versus 16% in one study and 42 versus 23% in another). There were acute severe reductions in visual acuity in 14 patients. Systemic adverse events that had a higher incidence with verteporfin compared with placebo, most of which were transient and mild or moderate, were injection site reactions (13 versus 5.6%), photosensitivity reactions (2.4 versus 0.3%), and infusion-related back pain (2.4 versus 0%).

Respiratory　Acute respiratory distress has been attributed to verteporfin (19^M).

- A 50-year-old woman with a history of food allergy was given intravenous verteporfin for a myopic choroidal neovascular membrane and 8 minutes later reported a feeling of warmness from her neck to the ears, and a throbbing sensation in

her throat causing a dry cough. Her face became red and sweaty while she was trying to swallow and breathe with difficulty. Her heart rate was 80/minute and her blood pressure 145/85 mmHg. She was thought to have laryngospasm and was given oxygen and intravenous chlorphenamine maleate 10 mg and betamethasone 4 mg. She recovered within a few minutes.

Nervous system　Loss of consciousness has been reported in a patient who had received intravenous verteporfin (20^A).

- An otherwise healthy 43-year-old woman underwent photodynamic therapy and 2 minutes after verteporfin infusion had begun felt light-headed and nauseated and subsequently lost consciousness and had a tonic–clonic seizure. The infusion was stopped immediately. She was cyanotic, had no palpable pulse, and was not breathing. She recovered after cardiopulmonary resuscitation. An electrocardiogram showed sinus rhythm without ischemic changes and cardiac enzymes were normal.

The authors thought that this incident may have been due to a severe vasovagal reaction, but the underlying mechanisms were uncertain.

Sensory systems　Choroidal ischemia and infarction can occur when photodynamic therapy affects normal blood vessels, which are usually less sensitive than new vessels. In a retrospective review of all patients who developed choroidal ischemia after photodynamic therapy with verteporfin there was choroidal ischemia in eight (2.1%) of 373 eyes of patients with choroidal neovascularization in age-related macular degeneration and in one (0.9%) of 114 eyes with pathological myopia (21^c). Choroidal infarction has been reported in eight patients with age-related macular degeneration after the use of photodynamic therapy with verteporfin (22^c). Although this complication is related to the dose of verteporfin and the intensity of light used, these were not excessive in these patients, and the authors suggested that these patients may have had especially sensitive vessels. Four of the eight patients had also received intravitreal triamcinolone and an interaction could not be ruled out.

Retinal pigment epithelium tears have been reported in two eyes after initial verteporfin therapy combined with intravitreal triamcinolone 4 mg in a prospective case series of 45 patients with choroidal neovascularization in age-related macular degeneration (23^c). A retinal pigment tear was also reported a few weeks after photodynamic therapy with verteporfin in a patient with choroidal neovascularization secondary to pathological myopia (24^A). In a retrospective review of 343 patients treated with photodynamic therapy, one had a serous pigment epithelial detachment and tear (25^c).

Large submacular hemorrhages have been reported after photodynamic therapy with verteporfin in 55 eyes of 52 patients with age-related macular degeneration and occult subfoveal choroidal neovascularization (26^c). Submacular hemorrhages, which precluded determining whether additional verteporfin therapy should be given, developed in five eyes. Visual acuity 3 months later was 8.5 lines worse than before treatment.

New subfoveal hemorrhage and its effect on visual acuity 2 weeks after verteporfin photodynamic therapy in predominantly classic subfoveal choroidal neovascularization secondary to age-related macular degeneration has been studied retrospectively in 104 eyes of 97 patients (27^c). New subfoveal hemorrhage was found in 22% (23/104) of the eyes; in 17% (4/23) of the eyes with new subfoveal hemorrhage there was moderate or severe loss of visual acuity. After 12 weeks there was considerable resorption of the new subfoveal hemorrhage and some improvement in visual acuity.

Skin   The incidence, duration, and time course of skin photosensitivity due to verteporfin has been studied in 17 healthy volunteers, 30 patients with skin cancers, and patients in three phase III trials (28^{Mc}). The frequency of photosensitivity was high at 1.5 hours after dosing and fell rapidly thereafter. The duration was dose-related, 2.0–6.7 days at doses of 6–20 mg/m^2. Photosensitivity reactions occurred in only 2.2% of patients in the phase III trials, including two severe events, one secondary to extravasation. All treatment-related reactions in the phase III trials occurred within the first 2 days after dosing, with the exception of two mild reactions and one moderate reaction that occurred 3 days after treatment.

Urinary tract   Nephrotic syndrome has been attributed to verteporfin (29^A).

- After four cycles of photodynamic therapy, general weakness with generalized edema developed in an otherwise healthy 66-year-old woman, resulting in dyspnea and ascites. There was heavy proteinuria, reduced serum total protein and albumin, and increased total cholesterol. Renal biopsy showed normal glomeruli and tubulointerstitium by light microscopy, with no deposition of immunoglobulins or complement. Transmission electron microscopy showed diffuse effacement of the foot processes of visceral epithelial cells, the characteristic finding in minimal change nephrotic syndrome.

Musculoskeletal   Infusion-related pain, usually back pain, occurs in 2–10% of patients. The mechanism may involve a high concentration of circulating thromboxane induced by the liposomal composition of verteporfin (30^C). It has also been suggested that it is associated with neutrophil margination (31^c). Prevention includes halving the infusion rate, non-steroidal anti-inflammatory drugs, and antihistamines (32^c). In one study of 250 patients, hydration had no preventive effect (33^C).

Immunologic   Hypersensitivity reactions to verteporfin are uncommon, but can be severe (34^c).

Drug–drug interactions   The risk of submacular hemorrhage may be increased by concomitant anticoagulant therapy. In a review of the charts of all patients who developed large submacular hemorrhages following photodynamic therapy for choroidal neovascular membranes secondary to age-related macular degeneration three met the criteria for a large submacular hemorrhage; all three had exudative age-related macular degeneration and were taking warfarin although the international normalized ratios were not excessively high (1.2–1.6) (35^c).

Management of adverse drug reactions   Although photodynamic therapy preferentially affects abnormal vessels, it can also damage the overlying retina. Brain-derived neurotrophic factor (BDNF) reportedly reduced this damage in adult rats (36^E). In another study the combination of brain-derived neurotrophic factor with ciliary neurotrophic factor (CNTF) was even more effective (37^E).

OTHER OCULAR MEDICAMENTS

Glucocorticoids

Sensory systems Intravitreal triamcinolone for the treatment of age-related macular degeneration can cause raised intraocular pressure and cataracts. In a longitudinal study in 111 phakic eyes, 57 were treated with intravitreal triamcinolone 4 mg and 54 were controls (38[c]). The eyes treated with triamcinolone that had no increase in intraocular pressure were unlikely to have posterior subcapsular cataracts (1%). In contrast, eyes in which intraocular pressure rose in response to triamcinolone had a high risk of accelerated progression to posterior subcapsular cataracts (51%).

Retinal breakage after intravitreal injection of triamcinolone acetonide has been reported in a 58-year-old man with proliferative diabetic retinopathy and diffuse macular edema (39[A]).

Phosphate-buffered eye drops

Corneal calcification is a complication of chronic eye diseases, such as uveitis, severe glaucoma, keratitis, and burns. In some cases of eye burns, corneal calcification has been found to be related to the use of calciferous caustic agents and phosphate-buffer-containing fluids. A total of 176 burnt eyes of 98 patients has therefore been retrospectively reviewed, and the following data were acquired: the type of caustic agent, the timing of exposure, the time and type of first-aid, the delay and type of immediate treatment, subsequent medications, the clinical grade, and sequelae (40[c]). Exposure to calciferous burning agents correlated with corneal calcification. Initial single rinsing with phosphate did not produce corneal calcification, but corneal calcification was correlated with chronically administered phosphate-buffered eye drops. Eye burns followed by calcification were of two different major patterns: either the corrosive substance contained calcium or phosphate-buffered eye drops were used in treatment. A proposed mechanism is the low content of calcium ion stabilizing proteins, such as hyaluronate or fetuin, in treatments for severe eye burns. Exceeding the solubility product of calcium and phosphate results in precipitation of calcium phosphate. In chronic corneal disturbance, it is recommended that phosphate-buffered medications should not be used.

References

1. Fung AE, Rosenfeld PJ, Reichel E. The International Intravitreal Bevacizumab Safety Survey: using the internet to assess drug safety worldwide. Br J Ophthalmol 2006;90:1344–9.

2. Yoganathan P, Deramo VA, Lai JC. Visual improvement following intravitreal bevacizumab (Avastin) in exudative age-related macular degeneration. Retina 2006;26:994–8.

3. Gomi F, Nishida K, Oshima Y, Sakaguchi H, Sawa M, Tsujikawa M, Tano Y. Intravitreal bevacizumab for idiopathic choroidal neovascularization after previous injection with posterior subtenon triamcinolone. Am J Ophthalmol 2007;143:507–10.

4. Chen CY, Wong TY, Heriot WJ. Intravitreal bevacizumab (Avastin) for neovascular age-related macular degeneration: a short-term study. Am J Ophthalmol 2007;143:510–2.

5. Spaide R. Ranibizumab according to need: a treatment for age-related macular degeneration. Am J Ophthalmol 2007;143:679–80.

6. Carvounis PE, Kopel AC, Benz MS. Retinal pigment epithelium tears following ranibizumab for exudative age-related macular degeneration. Am J Ophthalmol 2007;143:504–5.

7. Bakri SJ, Kitzmann AS. Retinal pigment epithelial tear after intravitreal ranibizumab. Am J Ophthalmol 2007;143:505–7.

8. Heier JS, Boyer DS, Ciulla TA, FOCUS Study Group. Ranibizumab combined with verteporfin photodynamic therapy in neovascular age-related macular degeneration: year 1 results of the FOCUS Study. Arch Ophthalmol 2006;124:1532–42.

9. Rosenfeld PJ, Brown DM, Heier JS, MARINA Study Group. Ranibizumab for neovascular age-

related macular degeneration. N Engl J Med 2006;355:1419–31.
10. Brown DM, Kaiser PK, Michels M. ANCHOR Study. Ranibizumab versus verteporfin for neovascular age-related macular degeneration. N Engl J Med 2006;355:1432–44.
11. Gaynes BI, Fiscella RG. Safety of verteporfin for treatment of subfoveal choroidal neovascular membranes associated with age-related macular degeneration. Expert Opin Drug Saf 2004;3(4):345–61.
12. Fenton C, Perry CM. Verteporfin: a review of its use in the management of subfoveal choroidal neovascularization. Drugs Aging 2006;23(5):421–45.
13. Lam DS, Chan WM, Liu DT, Fan DS, Lai WW, Chong KK. Photodynamic therapy with verteporfin for subfoveal choroidal neovascularisation of pathologic myopia in Chinese eyes: a prospective series of 1 and 2 year follow up. Br J Ophthalmol 2004;88(10):1315–9.
14. Browning AC, Chung AK, Ghanchi F, Harding SP, Musadiq M, Talks SJ, Yang YC, Amoaku WM, United Kingdom PDT Users Group. Verteporfin photodynamic therapy of choroidal neovascularization in angioid streaks: one-year results of a prospective case series. Ophthalmology 2005;112(7):1227–31.
15. Mauget-Faÿsse M, Mimoun G, Ruiz-Moreno JM, Quaranta-El Maftouhi M, De Laey JJ, Postelmans L, Soubrane G, Defauchy M, Leys A. Verteporfin photodynamic therapy for choroidal neovascularization associated with toxoplasmic retinochoroiditis. Retina 2006;26(4):396–403.
16. Fossarello M, Peiretti E, Zucca I, Perra MT, Serra A. Photodynamic therapy of pterygium with verteporfin: a preliminary report. Cornea 2004;23(4):330–8.
17. Schnurrbusch UEK, Jochmann C, Einbock W, Wolf S. Complications after photodynamic therapy. Arch Ophthalmol 2005;123(10):1347–50.
18. Azab M, Benchaboune M, Blinder KJ, Bressler NM, Bressler SB, Gragoudas ES, Fish GE, Hao Y, Haynes L, Lim JI, Menchini U, Miller JW, Mones J, Potter MJ, Reaves A, Rosenfeld PJ, Strong A, Su XY, Slakter JS, Schmidt-Erfurth U, Sorenson JA, Treatment of Age-Related Macular Degeneration with Photodynamic Therapy (TAP) Study Group, Verteporfin in Photodynamic Therapy (VIP) Study Group. Verteporfin therapy of subfoveal choroidal neovascularization in age-related macular degeneration: meta-analysis of 2-year safety results in three randomized clinical trials: Treatment Of Age-Related Macular Degeneration With Photodynamic Therapy and Verteporfin In Photodynamic Therapy Study Report no. 4. Retina 2004;24(1):1–12.
19. Fossarello M, Peiretti E. Acute respiratory distress due to verteporfin infusion for photodynamic therapy. Arch Ophthalmol 2006;124(10):1509–10.
20. Noffke AS, Jampol LM, Weinberg DV, Munana A. A potentially life-threatening adverse reaction to verteporfin. Arch Ophthalmol 2001;119(1):143.

21. Isola V, Pece A, Parodi MB. Choroidal ischemia after photodynamic therapy with verteporfin for choroidal neovascularization. Am J Ophthalmol 2006;142(4):680–3.
22. Klais CM, Ober MD, Freund KB, Ginsburg LH, Luckie A, Mauget-Faÿsse M, Coscas G, Gross NE, Yannuzzi LA. Choroidal infarction following photodynamic therapy with verteporfin. Arch Ophthalmol 2005;123(8):1149–53.
23. Michels S, Aue A, Simader C, Geitzenauer W, Sacu S, Schmidt-Erfurth U. Retinal pigment epithelium tears following verteporfin therapy combined with intravitreal triamcinolone. Am J Ophthalmol 2006;141(2):396–8.
24. Srivastava SK, Sternberg Jr P. Retinal pigment epithelial tear weeks following photodynamic therapy with verteporfin for choroidal neovascularization secondary to pathologic myopia. Retina 2002;22(5):669–71.
25. Sharp DM, Lai S, Markey CM. Photodynamic therapy with verteporfin for choroidal neovascularization due to age-related macular degeneration and other causes: a New Zealand outcomes study. Clin Experiment Ophthalmol 2007;35(1):24–31.
26. Do DV, Bressler NM, Bressler SB. Large submacular hemorrhages after verteporfin therapy. Am J Ophthalmol 2004;137(3):558–60.
27. Gelisken F, Inhoffen W, Karim-Zoda K, Grisanti S, Partsch M, Voelker M, Bartz-Schmidt KU. Subfoveal hemorrhage after verteporfin photodynamic therapy in treatment of choroidal neovascularization. Graefes Arch Clin Exp Ophthalmol 2005;243(3):198–203.
28. Houle JM, Strong HA. Duration of skin photosensitivity and incidence of photosensitivity reactions after administration of verteporfin. Retina 2002;22(6):691–7.
29. Kang SW, Kang SJ, Kim HO, Nam ES, Lee JH, Koh HJ. Photodynamic therapy using verteporfin-induced minimal change nephrotic syndrome. Am J Ophthalmol 2002;134(6):907–8.
30. Pece A, Vadala M, Manzi R, Calori G. Back pain after photodynamic therapy with verteporfin. Am J Ophthalmol 2006;141(3):593–4.
31. Spaide RF, Maranan L. Neutrophil margination as a possible mechanism for verteporfin infusion-associated pain. Am J Ophthalmol 2003;135(4):549–50.
32. Tornambe PE. Using intravenous diphenhydramine to minimize back pain associated with photodynamic therapy with verteporfin. Arch Ophthalmol 2002;120(6):872.
33. Borodoker N, Spaide RF, Maranan L, Murray J, Freund KB, Slakter JS, Sorenson JA, Yannuzzi LA, Guyer DR, Fisher YL. Verteporfin infusion-associated pain. Am J Ophthalmol 2002;133(2):211–4.
34. Doshi AB, Moshfeghi DM, Jack RL. Anaphylactoid reaction after verteporfin therapy. Am J Ophthalmol 2005;140(5):936–7.
35. Chaudhry NA, Lavaque AJ, Tom DE, Liggett PE. Large submacular hemorrhage following PDT

with verteporfin in patients with occult CNVM secondary to age-related macular degeneration. Ophthalmic Surg Lasers Imaging 2007;38(1):64–8.

36. Paskowitz DM, Nune G, Yasumura D, Yang H, Bhisitkul RB, Sharma S, Matthes MT, Zarbin MA, Lavail MM, Duncan JL. BDNF reduces the retinal toxicity of verteporfin photodynamic therapy. Invest Ophthalmol Vis Sci 2004;45(11):4190–6.

37. Paskowitz DM, Donohue-Rolfe KM, Yang H, Yasumura D, Matthes MT, Hosseini K, Graybeal CM, Nune G, Zarbin MA, Lavail MM, Duncan JL. Neurotrophic factors minimize the retinal toxicity of verteporfin photodynamic therapy. Invest Ophthalmol Vis Sci 2007;48(1):430–7.

38. Gillies MC, Kuzniarz M, Craig J, Ball M, Luo W, Simpson JM. Intravitreal triamcinolone-induced elevated intraocular pressure is associated with the development of posterior subcapsular cataract. Ophthalmology 2005;112(1):139–43.

39. Erol N, Topbas S, Sahin A. Retinal break following an intravitreal triamcinolone acetonide injection. Int Ophthalmol 2005;26(4–5):163–5.

40. Szebeni J. Relationship of eye burns with calcifications of the cornea? Graefe's Arch Clin Exp Ophthalmol 2005;243:443–9.

M.H. Pittler and E. Ernst

48

Treatments used in complementary and alternative medicine

Complementary and alternative medicine (CAM) remains popular with consumers and patients (1[R]). The often-voiced assumption that it is natural and therefore safe has for a long time hindered systematic research of its risks (2[R]). However, surveys suggest that adverse effects undoubtedly do occur (3[R]). As patients often do not discuss their use of complementary and alternative forms of medicine with doctors (4[R]) the risks are somewhat of a blind spot to both doctors and patients.

HERBAL MEDICINES   (SED-15, 1609; SEDA-27, 512; SEDA-28, 573; SEDA-29, 583)

Recent review articles have focused on the safety of herbal medicines, either in general (5[R]) or related to specific herbal traditions (6[R], 7[R]). Other reviews have addressed the potential of herbal medicines to damage specific organs, for example the kidneys (6[R], 7[R], 8[R], 9[R]), or during treatment of specific conditions (10[R]), or in defined populations, for example, children (7[R]). Several reviews have also addressed herb–drug interactions (11[R], 12[R], 13[R], 14[R]).

ASIAN HERBAL MEDICINES

A small survey of adverse events after routine practice of Chinese herbal medicine included

the data of 144 patients (15[c]). A total of 20 patients reported 32 adverse events associated with Chinese herbal medicines during the 4 weeks after treatment. There were no serious adverse events. The most commonly reported adverse events were *diarrhea, fatigue*, and *nausea*.

Shou wu pian

See *Polygonum multiflorum*.

Qing zhisan tain shou
(SEDA-29, 584)

Drug contamination   Asian herbal remedies are commonly adulterated with prescription drugs. Qing zhisan tain shou is used as a Chinese slimming aid and may contain the prescription-only medicine sibutramine, which can cause increased blood pressure (16[S]). Qing zhisan tain shou is supplied in a bicolored cream and a brown capsule formulation. The capsules are presented in a white and green carton with various lettering and imagery. Two other Chinese slimming products, Li da dai dai hua and Meizitang have also been found to contain sibutramine.

AYURVEDIC MEDICINES

Jambrulin

Drug contamination   Health Canada has issued an advisory notice to consumers, warning against the use of Jambrulin, an Ayurvedic

Side Effects of Drugs, Annual 30
J.K. Aronson (Editor)
ISSN: 0378-6080
DOI: 10.1016/S0378-6080(08)00048-2

medicinal product with a high content of lead (17^S). Jambrulin tablets are not authorized for sale in Canada and have not been found in the country's market. However, according to Health Canada, they can be purchased over the Internet, and travellers may have brought them into the country for personal use. Consumption of heavy metals, including lead, has potentially serious health risks because of accumulation in vital organs. Pregnant women, children, and infants are particularly susceptible to the toxic effects of lead.

SPECIFIC PLANTS

Agnus castus (Verbenaceae)
(SED-15, 3622)

Agnus castus is a deciduous shrub that is native to Mediterranean Europe and Central Asia. It has been used in the treatment of many female conditions, including menstrual disorders, premenstrual syndrome, corpus luteum insufficiency, hyperprolactinemia, infertility, acne, menopause, and disrupted lactation.

A systematic review of all clinical reports of adverse events in clinical trials, post-marketing surveillance studies, surveys, spontaneous reporting schemes, and to manufacturers and herbalist organizations has suggested that the adverse events are mild and reversible (18^M). The most frequent adverse events are *nausea, headache, gastrointestinal disturbances, menstrual disorders, acne, pruritus*, and *erythematous rashes*. No drug–drug interactions were reported.

Cannabis sativa (Cannabaceae)
(SED-15, 613)

See Chapter 4.

Cimicifuga (Actaea) racemosa (Ranunculaceae)   (SED-15, 3025; SEDA-27, 516; SEDA-28, 575; SEDA-29, 586)

Liver   *Cimicifuga racemosa* (or *Actaea racemosa*, common name black cohosh) is popular for menopausal problems (19^R). It has been reported to cause *hepatitis* (19^R, 20^R). However, evaluation of reports of acute liver disease is difficult, owing to the use of combination preparations and failure to analyse suspected products for purity and identity. Causality has not therefore been established.

Nevertheless, the Committee on Herbal Medicinal Products of the European Medicines Agency (EMEA) has reviewed case reports of hepatotoxicity in patients taking *Cimicifuga racemosa* root, and considers that there is a potential association between hepatotoxicity and herbal medicines containing *Cimicifuga* (21^S). The Committee reviewed 16 of the 42 case reports of hepatotoxicity to assess if Cimicifuga is linked to liver damage. Five cases were excluded, seven were thought to be unlikely to be related, and in four cases there was a temporal association between the start of *Cimicifuga* treatment and the occurrence of the hepatic reaction. EMEA has advised patients to stop using *Cimicifuga*, to consult their doctor immediately if symptoms of liver injury develop, and to inform their doctor if they are using herbal medicine products. EMEA has advised healthcare professionals to ask their patients about the use of *Cimicifuga*-containing products and to report suspected hepatic reactions to their national adverse reactions reporting schemes.

Citrus aurantium (Rutaceae)
(SED-15, 3087; SEDA-29, 586)

Citrus aurantium   (bitter orange) contains synephrine, which has ephedrine-like effects on the cardiovascular system (see Chapter 13).

- A 52-year-old woman developed a tachydysrhythmia shortly after taking 500 mg of an extract of *Citrus aurantium* titrated to contain 6% synephrine (22^A). The extract was withdrawn and she remained in good health until she again started taking the same herbal supplement. She was admitted to hospital with a tachydysrhythmia and was again treated and discharged. She had not taken any other medication, except levothyroxine. After 6 months follow up the patient was in good health.

Echinacea species (Asteraceae)

(SED-15, 363; SEDA-27, 516; SEDA-28, 576; SEDA-29, 587)

Echinacea is recommended for the prevention and treatment of the common cold. *Echinacea* species are native to North America, and the three most commonly used species are *E. angustifolia, E. pallida*, and *E. purpurea*.

A systematic review of all clinical reports of adverse events in clinical trials, post-marketing surveillance studies, surveys, spontaneous reporting schemes, and to manufacturers, the WHO, and national drug safety bodies has suggested that short-term use of *Echinacea* is associated with a relatively good safety profile, with a slight risk of transient, reversible, adverse events, of which *gastrointestinal upsets* and *rashes* occur most often (23[M]). In rare cases, *Echinacea* is associated with *allergic reactions*, which can be severe.

Ephedra   *(SED-15, 1221)*

See Chapter 13.

Eugenia caryophyllus (Myrtaceae; oil of cloves)

Oil of cloves contains about 80% eugenol, its active component. Initially used to treat gastrointestinal disturbances, it has more recently been used to treat toothache.

Liver   It has been suggested that eugenol-induced *hepatotoxicity* is similar to that seen with paracetamol poisoning.

- A 15-month-old boy accidentally took 10–20 ml of oil of cloves (24[A]). On arrival at the emergency department 1 hour later he was agitated and tachypneic, with biphasic stridor. Serial measurements of alanine transaminase activities showed evolving hepatic impairment 15 hours after ingestion. After 24 hours, the transaminase activity was in excess of 13 000 U/l, with blood urea and creatinine concentrations of 11.8 mmol/l and 134 µmol/l respectively, indicating evolving acute renal insufficiency. He improved slowly over the next 8 days, during which his urine output and blood urea returned to normal, although the transaminase activity remained moderately raised.

The authors pointed out that a substantial number of cases involving aromatherapy oils are on record. However, most are cases of poisoning, rather than true adverse effects following correct usage. Nevertheless, these cases do stress that such oils are not free of risks.

Ginkgo biloba (Ginkgoaceae; maidenhair tree)   *(SED-15, 1507; SEDA-27, 517; SEDA-28, 576; SEDA-29, 587)*

Hematologic   A few new cases of *bleeding* have been reported in patients undergoing a variety of surgical interventions after taking extracts of *Ginkgo biloba* regularly (25[c], 26[c], 27[c]). Contrary to previous belief, this augmented bleeding tendency may not be related to inhibition of platelet-activating factor by ginkgolides. The concentration required to inhibit PAF-mediated aggregation of human platelets exceeds by more than 100 times the peak values measured after the oral administration of *Ginkgo biloba* leaf extracts in recommended doses (28[c]).

In a systematic review of bleeding with *Ginkgo biloba* 15 reports were found in which there was a temporal association between administration and a bleeding event, including eight episodes of intracranial bleeding (29[M]). In 13 cases additional risk factors for bleeding were identified. In only six cases did the bleeding did not recur after *Ginkgo* was withdrawn. Bleeding times were measured in three patients only and were prolonged.

Drug–drug interactions   In an open, crossover, randomized study, 12 healthy men took a single dose of *warfarin* 25 mg either alone or after pretreatment with *Ginkgo biloba* for 7 days; *Ginkgo* did not significantly affect clotting or the pharmacokinetics or pharmacodynamics of warfarin (30[C]).

- A 55-year-old man with epilepsy had a fatal breakthrough seizure. He was considered to be compliant with his anticonvulsant therapy but the autopsy report showed subtherapeutic serum concentrations of sodium valproate and phenytoin. He had also taken herbal supplements, including *Ginkgo biloba* (31[A]).

Induction of CYP2C19 is one possible mechanism to explain the subtherapeutic concentrations of the anticonvulsant drugs in this case. *Ginkgo* nuts (but not the leaves) are also said to contain a potent neurotoxin, which can cause seizure activity.

Hypericum perforatum (Clusiaceae)
(SED-15, 842; SEDA-27, 517; SEDA-28, 577; SEDA-29, 587)

Drug–drug interactions   The effects of *Hypericum perforatum* on oral contraceptive therapy have been evaluated in 16 healthy women who took a low-dose *oral contraceptive* containing ethinylestradiol 20 micrograms and norethindrone acetate 1 mg or a placebo for two consecutive 28-day cycles in a single-blind sequential study (32^C). Treatment with *H. perforatum* 900 mg/day was added for two additional 28-day cycles and was associated with a significant 13–15% reduction in the dose exposure from the contraceptive. Breakthrough bleeding increased in the treatment cycles, as did evidence of follicle growth and probable ovulation. The authors suggest that *H. perforatum* is associated with increased metabolism of norethindrone and ethinylestradiol, breakthrough bleeding, follicle growth, and ovulation.

Morinda citrifolia (Rubiaceae)
(SED-15, 3085)

Liver   *Morinda citrifolia*, a Polynesian herbal remedy also known as noni, is a tropical fruit that has been implicated in liver damage.

- A 45-year-old man developed very high liver transaminase activities and raised lactate dehydrogenase activity (33^A). His medical history was unremarkable and he took no regular medications. There was no evidence of viral hepatitis, Epstein–Barr virus or cytomegalovirus infection, autoimmune hepatitis, Budd–Chiari syndrome, hemochromatosis, or Wilson's disease. The patient said that he had been drinking the juice of M citrifolia for prophylactic reasons for 3 weeks. A liver biopsy confirmed acute hepatitis and there was an inflammatory infiltrate with numerous eosinophils

in the portal tracts. Other causes were excluded and the histology suggested a causal role of the herb. He stopped taking noni and his transaminase activities normalized quickly and were within the reference ranges 1 month later.

Piper methysticum (Piperaceae)
(SED-15, 2837; SEDA-27, 518; SEDA-28, 578)

Preparations of *Piper methysticum* (kava) are used as anxiolytics and sedatives. However, they have been withdrawn from many European and North American markets because of safety concerns, and in particular *hepatotoxicity*. Depending on the preparation and dose used, adverse effects have been reported in 1.5–2.3% of subjects (34^R).

Cardiovascular   *Tachycardia* and *electrocardiographic abnormalities* have been reported in heavy users of kava (34^R). Whether these observations represent true adverse effects or are due to other factors is unclear.

Respiratory   Shortness of breath has been reported in heavy aboriginal kava users; *pulmonary hypertension* has been proposed as a possible cause (34^R).

Nervous system   Neurological adverse effects are uncommon after kava ingestion. However, *torticollis, oculogyric crises*, and *oral dyskinesias* in young to middle-aged people, *exacerbation of the symptoms of Parkinson's disease*, and three episodes of *abnormal body movements* have been reported (34^R). Three cases of *meningism* have been reported after kava consumption, two of them with focal manifestations (34^R).

Sensory systems   There has been a case of *impaired accommodation and convergence* following one-time use of kava (34^R).

Liver   A large number of cases implicating *P methysticum* in liver damage have been reported (SEDA-28, 578). These include *hepatitis, cirrhosis*, and *liver failure*. Although these reports are of varied quality and the association is not completely convincing, precautionary measures were taken and products were withdrawn from many European and North American markets.

The dose and duration of administration that increases the risk of liver damage is not clear. Pipermethystine, found in leaves and stem peelings, and kavalactones may contribute to the hepatotoxic effects (35[E]).

Gastrointestinal   Mild and infrequent *epigastric pain* and *nausea* have been reported with use of kava (34[R]).

Hematologic   *Increased erythrocyte volume, reduced platelet volume, reduced lymphocyte count*, and *reduced serum albumin* have been reported in chronic heavy kava users (34[R]). Kavain has antiplatelet effects, due to inhibition of cyclo-oxygenase and thromboxane synthesis.

Skin   "*Kava dermopathy*", a dry, scaly skin and/or yellow skin discoloration, which seems to be reversible after withdrawal, has been reported in chronic heavy users. It can cover underlying liver damage and therefore requires a thorough clinical assessment. Regular kava use can also cause *urticaria* (36[A]).

- A young boy who had not previously consumed kava developed an itchy urticarial rash a day after exposure; the rash dissipated in about 24 hours. A week later he again drank kava and again had marked urticaria the next morning. His skin was generally and markedly flushed and edematous, with raised itchy wheals on his arms and back. The eruption resolved 2–3 days after withdrawal.
- A kava bar owner was noted to be flushed with edematous skin and wheals on his arms. His eruption was itchy and he said that this skin reaction always developed after he consumed kava.

Musculoskeletal   *Rhabdomyolysis* has been reported after ingestion of the herbal combination preparation Guaranaginko Plus (37[A]). Each flacon contains guaraná 500 mg, *Ginko biloba* extract 200 mg, and kava 100 mg.

- A 29-year-old man took a combination preparation containing *Ginkgo biloba*, guaraná, and kava and developed rhabdomyolysis He had diffuse severe muscle pain and passed dark urine after an overnight fast. He had been a regular body builder from age 18 to age 27 years, had just resumed weight training at low intensities, and was taking Guaranaginko Plus. His creatine kinase activity was 100 500 IU/l and myoglobin 10 000 ng/ml. There were no renal complications, and the muscle pain and creatine kinase gradually subsided over 6 weeks. An underlying metabolic myopathy as the cause of myoglobinuria was excluded.

Polygonum multiflorum (Polygonaceae)   *(SED-15, 2890)*

Polygonum multiflorum is also known by the Chinese name He shou wu, and may be an ingredient of other traditional health products including, Shou wu pian, Shou wu wan, and Shen min. It is marketed for the relief of a variety of conditions, including early graying of the hair and baldness.

Liver   Although *Polygonum multiflorum* has been recommended for "enrichment of the liver" it has itself been implicated in *liver damage*.

- A 5-year-old previously healthy Caucasian girl developed jaundice, dark urine, and pale stools (38[A]). Liver biochemistry showed a raised serum bilirubin concentration and raised liver enzymes. After 1 month, the jaundice disappeared and the liver function tests normalized. However, 1 month later she relapsed with jaundice. Serum bilirubin and liver enzymes and were again raised. She had used Shou wu pian three tablets daily for 4 months before the first episode of jaundice and had stopped using it after the first presentation. However, she had again taken it in a lower dose for a further month. The remedy was withdrawn and after 5 months, her liver function normalized and she made an uneventful recovery.

After receiving several reports of liver disorders, including jaundice and hepatitis, the UK Medicines and Healthcare products Regulatory Agency (MHRA) issued a warning about the risks of using *Polygonum multiflorum*, advising members of the public who experience symptoms of liver disorders while taking products that contain *Polygonum multiflorum* to see their doctor and to stop taking the product immediately if a liver disorder is diagnosed (39[S]).

Zingiber officinale (Zingiberaceae; ginger)   *(SED-15, 3720)*

Ginger is used as a broad-spectrum antiemetic. However, although clinical and experimental studies suggest that it has some antiemetic properties, definitive clinical evidence is only available for pregnancy-related nausea and vomiting (40[R], 41[R]). Its anti-inflammatory properties (42[R]) have not been well studied clinically.

Pharmacokinetic data are only available for 6-gingerol and zingiberene. Preclinical safety data have not ruled out potential adverse effects, and therapy should be carefully monitored, especially during consumption of ginger over longer periods.

Systematic reviews   In a systematic review of 24 randomized controlled trials in 1073 patients ginger had no beneficial effects in postoperative nausea and vomiting (43[M]). Of 777 patients in 15 studies, 3.3% had mild adverse effects, mainly mild *gastrointestinal symptoms* and *sleepiness*, not requiring specific treatment. There was one serious adverse event, *abortion* in the 12th week of gestation, but that could not clearly be attributed to the ginger.

Pregnancy   Ginger and vitamin B_6 have been compared in the treatment of nausea and vomiting in pregnancy (44[c]). They were equally well tolerated but belching was more common in those who took ginger. The live birth rate was significantly lower in those who took vitamin B_6. The safety of ginger in pregnancy has been confirmed in a meta-analysis of six trials (45[M]).

PLANT TOXINS

Amygdalin

Amygdalin and laetrile (a synthetic form of amygdalin) have been used in the treatment of cancer.

Drug–drug interactions   An interaction of amygdalin with *vitamin C* has been suggested.

- A 68-year-old woman with cancer became comatose, with a reduced Glasgow Coma Score, seizures, and severe lactic acidosis, requiring intubation and ventilation shortly after taking amygdalin 3 g (46[A]). She also took vitamin C 4800 mg/day. She responded rapidly to hydroxocobalamin. The adverse drug reaction was rated probable on the Naranjo probability scale.

Vitamin C increases the in vitro conversion of amygdalin to cyanide and reduces body stores of cysteine, which detoxifies cyanide; the authors suggested that this was a plausible explanation for this adverse event.

Haematitium

Liver   *Haematitium*, a component of some herbal preparations, which contains zinc, tin, iron, magnesium, and diferric acid, has been implicated in *liver damage*.

- A 4-year-old boy was given a herbal mixture containing 20 g of burnt clay, ginger, licorice, mandarin skin, Chinese date, *Inula britannica*, bitter orange, *Codonopsis* root, and "haematitium" 10 ml tds for 3 days for vomiting (47[A]). The vomiting stopped for a few days but then recurred. He had jaundice and cervical lymphadenopathy. Investigations showed the pattern of acute hepatitis. Liver biopsy showed a severe acute hepatitis with portal-to-portal bridging necrosis and a significant number of eosinophils, raising the possibility of drug-induced hepatitis. He had signs of increasing liver dysfunction, with a worsening coagulopathy and an encephalopathy after 10 days. He underwent orthoptic liver transplant 19 days after the first onset of jaundice.

The authors reported a probable association between the hepatic failure and the herbal preparation, based on the World Health Organization definition of causality assessment.

Pyrrolizidine alkaloids
(SED-15, 2989)

Liver   Two sets of twins who were treated with traditional remedies developed liver disease (48[c]). One pair survived, albeit with hepatic damage. Of the other pair, one twin died within 24 hours and the second died 1 month after admission, with a diagnosis of *veno-occlusive liver disease*. In both cases, the pyrrolizidine alkaloid retrorsine was identified.

ACUPUNCTURE   *(SED-15, 890; SEDA-27, 520; SEDA-28, 581; SEDA-29, 589)*

Cardiovascular   *Vasovagal syncope* has been reported after routine use of acupuncture; the authors suggested that this is an uncommon complication (49[A]).

- A 72-year-old man visited an acupuncture clinic in Taipei, Taiwan because of pain over the right forearm for 5 months. He had no previous history of neurological deficits. He received six sessions of manual acupuncture with limited improvement. During the seventh session acupuncture and electro-acupuncture stimulation, 2 Hz, was applied at points of Li-11 and TP-5. After 5 minutes he complained of dizziness. He then experienced cold sweating and suddenly lost consciousness. Irregular tonic–clonic movements of the right arm, upward rolling of the eyes, and batting of both eyelids lasted 20–30 seconds after the attack of syncope. All needles were immediately removed. Strong needling stimulation at Du-26 (Renzhong) was performed. He remained confused for 2–3 minutes. About 10 minutes after this episode, his supine blood pressure was 144/82 mmHg with a pulse rate of 62/minute. He felt well, except for fatigue, after 40 minutes of rest. His laboratory tests, including blood chemistry, blood glucose, thyroid function, a complete blood count, and urinalysis, were normal. An electrocardiogram showed mild ST-T wave depression, implying myocardial ischemia. Further evaluation was suggested but he refused.

- A 63-year-old woman received acupuncture for pain over the left ankle for 5 days. She had been well in the past and denied systemic diseases and use of medications. She received manual needling at GB-34 and GB-40 points. After a 3-minute session she complained of dizziness and nausea, and then experienced cold sweating and suddenly lost consciousness. She had irregular tonic–clonic movements of the left arm with batting of both eyelids lasting for 10–15 seconds and lip cyanosis after the episode of syncope. All needles were immediately removed and she received strong needling stimulation at Du-26. The event lasted for 1 minute and she remained confused for 2–3 minutes. About 15 minutes after the episode, her supine blood pressure was 126/74 mmHg with a pulse rate of 56/minute. After 60 minutes of rest, she felt chest tightness and fatigue. She was referred to a cardiologist for further evaluation. Laboratory tests, including blood chemistry, blood glucose, thyroid function, a complete blood count, and urinalysis, were normal. Electroencephalography was also normal. However, electrocardiography showed mild ST-T depression in V3–5. A treadmill test was positive and 24-hour Holter monitoring showed intermittent ischemic ST segment depression.

CUPPING

Skin   Therapeutic cupping is a traditional treatment in Oriental countries, where it is used for treating low back pain, shoulder and leg pain, and cough and asthma. A jar is attached to the skin surface to cause local congestion through negative pressure, which is created by introducing heat.

- A 36-year-old woman developed a pruritic eruption on her back, with four annular, mildly erythematous macules (50[A]). One of the lesions was fibrotic at the edge and a diagnosis of keloid was made. There was no prior history of keloid formation on any other part of her body. She had been treated by cupping for a long-standing cough. She was given combination therapy, including cryotherapy, an intralesional glucocorticoid, and Contractubex gel (heparin, onion extract, allantoin). After four treatments the lesions became softer and less pruritic.

HOMEOPATHY   (SED-15, 892; SEDA-28, 582; SEDA-29, 591)

Observational studies   In an observational study of the adverse effects of homeopathic remedies in 181 patients, 50-millesimal dilutions were assessed (51[c]). The medicines prescribed were: *Pulsatilla pratensis, Lachesis mutus, Silicea terra*, sulfur, *Arsenicum album, Sepia officinalis*, and *Ignatia amara*, followed by *Natrum muriaticum, Lycopodium clavatum, Nux vomica*, and phosphorus. Nine adverse events were recorded, including one case of *allergy* to an excipient (lactose). The frequency of adverse reactions during classical homeopathic treatment was 2.7%. Adverse effects were generally mild and did not require specific treatment.

SPINAL MANIPULATION
(SED-15, 893; SEDA-27, 521; SEDA-28, 582; SEDA-29, 591)

Comparative studies   In 336 patients with neck pain who were randomized to manipulation or mobilization, the most common chiropractic treatments for neck pain, 85 patients reported 212 adverse events (52[R]). *Increased neck pain or stiffness* was the most common symptom, reported by 25%. Patients randomized to manipulation were more likely than those randomized to mobilization to have an adverse symptom within 24 hours of treatment.

The authors suggested that adverse reactions to chiropractic care for neck pain are common and are more likely to follow cervical spine manipulation than mobilization. Chiropractors should consider a conservative approach to manipulation, especially in patients with severe neck pain.

Sensory systems   In a systematic review of the recent literature (1995–2003) 14 case reports were found in which chiropractic upper spinal manipulation was associated with ophthalmological adverse effects (53[M]). The patients were of both sexes, usually middle-aged, and frequently healthy, who had consulted chiropractors for minor complaints. The ophthalmic consequences included *nystagmus, Wallenberg's syndrome, loss of vision, hemianopsia, ophthalmoplegia, diplopia, Horner's syndrome*, and *ptosis*. In many cases visual deficits were the first signs. The onset of symptoms was frequently instant. In several cases, the eventual clinical outcome entailed a permanent deficit. In most cases, causality between upper spinal manipulation and the ophthalmological adverse effect was certain or likely.

References

1. Saad B, Azaizeh H, Said O. Tradition and perspectives of Arab herbal medicine: a review. Evid Based Complement Alternat Med 2005;2(4):475–9.
2. Ernst E. The efficacy of herbal medicine—an overview. Fundam Clin Pharmacol 2005;19(4):405–9.
3. Cuzzolin L, Zaffani S, Benoni G. Safety implications regarding use of phytomedicines. Eur J Clin Pharmacol 2006;62(1):37–42.
4. Barraco D, Valencia G, Riba AL, Nareddy S, Draus CB, Schwartz SM. Complementary and alternative medicine (CAM) use patterns and disclosure to physicians in acute coronary syndromes patients. Complement Ther Med 2005;13(1):34–40.
5. Woodward KN. The potential impact of the use of homeopathic and herbal remedies on monitoring the safety of prescription products. Hum Exp Toxicol 2005;24(5):219–33.
6. Luyckx VA, Steenkamp V, Stewart MJ. Acute renal failure associated with the use of traditional folk remedies in South Africa. Ren Fail 2005;27(1):35–43.
7. Anochie IC, Eke FU. Acute renal failure in Nigerian children: Port Harcourt experience. Pediatr Nephrol 2005;20(11):1610–4.
8. Schetz M, Dasta J, Goldstein S, Golper T. Drug-induced acute kidney injury. Curr Opin Crit Care 2005;11(6):555–65.
9. Colson CR, De Broe ME. Kidney injury from alternative medicines. Adv Chron Kidney Dis 2005;12(3):261–75.
10. Ramkumar D, Rao SS. Efficacy and safety of traditional medical therapies for chronic constipation: systematic review. Am J Gastroenterol 2005;100(4):936–71.
11. Izzo AA, Di Carlo G, Borrelli F, Ernst E. Cardiovascular pharmacotherapy and herbal medicines: the risk of drug interaction. Int J Cardiol 2005;98(1):1–14.
12. Singh YN. Potential for interaction of kava and St John's wort with drugs. J Ethnopharmacol 2005;100(1–2):108–13.
13. Holstege CP, Mitchell K, Barlotta K, Furbee RB. Toxicity and drug interactions associated with herbal products: *Ephedra* and St John's wort. Med Clin North Am 2005;89(6):1225–57.
14. Marder VJ. The interaction of dietary supplements with antithrombotic agents: scope of the problem. Thromb Res 2005;117(1-2):7–13.
15. MacPherson H, Liu B. The safety of Chinese herbal medicine: a pilot study for a national survey. J Altern Complement Med 2005;11(4):617–26.
16. Anonymous. Qing zhisan tain shou. Presence of sibutramine. WHO Pharmaceuticals Newslett 2005;2:3.
17. Anonymous. Jambrulin. High lead content. WHO Newslett 2006;5:5.
18. Daniele C, Thompson Coon J, Pittler MH, Ernst E. *Vitex agnus castus*: a systematic review of adverse events. Drug Saf 2005;28(4):319–32.
19. Low Dog T. Menopause: a review of botanical dietary supplements. Am J Med 2005;118(Suppl 12B):98–108.
20. Mahady GB. Black cohosh (*Actaea/Cimicifuga racemosa*): review of the clinical data for safety and efficacy in menopausal symptoms. Treat Endocrinol 2005;4(3):177–84.
21. Anonymous. *Cimicifuga racemosa* (black cohosh). Concerns of liver injury. WHO Newslett 2006;4:1.
22. Firenzuoli F, Gori L, Galapai C. Adverse reaction to an adrenergic herbal extract (*Citrus aurantium*). Phytomedicine 2005;12(3):247–8.

23. Huntley AL, Thompson Coon J, Ernst E. The safety of herbal medicinal products derived from *Echinacea* species: a systematic review. Drug Saf 2005;28(5):387–400.

24. Janes SE, Price CS, Thomas D. Essential oil poisoning: N-acetylcysteine for eugenol-induced hepatic failure and analysis of a national database. Eur J Pediatr 2005;164(8):520–2.

25. Destro MW, Speranzini MB, Cavalheiro Filho C, Destro T, Destro C. Bilateral haematoma after rhytidoplasty and blepharoplasty following chronic use of Ginkgo biloba. Br J Plast Surg 2005;58:100–1.

26. Bebbington A, Kulkarni R, Roberts P. Ginkgo biloba: persistent bleeding after total hip arthroplasty caused by herbal self-medication. J Arthroplasty 2005;20:125–6.

27. Yagmur E, Piatkowski A, Groger A, Pallua N, Gressner AM, Kiefer P. Bleeding complication under Gingko biloba medication. Am J Hematol 2005;79:343–4.

28. Koch E. Inhibition of platelet activating factor (PAF)-induced aggregation of human thrombocytes by ginkgolides: considerations on possible bleeding complications after oral intake of Ginkgo biloba extracts. Phytomedicine 2005;12:10–6.

29. Bent S, Goldberg H, Padula A, Avins AL. Spontaneous bleeding associated with Ginkgo biloba: a case report and systematic review of the literature. J Gen Intern Med 2005;20:657–61.

30. Jiang X, Williams KM, Liauw WS, Ammit AJ, Roufogalis BD, Duke CC, Day RO, McLachlan AJ. Effect of ginkgo and ginger on the pharmacokinetics and pharmacodynamics of warfarin in healthy subjects. Br J Clin Pharmacol 2005;59:425–62.

31. Kupiec T, Raj V. Fatal seizures due to potential herb–drug interactions with Ginkgo biloba. J Anal Toxicol 2005;25:755–8.

32. Murphy PA, Kern SE, Stanczyk FZ, Westhoff CL. Interaction of St John's wort with oral contraceptives: effects on the pharmacokinetics of norethindrone and ethinyl estradiol, ovarian activity and breakthrough bleeding. Contraception 2005;71(6):402–8.

33. Millonig G, Stadlmann S, Vogel W. Herbal hepatotoxicity: acute hepatitis caused by a noni preparation (*Morinda citrifolia*). Eur J Gastroenterol Hepatol 2005;17(4):445–7.

34. Ulbricht C, Basch E, Boon H, Ernst E, Hammerness P, Sollars D, Tsourounis C, Woods J, Bent S. Safety review of kava (*Piper methysticum*) by the Natural Standard Research Collaboration. Expert Opin Drug Saf 2005;4(4):779–94.

35. Nerurkar PV, Dragull K, Tang CS. In vitro toxicity of kava alkaloid, pipermethystine, in HepG2 cells compared to kavalactones. Toxicol Sci 2004;79(1):106–11.

36. Grace R. Kava-induced urticaria. J Am Acad Dermatol 2005;53(5):906.

37. Donadio V, Bonsi P, Zele I, Monari L, Liguori R, Vetrugno R, Albani F, Montagna P. Myoglobinuria after ingestion of extracts of guarana, *Ginkgo biloba* and kava. Neurol Sci 2000;21(2):124.

38. Panis B, Wong DR, Hooymans PM, De Smet PA, Rosias PP. Recurrent toxic hepatitis in a Caucasian girl related to the use of Shou-Wu-Pian, a Chinese herbal preparation. J Pediatr Gastroenterol Nutr 2005;41(2):256–8.

39. Anonymous. *Polygonum multiflorum*. Risk of liver effects. WHO Newslett 2006;3:4.

40. Chrubasik S, Pittler MH, Roufogalis BD. *Zingiberis rhizoma*: a comprehensive review on the ginger effect and efficacy profiles. Phytomedicine 2005;12(9):684–701.

41. Boone SA, Shields KM. Treating pregnancy-related nausea and vomiting with ginger. Ann Pharmacother 2005;39(10):1710–3.

42. Grzanna R, Lindmark L, Frondoza CG. Ginger—an herbal medicinal product with broad anti-inflammatory actions. J Med Food 2005;8(2):125–32.

43. Betz O, Kranke P, Geldner G, Wulf H, Eberhart LH. Ist Ingwer ein klinisch relevantes Antiemetikum? Eine systematische Übersicht randomisierter kontrollierter Studien. Forsch Komplementärmed Klass Naturheilkd 2005;12(1):14–23.

44. Smith C, Crowther C, Hotham N, McMillan V. Ginger was as effective as vitamin B6 in improving symptoms of nausea and vomiting in early pregnancy. Obstet Gynecol 2004;103:639–45.

45. Borrelli F, Capasso R, Aviello G, Pittler MH, Izzo AA. Effectiveness and safety of ginger in the treatment of pregnancy-induced nausea and vomiting. Obstet Gynecol 2005;105(4):849–56.

46. Bromley J, Hughes BG, Leong DC, Buckley NA. Life-threatening interaction between complementary medicines: cyanide toxicity following ingestion of amygdalin and vitamin C. Ann Pharmacother 2005;39(9):1566–9.

47. Webb AN, Hardikar W, Cranswick NE, Somers GR. Probable herbal medication induced fulminant hepatic failure. J Paediatr Child Health 2005;41(9–10):530–1.

48. Conradie J, Stewart MJ, Steenkamp V. GC/MS identification of toxic pyrrolizidine alkaloids in traditional remedies given to two sets of twins. Ann Clin Biochem 42 (Pt 2) 2005:141–4.

49. Kung YY, Chen FP, Hwang SJ, Hsieh JC, Lin YY. Convulsive syncope: an unusual complication of acupuncture treatment in older patients. J Altern Complement Med 2005;11(3):535–7.

50. Birol A, Erkek E, Kurtipek GS, Kocak M. Keloid secondary to therapeutic cupping: an unusual complication. J Eur Acad Dermatol Venereol 2005;19(4):507.

51. Endrizzi C, Rossi E, Crudeli L, Garibaldi D. Harm in homeopathy: aggravations, adverse drug events or medication errors? Homeopathy 2005;94(4):233–40.

52. Hurwitz EL, Morgenstern H, Vassilaki M, Chiang LM. Frequency and clinical predictors of adverse reactions to chiropractic care in the UCLA neck pain study. Spine 2005;30(13):1477–84.

53. Ernst E. Ophthalmological adverse effects of (chiropractic) upper spinal manipulation: evidence from recent case reports. Acta Ophthalmol Scand 2005;83(5):581–5.

N.H. Choulis

49 Miscellaneous drugs, materials, medical devices, and techniques

Bisphosphonates *(SED-15, 523; SEDA-28, 590; SEDA-29, 602)*

Bisphosphonates and fractures

Bisphosphonates reduce the incidence of new fractures in patients with established osteoporosis (1^c, 2^c). They remain in the body for decades and are not metabolized, but are either excreted renally or deposited within the bones, accumulating with continued use. Since there is no known method of removing them from the bones, a major question is: can long-term inhibition of bone turnover be harmful? Two separate but related consequences of this inhibition are increased mineralization and accumulation of microdamage. As bone mineralization increases, the bone becomes brittle (3^M). This has been demonstrated by biomechanical measurements in bones with a wide range of mineralization. Brittle bones are more likely to fracture, but the optimal mineralization density for the human skeleton is not known. Microcracks occur in normal bone after the kind of stresses that are encountered in day-to-day life. These cracks are detected by the osteocytes, which initiate a bone-remodelling unit to repair the damage. If bone resorption is strongly inhibited, the damage cannot be repaired, because the osteoclasts won't dissolve the bone.

Thus, current knowledge of bone physiology suggests that bisphosphonates should increase bone strength by preventing trabecular plate perforation and improving bone mineralization in undermineralized bone. However, after prolonged severe suppression of bone formation,

negative effects could occur. Bone could become too brittle and/or accumulate microdamage. It is not known if or when these conditions occur in humans, but it is important to pay attention to reports that provide clues to long-term effects.

Nine patients sustained spontaneous non-spinal fractures while taking alendronate, six of whom had either delayed or absent fracture healing for 3 months to 2 years during therapy (4^c). Histomorphometric analysis of the cancellous bone showed markedly suppressed bone formation, with a reduced or absent osteoblastic surface in most cases. The osteoclastic surface was low or low-normal in eight patients and the eroded surface was reduced in four. Matrix synthesis was markedly reduced, with absence of double-tetracycline labelling and absent or reduced single-tetracycline labelling in all cases. The same trend was seen in the intracortical and endocortical surfaces. It is important to note that these patients did not have osteomalacia, as has been described with etidronate, a first-generation bisphosphonate. Instead, the biopsies resembled the "adynamic bone disease" that has been described in some patients with renal insufficiency.

These findings raise the possibility that severe suppression of bone turnover may develop during long-term alendronate therapy, resulting in increased susceptibility to, and delayed healing of, non-spinal fractures. Although co-administration of an estrogen or a glucocorticoid appears to be a predisposing factor, this apparent complication can also occur with monotherapy. These observations emphasize the need for increased awareness and monitoring for the potential development of excessive suppression of bone turnover during long-term alendronate therapy. Physicians should not be reassured that newer-generation bisphospho-

---

Side Effects of Drugs, Annual 30
J.K. Aronson (Editor)
ISSN: 0378-6080
DOI: 10.1016/S0378-6080(08)00049-4

nates are safe just because they don't cause osteomalacia.

R. Bisphosphonates and osteonecrosis of the jaw

DoTS classification:
Reaction: Bisphosphonates and osteonecrosis of the jaw
Dose-relation: ?Collateral
Time-course: Late
Susceptibility factors: Intravenous therapy, trauma, infection

In September 2003, painful bone exposure in the mandible, maxilla, or both, unresponsive to surgical and medical treatments, was reported in 36 patients who were receiving intravenous pamidronate or zoledronate (5[c]). Of these, 24 had received monthly pamidronate (Aredia) 90 mg intravenously, six had received pamidronate in the past but were receiving monthly zoledronate (Zometa) 4 mg intravenously at the time of presentation, and six had received only zoledronate; 22 were also taking dexamethasone, 24 were receiving maintenance chemotherapy, and four had received radiotherapy in the past. They presented with painful, exposed, avascular bone, simulating a dental abscess, in the mandible ($n = 29$), maxilla ($n = 5$), or both ($n = 2$). Removal of painful teeth was often the initiator of the exposed non-healing bone ($n = 28$); the other eight patients developed exposed bone spontaneously.

At about the same time, two other reports appeared. In one, published in September 2003, osteonecrosis was reported in three patients with breast cancers receiving pamidronate (6[A]). In the other, published in November 2003, five further cases of osteonecrosis of the jaw were reported in patients taking pamidronate or zoledronic acid. Three had spontaneous bone necrosis of the mylohyoid plate (internal posterior mandible) and two in the molar region after a tooth extraction (7[c]).

In retrospect, an early case of failure of dental implants to osseointegrate may have been due to osteonecrosis due to etidronate (8[A]), and there have also been reports in patients taking bisphosphonates other than pamidronate

and zoledronate, such as oral alendronate (9[c]), ibandronate (10[c]), and risedronate (11[c]). In a retrospective review of 63 patients aged 43–89 years (45 women), 57% were taking pamidronate, 31% zoledronate, and 12% other bisphosphonates; 24 had maxillary bone involvement (19 unilateral and five bilateral), 40 had mandibular bone involvement (37 unilateral and three bilateral), and one had exposed necrotic bone in all four quadrants (11[c]). All but nine had a history of a recent dentoalveolar procedure.

Many case series have been reported (12[c], 13[c], 14[c], 15[c], 16[c], 17[c], 18[c], 19[c]). About 96% of published cases were associated with intravenous pamidronate and zoledronate, about two dozen with alendronate, and only occasional cases with other bisphosphonates (20[AR]).

Incidence   The incidence of osteonecrosis is 9.4–10% among patients taking zoledronate and 4–14% among patients taking pamidronate (20[AR]). It can occur in any patient receiving a bisphosphonate, but the risk seems to be higher in patients with multiple myeloma than in those with solid tumors.

In a prospective study of 252 patients who had received bisphosphonates 17 (6.7%) developed osteonecrosis of the jaw: 11 of 111 (9.9%) with multiple myeloma, two of 70 (2.9%) with breast cancer, three of 46 (6.5%) with prostate cancer, and one of 25 (4%) with other neoplasms (21[C]). The median number of treatment cycles and time of exposure to bisphosphonates were 35 infusions and 39 months for patients with osteonecrosis compared with 15 infusions and 19 months in patients without osteonecrosis. The incidence increased with time to exposure, from 1.5% among patients treated for 4–12 months to 7.7% for treatment of 37–48 months. The cumulative hazard was significantly higher with zoledronic acid than with pamidronate alone or pamidronate and zoledronic acid sequentially. All but two patients with osteonecrosis had a history of dental procedures within the last year or used dentures.

Mechanism   The mechanisms whereby bisphosphonates cause osteonecrosis are not known, but some factors and processes are illustrated in Figure 1. Bisphosphonates inhibit bone remodelling (22[R]) and reduce intraosseous blood flow. They are taken up by

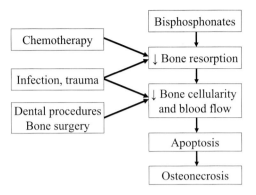

Fig. 1. Processes whereby bisphosphonates may cause osteonecrosis and some precipitating factors (adapted from (22ᶜ)).

osteoclasts and internalized in the cell cytoplasm, where they inhibit osteoclastic function and cause apoptosis (23ᴿ). They also inhibit osteoblast-mediated osteoclastic resorption and have antiangiogenic properties (24ᴿ). It is not clear why local damage is accentuated in the maxilla and mandible, but it may be related to constant stress from mastication (25ᴿ). Trauma caused by dental procedures and prosthodontic appliances can initiate the complication. However, it can occur in edentulous mouths.

Presentation   To date about 900 cases of bisphosphonate-related osteonecrosis have been reported. Bone involvement can be unilateral or bilateral; 63–68% of cases affect the mandible exclusively, 24–28% affect the maxilla exclusively, and 4.2% affect both jaws (20ᴬᴿ). The mean number of areas of exposed bone is 2.3 per affected patient, and each site averages 2 cm in size.

The most common presentation is absent or delayed hard-tissue and soft-tissue healing after dental extraction (26ᴿ). Discomfort in the mouth is common, and severe pain and paresthesia, sometimes due to nerve compression, can occur because of secondary infection. Progression can lead to exposure and dehiscence of bone. Bisphosphonate-associated osteonecrosis of the auditory canal has also been reported (27ᴬ).

Based on clinical observations in 141 patients the following staging system has been proposed (28ᶜ):

- Stage 1: Exposed necrotic bone that is asymptomatic.
- Stage 2: Exposed necrotic bone associated with pain and infection.
- Stage 3: Exposed necrotic bone in patients with pain, infection, and pathological fracture, extraoral fistula, or osteolysis extending to the inferior border.

The radiographic features of osteonecrosis have been demonstrated in 11 patients with conventional radiography, computed tomography, magnetic resonance image scanning, and bone scanning (29ᶜ). There were osteolytic lesions with involvement of cortical bone (plain X-ray) and the characteristic features of osteonecrosis and edema of the soft tissues (MRI). Both CT and MRI defined the extent of the lesions. Bone scanning was the most sensitive tool in detecting the osteonecrosis at an early stage.

Pathology   Bisphosphonate-induced osteonecrosis resembles infected osteoradionecrosis, and the two have been compared histologically in eight patients (30ᶜ). There were diffuse patchy areas of necrosis in bisphosphonate-induced osteonecrosis, while in infected osteoradionecrosis the necrosis was more widespread. In several cases there was pseudoepitheliomatous hyperplasia and numerous osteoclasts were seen close to regenerating bone. In all cases Actinomyces organisms were attached to the necrotic bone tissue.

Time course   Osteonecrosis is uncommon before 6 months after the start of therapy and the risk increases with duration of therapy (31ᶜ).

Susceptibility factors   All patients who are receiving bisphosphonates are at risk, and intravenous therapy carries a higher risk than oral (26ᴿ). About 80% of cases develop after a dental extraction. It has been suggested that hypocalcaemia and secondary hyperparathyroidism may also be predisposing factors (32ʳ).

Prevention and treatment   The following preventive measures have been recommended (26ᴿ):

- a dentist should see all patients before intravenous bisphosphonate therapy begins;

- *those who have been given an oral bisphos-phonate within the last 3 months should also undergo dental evaluation;*
- *all potential sites of infection must be elimi-nated;*
- *good oral and dental health should be achieved within 3–6 months.*

The following dental procedures are recom-mended:

- *comprehensive extraoral and intraoral exam-ination;*
- *full-mouth radiography, including panto-mography, to identify caries and periodontal disease;*
- *evaluation of third molars and identification of metastatic cancer and other bony pathol-ogy;*
- *periodontal health should be determined and appropriate therapy provided;*
- *plaque accumulation should be reduced;*
- *chronic periodontal inflammation and acute periodontal infections should be minimized;*
- *restorative dentistry should be performed to eliminate caries and defective restorations;*
- *extraction of teeth, if necessary, should be completed as soon as possible;*
- *the patient should be instructed about oral hygiene;*
- *the patient should be told about osteonecro-sis and its early signs;*
- *there should be periodic follow-up visits to reinforce the importance of oral hygiene and to monitor progress.*

Patients with asymptomatic exposed bone should be given systemic antimicrobial drugs, such as clindamycin or penicillin + metronida-zole, and an oral antimicrobial rinse, such as chlorhexidine gluconate (33[AR]). When there are purulent exudates or sinus tracts, culture and microbial sensitivity testing will guide therapy. Extensive debridement and local flap closure are generally unsuccessful, and can produce even larger areas of exposed and painful in-fected bone. Patients with draining sinuses, ex-tensive areas of necrotic bone, or large seques-tra may require extensive surgery.

Neodymium-YAG laser stimulation has been used to treat patients with bisphosphonate-induced osteonecrosis (34[c]). Six patients were treated with surgery plus antibiotics, six with

antibiotics only, six with laser stimulation as-sociated with antibiotics, and eight with laser stimulation after surgical debridement, removal of necrotic bone, and antibiotics. Of the 14 pa-tients who underwent laser stimulation, nine reported complete success (no pain, symptoms of infections, or signs of exposed bone or drain-ing fistulas), with a follow-up of 4–7 months. Only three patients reported no clinical im-provement.

Camphor   *(SED-15, 612)*

Anecdotal reports   Health Canada has warn-ed against the use of the Triaminic Vapour Patch, which contains camphor, eucalyptus oil, and menthol, because of serious adverse ef-fects that could occur if the product were ac-cidentally ingested by children (35[S]). Reported adverse effects from products that contain cam-phor or eucalyptus oils range from minor symp-toms, such as a *sensation of mouth burning, headache, nausea*, and *vomiting*, to more severe and life-threatening reactions, such as *seizures*. The Agency is aware of one child who had a seizure after chewing the patch. The product has been recalled and Health Canada has advised that consumers should stop using it; those who have used the patch and have health concerns should contact their physician or health-care practitioner. A nationwide voluntary recall of all Triaminic Vapour Patch products has also been conducted in the USA by Novartis Con-sumer Health.

Drug administration route   The systemic availability of camphor is very low after trans-dermal administration; the average C_{max} after the application of eight patches in eight subjects was only 41 ng/ml; the mean terminal half-life was 5.6 hours (36[c]).

Carbamates

Methomyl   (S-methyl-N((methylcarbamoyl)-oxy)thioacetimidate) is a water-soluble carba-mate insecticide that has a half-life in soil of about 6 weeks. It inhibits cholinesterases.

Drug contamination   Poisoning with methomyl through contamination in food has been reported.

Repeated attacks of *dizziness, nausea,* or *vomiting* occurred in 107 patrons of a Thai restaurant in central California and were attributed to methomyl (37[c]). The median latency period was 40 minutes from beginning eating to the first symptom and 2 hours to the onset of diarrhea. The median duration of symptoms was 6 hours. Patients reported *nausea* (95%), *dizziness* (72%), *abdominal cramps* (58%), *headache* (52%), *vomiting* (51%), *chills* (48%), and *diarrhea* (46%). In 51 cases (48%) *dizziness, lightheadedness,* or *a feeling of disequilibrium* was the initial symptom. The illness was statistically associated with several foods and ingredients, but no single dish or ingredient. However, there was an association with salt to the food, stronger with increasing amounts of salt. Methomyl was identified in a sample of vomitus (20 ppm) and in salt taken from containers in the storeroom (mean 5600 ppm) and the stovetop (mean, 1425 ppm). The oral toxic dose that caused illness in 50% of those exposed to methomyl was estimated to be 0.15 (range 0.09–0.31) mg/kg.

Of 124 diners who took ill while eating lunch at a seafood restaurant in the town of Chiching in the Kaohsiung municipality of Taiwan, 69 were sent to emergency departments (38[c]). The source of the outbreak was methomyl contamination. The median latent period from beginning eating to the first symptoms was 5 minutes. The most common clinical effects were general *weakness* (84%), *ataxia* (82%), *dizziness* (82%), *vomiting* (80%), *sweating* (75%), *a floating sensation* (71%), *headache* (69%), *dyspnea* (69%), and *blurred vision* (67%); 31 patients had residual symptoms 7 days after ingestion. Of the six residual symptoms reported, the most frequent were *dizziness* (40%), *poor appetite and dry mouth* (11%), and *gastrointestinal disturbances* (11%). The presence of residual symptoms correlated with the severity of the initial complaints. Almost all of the patients had eaten cooked rice (93%) and leaf vegetables stir-fried with crab claw (93%). High concentrations of methomyl were found in the leaf vegetables (380 ppm) and in fried mussels (1113 ppm).

Drug overdose   There have been reports of the effects of methomyl in cases of self-poisoning, including *acute pancreatitis,* an effect that the carbamate and organophosphorus insecticides share.

In 1995–96, the Occupational Medicine Service of the province of Ragusa, Sicily, examined all cases of pesticide poisoning in those who had been seen in two local emergency departments, and identified 86 cases of unintentional pesticide exposure (39[c]). Methomyl was involved in 51%. The most common symptoms were nausea and vomiting (48%), excessive sweating (33%), and dyspnea (16%), and 59 patients (69%) were hospitalized, five in intensive care. Methomyl poisoning was more common during the summer, while poisoning with all other pesticides showed no seasonal pattern.

- An 18-year-old Caucasian man developed a cholinergic crisis after taking an unknown amount of methomyl. His pseudocholinesterase activity was 2 kU/l (reference range: 5.4–13 kU/l) (40[A]). Two days later an abdominal CT scan showed blurring of the peripancreatic fat planes, inflammation and swelling of the pancreas, and a substantial amount of ascitic fluid in the left anterior pararenal space and pelvis. Paracentesis and analysis of the ascitic fluid showed it to be pancreatic ascites. After 11 days the pseudocholinesterase activity returned to normal, and an abdominal CT scan showed an intrapancreatic fluid collection, which was considerably smaller 1 month later.
- Two cases of acute pancreatitis complicating methomyl self-poisoning have been compared with five cases of pancreatitis after dichlorvos poisoning (41[c]). Both patients who took methomyl had deep coma and respiratory failure requiring mechanical ventilation. Acute pancreatitis occurred 24–72 hours after overdose and was characterized by painless abdominal paralytic ileus and vomiting. The clinical features and laboratory findings normalized by the fifth day. In one case an intrapancreatic fluid collection was found several days later.
- A 50-year-old man developed chest tightness, sweating, and vomiting 60 minutes after drinking a 30 ml volume nutrition supplement (42[A]). He had myosis and reduced serum cholinesterase activity. His serum methomyl concentration was 0.63 µg/ml and the urine concentration 0.10 µg/ml.
- A 35-year-old man died in cardiopulmonary arrest (43[A]). At autopsy his stomach contained 170 g of a greenish liquid with a small amount of shredded tobacco leaves. His serum cholinesterase activity was 47–90 IU (reference range 200–440 IU). There was nicotine (22 mg), methomyl (304 mg), and triazolam (1.7 mg) in his stomach. He had consumed tobacco leaves, Lannate™, which contains methomyl 45%, and Halcion™ tablets containing triazolam 0.25 mg. Methomyl concentrations

in blood were 3–8 ng/ml. There were substantial amounts of methomyl (2260–2680 ng/ml) in the cerebrospinal fluid and vitreous humor. Blood nicotine concentrations were 222–733 ng/ml. Small amounts of triazolam were detected in the bile (176 ng/ml) and liver (23 ng/g). The cause of death was respiratory paralysis produced by the additive effects of methomyl and nicotine shortly after consumption.

- In five cases of fatal ingestion of methomyl analysis of samples of blood plasma and serum showed more than 90% inhibition of cholinesterase (44[c]). The mean blood methomyl concentration was 27 (range 5.6–57) mg/l. These values are much higher than those previously reported in similar cases (0.57–1.4 mg/l). Methomyl concentrations in organs and tissues were significantly lower than those in blood and vitreous humor.

Methomyl has also been used for homicidal purposes (45[c]). Mean plasma cholinesterase activity in 105 healthy Thai children aged 5–6 years of age was 7417 U/l; it was lower in girls than in boys. Children whose parents were farmers had lower activity than those whose parents were employees, merchants, government officers, unemployed parents, or private business owners. Two victims of child homicide had cholinesterase activities 6 and 9% of average. The authors concluded that a plasma cholinesterase activity in a child lower than 10% of normal could suggest insecticide poisoning.

DYESTUFFS

Indocyanine green   *(SED-15, 2595)*

Sensory systems   Indocyanine green has been used to stain and visualize the internal limiting membrane during vitrectomy. *Visual field defects* on the nasal side can occur after the surgery by an unknown mechanism. In one patient nasal visual field defects occurred after indocyanine green-assisted peeling of the internal limiting membrane (46[A]).

- A 60-year-old woman with an epiretinal membrane in her right eye had indocyanine green-assisted peeling of the internal limiting membrane. The preoperative best corrected visual acuity was 20/60 in the right eye. Indocyanine green 25 mg was dissolved in distilled water 10 ml, which was further diluted with a viscoelastic material to give a 0.16% solution. To stain the internal limiting membrane, indocyanine green was injected into an air

filled eye and the dye was washed out 2 minutes later. There were no complications during surgery, but 17 days later she noticed nasal visual field loss, which worsened at 22 days. At 60 days detailed examination showed that the superior and inferior retinal nerve fibres were severely damaged.

In another study, 39 eyes of 38 patients with a macular hole underwent pars plana vitrectomy (47[c]). Indocyanine green-assisted peeling of the internal limiting membrane was performed on 22 eyes, using one of three techniques:

- indocyanine green 0.5%, with a 3-minute exposure to the retina (group 1; $n = 12$);
- indocyanine green 0.5%, with immediate washout (group 2; $n = 4$);
- indocyanine green 0.25%, with immediate washout (group 3; $n = 6$).

The other 17 eyes underwent vitrectomy without indocyanine green-assisted peeling of the internal limiting membrane (group 4). Postoperatively, all 12 eyes in group 1 and one of four eyes in group 2 had visual field defects. None of the eyes in group 3 had a visual field defect. Only one eye in group 4 had an inferotemporal defect. The visual field defects included nasal defects ($n = 10$), an inferotemporal defect ($n = 1$), and an extensive visual field defect ($n = 1$). These results suggest that visual field defects, specifically nasal defects, can occur after macular hole surgery with indocyanine green-assisted peeling of the internal limiting membrane, and that the risk depends on the concentration of indocyanine green and the retinal exposure time.

Isosulfan blue   *(SEDA-29, 607)*

Immunologic   Severe *anaphylactoid reactions* to isosulfan blue dye requiring resuscitation are reported to occur in 1.1% of patients with breast carcinoma undergoing sentinel lymphadenectomy. Of 1013 consecutive patients who underwent sentinel lymphadenectomy for breast carcinoma, 667 received prophylaxis and isosulfan blue dye, 33 received prophylaxis but no dye, 12 received dye but no prophylaxis, and 301 received no prophylaxis or dye (48[c]). Blue urticaria and facial edema were observed in 3 (0.5%) of 667 patients receiving prophylaxis and dye and in 1 (8.3%) of 12 patients receiving dye but no prophylaxis; prophylaxis was with a glucocorticoid, diphenhydramine, and famotidine intravenously just before or at induction of anesthesia. There were no episodes of hypotension, and no patients required vasopressors, ventilatory support, or intensive care observation. There were adverse reactions to agents other than blue dye in two of 667 patients who received prophylaxis and dye and in three of 301 who received no prophylaxis and no dye. Preoperative prophylaxis reduced the severity, but not the overall incidence, of adverse reactions to isosulfan blue dye. There were no life-threatening reactions in patients treated with preoperative prophylaxis. Based on these results, prophylaxis is now recommended for patients who receive isosulfan blue for lymphatic mapping and sentinel lymph node biopsy.

GLYCOLS *(SED-15, 1516)*

Diethylene glycol

Urinary tract   Several cases of *acute renal insufficiency*, many of them fatal, have recently been reported in Panama in patients taking lisinopril. The Panama Ministry of Health investigated these cases and has concluded that the reactions resulted from the concomitant use of a cough syrup that contained diethylene glycol and were not due to lisinopril at all, as had previously been feared (49[S]). Diethylene glycol is a highly toxic organic solvent that causes acute renal insufficiency and death. The US Congress passed the Federal Food, Medicines & Cosmetic Act in 1938 in reaction to toxicity due to diethylene glycol, which was used as a diluent for sulfanilamide (50[R]). The WHO issued an Alert in 1996 when several children died in Haiti after consuming diethylene glycol-contaminated paracetamol syrup (51[S]). The Panama Ministry of Health is currently performing a root-cause analysis of the events that led to the presence of a poisonous substance such as diethylene glycol in a pharmaceutical formulation for human consumption.

Polyethylene glycol *(SED-15, 1516; SEDA-29, 375)*

Comparative studies   There have been conflicting results regarding the adverse effects of established bowel cleansing regimens. In a comparison of the effects of three bowel cleansing regimens on subjective well-being, electrolyte balance, cardiac dysrhythmias, and the microscopic post-cleansing appearance of the colonic mucosa, 231 consecutive out-patients were randomly assigned to receive bowel preparation for colonoscopy with either polyethylene glycol 4 liters (PEG; group 1, $n = 76$); polyethylene glycol 2 liters plus bisacodyl 10 mg (group 2, $n = 71$); or sodium phosphate 90 ml (group 3, $n = 84$) (52[C]). Bowel preparation in group 2 was significantly poorer than in groups 1 and 3. The frequency of cardiac dysrhythmias and post-cleansing mucosal inflammation was similar in the three groups. There were *lower serum potassium* and *higher serum phosphate concentrations* in group 3. The authors concluded that there were no differences in the effectiveness and safety of bowel preparation with polyethylene glycol alone and sodium phosphate in individuals without cardiac, renal, or hepatic failure, despite a significantly larger effect of sodium phosphate on electrolyte balance.

Glycosaminoglycans *(SED-15, 239)*

Anecdotal reports   The Swedish Adverse Drug Reactions Database contains 86 reports of suspected adverse reactions associated with glucosamine products from 2001 until February 2006. The majority of these cases were reported after 2002, when the first glucosamine product, Artrox, was approved as a drug. According to the Agency, there are now just over 10 glucosamine products approved in Sweden, including Artrox, Glucosine, Glukosamin Copyfarm, and Glukosamin Pharma (53[S]). Previously unknown adverse reactions of particular interest included the following: *angioedema* ($n = 2$), *urticaria* ($n = 1$), *colitis* ($n = 2$), *gastric/duodenal ulceration* ($n = 3$), *edema/lower limb edema* ($n = 3$), *dizziness* ($n = 4$), *arthralgia* ($n = 2$), *bronchial asthma/bronchial* *asthma aggravated* (*n* = 3), *diabetes aggravated* (*n* = 2), and *hypercholesterolemia* (*n* = 2). There were also three cases of increased effect of *warfarin* during concomitant treatment with glucosamine.

Comparative studies   In a comparison of glucosamine hydrochloride 1200 mg/day and diclofenac 100 mg/day for 2 months in 54 patients with osteoarthrosis, glucosamine relieved pain, improved function of the affected joints, and reduced the need for NSAIDs; adverse effects were not observed (54^C).

Placebo-controlled studies   In a systematic review of double-blind, randomized, controlled trials in osteoarthritis of the knee glucosamine was more effective than placebo in delaying structural progression and caused no more adverse effects than placebo (55^M).

Lactose   *(SED-15, 3737)*

Skin   Lactose as an excipient in tablets has been associated with a *rash* (56^A).

- A 54-year-old woman taking cilazapril for hypertension, developed eyelid pruritus and a hyperpigmented edematous erythematous rash on both eyelids; she had had a similar eruption after consuming dairy products over at least 10 years. The lesions remitted after avoidance of cilazapril and administration of a glucocorticoid, but recurred after the separate administration of estriol for menopausal symptoms, clotiazepam for insomnia, and enalapril maleate for hypertension.

The single common excipient in these medications was lactose, and a subsequent oral provocation test with lactose provoked similar lesions on her eyelids after 24 hours. A fixed eruption was therefore diagnosed as being caused by the excipient lactose.

Menthol and peppermint oil

(SED-15, 2254; SEDA-26, 543; SEDA-29, 610)

Peppermint oil (*Menthae piperitae aetheroleum*) is obtained from the fresh leaves of peppermint, *Mentha piperita* L. by steam distillation. As a

calcium channel blocker, (–) menthol is responsible for the spasmolytic effect of peppermint oil. The FDA has listed peppermint and peppermint oil as being "generally recognized as safe" (57^S).

Gastrointestinal   *Heartburn* is one of the major adverse effects of oral peppermint oil, mostly because of inappropriate release of the oil in the upper gastrointestinal tract (58^C), resulting in relaxation of the lower esophageal sphincter, thus facilitating reflux. This effect is minimized by the use of modified-release formulations.

Drug administration route   The pharmacokinetics of peppermint oil and its effects on the gastrointestinal tract have been reviewed, with a focus on irritable bowel syndrome (59^M). In nine studies 269 subjects were exposed to peppermint oil either orally or by topical intraluminal (stomach or colon) administration in either single doses of 0.1–0.24 ml or daily for 2 weeks. With the exception of one study, in which peppermint oil potentiated neostigmine-stimulated colon activity (60^C), the data showed that it has a substantial spasmolytic effect. This effect begins as early as 0.5 minutes after topical (intestinal tract) administration and can last for up to 23 minutes. This is too short a duration of action for the treatment of, for example, irritable bowel syndrome. To expose the target organ, i.e. the large bowel, to a constant concentration of peppermint oil, in order to maintain the beneficial effect, a modified-release formulation is needed.

The systemic availability of menthol is very low after transdermal administration; the average C_{max} after the application of eight patches in eight subjects was only 30 ng/ml; the mean terminal half-life was 4.7 hours (30^c).

Drug interactions

Bupropion   In 600 African–American smokers taking part in a study of smoking cessation with bupropion, menthol (*n* = 471) and non-menthol (*n* = 129) smokers were compared (61^C). Menthol smokers were younger (41 versus 53 years), more likely to be female (74 versus 57%) and more likely to smoke their first cigarette within 30 minutes of waking up (82 versus 70%). Seven-day point-prevalence abstinence rates from smoking for menthol and non-menthol smokers respectively were 28 and 42% at 6 weeks and 21 and 27% at 6 months. Among those under 50 years old, non-menthol smokers were more likely to quit smoking (OR = 2.0; 95% CI = 1.03, 3.95) as those who took bupropion (OR = 2.12; 95% CI = 1.32, 3.39). The authors concluded that menthol attenuated the beneficial effects of bupropion.

Caffeine   The kinetics and effects of a single oral dose of caffeine 200 mg in coffee taken together with a single oral dose of menthol 100 mg or placebo capsules have been studied in a randomized, double-blind, two-way, crossover study in 11 healthy women (62[C]). Co-administration of menthol increased the t_{max} of caffeine 44 to 76 minutes but did not significantly reduce the C_{max}, AUC, terminal half-life, or oral clearance. Menthol reduced the reduction in heart rate due to caffeine. The authors concluded that a single oral dose of pure menthol 100 mg delayed caffeine absorption and blunted the heart rate response without altering caffeine metabolism.

Felodipine   The effects of menthol on a single oral dose of felodipine in a modified-release tablet (Plendil) 10 mg have been studied in a randomized, double-blind, two-way, crossover study in 10 healthy subjects (63[C]). Felodipine was given at the start of the study with menthol 100 mg or placebo, and menthol 50, 25, and 25 mg or placebo were given at 2, 5, and 7 hours respectively. Menthol co-administration did not significantly change the pharmacokinetics of felodipine or its effects on blood pressure and heart rate.

Warfarin   A possible interaction of menthol cough drops (Halls) with warfarin has been reported (64[A]).

- A 57-year-old white man awaiting cardioversion for atrial fibrillation was given warfarin. The dosage was adjusted to 7 mg/day and the target international normalized ratio (INR) was 2.28–2.68. About 1 week later his INR fell to 1.45. He reported that he had had a flu-like illness during the previous week and had used menthol cough drops. No other potential causes for the reduced INR were found. The dosage of warfarin was increased to 53 mg/week. After withdrawal of the menthol cough drops, the dosage of warfarin returned to what it had been before and the INR remained stable.

An objective causality assessment suggested that the reduced INR was possibly related to the use of menthol cough drops during warfarin therapy. The mechanism was not elucidated, but menthol may have slowed the absorption of warfarin.

Methylthioninium chloride (methylene blue)   *(SED-15, 2314; SEDA-27, 531; SEDA-28, 595; SEDA-29, 610)*

Interaction of methylthioninium chloride with selective serotonin reuptake inhibitors   ℞

There have been several recent case reports of encephalopathy in patients who were given methylthioninium chloride at the time of para-thyroid or thyroid surgery; in all cases the patients had also taken an SSRI (Table 1) (65[A], 66[A], 67[A], 68[A], 69[A], 70[A], 71[A], 72[C]). In one series of 132 patients who received an infusion of methylthioninium chloride at parathyroidectomy, 17 were taking medications that affected serotonin and five of them developed an encephalopathy postoperatively (Table 1); of the other 115, none developed an encephalopathy (72[c]). In a retrospective study of 193 patients, 12 had postoperative neurological sequelae (including confusion, agitation, delirium, hallucinations, reduced consciousness, blurred vision, loss of vision, sluggish pupils, inappropriate speech, singing, weak grip, tremor, and jerking limb movements); all 12 were taking an SSRI compared with only 16 (8.8%) of the other 181 (73[c]). There is also experimental evidence that methylthioninium potentiates the action of venlafaxine in mice (74[E]).

There are at least three possible mechanisms for this interaction, each of which might contribute:

- *Methylthioninium chloride inhibits nitric oxide synthase, reducing the amount of nitric oxide formed. Nitric oxide normally inhibits tryptophan hydroxylase, the rate-limiting enzyme in the synthesis of 5HT, so methylthioninium chloride could cause increased 5HT synthesis (75[E]).*

Table 1. *Twelve cases of encephalopathy after the administration of methylthioninium chloride to patients taking an SSRI*

Age, sex	Clinical circumstances	Dose	Time of onset and reaction	Duration and course	Concomitant SSRI treatment	Ref.
60, F	Parathyroidectomy for primary hyperparathyroidism	7.5 mg/kg pre-operatively	During recovery from anesthesia; confusion, nystagmus, myoclonic jerks, increased muscular tone in all limbs	48 hours	Fluoxetine	(64[A])
65, M	Parathyroidectomy secondary to renal insufficiency	7.5 mg/kg by intravenous infusion	During recovery from anesthesia; agitation, intense shivering, hyperpyrexia, consciousness reduced (Glasgow Coma score 7), hypercapnia, raised arterial pressure, tachycardia with extra beats, ST segment depression, left bundle branch block, raised potassium concentration (6.7 mmol/l)	Temperature fell after hemodialysis and infusion of dantrolene; mechanical ventilation discontinued on day 3; mental status returned to normal after 2 weeks	Citalopram	(65[A])
59, M	Parathyroidectomy for adenoma	700 mg (about 6 mg/kg) by intravenous infusion	During recovery from anesthesia; aphasia, slow speech, ?clonus, disorientation	48 hours (aphasia started improving much earlier); blue discoloration of urine persisted beyond 2 days	Paroxetine	(66[A])
50, F	Subtotal thyroidectomy	500 mg (5.5 mg/kg) intravenously	In post-anesthetic care unit; agitation, tachycardia, sweating, hypoxia (SpO$_2$ 88%), severe leg rigidity; required intubation	1 day	Sertraline	(67[A])
52, F	Parathyroidectomy for single adenoma	650 mg (7.5 mg/kg) pre-operatively by intravenous infusion	During recovery from anesthesia; delayed recovery from anesthesia, nystagmus, expressive aphasia, confusion, disinhibition	48 hours	Venlafaxine	(68[A])
48, F	Parathyroidectomy for adenoma	4 mg/kg (5 mg/kg intended) pre-operatively by intravenous infusion	2 hours after surgery; vomiting during infusion, generalized tonic–clonic seizure	Discharged taking antiepileptic treatment		(69[A])
65, F	Parathyroidectomy for adenoma	200 mg (1.75 mg/kg) intravenously during surgery	During recovery from anesthesia; agitation and restlessness, unable to speak or respond to verbal commands	Following slow improvement discharged after 7 days	Paroxetine	(69[A])
60, F	Parathyroidectomy for single adenoma	5 mg/kg by intravenous infusion	After 5 hours; vertigo, confusion, lethargy, expressive aphasia; required intubation	72 hours	Fluoxetine	(69[C])

(continued on next page)

Table 1. *(continued)*

Age, sex	Clinical circumstances	Dose	Time of onset and reaction	Duration and course	Concomitant SSRI treatment	Ref.
73, F	Parathyroidectomy for four-gland hyperplasia	5 mg/kg by intravenous infusion	After 5 hours; lethargy, expressive aphasia, reduced level of consciousness	48 hours	Escitalopram	(69[c])
60, F	Parathyroidectomy for a single adenoma	3 mg/kg by intravenous infusion	After 5 hours; agitation, confusion, expressive aphasia; required intubation	72 hours	Venlafaxine	(69[c])
48, F	Parathyroidectomy for single adenoma	3 mg/kg by intravenous infusion	After 3 hours; confusion, lethargy, vertigo	48 hours	Fluoxetine (also bupropion)	(74[c])
34, F	Parathyroidectomy for double adenoma	3 mg/kg by intravenous infusion	After 1 hour; confusion, disorientation	48 hours	Venlafaxine (also mirtazapine and quetiapine)	(69[c])

- 5HT receptors (apart from $5HT_3$ receptors) are G protein coupled receptors, and methylthioninium chloride inhibits guanylyl cyclase. It could thus increase the action of 5HT at its receptors. In mice methylthioninium chloride markedly enhanced head twitch (a serotonergic behaviour) induced by intracerebral injection of 5HT (76[E]).
- Methylthioninium chloride inhibits monoamine oxidase (77[E]).

It would be wise to withdraw drugs that affect serotonin at least a few days before the administration of methylthioninium chloride and to use a dose below 3 mg/kg.

Nicotine *(SED-15, 2508; SEDA-28, 596; SEDA-29, 610)*

Comparative studies   In a multicenter, community-based, prospective, longitudinal study of the safety of nicotine replacement therapy (NRT; $n = 370$), bupropion ($n = 413$), and the combination ($n = 121$) for smokers seeking to quit, adverse effects were reported by 3.8, 33, 22, and 5.7% of subjects at 15, 30, 60, and 90 days respectively (78[c]). Adverse effects were significantly more common in those who used the combination therapy or bupropion alone than in those who used NRT alone. A total of 83 smokers (9.3%) withdrew from treatment and 116 (13%) stopped temporarily because of adverse effects. There were no differences in the percentages of withdrawals among the different treatment options. Adverse effects were rarely severe ($n = 10$). Nevertheless, 41 subjects (4.5%) discontinued drug therapy indefinitely and 55 (6.1%) discontinued temporarily because of mild adverse effects. Pharmacological therapies for smoking cessation are safe as long as they are appropriately prescribed and supervised by clinicians according to clinical practice guidelines. Adverse effects are mostly mild, but may be unacceptable to patients.

Silicone *(SED-15, 3137; SEDA-29, 611)*

Observational studies   Silicone has been trialled as a sphincter-bulking agent. It was injected into the anal sphincter in 82 patients with severe fecal incontinence and low anal resting pressure (79ᶜ). Improvements were modest and follow up was limited. Long-term safety is not known.

Sodium metabisulfite   *(SEDA-29, 611)*

Respiratory   There is epidemiological evidence of an increased prevalence of occupational *asthma* among radiographers (80ᴿ, 81ᴿ). Symptoms in the eyes, nose, and airways (darkroom disease) suggest irritation or allergy caused by chemicals. However, these have not been defined.

- A 37-year-old female radiographer developed asthma 2 years after starting work in the department of radiology of a regional hospital (82ᴬᶜ). There was a complex exposure to powdered latex gloves, as well as various disinfectants, developers, and fixing agents. She had developed seasonal rhinitis 5 years earlier, which disappeared when work-related shortness of breath occurred. She noticed the asthma almost exclusively on exertion and while loading radiographic processing chemicals into an automatic processing machine in a small poorly ventilated darkroom. She left her job 6 years later because of increasing airway symptoms and medication with beta-adrenoceptor agonists. The diagnosis was made 2 years later when she had a positive immediate bronchial reaction on two separate days after inhalation of metabisulfite 48 and 96 mg.

The authors concluded that sodium metabisulfite exposure should be recognized as a cause of dark room asthma. Primary and secondary preventive measures should be taken. In industrialized countries, this occupational hazard will disappear with time owing to increasing use of digital radiography and dry laser imaging.

ANIMAL PRODUCTS

Bee sting venom

Management of adverse drug reactions   Immunotherapy of bee stings with venom can be associated with anaphylaxis. Of 1682 patients with *Hymenoptera* venom allergy seen during 34 months for immunotherapy, 11% had cardiovascular disease and 44 of these were taking a beta-blocker before immunotherapy (83ᴿ). In 31 of those, the drug was replaced before starting treatment. In three with coronary heart disease and one with severe ventricular dysrhythmias the drug was continued throughout immunotherapy. In nine it was reintroduced after reaching the maintenance dose. In another 12 patients, beta-blockers were newly started during immunotherapy. Of 25 patients who took beta-blockers during immunotherapy, three (12%) developed allergic adverse effects, compared with 23 (17%) of 117 with cardiovascular disease who were not taking beta-blockers. There were systemic allergic symptoms after re-exposure by sting challenge or field sting in one of seven (14%) with and four of 29 (14%) without beta-blockade. There were no severe reactions to treatment or sting re-exposure in patients taking beta-blockade. The authors concluded that beta-blockers might be beneficial in patients with severe cardiovascular disease receiving bee venom immunotherapy.

References

1. McClung MR, Geusens P, Miller PD, Zippel H, Bensen WG, Roux C, Adami S, Fogelman I, Diamond T, Eastell R, Meunier PJ, Reginster JY. Effect of risedronate on the risk of hip fracture in elderly women. Hip Intervention Program Study Group. N Engl J Med 2001;344:333–40.

2. Black DM, Cummings SR, Karpf DB, Cauley JA, Thompson DE, Nevitt MC, Bauer DC, Genant HK, Haskell WL, Marcus R, Ott SM, Torner JC, Quandt SA, Reiss TF, Ensrud KE. Randomized trial of effect of alendronate on risk of fracture in women with existing vertebral

fractures. Fracture Intervention Trial Research Group. Lancet 1996;348:1535–41.

3. Ott SM. Long-term safety of bisphosphonates. J Clin Endocrinol Metab 2005;90:1897–9.
4. Odvina CV, Zerwekh JE, Sudhaker Rao D, Maalouf N, Gottschalk FA, Pak CYC. Severely suppressed bone turnover: a potential complication of alendronate therapy. J Clin Endocrinol Metab 2005;90:1294–301.
5. Marx RE. Pamidronate (Aredia) and zoledronate (Zometa) induced avascular necrosis of the jaws: a growing epidemic. J Oral Maxillofac Surg 2003;61:1115–8.
6. Wang J, Goodger NM, Pogrel MA. Osteonecrosis of the jaws associated with cancer chemotherapy. J Oral Maxillofac Surg 2003;61(9):1104–7.
7. Migliorati CA. Bisphosphanates and oral cavity avascular bone necrosis. J Clin Oncol 2003;21:4253–4.
8. Starck WJ, Epker BN. Failure of osseointegrated dental implants after diphosphonate therapy for osteoporosis: a case report. Int J Oral Maxillofac Implants 1995;10(1):74–8.
9. Purcell PM, Boyd IW. Bisphosphonates and osteonecrosis of the jaw. Med J Aust 2005;182(8):417–8.
10. Sarathy AP, Bourgeois SL, Goodell GG. Bisphosphonate-associated osteonecrosis of the jaws and endodontic treatment: two case reports. J Endod 2005;31(10):759–63 [erratum, 835–6].
11. Ruggiero SL, Mehrotra B, Rosenberg TJ, Engroff SL. Osteonecrosis of the jaws associated with the use of bisphosphonates: a review of 63 cases. J Oral Maxillofac Surg 2004;62(5):527–34.
12. Schirmer I, Peters H, Reichart PA, Durkop H. Bisphosphonates and osteonecrosis of the jaw. Mund Kiefer Gesichtschir 2005;9(4):239–45.
13. Migliorati CA, Schubert MM, Peterson DE, Seneda LM. Bisphosphonate-associated osteonecrosis of mandibular and maxillary bone: an emerging oral complication of supportive cancer therapy. Cancer 2005;104(1):83–93.
14. Oltolina A, Achilli A, Lodi G, Demarosi F, Sardella A. Osteonecrosis of the jaws in patients treated with bisphosphonates. Review of the literature and the Milan experience. Minerva Stomatol 2005;54(7–8):441–8.
15. Carter G, Goss AN, Doecke C. Bisphosphonates and avascular necrosis of the jaw: a possible association. Med J Aust 2005;182:413–5.
16. Ficarra G, Beninati F, Rubino I, Vannucchi A, Longo G, Tonelli P, Pini Prato G. Osteonecrosis of the jaws in periodontal patients with a history of bisphosphonates treatment. J Clin Periodontol 2005;32(11):1123–8.
17. Marx RE, Sawatari Y, Fortin M, Broumand V. Bisphosphonate-induced exposed bone (osteonecrosis/osteopetrosis) of the jaws: risk factors, recognition, prevention, and treatment. J Oral Maxillofac Surg 2005;63(11):1567–75.
18. Bagan JV, Jimenez Y, Murillo J, Hernandez S, Poveda R, Sanchis JM, Diaz JM, Scully C. Jaw osteonecrosis associated with bisphosphonates: multiple exposed areas and its relationship to

teeth extractions. Study of 20 cases. Oral Oncol 2006;42(3):327–9.
19. Gibbs SD, O'Grady J, Seymour JF, Prince HM. Bisphosphonate-induced osteonecrosis of the jaw requires early detection and intervention. Med J Aust 2005;183(10):549–50.
20. Brooks JK, Gilson AJ, Sindler AJ, Ashman SG, Schwartz KG, Nikitakis NG. Osteonecrosis of the jaws associated with use of risedronate: report of 2 new cases. Oral Surg Oral Med Oral Pathol Oral Radiol Endod 2007;103(6):780–6.
21. Bamias A, Kastritis E, Bamia C, Moulopoulos LA, Melakopoulos I, Bozas G, Koutsoukou V, Gika D, Anagnostopoulos A, Papadimitriou C, Terpos E, Dimopoulos MA. Osteonecrosis of the jaw in cancer after treatment with bisphosphonates: incidence and risk factors. J Clin Oncol 2005;23(34):8580–7.
22. Ott SM. Long-term safety of bisphosphonates. J Clin Endocrinol Metab 2005;90:1897–9.
23. Russell RG, Rogers MJ, Frith JC, Luckman SP, Coxon FP, Benford HL, Croucher PI, Shipman C, Fleisch HA. The pharmacology of bisphosphonates and new insights into their mechanisms of action. J Bone Miner Res 1999;14(Suppl 2):53–65.
24. Rogers MJ, Watts DJ, Russell RG. Overview of bisphosphonates. Cancer 1997;80(Suppl 8):1652–60.
25. Wesselink PR, Beertsen W. Repair processes in the periodontium following dentoalveolar ankylosis: the effect of masticatory function. J Clin Periodontol 1994;21(7):472–8.
26. Migliorati CA, Casiglia J, Epstein J, Jacobsen PL, Siegel MA, Woo SB. Managing the care of patients with bisphosphonate-associated osteonecrosis: an American Academy of Oral Medicine position paper. J Am Dent Assoc 2005;136(12):1658–68.
27. Polizzotto MN, Cousins V, Schwarer AP. Bisphosphonate-associated osteonecrosis of the auditory canal. Br J Haematol 2006;132(1):114.
28. Ruggiero SL, Fantasia J, Carlson E. Bisphosphonate-related osteonecrosis of the jaw: background and guidelines for diagnosis, staging and management. Oral Surg Oral Med Oral Pathol Oral Radiol Endod 2006;102(4):433–41.
29. Chiandussi S, Biasotto M, Dore F, Cavalli F, Cova MA, Di Lenarda R. Clinical and diagnostic imaging of bisphosphonate-associated osteonecrosis of the jaws. Dentomaxillofac Radiol 2006;35(4):236–43.
30. Hansen T, Kunkel M, Weber A, James Kirkpatrick C. Osteonecrosis of the jaws in patients treated with bisphosphonates – histomorphologic analysis in comparison with infected osteoradionecrosis. J Oral Pathol Med 2006;35(3):155–60.
31. Durie BG, Katz M, Crowley J. Osteonecrosis of the jaw and bisphosphonates. N Engl J Med 2005;353(1):99–102.
32. Ardine M, Generali D, Donadio M, Bonardi S, Scoletta M, Vandone AM, Mozzati M, Bertetto O, Bottini A, Dogliotti L, Berruti A. Could the long-term persistence of low serum

calcium levels and high serum parathyroid hormone levels during bisphosphonate treatment predispose metastatic breast cancer patients to undergo osteonecrosis of the jaw? Ann Oncol 2006;17(8):1336–7.

33. Markiewicz MR, Margarone 3rd JE, Campbell JH, Aguirre A. Bisphosphonate-associated osteonecrosis of the jaws: a review of current knowledge. J Am Dent Assoc 2005;136(12):1669–74.

34. Vescovi P, Merigo E, Meleti M, Manfredi M. Bisphosphonate-associated osteonecrosis (BON) of the jaws: a possible treatment? J Oral Maxillofac Surg 2006;64(9):1460–2.

35. Anonymous. Triaminic vapour patch. Risk of ingestion. WHO Newslett 2006;4:4.

36. Martin D, Valdez J, Boren J, Mayersohn M. Dermal absorption of camphor, menthol, and methyl salicylate in humans. J Clin Pharmacol 2004;44(10):1151–7.

37. Buchholz U, Mermin J, Rios R, Casagrande TL, Galey F, Lee M, Quattrone A, Farrar J, Nagelkerke N, Werner SB. An outbreak of food-borne illness associated with methomyl-contaminated salt. JAMA 2002;288(5):604–10.

38. Tsai MJ, Wu SN, Cheng HA, Wang SH, Chiang HT. An outbreak of food-borne illness due to methomyl contamination. J Toxicol Clin Toxicol 2003;41(7):969–73.

39. Miceli G, Ravalli P, Settimi L, Ballard TJ, Bascherini S. Acute poisoning with methomyl and other pesticides in the province of Ragusa, Sicily. Ann Ist Super Sanita 2001;37(2):141–6.

40. Makrides C, Koukouvas M, Achillews G, Tsikkos S, Vounou E, Symeonides M, Christodoulides P, Ioannides M. Methomyl-induced severe acute pancreatitis: possible etiological association. JOP 2005;6(2):166–71.

41. Brahmi N, Blel Y, Kouraichi N, Abidi N, Thabet H, Amamou M. Acute pancreatitis subsequent to voluntary methomyl and dichlorvos intoxication. Pancreas 2005;31(4):424–7.

42. Kudo K, Hida Y, Zaitsu A, Inoue H, Tsuji A, Ishida T, Ikeda N. A case of poisoning in a man who drank a nutrition supplement containing methomyl, a carbamate pesticide. Fukuoka Igaku Zasshi 2005;96(7):305–10.

43. Moriya F, Hashimoto Y. A fatal poisoning caused by methomyl and nicotine. Forensic Sci Int 2005;149:167–70.

44. Tsatsakis AM, Tsakalof AK, Siatitsas Y, Michalodimitrakis EN. Acute poisoning with carbamate pesticides: the Cretan experience. Sci Justice 1996;36(1):35–9.

45. Ruangyuttikarn W, Phakdeewut T, Sainumtan W, Sribanditmongkol P. Children's plasma cholinesterase activity and fatal methomyl poisoning. J Med Assoc Thai 2001;84(9):1344–50.

46. Iriyama A, Yanagi Y, Uchida S, Tamaki Y, Aihara M, Obata R, Inoue Y. Retinal nerve fibre layer damage after indocyanine green assisted vitrectomy. Br J Ophthalmol 2004;88:1606–7.

47. Kanda S, Uemura A, Yamashita T, Kita H, Yamakiri K, Sakamoto T. Visual field defects after intravitreous administration of indocyanine

green in macular hole surgery. Arch Ophthalmol 2004;122:1447–51.

48. Raut CP, Hunt KK, Akins JS, Daley DM, Ross MI, Singletary SE, Marshall GD, Meric-Bernstam F, Babiera G, Feig BW, Ames FC, Kuerer HM. Incidence of anaphylactoid reactions to isosulfan blue dye during breast carcinoma lymphatic mapping in patients treated with preoperative prophylaxis. Wiley Intersci J 2005;104:692–9.

49. Anonymous. Diethylene glycol. Detected in cough syrup; fatalities reported. WHO Newslett 2006;5:2.

50. Wax PM. Elixirs, diluents, and the passage of the 1938 Federal Food, Drug and Cosmetic Act. Ann Intern Med 1995;122(6):456–61.

51. Junod SW. Diethylene glycol deaths in Haiti. Public Health Rep 2000;115(1):78–86.

52. Huppertz-Hauss G, Bretthauer M, Sauar J, Paulsen J, Kjellevold O, Majak B, Hoff G. Polyethylene glycol versus sodium phosphate in bowel cleansing for colonoscopy: a randomized trial. Endoscopy 2005;37:537–41.

53. Anonymous. Glucosamine products. 86 reports to date in Sweden. WHO Newslett 2006;3:3.

54. Svetlova MS, Ignat'ev VK. Experience with glucosamine hydrochloride in the treatment of patients with osteoarthrosis. Ter Arkh 2005;77(12):4–7.

55. Poolsup N, Suthisisang C, Channark P, Kittikulsuth W. Glucosamine long-term treatment and the progression of knee osteoarthritis: systematic review of randomized controlled trials. Ann Pharmacother 2005;39(6):1080–7.

56. Tsuruta D, Sowa J, Kobayashi H, Ishii M. Fixed food eruption caused by lactose identified after oral administration of four unrelated drugs. J Am Acad Dermatol 2005;52(2):370–1.

57. National Archives and Records Administration. Code of Federal Regulations. Title 21: Food and Drugs. Substances generally recognized as safe. 21.CFR. 182.10 and 21.CFR. 182.20. 1998; April 1.

58. Sigmund CJ, McNally EF. The action of a carminative on the lower esophageal sphincter. Gastroenterology 1969;56:13–8.

59. Grigoleit H-G, Grigoleit P. Gastrointestinal clinical pharmacology of peppermint oil. Phytomedicine 2005;12:607–11.

60. Rogers J, Tay HH, Misiewicz JJ. Peppermint oil. Lancet 1988:98–9.

61. Okuyemi KS, Ahluwalia JS, Ebersole-Robinson M, Catley D, Mayo MS, Resnicow K. Does menthol attenuate the effect of bupropion among African American smokers? Addiction 2003;98(10):1387–93.

62. Gelal A, Guven H, Balkan D, Artok L, Benowitz NL. Influence of menthol on caffeine disposition and pharmacodynamics in healthy female volunteers. Eur J Clin Pharmacol 2003;59(5–6):417–22.

63. Gelal A, Balkan D, Ozzeybek D, Kaplan YC, Gurler S, Guven H, Benowitz NL. Effect of menthol on the pharmacokinetics and pharmacodynamics of felodipine in healthy subjects. Eur J Clin Pharmacol 2005;60(11):785–90.

64. Arin MJ, Bate J, Krieg T, Hunzelmann N. Possible warfarin interaction with menthol cough drops. Ann Pharmacother 2005;39:S53–6.

65. Martindale SJ, Stedeford JC. Neurological sequelae following methylene blue injection for parathyroidectomy. Anaesthesia 2003;58:1041–2.

66. Mathew S, Linhartova L, Raghuraman G. Hyperpyrexia and prolonged postoperative disorientation following methylene blue infusion during parathyroidectomy. Anaesthesia 2006;61:580–3.

67. Bach KK, Lindsay FW, Berg LS. Prolonged postoperative disorientation after methylene blue infusion during parathyroidectomy. Anesth Analg 2004;99:1573–4.

68. Rosenbaum HK. January 2006 Case of the Month. Thyroidectomy—postop agitation and rigidity; serotonin syndrome. http://tinyurl.com/2k7xeh [last accessed 11 May 2007].

69. Majithia A, Stearns MP. Methylene blue toxicity following infusion to localise parathyroid adenoma. J Laryngol Otol 2006;120:138–40.

70. Patel AS, Singh-Ranger D, Lowery KA, Crinnion JN. Letter to the editor. Head Neck 2006;28:567–8.

71. Mihai R, Mitchell EW, Warwick J. Dose-response and postoperative confusion following methylene blue infusion during parathyroidectomy. Can J Anesth 2007;54:79–81.

72. Sweet G, Standiford SB. Methylene-blue–associated encephalopathy. J Am Coll Surg 2007;204:454–8.

73. Kartha SS, Chacko CE, Bumpous JM, Fleming M, Lentsch EJ, Flynn MB. Toxic metabolic encephalopathy after parathyroidectomy with methylene blue localization. Otolaryngol Head Neck Surg 2006;135(5):765–8.

74. Dhir A, Kulkarni SK. Involvement of l-arginine-nitric oxide-cyclic guanosine monophosphate pathway in the antidepressant-like effect of venlafaxine in mice. Prog Neuropsychopharmacol Biol Psychiatry 2007;31(4):921–5.

75. Wegener G, Volke V, Rosenberg R. Endogenous nitric oxide decreases hippocampal levels of serotonin and dopamine in vivo. Br J Pharmacol 2000;130(3):575–80.

76. Kim HS, Son YR, Kim SH. Nitric oxide synthase inhibitors enhance 5-HT2 receptor-mediated behavior, the head-twitch response in mice. Life Sci 1999;64(26):2463–70.

77. Aeschlimann C, Cerny T, Kupfer A. Inhibition of (mono)amine oxidase activity and prevention of ifosfamide encephalopathy by methylene blue. Drug Metab Dispos 1996;24(12):1336–9.

78. Sicari R, Palinkas A, Pasanisi EG, Venneri L, Picano E. Adverse effects of pharmacological therapy for nicotine addiction in smokers following a smoking cessation program. Nicotine Tobacco Res. 2005;7:2136–41.

79. Andrews C, Bharucha A. The aetiology, assessment and treatment of faecal incontinence. Nat Clin Pract 2005;2(11):516–25.

80. Smedley J, Inskip H, Wield G, Coggon D. Work-related respiratory symptoms in radiographers. Occup Environ Med 1996;53:450–4.

81. Dimich-Ward H, Wymer M, Kennedy S, Teschke K, Rousseau R, Chan-Yeung M. Excess of symptoms among radiographers. Am J Ind Med 2003;43:132–41.

82. Merget R, Korn M. Metabisulphite-induced occupational asthma in a radiographer. Eur Respir J 2005;25:386–8.

83. Muller UR, Haeberli G. Use of beta-blockers during immunotherapy for Hymenoptera venom allergy. J Allergy Clin Immunol 2005;115(3):606–10.

J.K. Aronson

50

Medication errors

Further reviews of medication errors have appeared (1[R], 2[R]).

Defining errors   In a two-stage Delphi study of errors in pediatric practice, using 40 scenarios that might be classified as prescribing errors, there was a consensus that 27 of the 40 scenarios should be included as prescribing errors, 10 should be excluded, and three might be considered to be errors depending on the individual clinical circumstances (3[c]). Failure to communicate essential information, transcription errors, and the use of drugs, formulations, or doses that were inappropriate for the individual patient were considered to be prescribing errors. Deviations from policies or guidelines, the use of unlicensed and off-label drugs, and omission of non-essential information were not considered to be prescribing errors.

Sources of medication errors   Errors in taking the medication history can lead to prescribing errors. In a systematic review of medication history errors described in articles published from 1966 to April 2005, 22 studies involving a total of 3755 patients (range 33–1053, median 104) were identified (4[M]). Errors in prescription medication histories occurred in up to 67% of cases: 10–61% had at least one error of omission (deletion of a drug used before admission), and 13–22% had at least one error of commission (addition of a drug not used before admission); 60–67% had at least one error of omission or commission. Only five studies (545 patients) explicitly distinguished between unintentional discrepancies and intentional therapeutic changes. In these studies 27–54% of patients had at least one medication history error and 19–75% of the discrepancies were unintentional. In six of the studies (588 patients),

the investigators estimated that 11–59% of the medication history errors were clinically important.

Transferring patients from one type of care to another can result in medication errors (5[c]). During 758 transfers of medications between primary and secondary care there were 142 medication errors, and on average there were two medication errors each time a patient was transferred. When patients were discharged from the hospital, the use of a specific medication dispensing system constituted a significant risk for medication errors. The most common error when patients were transferred to the hospital was inadvertent withdrawal of drugs. When patients left the hospital the most common error was erroneous addition of drugs. The authors suggested that improved documentation and transferring data about elderly patients' medications could reduce these errors. Specific medication dispensing systems did not seem to be useful in reducing the numbers of errors.

Frequency of errors

Hospital   In a study of 4951 prescriptions written during 25 weeks in a Croatian hospital, medication errors were classified as: incorrect dose, incorrect dose interval, duplication of therapy, and drug interactions (6[c]). The incidence of medication errors in the entire sample, including all potential drug interactions, was 15%. Excluding all but eight potentially serious interactions, the incidence was 7.7%. Dosage errors were the most frequent errors, followed by incorrect interval, drug duplication, and drug interactions. There was a large difference between the incidence of potential and clinically significant drug interactions (7.2 versus 0.2%).

In a UK eye hospital 144 out of 1952 prescription sheets (8%) had errors; 7% of the total errors were errors of prescription writing and 1% were drug errors (7[c]). Most of the errors were made by junior doctors and none was made by a senior doctor. The out-patient department had by far the highest prevalence of errors.

Side Effects of Drugs, Annual 30
J.K. Aronson (Editor)
ISSN: 0378-6080
DOI: 10.1016/S0378-6080(08)00063-9

In a cross-sectional study using three methods to detect medication errors, direct observation, unannounced control visits, and chart review in a medical and surgical department in Denmark, there were 1065 errors in 2467 opportunities for errors (43%) (8[c]). In the worst-case scenario 20–30% of all evaluated errors were assessed as potential adverse events. The frequencies of medication errors were as follows:

- ordering 167/433 (39%);
- transcription 310/558 (56%);
- dispensing 22/538 (4%);
- administration 166/412 (41%);
- discharge summaries 401/526 (76%).

The most common types of error throughout the medication process were: lack of drug form, unordered drug, omission of drug/dose, and lack of identity control.

Primary care   The Linnaeus Collaboration was formed in 2001 to study medical errors in primary care. General practitioners in six countries, Canada, Australia, England, the Netherlands, New Zealand, and the USA, anonymously reported errors in their practices between June and December 2001 (9[c]). In Canada, 15 family doctors reported 95 errors, of which 25 were treatment errors. In the other five countries, 64 doctors reported 413 errors, of which 85 were treatment errors. All countries reported similar proportions of laboratory and prescribing errors. Canadian doctors reported harm to patients from 39% of errors; doctors in other countries reported harm from 29% of errors. Canadian physicians considered errors "very serious" in 5.8% of instances; doctors in other countries thought them very serious in 7.1% of instances.

In a prospective cohort study of 1879 prescriptions from 1202 patients in four adult primary care practices in Boston, 661 were surveyed (10[c]). There were 143 prescribing errors (7.6%). Three led to preventable adverse events, 62 had a potential for harm, of which one was potentially life-threatening and 15 were serious. Errors in frequency ($n = 77$) and dose ($n = 26$) were common. The rates of medication errors and potential adverse events were not significantly different at basic computerized prescribing sites (4.3 versus 11%) compared

with handwritten sites. Advanced checks (including dose and frequency checking) could have prevented 95% of potential adverse events.

In 78 US practices both the culture and the structure of the practice affected prescription drug error rates (11[c]). Seeing more patients per hour, issuing more prescriptions per patient, and being cared for in a rural clinic were all strongly associated with more errors. Even by the strictest definition, there were about 13 errors per 100 prescriptions.

Of 77 511 prescriptions dispensed in primary health care in Bahrain, 5959 (7.7%; for 16 091 medication items) contained errors (12[c]). Minor errors of omission, such as absence of the physician's stamp (34%), date (9.8%), and information about the patient's address (3.8%), age (3.5%), and sex (0.5%) were not specified. Major errors of omission accounted for 93.6% and were as follows: strength/dose (31%), length of therapy/quantity (30%), dosage form (20%), and frequency of dosing (13%). In 6.3% errors of commission (incorrect information) the most common was strength/dose (3.3%), followed by frequency of dosing (2.6%), dosage form (0.3%), and length of therapy/quantity (0.1%). Major errors of omission associated with topical formulations were significantly more common than those with systemic formulations. However, prescriptions for systemic formulations had a higher rate of errors of commission. In 9.2% of prescriptions with errors, there were potential drug–drug interactions.

Children   Copies of 358 prescriptions written by residents in a pediatric emergency department during 6 months were matched with pediatric emergency department records (13[c]). In all, 212 prescriptions (59%) contained 311 errors. Minor omissions were the most common errors (62%), followed by incomplete directions (23%), dose/directions errors (6%), and unclear quantities to dispense (5%). Prescriptions written by pediatric residents were less likely to have an error (48%) than those written by emergency medicine residents (81%), family medicine residents (76%), or combined internal medicine/pediatrics residents (100%). Most of the errors (77%) were insignificant; under 5% were significant, and none was serious or severe.

In a prospective cohort study performed in a pediatric unit the hospital's computer clinical decision support system was modified so that doctors could choose the traditional prescription method or the enhanced method of computer calculated doses when prescribing paracetamol or promethazine (14^C). All prescriptions issued to children under 16 years of age in the out-patient clinic, in the emergency department, and at discharge from the in-patient service were analysed. A medication error was defined as an underdose (below the agreed value), an overdose (above the agreed value), no frequency of administration specified, no dose given, or an excessive total daily dose. Of 4274 prescriptions issued during 6 months the error rate in the emergency department was 16%, for out-patients 22%, and for discharge medication 24%. Most errors were the result of an underdose (64%). The computer-calculated dose error rate was 13% compared with the traditional prescription error rate of 28%. Calculated dose was an important and independent variable influencing the error rate (adjusted relative risk = 0.436, 95% CI = 0.336, 0.520). Other important independent variables were the type of drug prescribed and the seniority and pediatric training of the prescriber.

Elderly people   In a study of Dutch patients, aged 65 and over, for inappropriate prescriptions, the 1-year risk of receiving at least one inappropriate drug prescription was 17–19% according to the 1997 Beers criteria and 19–20% according to the updated criteria (15^c). The most frequently prescribed inappropriate drugs were nitrofurantoin, long-acting benzodiazepines, amitriptyline, promethazine, and cimetidine. Temazepam and zolpidem were mostly prescribed in supratherapeutic doses. Conventional NSAIDs in people with a history of peptic ulceration were the most frequently prescribed contraindicated drugs.

Renal insufficiency   Failure to reduce the dose of a drug that is eliminated by the kidneys in patients with chronic renal insufficiency can lead to drug toxicity. In a study of the electronic records of 224 patients with estimated creatinine clearance values below 50 ml/minute, 157 (70%) received one or more of 17 drugs with high rates of renal elimination (16^c). In all, 207 drugs requiring dose adjustment were prescribed, 52 in an inappropriately high dose. In 127 of the 224 patients (57%), chronic renal insufficiency was not documented. However, patients in whom it was documented were equally likely to be given an inappropriately high dose of a drug.

HIV infection   Of 400 medication errors that involved at least one single or combined HIV antiretroviral product that had been reported to a national medication error reporting program, 3% were harmful (17^C). Most of the errors (45%) were dispensing errors; the most frequent were wrong dose (38%) and wrong medication (32%). Similar brand and generic names were associated with many of the errors. Lamivudine (Epivir®) was the most common product involved. Errors were more likely in community hospitals than teaching hospitals.

In a retrospective study in 5473 HIV-infected patients the incidence of confirmed errors was 9.80 errors per 1000 new prescriptions dispensed for incorrect dosing, 9.51 errors per 1000 for contraindicated medications, and <1.00 for all other categories of error (18^c).

Preventing errors   The methods that have been used to prevent or reduce the risk of errors have been reviewed (19^R).

Computerized alerts can be used to prevent errors. However, practitioners sometimes override alerts because of poor specificity and excessive numbers of alerts (alert fatigue or overload). To tackle this, a system has been developed in which alerts were given only if they were related to potential effects of high severity, to which clinicians were required to respond (20^c). Over 6 months there were 18 115 potential drug alerts, of which 5182 (29%) were selected to be interruptive; 67% were accepted. The clinicians most commonly accepted duplicate drug class alerts (77%) and drug–disease alerts (53%), followed by drug–drug (42%), drug–laboratory (40%), and drug–pregnancy (10%) contraindication alerts.

Computerized entry without decision support has been compared with hand-written prescribing in an intensive care unit (21^c). The total proportion of errors was significantly lower with computerized entry (117 errors in 2429 prescriptions, 4.8%) than with hand-written prescribing (69 errors in 1036 prescriptions, 6.7%). The proportion of errors reduced with time after the introduction of computerized entry. Two errors in computerized entry led to patient harm, requiring an increased length of stay and, if they had been administered, three prescriptions with computerized entry could have led to permanent harm or death. There was a reduction in major/moderate patient outcomes with computerized entry when intercepted and non-intercepted errors were combined. However, the mean baseline APACHE II score did not differ significantly between the two methods.

In a sequential open comparison of electronic prescribing and traditional manual prescribing in two hospitals, errors regarding medications, diet, and/or nursing orders were assessed in four stages: medical prescription, pharmacy transcription/validation, nursing transcription, and dispensing (22[c]). With manual prescription there were 1576 errors in 18 539 orders (8.5%), and with electronic prescription there were 827 errors in 18 885 orders (4.38%). Pharmacy transcription/validation errors were significantly reduced (1.73 versus 0.13%), as were nursing transcription errors (2.54 versus 0.81%), and dispensing errors (2.13 versus 0.96%); however, the number of prescription errors increased (2.10 versus 2.40%).

In a prospective study of medication errors after experience for 2 years of a computerized entry system, 2268 orders were monitored (162 patients) (23[c]). There were 73 medication errors (22% of the patients) (59 prescribing errors and 14 monitoring errors). The most common prescribing errors were deficiencies related to the right class but wrong drug (28%), an incorrect dose (30%), and unclear orders (13%). Other errors related to incorrect frequency of administration (5%), maintenance of the intravenous route (5%), duplicated drug therapy (11.7%), drug interactions (1.7%), and length of therapy (3.3%). The 14 monitoring errors were failures to review a prescribed regimen for appropriateness and detection of problems. The authors concluded that although computerized entry has the potential to reduce medication errors, particularly those related to transcribing and patient identification, errors related to prescription and monitoring still occur.

As an alternative to computerized entry systems, computerized medication charts may be helpful in reducing errors. In a comparison of a traditional medication distribution system (611 prescriptions) with the use of a computerized medication chart updated daily by pharmacy assistants (598 prescriptions), the total prescription error rate was significantly higher with the computerized charts (50 versus 20%; OR = 3.80; 95% CI = 2.94, 4.90) (24[c]). However, this increase was caused by an increase in administrative prescription errors of low potential clinical significance (mainly omission of the prescriber's name and the prescription date). The error rate for errors with a potential clinical significance was significantly lower because of elimination of a specific error involving duplicate therapy (3.4% with the traditional medication chart versus 0% with the computerized chart). For errors in administration (1122 drugs before the intervention and 1175 drugs after), the total administration error rate was significantly lower after the intervention (6.1 versus 11%; OR = 0.61; 95% CI = 0.45, 0.84), as was the rate of errors with potential clinical significance. The contribution of handwritten medication orders to the total amount of medication orders was significantly reduced after the intervention (13 versus 21%) and the administration of a drug ordered by a handwritten order resulted in a significantly higher rate than with administration of a drug ordered by a printed order.

Medication errors might also be prevented by the use of standardized order forms. In a study of prescription of anti-emetics in oncology during two consecutive 4-month periods (control followed by test) a standardized form significantly reduced the number of prescribing errors, from 53 errors in 3592 medication orders in the control period to 12 errors in 3585 medication orders during the test period (25[c]).

A completely different approach to the problem of eliminating errors is hierarchical task analysis, which involves breaking a task down into its component parts. The so-called systematic human error reduction and prediction approach (SHERPA) has been applied in theory to medication errors, using the actions derived from a hierarchical task analysis as inputs, and showing how it could be possible to identify the likely causes of error and thus to eliminate them (26[c]).

Anecdotal reports   In a previous study there was large random variation in the administered dosage of intravenous infusions of N-acetylcysteine in patients with paracetamol self-poisoning (27[c]). Systematic calculation errors occur in about 5% of cases, and major errors in drawing up in a further 3%, with in-adequate mixing in 9%. However, there was no evidence that patients were adversely affected. In two patients errors in the administration of acetylcysteine have been reported (28[A]). In one patient, a 73-year-old woman, only 10% of the recommended doses were ordered for each of the infusion bags; the error was not detected until 40 hours after presentation, when it was corrected; she had a prolonged stay in the intensive care unit, complicated by aspiration pneumonia and sepsis, but recovered fully. In the other, a 28-year-old woman, a similar error occurred; she recovered without problems. The authors suggested that such problems could be avoided if acetylcysteine were prescribed in milliliters rather than mg/kg.

References

1. Guchelaar HJ, Colen HB, Kalmeijer MD, Hudson PT, Teepe-Twiss IM. Medication errors: hospital pharmacist perspective. Drugs 2005;65(13):1735–46.
2. Wheeler SJ, Wheeler DW. Medication errors in anaesthesia and critical care. Anaesthesia 2005;60(3):257–73.
3. Ghaleb MA, Barber N, Dean Franklin B, Wong IC. What constitutes a prescribing error in paediatrics? Qual Saf Health Care 2005;14(5):352–7.
4. Tam VC, Knowles SR, Cornish PL, Fine N, Marchesano R, Etchells EE. Frequency, type and clinical importance of medication history errors at admission to hospital: a systematic review. CMAJ 2005;173(5):510–5.
5. Midlöv P, Bergkvist A, Bondesson A, Eriksson T, Höglund P. Medication errors when transferring elderly patients between primary health care and hospital care. Pharm World Sci 2005;27(2):116–20.
6. Bacić Vrca V, Bećirević-Laćan M, Bozikov V, Birus M. Prescribing medication errors in hospitalised patients: a prospective study. Acta Pharm 2005;55(2):157–67.
7. Mandal K, Fraser SG. The incidence of prescribing errors in an eye hospital. BMC Ophthalmol 2005;5:4.
8. Lisby M, Nielsen LP, Mainz J. Errors in the medication process: frequency, type, and potential clinical consequences. Int J Qual Health Care 2005;17(1):15–22.
9. Rosser W, Dovey S, Bordman R, White D, Crighton E, Drummond N. Medical errors in primary care: results of an international study of family practice. Can Fam Physician 2005;51:386–7.
10. Gandhi TK, Weingart SN, Seger AC, Borus J, Burdick E, Poon EG, Leape LL, Bates DW. Outpatient prescribing errors and the impact of computerized prescribing. J Gen Intern Med 2005;20(9):837–41.
11. Kralewski JE, Dowd BE, Heaton A, Kaissi A. The influence of the structure and culture of med-ical group practices on prescription drug errors. Med Care 2005;43(8):817–25.
12. Al Khaja KA, Al-Ansari TM, Sequeira RP. An evaluation of prescribing errors in primary care in Bahrain. Int J Clin Pharmacol Ther 2005;43(6):294–301.
13. Taylor BL, Selbst SM, Shah AE. Prescription writing errors in the pediatric emergency department. Pediatr Emerg Care 2005;21(12):822–7.
14. Kirk RC, Li-Meng Goh D, Packia J, Min Kam H, Ong BK. Computer calculated dose in paediatric prescribing. Drug Saf 2005;28(9):817–24.
15. van der Hooft CS, Jong GW, Dieleman JP, Verhamme KM, van der Cammen TJ, Stricker BH, Sturkenboom MC. Inappropriate drug prescribing in older adults: the updated 2002 Beers criteria—a population-based cohort study. Br J Clin Pharmacol 2005;60(2):137–44.
16. Yap C, Dunham D, Thompson J, Baker D. Medication dosing errors for patients with renal insufficiency in ambulatory care. Jt Comm J Qual Patient Saf 2005;31(9):514–21.
17. Gray J, Hicks RW, Hutchings C. Antiretroviral medication errors in a national medication error database. AIDS Patient Care STDS 2005;19(12):803–12.
18. DeLorenze GN, Follansbee SF, Nguyen DP, Klein DB, Horberg M, Quesenberry Jr CP, Blick NT, Tsai AL. Medication error in the care of HIV/AIDS patients: electronic surveillance, confirmation, and adverse events. Med Care 2005;43(9 Suppl):III63–8.
19. Dean Franklin B, Vincent C, Schachter M, Barber N. The incidence of prescribing errors in hospital inpatients: an overview of the research methods. Drug Saf 2005;28(10):891–900.
20. Shah NR, Seger AC, Seger DL, Fiskio JM, Kuperman GJ, Blumenfeld B, Recklet EG, Bates DW, Gandhi TK. Improving override rates for computerized prescribing alerts in ambulatory care. AMIA Annu Symp Proc 2005:1110.
21. Shulman R, Singer M, Goldstone J, Bellingan G. Medication errors: a prospective cohort study

of hand-written and computerised physician order entry in the intensive care unit. Crit Care 2005;9(5):R516–21.

22. Delgado Sánchez O, Escrivá Torralva A, Vilanova Boltó M, Serrano López de las Hazas J, Crespí Monjo M, Pinteño Blanco M, Martínez López I, Tejada González P, Cervera Peris M, Fernández Cortés F, Puigventós Latorre F, Barroso Navarro MA. Estudio comparativo de errores con prescripción electrónica versus prescripción manual. Farm Hosp 2005;29(4):228–35.

23. Mirco A, Campos L, Falcão F, Nunes JS, Aleixo A. Medication errors in an internal medicine department. Evaluation of a computerized prescription system. Pharm World Sci 2005;27(4):351–2.

24. van Gijssel-Wiersma DG, van den Bemt PM, Walenbergh-van Veen MC. Influence of computerised medication charts on medication errors in a hospital. Drug Saf 2005;28(12):1119–29.

25. Sano HS, Waddell JA, Solimando Jr DA, Doulaveris P, Myhand R. Study of the effect of standardized chemotherapy order forms on prescribing errors and anti-emetic cost. J Oncol Pharm Pract 2005;11(1):21–30.

26. Lane R, Stanton NA, Harrison D. Applying hierarchical task analysis to medication administration errors. Appl Ergon 2006;37(5):669–79.

27. Ferner RE, Langford NJ, Anton C, Hutchings A, Bateman DN, Routledge PA. Random and systematic medication errors in routine clinical practice: a multicentre study of infusions, using acetylcysteine as an example. Br J Clin Pharmacol 2001;52(5):573–7.

28. Little M, Murray L, McCoubrie D, Daly FF. A potentially fatal prescribing error in the treatment of paracetamol poisoning. Med J Aust 2005;183(10):535–6.

Address list of national centers that participate in the WHO Drug Monitoring Programme

Editor's note: *The details given here were correct at the time of going to press in February 2008. However, details of this sort often change, and readers should contact the WHO Monitoring Programme at Uppsala if they are unable to reach any of the agencies listed using the information given. Countries whose names are in italics are provisional members.*

Algeria
Prof Abdelkader Helali
Tel: +213-21-96 5059
E-mail: pharmacomateriovigilancedz@
hotmail.com

Centre National de Pharmacovigilance et
    Matériovigilance
Ministère de la Santé et de la Population
BP 247, CHU de Bab El Oued
DA-16009 Alger, Algeria

Argentina
Dr Inés Bignone
Tel: +54-11-4340-0800, ext 1154
E-mail: ibignone@anmat.gov.ar

Departamento de Farmacovigilancia (ANMAT)
Avenida de Mayo 869, piso 11o
1084 Buenos Aires, Argentina

Armenia
Dr Anahit Ayvazyan
Tel: +374-1-584020, 584120
Fax: +374-1-542406
E-mail: anaida@pharm.am
Website: www.pharm.am

Department of Rational Therapy, Monitoring of
    Adverse Reactions, and Professional
    Information
Scientific Centre of Drug & Medical
    Technology Expertise
15 Moskovyan Street
Yerevan 375001, Armenia

Australia
Dr Gary Lacey
Tel: +61-2-6232 8310
Fax: +61-2-6232 8392
E-mail: gary.lacey@tga.gov.au

Adverse Drug Reactions Unit
Therapeutics Goods Administration
PO Box 100
Woden, ACT 2606, Australia

Austria
Dr Bettina Schade
Tel: +43-50555 36240
Fax: +43-50555 36207
E-mail: bettina.schade@ages.at

AGES PharmMed
Institut Pharmakovigilanz
Schnirchgasse 9
A-1030 Vienna, Austria

Bahrain
Ms Layla Abdur-Rahman
Tel: +973-25 86 68
Fax: +973-25 93 57
E-mail: lamousawi@hotmail.com

Ministry of Health
Pharmacy and Drug Control
PO Box 28136
Riffa, Bahrain

Belarus
Dr Gennady V Godovalnicov
Tel: +375-17-299 55 10
Fax: +375-17-299 53 58
E-mail: rcpl@rceth.nsys.by
Website: www.rceth.nsys.by

Ministry of Health
Center for Examinations and Test
Health Service Republican Unitary Enterprise
2-a Tovarishcheskij Per
22 0037 Minsk, Belarus

Belgium
Mr. Xavier De Cuyper
Tel: +32-2-5248005
Fax: +32-2-5248003
E-mail: xavier.decuyper@fagg-afmps.be
Website: www.afmps.be

Federal Agency for Medicines and Health
Victor Hortaplein 40, bus 40
B-1060 Brussels, Belgium

Bhutan
Mr Tashi Tobgay
Tel: +975-2-58668
Fax: +975-2-59357
E-mail: tashi_pharmacy@druknet.bt

National Pharmacovigilance Centre
Ministry of Health
Pharmacy Department
JDWNR Hospital, Thimphu, Bhutan

Bhutan
Mr Ugyen Dendup
Tel: +975-2-321 686
Fax: +975-2-324 215
E-mail: ntmpvc@druknet.bt

Traditional Medicines Pharmacovigilance Centre
Pharmaceutical and Research Unit
Institute of Traditional Medicine Service
Post Box 297, Thimphu, Bhutan

Botswana
Ms Motshegwana Olenkie Tebogo
Tel: +267-3632383
Fax: +267-3170169
E-mail: mtebogo@gov.bw

Drug Regulatory Unit
Ministry of Health
Private Bag 00355
Gaborone, Botswana

Brazil
Dr Anthony Wong
Tel: +55-11-3088 9431
Fax: +55-11-3088 9431
E-mail: anthwongbr@aol.com
Website: ceatox.com.br

CEATOX
Sao Paulo Regional Poison and
    Pharmacovigilance Centre
Inst. Crianca
Reference Centre
Av. Dr Enéas de Carvalho Aguiar 647
05403-903 Sao Paulo SP, Brazil

Brazil
Mr Murilo Freitas Dias
Tel: +55-61-448 1219
Fax: +55-61-448 1275
E-mail: murilo.freitas@anvisa.gov.br
Website: anvisa.gov.br/farmacovigilancia

Unidade de Farmacovigilância – UFARM
Agêncabal Nacional de Vigilânca Sanitária –
    ANVISA
SEPN 515 Bl.B Ed. Omega 2 Andar, Sala 2
CEP 70770-502 Brasilia DF, Brazil

Brunei Darussalam
Ms Asma A'tiyah Haji Abdul Hamid
Tel: +673-2-2242424, ext 569
Fax: +673-2-230001
E-mail: aatiyah@brunet.bn

Drug and Poison Information Section
Ministry of Health
RIPAS Hospital
Commonwealth Drive
Jalan Menteri Besar BB3910
Brunei Darussalam

Bulgaria
Dr Kapka Kaneva
Tel: +359-2-9446 999, ext 356
Fax: +359-2-9434 487
E-mail: kaneva@bda.bg
Website: www.bda.bg

Pharmacovigilance Unit
Bulgarian Drug Agency
26 Yanko Sakazov Boulevard
BG-1504 Sofia
Bulgaria

Canada
Dr Barbara Law
Tel: +1-613-952 9730
Fax: +1-613-998 6413
E-mail: barbara_law@hc-sc.gc.ca

Immunization & Respiratory Infections Division
Centre for Infectious Disease Prevention &
    Control, Public Health Agency of Canada
PL 0602C Bldg # 6, Tunney's Pasture 0603EI
Ottawa, Ontario K1A OK9, Canada

Canada
Ms Heather Sutcliffe
Tel: +1-613-946 1138 or 957 0337
Fax: +1-613-957 0335
E-mail: heather_sutcliffe@hc-sc.gc.ca
Website: hc-sc.gc.ca/hpb-dgps/therapeut/

Marketed Health Products Safety &
    Effectiveness Information Division
Marketed Health Products Directorate
Health Canada
Tunney's Pasture, A/L 0701C
Ottawa, Ontario K1A OK9, Canada

Chile
Dra Q F Cecilia Morgado-Cadiz
Tel: +56-2-239 8769
Fax: +56-2-239 8760
E-mail: cmorgado@ispch.cl

Jefa Centro Nacional de Informacion de
    Medicamentos y Farmacovigilancia –
    CENIMEF
Instituto de Salud Publica de Chile
Pharmacovigilance Centre
Avenida Marathon 1000, 3 piso, Nuñoa
Casilla 48 Santiago, Chile

China
Dr Shaohong Jin
E-mail: jinshh@nicpbp.org.cn

Division of ADR Monitoring
Center for Drug Reevaluation
State Food and Drug Administration
Building 11, Fa-Hua-Nan-Li
Chongwen District, Beijing 100061, China

Colombia
Dr José Rodrigo Valcárcel Vela
E-mail: invimafv@invima.gov.co

Grupo de Farmacovigilancia, Subdirección de
    Medicamentos y Productos Biológicos
Instituto Nacional de Vigilancia de
    Medicamentos y Alimentos – INVIMA
Carrera 68 D No. 17-11/21
Bogota, DC, Colombia

Congo, the Democratic Republic of the
Mr Franck Biayi Kanumpepa
Tel: +242-81-812 5838
E-mail: biayifranck@yahoo.fr

Centre National de Pharmacovigilance
Minisère de la Santé
c/o Programme d'Approvisionnement en
   Médicaments Essentiels
Avenue de Pharmacie No. 39
Barumbu
BP 3088 Kin 1
Kinshasa Gombe
Democratic Republic of the Congo

Costa Rica
Dr Adolfo Ortiz Barboza
Tel: +506-221 1662
Fax: +506-221 1167
E-mail: adolfoortizbarboza@yahoo.com

Ministero de Salud Oficinas Centrales
Dirección de Vigilancia de Salud
Centro Nacional de Farmacovigilancia
PO Box 10123-1000, San José, Costa Rica

Croatia
Dr Sinisa Tomic
Tel: +385-146 93 830
Fax: +385-146 73 175
E-mail: sinisa.tomic@almp.hr
Website: www.almp.hr

Croatian Agency for Medicinal Products and
   Medical Devices
Ksaverska Cesta 4
H 10000 Zagreb
Croatia

Cuba
Dra Giset Jiménez López
Tel: +53-7-2065603
Fax: +53-7-2023513
E-mail: giset@mcdf.sld.cu
Website: cdf.sld.cu/farmacovigilancia

Pharmacovigilance Department
Pharmacoepidemiology Development Center
Calle 44 esq. 5ta Ave No 502
Miramar, Playa, Havana CP 11300, Cuba

Cyprus
Dr. Christos Petrou
Tel: +357-22-407 179
Fax: +357-22-407 149
E-mail: cpetrou@phs.moh.gov.cy

Pharmaceutical Services
Ministry of Health
1475 Lefkosia
Cyprus

Czech Republic
Dr Jana Mladá
Tel: +42-2-72185848/72185111
Fax: +42-2-71432377/72185816
E-mail: farmakovigilance@sukl.cz
Website: www.sukl.cz

State Institute for Drug Control
Pharmacovigilance Unit
Srobarova 48
10041 Prague 10
Czech Republic

Denmark
Ms Elin Andersen
Tel: +45-44-88 92 87
Fax: +45-44-88 95 99
E-mail: ela@dkma.dk
Website: dkma.dk

Danish Medicines Agency
Medicines Control Division
Axel Heides gade 1
DK-2300 København
Denmark

Egypt
Dr Radwa Abou-Zeid
Tel: +20-354 5151
Fax: +20-354 5159
E-mail: dynamic1409@yahoo.com

Technical Research & Training Department
Central Administration of Pharmaceutical
   Affairs, Ministry of Health and Population
22 Falky street, Magles el Shaab-Cairo
Cairo, Egypt

Eritrea

Mr Seare Ghebreyesus
Tel: +291-1-120297/122429
Fax: +291-1-122899
E-mail: seareg@mon.gov.er

Drug Information Unit
Ministry of Health
PO Box 212
Asmara, Eritrea

Estonia

Dr Maia Uusküla
Tel: +372-7-374 140
Fax: +372-7-374 142
E-mail: maia.uuskula@sam.ee
Website: sam.ee

Ravimiamet
State Agency of Medicines
1 Nooruse Street
50411 Tartu
Estonia

Ethiopia

Mr Abraham Geberegiorgis Kahsay
Tel: +251-1-52 41 22
Fax: +251-1-52 13 92
E-mail: daca@telecom.net.et

Drug Administration and Control Authority of
  Ethiopia
ADR Monitoring & Promotion Control Division
PO Box 5681
Addis Ababa, Ethiopia

Fiji

Ms Vasiti Nawadra-Taylor
Fax: +679-33 88 003
E-mail: vnawadra@health.gov.fj

Pharmacy Department
Fiji Pharmaceutical Services
PO Box 106
Suva, Fiji

Finland

Prof Erkki Palva
Tel: +358-9-4733-4288/+358-50-5521154
Fax: +358-9-4733 4297
E-mail: erkki.palva@nam.fi
Website: www.nam.fi

National Agency for Medicines
Department of Safety & Drug Information
PO Box 55
Mannerheimintie 103B
SF-00301 Helsinki, Finland

France

Dr Carmen Kreft-Jaïs
Tel: +33-1-5587 3533
Fax: +33-1-5587 3532
E-mail: carmen.kreft-jais@afssaps.sante.fr
Website: afssaps.sante.fr

Agence Francaise de Securité Sanitaire des
  Produits de Santé
Unité de Pharmacovigilance
143-147 Boulevard Anatole France
F-93285 Saint-Denis, Cedex, France

Georgia

Pharmacological Committee
Tel: +995-99-563 451
Fax: +995-99-399 947
E-mail: pharmcom@posta.ge

Pharmacological Committee
29a Mitskevich Street
380060 Tbilisi, Georgia

Germany

Dr Ulrich Hagemann
Tel: +49-228-207-3480
Fax: +49-228-207-4636
E-mail: hagemann@bfarm.de
Website: www.bfarm.de

Federal Institute for Drugs and Medical Devices
Bundesinstitut für Arzneimittel und
  Medizinprodukte
Kurt-Georg-Kiesinger-Allee 3
DE-53175, Bonn, Germany

Germany
Dr Dirk Mentzer
Tel: +49-6103771011
E-mail: mendi@pei.de

Pharmacovigilance Unit
Facharzt für Kinderheilkunde
Paul Ehrlich Institut
Bundesamt für Sera und Impfstoffe
Paul Ehrlich Strasse 51-59
D-66235, Langen, Germany

Ghana
Mr Jonathan Martey
Tel: +233-21-67 30 90
Fax: +233-21-66 0389
E-mail: jmartey@qmail.com

Food and Drugs Board
PO Box CT 2783
Cantonments
Accra, Ghana

Greece
Ms Georgia Terzi-Vaslamatzi
Tel: +30-210-6507337
Fax: +30-210-6549585
E-mail: adr@eof.gr

Adverse Drug Reactions Department
National Organization for Medicines
284 Mesogeion Av
GR-155 62 Athens-Holargos, Greece

Guatemala
Dr José María Del Valle
Tel: +502-24752121-5, ext 136
Fax: +502-24406454
E-mail: jdelvalle@mspas.gob.gt
Website: www.mspas.gob.gt/farmacovigilancia

Programa Nacional de Farmacovigilancia
Asesoría de Medicamentos, MSPAS
6a. Avenida. 3-45 zona 11
Guatemala

Hungary
Dr Mariann Virányi
Tel: +36-1-266 6073
Fax: +36-1-266 6073
E-mail: viranyi.mariann@ogyi.hu

National Institute of Pharmacy
Adverse Drug Reactions Monitoring Centre
Zrínyi u. 3-1051
PO Box 450
H-1372 Budapest, Hungary

Iceland
Prof. Magnús Jóhannsson
Tel: +354-5-20 2114
Fax: +354-5-61 2170
E-mail: magnus.johannsson@lyfjastofnun.is
Website: ww.lyfjastofnun.is

Lyfjastofnun
The Icelandic Medicines Control Agency
Eidistorg 13-15
172 Seltjarnarnes
Iceland

India
Dr. M. Venkateshwarulu
Tel: +91-11-3018806
Fax: +91-11-23012648
E-mail: dci@nb.nic.in

Directorate General of Health Services
Nirman Bhawan
New Delhi 110011, India

Indonesia
Dra. Engko Sosialine M.
Tel: +62-21-4244744 Ext. 111
Fax: +62-21-42883485
E-mail: Indonesia-MESO-BadanPOM@
hotmail.com,
ditwas_dist_ptpkrt@pom.go.id
Website: pom.go.id

National Agency for Drug and Food Control
Jalan Percetakan Negara 23
Jakarta 10560, Indonesia

Iran, Islamic Republic of
Dr Kheirollah Gholami
Tel: +98-21-640 4223
Fax: +98-21-641 7252
E-mail: kheirollah_gholami_2000@yahoo.com

Ministry of Health and Medical Education
Research and Development Office
Iranian ADR Centre
Building no. 3, Fakhr-e-Razi Street, Enghlab Ave
Teheran 13145, Islamic Republic of Iran

Ireland
Ms Niamh Arthur
Tel: +353-1-676 4971
Fax: +353-1-676 2517
E-mail: niamh.arthur@imb.ie
Website: www.imb.ie

Pharmacovigilance Unit
Kevin O'Malley House
Irish Medicines Board
Earlsfort Centre
Earlsfort Terrace
Dublin 2, Ireland

Israel
Dr Dina Hemo
Tel: +972-2-568 1219
Fax: +972-2-672 58 20
E-mail: dina.hemo@moh.health.gov.il

Drug Monitoring Center
Department of Clinical Pharmacology
Ministry of Health
29 Rivka Street, PO Box 1176
Jerusalem 91010, Israel

Italy
Dr Mauro Venegoni
Tel: +39-6-596 841 16
Fax: +39-6-597 841 42
E-mail: m.venegoni@sanita.it

Ufficio Farmacovigilanza
AIFA
Via Sierra Nevada 60
IT-00144 Roma, Italy

Japan
Mr Tamaki Fushimi
E-mail: fushimi-tamaki@mhlw.go.jp

Safety Division
Pharmaceutical and Food Safety Bureau
Ministry of Health, Labour, and Welfare
1-2-2 Kasumigaseki, Chiyoda-Ku
Tokyo 100-8916, Japan

Jordan
Ms Nidaa Bawaresh
Tel. +962-6-4602000
Fax +962-6-4618425
E-mail: Nidaa.Bawaresh@jfda.jo

Jordanian Pharmacovigilance Centre
PO Box 811951, PC 11181
0096 Amman, Jordan

Kazakhstan
Dr Shinara Kulieva
Tel: +7-3172-317414
Fax: +7-3172-317594
E-mail: sh.kulieva@mz.gov.kz

Pharmacy Committee
Ministry of Health of the Republic of Kazakhstan
66 Moskovskaya St
437000 Astana, Kazakhstan

Korea, Republic of
Ms Kyoung-Min Myoung
Tel: +82-2-382 1658 60
Fax: +82-2-382-2870
E-mail: kendy@kfda.go.kr
Website: www.kfda.go.kr

Pharmaceutical Management Team
Korean FDA
231 Jinheungno
Eunpyeong-gu
Seoul 122-704, Republic of Korea

Kyrgyzstan
Dr Zamir Akaev
Tel: +996-312-54 29 10
Fax: +996-312-54 29 10
E-mail: ddp-me@elcat.kg
Website: www.pharm.med.kg

Drug Information Centre
Department of Drug Provision & Medical
  Equipment
Ministry of Health
Tretiya Liniya Street 25
720044 Bishkek, Kyrgyzstan

Latvia
Dr Inese Studere
Tel: +371-6-707 8442
Fax: +371-6-707 8428
E-mail: inese.studere@zva.gov.lv
Website: www.zva.gov.lv

ADR Monitoring Department
State Agency of Medicine of Latvia (SAM)
Jersikas St. 15
LV-1003 Riga
Latvia

Lithuania
Mindaugas Buta
Tel: +370-5-2124059
Fax: +370-5-2639265
E-mail: MindaugasButa@vvkt.lt
Website: www.vvkt.lt

Drug Safety and Information Division
State Medicines Control Agency
9/1 Traku Street
Vilnius, LT 01132
Lithuania

**Macedonia, the Former Yugoslav
Republic of**
Ms Vesna Nasteska-Nedanovska
Tel: +389-2-311 25 00
Fax: +389-2-323 08 57
E-mail: mgu@who.org.mk

Ministry of Health
UL 50 Divizija br 6
1000 Skopje
The Former Yugoslav Republic of Macedonia

Madagascar
Dr Donat P.E. Rakotomanana
Tel: +261-20-22 365 22
Fax: +261-20-22 365 22
E-mail: donat.agmed@blueline.mg

Agence du Médicament
Ex-Pharmacie Centrale
Tsaralalana BP 8145
Antananarivo 101, Madagascar

Malaysia
Mrs Tan Lie Sie

Pharmacovigilance
National Pharmaceutical Control Bureau
Ministry of Health
Malaysia

Malta
Dr Patricia Vella Bonanno
Tel: +356-23-43 91 10/12
Fax: +356-23-43 91 61/58
E-mail: patricia.vella@gov.mt

Medicines Authority
198 Rue D'Argens
Gzira GZR 03
Malta

Mexico
Dra Ma. Del Carmen Becerril Martinez
Tel: +52-55-551 485 81
Fax: +52-55-5080 5451
E-mail: mcbecerril@farmacopea.org.mx
Website: www.cofepris.gob.mx

Ministry of Health
Río Rhin No. 57 Col. Cuauhtémoc
Del. Cuauhtémoc
06700 Mexico City 06500, DF
Mexico

Moldova, Republic of
Dr Lucia Turcan
Tel: +373-22-73 7000
Fax: +373-22-73 7000
E-mail: pharmacovigilance@front.ru
Website: www.amed.md

Drug Authorization, Evaluation, and
   Pharmacovigilance Department
   of the Republic of Moldova Medicines Agency
Str. Korolenko 2/1
Chisinau 2028, Republic of Moldavia

Mongolia
Mrs Nanjaa Tsogzolmaa
Tel: +976-11-321 093
Fax: +976-11-320 633
E-mail: iltbih@yahoo.com

Department of Pharmacy and Medical Equipment
Government Building 8
Ministry of Health
Olimpic Street 2
Sukhbaatar district
Ulaanbaatar 210648, Mongolia

Morocco
Prof Rachida Soulaymani-Bencheikh
Tel: +212-37-6110 47 45 (gsm)
Fax: +212-37-77 71 79
E-mail: rsoulaymani@sante.gov.ma

Centre Anti Poisons et de Pharmacovigilance
Rue Lamfedel Cherkaoui
Rabat Institute
Al Irfane, BP 6671 Rabat, Morocco

Mozambique
Dr Esperanca Julia Sevene
Tel: +258-1-32 52 27 / 32 42 10
Fax: +258-1-32 52 55
E-mail: esevene@health.uem.mz

Drug Information Center (CIMed)
Faculty of Medicine, Department of
   Pharmacology
Eduardo Mondlane University
Av. Salvador Allende n. 702
PO Box 257, Maputo, Mozambique

Nepal
Mr Gajendra Bahadur Bhuju
Tel: +977-1-4780 432
Fax: +977-1-4780 572
E-mail: irishbhuju@hotmail.com
Website: www.dda.gov.np

Department of Drug Administration
Ministry of Health and Population
Bijulibazar, Nayabaneshwor
Kathmandu
Nepal

Netherlands
Prof. Dr A.C. van Grootheest
Tel: +31-73-646 9700
Fax: +31-73-642 6136
E-mail: ac.vangrootheest@lareb.nl
Website: www.lareb.nl

Netherlands Pharmacovigilance Centre Lareb
Goudsbloemvallei 7
NL-5237 MH 's-Hertogenbosch
The Netherlands

New Zealand
Dr Michael Tatley
Tel: +64-3-479 7247
Fax: +64-3-479 0509
E-mail: michael.tatley@stonebow.otago.ac.nz
Website: www.otago.ac.nz/carm

New Zealand Pharmacovigilance Centre
   (N2 PhuC)
Department of Preventive & Social Medicine
University of Otago
PO Box 913, Dunedin 9000
New Zealand

Nigeria
Mrs Adeline Osakwe
Tel: +234-09-6702823
Fax: +234-09-5241108
E-mail: nafdac_npc@yahoo.com
addyosakwe@yahoo.com

National Agency for Food & Drug
Administration and Control (NAFDAC)
Plot 2032 Olusegun Obasanjo Way
Wuse Zone 7
Abuja, Nigeria

Norway

Ms Ingebjorg Buajordet
Tel: +47-22-89 77 00
Fax: +47-22-89 77 99
E-mail: Ingebjorg.Buajordet@
legemiddelverket.no
Website: legemiddelverket.no

Norwegian Medicines Agency
Statens Legemiddelverk
Pharmacovigilance Section
Sven Oftedals vei 8
N-0950 Oslo
Norway

Oman

Dr Sawsan Ahmad Jaffar
Tel: +968-24-600 016
Fax: +968-24-602 287
E-mail: mohphar@omantel.net.om
Website: moh.gov.om

Directorate General of Pharmaceutical Affairs
    and Drug Control
Ministry of Health
PO Box 393
Muscat, PC-113, Sultanate of Oman, Oman

Pakistan

Prof Akhlaque Un-Nabi Khan
Tel: +92-21-588 2997/589 2801
Fax: +92-21-588 1444/589 3062

College of Physicians & Surgeons Pakistan
    (CPSP)
Department of Clinical Pharmacology
7th Central Street
Phase II, Defence Housing Authority
Karachi 75500, Pakistan

Panama

Indira Credidio
Tel: +507-2129404
Fax: +507-2129196
E-mail: icredidio@minsa.gob.pa

Ministerio de Salud
Calle Gorgas. Edificio 237
PO Box 2048
Panama, Panama

Peru

Dra Susana Vasquez Lezcano
Tel: +51-1-471 62 46
Fax: +51-1-470 59 97
E-mail: svasquez@digemid.gob.pe

Centro Nacional de Farmacovigilancia
Equipo de Farmacoepidemiologia
Coronel E odriozola N 103 – San Isidro
(Alt Cdra 32 Av Arequipa)
Lima 11, Peru

Philippines

Dr. Sonia Aqui
Tel: +63-2-8070700

Product Service Division
Bureau of Food and Drugs
Department of Health
Filinvest Corporate City, Alabang
Muntinlupa 1770, Philippines

Poland

Dr Agata Maciejczyk
Tel: +48-22-4921 300
Fax: +48-22-4921 309
E-mail: agata.maciejczyk@urpl.gov.pl
Website: www.urpl.gov.pl

Pharmacovigilence Unit
The Office for Registration of Medicinal
    Products, Medical Devices and Biocidal
    Products
41 Zabkowska Street
PL-03736 Warsaw, Poland

Portugal

Dr Regina Carmona
Tel: +351-21-798 7153
Fax: +351-21-798 7155
E-mail: regina.carmona@infarmed.pt
Website: www.infarmed.pt

National Pharmacovigilance Centre
INFARMED
Parque de Saúde de Lisboa
Avenida do Brasil, no. 53
1749-004 Lisboa, Portugal

Romania
Dr Iuliana Daniela Stanciu
Tel: +40-1-224 1102/224 1710
Fax: +40-1-2243 497
E-mail: daniela.stanciu@anm.ro
Website: www.anm.ro

Adverse Reactions Section
National Medicines Agency
Str Aviator Sanatescu no 48, Sector 1
R-71 324 Bucuresti, Romania

Russian Federation
Prof Victor Cheltsov
Tel: +7-095-1905 427/1903 490
Fax: +7-095-434 02 92
E-mail: ikolesnikova@regmed.ru

Department of Clinical Pharmacology
Miklukho-Maklay Street 8
117198 Moscow
Russian Federation

Serbia
Ms Milena Miljkovic
Tel: +381-11-395 1145
Fax: +381-11-395 1130
E-mail: milena.miljkovic@yahoo.com,
milena.miljkovic@alims.sr.gov.yu
Website: www.alims.sr.gov.yu

Medicines and Medical Devices Agency of Serbia
National Pharmacovigilance Center
Vojvode Stepe 458
11152 Belgrade, Republic of Serbia

Sierra Leone
Mr Wiltshire C.N. Johnson
Tel: +232-22-225983/228497
Fax: +232-22-224526
E-mail: infopharm_pbsl@yahoo.com

Drug Information and Pharmacovigilance Unit
Pharmacy Board of Sierra Leone
64 Siaka Steven Street
Freetown, Sierra Leone

Singapore
Ms Cheng Leng Chan
Tel: +65-6-866 3528
Fax: +65-6-478 9069
E-mail: chan_cheng_leng@hsa.gov.sg
Website: hsa.gov.sg/hsa/cpa/
CPA_pharma_about.htm

Pharmacovigilance Unit
Centre for Drug Administration
Health Sciences Authority
11 Biopolis Way, #11-03 Helios
Singapore 138667

Slovak Republic
Dr Pavol Gibala
Tel: +421-2-50701 239
Fax: +421-2-50701 237
E-mail: gibala@sukl.sk
Website: sukl.sk

Section of Drug Safety and Trials
State Institute for Drug Control
Kvetná 11
825 08 Bratislava 26, Slovak Republic

South Africa
Mr Mukesh Dheda
Tel: +27-12-3120526
E-mail: dhedam@health.gov.za

Pharmacovigilance Unit
Medicine Regulatory Affairs
National Department of Health
Private Bag X828
Pretoria 0001, South Africa

Spain
Dr Francisco José de Abajo
Tel: +34-91-822 5330
Fax: +34-91-822 5386
E-mail: fabajo@agemed.es
Website: www.agemed.es

Agencia Española de Medicamentos y
    Productos Sanitarios
División de Farmacoepidemiología y
    Farmacovigilancia
C/ Campezo 1, Edif. 8
E-28022 Madrid, Spain

Sri Lanka
Dr Shalini Sri Ranganathan
Tel: +94-1-695 300 ext 41 03 17
Fax: +94-1-695 300
E-mail: sshalini14@hotmail.com

Faculty of Medicine
University of Colombo
Kynsey Road, PO Box 271
Colombo 8, Sri Lanka

Suriname
Ms Naomi T Jessurun
Tel: +597-597 422 222, ext 376
Fax: +597-1-597 440 331
E-mail: hospitalpharmacy@azp.sr

Pharmacovigilance Centre Surinam
c/o Pharmacy Department
Academic Hospital Paramaribo
Flustraat
PO Box 389
Paramaribo, Surinam

Sweden
Dr Gunilla Sjölin-Forsberg
Tel: +46-18-17 47 98
Fax: +46-18-54 85 66
E-mail: gunilla.sjolin-forsberg@mpa.se
Website: www.mpa.se

Pharmacovigilance Unit
Medical Products Agency
Box 26
S-751 03 Uppsala, Sweden

Switzerland
Mr Ruedi Stoller
Tel: +41-31-322 0348
Fax: +41-31-322 0418
E-mail: Rudolf.Stoller@swissmedic.ch
Website: swissmedic.ch

Swissmedic
Schweizerisches Heilmittelinstitut
Pharmacovigilance Zentrum
Erlachstrasse 8
CH-3000 Bern 9, Switzerland

Tanzania, United Republic of
Mr. Adelard Bartholomew Mtenga
Tel: +255-22-245 0512 / 245 07 93
Fax: +255-22-245 0793
E-mail: amtengab@yahoo.com

Pharmacovigilance Unit
National ADR Monitoring Centre
The Tanzania Food and Drug Authority
PO Box 77150
Dar Es Salaam, United Republic of Tanzania

Thailand
Mrs Wimon Suwankesawong
Tel: +66-2-590 7261/53
Fax: +66-2-590 7269/591 8459
E-mail: wimon@fda.moph.go.th
Website: www.fda.moph.go.th

Thai National ADRM Centre
Food and Drug Administration
Ministry of Public Health
Ti-wa-nondh Road
Nonthaburi 11000, Thailand

Tunisia
Professor Chalbi Belkahia
Tel: +216-71-56 47 63/57 84 88
Fax: +216-71-57 13 90
E-mail: chalbi.belkahia@rns.tn

Centre National de Pharmacovigilance
9, Avenue Dr Zouheïr Essafi
1006 Tunis
Tunisia

Turkey
Mrs Demet Aydinkarahaliloglu
Tel: +90-312-309 1141/1192
Fax: +90-312-309 7118
E-mail: tufam@saglik.gov.tr
Website: www.iegm.gov.tr

Turkish Pharmacovigilance Center, TUFAM
Department of Quality Control
General Directorate of Pharmaceutical and
    Pharmacy, Ministry of Health
Cankiri Caddesi, No 57
06060 Diskapi, Ankara, Turkey

Uganda
Ms Helen Byomire-Ndagije
Tel: +256-41-347391/2
Fax: +256-41-342921/222469/222881
E-mail: hbyomire@nda.or.ug
Website: www.nda.or.ug

National Drug Authority
Plot 46/48 Lumumba Avenue
PO Box 23096
Kampala
Uganda

Ukraine
Prof Alexey Viktorov
Tel: +380-44249 7001
Fax: +380-44249 7001
E-mail: vigilance@pharma-center.kiev.ua
Website: www.pharma-center.kiev.ua

Pharmacovigilance Department
State Pharmacological Center
Ministry of Health of Ukraine
18 Chygorina Street, 01042 Kiev
Ukraine

United Kingdom
Dr June Raine
Tel: +44-20-7084 2400
Fax: +44-20-7084 2675
E-mail: june.raine@mhra.gsi.gov.uk
Website: www.mhra.gov.uk

Vigilance and Risk Management of Medicines
   Division
Medicines and Healthcare products Regulatory
   Agency
Market Towers
1 Nine Elms Lane
London SW8 5NQ, UK

United States of America
Dr M Miles Braun
Tel: +1-301-827 3974
Fax: +1-301-827 5218
E-mail: miles.braun@fda.hhs.gov

Division of Epidemiology, HFM-222
Center for Biologics Evaluation and Research
Food and Drug Administration
1401 Rockville Pike
Rockville, MD 20852, USA

United States of America
Dr Gerald Dal Pan
Tel: +1-301-827 3172
E-mail: dalpang@fda.hhs.gov

Office of Drug Safety
Center for Drug Evaluation and Research
Food and Drug Administration
5600 Fishers Lane, Room 15 B33
Rockville, MD 20857, USA

Uruguay
Dra Maria Cristina Alonzo
Tel: +598-2-4028032
Fax: +598-2-4028032
E-mail: farmacovigilancia@msp.gub.uy

Ministerio de Salud Publica
Direccion General de la Salud
Avenida 18 de Julio 1892, P. 2, Of. 219
CP 11.200 Montevideo, Uruguay

Uzbekistan
Dr Bakhtiyor Shoislamov
Tel: +998-711-444823
Fax: +998-711-444825
E-mail: bshaislamov@yandex.ru

Pharmacological Committee of HDDMEQC
Curator of Adverse Reaction Monitoring
   Commission
Usmankhodjaev St
K Umarov passage 16
700002 Tashkent, Uzbekistan

Venezuela
Drs María Aguilar
Tel: +58-212-662 4797
Fax: +58-212-693 1455
E-mail: liurdaneta@inhrr.gov.ve

Instituto Nacional de Higiene "Rafael Rangel"
Centro Nacional de Vigilancia Farmacológia
   (CENAVIF)
Ciudad Universitaria
Caracas 1010, Venezuela

Vietnam

Mrs. Nguyen Thu Thuy
Tel: +84-4-823 5812
Fax: +84-4-823 1253
E-mail: thuy_adr@yahoo.com

Centre of ADR Monitoring of Viet Nam
138 A – Glang Vo Street – Ba Dinh Dist.
Hanoi
Vietnam

Zambia

Dr Oscar O Simooya
Tel: +260-2-222206/231850/230562
Fax: +260-2-228319/222469/222881
E-mail: cbumed@zamnet.zm

Copperbelt University Health Services
PO Box 21692
Kitwe
Zambia

Zimbabwe

Ms. Gugu N. Mahlangu
Tel: +263-4-736981-5
Fax: +263-4-736980
E-mail: mcaz@africaonline.co.zw
Website: www.mcaz.co.zw

Medicines Control Authority
106 Baines Avenue
PO Box 10559
Harare, Zimbabwe

Index of drugs

Note. **Boldface** page numbers refer to main discussions.

5-aminosalicyclic acid
see mesalazine
6-mercaptopurine
potentiation, + mesalazine, 429
6-thioguanine
liver effects, **461**
during pregnancy, **461**

A

abacavir
immunologic effects, **348**
acarbose
liver effects, **496**
observational studies, **496**
vitamin B_6 concentration, 496
ACE inhibitors
see also specific drugs
angioedema, 234–235
diclofenac inhibition, 236
lithium toxicity, **26**
renal insufficiency, + aprotinin,
235
acebutolol
cutaneous lupus erythematosus,
223–224
acecainide
clearance, + levofloxacin, 300
acetaminophen
see paracetamol
acetazolamide
electrolyte balance, **255–256**
eye function, **255**
nervous system effects,
254–255
Stevens–Johnson syndrome,
256
acetylsalicylic acid
adverse reactions management,
129
end-stage renal disease,
128–129
gastrointestinal bleeding, +
SSRIs, 16–17
gastrointestinal effects, **128**
aciclovir
nervous system effects,
343–344
acitretin
dysphonia, 185
hyperostosis, 185
pseudoporphyria, 185
rectal bleeding, 185
sensorineural hearing loss, 185

acupuncture
cardiovascular effects, **556–557**
adalimumab
tumorigenicity, **439**
adapalene
see tazarotene
adefovir
observational studies, **344**
adenosine
comparative studies, **212**
sinus arrest, 213
adenosine receptor agonists
general effects, **213**
adrenaline (epinephrine)
cardiovascular effects, **170–171**
Agnus castus
general effects, **552**
airway anesthesia
laryngospasm, 152
ajmaline and derivatives
Brugada syndrome, 213
albendazole
eye pain, 364
pancytopenia, 364
albumin
general effects, **381**
albuterol
see salbutamol
alefacept
tumorigenicity, **440**
alemtuzumab
hematologic effects, **442–443**
infection risk, **443**
alfuzosin
general effects, **246**
aliskiren
see direct renin inhibitors
Allium sativum (garlic)
concomitant warfarin, **400**
alosetron
constipation, 423
alpha-glucosidase inhibitors
comparative studies, **496**
alprazolam
comparative studies, **49**
endocrine effects, **49–50**
psychological effects, **49**
withdrawal, **50**
aluminium
macrophagic myofasciitis, 262
susceptibility factors, **262–263**
aluminium adsorbent
general effects, **370–371**

ambrisentan
general effects, **245**
amfebutamone
see bupropion
aminolevulinic acid
nervous system effects, **184**
amiodarone
ataxia, 214
cardiovascular effects, **214**
comparative studies, **213–214**
diagnosis of reactions, **216**
eye function, 214–215
hepatic damage, 215
immunologic effects, **216**
low back pain, 216
metronidazole clearance, 216
respiratory effects, **214**
skin, **215–216**
susceptibility factors, **216**
amisulpride
clearance, + ciclosporin, 452
amlodipine
anasarca, 225–226
nails, **225**
amobarbital
ineffectiveness, + zonisamide,
100
amphetamines
cardiovascular effects, **1**
interactions, 2
nervous system effects, **1**
amphotericin B deoxycholate
(DAMB)
formulations, **319**
urinary tract, **319**
amphotericin B lipid complex
(ABLC)
monitoring therapy, **318–319**
susceptibility factors, **318**
urinary tract, **317–318**
amygdalin
interactions, **556**
toxicity, + vitamin C, 394
anagrelide
cardiovascular effects, **413**
renal tubular damage, 413
androgenic anabolic steroids
psychological effects, **478**
Angelica sinesis (dong quai)
concomitant warfarin, **400**
angiotensin converting enzyme
inhibitors
see ACE inhibitors

angiotensin II receptor
  antagonists
    see also specific drugs
  angioedema, 238–240
  cardiovascular effects, **240**
  fetotoxicity, **240–241**
anidulafungin
  concomitant antifungal azoles,
    320–321
  interactions, **330**
antacids
  absorption, + itraconazole, 321
  erlotinib absorption, 526
  fetotoxicity, **423**
anti-human CD40Mab chimeric
    5D12
  gastrointestinal effects, **443**
  observational studies, **443**
antiandrogens
  dosage regimens, **479**
antibiotics
  see also specific drugs and
    classes
  lithium toxicity, 26
anticholinergic drugs
  eyes, **177**
  nervous system effects, **177**
  psychological effects, **177**
anticoagulants
  gastrointestinal bleeding, +
    non-steroidal
    anti-inflammatory drugs
    (NSAIDs), 128
  hemorrhage, + epoprostenol,
    465
antidiarrheal agents
  placebo-controlled studies, **426**
antidysrhythmic drugs
  QT interval prolongation, 212
antiepileptic drugs
  see also specific drugs and
    classes
  effectiveness, + oral
    contraceptives, 78
  fractures, 78
antihistamines (H_1)
  ketoconazole clearance, 321
antihypertensives
  monitoring therapy, **234**
antimony
  cardiovascular effects, **263**
antipsychotic drugs
  cardiovascular effects, **56–57**
  comparative studies, **56**
  elderly patients, **59–61**
  endocrine effects, **58**
  metabolism effects, **58–59**
  nervous system effects, **57–58**
antiretroviral drugs
  dosage regimens, **347**
  observational studies, **347**
antithyroid drugs
  immunologic effects, **491**
  teratogenicity, **491–492**

apenems
  concentration, + valproic acid,
    283–284
aprinidine
  hematologic effects, **216–217**
aprotinin
  renal insufficiency, + ACE
    inhibitors, 235
arginine
  placebo-controlled studies, **396**
aripiprazole
  clearance, + itraconazole, 321
  formulations, **61**
  galactorrhea, 61
  placebo-controlled studies, **61**
aromatase inhibitors
  comparative studies, **475–476**
arsenic
  edema, 263
artemisinin
  nervous system effects, **338**
artesunate, **338**
articaine
  immunologic effects, **158**
  metabolism effects, **158**
ASA
  see acetylsalicylic acid
aspirin
  see acetylsalicylic acid
atazanavir
  metabolism effects, **351**
atenolol
  clearance, + rifampicin, 361
  concomitant itraconazole, 321
atorvastatin
  leukopenia, 516
  rhabdomyolysis, + fluconazole,
    322
azathioprine
  liver effects, **459–460**
  psychiatric effects, **459**
  susceptibility factors, **461**
azithromycin
  cardiovascular effects, **302**
  liver effects, **302**
  skin effects, **302**
aztreonam
  erythroderma, 286

B
Bacille Calmette–Guérin (BCG)
    vaccine
  BCG disease, 372
  susceptibility factors, **372**
baclofen
  concomitant propofol, 143
  overdose, **165**
  susceptibility factors, **165**
basiliximab
  infection risk, **444**
  susceptibility factors, **444**
BCG
  see Bacille Calmette–Guérin
    (BCG) vaccine

bee sting venom
  adverse reactions management,
    572
benzimidazoles
  comparative studies, **364**
benzocaine
  methemoglobinemia, 158–159
  tachycardia, 158
beta$_2$-adrenoceptor agonists
  cardiovascular effects, **200**
  respiratory effects, **198–199**
  susceptibility factors, **199–200,
    200**
beta-adrenoceptor antagonists
  cardiovascular effects, **223**
  formulations, **224**
  immunologic effects, **224**
  overdose, **224**
  respiratory effects, **223**
  sexual function, **224**
beta-lactam antibiotics
  contamination, **283**
  cross reactivity, **280–283**
  hematologic, **280**
  nervous system effects, **280**
bevacizumab
  observational studies, **544**
  skin, **444**
bicalutamide
  breasts, **480**
  endocrine effects, **479–480**
  tumorigenicity, **480**
biguanides
  altered vision, 497
  formulations, **497**
  liver effects, **497**
  overdose, **498**
  during pregnancy, **497**
  susceptibility factors, **497**
bile acids
  during pregnancy, **429**
bismuth
  urinary tract, **264**
bisoprolol
  benign prostatic hyperplasia
    exacerbation, 223
bisphosphonates
  osteonecrosis, **562–564**
bitter orange
  see Citrus aurantium
black cohosh
  see Cimicifuga racemosa
[beta]-blockers
  see [beta]-adrenoceptor
    antagonists
blood transfusion
  general effects, **381–382**
  immunologic effects, **382**
  infection risk, **383**
  purpura, 382
  susceptibility factors, **383**
  transfusion-related acute lung
    injury (TRALI), 382

bosentan
  general effects, **245**
botulinum toxins
  adverse reactions management,
    167–168
  immunologic effects, **167**
  myofascial necrosis, 166–167
  nervous system effects, **166**
  observational studies, **165–166**
  parasympathetic dysfunction of
    the visual system, 166
  skin, **166**
  susceptibility factors, **167**
  systemic reviews, **165**
  tolerance, **167**
brinzolamide
  metabolic acidosis, 256
brotizolam
  erythromycin concentration, 50
budesonide
  fetotoxicity, **193–194**
  formulations, **195–196**
  during pregnancy, **193**
  susceptibility factors, **194–195**
buprenorphine
  death, **119**
  Gamella morbillorum
    infection, 118–119
  gastrointestinal effects, **118**
  immunologic effects, **118**
  interactions, **119**
  during lactation, **119**
  liver effects, **118**
  placebo-controlled studies, **118**
  during pregnancy, **119**
  psychiatric effects, **118**
  respiratory depression, 118
  sexual function, **118**
  susceptibility factors, **119**
bupropion
  concentration, + erythromycin,
    303
  concomitant menthol, 568–569
  concomitant metamfetamine, 3
  CYP2D6 inhibition, 20
  hyponatremia, 20
  psychiatric effects, **20**

C

C1 inhibitor concentrate
  general effects, **383–384**
caffeine
  absorption, + menthol, 569
  overdose, **5**
calciferol
  see vitamin D
calcipotriol
  nails, **186**
  skin, **186**
calcitonin
  mineral balance, 507
calcium
  absorption, + gatifloxacin, 299

calcium channel blockers
  see also specific drugs
  overdose, **225**
calcium dobesilate
  hematologic, **231**
Camellia sinensis (green tea)
  concomitant warfarin, **401**
camphor
  general effects, **564**
candesartan
  cholestasis, 241
  hyperkalemia, +
    spironolactone, 241
  pancreatitis, 241
cannabinoids
  angle-closure glaucoma, 33
  cardiovascular effects, **31–32**
  fetotoxicity, **34**
  nervous system effects, 32
  psychiatric effects, **33**
  psychological effects, **32–33**
  respiratory effects, **33**
  tumorigenicity, **34**
carbamazepine
  asthenozoospermia, 79
  erythema multiforme, 79
  hyponatremia, 78–79
  interactions, **79**
  nervous system effects, **78**
  oxybutynin concentration, 178
  susceptibility factors, **79**
carbapenems
  valproate concentration, 97
cardiac glycosides
  cardiovascular effects, **209**
  diagnostic test interference,
    211
  interactions, **210–211**
  monitoring therapy, **211**
  necrotic enterocolitis, 209–210
  overdose, **210**
  platelet activation, 209
  susceptibility factors, **210**
caspofungin
  interactions, **330–331**
  observational studies, **330**
  susceptibility factors, **330**
caudal anesthesia
  susceptibility factors, **152**
cefaclor
  anaphylactic reaction, 284–285
cefepime
  nervous system effects, **285**
cefoperazone
  agranulocytosis, 285
cefprozil
  rash, 285
ceftroxone
  hemolytic anemia, 285
  immunologic effects, **286**
  nephrolithiasis, 285
  pseudotumor cerebri, 285
cefuroxime
  cardiovascular effects, **286**

  during lactation, **286**
celecoxib
  urinary tract, **130**
cephalosporins
  hemolytic anemia, 284
cetirizine
  interactions, **189**
Chinese wolfberry
  see Lycium barbarum
chiropractic
  see spinal manipulation
chloral hydrate
  susceptibility factors, **52–53**
chloramphenicol
  paroxysmal nocturnal
    hemoglobinuria, 298
chlorhexidine
  mouth, **278–279**
  placebo-controlled studies, **278**
chloroquine, + proguanil
  liver, **336**
chlorphenesin
  contact allergy, 279
chlorpromazine
  corneal deposits, **61**
chlorthalidone
  myopia, 257
chromium
  cardiovascular effects, **264**
cibenzoline
  Brugada syndrome, 217
ciclesonide
  metabolism effects, **196**
  placebo-controlled studies, **196**
ciclosporin
  adverse reactions management,
    453
  cardiovascular effects, **452**
  concentration, + orlistat, 430
  concentration, + vitamin E, 395
  concomitant anidulafungin,
    330
  concomitant caspofungin,
    330–331
  concomitant ketoconazole,
    321–322
  concomitant micafungin, 332
  interactions, **452–453**
  nervous system effects, **452**
  potassium channel syndrome,
    452
  seizures, + ketamine, 452–453
  urinary tract, **452**
cidofovir
  skin, **343**
  urinary tract, **343**
cilazapril
  hypotension, 235
  uremia, 235
cilostazol
  interactions, **231**
Cimicifuga racemosa (black
    cohosh)
  general effects, **552**

ciprofloxacin
  acute generalized
    exanthematous pustulosis
    (AGEP), 298
  acute renal insufficiency, 298
  eye function, **298**
  metabolism, +
    cyclophosphamide, 298
  musculoskeletal effects, **298**
  tonic-clonic seizures, 298
cisplatin
  valproate concentration, 96
citalopram
  psychological effects, **17–18**
citrate
  mineral balance, **399**
Citrus aurantium (bitter orange)
  general effects, **552**
clarithromycin
  digoxin concentration, 210
  drug–drug interactions, **302**
  hypotension, + nifedipine, 228
  myopathy, + statins, 517
  sensorineural hearing loss, 302
  skin, **302**
clindamycin
  skin, **302**
clomiphene
  teratogenicity, **474**
clonidine
  nervous system effects, **246**
  overdose, **246**
clopidogrel
  adverse reactions management,
    416–417
  concomitant statins, 517
  hematologic effects, **415–416**
  immunologic effects, **416**
  liver effects, **416**
  resistance, **416**
clove oil
  see Eugenia caryophyllus
clozapine
  cardiomyopathy, 62
  fluvoxamine concentration, 64
  hypersalivation, 63
  metabolism effects, **62–63**
  nervous system effects, **62**
  neutropenia, 63
  observational studies, **62**
  overdose, **63–64**
  susceptibility factors, **61–62,
    63**
  weight loss, + modafinil, 6
co-trimoxazole
  nervous system effects,
    338–339
cobalt
  device failure, 265
cocaine
  cochleovestibular deficit, 34
  concomitant modafinil, 7
  fetotoxicity, **35–36**
  liver effects, **35**

  overdose, **36**
  subarachnoid hemorrhage, 34
colchicine
  interactions, **133–134**
  myopathy, + statins, 517–518
  susceptibility factors, **133**
  treatment guidelines, 133
colestyramine
  thyroid hormone concentration,
    + propythiouracil, 492
colistin
  nervous system effects, **306**
  skin, **306**
  susceptibility factors, **306**
  urinary tract, **306**
combination vaccines
  safety profile, **369–370**
contrast media
  comparative studies, **533–534**
  fetotoxicity, **537–538**
  immunologic effects, **537**
  nephrotoxicity, **535–537**
copper
  general effects, 265
corticosteroids
  gastrointestinal bleeding, +
    non-steroidal anti-
    inflammatory drugs,
    128
cosmetics
  immunologic effects, **180–181**
  observational studies, **180**
  skin, **180**
coumarin anticoagulants
  concentration, +
    clarithromycin, 302
  gastrointestinal effects, **399**
  hematologic effects, **399–400**
COX-2 inhibitors (coxibs)
  see also celecoxib; rofecoxib
  concomitant opioids, 108–109
crack
  see cocaine
Cucurbita pepo
  concomitant warfarin, **401**
cupping
  skin, **557**
cyclophosphamide
  concomitant itraconazole, 322
  metabolism, + ciprofloxacin,
    298
  metabolism, + phenytoin, 86
  during pregnancy, **453**

D

dabigatran
  hematologic effects, **409**
daclizumab
  infection risk, **445**
  observational studies, **445**
dalbavancin
  comparative studies, **300–301**
danshen
  see Salvia mitiorrhiza

dapsone
  hematologic, **357**
daptomycin
  myopathy, **309**
  nervous system effects, **309**
  susceptibility factors, **310**
dasatinib
  dosage regimens, **523**
  pharmacokinetics, **523**
  skin, **524**
daunorubicin
  see anthracyclines
DDAVP
  see desmopressin
deferasirox
  general effects, **273**
deferiprone
  observational studies, **273–274**
deferoxamine
  during pregnancy, **274**
deflazacort
  see glucocorticoids
denileukin diftitox
  hematologic effects, **438**
dental anesthesia
  visual disturbances, 154
desflurane
  cardiac arrest, 137
  liver damage, 138
  malignant hyperthermia, 138
  respiratory effects, **138**
  sister chromatid exchange, 138
desloratadine
  biliary colic, 189
  susceptibility factors, **189**
desmopressin
  electrolyte balance, **512**
dexloxiglumide
  clearance, + ketoconazole, 322
dextrans
  cardiovascular effects, **384**
dextromethorphan
  formulations, **109**
  susceptibility factors, **109**
dextropropoxyphene
  overdose, **109–110**
diamorphine
  abuse, 110
  asthma, 110
  contamination, 110
  toxic leukoencephalopathy, 110
diazepam
  genotoxicity, **51**
  hypothalamic-pituitary-adrenal
    axis suppression, 50–51
  placebo-controlled studies, **50**
  self-aggressive behavior, 50
diclofenac
  ACE inhibitor inhibition, 236
didanosine
  concentration, + tenofovir, 348
  placebo-controlled studies, 348
diethylcarbamazine
  dosage regimens, **365**

diethylene glycol
  renal insufficiency, 567
digoxin
  concomitant exenatide, 500
diltiazem
  gingival enlargement, 226
  skin, **226**
dipeptidyl peptidase IV inhibitors
  metabolism effects, **498–499**
  observational studies, **498**
  pharmacokinetics, **498**
  placebo-controlled studies, **498**
diphenhydramine
  overdose, **189–190**
dipyridamole
  bronchospasm, 413
dipyrone
  agranulocytosis, 132–133
direct renin inhibitors
  clinical studies, **243**
  combination therapy, **243–244**
  general effects, **242–243**
  hyperkalemia, 244
  interactions, **244**
  mechanism of action, **243**
  pharmacokinetics, **243**
  during pregnancy, **244**
  susceptibility factors, **244**
disopyramide
  observational studies, **217**
diuretic sulfonamides
  hypersensitivity, **252–254**
diuretics
  open-angle glaucoma, 252
divalproex
  see also valproate
  vs. lithium, **24**
dobutamine
  ventricular tachycardia, 173
dofetilide
  torsade de pointes, 217
domperidone
  nervous system effects, **423**
donepezil
  cardiovascular effects, **9**
  comparative studies, **8–9**
  endocrine effects, **9–10**
  observational studies, **8**
  placebo-controlled studies, **9**
  susceptibility factors, **10**
dopamine receptor agonists
  gambling, 174–175
dorzolamide
  allergic contact dermatitis, 256
  anosmia, 256
  toxic epidermal necrolysis, +
    timolol, 224
doxazosin
  overdose, **246**
doxorubicin
  cardiovascular effects, **529**
doxycycline
  esophageal ulcers, 289–290
  nail discoloration, 290

placebo-controlled studies, **289**
  tooth discoloration, 289
drometrizole trisiloxane
  contact dermatitis, 184–185
droperidol
  concomitant morphine, 113
  general effects, **64**
drotrecogin alfa
  hematologic effects, **381**
duloxetine
  cardiovascular effects, **19**

E

Echinacea species
  general effects, **553**
echinocandins
  general effects, **329–330**
ecstasy
  cardiovascular effects, **39–40**
  cognitive deficits, 40
  death, **42**
  depression, 40–41
  epidemiology, **37–39**
  hyperthermia, 41–42
  immunosuppression, 41
  susceptibility factors, **43**
  tolerance, **42–43**
EDTA
  see ethylene diamine
    tetra-acetic acid (EDTA)
efalizumab
  cervical cancer, 445
  infection risk, **445**
  musculoskeletal effects, **445**
  skin, **445**
  thrombocytopenia, 445
efavirenz
  breasts, 350
  indinavir clearance, 351
  interactions, **350**
  metabolism effects, **349–350**
  nervous system effects, **349**
  susceptibility factors, **350**
eflornithine
  comparative studies, **341**
Eleutheroccus senticosus
  (Siberian ginseng)
  digoxin readings, 211
EMLA cream
  skin, **157**
enalapril
  allergic reaction, + sirolimus,
    236
  fetotoxicity, **236**
  hyperkalemia, 236
  pancreatitis, 236
  syndrome of inappropriate
    antidiuretic hormone
    secretion, 235
entacavir
  general effects, **344**
enteral nutrition
  comparative studies, **396**

Ephedra and ephedrine
  vasospasm, 171
epidural analgesia
  general effects, 108
epidural anesthesia
  hypersensitivity, 153
eplerenone
  susceptibility factors, **259**
epoetin
  see erythropoietins
epoprostenol
  hemorrhage, + anticoagulants,
    465
eprosartan
  general effects, **241**
erlotinib
  interactions, **526**
  pharmacokinetics, **526**
  rash, 526
ertapenem
  seizures, 284
erythromycin
  brotizolam concentration, 50
  interactions, **303**
  liver effects, **302–303**
erythropoietins
  cardiovascular effects, **389**
  general effects, **388**
  headache, 389
  hematologic effects, **389**
  peritonitis, 389
  skin, **389**
  tumorigenicity, **389**
escitalopram
  see citalopram
esomeprazole
  comparative studies, **424**
estrogens
  administration route, **469**
etanercept
  infection risk, **440**
ethambutol
  optic neuropathy, **358–359**
etherified starches
  general effects, **384**
ethylene diamine tetra-acetic acid
  (EDTA)
  general effects, **276**
etomidate
  endocrine effects, **141**
  nervous system effects,
    140–141
Eugenia caryophyllus
  liver effects, **553**
everolimus
  adverse reactions management,
    454
  clearance, + ketoconazole, 322
  comparative studies, **454**
  monitoring therapy, **454**
exenatide
  administration route, **500**
  concomitant digoxin, 210
  gastrointestinal effects, **499**

immunologic effects, **500**
interactions, **500**
metabolism effects, **499**
tumorigenicity, **500**
ezetimibe
liver effects, **515**

F

factor VIIa
cardiovascular effects, **387**
susceptibility factors, **387**
factor VIII
immunologic effects, **387–388**
factor IX
hematologic effects, **388**
immunologic effects, **388**
fanolesomab
marketing withdrawal, **446**
fat emulsions
general effects, **397**
felodipine
concomitant menthol, 569
gingival enlargement, 226
fenfluramines
overdose, 7
fentanyl
abuse, **111**
during breast feeding, **111**
gastrointestinal effects, **111**
hypothalamic-pituitary-adrenal
axis suppression, **111**
observational studies, **110–111**
respiratory effects, **111**
susceptibility factors, **111**
fexofenadine
clearance, + itraconazole,
322–323
general effects, **190**
fibrates
liver effects, **515**
filgrastim
see granulocyte
colony-stimulating factor
finasteride
breast effects, **483**
cataract, 482
comparative studies, **480–481**
endocrine effects, **482**
libido, reduced, 481
metabolism effects, **482**
myocardial infarction, 482
myopathy, 482
observational studies, **480**
pancreatic effects, **482**
psychosis, + sibutramine, 484
reproductive system effects,
483
sexual function, **482–483**
fish oils
cardiovascular effects, **515**
flecainide
monitoring therapy, **217–218**
neuropathy, 217
susceptibility factors, **217**

ventricular tachycardia, 217
fluconazole
concomitant statins, 518
erythema multiforme, 325
liver effects, **325**
rhabdomyolysis, + atorvastatin,
322
susceptibility factors, **325–326**
teratogenicity, 325
fluoroquinolones
hyperglycemia, 298
teratogenicity, **298**
flutamide
libido, reduced, 481
metabolism effects, **484–485**
fluticasone propionate
formulations, **197**
susceptibility factors, **197**
fluvoxamine
clearance, + sildenafil, 18
clozapine concentration, 64
lidocaine clearance, 218
neuroleptic malignant
syndrome, + quetiapine, 68
olanzapine clearance, 66
folinic acid
see leucovorin
fondaparinux
immunologic effects, **412**
formoterol
dosage regimens, **201**
formulations, **200–201**
fosmidomycin
susceptibility factors, **310**
fosphenytoin
see phenytoin
fresh frozen plasma
respiratory effects, **384**
furazolidone
anorexia, 341
fixed drug eruption, 341

G

G-CSF
see granulocyte-colony
stimulating factor
gabapentin
concomitant morphine, 113
overdose, **80**
placebo-controlled studies, **80**
gadolinium-based contrast agents
nephrogenic systemic fibrosis,
538–540
gallium
general effects, 265
garlic
see Allium sativum
gatifloxacin
absorption, + calcium, 299
availability, + multivitamins,
394
metabolism effects, **299**
susceptibility factors, **299**

gefitinib
adverse reactions management,
525
clearance, + ketoconazole, 323
diarrhea, 525
hair, **525**
nails, **525**
pharmacokinetics, **524**
respiratory effects, **524–525**
skin, **525**
gelatine
anaphylactic reactions, 371
gemfibrozil
atorvastatin clearance, 518
pioglitazone clearance, 501
gemtuzumab ozogamicin
cardiovascular effects, **446**
observational studies, **446**
gentamicin
retinal damage, 297
urinary tract, **297**
ginger
see Zingiber officinale
Ginkgo biloba
concomitant warfarin, **401**
hematologic effects, **553**
interactions, **553–554**
intracerebral bleeding, +
ibuprofen, 401
ginseng
see Panax ginseng
glibenclamide
during pregnancy, **501**
glimepiride
liver effects, **501**
globulins
comparative studies, **384–385**
lymphoproliferative disorder,
385
mucormycosis, 385
glucocorticoids
praziquantel concentration, 367
glucosamine
comparative studies, **568**
general effects, **567–568**
placebo-controlled studies, **568**
glyburide
see glibenclamide
glyceryl trinitrate
headache, 225
migraine, 225
oxygen desaturation, 225
glycoprotein IIb-IIIa inhibitors
hematologic effects, **414–415**
gold
dermatitis, 181
gold and gold salts
comparative studies, **265**
observational studies, **265**
gonadotropins
ovarian hyperstimulation,
468–469
during pregnancy, **469**
granulocyte colony-stimulating
factor (G-CSF)

cardiovascular effects, **435**
respiratory effects, **435**

H

H. pylori eradication regimens
general effects, **340–341**
observational studies, **425–426**
haematitium
liver effects, **556**
hair dyes
asthma, 181
genotoxicity, **181–182**
immunologic effects, **181**
teratogenicity, **182**
tumorigenicity, **182**
halogenated vapors
comparative studies, **137**
endocrine effects, **137**
metabolism effects, **137**
haloperidol
dyskinesia, 61
extrapyramidal symptoms, 69
he shou wu
see Polygonum multiflorum
Hemophilus influenzae vaccine
injury compensation, 373
heparins
cholesterol crystal embolism,
404
hematoma, 404
hyperkalemia, 404
immunologic effects, **408**
infection risk, **408–409**
observational studies, **404**
during pregnancy, **409**
skin, **407–408**
thrombocytopenia, 404–407
hepatitis B vaccine
injury compensation, 373
liver effects, **374**
heroin
see diamorphine
histamine H$_2$ receptor antagonists
tachyphylaxis, 423–424
HMG-CoA reductase inhibitors
dosage regimens, **517**
interactions, **517–518**
liver effects, **516**
musculoskeletal effects,
516–517
myopathy, + colchicine
toxicity, 134
observational studies, **516**
psychiatric effects, **516**
homeopathy
observational studies, **557**
hormonal contraceptives
essay, 468
hormone replacement therapy
(HRT)
administration route, **472–473**
cardiovascular effects, **469–470**
dosage regimens, **472**
hematologic effects, **470–471**

psychological effects, **470**
tumorigenicity, **471–472**
urinary tract, **471**
human papilloma virus vaccine
(HPV vaccine)
general effects, **374**
hydrazine
encephalopathy, + linezolid,
305
hydrochlorothiazide
angle-closure glaucoma, 257
necrotizing pancreatitis, 257
hydroxychloroquine
see also chloroquine
monitoring therapy, **337**
musculoskeletal effects, **337**
Hypericum perforatum (St. John's
wort)
concomitant warfarin, **401–402**
digoxin clearance, 210–211
interactions, **554**

I

ibuprofen
intracerebral bleeding, +
Ginkgo biloba, 401
imatinib
adverse reactions management,
523
cardiovascular effects, **521–522**
eye function, **522**
hematologic effects, **522**
interactions, **523**
levothyroxine availability, **490**
liver effects, **522**
pharmacokinetics, **520–521**
pustular eruption, +
voriconazole, 323
skin, **523**
imidapril
eosinophilic pleurisy, 236–237
pemphigus foliaceus, 236
imipenem
metabolism effects, **284**
observational studies, **284**
pure white cell aplasia, 284
immunoglobulins
cardiovascular effects, **386**
diagnosis test interference, **387**
dosage regimens, **386–387**
formulations, **386**
general effects, **385**
hematologic effects, **386**
liver effects, **386**
musculoskeletal effects, **387**
observational studies, **385**
placebo-controlled studies, **386**
stroke, **386**
indapamide
cardiovascular effects, **258**
indinavir
interactions, 351
indocyanine green
visual field defects, 566

infiltration anesthesia
hemodynamic changes, 155
nervous system effects, **155**
sensory system effects, **155**
infliximab
dosage regimens, **442**
immunologic effects, **440–441**
metabolism effects, **440**
observational studies, **440**
smoking, **442**
susceptibility factors, **441–442**
influenza vaccine
macrophagic myofasciitis, 374
infusion pumps
death, 107
inhaled glucocorticoids
local general effects, **193**
systemic availability, **193**
inhaled insulin
general effects, **495**
inhibitors of phosphodiesterase
type V
cardiovascular effects, **232**
hepatitis, 232
non-arteritic anterior ischemic
optic neuropathy (NAION),
232
orthostatic hypotention, 246
rash, 232
insulin
administration route, **494–495**
adverse reactions management,
495
cardiovascular effects, **494**
concomitant pramlintide, 497
hypoglycemia, 494
susceptibility factors, **494**
interferon
concomitant ribavirin, **344–347**
interferon alfa
adverse reactions management,
437
hematologic effects, **436–437**
nervous system effects, **436**
psychological effects, **436**
susceptibility factors, **437**
interferon beta
immunologic effects, **438**
nervous system effects, **437**
interferon, + ribavirin
adverse reactions management,
347
hematologic effects, **346**
interactions, **346–347, 348**
observational studies, **345–346**
skin, 346
interleukin-2 (IL-2)
dosage regimens, **438**
interleukin-11 (IL-11)
cardiovascular effects, **439**
hematologic effects, **439**
observational studies, **438–439**
interleukin-12 (IL-12)
immunologic effects, **439**

interpleural anesthesia
 bronchospasm, 155–156
intrauterine hormone replacement
 therapy (HRT)
 general effects, **472**
intravenous regional anesthesia
 rash, 156
iodine and iodides
 gastrointestinal effects, **490**
irbesartan
 angle-closure glaucoma, 241
 hepatitis, 241
 pancreatitis, 241
 toxicity, + lithium, 241–242
irinotecan
 concomitant ketoconazole, 323
iron salts
 immunologic effects, **265–266**
isoflurane
 hypertension, 138
 memory impairment, 138
isoniazid
 liver, **359**
isosulfan blue
 anaphylactic reaction, 566–567
isotretinoin
 hoarseness, 185
 port wine stain, 185–186
 psychiatric effects, **185**
ispaghula
 dry mouth, 426
itraconazole
 antacids absorption, 321
 clearance, + aripiprazole, 321
 clearance, + fexofenadine,
  322–323
 concomitant
  cyclophosphamide, 322
 immunologic effects, **326**
 liver failure, 326
 neuropathy, 326
 neurotoxicity, + vincristine,
  324
 tacrolimus concentration, **458**
ivermectin
 immunologic effects, **365**
 observational studies, **365**
 susceptibility factors, **365**
 vision disturbance, 365

J
jambrulin
 contamination, **551–552**
Japanese encephalitis vaccine
 general effects, 375

K
kava
 see Piper methysticum
ketamine
 abuse, **141–142**
 concomitant morphine, 113
 memory impairment, 141
 nervous system effects, **141**

overdose, **142**
 placebo-controlled studies, **141**
 seizures, + ciclosporin,
  452–453
 systemic reviews, **141**
ketoconazole
 antihistamines (H_1) clearance,
  321
 cardiovascular effects, **326**
 clearance, + dexloxiglumide,
  322
 clearance, + gefitinib, 323
 concomitant ciclosporin,
  321–322
 susceptibility factors, **327**
ketorolac
 concomitant morphine,
  113–114
khat
 contamination, **46**
 dependence, **45**
 epidemiology, **43**
 fertility, **45**
 fetotoxicity, **45**
 gastrointestinal effects, **45**
 lactation effects, **45**
 myocardial infarction, 44
 overdose, **46**
 psychiatric effects, **44–45**
 tumorigenicity, **45**

L
L-dopamine receptor agonists
 fibrotic reactions, 176
 metabolism effects, **175–176**
lactose
 skin, **568**
lactulose
 abdominal discomfort, 426
laetrile
 see amygdalin
lamivudine
 comparative studies, **344**
 liver, **344**
lamotrigine
 aseptic meningitis, 81
 comparative studies, **80**
 hematologic, **81**
 interactions, **81–82**
 interstitial pneumonitis, 81
 vs. lithium, 24
 observational studies, **80**
 placebo-controlled studies, **81**
 toxic epidermal necrolysis, 81
 visual impairment, 81
lapatinib
 cardiovascular effects, **527**
 interactions, **527**
 pharmacokinetics, **526–527**
lasofoxifene
 concomitant digoxin, 211
latanoprost
 coronary spasm, 465
 sweating, 4656

laxatives
 general effects, **426–427**
leflunomide
 gastrointestinal effects, **455**
 hair, **455**
 nervous system effects, **455**
 respiratory effects, **454–455**
 teratogenicity, **455**
lepirudin
 dosage regimens, **409–410**
 immunologic effects, **409**
 monitoring therapy, **410**
lercanidipine
 susceptibility factors, **226–227**
leukotriene modifiers
 Churg–Strauss syndrome, 203
leuprolide
 dosage regimens, **508**
 endocrine effects, **507**
 gestational diabetes, 508
 hematologic effects, **508**
 metabolism effects, **508**
 placebo-controlled studies, **507**
 skin, **508**
levalbuterol
 see levosalbutamol
levamisole
 comparative studies, **366**
 observational studies, **366**
 skin, **366**
 teratogenicity, **366**
levetiracetam
 comparative studies, **82–83**
 hyponatremia, 83
 interactions, **83**
 nervous system effects, **83**
 observational studies, **82**
levo-α-acetylmethadol (LAAM)
 interactions, 112
 QT interval prolongation, 111
levobupivacaine
 overdose, **160**
levocetirizine
 fixed drug eruption, 190
 susceptibility factors, **190**
levodopa
 dyskinesia, 174
levofloxacin
 anaphylactic reaction, 300
 clearance, + acecainide, 300
 clearance, + procainamide, 300
 hepatic failure, 299
 nervous system effects, **299**
 procainamide clearance, 219
 rhabdomyolysis, 300
 skin, **299**
levosalbutamol (levalbuterol)
 susceptibility factors, **201**
levothyroxine
 absorption, + orlistat, 430
li da dai dai hua
 contamination, 551
lidocaine (lignocaine)
 immunologic effects, **160**
 sensory system effects, 218

somnolence, 160
linezolid
    encephalopathy, + hydrazine,
        305
    hematologic, **304–305**
    interactions, **305**
    leukocytoclastic vasculitis, 305
    metabolism effects, **304**
    nervous system effects, **304**
    observational studies, **304**
    sensory system effects, **304**
    serotonin syndrome, + selective
        serotonin reuptake inhibitors,
        305
liposomal amphotericin (L-amB)
    liver effects, **319–320**
    observational studies, **319**
    susceptibility factors, **320**
liraglutide
    gastrointestinal effects, **500**
lisinopril
    toxicity, + lithium, 237
lithium
    amphetamine inhibition, 2
    anencephaly, **26**
    comparative studies, **23–24**
    death, **26**
    drug-procedure interactions, **27**
    endocrine effects, **25**
    fetotoxicity, **26**
    interactions, **26**
    monitoring therapy, **27**
    nephrogenic diabetes insipidus,
        25
    overdose, **26**
    parathyroid hormone increase,
        26
    pharmacogenetics, **23**
    placebo-controlled studies, **23**
    psychiatric effects, **24–25**
    QT interval prolongation, **24**
    toxicity, + irbesartan, 241–242
    toxicity, + lisinopril, 237
lobelline
    cough, 4
loop diuretics
    death, **259**
    fractures, 258–259
    mineral balance, **258**
    sensorineural hearing loss, 258
lopinavir
    clearance, + efavirenz, 350
lopinavir, + ritonavir
    interactions, **351–352**
lorazepam
    light-headedness, 51
lormetazepam
    dizziness, 51
lornoxicam
    gastrointestinal effects, **132**
losartan
    headache, 242
    hematologic, **242**
    zinc deficiency, 242

Lycium barbarum (Chinese
        wolfberry)
    concomitant warfarin, **402**

M

Ma-huang
    see Ephedra/ephedrine
magnesium salts
    adverse reactions management,
        267
    cardiovascular effects, **266**
    hematologic, **266**
    osteoporosis, 266–267
male hormonal contraception
    libido loss, 473–474
    sexual function, **474**
manganese
    parkinsonism, 267
mannitol
    hyperkalemia, 260
marijuana
    see cannabinoids
mazepine
    concentration, +
        clarithromycin, 302
MDMA
    see ecstasy
measles-mumps-rubella (MMR)
        vaccine
    psychiatric effects, **375–376**
measles vaccines
    injury compensation, 373
mebendazole
    liver effects, **364**
    teratogenicity, **364–365**
mefloquine
    clearance, + ketoconazole, 323
    comparative studies, **337**
    psychiatric effects, **337–338**
Meizitang
    contamination, 551
melarsoprol
    dosage regimens, **341**
meningococcal vaccine
    Guillain–Barré syndrome, 372
menthol
    see peppermint oil
meperidine
    see pethidine
mepivacaine
    allergic skin reactions, 160–161
mercury and mercurial salts
    gastrointestinal effects, **268**
    immunologic effects, **268**
mesalazine (mesalamine)
    formulations, **429**
    immunologic effects, **428**
    placebo-controlled studies, **428**
    potentiation, +
        6-mercaptopurine, 429
    rash, 428
    urinary tract effects, **428**
metamfetamine
    abuse, **2**

concomitant bupropion, 3
    management of adverse
        reactions, **3**
    nervous system effects, 2
metformin
    concentration, + orlistat,
        430–431
    concomitant sitagliptin, 499
methadone
    cardiovascular effects, **112**
    fetotoxicity, **113**
    immunologic effects, **113**
    observational studies, **112**
    psychiatric effects, **112**
methomyl
    general effects, **565**
    overdose, **565–566**
methotrexate
    concomitant piperacillin,
        287–288
methylene blue
    see methylthioninium chloride
methylenedioxymethamphetamine
    see ecstasy
methylergonovine
    cardiac arrest, 176
methylphenidate
    comparative studies, **4**
    overdose, **5**
    placebo-controlled studies, **4**
    susceptibility factors, **5**
methylthioninium chloride
    encephalopathy, + selective
        serotonin re-uptake
        inhibitors (SSRIs), **569–571**
methysergide
    scleroderma-like skin changes,
        176–177
metoprolol
    delirium, 223
metronidazole
    amiodarone clearance, 216
    interactions, **339–340**
    nervous system effects, **339**
    pancreatic effects, **339**
    teratogenicity, **339**
mexiletine
    hypersensitivity syndrome, 218
micafungin
    concomitant tacrolimus, **458**
    interactions, **331–332**
    observational studies, **331**
    susceptibility factors, **331**
midazolam
    comparative studies, **51–52**
    observational studies, **51**
    placebo-controlled studies, **52**
mifepristone (RU-486)
    gastrointestinal effects, **477**
    during pregnancy, **477**
milrinone
    hematologic effects, 212
    systemic review, 212

minocycline
  intracranial hypertension, 290
  lupus-like syndrome, 290–291
  mouth discoloration, 290
  pseudotumor cerebri, + lithium,
    26
  respiratory effects, **290**
  skin effects, **290**
minoxidil
  contact dermatitis, 183–184
mirtazapine
  agranulocytosis, 20–21
misoprostol
  infection risk, **466**
  observational studies, **466**
  uturine rupture, 466
MLN02
  immunologic effects, **447**
  infection risk, **447**
modafinil
  placebo-controlled studies, **6**
  weight loss, + clozapine, 6
molsidomine
  formulations, **225**
mometasone furoate
  adrenal suppression, 198
  comparative studies, **197**
  dosage regimens, **198**
montelukast
  immunologic effects, **203**
  susceptibility factors, **204**
Morinda citrifolia (noni)
  liver effects, **554**
morphine
  abuse, 114
  cognitive impairment, 114
  comparative studies, **113**
  death, 114
  dosage regimens, 115
  drug combination studies,
    113–114
  herpes simplex reactivation,
    107
  immunologic effects, 114
  pruritus, 107, 114
  susceptibility factors, 115
moxifloxacin
  coma, 300
  immunologic effects, **300**
  INR increase, + warfarin, 300
moxonidine
  general effects, **247**
[99m]Tc fanolesomab
  marketing withdrawal, 446
multivitamins
  gatifloxacin availability, 394
mumps vaccine
  see measles-mumps-rubella
    vaccine
  general effects, **376**
mupirocin
  general effects, **307**
mycophenolate mofetil
  clearance, + rifampicin, 361

gastrointestinal effects,
  455–456
  liver effects, **456**
mycophenolate sodium
  gastrointestinal effects, **456**
mycophenolic acid
  clearance, + norfloxacin, 300

N
N-deamino-8-d-arginine
  vasopressin
  see desmopressin
nalbuphine
  cardiovascular effects, **119**
nalmefene
  insomnia, **119**
naloxone
  placebo-controlled studies,
    119–120
naltrexone
  dependence, **120**
  formulations, **120**
  susceptibility factors, **120**
natalizumab
  marketing withdrawal, 447
nelfinavir
  concomitant zidovudine, 352
  metabolism effects, **352**
neomycin
  eighth nerve damage, 297
neuraminidase inhibitors
  systemic reviews, **352–353**
nevirapine
  concomitant fluconazole, 323
  indinavir clearance, +, 351
  during lactation, **351**
  observational studies, **350**
nicardipine
  pulmonary edema, 227
nickel
  immunologic effects, **268–269**
  skin, **268**
nicotine
  comparative studies, **570**
nifedipine
  gastrointestinal effects, **227**
  hypotension, + clarithromycin,
    228
  interactions, **228**
  during pregnancy, **227–228**
  shock, + clarithromycin, 302
nilotinib
  general effects, **524**
nitrofurantoin
  agranulocytosis, 303
  parotitis, 303
  respiratory effects, **303**
  skin, **303**
nitroglycerin
  see glyceryl trinitrate
nitrous oxide
  device interactions, **140**
non-steroidal anti-inflammatory
  drugs (NSAIDs)

  see also specific drugs
  gastrointestinal bleeding,
    125–127
  gastrointestinal bleeding, +
    SSRIs, 16–17
  lithium concentration, 26
  urinary retention, 128
noni
  see Morinda citrifolia
noradrenaline (norepinephrine)
  ventricular outflow tract
    obstruction, 171
norepinephrine
  see noradrenaline
norfloxacin
  clearance, + mycophenolic
    acid, 300
  toxic epidermal necrolysis, 300
NSAIDs
  see non-steroidal
    anti-inflammatory drugs

O
obstetric anesthesia
  fetotoxicity, **156**
octreotide
  gastrointestinal effects, **511**
  hematologic effects, **510**
  skin, **511**
  urinary tract, **511**
ocular anesthesia
  eyes, 156
ofloxacin
  Sweet's syndrome, 300
olanzapine
  adverse reactions management,
    67
  comparative studies, **64–65**
  fluvoxamine clearance, 66
  immunologic effects, **66**
  vs. lithium, **24**
  lithium concentration, 27
  monitoring therapy, **67**
  nervous system effects, **65–66**
  observational studies, **64**
  overdose, **66–67**
  placebo-controlled studies, **65**
  susceptibility factors, **66**
olsalazine
  diarrhea, 429
omalizumab
  general effects, **447**
omeprazole
  teratogenicity, **425**
  vitamin C plasma
    concentration, 425
opioids
  administration routes, **106–108**
  bone mineral density reduction,
    108
  concomitant COX-2 inhibitors,
    108–109
  interactions, **108–109**
oral contraceptives
  cardiovascular effects, **473**

clearance, + *Hypericum perforatum,* 554
effectiveness, + antiepileptic drugs, 78
erythema multiforme, 473
headache, 473
ineffectiveness, + zonisamide, 100
urinary tract infections, **473**
valproate concentration, 97
orlistat
  adverse reactions management, **431**
  comparative studies, **430**
  interactions, **430–431**
  levothyroxine availability, **490**
  liver failure, 430
  nutrition, **430**
  systemic reviews, **429–430**
oseltamivir
  observational studies, **353**
  susceptibility factors, **353**
otamixaban
  placebo-controlled studies, **412**
oxandrolone
  susceptibility factors, **478**
oxazepam
  tolerance, **52**
oxcarbazepine
  comparative studies, **84**
  hyponatremia, 84
  observational studies, **83–84**
  priapism, 84
  priapism, + lithium, 26
  susceptibility factors, **84–85**
  teratogenicity, **84**
oxybutynin
  carbamazepine concentration, 79, 178
oxycodone
  abuse, 115
oxytocin
  during pregnancy, **511**

P

paclitaxel
  concomitant ketoconazole, 323
Panax ginseng (ginseng)
  concomitant warfarin, **402**
pancreatic enzymes
  immunologic effects, **429**
papaverine
  cardiovascular effects, 115
  sexual function, 115
paracetamol (acetaminophen)
  absorption, + exenatide, 500
  asthma, 129–130, **129–130**
paraphenylenediamine
  allergic contact dermatitis, 182
parecoxib
  bronchospasm, 130
parenteral nutrition
  adverse reactions management, **396–397**

paroxetine
  fetal heart defects, 19
  metabolism effects, **18**
pazopanib
  general effects, **529**
PC-Spes
  concomitant warfarin, 403
pegfilgrastim
  see granulocyte colony-stimulating factor
pegvisomant
  liver effects, **510**
  metabolism effects, **510**
  tumorigenicity, **510**
penicillamine
  hematologic effects, **274–275**
  observational studies, **274**
  skin, **275**
penicillins
  jaundice, 286–287
  during lactation, **287**
pentoxifylline
  urticaria, 231
peppermint oil
  administration route, **568**
  heartburn, 568
  interactions, **568–569**
perfluorocarbons
  cerebral emboli, 383
perindopril
  pancreatitis, 237
  pulmonary eosinophilia, 237
pertussis vaccines
  injury compensation, 373
pethidine
  lactation effects, 116
  during pregnancy, 116
  vomiting, 115
phenobarbital
  susceptibility factors, **85**
phenylephrine
  cardiographic U waves, 172–173
phenylpropanolamine
  overdose, **173**
phenytoin
  anticonvulsant hypersensitivity syndrome, 85
  cognitive impairment, 85
  interactions, **86**
  teratogenicity, **86**
pholcodine
  hypersensitivity, 116
phosphate-buffered eye drops
  general effects, **548**
phosphates
  acute phosphate nephropathy, 427
  electrolyte balance, **427**
  susceptibility factors, **427–428**
photodynamic therapy
  see verteporfin
physostigmine
  concomitant morphine, 114

pimecrolimus
  placebo-controlled studies, **457**
pioglitazone
  interactions, **501**
  metabolism effects, **501**
Piper methysticum (kava)
  cardiovascular effects, **554**
  gastrointestinal effects, **555**
  hematologic effects, **555**
  liver effects, **554–555**
  musculoskeletal effects, **555**
  nervous system effects, **554**
  respiratory effects, **554**
  sensory system effects, **554**
  skin, **555**
piperacillin
  acute generalized exanthematous pustulosis (AGEP), 287
  concomitant methotrexate, 287–288
plasma substitutes
  coagulopathy, 384
pleconaril
  general effects, **353**
pneumococcal vaccine
  general effects, **372**
  injury compensation, 373
polio vaccine
  injury compensation, 373
poliomyelitis vaccine
  poliomyelitis, 376
polyethylene glycol
  comparative studies, **567**
  hypovolemia, 426
polyethylene glycol + electrolytes
  dizziness, 426
polygelines
  general effects, **384**
Polygonum multiflorum
  liver effects, **555**
polystyrene sulfonates
  abuse, **276**
  pneumonitis, 275–276
polyvinylpyrrolidone
  hypothyroidism, 279
posaconazole
  general effects, **327**
  susceptibility factors, **327–328**
postsynaptic α-adrenoceptor antagonists
  drug–drug interactions, **246**
pramlintide
  concomitant insulin, 497
  gastric emptying slowing, 496
  placebo-controlled studies, **496**
praziquantel
  concentration, + glucocorticoids, 367
  during pregnancy, **366–367**
pregabalin
  interactions, **88**
  nervous system effects, **88**
  placebo-controlled studies, **86–88**

pristinamycin
  skin effects, **307**
procainamide
  clearance, + levofloxacin, 300
  levofloxacin clearance, 219
  pure red cell aplasia, 219
progesterone antagonists, **477**
  observational studies, **477**
propafenone
  exanthematous pustulosis, 218
propofol
  formulations, **143**
  hypotension, 142
  interactions, **143**
  metabolism effects, **142–143**
  myopathy, 143
  nervous system effects, **142**
  pain on injection, **143–146**
  remifentanil effectiveness, 117
propranolol
  Brugada syndrome, 224
  mesenteric ischemia, 223
protamine
  coronary artery spasm, 417
proton pump inhibitors
  adenomatoid hyperplasia, 424
  adverse reactions management,
    424
  comparative studies, **424**
  immunologic effects, **424**
  susceptibility factors, **424**
  teratogenicity, **424**
pseudoephedrine
  *see also Ephedra/*ephedrine
  cardiovascular effects, **171–172**
  toxic epidermal necrolysis, 172
psilocybin
  hallucinogen persisting
    perception disorder (HPPD),
    46
psychotropic drugs
  clearance, + valproate, 97
psyllium
  anaphylactic reaction, 426
PTH
  see parathyroid hormone (PTH)
PUVA
  skin cancer, 184
pyrrolizidine alkaloids
  veno-occlusive liver disease,
    556

Q
qat
  see khat
qing zhisan tain shou
  contamination, **551**
quetiapine
  abuse, **68**
  auditory hallucinations, 68
  concentration, + erythromycin,
    303
  interactions, **68**
  vs. lithium, 24

nervous system effects, **68**
  observational studies, **67**
  placebo-controlled studies, **67**
  withdrawal, **68**
quilinggao
  concomitant warfarin, 403
quinapril
  skin, **237**
quinidine
  QT interval prolongation, 219
quinupristin/dalfopristin
  general effects, **307**

R
rabeprazole
  general effects, **425**
racivir
  general effects, **348–349**
raloxifene
  observational studies, **474**
ramipril
  agranulocytosis, **237–238**
  edema, 236
  hyperkalemia, 237
  polyserositis, 238
  sialadenitis, 238
ramoplanin
  gastrointestinal effects, **310**
ranibizumab
  observational studies, **545**
  placebo-controlled studies, **545**
ranolazine
  clearance, + ketoconazole, 323
rapamycin
  see sirolimus
reboxetine
  anorexia, 21
  weight loss, 21
remifentanil
  cardiovascular effects, **116**
  gastrointestinal effects, **117**
  hyperalgesia, 116
  observational studies, **116**
  during pregnancy, **117**
  propofol effectiveness, 117
  respiratory effects, **116**
  susceptibility factors, **117**
ribavirin
  concomitant interferon,
    344–347
rifampicin
  atorvastatin clearance, 518
  caspofungin clearance, 331
  comparative studies, **359**
  endocrine effects, **359–360**
  hematologic effects, **360**
  interactions, **361–362**
  liver effects, **360**
  mycophenolate sodium
    clearance, 456
  urinary tract, **360–361**
risperidone
  cardiovascular effects, **70**
  comparative studies, **69**

concentration, + itraconazole,
    324
  formulations, **70–71**
  hyperprolactinemia, 70
  overdose, **71**
  placebo-controlled studies, **69**
  rabbit syndrome, 70
  rabbit syndrome, + lithium, 27
  susceptibility factors, **70**
  tardive dyskinesia, 70
ritonavir
  see lopinavir, + ritonavir
  systemic glucocorticoids
    concentration, **465**
ritonavir/saquinavir
  concomitant rifampicin, 361
rituximab
  Merkel cell carcinoma, 448
rivaroxaban
  general effects, 411–412
  hematologic effects, 412
rivastigmine
  comparative studies, **10**
  placebo-controlled studies,
    10–11
rofecoxib
  immunologic effects, **131**
  inflammatory bowel disease,
    131
  oral lesions, 131
  Stevens–Johnson syndrome,
    131
  visual impairment, 130–131
ropivacaine
  tonic-clonic seizure, 161
  ventricular fibrillation, 161
rosiglitazone
  clearance, + trimethoprim,
    308–309
  fertility effects, **502**
  interactions, **502–503**
  liver effects, **502**
  mineral balance, **502**
  myopathy, 501–502
  sensory system effects, **502**
rotavirus vaccine
  intussusception, 377
  Kawasaki disease, 377
roxithromycin
  onycholysis, 303
RU-486
  see mifepristone
rubella vaccine
  see measles-mumps-rubella
    vaccine
  injury compensation, 373

S
salbutamol
  lactic acidosis, 201–202
salmeterol
  combinations, 202
Salvia mitiorrhiza (danshen)
  concomitant warfarin, **402–403**

saw palmetto
  headache, 481
selective serotonin reuptake
    inhibitors (SSRIs)
  concomitant digoxin, 211
  encephalopathy, +
    methylthioninium chloride,
    569–571
  gastrointestinal bleeding, +
    non-steroidal
    anti-inflammatory drugs, 128
  lactation effects, **16**
  liver effects, **16**
  serotonin syndrome, +
    linezolid, 305
  sexual dysfunction, 18
  teratogenicity, **16**
selenium
  general effects, **269**
serine protease inhibitors
  general effects, **389**
sertindole
  metabolism effects, **72**
sevoflurane
  hepatotoxicity, 140
  observational studies, **138**
  QT interval prolongation,
    138–139
  tonic convulsions, 139
shou wu pian
  see Polygonum multiflorum
sibutramine
  contamination of herbal
    medicines, 551
  during pregnancy, **8**
  psychosis, + finasteride, 484
sildenafil
  clearance, + fluvoxamine, 18
  concomitant itraconazole, 324
silicone
  observational studies, **571–572**
silver salts and derivatives
  argyria, 269–270
  renal insufficiency, 269
sirolimus (rapamycin)
  concomitant itraconazole, 324
  hepatotoxicity, 457
  infection risk, **458**
  interactions, **458**
  mycophenolate sodium
    clearance, 456
  pneumonitis, 457
  skin, **457**
  susceptibility factors, **458**
  urinary tract, **457–458**
sitagliptin
  concomitant metformin, 499
sitaxsentan
  general effects, **245**
smallpox vaccine
  general effects, **377**
sodium metabisulfite
  dark room asthma, 572

sodium stearoyl lactylate
  contact allergy, 183
somatostatin
  endocrine effects, **510**
somatropin (human growth
    hormone, hGH)
  cardiovascular effects, **508–509**
  death, **509**
  formulations, **509**
  musculoskeletal effects, **509**
  tumorigenicity, **509**
sorafenib
  cardiovascular effects, **528**
  endocrine effects, **528**
  interactions, **528–529**
  pharmacokinetics, **528**
sparfloxacin
  nails, **300**
spinal anesthesia
  hypotension, 153
  transient neurological
    symptoms, 153–154
spinal manipulation
  comparative studies, **557–558**
  sensory system effects, **558**
spironolactone
  endocrine effects, **259**
  gynecomastia, 259
  hyperkalemia, 259
  hyperkalemia, + candesartan,
    241
  susceptibility factors, **259–260**
SSRIs
  see selective serotonin reuptake
    inhibitors
St. John's wort
  see Hypericum perforatum
  voriconazole clearance, 324
statins
  see HMG-CoA reductase
    inhibitors
stavudine
  fetotoxicity, **349**
stem cells
  immunologic effects, **389–390**
streptokinase
  cardiovascular effects, **412–413**
  hematologic effects, **413**
  immunologic effects, **413**
sucralfate
  diarrhea, 425
sufentanil
  pruritus, 107
sulfamethoxazole
  see co-trimoxazole
sulfonylureas
  adverse reactions management,
    500
sunitinib
  hyperthyroidism, 527–528
  interactions, **527**
  pharmacokinetics, **527**
supercoumarins
  general effects, **404**

suramin
  observational studies, **367**
suxamethonium
  musculoskeletal effects, **164**
systemic glucocorticoids
  adverse reactions diagnosis,
    465
  cardiovascular effects, **463**
  concentration, + ritonavir, **465**
  endocrine effects, **464**
  fetotoxicity, **465**
  interactions, **465**
  nervous system effects, **463**
  osteoporosis, 464
  placebo-controlled studies, **463**
  during pregnancy, **464**
  psychological effects, **463–464**

T

tacalcitol
  general effects, **186**
tacrolimus
  concentration, +
    metronidazole, 340
  concomitant itraconazole, 324
  concomitant micafungin, 332
  flushing, 458
  interactions, **458**
tamoxifen
  cardiovascular effects, **476**
  comparative studies, **475–476**
  reproductive system, **475–476**
  susceptibility factors, **476**
tamsulosin
  intraoperative floppy iris
    syndrome (IFIS), 246
  overdose, **247**
tazarotene
  skin, **186**
tea (green)
  see Camellia sinensis
tegaserod
  diarrhea, 427
teicoplanin
  immunologic effects, **301**
telithromycin
  clearance, + itraconazole, 324
  concomitant verapamil, 301
  hypotension, + verapamil, 229
  observational studies, **301**
  placebo-controlled studies, **301**
  skin, **301**
telmisartan
  susceptibility factors, **242**
temazepam
  sedation, 52
temocapril
  syncope, 238
temsirolimus
  observational studies, **459**
  susceptibility factors, **459**
tenofovir
  clearance, + lopinavir, +
    ritonavir, 349

concomitant rifampicin,
361–362
didanosine concentration, 348
renal insufficiency, 349
terbinafine
interactions, **317**
skin effects, **316**
susceptibility factors, **316**
taste loss, 316
terlipressin
cardiovascular effects, **512**
testosterone
placebo-controlled studies, **478**
tumorigenicity, **478–479**
tetanus vaccines
injury compensation, 373
tetracaine
contact dermatitis, 161
tetracyclines
intracranial hypertension, 291
non-antimicrobial properties,
288–289
ocular pigmentation, 291
tooth staining, 291
theophylline
stuttering, **5–6**
thiazide diuretics
hypercalcemia, 256–257
thionamides
agranulocytosis, 490–491
thiopental sodium
hyperkalemia, 146
multiorgan failure, 147
thiopurines
tumorigenicity, **459**
thioridazine
risperidone concentration, 71
thiotepa
metabolism, + phenytoin, 86
thyroid hormones
interactions, **490**
musculoskeletal effects, **490**
psychiatric effects, **490**
tiagabine
gastric disturbances, 89
observational studies, **89**
tibolone
placebo-controlled studies, **485**
ticlopidine
hematologic, **417**
liver effects, **417**
tigecycline
comparative studies, **292**
food interactions, **292**
gastrointestinal effects, **292**
timolol
bronchial reactivity increase,
223
toxic epidermal necrolysis, +
dorzolamide, 224
tiotropium bromide
cardiovascular effects, **203**
comparative studies, **203**

titanium
general effects, 270
tobramycin
sensory system effects, **297**
urinary tract, **297–298**
tocopherols
see vitamin E
tolterodine
hyponatremia, 177–178
topical anesthesia
anosmia, 157
death, **158**
seizures, 157
topiramate
comparative studies, **89–90**
erectile dysfunction, 91
hyperthermia, 91–92
interactions, **92**
metabolic acidosis, 91
metabolism effects, **91**
observational studies, **89**
placebo-controlled studies, **90**
psychiatric effects, **91**
retrospective studies, **90**
vision effects, **90–91**
tramadol
comparative studies, **117**
pericarditis, 117–118
transdermal hormone replacement
therapy (HRT)
general effects, **472–473**
travoprost
abdominal cramp, 466
tretinoin
hypercalcemia, + voriconazole,
324
placebo-controlled studies, **186**
triamcinolone
eye function, **548**
tribavirin
see ribavirin
trichloroethylene
immunologic effects, **140**
overdose, **140**
teratogenicity, **140**
tricyclic antidepressants
mania, 15
overdose, **15–16**
trimethoprim
see also co-trimoxazole
aseptic meningitis, 308
clearance, + rosiglitazone,
308–309
endocrine effects, **308**
hematologic effects, **308**
liver effects, **308**
pancreatitis, 308
rosiglitazone concentration,
503
skin, **308**
triptans
serotonin syndrome, 232
triptorelin
polydactyly, 508

tyrosine kinase inhibitors
general effects, **520**
skin and hair, **520**

U
ultrasound contrast agents
cardiovascular effects, **540–541**
unfractionated heparin
interference, + abciximab, 415

V
vaccines
allergic disease, 370
formulations, **370–371**
Guillain–Barré syndrome, 370
injury compensation, **371–372,
373**
standardized case definitions,
371
valdecoxib
anuric renal insufficiency, 132
cardiovascular effects, **132**
carpal tunnel syndrome, 132
skin, **132**
valproate
administration route, **96**
adverse reactions management,
97–98
amphetamines inhibition, 2
color vision defects, 93
dosage regimens, **96**
hematologic effects, **93–94**
interactions, **96–97**
vs. lithium, **24**
observational studies, **92–93**
overdose, **96**
sialadenosis, 94
vitamin B_{12} concentration, 93
valproic acid
concentration, + apenems,
283–284
valsartan
pneumonitis, 242
vancomycin
immunologic effects, **301**
varicella vaccine
injury compensation, 373
vasopressin
hyponatremia, 511
venlafaxine
ejaculatory delay, 19
nervous system effects, **19**
verapamil
concomitant telithromycin, 301
cutaneous lupus erythematosus,
228
gingival enlargement, 228
hyperprolactinemia, 228
hypotension, + telithromycin,
229
interactions, **228–229**
overdose, **228**

verteporfin
  adverse reactions management,
    547
  eye function, **546–547**
  general effects, **545–546**
  hypersensitivity reaction, 547
  musculoskeletal effects, **547**
  nervous system effects, **546**
  photosensitivity, 547
  placebo-controlled studies, **546**
  respiratory effects, **546**
  submacular hemorrhage, +
    warfarin, 547
  urinary tract, **547**
vigabatrin
  visual field defects, 98–99
vincristine
  neurotoxicity, + itraconazole,
    325
virginiamycin
  tolerance (antibacterial
    resistance), **307**
vitamin A (retinoids)
  teratogenicity, **185**
vitamin C
  amygdalin metabolism effects,
    556
  amygdalin toxicity, 394
vitamin D analogues
  mineral metabolism, **394**
vitamin E
  cardiovascular effects, **395**
  ciclosporin concentration, 395
  interactions, **395**

during pregnancy, **395**
vitamins
  ciclosporin concentration, 453
von Willebrand factor
  formulations, **388**
voriconazole
  comparative studies, **328**
  hypercalcemia, + tretinoin, 324
  monitoring therapy, **329**
  peripheral neuropathy, 328
  pustular eruption, + imatinib,
    323
  skin, **328**
  susceptibility factors, **329**

W

warfarin
  clearance, + St. John's wort,
    401–402
  concomitant *Ginkgo biloba*,
    553
  gastrointestinal bleeding, +
    SSRIs, 16–17
  herbal interactions, **400–403**
  inhibition, + menthol, 569
  INR increase, + moxifloxacin,
    300
  submacular hemorrhage, +
    verteporfin, 547
water-soluble intravascular
    iodinated contrast agents
  comparative studies, **533–534**
  fetotoxicity, **537–538**
  immunologic effects, **537**

X

ximelagatran
  comparative studies, **410**
  hematologic effects, **410**
  hepatotoxicity, 411
  product withdrawal, **410**

Z

zaleplon
  observational studies, **53**
zidovudine
  concomitant nelfinavir, 352
zinc
  copper deficiency, 270
Zingiber officinale (ginger)
  concomitant warfarin, **403**
  during pregnancy, **556**
  systemic reviews, **556**
ziprasidone
  comparative studies, **72**
  lithium toxicity, 27
  observational studies, **72**
  overdose, **74**
  rhabdomyolysis, 72–73
zolpidem
  postural sway, 53
zonisamide
  concomitant valproate, 96–97
  dosage regimens, **99–100**
  interactions, **100**
  placebo-controlled studies, 99,
    99
  renal calculi, 99
  susceptibility factors, **99**

Index of adverse effects

A

abdominal cramp
cefaclor, 284
travoprost, 466
abdominal discomfort
lactulose, 426
rofecoxib, 131
abdominal distension
alpha-glucosidase inhibitors,
496
diltiazem, 226
abdominal pain
adenosine receptor agonists,
213
anti-human CD40 Mab
chimeric 5D12, 443
biguanides, 497
clarithromycin + colchicine,
133
desloratadine, 189
diuretic sulfonamides, 252
fosmidomycin, 310
H. pylori eradication regimens,
425, 426
lamotrigine, 80
mesalazine, 428, 429
methylphenidate, 5
micafungin, 331
misoprostol, 466
montelukast, 203
orlistat, 429, 430
phosphates, 427
proton pump inhibitors, 424
rabeprazole, 425
ramoplanin, 310
rofecoxib, 131
telithromycin, 301
warfarin, 399
abdominal tenderness
ofloxacin, 300
abdominal tightness
phosphates, 427
abnormal thoughts
pregabalin, 87, 88
abrasions
bevacizumab, 544
abruptio placenta
misoprostol, 466
absence seizure
valproate, 96
acantholytic dermatitis
interferon + ribavirin, 346
acanthosis
penicillamine, 275
accidental injuries
pregabalin, 87

accidents
rivastigmine, 10
accommodation impairment
Piper methysticum, 554
acid regurgitation
mycophenolate sodium, 456
acne
Agnus castus, 552
sirolimus (rapamycin), 457
acneiform eruption
sirolimus (rapamycin), 457
acute coronary syndrome
cannabinoids, 31
**acute generalized
exanthematous pustulosis
(AGEP)**
ciprofloxacin, 298
piperacillin, 287
terbinafine, 316
**acute hemolytic transfusion
reaction**
blood transfusion, 381
acute leukemia
valproate, 94
acute phosphate nephropathy
phosphates, 427
acute reactive encephalopathy
melarsoprol, 341
acute renal insufficiency
ciprofloxacin, 298
rifampicin, 360–361
acute respiratory distress
verteporfin, 546
**acute respiratory distress
syndrome (ARDS)**
cocaine, 35
immunoglobulins, 385
lamotrigine, 81
acute tubular necrosis
colistin, 306
gentamicin, 297
adenomatoid hyperplasia
proton pump inhibitors, 424
adenovirus infection
alemtuzumab, 443
adrenal insufficiency
etomidate, 141
adrenal suppression
budesonide, 194
mometasone furoate, 198
**adult respiratory distress
syndrome**
see acute respiratory distress
syndrome
after-taste
naltrexone, 120

AGEP
see acute generalized
exanthematous pustulosis
(AGEP)
aggression
androgenic anabolic steroids,
478
diamorphine, 110
levamisole, 366
levetiracetam, 82
agitation
ketamine, 141
metformin + orlistat, 431
methylphenidate, 5
methylthioninium chloride +
statins, 569, 570, 571
rivastigmine, 10
zonisamide, 99
agnosia
cannabinoids, 32
agranulocytosis
see also leukopenia,
neutropenia
antithyroid drugs, 216
calcium dobesilate, 216
cefoperazone, 285
clarithromycin + colchicine,
133
dipyrone, 132–133
mirtazapine, 20–21
nitrofurantoin, 303
ramipril, 237–238
thionamides, 490–491
ticlopidine, 216, 417
airway obstruction
ACE inhibitors, 235
akathisia
olanzapine, 65
alertness
khat, 44
allergic contact dermatitis
dorzolamide, 256
paraphenylenediamine, 182
valdecoxib, 132
allergic disease
vaccines, 370
allergic granulomatous angiitis
proton pump inhibitors, 424
allergic rash
clopidogrel, 416
allergic reaction
blood transfusion, 382
botulinum toxins, 166
chlorhexidine, 278
Echinacea species, 553
lepirudin, 409

penicillins, 287
telithromycin, 301
allergic skin reaction
hair dyes, 181
mepivacaine, 160–161
allergy
homeopathy, 557
allergy-like reaction
water-soluble intravascular
iodinated contrast agents,
533, 537
allo-antibody formation
blood transfusion, 382
alopecia
see hair loss
alveolar hemorrhage
anticoagulants + epoprostenol,
465
amblyopia
pregabalin, 87, 88
tiagabine, 89
amenorrhea
leuprolide, 507
amnesia
pregabalin, 88
tiagabine, 89
anal irritation
phosphates, 427
anaphylactic reaction
caspofungin, 330
cefaclor, 284–285
etherified starches, 384
gelatine, 371
iron salts, 266
isosulfan blue, 566–567
levofloxacin, 300
polygelines, 384
psyllium, 426
anaphylactic shock
beta-lactam antibiotics, 281
anaphylaxis
bee sting venom, 572
beta-adrenoceptor antagonists,
224
blood transfusion, 382
proton pump inhibitors, 424
tetanus vaccines, 373
anasarca
amlodipine, 225–226
ANCA
see antineutrophil cytoplasmic
antibodies (ANCA)
anemia
antiandrogens, 479
clopidogrel, 415
cyclophosphamide, 453
interferon + ribavirin, 345, 346,
347
linezolid, 304, 305
nevirapine, 350
sunitinib, 527
supercoumarins, 404
suramin, 367
ticlopidine, 417
trimethoprim, 308

anencephaly
biguanides, 497
omeprazole, 425
anesthesia prolongation
spinal anesthesia, 154
angina
see also cardiac ischemia
cefuroxime, 286
latanoprost, 465
oseltamivir, 353
angioedema
ACE inhibitors, 234–235
acetylsalicylic acid, 129
amiodarone, 216
angiotensin II receptor
antagonists, 238–240
cefaclor, 284
glucosamine, 567
iron salts, 266
itraconazole, 326
MLN02, 447
pholcodine, 116
ramipril, 238
sirolimus (rapamycin), 457
streptokinase, 413
topical anesthesia, 157
tramadol, 118
angle-closure glaucoma
acetazolamide, 255
cannabinoids, 33
hydrochlorothiazide, 257
irbesartan, 241
topiramate, 90–91
ankle edema
levetiracetam, 82
anophthalmia
biguanides, 497
anorexia
see appetite loss
anorgasmia
levetiracetam, 82
anosmia
dorzolamide, 256
topical anesthesia, 157
antibody production
erythropoietins, 389
exenatide, 500
factor VIII, 387
infliximab, 440–441
interferon beta, 438
lepirudin, 409
**anticonvulsant hypersensitivity
syndrome**
phenytoin, 85
antihuman antibodies
MLN02, 447
**antineutrophil cytoplasmic
antibody (ANCA)-positive
vasculitis**
antithyroid drugs, 491
antiphospholipid syndrome
heparins, 407
anuric renal insufficiency
valdecoxib, 132

anxiety
ketamine + morphine, 113
levetiracetam, 82
mefloquine, 337
modafinil, 6
quetiapine, 68
risperidone, 71
ziprasidone, 72
aphasia
adrenaline (epinephrine), 170
cannabinoids, 32
methylthioninium chloride +
statins, 570, 571
aphthous ulceration
sirolimus (rapamycin), 457
aplasia cutis congenita
antithyroid drugs, 491
aplastic anemia
dapsone, 357
apnea
combination vaccines, 369
ecstasy, 41
fentanyl, 111
immunoglobulins, 386
levetiracetam, 82
obstetric anesthesia, 156
sevoflurane, 139
appetite, poor
methomyl, 565
appetite increase
olanzapine, 64, 65
risperidone, 69
appetite loss
articaine, 158
biguanides, 497
furazolidone, 341
H. pylori eradication regimens,
340, 426
interferon + ribavirin, 345
ivermectin, 365
khat, 45
lamotrigine, 80
methylphenidate, 4
modafinil, 6
mycophenolate sodium, 456
naltrexone, 120
pramlintide, 496
reboxetine, 21
rifampicin, 361
rofecoxib, 131
suramin, 367
terbinafine, 316–317
topiramate, 89, 90
ziprasidone, 65
zonisamide, 99
ARDS
see acute respiratory distress
syndrome
areflexia
cocaine, 34
argyria
silver salts and derivatives,
269–270

arterial thrombosis
bevacizumab, 444
arthralgia
anti-human CD40 Mab
chimeric 5D12, 443
antithyroid drugs, 491
ceftroxone, 285
deferiprone, 274
everolimus, 454
glucosamine, 567
H. pylori eradication regimens,
426
interferon + ribavirin, 346
micafungin, 331
minocycline, 290
montelukast, 203
proton pump inhibitors, 424
quinupristin/dalfopristin, 307
arthritis
rubella vaccine, 373
ascites
methomyl, 565
verteporfin, 547
aseptic meningitis
ciprofloxacin, 299
immunoglobulins, 386
lamotrigine, 81
mumps vaccine, 376
trimethoprim, 308
Aspergillus infection
gemtuzumab ozogamicin, 446
asterixis
pregabalin, 88
asthenozoospermia
carbamazepine, 79
asthma
adalimumab, 439
beta$_2$-adrenoceptor agonists,
198–199
diamorphine, 110
glucosamine, 567
hair dyes, 181
paracetamol, 129–130
sodium metabisulfite, 572
asystole
olanzapine, 67
ataxia
acetazolamide, 255
amiodarone, 214
artemisinin, 338
colistin, 306
methomyl, 565
pregabalin, 87, 88
tiagabine, 89
valproate, 92
zonisamide, 99
atherosclerosis
insulin, 494
atrial dysrhythmia
formoterol, 200
atrial fibrillation
cannabinoids, 31
donepezil, 9

atrial flutter
amiodarone, 214
atrioventricular block
cannabinoids, 31
donepezil, 9
auditory disturbance
see entries at hearing-
auditory hallucination
quetiapine, 68
autism
manganese, 268
measles-mumps-rubella
vaccine, 375

B
back pain
fentanyl, 111
liposomal amphotericin
(L-amB), 320
proton pump inhibitors, 424
systemic glucocorticoids, 463
verteporfin, 546, 547
backache
immunoglobulins, 385
bacteremia
heparins, 408–409
Bartter-like syndrome
gentamicin, 297
BCG disease
Bacille Calmette–Guérin
(BCG) vaccine, 372
behavior, disturbed
lamotrigine, 81
behavior change
androgenic anabolic steroids,
478
diamorphine, 110
levetiracetam, 82
behavior problem
cocaine, 36
topiramate, 91
belching
Zingiber officinale, 556
**benign prostatic hyperplasia
exacerbation**
bisoprolol, 223
bezoar
nifedipine, 227
biliary colic
desloratadine, 189
biliary sludge
ceftroxone, 285
birth weight reduction
cocaine, 35
khat, 45
bitter taste
H. pylori eradication regimens,
425
bleeding
amiodarone, 214
anticoagulants + epoprostenol,
465
bevacizumab, 444
dabigatran, 409

danshen + warfarin, 402
drotrecogin alfa, 381
garlic, 400
Ginkgo biloba, 553
glycoprotein IIb-IIIa inhibitors,
415
heparins, 405
leuprolide, 508
streptokinase, 413
sunitinib, 527
ximelagatran, 410
bleeding, postoperative
rivaroxaban, 412
blepharoconjunctivitis
imatinib mesylate, 522
blistering
water-soluble intravascular
iodinated contrast agents,
534
bloating
mesalazine, 429
phosphates, 427
blood pressure increase
see also hypertension
amphetamines, 1
bevacizumab, 544
duloxetine, 19
ecstasy, 39
fluvoxamine + quetiapine, 68
ketamine, 141
olanzapine, 64
pseudoephedrine, 171
BNP increase
digoxin, 211
body movements
desflurane, 138
bone ache
imatinib mesylate, 523
bone marrow suppression
hydroxychloroquine, 337
penicillamine, 274
ticlopidine, 417
bone mineral density reduction
opioids, 108
thyroid hormones, 490
Bong lung
cannabinoids, 33
brachial neuritis
tetanus vaccines, 373
bradycardia
beta-adrenoceptor antagonists,
223
bupivacaine, 159
cannabinoids, 32
chloral hydrate, 52–53
combination vaccines, 369
dextrans, 384
immunoglobulins, 386
levobupivacaine, 160
methadone, 112
obstetric anesthesia, 156
phosphates, 427
propafenone, 218
propofol, 142

remifentanil, 116
tamsulosin, 247
ultrasound contrast agents, 540
brain edema
pregabalin, 88
brainstem encephalopathy
artemisinin, 338
brainstem herniation
acetazolamide, 255
breast cancer
bicalutamide, 480
hormone replacement therapy,
471
breast enlargement
finasteride, 484
breast pain
bicalutamide, 480
breast tenderness
finasteride, 484
breathing difficulty
suxamethonium, 164
broad complex tachycardia
cardiac glycosides, 209
bronchial reactivity increase
timolol, 223
bronchiectasis
rabeprazole, 425
bronchitis
zanamivir, 353
bronchoconstriction
colistin, 305
bronchospasm
dipyridamole, 413
interpleural anesthesia,
155–156
mesalazine, 429
parecoxib, 130
zanamivir, 352
Brugada syndrome
ajmaline and derivatives, 213
cibenzoline, 217
propranolol, 224
bruising
botulinum toxins, 165
heparins, 408
inhaled glucocorticoids, 193
interferon alfa, 436, 437
quilinggao + warfarin, 403
supercoumarins, 404
bullae
pseudoephedrine, 172
bundle branch block
methylthioninium chloride +
statins, 570
burning
aminolevulinic acid, 184
chlorhexidine, 279
cosmetics, 180
tacalcitol, 186

C
calcifying panniculitis
heparins, 408
calcinosis cutis
heparins, 408

candidiasis
fluconazole, 326
fluticasone propionate +
salmeterol, 202
mometasone furoate, 198
capillary leak syndrome
granulocyte colony-stimulating
factor, 435
cardiac
see also entries at coronary-,
heart-
cardiac arrest
see also myocardial
infarction
antipsychotic drugs, 60
cannabinoids, 31
cardiac glycosides, 209
desflurane, 137
methylergonovine, 176
phosphates, 427
cardiac rupture
ultrasound contrast agents,
540–541
cardiac toxicity
gemtuzumab ozogamicin, 446
cardiographic U waves
phenylephrine, 172–173
cardiomegaly
interleukin-11, 439
cardiomyopathy
clozapine, 62
sibutramine, 7
systemic glucocorticoids, 463
cardiovascular collapse
bismuth, 264
bupivacaine, 159
carotid sinus syndrome
donepezil, 9
carpal tunnel syndrome
valdecoxib, 132
cataract
finasteride, 482
triamcinolone, 548
cataract progression
bevacizumab, 544
cauda equina syndrome
spinal anesthesia, 154
cecocentral scotomata
linezolid, 304
central retinal artery occlusion
bevacizumab, 544
cerebral edema
acetazolamide, 255
ecstasy, 42
cerebral hemorrhage
coumarin anticoagulants, 399
cerebral vasculitis
metamfetamine, 2
cerebrovascular disease
cannabinoids, 32
cheilitis
voriconazole, 328
chest pain
adenosine receptor agonists,
213

adrenaline (epinephrine), 170
botulinum toxins, 166
cannabinoids, 31
diamorphine, 110
gemtuzumab ozogamicin, 446
infliximab, 440
triptans, 232
verteporfin, 546
chest tightness
acupuncture, 557
colistin, 305
ecstasy, 40
immunoglobulins, 385
levetiracetam, 82
methomyl, 565
chills
aztreonam, 286
efalizumab, 445
immunoglobulins, 385, 386
levamisole, 366
methomyl, 565
choanal atresia
antithyroid drugs, 491
cholelithiasis
see gall stones
cholestasis
candesartan, 241
fluvoxamine, 16
parenteral nutrition, 396–397
cholestatic hepatitis
rosiglitazone, 502
ticlopidine, 417
cholesterol crystal embolism
heparins, 404
cholesterol increase
paroxetine, 18
chorea
co-trimoxazole, 338
choreoathetosis
levetiracetam, 82
olanzapine, 66, 67
choroidal infarction
verteporfin, 546
choroidal ischemia
verteporfin, 546
**chronic obstructive pulmonary
disease (COPD)**
beta-adrenoceptor antagonists,
223
paracetamol (acetaminophen),
130
chronic pulmonary fibrosis
gefitinib, 524
chrysiasis
gold and gold salts, 265
Churg–Strauss syndrome
leukotriene modifiers, 203
**circulatory transfusion
reactions**
blood transfusion, 382
cirrhosis
fibrates, 515
Piper methysticum, 554
cleft palate
valproate, 95

clonus
methylthioninium chloride +
statins, 570
coagulation activation
factor IX, 388
coagulopathy
drotrecogin alfa, 381
etherified starches, 384
leuprolide, 508
plasma substitutes, 384
cochleovestibular deficit
cocaine, 34
cognitive deficit
cannabinoids, 33
cognitive impairment
interferon alfa, 436
ketamine, 141
morphine, 114
phenytoin, 85
tiagabine, 89
topiramate, 90
valproate, 95
cogwheel rigidity
manganese, 267–268
cold sensation
valproate, 96
colitis
glucosamine, 567
levetiracetam, 82
pregabalin, 88
rofecoxib, 131
color vision impairment
ethambutol, 358
linezolid, 304
metronidazole, 339
valproate, 93
coma
amitriptyline, 15
carbamazepine, 78
ecstasy, 41
methomyl, 565
moxifloxacin, 300
olanzapine, 67
trichloroethylene, 140
compartment syndrome
streptokinase, 413
concentration impairment
carbamazepine, 78
efavirenz, 349
interferon alfa, 436
topiramate, 89, 90
confusion
adrenaline (epinephrine), 170
carbamazepine + oxybutynin,
178
colistin, 306
diamorphine, 110
ketamine + morphine, 113
metformin + orlistat, 431
methadone, 112
methylthioninium chloride +
statins, 569, 570, 571
naltrexone, 120
olanzapine, 64

oseltamivir, 353
pregabalin, 88
tiagabine, 89
venlafaxine, 19
congenital heart defect
fluconazole, 325
congestion
acitretin, 185
congestive heart failure
adalimumab, 439
infliximab, 440
conjunctival cyst
ocular anesthesia, 156
conjunctival hemorrhage
chloroquine + proguanil, 336
conjuctival injection
interleukin-11, 439
conjunctival swelling
bevacizumab, 544
consciousness, loss of
cefaclor, 285
verteporfin, 546
consciousness alteration
silver salts and derivatives, 269
constipation
alosetron, 423
clozapine, 62
dalbavancin, 301
daptomycin, 309
dextromethorphan, 109
fentanyl, 111
gabapentin + morphine, 113
H. pylori eradication regimens,
425, 426
interleukin-2, 438
ivermectin, 365
khat, 45
levetiracetam, 82
methadone, 112
naltrexone, 120
sibutramine, 7
contact allergy
corticosteroids, topical, 183
cosmetics, 180
sodium stearoyl lactylate, 183
contact dermatitis
see also allergic contact
dermatitis
colophony, 183
hair dyes, 181
minoxidil, 183–184
nickel, 268, 269
paraphenylenediamine, 182
tetracaine, 161
contact hypersensitivity
aluminium adsorbent, 370
convulsions
calcitonin, 507
colistin, 306
combination vaccines, 369
levamisole, 366
obstetric anesthesia, 156
ropivacaine, 161
statins, 16

coordination impairment
metronidazole, 339
copper deficiency
zinc, 270
cornea verticillata
amiodarone, 214
corneal calcification
phosphate-buffered eye drops,
548
corneal deposits
chlorpromazine, 61
corneal edema
acetazolamide, 255
cannabinoids, 33
coronary
see also entries at cardi-, heart-
coronary artery disease
cannabinoids, 31
coronary artery spasm
ecstasy, 39–40
latanoprost, 465
protamine, 417
pseudoephedrine, 172
coronary syndrome, acute
cannabinoids, 31
cortisol concentration
alprazolam, 49
cough
ACE inhibitors, 234
arsenic, 263
colistin, 305
desflurane, 138
erlotinib, 526
fentanyl, 111
interferon + ribavirin, 345
lobelline, 3
nitrofurantoin, 303
oseltamivir, 353
verteporfin, 546
zanamivir, 353
cramps
imatinib mesylate, 523
phosphates, 427
progesterone antagonists, 477
somatropin, 509
craniopharyngioma
somatropin, 509
crush fractures
lopinavir + ritonavir, 351
Cushing's syndrome
lopinavir + ritonavir, 351
systemic glucocorticoids, 464
cutaneous lupus erythematosus
acebutolol, 223–224
terbinafine, 316
verapamil, 228
cutaneous sarcoidosis
interferon + ribavirin, 346
cyanosis
acupuncture, 557
cystitis
proton pump inhibitors, 424
rabeprazole, 425

cytomegalovirus infection
  MLN02, 447
cytomegalovirus reactivation
  alemtuzumab, 442, 443
cytopenia
  clopidogrel, 416

D
dark room asthma
  sodium metabisulfite, 572
dark urine
  chloroquine + proguanil, 336
deafness
  cocaine, 34
death
  antipsychotic drugs, 60–61
  beta$_2$-adrenoceptor agonists,
    198–199
  bevacizumab, 544
  caffeine, 5
  infusion pumps, 107
  loop diuretics, 259
  ^{99m}Tc fanolesomab, 446
  opioids, 107
  propofol, 142
  somatropin, 509
deep vein thrombosis
  interleukin-2, 438
dehydration
  cilazapril, 235
  clarithromycin + colchicine,
    133
delirium
  bupropion, 20
  ketamine, 141
  lithium, 24
  methylthioninium chloride +
    statins, 569
  metoprolol, 223
  olanzapine, 67
  pregabalin, 88
  risperidone, 71
delusions
  bupropion, 20
dementia
  lithium, 24–25
demyelinating disease
  infliximab, 440
depersonalization
  psilocybin, 46
depression
  ecstasy, 40–41
  finasteride, 482
  HMG-CoA reductase
    inhibitors, 516
  interferon alfa, 436
  levetiracetam, 82
  mefloquine, 337
  risperidone, 71
  temsirolimus, 459
  tiagabine, 89
  topiramate, 91

derealization
  psilocybin, 46
dermatitis
    see also contact dermatitis,
      exfoliative dermatitis
  efalizumab, 445
  gold, 181
  gold and gold salts, 265
  interferon + ribavirin, 345, 346
  nail cosmetics, 183
  sunitinib, 527
desquamation
  ceftroxone, 285
  diltiazem, 226
  voriconazole, 328
**desquamation of the oral
  mucosa**
  chlorhexidine, 278–279
device failure
  cobalt, 265
diabetes mellitus
  antipsychotic drugs, 58
  flutamide, 484
  glucosamine, 568
  risperidone, 71
diabetes, gestational
  leuprolide, 508
diabetic ketoacidosis
  antipsychotic drugs, 58
  insulin, 494
diarrhea
  azithromycin, 302
  biguanides, 497
  cefaclor, 284
  citalopram, 17
  clarithromycin + colchicine,
    133
  dalbavancin, 301
  daptomycin, 309
  dextromethorphan, 109
  direct renin inhibitors, 244
  donepezil, 9
  erlotinib, 526
  gefitinib, 525
  H. pylori eradication regimens,
    340, 425, 426
  imatinib mesylate, 523
  interleukin-11, 439
  ivermectin, 365
  leflunomide, 455
  legaserod, 427
  mesalazine, 428, 429
  methomyl, 565
  micafungin, 331
  mycophenolate sodium, 456
  naltrexone, 120
  octreotide, 511
  olsalazine, 429
  omeprazole, 425
  orlistat, 430
  oseltamivir, 353
  pazopanib, 529
  pregabalin, 86, 88
  proton pump inhibitors, 424

  ramoplanin, 310
  rivastigmine, 10
  rofecoxib, 131
  sorafenib, 528
  sucralfate, 425
  sunitinib, 527
  telithromycin, 301
  terbinafine, 317
  tigecycline, 292
  topiramate, 90
  trichloroethylene, 140
  water-soluble intravascular
    iodinated contrast agents,
    534
  zanamivir, 353
DIC
    see disseminated intravascular
      coagulation (DIC)
**diffuse venous
  thromboembolism**
  immunoglobulins, 386
diplopia
  artemisinin, 338
  citalopram, 17
  pregabalin, 87
  spinal manipulation, 558
  suxamethonium, 164
discolored stools
  chloroquine + proguanil, 336
disinhibition
  levetiracetam, 82
  methylthioninium chloride +
    statins, 570
disorientation
  diamorphine, 110
  methylthioninium chloride +
    statins, 570, 571
**disseminated intravascular
  coagulation (DIC)**
  immunoglobulins, 385, 386
disturbed dreaming
  ketamine, 141
dizziness
  acupuncture, 557
  adenosine receptor agonists,
    213
  alfuzosin, 246, 481
  baclofen, 165
  carbamazepine + oxybutynin,
    178
  cefaclor, 284
  citalopram, 17
  colistin, 306
  dextromethorphan, 109
  direct renin inhibitors, 244
  efavirenz, 349
  endothelin receptor
    antagonists, 245
  fentanyl, 110, 111
  fluticasone propionate +
    salmeterol, 202
  gabapentin, 80
  glucosamine, 567
  H. pylori eradication regimens,
    425

human papilloma virus vaccine, 374
interleukin-2, 438
iron salts, 266
ivermectin, 365
lamotrigine, 80
levetiracetam, 82
lormetazepam, 51
mesalazine, 429
metformin + orlistat, 431
methomyl, 565
modafinil, 6
naltrexone, 120
nifedipine, 228
oxcarbazepine, 85
oxybutynin, 177
pethidine, 116
polyethylene glycol + electrolytes, 426
pregabalin, 86, 87, 88
progesterone antagonists, 477
quetiapine, 68
rivastigmine, 10
tamsulosin, 247
terbinafine, 317
tiagabine, 89
topiramate, 89, 91
valproate, 96
zanamivir, 352
ziprasidone, 72
zonisamide, 99
dream disturbance
donepezil, 9
ketamine, 141
dreams, abnormal
efavirenz, 349
dreams, vivid
ketamine + morphine, 113
DRESS
see drug rash with eosinophilia and systemic symptoms (DRESS)
drowsiness
dextromethorphan, 109
doxazosin, 246
ivermectin, 365
levetiracetam, 82
naltrexone, 120
oxcarbazepine, 84
penicillamine, 274
topiramate, 90
drug hypersensitivity syndrome
water-soluble intravascular iodinated contrast agents, 537
drug rash with eosinophilia and systemic symptoms (DRESS)
erythropoietins, 389
dry mouth
citalopram, 17
dextromethorphan, 109
gabapentin + morphine, 113
ispaghula, 426
mefloquine, 337

methomyl, 565
methylphenidate, 4
modafinil, 6
naltrexone, 120
pregabalin, 86, 87
terbinafine, 317
tiotropium bromide, 203
dry skin
finasteride, 481
interferon + ribavirin, 345
Piper methysticum, 555
duodenal ulcer
khat, 45
dysarthria
acetazolamide, 255
artemisinin, 338
manganese, 267–268
metronidazole, 339
dysesthesia
cefaclor, 285
linezolid, 304
dyskinesia
haloperidol, 61
levodopa, 174
dyslipidemia
atazanavir, 351
dysmorphic facial features
fluconazole, 325
dyspepsia
inhibitors of phosphodiesterase type V, 232
interferon + ribavirin, 345
mycophenolate sodium, 456
omeprazole, 425
ramoplanin, 310
tigecycline, 292
dysphagia
see swallowing difficulty
dysphonia
acitretin, 185
fluticasone propionate + salmeterol, 202
inhaled glucocorticoids, 193
mometasone furoate, 198
dysphoria
mefloquine, 337
topiramate, 90
dyspnea
adenosine receptor agonists, 213
amiodarone, 214
arsenic, 263
caspofungin, 330
cefaclor, 284, 285
diuretic sulfonamides, 254
erlotinib, 526
gefitinib, 524
infliximab, 440, 441
interferon + ribavirin, 345
lidocaine, 160
methomyl, 565
nitrofurantoin, 303
suramin, 367
verteporfin, 547

zanamivir, 352
dysrhythmia
antipsychotic drugs, 56
botulinum toxins, 166
hormone replacement therapy, 470
interleukin-11, 439
olanzapine, 66
oseltamivir, 353
propofol, 142
zanamivir, 352
dystonia
cannabinoids, 32
levetiracetam, 83
olanzapine, 67
ziprasidone, 65

E
ear infection
oxcarbazepine, 83
ecchymosis
see bruising
ectopic contact dermatitis
nail cosmetics, 183
eczema
calcipotriol, 186
corticosteroids, topical, 183
EMLA cream, 157
H. pylori eradication regimens, 426
interferon + ribavirin, 346
edema
aminolevulinic acid, 184
arsenic, 263–264
articaine, 158
ceftroxone, 285
everolimus, 454
glucosamine, 567
granulocyte colony-stimulating factor, 435
imatinib mesylate, 521, 522
interleukin-11, 439
isosulfan blue, 566
lactose, 568
quinupristin/dalfopristin, 307
sirolimus (rapamycin), 457
streptokinase, 413
tobramycin, 297
verteporfin, 547
water-soluble intravascular iodinated contrast agents, 537
zanamivir, 352
eighth nerve damage
neomycin, 297
ejaculatory delay
venlafaxine, 19
ejaculatory disorder
citalopram, 17
finasteride, 481, 483, 484
elastosis perforans serpiginosa
penicillamine, 275
electrolyte abnormality
amphotericin, 317

polystyrene sulfonates, 276
embryopathy
  fluconazole, 325
  valproate, 95–96
emergence reaction
  ketamine, 141
emesis
  see vomiting
emotional instability
  levetiracetam, 82
emotional lability
  topiramate, 89
emphysema
  cannabinoids, 33
encephalitis
  pertussis vaccines, 373
encephalitis-like syndrome
  Japanese encephalitis vaccine, 375
encephalopathy
  cefepime, 285
  hydrazine + linezolid, 305
  methylthioninium chloride + statins, 569–571
  pertussis vaccines, 373
  pregabalin, 88
encephalopathy, acute reactive
  melarsoprol, 341
end-stage renal disease
  acetylsalicylic acid, 128–129
endocarditis
  beta-lactam antibiotics, 280
endometrial cancer
  hormone replacement therapy, 471–472
endometritis
  misoprostol, 466
endophthalmitis
  bevacizumab, 544
  ranibizumab, 545
enthesitis
  acitretin, 185
eosinophilia
  epidural anesthesia, 153
  leukotriene modifiers, 203
  vancomycin, 301
  water-soluble intravascular iodinated contrast agents, 537
eosinophilic pleurisy
  imidapril, 236–237
eosinophilic pneumonia
  minocycline, 290
epidermal hematoma
  clopidogrel, 416
epididymitis
  botulinum toxins, 166
epigastralgia
  mycophenolate sodium, 456
epigastric pain
  Piper methysticum, 555
epistaxis
  heparins, 405
  micafungin, 331

quilinggao + warfarin, 403
  sirolimus (rapamycin), 457
  sunitinib, 527
  supercoumarins, 404
  topiramate, 90
erectile dysfunction
  beta-adrenoceptor antagonists, 224
  finasteride, 481, 482
  topiramate, 91
erythema
  Agnus castus, 552
  aminolevulinic acid, 184
  articaine, 158
  aztreonam, 286
  beta-lactam antibiotics, 281
  clarithromycin, 302
  clopidogrel, 416
  dasatinib, 524
  epidural anesthesia, 153
  fondaparinux, 412
  gefitinib, 525
  lactose, 568
  manganese, 268
  somatropin, 509
  tobramycin, 297
  trimethoprim, 308
  tyrosine kinase inhibitors, 520
  voriconazole, 328
erythema multiforme
  carbamazepine, 79
  erythropoietins, 389
  fluconazole, 325
  oral contraceptives, 473
  terbinafine, 316
  vancomycin, 301
erythema-multiforme-like reaction
  diltiazem, 226
erythema toxicum
  terbinafine, 316
erythroderma
  aztreonam, 286
  ceftroxone, 285
  diltiazem, 226
esophageal reflux
  botulinum toxins, 166
esophageal ulcer
  doxycycline, 289–290
esophagitis
  khat, 45
esotropia
  tetracycline, 291
euphoria
  khat, 44
  pregabalin, 86
exanthema
  corticosteroids, topical, 183
  nickel, 269
  terbinafine, 316
  valdecoxib, 132
exanthematous eruption
  diltiazem, 226

exanthematous pustulosis
  propafenone, 219
exfoliative dermatitis
  diltiazem, 226
extrapyramidal disorder
  olanzapine, 64
extrapyramidal effect
  cannabinoids, 32
extrapyramidal movement
  citalopram, 17
extrapyramidal symptom
  amisulpride, 64
  fluvoxamine + quetiapine, 68
  haloperidol, 69
  quetiapine, 67
  risperidone, 69
eye function
  amiodarone, 214–215
  anticholinergic drugs, 177
eye pain
  albendazole, 364
eyelid edema
  imatinib mesylate, 522

                                 F
facial paralysis
  bismuth, 264
  infiltration anesthesia, 155
factor VIII inhibitor production
  interferon alfa, 436
fainting
  acupuncture, 556–557
  alfuzosin, 246
  antimony, 263
  azithromycin, 302
  beta-adrenoceptor antagonists, 223
  dextrans, 384
  donepezil, 9
  human papilloma virus vaccine, 374
  indapamide, 258
  latanoprost, 465
  methadone, 112
  temocapril, 238
  zanamivir, 352
Fanconi syndrome
  valproate, 93–94
fat necrosis
  heparins, 407–408
fatigue
  see also hyposthenia, malaise, tiredness, weakness
  acupuncture, 557
  articaine, 158
  azithromycin, 302
  biguanides, 497
  carbamazepine, 78
  chloroquine + proguanil, 336
  deferiprone, 274
  dextromethorphan, 109
  gabapentin, 80
  interferon + ribavirin, 345

interleukin-2, 438
lamivudine, 344
lamotrigine, 80
lapatinib, 526
levetiracetam, 82
methadone, 112
oseltamivir, 353
oxcarbazepine, 85
pazopanib, 529
phosphates, 427
sibutramine, 7
somatropin, 509
sorafenib, 528
sunitinib, 527
suramin, 367
topiramate, 89, 90, 91
valproate, 92, 96
febrile transfusion reaction
blood transfusion, 381
fecal incontinence
orlistat, 429
fecal spotting
orlistat, 429
fetal death
leflunomide, 455
nifedipine, 227
fetal distress
antacids, 423
fetal growth impairment
angiotensin II receptor
antagonists, 240
cannabinoids, 34
fetal heart defect
paroxetine, 19
fever
see also hyperthermia
antithyroid drugs, 491
botulinum toxins, 165
carbamazepine, 79
ceftroxone, 285
clarithromycin + colchicine,
133
clopidogrel, 416
cocaine, 35
colistin, 306
combination vaccines, 369
dalbavancin, 301
efalizumab, 445
fluvoxamine + quetiapine, 68
immunoglobulins, 385
infliximab, 441
levamisole, 366
levofloxacin, 299
measles-mumps-rubella
vaccine, 375, 376
melarsoprol, 341
minocycline, 290
ofloxacin, 300
penicillamine, 275
phenytoin, 85
propofol, 143
thiopental sodium, 147
vancomycin, 301

water-soluble intravascular
iodinated contrast agents,
534
fibrinolysis
hormone replacement therapy,
471
fibrosis
nitrofurantoin, 303
fibrotic reaction
dopamine receptor agonists,
176
fixed drug eruption
clarithromycin, 302
furazolidone, 341
levocetirizine, 190
flank pain
supercoumarins, 404
flares
penicillins, 287
flashback
psilocybin, 46
flatulence
alpha-glucosidase inhibitors,
496
phosphates, 427
pregabalin, 86
ramoplanin, 310
flatus
botulinum toxins, 166
orlistat, 429
floating sensation
methomyl, 565
flu-like symptoms
botulinum toxins, 166
efalizumab, 445
interferon + ribavirin, 345
minocycline, 290
olanzapine, 65
tiagabine, 89
topiramate, 90
fluid retention
imatinib mesylate, 521
flushing
adenosine receptor agonists,
213
calcitonin, 507
immunoglobulins, 386
infliximab, 440
inhibitors of phosphodiesterase
type V, 232
nifedipine, 228
tacrolimus, 458
focal brain edema
pregabalin, 88
folliculitis
gefitinib, 525
tyrosine kinase inhibitors, 520
foot drop
adalimumab, 439
fracture
antiepileptic drugs, 78
bisphosphonates, 561
loop diuretics, 258–259
lopinavir + ritonavir, 351

fulminant hepatic failure
Ephedra and ephedrine, 171
***Fusobacterium* infection**
gemtuzumab ozogamicin, 446

G
gait disturbance
interferon alfa, 436
levetiracetam, 83
ziprasidone, 72
galactorrhea
amisulpride, 64
antipsychotic drugs, 58
aripiprazole, 61
risperidone, 69
gallstones
ceftroxone, 285
octreotide, 511
parenteral nutrition, 396–397
gambling
dopamine receptor agonists,
174–175
***Gamella morbillorum* infection**
buprenorphine, 118–119
gastric disturbance
tiagabine, 89
gastric/duodenal ulceration
glucosamine, 567
gastric emptying slowing
pramlintide, 496
gastric mucosal damage
iodine, 490
gastritis
khat, 45
gastroenteritis
montelukast, 203
rabeprazole, 425
gastrointestinal bleeding
acetylsalicylic acid, 128
clopidogrel, 415
coumarin anticoagulants, 399
non-steroidal
anti-inflammatory drugs,
125–127
risperidone, 71
statins, 16
gastrointestinal discomfort
deferiprone, 274
gastrointestinal disturbance
Agnus castus, 552
hydroxychloroquine, 337
linezolid, 304
pristinamycin, 307
gastrointestinal effects
quinupristin/dalfopristin, 307
gastrointestinal perforation
bevacizumab, 444
gastrointestinal symptoms
Zingiber officinale (ginger),
556
gastrointestinal upsets
Echinacea species, 553
genital tumors
UVB, 184

gestational diabetes
leuprolide, 508
giddiness
antimony, 263
cocaine, 34
gingival bleeding
quilinggao + warfarin, 403
supercoumarins, 404
gingival enlargement
diltiazem, 226
felodipine, 226
verapamil, 228
gingivitis
sirolimus (rapamycin), 457
glaucoma, open-angle
diuretics, 252
glioblastoma multiforme
hair dyes, 182
glioma
hair dyes, 182
glomerular nephrotoxicity
amphotericin B deoxycholate
(DAMB), 319
glove-and-stocking neuropathy
linezolid, 304
graft-versus-host disease
stem cells, 389–390
granulocytopenia
ticlopidine, 417
granulomatous reaction
leuprolide, 508
ground-glass attenuation
gefitinib, 524
ground-glass opacity
amiodarone, 214
arsenic, 263
leflunomide, 454
valsartan, 242
growth delay
budesonide, 194–195
**growth hormone insensitivity
syndrome**
insulin, 495
Guillain–Barré syndrome
meningococcal vaccine, 372
vaccines, 370
gynecomastia
antipsychotic drugs, 58
bicalutamide, 480
efavirenz, 350
finasteride, 481
risperidone, 69, 71
spironolactone, 259

H
hair depigmentation
pazopanib, 529
sunitinib, 527
hair loss
botulinum toxins, 166
leflunomide, 455
tyrosine kinase inhibitors, 520
valproate, 94
voriconazole, 329

hallucinations
ketamine + morphine, 113
methylthioninium chloride +
statins, 569
propofol, 142
topiramate, 90
tramadol, 118
voriconazole, 328
**hallucinogen persisting
perception disorder (HPPD)**
psilocybin, 46
halo dermatitis
interferon + ribavirin, 346
hand-foot skin reactions
sorafenib, 528
headache
adenosine receptor agonists,
213
adrenaline (epinephrine), 170
Agnus castus, 552
alfuzosin, 481
anti-human CD40 Mab
chimeric 5D12, 443
botulinum toxins, 165
camphor, 564
cannabinoids, 33
ceftroxone, 285
chloroquine + proguanil, 336
daptomycin, 309
desmopressin, 512
dextromethorphan, 109
direct renin inhibitors, 244
efalizumab, 445
endothelin receptor
antagonists, 244, 245
erythropoietins, 389
esomeprazole, 424
finasteride, 482
fluticasone propionate +
salmeterol, 202
formoterol, 200
gabapentin, 80
gatifloxacin, 299
glyceryl trinitrate, 225
H. pylori eradication regimens,
425, 426
immunoglobulins, 385, 386
inhibitors of phosphodiesterase
type V, 232
irbesartan, 241
ivermectin, 365
khat, 44
lamotrigine, 80, 90
levetiracetam, 82
losartan, 242
melarsoprol, 341
mesalazine, 428, 429
methomyl, 565
micafungin, 331
molsidomine, 225
mometasone furoate, 197
nifedipine, 228
olanzapine, 65
oral contraceptives, 473

oseltamivir, 353
oxcarbazepine, 84, 85
phosphates, 427
pregabalin, 86, 87, 88
progesterone antagonists, 477
proton pump inhibitors, 424
quetiapine, 68
quinupristin/dalfopristin, 307
rabeprazole, 425
risperidone, 71
saw palmetto, 481
sibutramine, 8
somatropin, 509
tamsulosin, 247
terbinafine, 316
tiagabine, 89
topiramate, 89, 91
valproate, 92
zanamivir, 352
ziprasidone, 72
zonisamide, 99
hearing impairment
clarithromycin, 302
loop diuretics, 258
psilocybin, 46
tacrolimus, 458
heart
see also entries at coronary-,
cardi-
heart attack
risperidone, 71
heart beat
see cardiac dysrhythmias,
tachycardia; *specific
conditions, such as* sinus
node dysfunction
heart block
nifedipine, 228
heart failure
anagrelide, 413
imatinib mesylate, 521
vitamin E, 395
heart failure worsening
beta-adrenoceptor antagonists,
223
heart rate increase
desflurane, 138
duloxetine, 19
pseudoephedrine, 171
heartburn
H. pylori eradication regimens,
426
peppermint oil, 568
heat sensation
water-soluble intravascular
iodinated contrast agents,
534
heavy eyelids
suxamethonium, 164
hemangioma
valproate, 95
hematoma
botulinum toxins, 166
clopidogrel, 415

coumarin anticoagulants, 399
heparins, 404, 405
leuprolide, 508
streptokinase, 413
supercoumarins, 404
hematuria
coumarin anticoagulants, 399
penicillamine, 274
supercoumarins, 404
hemianopsia
spinal manipulation, 558
hemiparesis
cannabinoids, 32
pregabalin, 88
hemodynamic changes
infiltration anesthesia, 155
hemoglobinuria
chloramphenicol, 298
hemolysis
blood transfusion, 382
immunoglobulins, 385
interferon + ribavirin, 346
hemolytic anemia
ceftroxone, 285
cephalosporins, 284
interferon + ribavirin, 346
penicillamine, 274
streptokinase, 413
**hemolytic transfusion reaction,
acute**
blood transfusion, 381
hemolytic-uremic syndrome
everolimus, 454
hemorrhage
anticoagulants + epoprostenol,
465
clopidogrel, 415–416
coumarin anticoagulants, 399
supercoumarins, 404
hepat-
see also entries at liver-
hepatic damage
amiodarone, 215
hepatic decompensation
lamivudine, 344
hepatic failure
levofloxacin, 299
thiopental sodium, 147
hepatic insufficiency
clarithromycin + colchicine,
133
hepatic necrosis
cocaine, 35
coumarin anticoagulants, 399
hepatitis
buprenorphine, 118
cocaine, 35
coumarin anticoagulants, 399
ezetimibe, 515
granulocyte colony-stimulating
factor, 435
haematitium, 556
imatinib mesylate, 521, 522
inhibitors of phosphodiesterase
type V, 232

irbesartan, 241
oseltamivir, 353
Piper methysticum, 554
rofecoxib, 131
ticlopidine, 417
vancomycin, 301
hepatitis B infection
blood transfusion, 383
hepatitis E infection
blood transfusion, 383
hepatocellular carcinoma
valproate, 94
hepatocytolysis
fluvoxamine, 16
hepatosplenomegaly
stem cells, 390
hepatotoxicity
6-thioguanine, 461
azathioprine, 459
biguanides, 497
bosentan, 245
chloroquine + proguanil, 336
clopidogrel, 416
gemtuzumab ozogamicin, 446
glimepiride, 501
imatinib mesylate, 522
isoniazid, 359
liposomal amphotericin
(L-amB), 319–320
mycophenolate mofetil, 456
nevirapine, 350
sevoflurane, 140
sirolimus (rapamycin), 457
statins, 16
ximelagatran, 411
herpes simplex reactivation
morphine, 107
herpes zoster infection
leflunomide, 455
stem cells, 390
HGV infection
blood transfusion, 383
hiccups
epidural anesthesia, 152–153
hidradenitis suppurativa
sirolimus (rapamycin), 457
high-output heart failure
anagrelide, 413
HIV infection
blood transfusion, 383
hives
MLN02, 447
hoarseness
ciclesonide, 196
fluticasone propionate +
salmeterol, 202
inhaled glucocorticoids, 193
isotretinoin, 185
streptokinase, 413
Horner's syndrome
spinal manipulation, 558
hot flushes
leuprolide, 507

Hutchinson's sign
amlodipine, 225
hydrocephalus
metronidazole, 339
omeprazole, 425
hydrops
enalapril, 236
hypacusis
interferon alfa, 436
hyperalgesia
remifentanil, 116
hyperammonemia
acetazolamide, 255
valproate, 96, 97–98
hyperbilirubinemia
gemtuzumab ozogamicin, 446
quinupristin/dalfopristin, 307
hypercalcemia
calcitonin, 507
gentamicin, 297
thiazide diuretics, 256–257
tretinoin + voriconazole, 324
hypercalciuria
gentamicin, 297
hypercapnia
methylthioninium chloride +
statins, 570
hyperchloremia
valproate, 93
hypercholesterolemia
efavirenz, 350
glucosamine, 568
verteporfin, 546
hyperexcitability
ketamine, 141
hyperglycemia
efavirenz, 350
fluoroquinolones, 298
formoterol, 201
gatifloxacin, 299
immunoglobulins, 387
risperidone, 69, 71
suramin, 367
temsirolimus, 459
hyperkalemia
candesartan + spironolactone,
241
cilazapril, 235
direct renin inhibitors, 244
enalapril, 236
heparins, 404
losartan + spironolactone, 242
mannitol, 260
propofol, 143
spironolactone, 259
stavudine, 349
thiopental sodium, 146
hyperkinesia
lamotrigine, 80
hyperlactatemia
linezolid, 304
hyperlipidemia
antipsychotic drugs, 58
clozapine, 63

everolimus, 454
propofol, 143
temsirolimus, 459
hypermagnesiuria
gentamicin, 297
hypernatremia
valproate, 93
hyperostosis
acitretin, 185
hyperparathyroidism
lithium, 25
hyperphosphatemia
phosphates, 427, 428
vitamin D analogues, 394
hyperpigmentation
gold and gold salts, 265
hyperprolactinemia
antipsychotic drugs, 58
risperidone, 70, 71
verapamil, 228
hyperpyrexia
methylthioninium chloride +
statins, 570
hyper-reflexia
ecstasy, 43
hypersalivation
clozapine, 62, 63
hypersensitivity reaction
amiodarone, 216
antithyroid drugs, 491
ceftroxone, 285
clopidogrel, 416
colistin, 306
diuretic sulfonamides, 252–254
epidural anesthesia, 153
heparins, 408
interferon + ribavirin, 348
iron salts, 265–266
lidocaine, 160
mesalazine, 428
mexiletine, 218
olanzapine, 66
pholcodine, 116
polygelines, 384
vancomycin, 301
verteporfin, 547
hypersomnia
levetiracetam, 83
hypertelorism
fluconazole, 325
valproate, 95
hypertension
see also blood pressure
increase
acetazolamide, 255
adrenaline (epinephrine),
170–171
bevacizumab, 444
cannabinoids, 32
erythropoietins, 388
fluvoxamine + quetiapine, 68
immunoglobulins, 386
infliximab, 440
isoflurane, 138

leflunomide, 454
melarsoprol, 341
methadone, 112
pazopanib, 529
polystyrene sulfonates, 276
pseudoephedrine, 172
sorafenib, 528
statins, 16
sunitinib, 527
venlafaxine, 19
hyperthermia
see also fever
ecstasy, 41–42
ketamine, 141
khat, 46
topiramate, 91–92
hyperthyroidism
amiodarone, 215
sunitinib, 527–528
hypertonia
beta$_2$-adrenoceptor agonists,
200
fenfluramine, 7
obstetric anesthesia, 156
hypertriglyceridemia
efavirenz, 349–350
propofol, 142–143
hyperviscosity
immunoglobulins, 385, 386
hypesthesia
adenosine receptor agonists,
213
interferon alfa, 436
topiramate, 90
hyphema
aspirin + *Ginkgo biloba*, 401
hypocalcemia
citrate, 399
methadone, 112
phosphates, 427, 428
hypocapnia
acetazolamide, 255
hypoestrogenism
antipsychotic drugs, 58
hypoglycemia
biguanides, 498
exenatide, 499
gatifloxacin, 299
glibenclamide, 501
insulin, 494
leuprolide, 508
statins, 16
stavudine, 349
hypokalemia
formoterol, 200, 201
gentamicin, 297
liposomal amphotericin
(L-amB), 320
methadone, 112
valproate, 93
hypomagnesemia
gentamicin, 297
hypomania
androgenic anabolic steroids,
478

topiramate, 91
hyponatremia
bupropion, 20
carbamazepine, 78–79
desmopressin, 512
levetiracetam, 83
oxcarbazepine, 84
phosphates, 427
tolterodine, 177–178
vasopressin, 511
hypophosphatemia
imatinib mesylate, 522
micafungin, 331
valproate, 93
hypopigmentation
imatinib mesylate, 523
hypoplastic midface
valproate, 95
hyposthenia
see also fatigue, malaise,
tiredness, weakness
botulinum toxins, 165
hypotension
alfuzosin, 481
beta-adrenoceptor antagonists,
223
bupivacaine, 159
cannabinoids, 32
cefaclor, 284, 285
cilazapril, 235
clarithromycin + colchicine,
133
clarithromycin + nifedipine,
228
cocaine, 35
cocaine + modafinil, 7
dextrans, 384
doxazosin, 246
etherified starches, 384
fentanyl, 111
infliximab, 440
inhibitors of phosphodiesterase
type V, 232
levobupivacaine, 160
misoprostol, 466
molsidomine, 225
nifedipine, 227–228
obstetric anesthesia, 156
polygelines, 384
propafenone, 218
propofol, 142
protamine, 417
remifentanil, 116
spinal anesthesia, 153
tamsulosin, 247
telithromycin + verapamil, 229
terlipressin, 512
trichloroethylene, 140
ziprasidone, 65
**hypothalamic-pituitary-adrenal
axis activation**
alprazolam, 50
**hypothalamic-pituitary-adrenal
axis suppression**
diazepam, 50–51

fentanyl, 111
systemic glucocorticoids, 464
hypothermia
statins, 16
hypothyroidism
lithium, 25
polyvinylpyrrolidone, 279
rifampicin, 359
somatostatin, 510
hypotonia
antacids, 423
hypouricemia
valproate, 93
hypovolemia
polyethylene glycol, 426
hypoxemia
amiodarone, 214
gefitinib, 524
hypoxia
gemtuzumab ozogamicin, 446
granulocyte colony-stimulating
factor, 435
methylthioninium chloride +
statins, 570
remifentanil, 116
sevoflurane, 138

I

IBCT
see incorrect blood component
transfusion (IBCT)
IFIS
see intraoperative floppy iris
syndrome (IFIS)
immunosuppression
ecstasy, 41
impotence
finasteride, 481, 484
incoordination
pregabalin, 86, 88
**incorrect blood component
transfusion (IBCT)**
blood transfusion, 382
indigestion
H. pylori eradication regimens,
426
phosphates, 427
induration of the skin
heparins, 408
inebriation
levetiracetam, 82
infarction
see cerebral infarction,
myocardial infarction
infection
adalimumab, 439
epidural analgesia, 108
pregabalin, 87
tiagabine, 89
inflammatory bowel disease
rofecoxib, 131
infusion reactions
amphotericin, 317
infliximab, 440, 441

infusion-related pain
verteporfin, 547
infusion-site reaction
quinupristin/dalfopristin, 307
injection site pain
naltrexone, 120
propofol, 143
risperidone, 71
ziprasidone, 72
injection site reaction
daptomycin, 309
heparins, 405
human papilloma virus
vaccine, 374
omalizumab, 447
verteporfin, 546
injection site trauma
botulinum toxins, 166
injuries, accidental
pregabalin, 87
INR decrease
ginseng + warfarin, 402
green tea + warfarin, 401
menthol + warfarin, 568
St. John's wort + warfarin, 401
INR increase
dong quai + warfarin, 400
garlic + warfarin, 400
insomnia
citalopram, 17
dextromethorphan, 109
interferon + ribavirin, 345
methadone, 112
micafungin, 331
nalmefene, 119
naltrexone, 120
oseltamivir, 353
oxcarbazepine, 84
phosphates, 427
proton pump inhibitors, 424
risperidone, 71
tiagabine, 89
topiramate, 89
ziprasidone, 65, 72
insulin resistance
antipsychotic drugs, 58
interstitial nephritis
celecoxib, 130
rofecoxib, 131
vancomycin, 301
interstitial pneumonia
leflunomide, 454
nitrofurantoin, 303
interstitial pneumonitis
lamotrigine, 81
intestinal pseudo-obstruction
diltiazem, 226
intracerebral bleeding
Ginkgo biloba + ibuprofen, 401
intracranial hemorrhage
coumarin anticoagulants, 399
glycoprotein IIb-IIIa inhibitors,
415

intracranial hypertension
minocycline, 290
tetracycline, 291
intracranial pressure, increase
acetazolamide, 255
intraocular inflammation
ranibizumab, 545
**intraoperative floppy iris
syndrome (IFIS)**
tamsulosin, 246
intravascular hemolysis
hydroxychloroquine, 337
immunoglobulins, 386
intussusception
rotavirus vaccine, 377
vaccines, 373
irritability
efavirenz, 349
levetiracetam, 82
methylphenidate, 5
oxcarbazepine, 83, 84
irritation
calcipotriol, 186
ischemic stroke
metamfetamine, 2
itching
Agnus castus, 552
aluminium, 262
aluminium adsorbent, 370
aminolevulinic acid, 184
aztreonam, 286
calcipotriol, 186
cefaclor, 285
ceftroxone, 285
clarithromycin, 302
clopidogrel, 416
colistin, 306
cosmetics, 180
cupping, 557
diltiazem, 226
epidural analgesia, 108
etherified starches, 384
fentanyl, 110
fondaparinux, 412
gold and gold salts, 265
hydroxychloroquine, 337
infliximab, 441
interferon + ribavirin, 345, 346
ivermectin, 365
ketamine + morphine, 113
lamotrigine, 80
levamisole, 366
levocetirizine, 190
levofloxacin, 299
lidocaine, 160
manganese, 268
mepivacaine, 161
morphine, 107, 114, 115
omalizumab, 447
penicillins, 287
proton pump inhibitors, 424
quinupristin/dalfopristin, 307
rofecoxib, 131
sufentanil, 107

tacalcitol, 186
telithromycin, 301
temsirolimus, 459
tramadol, 118
vancomycin, 301

J

jaundice
azithromycin, 302
biguanides, 497
ceftroxone, 285
ciclosporin, 321
clopidogrel, 416
cocaine, 35
glimepiride, 501
haematitium, 556
hepatitis B vaccine, 374
penicillins, 286–287
Polygonum multiflorum, 555
rofecoxib, 131
rosiglitazone, 502
ticlopidine, 417
jitteriness
statins, 16
joint pain
levofloxacin, 299
ofloxacin, 300

K

Kawasaki disease
rotavirus vaccine, 377
kidney
see also entries at nephro-,
renal-
kidney stones
ceftroxone, 285
topiramate, 89
Kounis syndrome
cefuroxime, 286

L

lacrimation
vancomycin, 301
lactation reduction
khat, 45
lactic acidosis
amygdalin, 556
biguanides, 498
salbutamol, 201–202
laryngeal dystonia
antipsychotic drugs, 57–58
laryngospasm
airway anesthesia, 152
verteporfin, 546
left bundle branch block
methylthioninium chloride +
statins, 570
left ventricular dysfunction
imatinib mesylate, 521
lens injury
bevacizumab, 544
lethargy
entacavir, 344

levetiracetam, 82, 83
methylthioninium chloride +
statins, 570, 571
leukemia, acute
valproate, 94
leukocytoclastic vasculitis
linezolid, 305
montelukast, 203
sirolimus (rapamycin), 457
teicoplanin, 301
leukocytosis
carbamazepine, 79
minocycline, 290
vancomycin, 301
leukopenia
see also agranulocytosis,
neutropenia
atorvastatin, 516
clarithromycin + colchicine,
133
denileukin diftitox, 438
H. pylori eradication regimens,
426
interferon + ribavirin, 345
linezolid, 304
penicillamine, 275
suramin, 367
temsirolimus, 459
ticlopidine, 417
libido loss
finasteride, 481, 482, 483, 484
flutamide, 481
male hormonal contraception,
473–474
methadone, 112
lichenoid lesions
inhibitors of phosphodiesterase
type V, 232
lightheadedness
efavirenz, 349
lorazepam, 51
methomyl, 565
line migration
epidural analgesia, 108
lingual paresthesia
lidocaine (lignocaine), 218
lipoatrophy
octreotide, 511
lipohypertrophy
exenatide, 500
liver
see also entries at hepat-
liver damage
alosetron, 423
desflurane, 138
liver dysfunction
carbamazepine, 79
liver failure
itraconazole, 326
orlistat, 430
Piper methysticum, 554
trimethoprim, 308
longitudinal melanonychia
amlodipine, 225

loose stools
orlistat, 429
low back pain
amiodarone, 216
rabeprazole, 425
rifampicin, 361
lung injury
arsenic, 263
lupus erythematosus, cutaneous
acebutolol, 223–224
terbinafine, 316
verapamil, 228
lupus-like syndrome
adalimumab, 439
antithyroid drugs, 491
infliximab, 440
minocycline, 290–291
nitrofurantoin, 303
lupus pernio
heparins, 408
lymphocele
everolimus, 454
lymphocytosis
carbamazepine, 79
lymphoma
adalimumab, 439
pimecrolimus, 457
thiopurines, 459
lymphopenia
denileukin diftitox, 438
suramin, 367
lymphoproliferative disorder
alefacept, 440
everolimus, 454
globulins, 385

M

macrophagic myofasciitis
aluminium, 262
influenza vaccine, 374
macular edema
rosiglitazone, 502
macular rash
melarsoprol, 341
terbinafine, 316
maculopapular eruption
manganese, 268
temsirolimus, 459
water-soluble intravascular
iodinated contrast agents,
537
maculopapular lesions
nickel, 269
maculopapular rash
mepivacaine, 161
micafungin, 331
pseudoephedrine, 172
trimethoprim, 308
vancomycin, 301
madarosis
botulinum toxins, 166
malaise
see also fatigue, hyposthenia,
tiredness, weakness

6-thioguanine, 461
alfuzosin, 481
alosetron, 423
aztreonam, 286
cannabinoids, 33
H. pylori eradication regimens, 425
ivermectin, 365
lamivudine, 344
rofecoxib, 131
suramin, 367
malar hypertrichosis lanuginosa
interferon + ribavirin, 346
male breast cancer
bicalutamide, 480
malignant hyperthermia
desflurane, 138
mania
antidepressants, 15
systemic glucocorticoids, 464
thyroid hormones, 490
manic psychosis
isotretinoin, 185
marrow hypoplasia
alemtuzumab, 442
mask-like face
manganese, 267–268
venlafaxine, 19
measles inclusion-body encephalitis (MIBE)
measles-mumps-rubella vaccine, 375–376
melena
coumarin anticoagulants, 399
memory impairment
alprazolam, 49
cannabinoids, 32
carbamazepine, 78
diamorphine, 110
isoflurane, 138
ketamine, 141
systemic glucocorticoids, 463
valproate, 92
zolpidem, 53
meningioma
interferon beta, 437
menorrhagia
supercoumarins, 404
menstrual abnormality
Agnus castus, 552
antipsychotic drugs, 58
valproate, 94–95
Merkel cell carcinoma
rituximab, 448
mesenteric ischemia
propranolol, 223
metabolic acidosis
acetazolamide, 255
brinzolamide, 256
clarithromycin + colchicine, 133
gentamicin, 297
granulocyte colony-stimulating factor, 435

linezolid, 304
propofol, 142, 143
thiopental sodium, 147
topiramate, 91
valproate, 93
metallic taste
H. pylori eradication regimens, 425, 426
methemoglobinemia
benzocaine, 158–159
dapsone, 357
methicillin-resistant *Staphylococcus aureus* (MRSA)
etanercept, 440
Meyerson's syndrome
interferon + ribavirin, 346
MI
see myocardial infarction
MIBE
see measles inclusion-body encephalitis
microangiopathy
cocaine, 35
microchimerism
blood transfusion, 382
migraine
glyceryl trinitrate, 225
milia
interferon + ribavirin, 346
miosis
fentanyl, 111
mood change
efavirenz, 349
hormone replacement therapy, 470
mood disorder
fluticasone propionate + salmeterol, 202
mood lability
topiramate, 91
moodiness
methylphenidate, 4
motor block
epidural analgesia, 108
motor effects
ketamine, 141
motor polyneuropathy
aminolevulinic acid, 184
mouth burning
camphor, 564
mouth discoloration
minocycline, 290
MRSA
see methicillin-resistant *Staphylococcus aureus*
mucinosis
adalimumab, 439
mucormycosis
globulins, 385
mucositis
temsirolimus, 459
multifocal leukoencephalopathy
interferon alfa, 436

multiorgan dysfunction
thiopental sodium, 147
multiorgan failure
nifedipine, 228
muscle cramps
see also cramps
imatinib mesylate, 523
muscle pain
daptomycin, 309
human papilloma virus vaccine, 374
interferon alfa, 436
Piper methysticum, 555
muscle rigidity
ecstasy, 43
venlafaxine, 19
muscle rupture
ciprofloxacin, 298
myalgia
anti-human CD40 Mab chimeric 5D12, 443
ceftroxone, 285
efalizumab, 445
immunoglobulins, 386
ivermectin, 365
quinupristin/dalfopristin, 307
somatropin, 509
suxamethonium, 164
Mycobacterium hominis infection
basiliximab, 444
Mycobacterium xenopi infection
sirolimus (rapamycin), 458
mycosis fungoides
alefacept, 440
myelodysplasia
alemtuzumab, 442
myelopathy
nitrous oxide, 140
myelosuppression
H. pylori eradication regimens, 426
imatinib mesylate, 522
interferon + ribavirin, 346
linezolid, 304
myelotoxicity
H. pylori eradication regimens, 340
myocardial infarction
see also cardiac arrest
botulinum toxins, 165, 166
cefuroxime, 286
cocaine, 35
finasteride, 482
gemtuzumab ozogamicin, 446
immunoglobulins, 385
khat, 44
myocardial ischemia
ultrasound contrast agents, 540
myoclonic jerk
methylthioninium chloride + statins, 570
myoclonic movement
etomidate, 140
propofol, 142

myoclonic seizure
pregabalin, 88
myoclonus
ecstasy, 41
olanzapine, 66
tiagabine, 89
myofascial necrosis
botulinum toxins, 166–167
myopathy
ciclosporin, 452
clarithromycin + statins, 517
colchicine + statins, 134,
517–518
daptomycin, 309
finasteride, 482
HMG-CoA reductase
inhibitors, 516
hydroxychloroquine, 337
propofol, 143
rosiglitazone, 501–502
myopia
acetazolamide, 255
chlorthalidone, 257
topiramate, 90
myosis
methomyl, 565

N

nail discoloration
doxycycline, 290
sparfloxacin, 300
NAION
see non-arteritic anterior
ischemic optic neuropathy
(NAION)
nasal congestion
endothelin receptor
antagonists, 245
inhibitors of phosphodiesterase
type V, 232
nasopharyngitis
naltrexone, 120
nausea
acupuncture, 557
Agnus castus, 552
alosetron, 423
baclofen, 165
biguanides, 497
bismuth, 264
calcitonin, 507
camphor, 564
cefaclor, 284
ceftroxone, 285
chloroquine + proguanil, 336
citalopram, 17
clopidogrel, 416
cocaine + modafinil, 7
cosmetics, 180
daptomycin, 309
deferiprone, 274
desloratadine, 189
desmopressin, 512
dextrans, 384
dextromethorphan, 109

diuretic sulfonamides, 252
donepezil, 9
droperidol + morphine, 113
epidural analgesia, 108
etherified starches, 384
exenatide, 499
fentanyl, 111
gabapentin, 80
H. pylori eradication regimens,
340, 425, 426
imatinib mesylate, 521, 523
immunoglobulins, 386
interferon + ribavirin, 345
irbesartan, 241
iron salts, 266
ivermectin, 365
ketamine + morphine, 113
lamotrigine, 80
lapatinib, 526
levetiracetam, 82
liraglutide, 500
mefloquine, 337
methomyl, 565
modafinil, 6
morphine, 107, 115
mycophenolate sodium, 456
naltrexone, 120
nifedipine, 228
opioids, 107
orlistat, 429
oseltamivir, 353
oxcarbazepine, 85
pazopanib, 529
pethidine, 116
phosphates, 427
physostigmine, 114
pramlintide, 496
pregabalin, 87
progesterone antagonists, 477
pseudoephedrine, 172
quetiapine, 68
rabeprazole, 425
ramoplanin, 310
sunitinib, 527
suramin, 367
telithromycin, 301
temsirolimus, 459
terbinafine, 317
tiagabine, 89
tigecycline, 291, 292
topiramate, 89, 90
valproate, 92, 96
verteporfin, 546
voriconazole, 329
water-soluble intravascular
iodinated contrast agents,
534
zanamivir, 353
ziprasidone, 72
zonisamide, 99
neck pain
spinal manipulation, 557
necrotic enterocolitis
cardiac glycosides, 209–210

necrotizing pancreatitis
hydrochlorothiazide, 257
necrotizing vasculitis
minocycline, 291
nephr-
see also entries at kidney-,
renal-
nephritis, interstitial
celecoxib, 130
rofecoxib, 131
vancomycin, 301
nephrogenic diabetes insipidus
lithium, 25
nephrogenic systemic fibrosis
gadolinium-based contrast
agents, 538–540
nephrolithiasis
see kidney stones
nephropathy, acute
phosphates, 427
nephrotic syndrome
celecoxib, 130
verteporfin, 547
nephrotoxicity
aminoglycoside antibiotics +
colistin, 297
amphotericin, 317
amphotericin B deoxycholate
(DAMB), 319
ciclosporin, 452
colistin, 306
contrast media, 535–537
mesalazine, 428
sirolimus (rapamycin), 457
nervousness
efavirenz, 349
lamotrigine, 80
levamisole, 366
naltrexone, 120
pregabalin, 88
topiramate, 90, 91
neuroblastoma
hair dyes, 182
**neuroleptic malignant
syndrome**
fluvoxamine + quetiapine, 68
olanzapine, 65
venlafaxine, 19
neurological soft signs
antipsychotic drugs, 57
neuromuscular blockade
colistin, 306
neuropathy
ciclosporin, 452
daptomycin, 309
flecainide, 217
itraconazole, 326
neuropsychiatric disorder
efavirenz, 349
neurosensory deafness
proton pump inhibitors, 424
neurotoxicity
aciclovir, 343
itraconazole + viricristine, 325

metronidazole, 339
neutropenia
    see also agranulocytosis,
        leukopenia
    alemtuzumab, 442, 443
    beta-lactam antibiotics, 280
    clopidogrel, 416
    cyclophosphamide, 453
    dasatinib, 523
    deferiprone, 274
    gemtuzumab ozogamicin, 446
    imatinib mesylate, 522
    immunoglobulins, 386
    interferon + ribavirin, 346
    levamisole, 366
    linezolid, 304
    nevirapine, 350
    nilotinib, 524
    stavudine, 349
    sunitinib, 527
    trimethoprim, 308
nodal rhythm
    levobupivacaine, 160
nodules
    aluminium, 262
    aluminium adsorbent, 370
    dasatinib, 524
    minocycline, 290
**non-arteritic anterior ischemic
    optic neuropathy (NAION)**
    inhibitors of phosphodiesterase
        type V, 232
numbness
    donepezil, 9
nystagmus
    acetazolamide, 255
    carbamazepine + oxybutynin,
        178
    cocaine, 34
    fenfluramine contamination, 7
    methylthioninium chloride +
        statins, 570
    spinal manipulation, 558

O

obesity
    antipsychotic drugs, 58–59
obsessive-compulsive symptoms
    azathioprine, 459
    topiramate, 91
obstructive cardiomyopathy
    systemic glucocorticoids, 463
obstructive ileus
    montelukast, 203
ocular pigmentation
    tetracycline, 291
ocular pruritus
    tobramycin, 297
oculogyric crisis
    cannabinoids, 32
    Piper methysticum, 554
OHSS
    see ovarian hyperstimulation

oily discharge
    orlistat, 429
oligohydramnios
    angiotensin II receptor
        antagonists, 240
    enalapril, 236
oligospermia
    male hormonal contraception,
        474
oliguria
    rifampicin, 361
    silver salts and derivatives, 269
onycholysis
    roxithromycin, 303
onychopathy
    sirolimus (rapamycin), 457
open-angle glaucoma
    diuretics, 252
ophthalmoplegia
    spinal manipulation, 558
optic neuropathy
    amiodarone, 215
    ethambutol, 358–359
    linezolid, 304
oral candidiasis
    budesonide, 195
    ciclesonide, 196
    dalbavancin, 301
    fluticasone propionate, 196
    fluticasone propionate +
        salmeterol, 202
    H. pylori eradication regimens,
        340
    inhaled glucocorticoids, 193
    mometasone furoate, 197
oral dyskinesia
    Piper methysticum, 554
oral epithelial dysplasia
    adalimumab, 439
oral lesions
    rofecoxib, 131
oral mucositis
    H. pylori eradication regimens,
        426
oral sores
    esomeprazole, 424
orbital cellulitis
    ocular anesthesia, 156
orbital swelling
    ocular anesthesia, 156
orgasmic dysfunction
    finasteride, 483
orthostatic hypotension
    alfuzosin, 481
    inhibitors of phosphodiesterase
        type V, 246
    quetiapine, 67
    tamsulosin, 247
osteonecrosis of the jaw
    bisphosphonates, 562–564
osteoporosis
    antipsychotic drugs, 58
    lopinavir + ritonavir, 351
    magnesium salts, 266–267

systemic glucocorticoids, 464
otalgia
    tacrolimus, 458
out-of-body experience
    ketamine, 141
ovarian hyperstimulation
    gonadotropins, 468–469
oxygen desaturation
    glyceryl trinitrate, 225

P

pain
    efalizumab, 445
    interleukin-11, 439
palpitation
    adenosine receptor agonists,
        213
    cannabinoids, 31
    diamorphine, 110
    ecstasy, 40
    formoterol, 200
    indapamide, 258
    infliximab, 440
    ivermectin, 365
    nifedipine, 227, 228
pancreatitis
    enalapril, 236
    hydrochlorothiazide, 257
    irbesartan, 241
    lisinopril, 237
    methomyl, 565
    metronidazole, 339
    perindopril, 237
    propofol, 143
    trimethoprim, 308
    water-soluble intravascular
        iodinated contrast agents,
        534
pancytopenia
    adalimumab, 439
    albendazole, 364
    clarithromycin + colchicine,
        133
    linezolid, 304
    ticlopidine, 417
panic attack
    azathioprine, 459
panniculitis
    dasatinib, 524
    minocycline, 291
papilledema
    interleukin-11, 439
parakeratosis
    interferon + ribavirin, 346
    penicillamine, 275
paralytic ileus
    clarithromycin + colchicine,
        133
    methomyl, 565
paranoia
    bupropion, 20
    ketamine, 141
    khat, 44
paraplegia
    somatropin, 509

parasympathetic dysfunction of the visual system
  botulinum toxins, 166
parathyroid hormone increase
  lithium, 26
paresthesia
  adalimumab, 439
  colistin, 306
  epidural analgesia, 108
  linezolid, 304
  metronidazole, 339
  topiramate, 89, 90, 91
  valproate, 96
parkinsonism
  antipsychotic drugs, 57
  levetiracetam, 83
  manganese, 267–268
  valproate, 93
paronychia
  tyrosine kinase inhibitors, 520
paronychial inflammation
  gefitinib, 525
parotitis
  nitrofurantoin, 303
paroxysmal nocturnal hemoglobinuria
  chloramphenicol, 298
pedal edema
  rifampicin, 361
pemphigus foliaceus
  imidapril, 236
  penicillamine, 275
  quinapril, 237
pemphigus vulgaris
  quinapril, 237
pericardial effusion
  nickel, 269
  nilotinib, 524
  ramipril, 238
pericarditis
  nickel, 268–269
  tramadol, 117–118
perineal anesthesia
  linezolid, 304
periosteal bone change
  interleukin-11, 439
peripheral edema
  endothelin receptor antagonists, 245
  polystyrene sulfonates, 276
  pregabalin, 86, 87, 88
  suramin, 367
peripheral neuropathy
  leflunomide, 454
  linezolid, 304
  melarsoprol, 341
  voriconazole, 328
peritonitis
  erythropoietins, 389
periungual infections
  sirolimus (rapamycin), 457
periungual irritation
  calcipotriol, 186

periungual pigmentation
  amlodipine, 225
persistent pulmonary hypertension
  statins, 16
personality change
  levamisole, 366
petechiae
  arsenic, 263
  ceftroxone, 285
  heparins, 405
  interferon alfa, 437
  omalizumab, 447
Peyronie's disease
  beta-adrenoceptor antagonists, 224
pharyngitis
  interferon + ribavirin, 345
  mometasone furoate, 197, 198
  oxcarbazepine, 83
  tiagabine, 89
  vancomycin, 301
  zonisamide, 99
phosphate nephropathy, acute
  phosphates, 427
photoageing
  voriconazole, 328
photophobia
  vancomycin, 301
photosensitivity
  entacavir, 344
  verteporfin, 546, 547
  voriconazole, 329
photosensitization
  voriconazole, 328
phototoxicity
  amiodarone, 216
pigmentation
  minocycline, 290
platelet activation
  cardiac glycosides, 209
pleural effusion
  arsenic, 263
  dasatinib, 523
  nilotinib, 524
  nitrofurantoin, 303
  ramipril, 238
pleurocarditis
  minocycline, 290
pneumonia
  botulinum toxins, 165
  leflunomide, 454
  minocycline, 290
  nitrofurantoin, 303
  MLN02, 447
pneumonitis
  lamotrigine, 81
  sirolimus (rapamycin), 457
  valsartan, 242
pneumothorax
  cannabinoids, 33
polio
  polio vaccine, 373

poliomyelitis
  poliomyelitis vaccine, 376
polyarteritis nodosa
  minocycline, 290
polyarthropathy
  immunoglobulins, 387
polydactyly
  leuprolide, 508
polyps
  lornoxicam, 132
polyserositis
  ramipril, 238
poor attention
  diamorphine, 110
porphyria cutanea tarda
  interferon + ribavirin, 346
port wine stain
  isotretinoin, 185–186
postural sway
  zolpidem, 53
posturing
  venlafaxine, 19
potassium channel syndrome
  ciclosporin, 452
priapism
  inhibitors of phosphodiesterase type V, 232
  lithium + oxcarbazepine, 26
  oxcarbazepine, 84
progressive multifocal leukoencephalopathy
  interferon + ribavirin, 346
  natalizumab, 447
prolonged QT interval
  see QT interval prolongation
propofol infusion syndrome
  propofol, 142
proptosis
  rosiglitazone, 502
prostate cancer
  testesterone, 478–479
proteinuria
  bevacizumab, 444
  everolimus, 454
  sirolimus (rapamycin), 458
  verteporfin, 547
pruritus
  see itching
pseudo-pseudoxanthoma elasticum
  penicillamine, 275
pseudomembranous colitis
  oseltamivir, 353
pseudoporphyria
  acitretin, 185
  voriconazole, 328
pseudotumor cerebri
  ceftroxone, 285
  lithium + minocycline, 26
psoriasis
  calcipotriol, 186
psychiatric symptom worsening
  lamotrigine, 81

psychomotor slowing
topiramate, 90
psychosis
cannabinoids, 33
finasteride + sibutramine, 484
isotretinoin, 185
ketamine, 141
khat, 44
thyroid hormones, 490
topiramate, 91
ptosis
botulinum toxins, 166
fluconazole, 325
imatinib mesylate, 522
spinal manipulation, 558
pulmonary capillaritis
antithyroid drugs, 491
pulmonary congestion
ecstasy, 41
granulocyte colony-stimulating
factor, 435
pulmonary edema
ecstasy, 42
gemtuzumab ozogamicin, 446
magnesium salts, 266
nicardipine, 227
nilotinib, 524
phenylpropanolamine, 173
silver salts and derivatives, 269
pulmonary embolism
botulinum toxins, 165
fresh frozen plasma, 384
heparins, 405
tamoxifen, 476
pulmonary eosinophilia
perindopril, 237
pulmonary hemorrhage
antithyroid drugs, 491
glycoprotein IIb-IIIa inhibitors,
415
pulmonary hypertension
Piper methysticum, 554
statins, 16
pulmonary hypoplasia
angiotensin II receptor
antagonists, 240
pulmonary infiltrates
granulocyte colony-stimulating
factor, 435
valsartan, 242
pupillary dilatation
fenfluramine, 7
pure red cell aplasia
dapsone, 357
erythropoietins, 389
procainamide, 219
pure white cell aplasia
imipenem, 284
purpura
blood transfusion, 382
EMLA cream, 157
montelukast, 203
teicoplanin, 301
trimethoprim, 308

valdecoxib, 132
pustular eruption
imatinib + voriconazole, 323
terbinafine, 316
pustular psoriasis
calcipotriol, 186
pustulosis
corticosteroids, topical, 183
**pustulosis, acute generalized
exanthematous (AGEP)**
ciprofloxacin, 298
piperacillin, 287
pyrexia
anti-human CD40 Mab
chimeric 5D12, 443
oseltamivir, 353
oxcarbazepine, 83

Q
QT interval prolongation
antidysrhythmics, 212
antihistamines (H_1) +
ketoconazole, 321
antimony, 263
antipsychotic drugs, 56, 57
diphenhydramine, 189–190
disopyramide + fluconazole,
322
hormone replacement therapy,
470
indapamide, 258
inhibitors of phosphodiesterase
type V, 232
ketoconazole, 326
levo-α-acetylmethadol
(LAAM), 111
lithium, 24
methadone, 112
phosphates, 427
quinidine, 219
sevoflurane, 138–139
telithromycin, 301

R
rabbit syndrome
citalopram, 17
lithium + risperidone, 27
risperidone, 70
rash
Agnus castus, 552
amisulpride, 64
antithyroid drugs, 491
azithromycin, 302
botulinum toxins, 166
caspofungin, 330
cefprozil, 285
ciprofloxacin, 299
clarithromycin, 302
clopidogrel, 416
colistin, 306
daptomycin, 309
dasatinib, 524
diuretic sulfonamides, 254
Echinacea species, 553

ecstasy, 43
EMLA cream, 157
erlotinib, 526
fentanyl, 110
finasteride, 484
gatifloxacin, 299
heparins, 405
hydroxychloroquine, 337
imatinib mesylate, 523
infliximab, 441
inhibitors of phosphodiesterase
type V, 232
interferon + ribavirin, 345
intravenous regional
anesthesia, 156
lactose, 568
lamotrigine, 80
lapatinib, 526
levamisole, 366
levofloxacin, 299
linezolid, 304
manganese, 268
measles-mumps-rubella
vaccine, 376
melarsoprol, 341
mepivacaine, 160, 161
mesalazine, 428
micafungin, 331
nevirapine, 350
ofloxacin, 300
omalizumab, 447
oseltamivir, 353
oxcarbazepine, 84, 85
penicillamine, 274
phenytoin, 85
pregabalin, 88
proton pump inhibitors, 424
pseudoephedrine, 172
quinupristin/dalfopristin, 307
sirolimus (rapamycin), 457
suramin, 367
telithromycin, 301
temsirolimus, 459
tiagabine, 89
trimethoprim, 308
valproate, 92
water-soluble intravascular
iodinated contrast agents,
534, 537
zanamivir, 352
rectal bleeding
acitretin, 185
rofecoxib, 131
supercoumarins, 404
rectal burning
phosphates, 427
rectal hemorrhage
mesalazine, 429
red eyes
irbesartan, 241
reflux symptoms
H. pylori eradication regimens,
425
REM sleep reduction
sibutramine, 8

renal
see entries at kidney-, nephr-
renal disease, end-stage
acetylsalicylic acid, 128–129
renal dysfunction
etherified starches, 384
liposomal amphotericin
(L-amB), 320
renal impairment
cilazapril, 235
granulocyte colony-stimulating
factor, 435
renal insufficiency
ACE inhibitors + aprotinin, 235
amphotericin B deoxycholate
(DAMB), 319
angiotensin II receptor
antagonists, 240
antithyroid drugs, 491
bismuth, 264
ciprofloxacin, 298
colistin, 306
diethylene glycol, 567
enalapril, 236
immunoglobulins, 385, 386
rifampicin, 360–361
silver salts and derivatives, 269
tenofovir, 349
thiopental sodium, 147
tobramycin, 297
valdecoxib, 132
renal pain
topiramate, 90
renal tubular damage
anagrelide, 413
respiratory arrest
botulinum toxins, 165
bupivacaine, 159
respiratory depression
buprenorphine, 118
dextropropoxyphene, 110
epidural analgesia, 108
ketamine, 142
morphine, 107
risperidone, 71
respiratory difficulty
streptokinase, 413
respiratory distress
anticoagulants + epoprostenol,
465
cyclophosphamide, 453
water-soluble intravascular
iodinated contrast agents,
537
verteporfin, 546
**respiratory distress syndrome,
acute (ARDS)**
cocaine, 35
immunoglobulins, 385
lamotrigine, 81
respiratory failure
colistin, 306
infiltration anesthesia, 155
methomyl, 565

trichloroethylene, 140
respiratory infection
proton pump inhibitors, 424
restless legs
interferon alfa, 436
restlessness
methylthioninium chloride +
statins, 570
naltrexone, 120
retinal breakage
triamcinolone, 548
retinal damage
gentamicin, 297
retinal detachment
bevacizumab, 544
retinal edema
imatinib mesylate, 522
retinal pigment epithelial tears
bevacizumab, 544
ranibizumab, 545
verteporfin, 546–547
retinal toxicity
hydroxychloroquine, 337
retrosternal pain
cannabinoids, 31
rhabdomyolysis
atorvastatin + fluconazole, 322
HMG-CoA reductase
inhibitors, 516–517
ketamine, 142
levofloxacin, 300
phenytoin, 85
Piper methysticum, 555
propofol, 142
thiopental sodium, 147
ziprasidone, 72–73
rhinitis
interleukin-11, 439
rhinorrhea
mupirocin, 307
right upper quadrant pain
alosetron, 423
rigidity
ecstasy, 43
levetiracetam, 83
venlafaxine, 19
rigor
levamisole, 366
risky behavior
alprazolam, 49
cannabinoids, 33
dopamine receptor agonists,
174–175

S

sadness
efavirenz, 349
sarcoidosis, cutaneous
interferon + ribavirin, 346
scalp folliculitis
sirolimus (rapamycin), 457
scleral bleeding
interferon alfa, 436

scleroderma-like skin changes
methysergide, 176–177
scotoma
ethambutol, 358
linezolid, 304
sedation
chloral hydrate, 52
methadone, 112
olanzapine, 64, 65
quetiapine, 67
risperidone, 69
ziprasidone, 72
seizure
amitriptyline, 15
baclofen, 165
baclofen + propofol, 143
botulinum toxins, 165
bupropion, 20
cannabinoids, 32
ciprofloxacin, 298
desmopressin, 512
ecstasy, 43
ertapenem, 284
ketamine, 142
levofloxacin, 299
olanzapine, 65
oseltamivir, 353
topical anesthesia, 157
valproate, 96
water-soluble intravascular
iodinated contrast agents,
534
zanamivir, 352
seizure aggravation
topiramate, 90
seizure increase
zonisamide, 99
self-aggressive behavior
diazepam, 50
semen volume reduction
khat, 45
sensorimotor polyneuropathy
interferon alfa, 436
leflunomide, 455
sensorineural hearing loss
acitretin, 185
clarithromycin, 302
loop diuretics, 258
sensory neuropathy
interleukin-2, 438
sepsis
propofol, 143
septic arthritis
basiliximab, 444
septic shock
beta-lactam antibiotics, 280
serotonin syndrome
linezolid + statins, 305
triptans, 232
venlafaxine, 19
sexual dysfunction
risperidone, 71
statins, 18

shivering
methylthioninium chloride +
statins, 570
shock
beta-blockers + verapamil, 228
nifedipine, 228
shortness of breath
cannabinoids, 31
diamorphine, 110
immunoglobulins, 385
ivermectin, 365
Piper methysticum, 554
SIADH
see syndrome of inappropriate
antidiuretic hormone
secretion (SIADH)
sialadenitis
levamisole, 366
ramipril, 238
sialadenosis
valproate, 94
sick sinus syndrome
beta-adrenoceptor antagonists,
223
SILENT
see syndrome of irreversible
lithium-induced
neurotoxicity (SILENT)
singing
methylthioninium chloride +
statins, 569
sinus arrest
adenosine, 213
sinus brachycardia
cannabinoids, 31
methadone, 112
phosphates, 427
sinus node dysfunction
donepezil, 9
sinus tachycardia
beta$_2$-adrenoceptor agonists,
200
cannabinoids, 31
diphenhydramine, 189–190
ecstasy, 43
sister chromatid exchange
desflurane, 138
skeletal anomaly
fluconazole, 325
skin cancer
pimecrolimus, 457
PUVA, 184
UVB, 184
skin eruption
carbamazepine, 79
skin necrosis
coumarin anticoagulants, 399
heparins, 405, 406
slate-grey discoloration
amiodarone, 216
sleep disorder
H. pylori eradication regimens,
425

sleep disturbance
lamotrigine, 80, 90
levetiracetam, 82
mefloquine, 337
sleepiness
Zingiber officinale (ginger),
556
small bowel obstruction
nifedipine, 227
warfarin, 399
somnolence
baclofen, 165
citalopram, 17
dextromethorphan, 109
efavirenz, 349
fentanyl, 111
gabapentin, 80
levetiracetam, 82, 83
lidocaine, 160
methylphenidate, 5
oxcarbazepine, 83, 85
oxybutynin, 177
pregabalin, 86, 87, 88
temsirolimus, 459
tiagabine, 89
topiramate, 89
ziprasidone, 72
zonisamide, 99
sore throat
mirtazapine, 20
soreness
vancomycin, 301
speech difficulty
topiramate, 90
sperm count, reduced
khat, 45
sperm motility reduction
khat, 45
spinal cord infarction
infiltration anesthesia, 155
spinal epidural lipomatosis
systemic glucocorticoids, 463
splenic rupture
glycoprotein IIb-IIIa inhibitors,
414
spongiosis
interferon + ribavirin, 346
ST segment depression
cannabinoids, 31
ecstasy, 40
ST segment elevation
cannabinoids, 31
startle reaction
quetiapine, 67
status epilepticus
measles-mumps-rubella
vaccine, 375
olanzapine, 66
steatohepatitis
valproate, 94
steatosis
cocaine, 35
ecstasy, 41

Stevens–Johnson syndrome
acetazolamide, 256
azithromycin, 302
clarithromycin, 302
nitrofurantoin, 303
phenytoin, 85
rofecoxib, 131
terbinafine, 316
stinging
aminolevulinic acid, 184
stomach ache
terbinafine, 317
stomatitis
gold and gold salts, 265
khat, 45
sunitinib, 527
stools, discolored
chloroquine + proguanil, 336
stridor
caspofungin, 330
Eugenia caryophyllus, 553
stroke
adrenaline (epinephrine), 170
antipsychotic drugs, 59–60
bevacizumab, 544
botulinum toxins, 165
cannabinoids, 32
immunoglobulins, 386
pseudoephedrine, 172
ranibizumab, 545
risperidone, 71
streptokinase, 413
stuttering
theophylline, 5
subarachnoid hemorrhage
cocaine, 34
subcutaneous calcinosis
heparins, 408
subfoveal hemorrhage
verteporfin, 547
subileus
anti-human CD40 Mab
chimeric 5D12, 443
submacular hemorrhage
verteporfin, 547
verteporfin + warfarin, 547
subretinal hemorrage
bevacizumab, 544
sudden cardiac death
antipsychotic drugs, 56
sudden infant death
hexavalent vaccines, 370
suicidal ideation
khat, 44
lithium, 25
suicide
HMG-CoA reductase
inhibitors, 516
supraventricular tachycardia
cannabinoids, 31
hormone replacement therapy,
470
levobupivacaine, 160

swallowing difficulty
botulinum toxins, 166
diuretic sulfonamides, 254
mirtazapine, 20
quetiapine, 67
suxamethonium, 164
tramadol, 118
venlafaxine, 19
sweating
acupuncture, 557
infliximab, 440
latanoprost, 466
methadone, 112
methomyl, 565
methylthioninium chloride +
statins, 570
nefopam, 113
pseudoephedrine, 172
tramadol, 118
Sweet's syndrome
minocycline, 290
ofloxacin, 300
swelling
combination vaccines, 369
syncope
see fainting
**syndrome of inappropriate
antidiuretic hormone
secretion (SIADH)**
enalapril, 235
**syndrome of irreversible
lithium-induced
neurotoxicity (SILENT)**
lithium, 24
synostosis
fluconazole, 325
systolic murmur
systemic glucocorticoids, 463

T
T wave inversion
ecstasy, 40
TA-GVHD
see transfusion associated
graft-versus-host disease
tachycardia
acetazolamide, 255
amiodarone, 214
benzocaine, 158
$beta_2$-adrenoceptor agonists,
200
cannabinoids, 32
clopidogrel, 416
doxazosin, 246
fluvoxamine + quetiapine, 68
immunoglobulins, 386
interleukin-11, 439
ketamine, 141
methylphenidate, 5
methylthioninium chloride +
statins, 570
modafinil, 6
nefopam, 113

nifedipine, 227
Piper methysticum, 554
systemic glucocorticoids, 463
trichloroethylene, 140
ultrasound contrast agents, 540
valproate, 96
venlafaxine, 19
tachydysrhythmia
Citrus aurantium, 552
tachyphylaxis
histamine H_2 receptor
antagonists, 423–424
tachypnea
cocaine, 36
Eugenia caryophyllus, 553
tardive dyskinesia
antipsychotic drugs, 57
metoclopramide, 423
risperidone, 70
taste disturbance
H. pylori eradication regimens,
426
omeprazole, 425
topiramate, 90
temperature change
immunoglobulins, 386
teratogenicity
bosentan, 245
tetany
polystyrene sulfonates, 276
tetraplegia
infiltration anesthesia, 155
thoughts, abnormal
pregabalin, 87, 88
thoughts, racing
modafinil, 6
throat irritation
colistin, 305
fluticasone propionate +
salmeterol, 202
thrombocytopenia
alemtuzumab, 442
blood transfusion, 382
clarithromycin + colchicine,
133
clopidogrel, 415
dasatinib, 523
deferiprone, 274
drotrecogin alfa, 381
efalizumab, 445
gemtuzumab ozogamicin, 446
glycoprotein IIb-IIIa inhibitors,
414
H. pylori eradication regimens,
426
heparins, 404–407
interferon + ribavirin, 345, 346
interferon alfa, 437
interleukin-11, 439
linezolid, 304, 305
nilotinib, 524
rifampicin, 360
sunitinib, 527
suramin, 367

temsirolimus, 459
ticlopidine, 417
trimethoprim, 308
thrombocytopenic purpura
measles vaccines, 373
thromboembolism
oral contraceptives, 473
tamoxifen, 476
thrombosis
erythropoietins, 389
hormone replacement therapy,
470
infliximab, 440
octreotide, 510
tamoxifen, 476
**thrombotic thrombocytopenia
purpura**
ticlopidine, 417
thyroid dysfunction
interferon beta, 437
tinnitus
cocaine, 34
lidocaine (lignocaine), 218
tacrolimus, 458
tiredness
see also fatigue, hyposthenia,
malaise, weakness
carbamazepine, 78
valproate, 92
tongue edema
ACE inhibitors, 235
tongue swelling
tramadol, 118
tonic-clonic movements
acupuncture, 557
sevoflurane, 139
tonic-clonic seizures
ciprofloxacin, 298
cocaine, 35
ecstasy, 41
methylthioninium chloride +
statins, 570
ropivacaine, 161
verteporfin, 546
tonic convulsions
sevoflurane, 139
tooth discoloration
chlorhexidine, 278
doxycycline, 289
tetracycline, 291
torsade de pointes
amiodarone, 214
antipsychotic drugs, 56
indapamide, 258
ketoconazole, 326
methadone, 112
sevoflurane, 138
torticollis
Piper methysticum, 554
toxic epidermal necrolysis
dorzolamide + timolol, 224
inhibitors of phosphodiesterase
type V, 232
lamotrigine, 81

levofloxacin, 299
nitrofurantoin, 303
norfloxacin, 300
oseltamivir, 353
phenytoin, 85
pristinamycin, 307
pseudoephedrine, 172
terbinafine, 316
trimethoprim, 308
water-soluble intravascular
    iodinated contrast agents,
    534
toxic leukoencephalopathy
diamorphine, 110
toxic optic neuropathy
linezolid, 304
toxic shock syndrome
misoprostol, 466
**transfusion associated
    graft-versus-host disease
    (TA-GVHD)**
blood transfusion, 381–382,
    382
**transfusion-related acute lung
    injury (TRALI)**
blood transfusion, 381, 382
immunoglobulins, 385
transient ischemic attack
bevacizumab, 544
cannabinoids, 32
interleukin-11, 439
**transient neurological
    symptoms**
spinal anesthesia, 153–154
tremor
co-trimoxazole, 338
formoterol, 200
levetiracetam, 83
manganese, 267–268
mefloquine, 337
melarsoprol, 341
methylthioninium chloride +
    statins, 569
naltrexone, 120
olanzapine, 65
pregabalin, 88
tiagabine, 89
topiramate, 90
valproate, 92, 93, 96
venlafaxine, 19
tuberculosis reactivation
adalimumab, 439
tubular necrosis, acute
colistin, 306
gentamicin, 297
tumor growth
erythropoietins, 389
type 2 diabetes mellitus
antipsychotic drugs, 58

U

ulcer, aphthous
mirtazapine, 20

ulcer, gastroduodenal
acetylsalicylic acid, 128
upper quadrant pain
fluvoxamine, 16
upper respiratory symptoms
modafinil, 6
**upper respiratory tract
    infection**
dextromethorphan, 109
naltrexone, 120
topiramate, 90
**upper respiratory tract
    inflammation**
proton pump inhibitors, 424
uremia
cilazapril, 235
urinary incontinence
hormone replacement therapy,
    471
urinary retention
morphine, 107
non-steroidal
    anti-inflammatory drugs, 128
spinal anesthesia, 154
urinary tract infection
modafinil, 6
urine, dark
chloroquine + proguanil, 336
urticaria
antithyroid drugs, 491
beta-lactam antibiotics, 281
cefaclor, 284
ciprofloxacin, 299
colistin, 306
etanercept, 440
glucosamine, 567
isosulfan blue, 566
itraconazole, 326
lidocaine, 160
mepivacaine, 160
pentoxifylline, 231
Piper methysticum, 555
trimethoprim, 308
water-soluble intravascular
    iodinated contrast agents,
    537
zanamivir, 352
urticarial vasculitis
trimethoprim, 308
uterine hyperstimulation
misoprostol, 466
uterine rupture
misoprostol, 466
uveitis
bevacizumab, 544
ranibizumab, 545

V

vacuolar myopathy
hydroxychloroquine, 337
vaginal bleeding
phenytoin, 85
**variant Creutzfeldt–Jakob
    disease**
blood transfusion, 383

Varicella zoster **reactivation**
ecstasy, 41
vasculitis
antithyroid drugs, 491
leukotriene modifiers, 203
levamisole, 366
linezolid, 305
montelukast, 203
teicoplanin, 301
trimethoprim, 308
vasoconstriction
glyceryl trinitrate, 225
triptans, 231–232
vasodilatation
acetazolamide, 255
vasospasm
cocaine, 34
Ephedra and ephedrine, 171
vasovagal syncope
acupuncture, 556–557
veno-occlusive disease
gemtuzumab ozogamicin, 446
pyrrolizidine alkaloids, 556
**venous access device
    complications**
amphotericin, 317
venous thromboembolism
antipsychotic drugs, 60
immunoglobulins, 386
ventricular asystole
pregabalin, 88
ventricular bigeminy
nifedipine, 227
ventricular dysfunction
imatinib mesylate, 521
ventricular dysrhythmia
antipsychotic drugs, 60
bee sting venom, 572
nifedipine, 227
ventricular extra beats
cannabinoids, 31
nifedipine, 227
ventricular fibrillation
amitriptyline, 15
cannabinoids, 31
indapamide, 258
ropivacaine, 161
ventricular hypertrophy
systemic glucocorticoids, 463
**ventricular outflow tract
    obstruction**
noradrenaline
    (norepinephrine), 171
systemic glucocorticoids, 463
ventricular tachycardia
amitriptyline, 15
antimony, 263
azithromycin, 302
cardiac glycosides, 209
dobutamine, 173
fish oils, 515
flecainide, 217

indapamide, 258
inhibitors of phosphodiesterase
  type V, 232
methadone, 112
olanzapine, 67
thiopental sodium, 146
vertigo
colistin, 306
H. pylori eradication regimens,
  425
interferon alfa, 436
methylthioninium chloride +
  statins, 570, 571
oseltamivir, 353
pregabalin, 87
rabeprazole, 425
telithromycin, 301
topiramate, 89, 90
tramadol, 118
vestibular damage
tobramycin, 297
vigilance impairment
citalopram, 18
zolpidem, 53
violent death
HMG-CoA reductase
  inhibitors, 516
vision, blurred
cannabinoids, 33
ethambutol, 358
irbesartan, 241
lamotrigine, 81
metformin + orlistat, 431
methomyl, 565
methylthioninium chloride +
  statins, 569
naltrexone, 120
pregabalin, 86, 87
suxamethonium, 164
vision disturbance
biguanides, 497
botulinum toxins, 165
colistin, 306
dental anesthesia, 154
ivermectin, 365
ketamine, 141
linezolid, 304
nifedipine, 228
psilocybin, 46
rofecoxib, 130–131
topiramate, 90
verteporfin, 546
voriconazole, 328
vision loss
bevacizumab, 544
methylthioninium chloride +
  statins, 569
spinal manipulation, 558
visual field constriction
lamotrigine, 81
visual field defects
indocyanine green, 566
vigabatrin, 98–99

visual obstruction
imatinib mesylate, 522
vitamin B$_6$ concentration
acarbose, 496
vitamin B$_{12}$ concentration
valproate, 93
vitamin C plasma concentration
omeprazole, 425
vitreous hemorrhage
infliximab, 440
vocal cord edema
acitretin, 185
voice changes
suxamethonium, 164
vomiting
adrenaline (epinephrine), 170
baclofen, 165
biguanides, 497
bismuth, 264
camphor, 564
cefaclor, 284
ceftroxone, 285
chloroquine + proguanil, 336
clopidogrel, 416
cocaine, 35
deferiprone, 274
desloratadine, 189
diuretic sulfonamides, 252
droperidol + morphine, 113
epidural analgesia, 108
fentanyl, 110, 111
fluvoxamine, 16
gabapentin, 80
gatifloxacin, 299
H. pylori eradication regimens,
  340, 425
immunoglobulins, 386
ivermectin, 365
liraglutide, 500
mesalazine, 428
methomyl, 565
methylphenidate, 5
micafungin, 331
montelukast, 203
morphine, 107, 114, 115
naltrexone, 120
nifedipine, 228
orlistat, 429
oseltamivir, 353
oxcarbazepine, 85
pethidine, 115, 116
phosphates, 427
physostigmine, 114
rifampicin, 361
rivastigmine, 10
sevoflurane, 138
telithromycin, 301
tigecycline, 291, 292
valproate, 92, 96
warfarin, 399
zanamivir, 353
vortex keratopathy
amiodarone, 214

W
Wallenberg's syndrome
spinal manipulation, 558
watershed infarct
acetazolamide, 255
weakness
  see also fatigue, hyposthenia,
    malaise, tiredness
articaine, 158
botulinum toxins, 165, 166
cocaine, 35
colistin, 306
daptomycin, 309
interferon + ribavirin, 345
interferon alfa, 436
lamotrigine, 80
levetiracetam, 82
mefloquine, 337
metformin + orlistat, 431
methomyl, 565
olanzapine, 64
polystyrene sulfonates, 276
pregabalin, 87, 88
progesterone antagonists, 477
suramin, 367
suxamethonium, 164
tiagabine, 89
verteporfin, 546, 547
weight gain
clozapine, 62–63
escitalopram + quetiapine, 68
levetiracetam, 82
olanzapine, 64, 65, 66
oxcarbazepine, 84
paroxetine, 18
polystyrene sulfonates, 276
pregabalin, 87, 88
quetiapine, 67
risperidone, 69, 71
rosiglitazone, 502
sibutramine, 7
valproate, 92
weight loss
arsenic, 263
clozapine + modafinil, 6
exenatide, 499
leflunomide, 454, 455
mefloquine, 337
reboxetine, 21
rofecoxib, 131
topiramate, 89, 90, 91
wheal
beta-lactam antibiotics, 281
penicillins, 287
wheeze
cefaclor, 284
influenza vaccine, 374
streptokinase, 413
wind
  see flatulence
working memory perfomance
amphetamines, 1
wound healing complications
bevacizumab, 444

X

xerosis
  interferon + ribavirin, 346

Y

***Yersinia enterocolitica* infection**
  blood transfusion, 383

Z

zinc deficiency
  losartan, 242